The Life Extension Foundation's

Disease Prevention and Treatment

Expanded Third Edition

The Life Extension Foundation's

Disease Prevention and Treatment

Scientific Protocols That Integrate Mainstream and Alternative Medicine

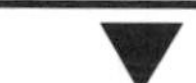

Expanded Third Edition

Based upon Thousands of Research Studies and the Clinical Experience of Physicians Around the World

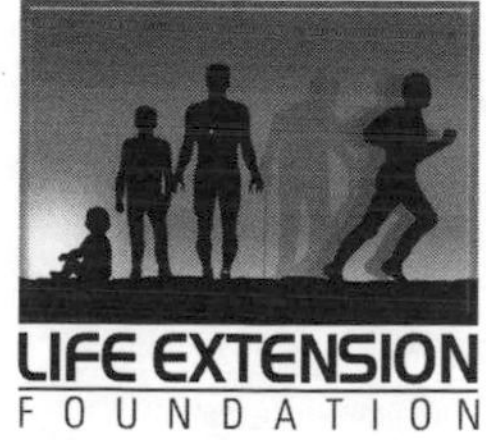

Editor: Melanie Segala

On-line Research Coordinator: Amber Needham

Page Design & Production: Publication Services

Cover Design: Roy Rauschenberg/Jato Design

Life Extension Foundation books may be purchased for personal, educational, business, or sales promotional use. For information, please write: The Life Extension Foundation, P.O. Box 229120, Hollywood, Florida 33022-9120.
Web site: www.lef.org

THIRD EDITION

ISBN 0-9658777-4-4

PREFACE

Progress in medicine is occurring rapidly, but there are lengthy delays between the time a medical discovery is made and when it actually becomes available to the public. The purpose of this book is to bridge the information gap between the research community and the practice of medicine.

In the last few years, the Life Extension Foundation has been seeking to establish a Life Extension Medical Center where the best medical care, based upon the latest scientific evidence, would be available to patients, without regard to the views of medical and political authorities. This book describes some of the innovative treatments that would be implemented at such a medical center.

While this book provides practical advice for those suffering from difficult-to-treat diseases, the long-term objective of this work is to reform an obsolete healthcare system that hinders medical progress.

Among the reasons for the time lag in delivering medical advances are bureaucratic delays caused by the FDA and other government agencies; delays in publishing new findings in peer-reviewed journals; the excessive influence of the large pharmaceutical companies; excessive conservatism on the part of doctors, medical centers, and insurance companies; and lack of cooperation, creativity, and coordination among all the components of the medical system.

Whatever the reasons, it is a fact that few patients, rich or poor, are provided with the best available health and medical care, and that many lives are impaired or lost because of the lack of availability of the latest medical advances.

One problem with today's system of disease treatment is that practicing physicians cannot keep up with the exponential growth of scientific knowledge. A common complaint directed at doctors is that they are not staying informed about the latest medical findings. The reality is that there are far too many new research findings about disease therapies appearing in the scientific literature for doctors to keep up with them all.

Just look at a typical doctor's schedule. His or her day begins early with hospital rounds and/or supervised medical testing. The doctor then sees patients back-to-back during office hours and spends evening hours reviewing test results and making late-night hospital rounds. If the doctor is lucky, he or she will enjoy a night of uninterrupted sleep before embarking on the next hectic day. It is difficult to imagine how a doctor maintaining this kind of schedule can stay current with the hundreds of new scientific studies that appear every day, yet people still expect their doctors to master the latest advances in medicine.

At the Life Extension Foundation, we have long recognized the limitations of practicing medicine and have taken aggressive steps to assist Foundation members in obtaining access to the best medical therapies available worldwide. Since 1980, we have sought to integrate conventional medical practice with novel therapies substantiated by published scientific studies. We believe that optimal clinical practice should consist of the primary physician networking with a team of researchers to develop multi-modal treatment strategies tailored to the needs of individual patients.

The public too often hears about a new life-saving therapy, only to be told that the treatment won't be available for many years. The need to change the way medicine is practiced has reached a critical stage. Too much vital knowledge is being overlooked by clinical physicians who cannot possibly keep up with it all. Patients needlessly suffer and die, although effective therapies that have not yet been accepted by mainstream medicine may already exist. This book has been written to help document the need to radically change the practice of medicine and to save as many lives as possible.

The information in this book is not intended to replace the attention or advice of a physician or other health care professional. Anyone who wishes to embark on any dietary, drug, exercise, or other lifestyle change intended to prevent or treat a specific disease or condition should consult with, and seek clearance and guidance from, a qualified health care professional. The book offers suggestions based upon scientific evidence. Patients need to be treated in an individual manner by their own personal physicians. The information in this book must not be considered a substitute for the individual attention of a personal physician.

For additional information on the therapies discussed in these protocols, and to examine the thousands of scientific abstracts that document their value, please pay a visit to the Life Extension Foundation Web site at www.lef.org Just click on *Disease Therapies* on our home page. The protocols in this book are updated regularly on the Foundation's Web site.

Saul Kent and William Faloon
The Life Extension Foundation
November 1999

ACKNOWLEDGMENTS

Many individuals contributed to the expanded 3rd edition of *Disease Prevention and Treatment*. The Life Extension Foundation publishers wish to thank the medical professionals, researchers, and writers who collaborated on the editorial development of this endeavor. Of note, Andrew Baer, M.D., provided insight into clinical applications of several disease protocols. Ronald Kelsey, Ph.D., synthesized research and integrated traditional and alternative treatment approaches. The Advisory Staff made many valuable suggestions on the inclusion of new topics based upon the needs and concerns of Life Extension Foundation members.

MEDICAL ADVISORY BOARD

Andrew M. Baer, M.D. (McLean, Virginia) focuses on anti-aging and mind/body medicine, consciousness technology, degenerative diseases, and the treatment of age-associated memory impairment.

Gustavo Tovar Baez, M.D., operates the Life Extension Clinic in Caracas, Venezuela. He is the first physician in Caracas to specialize in anti-aging medicine.

Sam Baxas, M.D., head of the Baxamed Medical Center for Youth Restoration in Basel, Switzerland, has developed cell therapy and growth hormone therapies for a variety of diseases, including Parkinson's disease and arthritis.

Ricardo Bernales, M.D., is a general practitioner in Chicago focusing on allergies, bronchial asthma, and immunodeficiency, and is a board-certified pediatrician.

Thomas F. Crais, M.D., F.A.C.S., a board-certified plastic surgeon, is medical director of the microsurgical research and training lab at Southern Baptist Hospital, New Orleans.

Martin Dayton, M.D., D.O., practices at the Sunny Isles Medical Center in North Miami Beach, Florida. His focus is on nutrition, aging, chelation therapy, holistic medicine, and oxidative medicine.

Arnold Fox, M.D., is an internist, cardiologist, and practicing physician in Beverly Hills, California, specializing in anti-aging medicine using nutritional and hormone therapies. He is the author of *The Fat Blocker Diet*.

Carmen Fusco, M.S., R.N., C.N.S., is a research scientist and clinical nutritionist in New York City who has lectured and written numerous articles on the biochemical approach to the prevention of aging and degenerative diseases.

Miguelangelo Gonzalez, M.D., is a certified plastic and reconstructive surgeon at the Plastic and Reconstructive Surgery Institute of Jalisco, Guadalajara, Mexico.

Garry F. Gordon, M.D., D.O. (Payson, Arizona) researches alternative medical approaches for medical problems unresponsive to traditional therapies. He is president of the International College of Advanced Longevity Medicine.

Richard Heifetz, M.D., is a board-certified anesthesiologist in Santa Rosa, California, specializing in the delivery of anesthesia for office-based plastic/cosmetic surgery, chelation therapy, and pain management.

Maurice D. Marholin, D.O., D.C., a fellow in nutrition under a grant from the National Cancer Institute, focuses on internal medicine at the University of Alabama.

Herbert Pardell, D.O., operates an anti-aging clinical practice in North Miami, Florida, that specializes in hyperbaric oxygen, chelation, and alternative medicine. He is medical director of the Life Extension Foundation.

Lambert Titus K. Parker, M.D., practices internal medicine at Schuyler Hospital in Montour Falls, New York, and is director of the clinic's intensive care unit.

Ross Pelton, R.Ph., Ph.D., C.C.N., is director of education for Natural Health Resources, writes a monthly column for *American Druggist*, has authored four books, and teaches continuing education courses.

Joseph P. Pepping, Pharm.D., is a nutritional medicine and pain management consultant at Kaiser Permanente in Honolulu, Hawaii, and author of several review articles in nutritional pharmacology.

Patrick Quillan, Ph.D., R.D., C.N.S. (Tulsa, Oklahoma) promotes rational healing principles in world health care. He has served as vice president of nutrition for Cancer Treatment Centers of America.

Marc R. Rose, M.D., practices ophthalmology in Los Angeles and is president of the Rose Eye Medical Group. He is on the staff of Pacific Alliance Medical Center, Los Angeles, and other area hospitals.

Michael R. Rose, M.D., a board-certified ophthalmologist with the Rose Eye Medical Group in Los Angeles, is on the staff of the University of Southern California and UCLA.

Roman Rozencwaig, M.D., is a pioneer in research on melatonin and aging. Dr. Rozencwaig practices in Montreal, Canada, and is on the staff at Reddy Memorial Hospital and Bishop Medical Centre.

Carol Ann Ryser, M.D., F.A.A.P., medical director of Health Centers of America, in Kansas City, Missouri, focuses on pediatrics and mental health.

E.K. Schandl, Ph.D., is a clinical biochemist and oncobiologist with the Center for Metabolic Disorders, director of American Metabolic Laboratories in Hollywood, Florida, and scientific director of the Life Extension Foundation.

Michael D. Seidman, M.D., is the regional coordinator of Otolaryngology–Head and Neck Surgery for the Bloomfield Satellite of HFHS, co-director of the Tinnitus Center, and co-chair of the Complementary/Alternative Medicine Initiative for HFHS.

Herbert R. Slavin, M.D., is medical director of the Institute of Advanced Medicine in Lauderhill, Florida, specializing in anti-aging medicine, disease prevention, chelation therapy, and natural hormone replacement therapy.

R. Arnold Smith, M.D., is a clinical radiation oncologist who specializes in using immunotherapy to enhance the safety and efficacy of conventional cancer therapies.

Stephen L. Smith, M.D. (Richland, Washington), who focuses on treating allergies, is a member of the American Society for Lasers in Medicine and Surgery.

Stephen Strum, M.D., is a medical oncologist who specializes in the treatment of prostate cancer. He practices at Healing Touch Oncology in Marina del Rey, California.

Javier Torres, M.D., is a member of the American Academy of Physical Medicine and Rehabilitation and is on the medical staffs of Sunrise Hospital, Desert Springs Hospital, Valley Hospital, and Mountain View Hospital, all in Las Vegas, Nevada.

Charles E. Williamson, M.D., of the Institute for Integrative Medicine in Boca Raton, Florida, focuses on anti-aging, longevity, and pain management.

Jonathan V. Wright, M.D., is a family practitioner at the Tahoma Clinic in Kent, Washington. Dr. Wright is also a board member of the Vitamin C Foundation and the American Preventive Medical Association, among many other groups.

FOREWORD

What Is The Life Extension Foundation?

Before you consider making use of the disease prevention and treatment protocols in this book, you should know something about the organization that developed them.

The Life Extension Foundation is the world's largest organization dedicated to the investigation of scientific methods of preventing and treating disease, aging, and death. In addition to developing specific disease treatment protocols, the Foundation funds pioneering scientific research aimed at achieving an indefinitely extended healthy human life span.

Life Extension Foundation members believe in taking advantage of documented scientific therapies to prevent disease and slow premature aging today. The medical literature contains thousands of papers on the use of nutrient supplements, hormone modulation, and other therapies that have been shown to improve the quality of life. Life extensionist members attempt to use this scientific information, in conjunction with their physicians, to improve their chances of living longer in good health.

Laboratory research supported by the Life Extension Foundation (LEF) has documented the value of various nutrients, hormones, and drugs in preventing and reversing cell damage caused by oxidation, inflammation, excitotoxicity, and other lethal processes. This research has succeeded in blocking many types of damage caused by ischemia (reduced blood flow). Ischemia can be caused by blockage of a coronary artery, leading to a heart attack, or blockage of a cerebral artery, leading to a stroke. Ischemia is an underlying cause of damage in patients who suffer from all types of degenerative diseases, accidents, and the aging-related deterioration of the brain and other organs. Scientists funded by LEF have successfully restored dogs to life and healthy function after up to 17 minutes without oxygen at normal body temperature. This type of research is leading to the ability to save the lives of millions of people who would otherwise die, and to improve the quality of life for all of us as we grow older.

LEF also funds the only scientific program in the world dedicated to the development of new medical uses for advanced low-temperature technologies. Fundamental breakthroughs in cryobiology and ice control made by LEF-funded scientists are leading to remarkable new methods of cryopreserving cells, tissues, and organs for transplantation. Over the next 10 to 20 years, the use of cryopreserved tissues—both natural and artificial—for the treatment of aging and degenerative diseases will revolutionize the practice of medicine. The long-term goal of LEF's low-temperature research program is the development of perfected human suspended animation, which will, eventually, enable physicians to transport dying patients through time for treatment by the super-advanced medical scientists of the future.

At the heart of LEF's efforts to extend the healthy human life span are its unique research programs to identify, measure, and develop advanced, new therapies to slow, reverse, and ultimately eliminate the across-the-board deterioration characteristic of the aging process in humans. Today, aging is the underlying cause of most deaths in the United States and other developed countries. Killers such as heart disease, stroke, cancer, and Alzheimer's disease are caused in large part by the progressive decline in structure and function associated with aging. The control of human aging will reduce and eventually eliminate degenerative diseases, enabling us to remain healthy and vigorous at any age, and will allow us to live in good health for centuries.

LEF is funding a highly innovative high-tech research program that aims to pinpoint the genetic and biochemical changes associated with aging. Our objective is to use these data to develop a validated method to measure aging over short periods of time. This method will then be used to screen and evaluate very rapidly the safety and effectiveness of vast numbers of therapies with anti-aging potential.

LEF is currently the only source of funding on earth for life span studies in mice to determine the effects of potential anti-aging therapies on aging and life span. These studies are being conducted by experimental gerontologists at the University of Wisconsin in Madison, the University of California in Riverside, and the University of Arkansas in Little Rock. The studies have been designed to test the anti-aging potential of vitamins, drugs, and hormones now being used by life extensionists to counteract biochemical processes proposed (by gerontologists) as primary causes of aging. Some of these mechanisms of aging include oxidative stress (induced by free radicals), declining energy production (mitochondrial disorder), glycosylation (pathological binding of protein and glucose molecules), and loss of methylation capacity (required for DNA maintenance-and-repair enzymatic actions).

As the Foundation's revolutionary research programs lead to the discovery of authentic anti-aging therapies, we will seek to incorporate these therapies into clinical medicine as quickly as possible. We will accelerate the pace of our unique, anti-aging research programs until we achieve total control over aging and have the ability to extend the healthy human life span for hundreds—even thousands—of years!

Every month, members of the Life Extension Foundation receive a 96-page magazine that brings them up to date on the latest medical breakthroughs from around the world. In addition to learning about lifesaving therapies first, LEF members can obtain pharmaceutical-quality supplements through a unique wholesale "buyers club" discount program that is available only to Foundation members. New members receive free books that contain highlights of what the Foundation has published since 1980.

The Foundation monitors thousands of scientific studies every week to ensure that its disease prevention and treatment protocols are as up to date as possible. LEF interacts with the foremost medical and anti-aging researchers in the world in order to obtain inside information about the latest life extension breakthroughs. Foundation members often gain access to disease-preventing, anti-aging findings before they are published in science and medical journals.

The Life Extension Foundation was incorporated in 1980, but its founders have been writing about and financially supporting anti-aging research since the 1960's. A summary of the life-saving medical discoveries the Foundation has introduced over the last 20 years appears on the next page.

New medical information is being uncovered at an exponential rate. The first edition of this book, which was published in1996, contained 327 pages and was based on 2500 scientific abstracts. In this third edition, the Life Extension Foundation's protocols have been expanded to over 900 larger pages, which are based on more than 8000 scientific abstracts.

The Life Extension Foundation can assist you in finding offshore pharmacies that will sell you advanced European and Asian medications that may be 5 or more years ahead of FDA-approved drugs. The Foundation is the foremost organization in the United States protecting the rights of Americans to import lifesaving medications for their own personal use. The Foundation maintains a directory of innovative practicing physicians who can assist you in implementing the advanced therapies recommended in this book.

For membership information, call the Life Extension Foundation at (800) 841-5433 or visit the Foundation's Web site at www.lef.org

LIFE-SAVING MEDICAL DISCOVERIES INTRODUCED BY THE FOUNDATION

1980 The Foundation recommended antioxidants to prevent disease.

1981 The Foundation recommended lowering blood homocysteine levels for prevention of cardiovascular disease.

1981 The Foundation introduced DHEA as a disease-preventing therapy.

1983 The Foundation recommended low-dose aspirin to prevent heart attacks.

1983 The Foundation introduced coenzyme Q10 to prevent and treat heart disease.

1983 The Foundation warned that excess iron causes cancer and heart disease.

1985 The Foundation made lycopene available to prevent cancer.

1986 The Foundation recommended deprenyl as an anti-aging drug.

1988 The Foundation made phosphatidylserine available to slow brain aging.

1991 The Foundation sued the FDA for quicker approval of lifesaving drugs.

1992 The Foundation funded the first critical care research facility where antioxidant drugs, nutrients, and hormones were used to protect against the cell damaging effects of cerebral ischemia.

1992 The Foundation introduced melatonin for sleep and disease prevention.

1995 The Foundation introduced the first anti-aging drug formula in the world.

1996 The Foundation founded the first mail-order blood testing laboratory that offered state-of-the-art medical testing directly to the lay public.

1996 The Foundation introduced 110 disease prevention and treatment protocols that integrated conventional with alternative medicine.

1997 The Foundation introduced Americans to a safe and effective antidepressant, SAMe, used in Europe.

1997 The Foundation informed its members about the dangers of taking only the "alpha" form of Vitamin E.

1997 The Foundation introduced Americans to the *Urtica dioica* extract used in Germany to treat benign prostate enlargement.

1997 The Foundation introduced the first soy extract that contained 40% isoflavones.

1998 The Foundation exposed the FDA's fraudulent suppression of a breast cancer therapy that was shown to reduce mortality rates by 75% over a three-year period.

1998 The Foundation documented that high estrogen levels in men are a primary cause of prostate disease.

1998 The Foundation introduced a form of vitamin B_{12} (methylcobalamin) that is used as a drug in Japan to treat neurological disorders.

1998 The Foundation introduced the concept of slowing aging by protecting against "mitochondrial disorder."

1998 The Foundation exposed a lethal misconception among vitamin supplement takers that folic acid adequately suppresses homocysteine levels.

1999 The Foundation exposed the FDA's underhanded approval of a dangerous drug (tamoxifen) for use by healthy women.

1999 The Foundation showed how vitamin C could be used to prevent nitroglycerin drug intolerance in patients with coronary artery disease.

1999 The Foundation showed how FDA-approved estrogen drugs do not protect against heart disease.

1999 The Foundation introduced natural agents used in Europe to safely suppress tumor necrosis factor and cyclooxygenase-2.

A BIT OF MEDICAL HISTORY

In 1928, Dr. Alexander Fleming discovered penicillin. His work was published the very next year in the *British Journal of Experimental Pathology.* Nevertheless, the medical profession did not begin treating humans with this lifesaving therapy until 1941, and the general population did not gain access to penicillin until 1946.

Millions of people suffered and died from bacterial/infectious diseases when a cure (penicillin) had already been discovered and published in a respected medical journal. For 18 years, millions of people could only watch helplessly as their loved ones suffered and died from a host of bacterial diseases that penicillin could have cured.

The leading cause of death and disability today is ignorance about therapies to prevent and treat the degenerative diseases of aging. This book is dedicated to eradicating the ignorance that is causing humans to suffer and die from diseases that may already have cures or effective palliative therapies. Almost every therapy discussed in this book is documented extensively by findings from peer-reviewed, published studies from eminent medical journals around the world. Despite this scientific evidence, however, many of these therapies are being largely ignored by the medical establishment.

The protocols in this book are also available on the Life Extension Foundation's Web site at www.lef.org where you can find thousands of scientific abstracts that support the use of the therapies in these protocols.

How to Keep Up-To-Date

The information in this book is only as current as the day the book was sent to the printer. However, hundreds of new studies have appeared in the peer-reviewed scientific literature since that day.

The best way to keep informed about the latest medical findings regarding any medical condition that concerns you is to check out the Life Extension Foundation's Web site at www.lef.org on a regular basis.

The Foundation regularly updates all of its disease prevention and treatment protocols and posts this information on its Web site. You will also find additional health and medical information on the Foundation's site that could improve your health and save your life! Your entree into the world of innovative medical therapies is available 24 hours a day at www.lef.org

TABLE OF CONTENTS

ACETAMINOPHEN POISONING (ANALGESIC TOXICITY)

Most people are under the notion that over-the-counter (OTC) medications—in particular, nonnarcotic analgesic drugs (pain killers)—must be safe or else they would require a prescription. These drugs include acetaminophen (Tylenol), aspirin, and a group called nonsteroidal anti-inflammatory drugs (NSAIDs) such as ibuprofen (Motrin, Advil). Many people either use these drugs chronically or take higher than recommended doses and do not realize that they are causing stomach, liver, and kidney damage. The chronic use of these medications can cause other problems as well.

Aspirin and NSAIDs

A few things should be mentioned about nonnarcotic pain killers, or analgesic medication, as your doctor would call them. These medications are usually prescribed for mild to moderate pain mostly associated with inflammation. The method of action involves the effect these medications have on a group of substances called prostaglandins which have many functions including contributing to inflammation and bleeding. Tylenol, however, works differently and does not cause bleeding.

The effect of aspirin and NSAIDs on bleeding is of concern if a person is about to undergo surgery. Platelets, which are responsible for preventing bleeding, are affected by aspirin and NSAIDs. The turnover of platelet creation is about 2 weeks. Once exposed to these drugs, their ability to stop bleeding is decreased. That is why aspirin and NSAIDs should not be taken for 2 weeks prior to surgery. NSAIDs have been associated with ulcers and gastrointestinal bleeding even in patients who have achlorhydria, which is a marked decrease or absence of stomach acid. NSAIDs may also increase the risk of the development of gastric infection from *H. pylori,* as a study suggests. *H. pylori* has also been shown to cause gastric ulcer disease.

Additionally, chronic NSAID use has been shown to be one of the causes of increased intestinal permeability, which can cause T-cell mediated allergy, which may contribute to autoimmune and other diseases. (*See the Allergies and Autoimmune Diseases protocols.*)

Acetaminophen

Acetaminophen (Tylenol) is perhaps one of the more potentially dangerous analgesic drugs. An intentional overdose can be fatal, and chronic dosing may cause liver and kidney damage as well. When a person takes acetaminophen, it is metabolized by a number of metabolic systems in the liver, including one called the P450 system. This results in an intermediate byproduct, or metabolite, that is very reactive and can kill liver cells. This intermediate metabolite is normally converted to a harmless final metabolite by an antioxidant in the liver called glutathione. Antioxidants prevent damage caused by free radicals, which are very reactive chemical entities created biochemically in our bodies as a result of many different reactions, including the metabolism of drugs.

However, when too much acetaminophen is taken, there is not enough glutathione available, and the toxic metabolite accumulates, resulting in liver failure and death. Alcoholics and those on certain medications which stimulate the P450 system are at particular risk because with increased P450 activity, more of the toxic intermediate is created than there is glutathione available to further metabolize it to something harmless. Although not fatal, chronic acetaminophen use decreases the functional capacity of the liver.

If a person attempts to commit suicide by taking an entire bottle of acetaminophen, the emergency room doctor will administer an antioxidant drug called Mucosil (Mucomyst). If administered in time, Mucosil can save the patient's life by inhibiting free-radical damage to the liver caused by acetaminophen-induced depletion of hepatic glutathione. The active ingredient in Mucosil is the nutrient *N*-acetylcysteine (NAC). NAC suppresses the toxic free radicals generated by ingested acetaminophen. If you have to take acetaminophen, we suggest you take the amino acid *N*-acetylcysteine or *L*-cysteine along with at least 1 gram of vitamin C with each dose of acetaminophen.

Another approach to protecting against acetaminophen-induced free-radical liver damage is to take one capsule of a multinutrient formula that contains glutathione, vitamin C, and cysteine with each dose of acetaminophen. This antioxidant formula will provide significant protection to the liver. Additionally, for those who must take acetaminophen chronically, the herb milk thistle (silymarin) may offer some liver protection by increasing the amount of the protective antioxidant glutathione. For those whose liver function has been compromised by analgesics or other toxins, treatment with SAMe (*S*-adenosylmethionine) may help to repair the liver.

Acetaminophen can also cause permanent kidney damage when taken over extended periods of time. This damage can be lethal to those with underlying kidney disease. There are no nutrient supplements known to protect against acetaminophen-induced kidney damage, although the amino acid taurine (1000 mg to 3000 mg a day) and high doses of vitamin E succinate (800 to 1200 IU a day) might be helpful.

The Food and Drug Administration does not require the manufacturers of Tylenol and other brands of acetaminophen to adequately warn people with kidney disease to avoid this pain medication. However, for those in chronic pain who cannot find relief from natural pain relief therapies (see Pain and Arthritis protocols), it is suggested that Tylenol and other brands of acetaminophen be used sparingly.

Some people alternate other types of OTC pain-relieving drugs, such as aspirin, Advil, and Naprosyn, to avoid using acetaminophen on a daily basis. Although these drugs also have dangerous side effects, alternating their use may help to reduce their toxicity.

To illustrate how dangerous acetaminophen can be, one study showed that people who used acetaminophen with other pain relievers on a regular basis had a three- to eightfold increase in their risk of kidney cancer. Kidney cancer is very difficult to treat. The liver/kidney/heart muscle toxicities and the cancer risks of analgesic drugs have not been reported by most media, which reap tremendous profits from the advertising of pain-relief products.

When using the drug Mucosil (*N*-acetylcysteine) to treat acute liver failure from acetaminophen overdose, it is crucial that the drug be administered immediately and that it be continued for at least 36 hours in all cases. Optimal results occur when NAC is administered within 10 hours of acetaminophen overdose. NAC is also effective when given after 15 hours of acetaminophen poisoning. Treatment with *N*-acetylcysteine (NAC) should not be discontinued until all clinical signs of toxicity have subsided. Permanent liver injury can occur if NAC therapy is discontinued too soon. Patients who develop chronic liver failure should be treated with a prolonged course of NAC under a physician's care.

Headache and Analgesic Rebound

One of the more common reasons for chronic analgesic use is for the treatment of headache. Many patients suffer from chronic headaches for years, some over 10 years in duration. These patients have seen numerous physicians, including neurologists and pain specialists and have received countless studies, including MRIs and CTs of the brain. They have also had several diagnoses over the course of their treatment. A large proportion of these patients suffered from a condition that has been described in the literature as analgesic rebound. Simply stated, the problem began when the patients first experienced a few headaches in succession and began taking analgesic medications. They quickly increased the dose and found that they could not survive without the medications. However, the medications failed to totally relieve their headaches. The treatment, from the doctor's perspective, is simple; stop taking all pain medications. The cause of the headaches is a rebound effect from stopping large doses of analgesic medications. If the patient can get through several weeks of totally ceasing the use of all analgesic medications, the headaches will cease. Needless to say, it is not surprising how difficult it is to convince the patient of this.

Physicians may attempt various types of treatment to help break the cycle, including acupuncture, orthomolecular doses of intravenous vitamin C, intravenous dimethyl sulfoxide (DMSO), and short-time low-dose corticosteroid administration. Ultimately, it may be the cessation of all analgesic drug use that rids the patient of the headache. However, to help the patient deal with the pain during the two-week treatment program, the administration of intravenous DMSO or short-term corticosteroid has been most helpful. Next to "cold turkey," intravenous DMSO is probably the best way to go. (*See the Migraine protocol.*)

Summary

1. Aspirin, Tylenol, and NSAIDs, while generally safe for short-term use, can cause problems with long-term administration. These include liver and kidney damage, gastrointestinal bleeding. Those who drink excessive alcohol are at risk and should not take Tylenol at all.
2. Those who must chronically take acetaminophen drugs should take vitamin C, NAC, *L*-cysteine, taurine, vitamin E succinate, and milk thistle. Those who develop liver damage should consider taking SAMe. They should also consider the intravenous administration of vitamin C and glutathione by a physician experienced with this treatment.

WARNING: Known acetaminophen overdose is an emergency requiring hospitalization. If the amount of acetaminophen taken is unclear, do not wait until symptoms develop to make a decision to seek hospital care. By that time it is too late and death may be likely. Do not attempt to treat this at home with oral Mucosil (*N*-acetylcysteine.) Hospital monitoring is essential.

3. Chronic use of analgesic drugs to treat headaches may actually be the cause of the headaches. Under a physician's care, try stopping all use of these drugs. If this proves to be very difficult, consult with a physician who utilizes intravenous DMSO or would consider short-term administration of corticosteroids. Contact the American Academy for Advancement of Medicine, (800) 532-3688, to find such a physician in your area.

Product availability. Glutathione, vitamin C, cysteine capsules, NAC (*N*-acetylcysteine) caps, taurine, vitamin E succinate caps, and vitamin C caps are available from the Life Extension Foundation at (800) 544-4440, or order on-line at www.lef.org.

ACNE

Acne is an inflammatory disease of the oil glands. The oil glands, mainly located on the face, chest, back, and upper arms, are called sebaceous glands. The thick, oily material they secrete is called sebum. During puberty, hormonal changes stimulate secretion of the oil glands and also cause their enlargement. As a person approaches adolescence, the oil glands are activated. The causes of acne are unknown, and there is much to be learned about the elements which influence its development.

Types of Acne

1. Superficial pustules (pus at follicular opening)
2. Nodules (pus deep in dermis)
3. Cysts (nodules that fail to discharge to surface of skin)
4. Large deep pustules (nodules that break down, leading to scars)
5. Open comedones (blackheads), dilated follicles with central dark, horny plugs
6. Closed comedones (whiteheads), inflammatory changes of small follicular papules with or without red papules.

Acne-like lesions can occur in response to a variety of compounds: corticosteroids, halogens, isonicotinic acid, diphenylhydantoin, and some psychotropics. Exposure to various industrial pollutants such as oils, coal tar derivatives, tobacco smoke, and chlorinated hydrocarbons also causes acne. Other factors can include cosmetics, facial creams, over-washing, and repetitive touching.

Oil gland plugs are visible as black or white dots at the skin surface. When the oil builds up, the swollen gland usually appears as a white blemish called a whitehead. The primary problem is plugging of the oil gland openings caused by a build-up in the tiny orifices, which conduct oil to the surface. This irritation increases, producing the red spots we see as acne blemishes. Bacteria within the blemish cause the oil to "alter," giving rise to infectious irritation (inflammation) of the oil gland wall. Eventually breakage of the gland occurs below the skin.

Young people tend to have small red blemishes (papules), pus-filled yellowish blemishes (pustules), larger hard blemishes (nodules), and sometimes cystic lesions under the skin. These last-mentioned cysts are the most difficult of all acne spots, and pose the greatest threat of scarring. They become ruptured oil glands walled off by the skin. The primary reason for treating acne is to prevent scarring.

As the redness due to facial blemishes improves, the blemishes turn a lighter purplish color as healing begins. Most blemishes will fade with time. Cosmetics wearers should use only water-based foundation and powder blush. Generic medications produce unpredictable and inconsistent results. Sun exposure can actually make acne worse, and may be a cause of skin cancer later in life. A false notion is that acne is an infection. Acne cannot be transmitted to others. It is not an allergy and, despite common thinking, foods have little or no effect on it.

Rosacea is a rash commonly confused with acne. The cause is unknown, but it occurs most frequently in women with a fair complexion who are over 30. Symptoms include a swollen red nose, puffy cheeks, and a persistent blush on other parts of the face. Oral antibiotics such as tetracycline are effective in the treatment, as are topical antibiotics such as metronidazole gel.

Use of Cosmetics

Regular cosmetics can block oil glands and cause new lesions. Cold creams can cause obstruction of oil glands and create new acne. Hypoallergenic, oil-free, water-based foundations and powder blush are better for the skin.

Sex Hormones and Acne

Sexual activities have absolutely nothing to do with the development or remission of acne lesions. Some women do notice a flareup of acne symptoms a few days to a week before the onset of their menstrual periods. This can be handled adequately with adjustment of the acne treatments, including increasing the dosage of the medicines you'll be using around that time.

Androgens are male sex hormones. Acne is considered to be an androgen-dependent condition. Androgen excess, either systemic or local, is associated with more severe forms of the disease. Androgens control sebaceous gland secretion and exacerbate the development of abnormal follicular epithelium.

The endocrine glands are any of various glands, such as the thyroid, adrenal, and pituitary, that secrete hormones directly into the blood or lymph. Endocrine disorders producing excess androgens are important etiological factors in the onset of acne. These include idiopathic adrenal androgen excess, partial defect in 21-hydroxylase, and polycystic ovarian syndrome. Free testosterone, dehydroepiandrosterone (DHEA), dehydroepiandrosterone sulfate (DHEA-S), and low sex-hormone-binding globulin levels have all been implicated. The skin of acne patients shows greater activity of 5-alpha-reductase, the enzyme converting testosterone to the more potent androgen, dihydrotestosterone. This increased activity is independent of systemic levels of androgens and may explain the poor correlation between systemic levels of androgens and the severity of the acne lesions.

Acne Treatments

There are about as many ways to treat acne patients as there are patients who have acne. Most external treatments dry the face to some extent and cause some degree of mild peeling that loosens plugs in oil glands. Peeling smooths the face and resolves the old and new lesions. Most patients receive some sort of topical drying therapy to promote healing. External medications can be irritating and may need a period of adjustment. Some minor irritation often occurs, especially at the start of therapy.

Antibiotics

Other major ways in which acne is treated include oral antibiotics to prevent the formation of new blemishes while externally applied medications are working to resolve the old and the new blemishes. Antibiotics prevent new blemishes in at least two ways: (1) by killing bacteria which make an enzyme that changes oil into a substance called "free fatty acid" (FFA). FFA is very irritating and can cause the rupture of oil glands, making what we normally see as a red acne blemish. (2) The other advantage of antibiotics is that they inhibit the enzyme that breaks down sebum into FFA. Some generic antibiotics however, can suppress and may compromise your immune system if used for prolonged periods of time.

Antibiotics, including topical ones, should not be used during pregnancy.

WARNING: Studies have shown that prolonged used of antibiotics may cause fetal damage, mental retardation, and even autism after birth; they should not be used in pregnancy unless approved by your obstetrician.

There have been a few studies that show possible decreased effectiveness of birth control pills when a patient is on oral antibiotics.

It is important to follow dosing recommendations for various antibiotics. Tetracycline (Sumycin tablets, Achromycin, Panmycin) needs to be taken on an empty stomach, which means an hour before meals or two hours after meals. Minocycline (Minocin) may be taken with or without meals, though it may be slightly more effective if taken on an empty stomach. Erythromycin (EES-400, PCE, E-mycin) should be taken with meals, since it may upset the stomach and cause stomach pain in some patients if taken on an empty stomach.

Isotretinoin

If antibiotics are ineffective in the treatment of cystic acne conditions, physicians will often prescribe isotretinoin (Accutane) capsules. Accutane is a retinoid which inhibits sebaceous gland function and keratinization. It is prescribed with caution in women of child-bearing age because of the high risk of fetal deformity if taken even for short periods while pregnant. Regular blood testing is given to determine the presence of liver damage. Dry eyes, chapped lips, and dryness of the vaginal lining and penis have been reported. Treatment may last for up to 20 weeks. Treatment should be discontinued for 4 months before restarting therapy.

Diet and Nutrition

Western medicine now believes that acne is not a food-related problem and seldom asks patients to change their diets as a means of reducing outbreaks. Some alternative therapists, however, make a change in diet on the basis of treatment. Experts in both schools of thought concede that chocolate, fats, and other foods don't cause acne, but they are unsure of whether they can aggravate the condition.

Subjects fed a high-protein diet (44% protein, 35% carbohydrate, and 21% fat) show substantially less 5-alpha-reduction of testosterone and enhanced cytochrome p-450 hydroxylation of estradiol, both therapeutic goals. A high carbohydrate diet (10% protein, 70% carbohydrate, and 20% fat) had the opposite effect.

Foods high in iodine should be eliminated and milk consumption (due to high hormone content) should be limited. Trans-fatty acids and high-fat foods should also be eliminated. Meats and poultry that originated from hormone-raised animals should be avoided at all costs.

Where diet is concerned in the treatment of acne, the safest thing is to avoid and eliminate all refined or concentrated carbohydrates and limit high-fat and high-carbohydrate foods. Focus on avoiding foods containing trans-fatty acids and iodine.

Sugar, Insulin, and Chromium

Many dermatologists have reported that insulin is effective in the treatment of acne, suggesting impaired cutaneous glucose tolerance and/or insulin insensitivity. The insulin was given either systemically (5 to 10 units 2 to 3 times a week) or injected directly into the lesion.

One study comparing the results of oral glucose tolerance tests in acne patients showed no differences from controls. However, repetitive skin biopsies revealed that the acne patients' skin glucose tolerance was significantly impaired. One researcher, in discussing the role of glucose tolerance in acne, coined the term *skin diabetes* to describe the disorder of acne.

Considering the known immuno-suppressive effects of sugar, all concentrated carbohydrates should be strictly eliminated. High-chromium yeast is known to improve glucose tolerance and enhance insulin sensitivity. In an uncontrolled study, chromium was reported to induce rapid improvement in patients with acne.

Herbs, Vitamins, and Minerals

Some alternative therapies for acne attempt to reduce inflammation and fight infection. Other approaches use herbal or dietary measures to control factors, such as stress, that may promote acne. For mild or moderate acne, these approaches may make sense, but acne vulgaris and rosacea respond much more slowly than most other ailments to any therapy. Many acne treatments take up to a year to produce results.

Among vitamin and mineral supplements, nutritionists generally suggest zinc (methionate is best), which plays a part in how the body processes hormones. A 50-mg zinc supplement daily may contribute to reducing inflammation and healing damaged skin. Chromium supplements are said to boost the body's ability to break down glucose.

Vitamin B_6, which aids in the metabolism of hormones, can be particularly effective for women suffering from premenstrual acne; 50 mg daily is a typical dosage. Vitamin E, an antioxidant, may also be included at doses of 200 to 400 IU daily.

Other skin-supporting nutrients include water, fiber, vitamin A, beta carotene, vitamin C, calcium, selenium, silica, B vitamins, vitamin B_6, biotin, essential fatty acids, olive oil, cod liver oil, linseed oil, omega-3 fatty acids (EPA), gamma-linolenic acid (GLA), all amino acids, *L*-cysteine, and *L*-proline.

Vitamin A

Vitamin A retinols, including oral vitamin A, have been shown in many studies to reduce sebum production and the hyperkeratosis of sebaceous follicles. Retinol has been shown to be effective in treating acne.

CAUTION: Although dosages of vitamin A below 300,000 IU a day for a few months rarely cause toxicity symptoms, early recognition is important.

Cheilitis (chapped lips) and xerosis (dry skin) will generally occur in the majority of patients, particularly in dry weather. Refer to Appendix A for complete information about using high-potency vitamin A supplements.

Herbal Therapies

Some herbs heal the skin and soothe inflammation and itching. Chinese herbalists may recommend echinacea, calendula, tea tree oil, and goldenseal tincture or blue flag, which works well with echinacea. Drinking tea of nettles and cleavers tincture may be effective. Never use any herbal preparation on newborns without consulting your doctor.

If stress may be contributing to your acne, relax with a cup of lavender or chamomile tea. A facial steam treatment with these herbs two or three times a week may help.

Topical treatments with bentonite masks three times a week, use of calendula soap, and the draining of comedones with a comedo extractor will help.

At-Home Remedies

- ▼ Wash your face gently with unscented, oil-free soap and keep your skin clean; however, scrubbing an inflamed skin condition only makes acne worse.
- ▼ Control the urge to pop pimples; let them pop when they're ready.
- ▼ For mild to moderate acne, try treatments that contain benzoyl peroxide.
- ▼ Do not overexpose your acne to sunlight; do so only in moderation.
- ▼ Young men with moderate to severe acne should use new razor blades every time they shave to lessen the risk of infection.
- ▼ Avoid alcohol-based after-shaves; use herbal alternatives that include essential oils of lavender, chamomile, or tea tree oil.

Prevention

Because of acne's association with fluctuating hormone levels and possible genetic influences, many doctors believe there is no way to prevent it. Although the accepted wisdom is that neither good hygiene nor diet can prevent outbreaks, the diet and nutrition recommendations may be helpful. Good general hygiene and sensible skin care are especially important during adolescence. The basics include a daily bath or shower, and washing face and hands with unscented or mildly antibacterial soap. Teenage girls are better off not using cosmetics regularly. Despite claims to the contrary, few if any commercial skin medications have any beneficial effect on acne.

Summary

1. Over-exposure to the sun may worsen the condition.
2. Only hypoallergenic, oil-free cosmetics should be used.
3. Oral and topical antibiotics may prevent new blemishes by killing bacteria and breaking down sebum into FFA.
4. Foods high in fat, hormones, and iodine should be eliminated.
5. Chromium may improve glucose tolerance, thus improving an acne condition.
6. Zinc, 50 mg daily, may be taken to reduce inflammation and heal damaged skin.
7. Vitamin B_6, 50 mg daily, may be taken to aid in hormone metabolism.
8. Vitamin E, 200 to 400 IU daily, is suggested for its antioxidant properties.
9. Vitamin A, below 300,000 IU daily, should be taken to reduce sebum production.
10. Bentonite masks should be applied three times a week, and regular washing with calendula soap may be helpful.

For more information. Contact the American Academy of Dermatology, 708-330-0230.

Product availability. Chromium capsules, zinc supplements, complete B-Complex vitamins, vitamin E, and the complete multi-nutrient Life Extension Mix can be ordered by calling (800) 544-4440 or order on-line at www.lef.org.

ADRENAL DISEASE

The adrenals are two relatively crescent-shaped glands that are found lying over the upper pole of each kidney. Each adrenal gland consists of internal layers that produce different substances. The inner part, or adrenal medulla, manufactures epinephrine and norepinephrine, more commonly known as adrenaline and noradrenaline. These hormones are the "fight or flight" hormones that are released in potentially "life or death" situations. Their release increases heart rate and blood pressure and diverts more blood to the brain, heart, and skeletal muscles. This is important when discussing stress (*see Anxiety and Stress protocol*) as well as adrenal fatigue.

The adrenal cortex lies outside the adrenal medulla and responds to a different type of stress. This is where the steroid hormones are made. These include cortisone, hydrocortisone, testosterone, estrogen, 17-hydroxy-ketosteroids, DHEA, DHEA sulfate, pregnenolone, aldosterone, androstenedione, progesterone, and some other hormones which are intermediates in production. Many of these hormones are also made elsewhere in the body, but aldosterone, cortisone, and hydrocortisone are made only in the adrenal glands.

The hormone aldosterone, in concert with the kidneys, regulates the balance of sodium and potassium in the body. This regulation is critical to many areas of physiological function, including the ability to react to stress and to maintain fluid balance. It even contributes to maintenance of blood pressure.

Supplemental Steroids and Adrenal Disease

Cortisone and hydrocortisone regulate the body's glucose. Most readers are familiar with the administration of corticosteroids to suppress the immune system. Corticosteroids became available in the late 1940s and were heralded as a miraculous treatment for rheumatoid arthritis. It did not take long to find out that there was a serious price to pay for chronic corticosteroid use. Patients developed symptoms, and physical findings such as the development of Cushing's syndrome resulted from the body's overexposure to corticosteroids.

Patients with Cushing's syndrome usually have central obesity, sparing the arms and legs, a reddish "moon face," "buffalo hump," protuberant abdomen, and thin extremities. Additionally, women may have less frequent menses or lose them altogether. Men may become impotent. There is also weakness, headache, high blood pressure, acne, and thinning of the skin. Patients may develop diabetic symptoms and easy bruisability as well as other problems. Wound healing is impaired and patients are susceptible to infections. Mental symptoms may range from increased fluctuation of mood to psychosis.

Out of these findings, an irrational approach developed to the question of relative adrenal function. A person who suffers from total failure of the adrenal glands is said to have Addison's disease. So physicians approach patients as normal, or as suffering from Addison's disease or Cushing's syndrome. (It should be noted that low steroid levels can also be caused by failure of the hypothalamus, thalamus, and pituitary areas of the brain. In this case, the adrenal glands still function.) This discussion is directed only at the function of the adrenal glands.

The result is that, when a physician evaluates a patient relying solely upon laboratory data, the patient is considered either "normal" or having one of the conditions mentioned. There is no in between. However, just as in thyroid dysfunction (*see Thyroid Deficiency protocol*), normal laboratory tests do not exclude what many physicians call adrenal fatigue.

Adrenal Fatigue

The main cause of adrenal fatigue is continual low-level stress, which taxes the adrenal glands, limiting their reserve. This low-level stress may be caused by emotional or physical upsets or even loss of sleep. Essentially, "the tank, running on empty, does not have enough gas to get you home." Clinically, this manifests in the development of exhaustion after stress that does not become resolved. Days after hearty exercise, a person may complain of exhaustion. So, if a person who could normally walk several blocks to go shopping suddenly complains that this makes him or her exhausted, adrenal fatigue should be considered before anything else.

Another interesting and common symptom is that people may note that they are relatively more alert, energetic, and "with it," later in the day. They may get to sleep later than normal and the sleep is not restful. They find that sleeping in late is when they get the most restorative sleep.

The association with impaired immune function and the administration of corticosteroids has blurred an important fact. Decreased levels of corticosteroids also impair immune function. What further complicates the matter is the fact that it is now thought that continual overproduction of cortisol, not in the range that would produce Cushing's syndrome, contributes to immune suppression, atherosclerosis, brain cell injury, and accelerated aging.

According to the experience of many physicians who practice complementary medicine, certain conditions can be benefited from treating adrenal fatigue. Some of these conditions are acute viral illness, allergies, gastritis, osteoarthritis, rheumatoid arthritis, eczema, contact dermatitis, urticaria (hives), psoriasis, and allergic rhinitis, to name the more common examples.

Treatment of Adrenal Fatigue

It is most important to make certain that full-blown Addison's disease is not the problem, since it must be treated vigorously. The patient should be evaluated by a physician with experience in recognizing and treating adrenal fatigue. A resource for finding such a physician is noted at the end of this protocol.

The goal is to relieve the stressful situation causing the problem and, while this is being done, supply additional corticosteroid. This may be done in a number of ways. Many physicians familiar with complementary medicine suggest beginning with adrenal glandular concentrates, which may be found at your health store. In combination with this, or taken alone, glycyrrhiza, which comes from licorice and may be taken in a variety of ways, including as a tea, may be helpful. It reduces the amount of hydrocortisone broken down by the liver, thereby reducing the workload of the adrenal glands.

Some patients may require more potent measures. In addition to the previous recommendations, some physicians utilize adrenal cortical extract (ACE), which contains all the corticosteroids in the proper proportions. It used to be widely available in this country, but at the present time it is not. Again, complementary physicians may have experience with it. If ACE is unobtainable, off-the-shelf brands of hydrocortisone may be given in physiologic dosages of 5 to 10 mg four times a day. When hydrocortisone was first used, the doses were 100 mg and up, which resulted in the development of the problems that have made conventional physicians fearful of administering corticosteroids on a short-term basis. Prednisone, which must be converted in the liver to become active, is not recommended.

Adrenal Function and Aging

Aging and the diseases of aging can cause a decline in critical hormones produced by the adrenal glands. Pregnenolone is converted into crucial anti-aging hormones such as DHEA (dehydroepiandrosterone), estrogen, progesterone and testosterone. Pregnenolone supplementation may help to rectify hormone imbalances caused by aging-induced adrenal insufficiency.

Additionally, pregnenolone or DHEA supplementation may protect against the over-production of cortisol from the adrenal glands. Too much cortisol may accelerate aging and a host of other degenerative diseases. Vitamin C and aspirin may block excessive cortisol production as well. As both pregnenolone and DHEA are presently thought to have anti-aging and nootropic properties, experienced physicians often prescribe both (*see protocol on Age-Associated Mental Impairment for a discussion on nootropic agents*). (*See also Precautions under the DHEA Replacement Therapy protocol.*)

At times of increased stress, the addition of adrenal glandulars may be advisable. Long-term use is not recommended.

The European drug KH3 (the active ingredient is procaine) can block some of the cell-damaging effects of cortisol. To help protect against cortisol toxicity, take one to two KH3 capsules in the morning on an empty stomach and one to two KH3 capsules in mid-afternoon on an empty stomach.

CAUTION: Addison's disease requires expert physician intervention. Glucocorticoid and mineralocorticoid drugs are prescribed for Addison's disease. Once cortisol levels are stabilized, serum levels of DHEA should be evaluated to determine if DHEA replacement therapy is warranted. In 80% of cases, Addison's disease is caused by an autoimmune attack on the adrenal glands.

(Before taking DHEA or pregnenolone, refer to the Foundation's precautions in the DHEA Replacement Therapy protocol. Also refer to the Autoimmune Diseases protocol for additional suggestions.)

Summary for Treating Adrenal Fatigue

1. Get physician evaluation to rule out Addison's disease.
2. Identify and relieve sources of stress.
3. Take licorice tea or its equivalent 4 times a day.
4. Consider physician-administered ACE (adrenal cortical extract) injections for 3 to 7 days.
5. Consider hydrocortisone tablets, 5 to 10 mg, 4 times a day for 3 to 7 days.

Summary for Maintaining Corticosteroid Balance to Prevent Aging

1. Obtain baseline corticosteroid and DHEA levels.
2. Begin with 50 mg of pregnenolone a day and follow with lab tests.
3. Consider the addition of DHEA. Dosage may range from 5 to 100 mg a day and must be followed by lab tests (*see DHEA Replacement Therapy precautions*).
4. Consider ¼ tablet of aspirin daily, taken with a heavy meal.
5. Consider vitamin C, 3000 mg a day in divided doses.
6. Take adrenal glandulars at times of increased stress.
7. Consider KH3, 1 capsule in the morning and 1 to 2 in the afternoon.

For more information. Contact the American College for Advancement in Medicine, (800) 532-3688, for a physician in your area who practices complementary medicine.

Product availability. Pregnenolone capsules, DHEA, vitamin C powder and capsules, and ¼ aspirin tablets (Healthprin) can be ordered by phoning (800) 544-4440, or order on-line at www.lef.org. The Life Extension Foundation does not carry KH3, but can provide a list of companies abroad that sell KH3 to Americans for personal use.

AGE-ASSOCIATED MENTAL IMPAIRMENT (COGNITIVE ENHANCEMENT)

Aging precipitates a progressive decline in overall cognitive function. It causes us to lose our ability to store and retrieve from short-term memory and to learn new information. Many neurological diseases are directly related to aging. Aging impacts cognitive function in several ways, including

- Damaging effects from years of free-radical exposure
- Changes in lifestyle, diet, and nutrient absorption, leading to deficiencies
- Decreases in levels of key hormones
- Decreases in oxygen available to brain cells because of impaired circulation due to pathology (for example, atherosclerosis or heart disease) or a lifetime of poor health habits (for example, smoking, drinking, drug abuse, limited exercise, poor diet, or stress)
- Declining energy output of brain cells

The Life Extension Foundation has evaluated thousands of published studies showing that brain aging can be controlled, at least in part. Some of these studies demonstrate a preventive effect, whereas others show a benefit in reversing the cognitive impairment caused by normal aging or by a specific disease of aging, such as stroke.

This protocol has been designed specifically for those experiencing age-associated mental impairment due either to aging itself or to an age-related disease. Younger people, or parents who are concerned about possible cognitive deficits in their children, should consult the *Attention Deficit Disorder* protocol.

Forms

Age-associated neurological impairment can take a variety of forms, including memory loss, senility, and dementia. Dementia, a general term for diseases involving nerve cell deterioration, is defined as a loss in at least two areas of complex behavior—areas include language, memory, visual and spatial abilities, and judgment—so as to interfere with a person's daily living. Dementia, the most serious form of age-associated mental impairment, is often a slow, gradual process that may take months or even years to become noticeable. Symptoms vary depending on which areas of the brain are affected.

It is important to distinguish normal, age-associated mental impairment from conditions such as dementia that signal a disease process. Not all memory difficulties or cognitive complaints indicate the presence of Alzheimer's disease or any mental disorder. Many memory changes are temporary and are linked to environmental factors such as stress rather than to physiological (bodily) processes. It is also common for older people and those around them to notice memory lapses and to be more concerned about them than younger people, when in fact those lapses may not be any different from those of a younger person who misplaces her keys.

At the same time, serious cognitive difficulties should not be dismissed as unavoidable consequences of aging. A helpful guideline is that many people with serious mental impairment do not recognize or will not admit that they have a problem, while it is obvious to those around them. The recommendations given in this protocol can help age-associated mental impairment of any form or cause, but significant impairment arising from diseases such as stroke should be treated with the help of medical professionals.

Causes

Age-associated mental impairment can have a variety of causes beyond overall aging. Conditions that affect the brain and result in intellectual, behavioral, and psychological dysfunction include the following:

Medication side effects. Adverse side effects can result from too high or too low a dosage of medications, unusual reactions to medications, or combinations of medications. It is especially common in the older population for individuals to be taking many different medications prescribed by different doctors, in addition to over-the-counter supplements. Be certain that your primary physician is aware of all prescription and nonprescription medications that you take.

Substance abuse. Abuse of drugs (legal or illegal) and alcohol can cause mental impairment. Older people are less able to tolerate and recover from the use of such substances. Alcohol also causes liver damage, increasing the risk of liver disease, which often leads to dementia.

Metabolic disorders. Thyroid problems, anemias, and nutritional deficiencies—common in older people who have less appetite and less energy to cook and shop, and who absorb fewer nutrients from the food they eat—have a negative impact on mental function. These problems may go undetected in older people when symptoms are attributed to aging.

Neurological disorders. Multiple sclerosis (*see Multiple Sclerosis protocol*) and normal-pressure hydrocephalus (increased fluid in the brain) are examples of conditions that affect mental function.

Infections. The brain is susceptible to viral, bacterial, and fungal infections. One extremely rare infection of the brain that causes dementia is Creutzfeldt-Jakob disease, transmitted by a special protein (prion) that damages tissue as it replicates.

Trauma. Head trauma can result in transient (concussion) or lasting mental impairment. Trauma is obvious in most cases based on history and examination. One type of head trauma frequent in older people, however, is not always obvious. It is called a subdural hematoma, which means that blood is leaking into the tissues around the brain. This type of injury can occur after very minimal trauma, and its onset can be very gradual if the leak is small. Symptoms—headache, confusion, and lethargy—are often nonspecific. (*See also Trauma protocol.*)

Toxic factors. Exposure to substances such as carbon monoxide and methyl alcohol can cause mental impairment.

Hormonal changes. Medicine is only beginning to understand the hormonal changes that accompany aging. In women a fairly sudden drop in the hormone estradiol leads to menopause (*see Menopause protocol*). In addition to symptoms such as hot flashes, decreased bone density, and vaginal dryness, symptoms of altered mental function such as mood swings, nervousness, and fatigue are common. In men, testosterone levels decrease gradually over time, leading to decreased muscle tissue and bone density, increased abdominal fat and cholesterol, deteriorating heart function, and psychological and sexual changes that can impact mental function. In both sexes, the level of the hormone dehydroepiandrosterone (DHEA) falls precipitously with age.

Tumors. Abnormal tissue growth (tumors) in the brain can be either primary (originating in the brain itself) or metastatic ("seeds" of tissue that originated in a tumor in another part of the body, and that have traveled to the brain and begun to grow). Metastatic tumors are more common. Approximately 70% of brain tumors are benign. (*See also Cancer protocols.*)

Depression

Depression, stress, and grief are common causes of mental impairment that are transient and treatable (*see Anxiety and Stress protocol and Depression protocol*). Depression in older people is often overlooked because symptoms are confused with those of a medical illness. Depression is also considered a normal part of aging: the National Mental Health Association reports that over 58% of older adults believe depression accompanies aging. Although older adults may have difficult experiences such as changes in health status, relocation, or loss of loved ones, if the sadness that follows one of these life changes lingers for a long period of time, it may be diagnosed as clinical depression (*see Depression protocol*). Late-life depression affects about 6 million people, most of them women, but only about 10% of them ever receive treatment for their condition. Depression has serious consequences. It takes the pleasure out of daily life, aggravates other medical conditions, and can lead to suicide. In fact, older adults are considered the group most at risk for suicide. (The suicide rate in older adults is more than 50% higher than the rate for the nation as a whole.) Mental illnesses can also impair mental functioning.

Circulatory Disorders

Circulatory disorders, such as heart problems (*see Atherosclerosis and Congestive Heart Failure protocols*) or stroke can restrict the oxygen available to brain cells by reducing blood flow. Also, many people who feel fine may have a buildup of plaque in their arteries (atherosclerosis), which can eventually limit the oxygen supply to the brain. The most common type of stroke is called an ischemic stroke. This means that a blood clot has traveled to the brain, where it has lodged in a vessel so that brain cells have died from lack of oxygen.

In a hemorrhagic stroke, a vessel bursts, flooding brain cells with blood. Transient ischemic attacks (TIAs) are miniature strokes caused when blood flow is blocked to a variable extent for a few hours or a day but is then restored, causing no permanent damage. TIAs are an important warning signal that treatment is necessary to prevent a more serious stroke.

Strokes occur most often in older people: three fourths occur in people over age 65. Symptoms depend on the part of the brain affected, but can include difficulty moving, talking, and thinking. The Stroke protocols describe the acute care of strokes, in other words, what to do right after a stroke has occurred. The recommendations contained in these protocols will help to improve long-term recovery of mental function, such as memory, attention, and learning. It should be noted that normal aging creates a perfusion (circulation) deficit in the brain, so nutrients and drugs that improve cerebral circulation are of critical importance to even healthy humans as they grow older.

Mid-Life Blood Pressure: A New Risk Factor

A 30-year study of male twins showed that elevated blood pressure in mid-life predisposed men to accelerated brain aging and an increase in stroke later in life. Men with even mildly elevated blood pressure 25 years before showed smaller brain volumes and more strokes compared to their twin brothers who did not have the elevation in blood pressure. This study, published in the journal *Stroke* (1999;30), emphasized the importance of aggressively treating elevated blood pressure even if it is not grossly abnormal. Refer to the Foundation's *Hypertension protocol* for information about blood pressure control therapies and diets.

Behavioral Treatments

Taking steps to improve overall health is highly recommended to prevent or minimize age-associated mental impairment. For example, exercising regularly, not smoking, and monitoring blood cholesterol level can reduce the risk of stroke and heart disease and keep arteries open, supplying the brain with oxygen and nutrients. Regular exercise improves some mental abilities by an average of 20 to 30%. Abstaining from alcohol or drug use, or minimizing it, can also help preserve mental function. Since people tend to eat less food as they age, the use of low-fat, nutrient-rich foods is recommended. Such a diet will help prevent nutrient deficiencies, which can impair mental function through physical illness.

Pharmacological and Nutritional Supplements

Memory-Enhancing Nutrients

The most commonly used memory-enhancing nutrients are choline, lecithin, and phosphatidylcholine, which are precursors to the chemical neurotransmitter acetylcholine, which carries messages between brain cells. Because acetylcholine helps brain cells communicate with each other, it plays an important role in learning and memory. One recent study found that phosphatidylcholine administered with vitamin B_{12} improved the memory of rats in whom brain damage had caused memory impairment. Acetylcholine deficiency can predispose a person to a wide range of neurological diseases, including Alzheimer's disease and stroke. Supplement choline, lecithin, and phosphatidylcholine early in the day to maximize improvement in brain productivity throughout the day. Suggested dosage ranges are 2,500 to 10,000 mg a day of choline or 10,000 to 15,000 g a day of lecithin, and/or 1,200 to 6,000 mg a day of phosphatidylcholine.

Brain Cell Energy Boosters

Another memory enhancement technique involves boosting the energy output of brain cells. With aging there is a decline in the ability of neurons to take up glucose (fuel) and to produce energy. This energy production decline not only causes memory and cognitive deficits but also results in the accumulation of cellular debris, which eventually kills brain cells. When enough brain cells have died from accumulated cellular debris, senility is usually diagnosed. Stroke and head trauma victims are especially in need of brain cell energy boosters, though everyone who undergoes normal aging will suffer from cerebral circulatory deficits and reduced brain cell energy output.

Ginkgo biloba extract (120 mg a day). This extract from the "maidenhair tree" improves blood flow, protects against free radicals, and is believed to improve memory. Ginkgo biloba is approved in Germany for the treatment of dementia. A scientific review found that the activities of the secondary metabolites of ginkgo biloba (the molecules into which it gets broken) are responsible for its cognition-enhancing and anti-aging activity, including neuroprotective effects.

In a study of 236 Alzheimer's patients, ginkgo biloba extract was found to stabilize or ameliorate dementia. In another study, patients with memory disturbances were supplemented with ginkgo biloba. Following ginkgo treatment, 15% of patients reported the total absence of memory disturbance symptoms, and 62% reported remaining symptoms as being mild to moderate. A study at the National Institutes of Health demonstrated that ginkgo biloba protects against the neurotoxic effects of reperfusion (the return of blood flow) following ischemia (the stopping of blood flow, as in a stroke) in rats.

Treatment with ginkgo biloba extract can also partially prevent certain harmful, age-related structural changes as well as free-radical damage to the mitochondria (where energy is produced in a cell) in the brains of old rats. In fact, another study showed that treating rats with ginkgo biloba extract not only improved their brain function (learning and memory) but also significantly extended their lifespan. There are over 1200 published studies in the scientific literature on ginkgo biloba extract.

Acetyl-L-carnitine (1000 to 2000 mg a day). About 95% of cellular energy occurs in the mitochondria, and diseases of aging are increasingly being referred to as "mitochondrial disorders." Acetyl-*L*-carnitine is the biologically active amino acid involved in the transport of fatty acids into the cell's mitochondria for the purpose of producing energy. Acetyl-*L*-carnitine is sold as an expensive drug in Europe to treat heart and neurological disease. It can increase muscle mass and convert body fat into energy. Acetyl-*L*-carnitine has been shown to protect brain cells against aging-related degeneration and to improve mood, memory, and cognition. Many people use acetyl-*L*-carnitine to maintain immune competence and reduce the formation of the aging pigment lipofuscin. The most important effect of acetyl-*L*-carnitine, however, is to maintain the function of the cell's energy powerhouse, the mitochondria.

A recently published article reported on research that showed that acetyl-*L*-carnitine modulated the use of glucose in the brain of rats. A Stanford University study of patients with Alzheimer's disease found that acetyl-*L*-carnitine slowed the progression of the disease in younger subjects.

Coenzyme Q_{10} (CoQ_{10}) (100 to 300 mg a day). When CoQ_{10} is orally administered, it is incorporated into the mitochondria of cells throughout the body, where it facilitates and regulates the oxidation of fats and sugars into energy. Heart cells have a high energy demand, and initial clinical studies investigated the effect of CoQ_{10} on cardiac mitochondrial function. Therapeutic efficacy was shown in double-blind studies when CoQ_{10} was used in the treatment of congestive heart disease, coronary artery disease, and valvular disorders. Scientists are now looking at the effects of CoQ_{10} on another organ whose cells also require a high level of energy metabolism—the brain!

Here are the highlights from a study published in the *Proceedings of the National Academy of Sciences* (1998; 95):

> When coenzyme Q_{10} was administered to middle-age and old rats, the level of CoQ_{10} increased by 10% to 40% in the cerebral cortex region of the brain. This increase was sufficient to restore levels of CoQ_{10} to those seen in young animals.
>
> After only two months of CoQ_{10} supplementation, mitochondrial energy expenditure in the brain increased by 29% compared to the group not getting CoQ_{10}. The human equivalent dose of CoQ_{10} to achieve parallel results was 100–200 mg a day.
>
> When a neuro-toxin was administered, CoQ_{10} helped protect against damage to the striatal region of the brain where dopamine is produced.
>
> When CoQ_{10} was administered to rats genetically bred to develop ALS (Lou Gehrig's disease), a significant increase in survival time was observed.

The scientists concluded that

> CoQ10 can exert neuroprotective effects that might be useful in the treatment of neurodegenerative diseases.

This study showed that short-term supplementation with moderate amounts of CoQ_{10} produced profound anti-aging effects in the brain. Previous studies had shown that CoQ_{10} may protect the brain via several mechanisms, including reduction in free radical generation and protection against glutamate-induced excitotoxicity. This study documented that orally supplemented CoQ_{10} specifically enhanced metabolic energy levels of brain cells. While this effect in the brain had been postulated previously, the new study provides solid evidence.

Based on the types of brain cell injury against which CoQ_{10} protected, the scientists suggested that it might be useful in the prevention or treatment of Huntington's disease and Lou Gehrig's disease (amyotrophic lateral sclerosis). It was noted that, although, vitamin E delays the onset of Lou Gehrig's disease in mice, it does not increase survival time. CoQ_{10} was suggested as a more effective treatment strategy for neurodegenerative disease than vitamin E because survival time was increased in mice treated with CoQ_{10}.

CoQ_{10} might be effective in the prevention and treatment of Parkinson's disease *(reference: Annals of Neurology,* 1997 August). A study showed that the brain cells of Parkinson's patients have a specific impairment that causes the disruption of healthy mitochondrial function. It is known that "mitochondrial disorder" causes cells in the substantia nigra region of the brain to malfunction and die, thus creating a shortage of dopamine.

An interesting finding was that CoQ_{10} levels in Parkinson's patients were 35% lower than age-matched controls. This deficit of CoQ_{10} caused a significant reduction in the activity of enzyme complexes that are critical to the mitochondrial function of the brain cells affected by Parkinson's disease.

The ramifications of this study are significant. Parkinson's disease is becoming more prevalent as the human life span increases. The new study confirms previous studies that Parkinson's disease may be related to CoQ_{10} deficiency. The conclusion of the scientists was that

> The causes of Parkinson's disease are unknown. Evidence suggests that mitochondrial dysfunction and oxygen free radicals may be involved in its pathogenesis. The dual function of CoQ_{10} as a constituent of the mitochondrial electron transport chain and a potent antioxidant suggest that it has the potential to slow the progression of Parkinson's disease.

CoQ_{10} levels decrease with aging. Depletion is caused by reduced synthesis of CoQ_{10} in the body along with increased oxidation of CoQ_{10} in the mitochondria. A CoQ_{10} deficit results in the inactivation of enzymes needed for mitochondrial energy production, whereas supplementation with CoQ_{10} preserves mitochondrial function.

Aged humans have only 50% of the CoQ_{10} present in young adults, thus making CoQ_{10} one of the most important nutrients for people to supplement.

CoQ_{10} is one of the most important supplements on this list to take on a daily basis. Thousands of published studies show that ginkgo, acetyl-*L*-carnitine, and CoQ_{10} play a critical role in brain cell energy metabolism, not only in healthy people, but also in those suffering from neurological diseases.

Phosphatidylserine (PS) (100 to 300 mg a day). PS plays an important role in maintaining the integrity of brain cell membranes. The breakdown of brain cell membranes prevents glucose and other nutrients from entering the cell. By protecting the integrity of brain cell membranes, phosphatidylserine facilitates the efficient transport of energy-producing nutrients into cells, enhancing brain cell energy metabolism. Abnormalities in the composition of phosphatidylserine have been found in patients with Alzheimer's disease.

Vinpocetine. Vinpocetine was introduced into clinical practice 22 years ago, in Hungary, for the treatment of cerebrovascular disorders and symptoms related to senility. Since then, it has been used increasingly throughout the world in the treatment of cognitive deficits related to normal aging. Vinpocetine is a pharmaceutical extraction from the periwinkle plant.

It is well established that normal aging results in a reduction of blood flow to the brain and a decrease in the metabolic activity of brain cells. Vinpocetine functions via several important mechanisms to correct known multiple causes of brain aging. The biological actions of vinpocetine initially showed that it enhances circulation and oxygen utilization in the brain, increases tolerance of the brain toward diminished blood flow, and inhibits abnormal platelet aggregation that can interfere with circulation or cause a stroke.

More recent studies demonstrate that vinpocetine offers significant and direct protection against neurological damage caused by aging. The molecular evidence indicates that the neuroprotective action of vinpocetine is related to the ability to maintain brain cell electrical conductivity and to protect against damage caused by excessive intracellular release of calcium.

Vinpocetine enhances cyclic GMP levels in the vascular smooth muscle, leading to reduced resistance of cerebral vessels and increased cerebral blood flow. In one double-blind clinical trial, vinpocetine was shown to effect significant improvement in elderly patients with chronic cerebral dysfunction. Forty-two patients received 10 mg of vinpocetine 3 times a day for 30 days, then 5 mg 3 times a day for 60 days. Placebo tablets were given to another 42 patients for the 90-day trial period. Patients on vinpocetine scored consistently better in all evaluations of the effectiveness of treatment, including measurements on the Clinical Global Impression (CGI) scale, the Sandoz Clinical Assessment–Geriatric (SCAG) scale, and the Mini-Mental Status Questionnaire (MMSQ). There were no serious side effects related to the treatment drug.

In another double-blind study, 22 elderly patients with central nervous system degenerative disorders were treated with vinpocetine or placebo. Patients received 10 mg of vinpocetine 3 times a day for 30 days, then 5 mg 3 times a day for 60 days. Another 18 elderly patients were given matching placebo tablets for the 90-day trial. Vinpocetine-treated patients scored consistently better in all evaluations of the effectiveness of treatment, including measurements on the CGI and SCAG scales, and the MMSQ.

According to CGI assessments, severity of illness decreased in 73% of the patients in the vinpocetine group at day 30 and in 77% of patients at day 90. Improvement was seen in 77% and 87% of the patients at days 30 and 90, respectively. Patients also showed statistically significant improvement for all SCAG items except one at days 30 and 90. The physician rated the improvement in 59% of the vinpocetine-treated patients as "good" to "excellent." There were no serious side effects associated with the treatment drug.

Vinpocetine safety and efficacy were demonstrated in a study of infants who suffered severe brain damage caused by birth trauma. Vinpocetine caused a significant reduction or disappearance of seizures. The vinpocetine group also showed a decrease of the phenomena of intracranial hypertension and normalization of psychomotor development.

In a study to ascertain how vinpocetine boosts cognition, scientists measured the electrical firing effects in the neurons of anesthetized rats. The administration of vinpocetine produced a significant increase in the firing rate of neurons. The scientists noted that the dose of vinpocetine used to increase electrical firing corresponded to the dose range that produced memory-enhancing effects. These results provided direct electrophysiological evidence that vinpocetine increases the activity of ascending noradrenergic pathways and that this effect can be related to the cognitive-enhancing characteristics of the compound.

Life Extension Foundation members learned about the damaging effects of glutamate-induced excitotoxicity earlier this year. A vitamin B_{12} metabolite called methylcobalamin was shown to specifically protect against this type of neuronal injury. Vinpocetine has been documented to partially protect against excitotoxicity induced by a wide range of glutamate-related neurotoxins.

The effect of vinpocetine on memory functions was studied in 50 patients with disturbances of cerebral circulation. Improvement of cerebral circulation was observed after i.v. and oral administration of vinpocetine. Blood flow was most markedly increased in the gray matter of the brain. Improvement of memorizing capacity evaluated by psychological tests was recorded after 1 month of vinpocetine treatment. Longer-term use was associated with alleviation or complete disappearance of symptoms of neurological deficit. No side effects attributable to the drug were observed. The doctors stated that vinpocetine is indicated in the treatment of ischemic disorders of the cerebral circulation, particularly in chronic vascular insufficiency.

The benefits of vinpocetine are not restricted to the brain. One study showed beneficial effects in protecting the retina against uveretinal pathology caused by the hepatitis B virus. While hepatitis viruses primarily affect the liver, most people don't know that these viruses can also infect the heart muscle, retina, and other parts of the body.

Another study showed that vinpocetine administered to rats inhibited the development of gastric lesions induced by ethanol. Pretreatment with the non-steroidal anti-inflammatory drug indomethacin counteracted the protective action of vinpocetine against ethanol-induced damage. This study showed that vinpocetine protected against a wide range of gastric insults and ulceration, indicating its potential clinical value as a gastroprotective agent. In Russia, vinpocetine is a popular drug used by alcoholics to recover from gastric and neurological ethanol-induced toxicity.

Space motion sickness has been a perplexing problem in both the Soviet and U.S. manned space programs. Both the sensory conflict theory (neuronal signal mismatch) and the cephalic fluid shift concept explain the mechanism. Vinpocetine has been used successfully in offsetting space motion sickness in experimental test subjects.

Piracetam (2400 to 4800 g a day). According to the scientific literature, piracetam is known to improve a whole series of mental activities and especially higher cortical functions. In animal experiments and in single-photon-emission tomography studies of patients with acute ischemic stroke, piracetam improved microcirculation and neuronal metabolism, and enhanced transmitter functions. One study demonstrated that piracetam facilitates learning and memory in chicks by causing increased plasma levels of corticosterone, which acts on the brain to preserve long-term memories. Another study found that piracetam provides neurological and functional protection against deficits resulting from a moderate or severe stroke when administered within a few days. The study also noted that piracetam is well tolerated and is effective when taken orally and that other treatments have very limited efficacy. Research has demonstrated that piracetam's effect on circulation in the brain translates into improvements in aphasia (inability to speak) and level of consciousness, as well as fewer deaths.

Centrophenoxine (250 to 1000 mg a day). Centrophenoxine is used widely in Europe in combination with piracetam to improve memory and enhance mental energy.

Picamilon (50 to 100 mg three times a day). This Russian drug improves blood flow to cerebral vessels and enhances energy levels.

Pyritinol (200 mg three times a day). Pyritinol has been used in Europe to enhance neuronal metabolism in order to help restore youthful cognitive function.

Hydergine (4 to 10 mg a day). Hydergine is approved by the FDA to treat individuals over age 60 who manifest signs or symptoms of mental incapacity. When one study showed that Hydergine was not effective in treating Alzheimer's disease, American physicians virtually stopped prescribing Hydergine, even though the drug had never been approved as an Alzheimer's therapy.

Protection against brain aging with Hydergine

Hydergine remains a popular supplement among health-conscious people seeking to slow age-related mental decline. Recent studies reveal new mechanisms by which Hydergine protects against brain aging.

A study (*European Neuropsychopharmacology*, 1998, Vol. 8, Issue 1, 13–16) showed that Hydergine causes an increase of superoxide dismutase (SOD) and catalase in the brain while decreasing toxic levels of monoamineoxidase (MAO).

What was interesting about this study is that Hydergine was administered for only 20 days, but its effects in the brains of the rats was dramatic. Hydergine specifically increased SOD in the hippocampus and in the corpus striatum regions. These regions of the brain suffer severe oxidative damage from hydrogen peroxide and other free radical generating agents. Hydergine caused catalase levels to increase throughout the brain.

SOD and catalase are the body's natural antioxidants and are considered among the most effective free radical scavengers. Orally ingested SOD and catalase have not proven efficacious because these antioxidant enzymes are broken down in the stomach. Scientists have therefore concentrated on ways of prompting the body to produce its own cellular SOD and catalase. This study showed that Hydergine can increase brain levels of SOD and catalase after only short-term administration.

Another cause of brain aging is the elevation of an enzyme in the brain called monoamine oxidase (MAO). Elevated MAO levels damage brain cells and are a specific cause of age-related neuronal deterioration. Too much MAO has also been shown to cause pathological disorders such as Parkinson's disease.

Age-related depression has been linked to excessive production of MAO that occurs in the elderly. Drugs that inhibit MAO were widely used in the past to effectively treat depression. MAO-inhibiting drugs are seldom used today because of potential toxicity. Hydergine appears to safely inhibit MAO levels, as extensive human testing has not found any of the classic toxic signs of excessive MAO inhibition.

The scientists who conducted this study concluded by stating that

> Decreasing MAO levels and supporting the antioxidant enzymes may underlie the efficacy of Hydergine in the treatment of age related cognitive decline.

Another study showed a mechanism of how Hydergine protects against brain aging and the development of Alzheimer's disease (*Life Sciences*, Vol. 58, No. 8, 1996). This study identified a defect that occurs in brain cell membranes and showed that Hydergine could inhibit these degenerative changes. The scientists who authored the *Life Sciences* study identified specific antibodies that bind to brain cell membranes and then target the cell for destruction and removal by the immune system.

Young brains have significantly lower levels of these destructive antibodies compared to old brains. Hydergine-treated mice showed a reduction in these destructive antibodies, suggesting that middle-aged people who take Hydergine could retard the development of senile dementia caused by programmed immune destruction. The animals receiving Hydergine in middle-age maintained healthy brain cell metabolic activities compared to the control group who did not receive Hydergine. The scientists concluded that Hydergine therapy begun in middle age could protect against the initiation of the cascade that leads to Alzheimer's disease.

The scientists emphasized that once the Alzheimer's disease cascade begins, Hydergine would be of little value as the brain cells have already been inevitably marked and targeted for immune destruction.

The Life Extension Foundation has long advocated the use of Hydergine by people of all ages to *prevent* the degenerative changes that lead to brain cell aging and Alzheimer's disease. Hydergine appears frequently in the scientific literature as therapy for a wide range of diseases ranging from asthma to stroke. Hydergine may be the most under-utilized drug in the United States because of its failure to treat advanced Alzheimer's disease.

Earlier published studies showed that Hydergine can

- ▼ Improve blood supply to the brain.
- ▼ Increase the amount of oxygen delivered to the brain.
- ▼ Increase oxygen use by the brain.
- ▼ Enhance metabolism in brain cells.
- ▼ Protect the brain from damage during periods of decreased or insufficient oxygen supply.
- ▼ Slow the deposit of age pigment (lipofuscin) in the brain.
- ▼ Prevent free radical damage in brain cells.
- ▼ Increase intelligence, memory, learning, and recall.

- Enhance the use of glucose by brain cells.
- Increase ATP levels in the brain.
- Stop blood from becoming sticky.
- Raise the brain levels of serotonin.

Hydergine is a popular "smart drug" that people of all ages use to boost cognitive productivity now, and to protect against brain aging in the future.

How to use deprenyl and Hydergine

Low-dose deprenyl is thought to protect against brain aging by specifically inhibiting monoamine oxidase B (MAO B) in the brain. The ideal human dose of deprenyl to slow brain aging has been estimated to be about 1.5 mg a day by scientists who have conducted life span studies on the drug. Since deprenyl is usually sold in 5-mg tablets, and has a long-acting effect on the brain, most life extenders take the low dose of 5 mg of deprenyl twice a week.

Hydergine, on the other hand, seems to be more effective when higher doses are used. European doctors often prescribe 4.5 to 20 mg a day of Hydergine without concern for toxicity.

High-dose Hydergine and low-dose deprenyl have been used together for more than 10 years by people seeking to protect against neurological aging and boost cognitive function. No adverse effects have been reported when using these two medications together.

For middle-aged people who have a family history of Alzheimer's disease, a daily dose of 10 mg to 20 mg of Hydergine is suggested. For middle-aged people seeking to slow their rate of brain cell aging, a daily dose of 5 mg to 10 mg of Hydergine is suggested.

In 5% of people, Hydergine can induce a mild state of nausea. These people should use Sandoz brand Hydergine LC, an enterically coated capsule that bypasses the stomach and prevents nausea. The problem with these capsules is that they only come in strengths of 1 mg. For the remaining 95% of people for whom Hydergine does not cause nausea, European suppliers sell 5 mg Hydergine tablets that make taking high doses of Hydergine convenient and very economical.

Nimodipine (30 mg three times a day). Especially recommended for head trauma victims, nimodipine (brand name Nimotop) is a calcium channel blocker specific to the central nervous system. It prevents movement of calcium into the cells of blood vessels, thereby relaxing the vessels and increasing the supply of blood and oxygen. It dramatically improves cerebral blood flow. Nimodipine is an FDA-approved drug used to prevent and treat problems caused by a burst blood vessel around the brain but has been ignored by most neurologists treating victims of stroke and other age-related neurological diseases.

Nicotinamide adenine dinucleotide (NADH) (5 to 10 mg a day). NADH is a coenzyme that acts as an electron carrier in the body. One recent study concluded that nicotinamide enhances brain choline concentrations by mobilizing choline from choline-containing phospholipids.

Hormones

Hormones are required to facilitate brain cell energy, maintain proper levels of acetylcholine, and protect brain cell membrane function. Neurohormones help restore youthful synchronization within the aging brain. Hormone supplementation is often required to achieve the requisite levels of the neuro-hormones.

Pregnenolone and **DHEA** improve brain cell activity and enhance memory. (Pregnenolone is converted into DHEA in the body.) DHEA is the most plentiful steroid hormone in the human body, but its exact function is unknown. What is known is that its concentration plummets with age: its daily production drops from 30 mg at age 20 to less than 6 mg at age 80. DHEA is naturally synthesized in abundance in young people from pregnenolone in the brain and the adrenal glands. It is known to affect the excitability of neurons in the hippocampus, the part of the brain responsible for memory.

Current findings suggest that DHEA enhances memory by facilitating the induction of neural plasticity, the condition that permits the neurons (nerve cells of the brain) to change in order to record new memories. Studies have shown that DHEA not only improves memory deficits, but also relieves depression in older people and increases perceived physical and psychological well-being. DHEA has been shown to help preserve youthful neurological function. Together, pregnenolone and DHEA help to maintain the brain cells' ability to store and retrieve information in short-term memory.

Pregnenolone initiates the memory storage process by stimulating the activity of an important molecule known as *adenylate cyclase,* which is needed to activate and regulate enzymes crucial to cellular energy production. Pregnenolone then regulates the sequential flow of calcium ions through the cell membrane. The pattern of calcium ion exchange may determine how memories are encoded by neurons. Pregnenolone also modulates chemical reactions, calcium-protein binding, gene activation, protein turnover, and enzymatic reactions involved in the storage and retrieval of memory.

The suggested supplementation range for pregnenolone is 50 to 150 mg a day in three equal doses. The recommended dosage for DHEA is 25 to 50 mg a day. Women usually need less DHEA than men. Five capsules of a multi-nutrient formula for the aging brain called *Cognitex* contain the suggested daily doses of pregnenolone, choline, vitamin B5, phosphatidylserine, and vinpocetine. Vinpocetine functions in a similar way to the drugs piracetam, Pyritinol, Picamilon, and Hydergine. Refer to the *DHEA Replacement Therapy protocol* before using pregnenolone or DHEA.

The hormones testosterone and estrogen play an important role in maintaining neurological function. Refer to the *Male Hormone Modulation Therapy protocol* or *Female Hormone Modulation Therapy protocol* for further information about how to safely adjust sex steroid hormones to improve cognitive function and mood.

Melatonin, a naturally occurring hormone produced in the brain's pineal gland, also enhances cognitive function. It is one of the body's most potent natural antioxidants, making it ideal to prevent age-related dementias such as Alzheimer's disease that are thought to be caused, or at least exacerbated, by a lifetime of free-radical damage, especially since melatonin easily enters the brain from the bloodstream. Melatonin is also the primary regulator of brain cell synchronization, the body's internal clock, and is being researched as a possible treatment for various psychological conditions. Abnormally low levels of melatonin have been discovered in patients suffering from some kinds of depression. The suggested level of melatonin supplementation for enhancing neurological function in those over age 35 is 500 micrograms to 3 milligrams a night, one half hour before going to bed (melatonin has a sedative effect). Those over age 50 can take up to 6 milligrams before bedtime.

Vitamins

Vitamins can protect and enhance cognitive function. B vitamins in particular play an integral role in the functioning of the nervous system and help the brain synthesize chemicals that affect moods. A balanced complex of the B vitamins is also essential for energy and for balancing hormone levels. One recent study determined not only that low folate (a B vitamin) levels are associated with cognitive deficits, but also that patients treated with folic acid for 60 days showed a significant improvement in both memory and attention efficiency.

In a 6-year study to determine the relationship between nutritional status and cognitive performance in 137 elderly people, several significant associations were observed between cognition and vitamin status. Higher present and past intake of vitamins A, C, E, and B complex were significantly related to better performance on abstraction and visuospatial tests.

In addition to a direct effect, vitamins indirectly impact mental function by altering the levels of harmful or beneficial substances in the body. For instance, elevated homocysteine (an amino acid) levels have been linked to heart disease and poorer cognitive function. In one study, vitamin B_6 and folate, taken at higher-than-recommended dosages, reduced blood levels of homocysteine. Another study showed that less-than-optimal levels of vitamin B_6, B_{12}, and folic acid lead to a deficiency of *S*-adenosylmethionine (SAMe). SAMe deficiency can cause depression, dementia, or demyelinating myelopathy (a degeneration of the nerves).

The typical American diet does not always provide these essential vitamins, at least in high doses. Because vitamin C and the B complex are water soluble and excreted from the body daily, they must be replenished daily. Older people are at greater risk for vitamin deficiency because they tend to eat less of a variety of foods, although their requirements for certain vitamins such as B_6 are actually higher. Older people may also have problems with efficient nutrient absorption from food. Even healthy older people often exhibit deficiencies in vitamin B_6, vitamin B_{12}, and folate, as well as zinc. The Life Extension Mix (dosage: 3 tablets with breakfast, 3 tablets with lunch, 3 tablets with dinner) provides high levels of the vitamins shown to significantly improve mental function. Because vitamin B_{12} deficiency is a special concern in the elderly and has been linked to neurological impairment, sublingual vitamin B12 tablets can add an additional 1000 to 2000 micrograms a day of this critical nutrient.

Antioxidants

Free radicals are atoms or groups of atoms that can cause damage to cells by a process known as oxidation, which impairs the immune system and leads to infections and degenerative diseases. Free radicals occur in air pollutants, smoke, radiation, environmental toxins, and processed foods, and are also released in the human body through sun exposure and stress. Antioxidants neutralize free radicals and help prevent such free-radical damage as normal brain aging. Their destructive activity has been implicated in many disease processes, including stroke and heart disease.

A recent study published in a premier American medical journal compared groups of older people over time and at a given moment with regard to antioxidant intake and memory performance. The study found that free recall, recognition, and vocabulary were significantly related to vitamin C and beta carotene levels. The levels of these antioxidants were found to be significant predictors of cognitive function even after controlling for possible confounding variables such as differences in education, age, and gender.

Life Extension Mix is a multi-nutrient formula that contains the ideal potencies of antioxidants, vitamins C and E, and beta carotene. It provides an easy and cost-effective way to supplement the optimal combination of vitamins, minerals, amino acids, and antioxidants.

Conclusion

Age-associated mental impairment can range in severity from forgetfulness to senility to dementia. It can be caused by a wide variety of specific disease processes, many of which are treatable, or by life events, such as the loss of a loved one. It can also result from brain aging. Whatever its form or cause, it need not be accepted as a consequence of growing older.

Behavioral modifications, such as increased physical and mental activity and a healthy diet, can improve mental function both directly and indirectly by enhancing overall health. Memory can also be improved by using aids such as lists and routines, and by making connections to existing knowledge. Age-associated mental impairment can be treated safely and effectively with memory-enhancing nutrients that increase available acetylcholine, brain cell energy boosters (including naturally occurring substances like acetyl-*L*-carnitine, ginkgo biloba extract, Coenzyme Q_{10}, NADH, and phosphatidylserine, as well as FDA-approved and offshore drugs), hormones, and vitamins that become deficient (especially in older people), and antioxidants. It is advisable to consult your physician prior to any treatment program and to inform your physician of all supplements you take.

Summary

1. Determine the severity and duration of the mental impairment and consult a physician if it interferes with daily functioning or has lasted a long time.
2. Determine whether the mental impairment is the result of a specific disease process, which may be treatable, or life event, such as bereavement.

3. Behavioral modifications, such as increased physical and mental activity and a healthy diet, may be helpful. Correct any hearing or vision deficits that interfere with activity.
4. Utilize memory aids such as lists, routines, and actively making connections to existing knowledge.
5. Choline (2,500 to 10,000 mg a day) or lecithin (10,000 to 15,000 mg a day), and/or phosphatidylcholine (1,200 to 6,000 mg a day) should be taken early in the day. (Five Cognitex capsules a day supply the minimum dose of these choline-based nutrients.)
6. Take ginkgo biloba extract (120 mg a day), acetyl-*L*-carnitine (1,000 to 2,000 mg a day), and Coenzyme Q_{10} (100 to 200 mg a day).
7. Take Cognitex (5 capsules a day), which supplies pregnenolone, choline, vitamin B5, phosphatidylserine, and vinpocetine. **Refer to DHEA Replacement Therapy protocol before using pregnenolone.**
8. Take DHEA (25 to 50 mg a day). **Refer to DHEA Replacement Therapy protocol before initiating DHEA or pregnenolone replacement.**
9. Take melatonin (500 micrograms to 3 mg a night to maintain neurological function; 3 to 10 mg a night for those who have an age-related degenerative brain disease) one half hour before bedtime.
10. Take Life Extension Mix (3 tablets with breakfast, 3 tablets with lunch, 3 tablets with dinner) to provide vital antioxidants and vitamins.
11. Take one or a combination of the following drugs: Picamilon (50 to 100 mg three times a day), Pyritinol (200 mg three times a day), piracetam (2,400 to 4,800 mg a day), centrophenoxine (250 to 1,000 mg a day), Hydergine (4 to 10 mg a day), and nimodipine (30 mg three times a day). Take nimodipine under the care of a physician.

For more information. Contact the National Institute on Aging, (800) 222-2225; the Alzheimer's Association, (800) 272-3900; and the National Institute of Neurological Disorders and Stroke, (800) 352-9424.

Product availability. Lecithin, ginkgo biloba extract, acetyl-*L*-carnitine, coenzyme Q_{10}, NADH, pregnenolone, DHEA, Cognitex, melatonin, and Life Extension Mix are available from the Life Extension Buyers' Club by calling (800) 544-4440, or order on-line at www.lef.org. Piracetam, Picamilon, Pyritinol, and centrophenoxine are available from overseas companies for personal use only. Ask the Foundation for a list of these companies. A physician must prescribe Hydergine and nimodipine.

AIDS

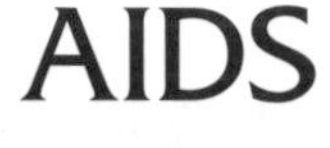

See HIV and Aids (Acquired Immune Deficiency)

ALCOHOL-INDUCED HANGOVER: PREVENTION

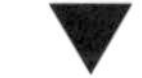

If you are reading this book, you are probably interested in life extension and anti-aging concepts. Because alcohol consumption produces toxic compounds, in the best of all possible worlds it would be better not to drink alcohol at all. For those who still want to drink, it is possible to do so more safely. The first piece of advice would be to drink only moderately and follow this protocol.

WARNING: What follows is for those who choose to drink moderately. This advice is not for those who suffer from alcoholism. Simply put, an alcoholic has "lost the power of choice in drink" and is "without defense against the first drink." In short, an alcoholic cannot drink safely. The Foundation is all too aware that an alcoholic may easily misinterpret the following information as a license to drink. It is not. It is only for those who drink by choice and who do so in moderation.

The consumption of alcohol results in the formation of two very toxic compounds: acetaldehyde and malondialdehyde. These compounds generate massive free radical damage to cells throughout the body. The free radical damage generated by these alcohol metabolites creates an effect in the body similar to radiation poisoning. That is why people feel so sick the day after consuming too much alcohol. If the proper combination of antioxidants is taken at the time the alcohol is consumed or before the inebriated individual goes to bed, the hangover and much of the cellular damage caused by alcohol may be prevented.

Aging makes us increasingly vulnerable to alcohol-induced hangover, liver injury, and damage to the central nervous system. In the elderly, alcohol- and drug-induced injury are more common and more serious, and recovery is more difficult.

Nutrients that neutralize alcohol by-products and protect cells against the damaging effects of alcohol include vitamin C, vitamin B_1, the amino acids cysteine and glutathione, vitamin E, and selenium. There are several commercial preparations that can be taken at the time the alcohol is consumed or before bedtime to help prevent a hangover. One of these is called *Anti-Alcohol Antioxidants.* Six capsules of this formula contain the proper amounts of antioxidant nutrients to help prevent a hangover.

Another product drinkers use is Kyolic Garlic Formula 105. Garlic contains *S*-allyl-cysteine; this particular kyolic-brand formula also contains vitamins C and E, beta-carotene, and selenium. Since the heavy consumption of alcohol produces many deleterious effects within the body, including an increased risk of cancer, liver disease, and neurological disease, it is suggested that hangover-prevention formulas such as Kyolic Garlic Formula 105 and/or Anti-Alcohol Antioxidants be taken any time alcohol is consumed.

Free radical damage is a major mechanism by which ethanol damages the liver. As has already been discussed, supplementing with the right antioxidants while consuming ethanol significantly reduces damage to cells throughout the body, including damage to the liver. Ethanol also damages the liver by depressing an enzyme required to convert methionine into *S*-adenosylmethionine (SAMe). A deficiency of SAMe can predispose an alcoholic to develop liver cirrhosis. An alcohol-induced depletion of SAMe can be overcome by SAMe supplementation, which restores hepatic SAMe levels and significantly attenuates parameters of ethanol-induced liver injury.

Supplementation with 400 to 800 mg of SAMe twice a day may help to reverse alcoholic cirrhosis. For those alcoholics who cannot afford SAMe, supplementation with 500 mg of trimethylglycine (TMG, also known as glycine betaine), 800 micrograms of folic acid, and 500 micrograms of vitamin B_{12}, twice a day could help the liver to synthesize *S*-adenosylmethionine. Phosphatidylcholine supplementation, at a dose of 2000 mg a day, may protect against alcohol-induced septal fibrosis, cirrhosis, and lipid peroxidation.

Chronic alcohol consumption can constrict arteries in the brain and lead to neurological deficit. Supplementation with 500 mg to 1500 mg a day of magnesium could help keep cerebral blood vessels open by blocking excess infiltration of calcium into endothelial cells. European medications such as Picamilon (50 mg, three times a day) and Pyritinol (200 mg, three times a day) could help prevent and restore neurological function lost because of chronic ethanol intake. An expensive prescription drug called Nimotop (nimodipine), in the dose of 30 mg, three to four times a day, can slowly repair central nervous system damage caused by excess alcohol intake.

Those who drink routinely might consider taking 500 mg a day of milk thistle extract (silymarin), which may have a protective effect upon the liver. Alcohol depletes many vitamins and minerals from the body, so taking high-potency vitamin-mineral supplements throughout the day is very important. For protecting and restoring liver function lost because of alcohol insult, refer to the *Liver protocol*.

Summary

1. Drink in moderation if at all.
2. Take 6 capsules of Anti-Alcohol Antioxidants or 6 capsules of Kyolic Garlic Formula 105, every 2 hours that alcohol is being consumed.
3. At a minimum, take 6 capsules of Anti-Alcohol Antioxidants or 6 capsules of Kyolic Garlic Formula 105 before falling asleep.
4. Take supplements to replenish nutrients depleted by excessive alcohol consumption.

Product availability. The Anti-Alcohol Antioxidant formula, Kyolic Garlic Formula 105, magnesium, vinpocetine, and *S*-adenosylmethionine can be obtained from the Life Extension Buyers Club by calling (800) 544-4440, or order on-line at www.lef.org. The Foundation can also refer you to suppliers of offshore medications such as Picamilon and Pyritinol.

ALLERGIES

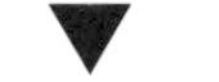

by Daniel N. Tucker, M.D.

Allergies are abnormal immune reactions to specific agents known as antigens or allergens. Examples of common allergens are foods, drugs, pollens, dust mites, mold spore, animal danders, feathers, and insect venoms, as well as other substances which nonallergic people find relatively nondangerous with usual exposure.

Allergies may also develop when an otherwise innocent substance has significant contact with an already inflamed surface (sensitization), such as from a viral infection or exposure to irritants, and becomes involved in the immune response. Thereafter, repeat exposure to such a substance may evoke an allergic response with the release of a histamine and a variety of pro-inflammatory substances, including enzymes, leukotrienes, and interleukins, and the creation of damaging free radicals. The multiplicity of these pro-inflammatory substances explains why single medications such as antihistamines often fail to completely control symptoms.

Types of Reactions

Allergic reactions may involve any part of the body, but they typically involve the body surfaces, which serve as exposure points and gateways. Reactions include hay fever, allergic rhinitis, allergic sinusitis, allergic conjunctivitis, itchy throats, itchy ears, plugged up ears, asthma, hives, giant hives (angioedema), allergic gastrointestinal symptoms, and various types of allergic dermatitis and rashes. Headaches, dizziness, fatigue, joint and muscle pains, and many other symptoms can also be allergic in nature.

The most severe, life-threatening reaction is anaphylaxis, or anaphylactic shock. This may include any or all of the above symptoms to an extreme degree plus vascular collapse or swelling sufficient to occlude airways, including the mouth and throat. Such a severe reaction is an absolute medical emergency and requires prompt emergency care. Anyone who has ever experienced such a reaction should go to all extremes to prevent a recurrence and should carry medications for prompt self-administration. Should there be a recurrence, the person should go straight to the nearest medical facility, even if the self-administered medication seems to give temporary relief. Anyone who has had a significant reaction to a medication should know the name of the medication and, along with the names of close relatives, carry this information at all times. A medallion or bracelet is easy identification for medical personnel to find.

Immunological reactions are divided into four types or categories:

Type I reactions include anaphylactic shock, as noted above, as well as allergic rhinitis, allergic asthma, and many acute skin reactions such as acute drug reactions. In this type of reaction, an antigen (allergen) binds to IgE antibodies on the surface of mast cells or basophils as well as the tissues that release histamine and the other mediators that produce tissue damage and symptoms.

Type II reactions include autoimmune processes such as immune hemolytic anemia and RH hemolytic disease of a newborn as well as other multiple examples of antibody (IgG and/or IgM) directed against antigens (including normal receptor sites) on our own tissue. Autoimmune antibodies are far more common than generally appreciated and tend to increase with age. Their activity is generally a factor in many age-related problems. Many bacteria, including some normally found in our gastrointestinal tract, share antigens similar to those located on some human cells. Significant exposure to an immune response such as these bacterial antigens can evoke autoimmune diseases. An example of this is the role of the intestinal organism klebsiella in precipitating ankylosing spondylitis in genetically susceptible people. This becomes a significant concern in leaky gut syndrome.

Type III reactions are immune complex reactions. When an antigen and an antibody combine in large enough amounts, complexes may be formed which can be deposited in tissues and blood vessels, resulting in tissue injury. This may be seen in some types of nephritis, arthritis, drug reactions, and some infections, as well as in leaky gut syndrome.

Type IV reactions are termed delayed hypersensitivity and, unlike the first three types, are not related to humoral antibodies (water soluble proteins generated by the body, termed immunoglobulins) by the T-lymphocytes (CD4) which, as the name implies, require longer to respond in a sensitized person. Examples include contact dermatitis (poison ivy type), graft rejection, elimination of tumor cells, and the immune response to fungal, viral, and intercellular bacterial infections. The well-known TB skin test is an example of Type IV delayed hypersensitivity reaction; i.e., other responses in a previously sensitized individual can take from minutes to hours for manifestation, but Type IV reactions can be thought of as taking from hours to days.

Avoidance of Allergens

The best therapy for an allergic problem is to, wherever possible, avoid the offending substance or substances. The environment of an allergic person should be kept as free of known allergens or potential allergens as possible. Allergy-proof and mite-proof covers should be used on all pillows, mattresses, and box springs in the sleeping area, and all bedding should be washed in very hot (135°F) water, weekly. Mold exposure is to be avoided by eliminating moisture-laden growth areas, and any new growth must be eliminated promptly. Pets should be kept out of the sleeping area. Cats and dogs should be bathed frequently to reduce the amount of surface allergens on their bodies. Air conditioning is helpful for pollen allergies, but filters must be changed regularly. Food allergies are commonly recognized by the allergic individual's tracking exposure to an offending food or may be identified through the use of elimination diets with cautious reintroduction of suspected foods.

Therapeutic Options

Adequate supplements of essential fatty acids with both omega-6 and omega-3 types should be taken since these have an anti-inflammatory effect when taken together. One pro-inflammatory effect of some omega-6 fatty acids is the over-production of arachidonic acid. This pro-inflammatory effect is blocked by the omega-3 fatty acids, so both must be used together.

The most potent anti-inflammatory, omega-6 fatty acid, is GLA (gamma-linolenic acid), which can be obtained from primrose, black currant seed, or borage oils. A suggested dose would be about 1500 mg daily of GLA from these oils. Borage oil provides the highest concentration, thereby requiring fewer capsules to be swallowed. This should be balanced with approximately twice as much of the omega-3 essential fatty acids EPA (eicosapentaeonoic acid) and DHA (docosahexaenoic acid) found in the oil from fatty fish (Mega EPA), flaxseed oil, or perilla oil, at about 3000 mg daily. A good balanced product with the correct ratio is Udo's Choice Perfected Oil, two capsules three times daily. Oil supplements should be taken at the beginning of a meal to reduce heartburn and aftertaste.

Coenzyme Q_{10} (CoQ_{10}), an oil-based supplement with tocotrienols, should be taken in the dose of one to three 30-mg capsules a day. CoQ_{10} penetrates the mitochondrial membrane and is one of the few antioxidants which can do so. Tocotrienols are relatives of tocopherols, or vitamin E, and are particularly effective free-radical fighters at the cell membrane level.

An intake of magnesium supplements from 500 to 1000 mg daily is particularly helpful in many conditions such as asthma. The dose should be kept below the diarrhea level. Magnesium should be accompanied by 900 to 1000 mg a day of elemental calcium in a tablet or capsule that completely dissolves. Calcium has a constipating effect which tends to offset the magnesium. Calcium and magnesium supplements should not be taken at the exact same time as the essential fatty acids since they will tend to interfere with absorption.

Allergic reactions can be mitigated and sometimes eliminated by maintaining high levels of antioxidants in the tissue. For allergy sufferers, we suggest three tablets of Life Extension Mix with meals three times a day, a total of nine tablets daily.

A number of agents included in the Life Extension Mix may be helpful if taken in higher individual doses. In particular, vitamin C is a natural antihistamine and may be taken at doses of up to 12,000 mg daily provided the dose is kept below the diarrhea level. Extra polyphenols, a group which includes the bioflavonoids, may also be beneficial by teaming up with vitamin C to further suppress allergic reactions. An excellent source of this is grape seed-skin extract, 100 mg, one to three times a day. Extra doses of the potent antioxidant *N*-acetyl-cysteine (NAC), 600 mg daily in addition to that already in the Life Extension Mix, is often helpful and may be supplemented with the potent antioxidant alpha-lipoic acid, at doses of 250 mg twice a day.

L-Glutathione may also be taken as a supplement; however, the NAC is a precursor to the glutathione and may naturally raise glutathione to optimal levels.

Extracts from the stinging nettle leaf are especially useful when taken with vitamin C and bioflavonoids in reducing symptoms of allergies. Several other herbal products have established anti-allergy properties. These include ginkgo biloba and angelica. DHEA can modulate autoimmune reactions. The dose varies, but 25 mg twice a day is usually suggested. Refer to the *DHEA Replacement Therapy protocol* for additional dosing and safety precautions before using DHEA.

Leaky gut syndrome may be addressed through the use of friendly bacteria such as Life Flora, one capsule with meals three times a day for 4 to 5 days, then once a day or more as needed. This should be supplemented with the use of an indigestible fiber, such as fructosoligosaccarides (FOS), that stimulates the growth of beneficial bacteria. The amino acid glutamine is a major factor in preserving the integrity of the cells of the gastrointestinal tract in keeping the toxins and antigens from entering the bloodstream. It is a major source of energy for cells in the gastrointestinal tract. Although present in most proteins, additional supplements of glutamine are very helpful in treating leaky gut syndrome and should be taken in a dose of 1000 mg daily when symptoms improve.

For allergy problems with symptoms not relieved by personal measures, a health care professional trained in allergies should be consulted for allergen identification, assistance in allergen avoidance, and symptomatic treatment. Many allergy problems may be treated by a professional with allergen-immunotherapy (desensitization), a series of treatments which can make you less sensitive to some allergens. Women who are pregnant or may become so and persons with other significant medical problems should seek guidance from a health care professional before using the above supplements and herbs as should parents before using these products on children.

Additional Suggestions by Professor Carmen Fusco

Carmen Fusco is a registered nurse and college professor who treats patients using alternative therapies at her practice in New York City.

Professor Fusco recommends 300 to 500 mg twice a day of pantothenic acid (vitamin B_5) in the form of calcium pantothenate. Pantothenic acid helps both the adrenals and the thymus gland in the fight against allergies. She also suggests Drenamin, which helps in most allergies, and Antronex, which contains an antihistamine produced by the liver, in alleviating nasal allergies.

Stress often precipitates allergies, so any nutrient such as vitamins B_5 and C that helps buffer stress will help against allergies. Studies have shown that the thymus, the gland most responsible for cell-mediated immunity, is also responsive to various levels of pantothenic acid. This becomes particularly important in cell allergies and the more severe autoimmune conditions.

Pantothenic acid is virtually nontoxic in higher doses. Unlike other B vitamins, it does not imbalance or increase the requirements of the other B vitamins. The Life Extension Mix formula, which has been used by so many to alleviate allergy problems, provides 600 mg of pantothenic acid in each daily dose.

Summary

The number of supplements required to suppress allergy symptoms can appear daunting, but the health benefits of consuming these nutrients include reductions in the risk of cardiovascular disease, cancer, dementia, osteoporosis, arthritis, and a host of degenerative diseases associated with normal aging. Therefore, while the objective of the allergy patient is immediate relief, the use of nutritional supplements can provide a long-term solution in treating the underlying cause of the chronic allergy problem and helping to maintain an optimal state of health.

I suggest that one or more of the following nutritional supplements should be tried by the allergy sufferer for at least 2 months:

1. Life Extension Mix, 3 tablets, 3 times a day.
2. GLA from borage oil, 1500 mg a day, along with at least 3000 mg a day of the omega-3 fatty acids from fish, flax, or perilla oils. (Six to twelve capsules a day of Udo's Choice multi-oil blend may also be used.)
3. CoQ_{10} with tocotrienols, 30 mg, 3 times a day.
4. Vitamin C, 3000 to 9000 mg a day (Life Extension Mix provides about 2500 mg of vitamin C).
5. Magnesium, 500 to 1500 mg a day, taken with 900 to 1000 mg of calcium,
6. DHEA, 25 mg, twice a day (refer to *DHEA Replacement Therapy protocol* for safety precautions).
7. NAC, 600 mg a day, in addition to the 600 mg already contained in Life Extension Mix.
8. Life Flora, 1 capsule 3 times a day for a week, then reduce dose to 1 capsule a day thereafter. Supplementation with 5000 mg of FOS powder will help protect the beneficial bacterial contained in Life Flora in your gut.
9. Grape seed-skin extract, 100 mg, 3 times a day.
10. Nettle leaf extract, 750 mg a day.

For more Information. Contact the Asthma & Allergy Foundation of America, (800) 7 ASTHMA.

Product availability. Life Extension Mix, *N*-Acetyl-Cysteine, perilla oil, Udo's Choice, DHEA, Life Flora, grape seed-skin extract, Super CoQ_{10}, calcium, magnesium, vitamin C, Mega GLA, and Super Max EPA may be ordered by calling (800) 544-4440 or order on-line at www.lef.org.

ALZHEIMER'S DISEASE

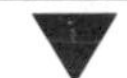

by Ben Best

Incidence and Symptoms

Alzheimer's disease is the leading cause of dementia in the elderly and is the fourth leading cause of death in developed nations (after heart disease, cancer, and stroke). Up to 70% of dementia cases are due to Alzheimer's disease, with blood vessel disease (stroke, atherosclerosis) being the second most common cause. The frequency of Alzheimer's among 60-year-olds is about 1%. The incidence doubles approximately every 5 years, becoming 2% at age 65, 4% at 70, 8% at 75, 16% at 80, and 32% at 85. It is estimated that as many as two thirds of those in their 90s suffer from some form of dementia. For those who aspire to live a very long life, dementia is a threat second only to death—or *is* death in another form.

Alzheimer's disease is incurable. It leads to death within an average of 8 years after diagnosis, the last 3 of which are typically spent in an institution. Besides memory loss, Alzheimer's patients show dramatic personality changes, disorientation, declining physical coordination, and an inability to care for themselves. In the final stages, victims are bedridden, lose urinary and bowel control, and suffer epileptic attacks. Death is usually due to pneumonia or urinary tract infection.

Therapy and Prevention

Current therapies cannot stop or eliminate Alzheimer's disease, but they can slow the progress and temporarily reverse symptoms. Moreover, diagnosis of the disease is only 85 to 90% accurate, and the diagnosis is only confirmed by brain biopsy after death. Alzheimer's-like symptoms can be manifested by brain cancer, meningitis, neurosyphilis, hypothyroidism, hypoglycemia, congestive heart failure, AIDS, vascular disease, Parkinson's disease, Huntington's disease, multiple sclerosis, subdural hematoma, and liver or kidney dysfunction. Many of these conditions are curable. Nutritional deficiencies of vitamin E, magnesium, and B vitamins (B_{12}, folic acid, niacin, and thiamine) can also produce symptoms which might be mistaken for dementia.

The neurons in the cerebral cortex are the focal site of cellular degeneration in Alzheimer's, but lower brain nuclei that send modulating neurotransmitters to the cortex are also severely affected. Serotonin, GABA, somatostatin, norepinephrine and acetylcholine are reduced 50% or more. The most striking symptoms are produced by acetylcholine depletion—which contributes significantly to loss of memory and loss of capacity for attentiveness.

Feeding lecithin (phosphatidylcholine) to animals increases brain acetylcholine levels, but clinical trials using lecithin on Alzheimer's patients has shown little or no improvement. Likewise, attempts to treat patients with drugs that stimulate acetylcholine receptors have been a failure. But acetylcholinesterase inhibitors have proven to be of therapeutic value.

Neurons send signals to other neurons by releasing chemicals into synapses. But signals are only effective when they have a beginning and an end. You can't send Morse code by applying constant pressure on a telegraph key. Acetylcholinesterase, the enzyme that breaks down acetylcholine, ends the chemical signal that begins when acetylcholine is released into a synapse and then connects with a receptor. The memory loss effect that acetylcholinesterase plays in Alzheimer's may be due to amplification of signals which would have been weakened by neurodegeneration.

The only two FDA-approved drugs for treatment of Alzheimer's disease are both acetylcholinesterase inhibitors: tacrine (Cognex) and donepezil (Aricept). Huperzine-*A*, metrifonate, and rivastigmine are also acetylcholinesterase inhibitors—and the last two may receive FDA approval soon. Huperzine-*A* has been used for centuries in China as an herbal medicine prepared from the moss *Huperzia serrata*. Side effects from tacrine, including liver toxicity, make donepezil (Aricept) the first drug of choice.

Currently, the most respected standard for assessing the neuropsychological status of Alzheimer's patients is the Alzheimer's Disease Assessment Scale-Cognitive Subscale (ADAS-Cog). Memory, orientation, language, and functionality are measured on a 70-point scale that increases (on average) by 7 to 10 points per year as the patient's cognition worsens. An improvement of 4 points (4 point decline in score) corresponds to a clinically significant reversal of symptoms of nearly half a year.

Patients receiving 160 mg/day of tacrine in a 30-week double-blind, placebo-controlled study showed an ADAS-Cog improvement of 4.1 points if they completed the trial. But only 27% of the patients completed the trial, largely because tacrine is so toxic to the liver and causes other severe side effects. A clinical trial with donepezil (Aricept) (5 or 10 mg/day) showed a 3.1 point ADAS-Cog improvement, with only 12% dropping out due to side effects. Rivastigmine's side effects are comparable to those of donepezil, but the ADAS-Cog is 4.9. Metrifonate has shown a 2.8 point ADAS-Cog improvement, with very few side effects. Clinical trials with higher doses of metrifonate are underway. Less than half of patients show any benefit at all from acetylcholinesterase inhibitors, even when there are no side effects, so the ADAS-Cog scores may greatly under-represent the improvement seen in patients who do benefit.

Although acetylcholinesterase inhibitors can apparently reverse symptoms by several months, they have not been shown to slow the progress of neuron degeneration. By contrast, a double-blind, placebo-controlled clinical trial with daily doses of 10 mg deprenyl (selegiline), 2000 IU vitamin E, or both showed a 25% slowing of the progress of the disease—but without any cognitive improvement. There was no advantage to using both deprenyl and vitamin E, so vitamin E alone would be a less expensive and more convenient therapy for most patients.

Treatment of cultured neurons with vitamin E has been shown to protect them from beta-amyloid toxicity. This suggests that vitamin E and other antioxidants such as vitamin C (which regenerates vitamin E) and Coenzyme Q_{10} may be of value in preventing Alzheimer's disease. In fact, melatonin has been shown to protect cell cultures from beta-amyloid toxicity. *N*-acetylcysteine has protected cultured cells from oxidative stress due to AGE-modified tau-protein. (Advanced Glycation End-Products, AGEs, lead to the formation of toxic hydroxyl free radicals and impaired ion and glucose transport, which cause neuron degeneration. This is discussed in detail further in the text.)

Gingko biloba not only has antioxidant properties, but is anti-inflammatory and promotes cerebral circulation. One double-blind, placebo-controlled trial with gingko biloba showed an ADAS-Cog of 1.4 points above placebo, although a meta-analysis of many such studies showed only a modest ADAS-Cog improvement.

The protective effect of estrogen against Alzheimer's is well-documented, but remains controversial. Studies of 2529 women in the Leisure World Retirement Community cohort, 472 women in the Baltimore Longitudinal Study of Aging, and 1124 women in a Manhattan cohort showed a 30%, 50%, and 60% lower risk, respectively, for Alzheimer's disease among post-menopausal women taking estrogen-replacement therapy over those who were not. Animal experiments show that removal of the ovary can reduce choline uptake in the frontal cortex and hippocampus by 24% and 34%—and cause a 45% decline in mRNA for Nerve Growth Factor (NGF) in the frontal cortex. Estrogen replacement mostly reverses these effects. The controversy is partly due to studies which have shown an increase in breast cancer incidence of 25% with estrogen replacement therapy. But other studies have shown colon cancer is reduced 50%, hip fractures (and osteoporosis) are reduced 40%, and risk of heart attack may also be reduced. A pilot study has shown significant ADAS-Cog improvement with tacrine and estrogen over tacrine alone. Large clinical trials with estrogen are currently in progress.

A 50% reduction of risk against Alzheimer's disease is seen in elderly arthritic patients who have been taking Non-Steroidal Anti-Inflammatory Drugs (NSAIDs) such as ibuprofen and indomethicin. Aspirin was only effective in dosages over 2.4 grams/day. A clinical trial of 100 to 150 mg/day of indomethicin for 6 months resulted in a 14-point ADAS-Cog improvement among the 79% of patients who did not drop out due to gastrointestinal side effects. Inflammation apparently contributes significantly to the final neurodegenerative processes which are initiated by beta-amyloid and neurofibrillary tangles.

A meta-analysis of studies using Hydergine (ergoloid mesylates) showed modest improvement for Alzheimer's symptoms, but only in dosages of 4 to 9 mg/day, rather than the typical dose of 3 mg/day. So-called nootropics (Greek for "toward mind") such as piracetam are usually ineffective because most Alzheimer's patients have elevated corticosteroids, which suppresses the memory-improving effects.

Some, but not all, studies have shown a reduced incidence of Alzheimer's disease among light smokers (fewer than 10 cigarettes per day), but an increased incidence of the disease among heavy smokers (more than 20 cigarettes per day). A pilot study with six patients using nicotine patches (to avoid the effects of the other toxic chemicals in cigarette smoke) showed some improvement in a learning task, but no effect on global cognition or short-term memory. Metanicotine is less toxic than nicotine and causes nearly the same acetylcholine release as nicotine.

Studies with 2 or 3 grams a day of acetyl-*L*-carnitine have shown a reduced rate of disease progression for Alzheimer's patients. Acetyl-*L*-carnitine reduces lipofuscin in neurons. Although lipofuscin is cellular debris from glycation and oxidation, detrimental effects in general and a contribution to Alzheimer's disease in particular have not been shown. The (modest) benefits of acetyl-*L*-carnitine are more likely due to its ability to normalize cell metabolism, increase NGF utilization, and increase acetylcholine synthesis.

The Japanese drug idebenone not only acts as an antioxidant, but it increases NGF and thereby improves cortical acetylcholine levels. Some improvement was also seen with 300 mg/day of phosphatidylserine. Desferrioxamine (which binds to aluminum and iron) given by intramuscular injection to a small group of Alzheimer's patients reduced the rate of decline of daily living skills to half that of the no-treatment group. Aminoguanidine could be of value in reducing AGEs in Alzheimer's patients. There are many such therapies that have shown some promise in small isolated studies, but which require large clinical trials if their merit is to be established with certainty.

Future Prospects for Therapy

Acetylcholinesterase inhibitors with more effectiveness and fewer side effects than tacrine or donepezil are likely to be on the market soon. NSAIDs which inhibit the enzyme cyclooxygenase-2 show great promise of being selectively advantageous for Alzheimer's disease immune/inflammatory response, with fewer side effects than current NSAIDs.

Nonetheless, all current and near-term future therapies treat symptoms or slow the disease, at best. More advanced therapies in the future may inhibit beta-amyloid formation, toxicity, and/or aggregation—or remove/destroy beta-amyloid. Replacement or regrowth of neuromodulatory nuclei-producing acetylcholine, serotonin, dopamine and noradrenaline may become feasible. Although reversal of neuron degeneration in the cerebral cortex is not currently possible, improved means of early disease detection and the ability to stop the disease entirely would be nearly as good as finding a cure.

An ounce of prevention is worth more than a ton of cure in the case of Alzheimer's disease, since the disease may remain incurable in the foreseeable future. Much is already known about risk factors for the disease, and there are many steps which prudent people can take to reduce the likelihood of the disease—or to delay its onset.

Treatment Protocols

The fact that a physician is required for protocol number one (next page) should not be taken to imply that a physician's advice would not be useful for other protocols. The first protocol (below) has a greater proven effectiveness than the second or third. Although deprenyl plus vitamin E has proven to be no better than vitamin E alone, other combinations of antioxidants are recommended because the antioxidant effect occurs at different locations and against different free radicals for different antioxidants.

Protocol Number 1. For treatment of the disease by physician's prescription and active monitoring, use the following:

- Donepezil (Aricept), 5 or 10 mg daily.
- Indomethacin, 100 to 150 mg daily or aspirin if over 2.4 grams daily.
- Estrogen replacement therapy, as directed by physician. (For postmenopausal women only. Estrogen does not work on male Alzheimer's patients.)
- Vitamin E, 1000 mg daily of alpha-tocopherol and 100 mg daily of gamma-tocopherol. Vitamin E can increase prothrombin time, so patients who take warfarin or have vitamin K

deficiency should consider using deprenyl, 10 mg daily instead of high-dose vitamin E. Kelp may be advisable to prevent vitamin K deficiency in many cases.

Protocol Number 2. For treatment of the disease by means that may supplement those provided by a physician, use the following:

- Acetyl-*L*-carnitine, 1000 mg in the morning and 1000 mg in the afternoon.
- *N*-acetyl-cysteine, 600 mg 3 times daily.
- Melatonin, 10 mg at bedtime.
- Gingko biloba, 120 mg in the morning.
- Vitamin C, 1000 mg 3 times daily.
- Coenzyme Q_{10}, 100 mg 3 times daily.

Protocol Number 3. Additional treatments which may provide some additional benefit are as follows:

- Cognitex, 5 capsules in the morning and 5 in the afternoon (Cognitex contains phosphatidylserine and acetylcholine precursors).
- Hydergine, 5 mg in the morning and 5 mg in the afternoon.
- Piracetam, 1600 mg in the morning and 1600 mg in the afternoon (only of possible benefit in early stages of the disease, and only if cortisol levels are not elevated).
- Aminoguanidine, initial dose of 300 mg a day. Toxicity may occur with higher doses, but some people may tolerate up to 600 mg a day.
- Vitamin B_{12}, 2000 mg a day in sublingual form (under the tongue) or by injection. Although this is not a specific treatment for Alzheimer's, it may treat deficiency mistaken for or co-existing with Alzheimer's disease. The ideal form of vitamin B_{12} to treat neurological disease is methylcobalamin.

Protocol Number 4. For prevention in people who have not been diagnosed with the disease, use the following:

- Estrogen replacement therapy, as directed by physician (postmenopausal women only).
- Vitamin E, as directed in Protocol Number 1, with half the dosage and all of the warnings.
- All of Protocol Number 2, with half the dosage.
- Life Extension Mix and Life Extension Booster.
- Avoid high levels of blood sugar, since this can increase glycation.
- Reduce consumption of omega-6 fatty acids, such as are found in safflower and sunflower seed oil, and increase consumption of omega-3 fatty acids, such as are found in perilla oil, linseed oil, and fish oil. Arachidonic acid from excessive omega-6 can worsen oxidative damage in the brain and increase inflammation, whereas the omega-3 fatty acids will have the opposite effect.
- Do not plan for mental decline with advancing age by avoiding challenges. To plan for mental decline is to arrange for mental decline. People with active minds, more education, and challenging occupations are more resistant to Alzheimer's disease.

Molecular Causes of the Disease

For over a hundred years neuroscientists have debated whether the accumulation of lipofuscin (age pigments) in neurons is a cause of dementia. It has been argued that lipofuscin is formed by lipid peroxidation, but this seems unlikely insofar as these pigments are primarily composed of protein and carbohydrate. Recent evidence has shown that glycation (protein cross-linking by sugar) is probably a greater cause of lipofuscin formation than lipid peroxidation. Although a role for lipofuscin cannot definitely be ruled out, few neurologists today believe that it is a central factor in Alzheimer's disease.

CAUTION: This section is highly technical. It is written for the benefit of the physician or knowledgeable layperson. It is not necessary that you understand this section to benefit from the treatment protocols that have been suggested.

In the 1970s many neurologists became convinced that Alzheimer's disease is due to degeneration of the basal forebrain neurons which send the neurotransmitter acetylcholine to the cerebral cortex. There are less than half a million acetylcholine-producing neurons in the basal forebrain nuclei, but these neurons specifically innervate areas of the cerebral cortex that play a key role in memory formation—the hippocampus, in particular. Most neurologists now believe, however, that degeneration of cholinergic neurons in Alzheimer's disease is only one manifestation of widespread degeneration of cognitively important neurons in the cerebral cortex and associated areas of the brain.

The most characteristic features of Alzheimer's disease are senile plaques of beta-amyloid peptide, neurofibrillary tangles, loss of synapses, and (ultimately) death of neurons. Although neurofibrillary tangles are more closely associated with neuron death than beta-amyloid, the evidence is becoming convincing that beta-amyloid is the factor most responsible for starting the degenerative processes of Alzheimer's disease.

Both neurofibrillary tangles and beta-amyloid senile plaques are due to protein abnormalities. The beta-amyloid peptide present in the core of senile plaques is a 42 amino-acid chain produced by cleavage of a larger protein known as Amyloid Precursor Protein (APP). APP is normally found embedded in neural membranes and is thought to contribute to stabilizing contact points between synapses. Beta-amyloid resists the degradation enzymes that normally recycle cellular proteins. Aggregates of beta-amyloid accumulate throughout brain tissue in normal aging, but do not cause pathology as long as the aggregates are diffused throughout the cell. The damage begins when the beta-amyloid becomes concentrated in senile plaques.

Neurons—and in particular the axons of neurons—use microtubules to transport substances between the center of the neuron and its outer portions. The assembly and structural integrity of microtubules are dependent upon several proteins, the most important of which is a protein called "tau." When tau is abnormally phosphorylated, it forms the paired helical filaments known as neurofibrillary tangles. Why this abnormal phosphorylation occurs is unknown, but the loss of microtubule transport is particularly damaging in neurons that produce and release large amounts of neurotransmitter. The large pyramidal neurons of the cortex and the forebrain acetylcholine neurons (among others) that are important for cognition have more microtubules than other neurons—and these large neurons have the most neurofibrillary tangles in Alzheimer's disease.

Genetic mutations account for less than 5% of Alzheimer's disease patients, but these genetic abnormalities have contributed significantly to understanding what causes the disease. The first gene linked to inherited Alzheimer's was the APP gene on chromosome 21. (Down syndrome victims, who invariably develop Alzheimer's if they live beyond 40, have three copies of chromosome 21.) Most other genes associated with Alzheimer's are either linked to beta-amyloid production or are of unknown function. But the gene on chromosome 17 that encodes tau polypeptides is not associated with inherited forms of the disease.

The second gene discovered to be responsible for an inherited form of Alzheimer's disease was the gene on chromosome 19 responsible for cholesterol transport protein: apolipoprotein-*E* (apoE). People with the ApoE4 gene on both copies of chromosome 19 are eight times more likely to develop Alzheimer's than people with two copies of ApoE2 or ApoE3. Beta-amyloid binds most readily to ApoE4. ApoE4 facilitates the transformation of beta-amyloid from the diffuse form to the aggregated form.

Free radical damage is probably the most significant cause of biological aging. The second most significant cause of aging is probably the nonenzymatic cross-linking of proteins by sugars—a process known as *glycation*. The body protects itself from glycation by periodic degradation and replenishment of proteins. But long-lived proteins like collagen are particularly vulnerable to glycation, which is why our tissues become more fibrous and less resilient as we age.

Insoluble proteins like aggregated beta-amyloid and phosphorylated tau are especially liable to form Advanced Glycation End-Products (AGEs). The cross-linking further increases insolubility and also leads to protein-binding of metals such as iron and copper, which generates toxic hydroxyl free radicals. Glycated proteins produce nearly 50 times more free radicals than non-glycated proteins. Lipid peroxidation caused by beta-amyloid results in an aldehyde called 4-hydroxynonenal that binds to proteins involved in transport of ions and binds to proteins that transport glucose. With impaired ion and glucose transport, neurons begin to degenerate.

Beta-amyloid can also bind to complement protein C1, thereby leading to an immune-inflammatory response. The resulting cytokines are thought to trigger more beta-amyloid cleavage from APP. When beta-amyloid is added to cultured neurons or injected into the cerebral cortex of nonhuman primates, it leads to the appearance of the phosphorylated tau-protein of neurofibrillary tangles.

To summarize the current hypothesis: It appears that Alzheimer's disease begins with gradual accumulation of beta-amyloid peptide in the form of diffuse plaques which, through glycation and oxidation evolve into senile plaques. Certain neurons with high metabolic demands or special sensitivity to beta-amyloid develop neurofibrillary tangles, which are even more destructive than beta-amyloid deposits. These neurons may include those in nuclei outside of the cerebral cortex which activate the cortex with modulatory neurotransmitters such as acetylcholine, serotonin, and noradrenaline. Such nuclei are normally nurtured by Nerve Growth Factor (NGF) traveling down the axons, but the NGF may be replaced by beta-amyloid, which leads to neurofibrillary tangles. Degenerating neurons activate the immune/inflammatory system which activates cytokines, such as interleukin-1 and interleukin-6. Interleukin-1 increases the toxicity and interleukin-6 increases the production of beta-amyloid. A vicious cycle of inflammation and beta-amyloid production—along with glycation and oxidation of tau-protein and beta-amyloid—ultimately results in the destruction of large numbers of brain cells.

Summary

Alzheimer's disease is a progressive form of dementia primarily affecting people over 60. The disease is incurable and leads to death within about 8 years. The acetylcholinesterase inhibitors, tacrine and donepezil, are the only currently approved drugs by the FDA in the treatment of Alzheimer's disease. Both drugs can reverse symptoms by several months but cannot slow the progress of neuron degeneration. Certain natural supplements taken in combination with and without prescription medication may reduce the likelihood of the disease or delay its onset, or slow its progress. Treatment Protocols 1 to 4 provide recommendations on the use of several natural substances, including the following:

1. Vitamins E, C, Coenzyme Q_{10}, and melatonin to protect against free-radical beta-amyloid activity.
2. Gingko biloba for antioxidant, anti-inflammatory, and cerebral circulation properties.
3. Estrogen replacement in post-menopausal women only, to reverse the effects of reduced choline uptake in the frontal cortex and hippocampus and a decline in mRNA for Nerve Growth Factor.
4. NSAIDs to reduce inflammation leading to final neurodegenerative processes.
5. Acetyl-*L*-carnitine to reduce disease progression by means of normalizing cell metabolism, increasing NGF utilization, and increasing acetylcholine synthesis.

For more information. Contact the Alzheimer's Disease Education and Referral Center, (800) 438-4380.

Product Availability. Cognitex, ginkgo caps, Life Extension Mix, acetyl-*L*-carnitine, NADH, Coenzyme Q_{10}, vitamin B_{12}, phosphatidylserine, DHEA, pregnenolone, lecithin, and melatonin can be obtained by calling (800) 544-4440, or order online at www.lef.org. THA and Aricept are FDA-approved prescription drugs that must be prescribed by a physician. Piracetam, Hydergine, deprenyl, aminoguanidine, and centrophenoxine are available from overseas companies for personal use only. Ask the Foundation for a list of companies offering these products when you call the above number.

AMNESIA

Amnesia is a term describing a group of disorders involving partial or total inability to remember past experiences. Memory can be divided into three major components: immediate, covering the past few seconds; intermediate, covering the duration from a few seconds past to a few days past; and remote or long-term, extending further back in time. One of the more common types of amnesia occurs after head trauma. Amnesia is said to be retrograde when the memory loss is for events prior to the injury. It is anterograde when the loss is for events after the injury. Head trauma may result in one or both types.

Many aging persons gradually develop noticeable difficulties in memory, at first for names, then for events, and sometimes even occasionally for spatial relationships. This widely experienced, so-called benign forgetfulness bears no proven relationship to degenerative dementia, but may be a forewarning, since some similarities are hard to overlook. The most common causes of severe memory loss are the degenerative dementia, severe head trauma, brain anoxia (lack of oxygen) or ischemia (lack of blood), alcoholic-nutritional disease, and various drug intoxications.

Transient global amnesia is the sudden appearance of severe, forgetful confusion lasting from as little as 30 to 60 min to as long as 12 hours or more. It is an unusual but not uncommon syndrome. During severe attacks there is total disorientation except for one's identity, combined with a retrograde memory deficit that can extend back for several years, but which gradually resolves as the attack subsides. Patients generally have a rapid, total recovery, therefore no treatment is indicated. However, since this may involve potential poor cerebral circulation due to atherosclerosis, a work-up may be indicated. If there is a personal or family history of cerebrovascular disease, it is suggested that the atherosclerosis protocol be followed and a consideration given to chelation therapy.

Amnesia can also be caused by acute or long-term alcohol use. In particular, heavy alcohol consumption with poor diet and low intake of thiamine leads to an irreversible syndrome called Wernicke-Korsakoff syndrome, which is an encephalopathy (diffuse brain disorder) and psychosis.

An interesting modality called cranio-electro-neuro-stimulation (CES) has actually been around for years but is not widely known. It involves the passage of a low-voltage, low-current, 100-Hz current laterally between the ears. Studies have shown it to be beneficial for treating the cognitive impairment associated with long-term alcohol use. However, this does not include the defects associated with Wernicke-Korsakoff syndrome.

Benzodiazepines are a class of drugs which are primarily used to treat anxiety and insomnia. They are one of the most commonly prescribed classes of drugs sold. One of the problems associated with long-term use of these drugs, particularly in the elderly, is memory loss. Since aging is inherently associated with some degree of increasing memory impairment and the elderly population is prone to insomnia, prescribing benzodiazepines is problematic. (*See the Insomnia protocol.*) In fact, benzodiazepines are specifically administered to patients prior to surgery because they cause anterograde amnesia. Patients who have not been given a benzodiazepine pre-operatively have complained of remembering surgery, and this resulted in law suits. The point is that the amnesia caused by benzodiazepines is not a side effect, but an anticipated effect exploited in this situation. Therefore, the routine use of benzodiazepines is not recommended.

So what can be done for patients recovering from amnesia resulting from trauma? European doctors use the drugs piracetam and vasopressin to help people suffering from amnesia recover their memories. Published studies show that the recovery of memory in amnesia patients can take from several hours to a few days when vasopressin and/or piracetam are used.

The recommended dosage of vasopressin is at least 16 IU per day, usually in the form of a nasal spray, though physicians may prescribe higher amounts to treat acute amnesia. The recommended dose of piracetam is 4800 mg per day until memory is restored.

Gingko biloba and supplements such as vitamin B_{12} may also be helpful in treating memory loss. Additional agents which may be helpful can be found in the *Age-Associated Memory Impairment protocol*.

Summary

1. See the Age-Associated Memory Impairment protocol.
2. Consider chelation therapy.
3. Consider vasopressin, 16 IU per day until memory is restored.
4. Consider piracetam, 4800 mg per day, or vinpocetine, 30 mg per day until memory is restored.
5. Gingko biloba, 120 mg per day.
6. For alcoholic cognitive impairment and possibly for memory loss from other causes, CES 3 times per day for 45 minutes.
7. Avoid benzodiazepine drugs.
8. Make sure you are taking adequate vitamin supplements.

For more information. Call the American College for the Advancement of Medicine, (800) 532-3688, for the location and phone number of a physician in your area who specializes in complementary medicine and has a familiarity with chelation therapy.

Product availability. Vasopressin (Novartis) is a prescription drug produced by the Sandoz pharmaceutical company. You must see a physician and get a prescription for this medication. Piracetam is an unapproved drug that has to be ordered from offshore pharmacies. For a list of such pharmacies, call (800) 544-4440.

AMYOTROPHIC LATERAL SCLEROSIS (ALS)

Description

Amyotrophic lateral sclerosis (ALS), also known as Lou Gehrig's Disease, is a rapidly progressive, fatal neuromuscular disease caused by the destruction of nerve cells in the brain and spinal cord. This causes loss of nervous control of the voluntary muscles, resulting in the degeneration of the muscles, which in turn leads to death from respiratory complications. ALS is always progressive, and the rate of progression varies for each person.

People afflicted with ALS do not lose their ability to see, hear, touch, smell, or taste. The bladder and muscles of the person's eyes are not affected either, nor are sexual drive and function. The disease does not affect the person's mind. The average life expectancy for a newly diagnosed person is 2 to 5 years, although improved medical care is resulting in persons living longer. ALS frequently takes its toll before being diagnosed, causing the people who have the disease to be significantly debilitated before they learn they have it.

Causes

The causes of ALS are unknown. There are three types of ALS: (1) sporadic, the most common form of the disease; (2) familial, the inherited form of ALS, of which only a small number of cases occur; and (3) Guamian, named after Guam because of the large number of cases that occur in Guam and other territories of the Pacific.

Because there are high numbers of ALS patients in Guam, in Western New Guinea, and in Japan, there is a theory that ALS might be caused by environmental problems. These areas have large amounts of heavy metals such as lead, mercury, and aluminum. These metals can poison the body and cause ALS symptoms. Even though men make up the majority of those who contract ALS, women also get the disease. Race, ethnicity, or socioeconomic boundaries make no difference as to who will come down with ALS. Most of those who get the disease are usually between the ages of 40 and 70, but people in their 20s and 30s can also get it.

Symptoms

ALS symptoms vary from one person to another according to which group of muscles are affected by the disease. Tripping, dropping things, abnormal fatigue in the arms and/or legs, slurred speech, difficulty in talking loudly, uncontrollable bouts of laughing or crying, and muscle cramps and twitches are symptoms of ALS. ALS usually starts first in the hands and will cause problems in dressing, bathing, or other simple tasks. It may progress more on one side of the body and generally proceeds up the arm or leg. If it starts in the feet, walking will become difficult. ALS can also start in the throat, causing trouble with swallowing.

Assessment and Treatment

Neurologists use clinical tests such as blood testing, electromyograms (EMG), magnetic resonance imagings (MRI), CT scans, and nerve biopsies to establish a profile when diagnosing ALS. These profiles will eliminate other possibilities as to what the person might be suffering from.

There is no cure for ALS. There are, however, things that can be done to improve or maintain the lifestyle of a person who is suffering from the disease. First, the patient should continue his or her usual daily activities, stopping just before getting tired. Physicians often will give the patient exercises, such as breathing exercises and/or exercises to strengthen the muscles that are not affected with the disease. Foot braces, hand splints, or wheelchairs, combined with exercise, will enable the patient to remain as independent as possible for as long as possible.

Counseling can be of help to ease the mental anguish brought on by this disease. Family counseling can also be helpful to the person with ALS as well as the family.

One of the side effects of this disease is uncontrolled muscle contractures or spasms. Physical therapy cannot restore normal muscle function, but may help in preventing painful contractures of the muscles and in maintaining normal muscle strength and function. The physical therapist should show family members how to perform these exercises so they can help maintain this therapy for the person with ALS.

Speech therapy may also be helpful in maintaining the person's ability to speak. Swallowing therapy is important as well, to assist with the problems of swallowing and drinking. This treatment helps prevent choking. It is recommended that the patient adopt a new head posture and positioning of the tongue. The patient should also change the consistency of the food to aid swallowing accordingly as the disease progresses.

Occupational therapy is also important. The therapist will come to the person's home and recommend where to move furniture to make it easier for the patient to move around her house. The therapist will also place kitchen appliances in areas where making meals will be easier. The occupational therapist will also bring devices that will help the person in making the telephone, computer, and other devices easier to use.

When the ability to breathe decreases, a respiratory therapist is needed to measure the breathing capacity. These tests should take place on a regular basis. To make breathing easier, the patient should not lie down immediately after eating; the patient should not eat large meals, because they can increase abdominal pressure and prevent the diaphragm from expanding; and when sleeping, the head should be elevated 15 to 30 degrees to keep the abdominal organs away from the diaphragm. When breathing capacity falls below 70%, noninvasive ventilatory assistance should be provided. This involves a nasal mask connected to a mechanical ventilator. When the breathing capacity falls below 50%, a permanent hook-up to a ventilator should be considered.

People suffering with ALS should avoid eating processed foods (foods with preservatives and artificial ingredients) and only eat fresh, natural foods. Fresh fruits and vegetables are good because they provide vitamins and antioxidant substances, as well as meat, fish, eggs, and cheese, which contain protein. Nutrient-dense foods should be eaten. These are foods a person can eat much less of to get the adequate amount of nutrition; thus, the patient does not have to waste a lot of energy eating. Foods containing fiber are also good to eat because they prevent constipation.

Various medications can be given to the patient as ALS progresses. Baclofen will relieve stiffness in the limbs and throat. Nutritional supplements called branched-chain amino acids can slow down weight loss and muscle decline. Quinine will ease the cramps. Tricyclic antidepressants can control the production of excess saliva. Riluzole, the only FDA-approved drug to treat ALS, reduces the presynaptic release of glutamate. A number of nutrients, from vitamins and minerals to herbs, are natural antioxidants, which help slow the breakdown of motor neurons. Vitamins A, C, and E, along with beta-carotene, Coenzyme Q_{10}, grapeseed extract, green tea, melatonin, garlic, zinc, and selenium are helpful.

New Research Results on ALS

Pigment epithelium-derived factor (PEDF), a natural substance produced by the body, was located for the first time in the spinal cord and skeletal muscles of humans, monkeys, and rats. Previously, scientists believed that PEDF was found only in the pigmented layer of cells beneath the retina. Using slices of rat spinal cords kept alive in culture, PEDF showed a dramatic ability to protect cells from the toxic effects of threohydroxyaspartate (THA), a drug that mimics the effects of ALS, causing slow death of motor neurons. The PEDF-treated sections showed a near-normal neuron count compared with untreated cultures. According to Dr. Ralph Kuncl, who led the Johns Hopkins research team, protection of the spinal cord nerves in culture by PEDF was nearly complete. He went on to state that ". . . If we had this same level of protection in patients with ALS, they'd experience slight muscle weakness at most." The effectiveness of PEDF will be tested next on transgenic mouse models.

The same research team recently reported (in the May 1999 issue of *Molecular and Cellular Neuroscience*) on another natural compound known as neurturin, a neurotrophic substance that will stimulate regeneration of damaged nerve cells. Neurotrophic factors including PEDF and neurturin are believed to protect healthy cells from the damaging effects of glutamate, a neurotransmitter that gluts the spaces between motor nerve cells, causing overstimulation and contributing to the progression of the disease. Although riluzole mildly restrains the immediate release of glutamate, it provides minimal protection to motor neurons, as do PEDF and neurturin. The researchers predict the development of an "ALS cocktail," drug combinations containing neurotrophic factors, each working at a different point in the process.

A study published in the journal *Nature (Medicine)* found the amino acid creatine more effective than riluzole in extending the survival of mice with an ALS-type disease. The scientists reported that with 1% creatine administration, survival was extended by 13 days, and with 2% administration of creatine, survival doubled to 26 days. These scientists note that riluzole alone extends survival rate by 13 days (in mice). The supplemented creatine protected the mice from the loss of motor neurons and also improved movement. This study proposed that creatine could help reverse the effects of ALS at the cellular level. This is done by stabilizing the enzymes in the mitochondria, the "powerhouses" of the cell that store energy, thus slowing the cell death process.

A recent study in *Nature Medicine* also suggests that creatine may be more effective than prescription therapy for ALS. After taking creatine, patients with muscular dystrophy also showed a 10% increase in strength, according to a study in *Neurology*. "Creatine is well tolerated, . . . and harnessing its apparent ability to buffer and stabilize the production and transportation of energy within cells could yield important health benefits for people with ALS and other progressive diseases," explains Leon Charash, M.D., who chairs the medical advisory committee of the Muscular Dystrophy Association.

Promising Study on CoQ_{10}

In a study published in the *Proceedings of the National Academy of Sciences* (1998; 95), when CoQ_{10} was administered to rats genetically bred to develop ALS, a significant increase in survival time was observed. After only 2 months of CoQ_{10} supplementation, mitochondrial energy expenditure in the brain increased by 29% compared to the group not getting CoQ_{10}. The human equivalent dose of CoQ_{10} to achieve these results was 100 to 200 mg a day.

The conclusion by the scientists was that "CoQ_{10} can exert neuroprotective effects that might be useful in the treatment of neurodegenerative diseases."

This study documented that orally supplemented CoQ_{10} specifically enhanced metabolic energy levels of brain cells. While this effect in the brain has been previously postulated, this study provides hard-core evidence. Based on the types of brain cell injury that CoQ_{10} protected against, the scientists suggested that it may be useful in the prevention or treatment of Huntington's disease and ALS. It was noted that while vitamin E delays the onset of ALS in mice, it does not increase survival time. CoQ_{10} was suggested as a more effective treatment strategy for neurodegenerative disease than vitamin E, because survival time was increased in mice treated with CoQ_{10}.

About 95% of cellular energy is produced from structures in the cell called *mitochondria*. The mitochondria have been described as the cell's "energy powerhouse," and the diseases of aging are increasingly being referred to as "mitochondrial disorders." When Coenzyme Q_{10} is administered orally, it is incorporated into the mitochondria of cells throughout the body where it facilitates and regulates the oxidation of fats and sugars into energy.

CoQ_{10} levels decrease with age. Depletion is caused by reduced synthesis of CoQ_{10} in the body along with increased oxidation of CoQ_{10} in the mitochondria. A CoQ_{10} deficit results in the inactivation of enzymes needed for mitochondrial energy production, whereas supplementation with CoQ_{10} preserves mitochondrial function.

Based on this very preliminary research, ALS patients might want to take 100 mg of an oil-based Coenzyme Q_{10} supplement 3 times a day. CoQ_{10} absorbs best when taken with fat, so oil-based supplements of CoQ_{10} can markedly improve systemic absorption.

Soy Supplementation

The phytoestrogen genistein, found in soy products, may also help the survival rate in ALS patients, according to research results in the journal *Biochemical and Biophysical Research Communications*.

Researchers at the Hughes Institute in Minnesota studied the effects of genistein on male and female mice with familial ALS. The researchers propose that the higher incidence of the disease and earlier onset in the male mice could be related to the presence of estrogen in females. Results of the study indicated that the genistein provided neuroprotective effects that were both estrogen dependent and independent. Genistein warrants further study as a preventive agent against conditions such as ALS and stroke. Because there are insufficient research studies on humans, a physician must be consulted for dosage and prophylactic effectiveness.

Free Radicals Implicated

In a study published in *Neurochemical Research* (April 1997; 22 [4]:535–39), several parameters indicative of oxidative stress were evaluated in blood from individuals with the sporadic form of amyotrophic lateral sclerosis (SALS) and were compared to healthy controls. Plasma levels of 2-thiobarbituric-reactive substances (TBARS), products of lipid peroxidation, were significantly higher ($p < 0.03$) in the SALS patients compared to controls. The ratio TBARS/alpha-tocopherol was 47% higher in the SALS individuals than in controls. This indicates that supplementation with antioxidants like vitamin E, selenium, ascorbyl palmitate, and grape-seed extract might be of some benefit.

The Neurologically Active Form of Vitamin B_{12}

One cause of brain cell death is glutamate toxicity. Brain cells use glutamate as a neurotransmitter, but unfortunately glutamate is a double-edged sword in that it can also kill aging brain cells. The release of glutamate from the synapses is the usual means by which neurons communicate with each other. Effective communication means controlled release of glutamate at the right time to the right cells. But when glutamate is released in excessive amounts, intercellular communication ceases. It is like replacing radio signals with x-rays. The flood of glutamate onto the receiving neurons drives them into hyperactivity and the excessive activity leads to cellular degradation.

It may be possible to protect brain cells against glutamate toxicity by taking methylcobalamin supplements. In a study published in the *European Journal of Pharmacology* (Sept. 7, 1993; 241 [1]:1–6), it was shown that chronic exposure of rat cortical neurons to methylcobalamin protected against glutamate-, aspartate-, and nitroprusside-induced neurotoxicity. This study also showed that *S*-adenosyl-methionine (SAMe) protected against neurotoxicity. In a study published in *Investigational Ophthalmology Visual Sciences* (April 1997; 38 [5]:848–54), a combination of methylcobalamin and SAMe was used to protect against retinal brain cell toxicity caused by glutamate and nitroprusside. The mechanism by which methylcobalamin protected against neurotoxicity was postulated by the researchers to be enhancement of brain cell methylation. The scientists who conducted these studies emphasized that chronic exposure of methylcobalamin was necessary to protect against neurotoxicity. This indicates that for methylcobalamin to be effective in protecting against neurological disease, daily supplementation may be required. An appropriate dose for an ALS patient to take would be 20 to 60 mg a day taken sublingually. Re-methylation nutrients such as folic acid and TMG (trimethylglycine) are being studied as possible therapies to treat Alzheimer's disease, and the same mechanism of action might have a beneficial effect against ALS.

A study published in the journal *Internal Medicine* (Feb 1994; 33 [2]:82–86) investigated the daily administration of 60 mg of methylcobalamin to patients with chronic progressive MS, a disease that has a poor prognosis and widespread demyelination in the central nervous system. Although motor disability did not improve, there were clinical improvements in visual and auditory MS-related disabilities. The scientists stated that methylcobalamin might be an effective adjunct to immunosuppressive treatment for chronic progressive MS. This again suggests a potential benefit, but no clinical studies on ALS patients using methylcobalamin have been conducted.

The effects of methylcobalamin were studied on an animal model of muscular dystrophy. This study, published in *Neuroscience Letters* (March 28, 1994; 170 [1]:195–97), looked at the degeneration of axon motor terminals. In mice receiving methylcobalamin, nerve sprouts were more frequently observed and regeneration of motor nerve terminals occurred in sites that had previously been in a degenerating state.

In a study published in the *Journal of Neurological Science* (April 1994; 122 [2]:140–43), scientists postulated that methylcobalamin could up-regulate protein synthesis and help regenerate nerves. The scientists showed that very high doses of methylcobalamin produced nerve regeneration in laboratory rats. The scientists stated that ultra-high doses of methylcobalamin might be of clinical use for patients with peripheral neuropathies. The human equivalent dose to duplicate this study would be about 40 mg of sublingually administered methylcobalamin.

In humans, a subacute degeneration of the brain and spinal cord can occur by the demyelination of nerve sheaths caused by a folic acid or vitamin B_{12} deficiency. In a study published in the *Journal of Inherited Metabolic Diseases* (1993; 16 [4]:762–70), it was shown that some people have genetic defects that preclude them from naturally producing methylcobalamin. The scientists stated that a deficiency of methylcobalamin directly caused demyelination disease in people with this inborn defect that prevents the natural synthesis of methylcobalamin.

An early study published in the Russian journal *Farmakol Toksikol* (November 1983; 46 [6]:9–12) showed that the daily administration of methyl cobalamin in rats markedly activated the regeneration of mechanically damaged axons of motor neurons. An even more pronounced effect was observed in laboratory rats whose sciatic nerves were mechanically crushed. Two studies published in the Japanese journal *Nippon Yakurigaku Zasshi* (March 1976; 72 [2]:269–78) showed that the administration of methylcobalamin caused significant increases in the *in vivo* incorporation of the amino acid leucine into the crushed sciatic nerve, and this resulted in a stimulating effect on protein synthesis repair and neural regeneration.

Based on its unique mechanisms of action, methylcobalamin could be effective in slowing the progression of diseases such as ALS. Since methylcobalamin is not a drug, there is little economic incentive to conduct expensive clinical studies on it, so it may be a long time before we know just how effective this vitamin B_{12} analog is in slowing the progression of ALS.

Additional Suggestions for Nutritional Supplementation

Acetyl-*L*-carnitine has produced dramatic results in protecting neurons in a wide range of disease states. We therefore suggest that ALS patients take 3000 mg a day of acetyl-*L*-carnitine. Neuron damage can be caused by degeneration of the myelin sheath, a fatty layer that wraps the signal-moving neuronal fibers. Taking 2 tablespoons a day of Udo's Choice Essential Fatty Acids will provide omega-3 and omega-6 fatty acids, which may help to repair the myelin sheath required for proper neuron conduction.

Since pregnenolone and DHEA are involved in the regulation of neurologic function, supplementation with 50 mg 3 times a day of pregnenolone, and/or 25 mg 2 to 3 times a day of DHEA should be considered.

Innovative drug therapies for ALS also might include 10 to 20 mg a day of Hydergine, 40 mg a day of vinpocetine, and testosterone and human growth hormone replacement therapy.

To help protect against respiratory dysfunction, 600 mg of *N*-acetylcysteine (NAC) and 1000 mg of vitamin C, 3 times a day, are suggested.

Free-radical damage has been implicated in the ALS disease process, so the standard dose of Life Extension Mix, which is 3 tablets 3 times a day, might be helpful. While Life Extension Mix contains a considerable amount of magnesium, 500 mg a day of additional magnesium also is suggested.

Alpha-lipoic acid is a potent antioxidant that is especially effective in preventing diabetic neuropathy. Therefore, we suggest a dose of 250 mg 3 times a day of alpha-lipoic acid to protect the neurons affected by ALS.

Nutritionist Carmen Fusco reports that, while under her care for ALS, Senator Jacob Javits seemed to improve enough to reduce his hospital admissions with the following nutrients: octocosonol as it occurs in raw wheat germ oil; mega doses of pantothenic acid (vitamin B_5, the "stress vitamin"); and DMG sublingual. Fusco also has used the branch-chain amino acids and sublingual vitamin B_{12}. Dr. Benjamin Frank recommended the coenzyme form of the B vitamins, which were administered intramuscularly by injection.

Summary

Physical, occupational, and speech therapies are important to the patient with ALS to make it easier to live their lives. Wheelchairs, foot braces, and other devices that can make it easier to use the telephone and computer are helpful in making the patient as independent as possible.

Some supplements that may be beneficial to ALS patients are

1. Coenzyme Q_{10}, 100 mg (in an oil base for maximum absorption), 3 times a day.
2. Methylcobalamin, 20 mg, 2 to 3 times a day.
3. Vitamin C, 1000 mg 3 times a day.
4. Vitamin E, 800 units 3 times a day.
5. Beta carotene, 20,000 units a day.
6. Creatine, 5 grams a day on an empty stomach.
7. Zinc, 30 mg with food.
8. Magnesium, 500 mg a day.
9. Alpha-lipoic acid, 250 mg 2 to 3 times a day.
10. Acetyl-*L*-carnitine, 3000 mg a day.
11. Udo's Choice Essential Fatty Acids, 2 tablespoons a day.
12. Pregnenolone, 50 mg 3 times a day.
13. DHEA, 25 mg 3 times a day.
14. Selenium 300 mcg a day.
15. Grape-seed extract 100 to 300 mg a day.

For more information. Contact the ALS Association National Office, 21021 Ventura Blvd., Suite 321, Woodland Hills, CA 91364; (818) 340-7500; patient hotline: (800) 782-4747; e-mail, alsinfo@alsa-national.org. This association is a nonprofit voluntary national health organization committed solely to the fight against ALS through research, patient support, information, advocacy, and public awareness.

Contact the Family Caregiver Alliance, 690 Market Street, Suite 600, San Francisco, CA 94104; (415) 434-3388; Web site http://www.caregiver.org; e-mail, info@caregiver.org. The Family Caregiver Alliance supports and assists caregivers of brain-impaired adults through education, research, services, and advocacy.

Product availability. For a listing of physicians in your area who might be knowledgeable in these innovative approaches, call (800) 544-4440. Acetyl-*L*-carnitine, alpha-lipoic acid, *N*-acetylcysteine, pregnenolone, DHEA, Life Extension Mix, and magnesium are available by calling (800) 544-4440 or ordering on-line at www.lef.org. Hydergine is available by prescription in the United States or from overseas pharmacies.

ANEMIA/ THROMBOCYTOPENIA/ LEUKOPENIA

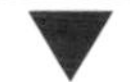

Referred to as the *hidden hunger* by The World Health Organization, anemia poses a significant health risk worldwide. Approximately 5 million people suffer from anemia in the United States. Additionally, 20% of all premenopausal women in the United States suffer from anemia. The incidence of anemia is far greater in second- and third-world countries, where the death rate is still 100% for some forms of anemia.

This protocol deals with the following three distinct blood diseases: anemia, thrombocytopenia, and leukopenia.

ANEMIA

Generally defined as a decrease in the number of red blood cells or quantity of hemoglobin or hematocrit. This reduced blood cell count reduces the amount of oxygen the blood can carry to the body.

THROMBOCYTOPENIA

A condition that occurs when the body does not have enough blood platelets, or the platelets are damaged. A person may bleed uncontrollably from a large vessel or from small capillaries. Often this bleeding into tissue becomes visible as a bruise or red marks on the skin.

LEUKOPENIA

An abnormal decrease in the number of white blood cells, often reducing immune system function.

ANEMIA

General Causes of Anemia

Researchers studying the management of common forms of anemia at Wright State University School of Medicine at Dayton, Ohio, advised in a 1999 study that

> Anemia is a prevalent condition with a variety of underlying causes. Once the etiology has been established, many forms of anemia can be easily managed by the family physician. Iron deficiency, the most common form of anemia, may be treated orally or, rarely, parenterally. Vitamin B_{12} deficiency has traditionally been treated with intramuscular injections, although oral and intranasal preparations are also available. The treatment of folate deficiency is straightforward, relying on oral supplements. Folic acid supplementation is also recommended for women of child-bearing age to reduce their risk of neural tube defects. *Journal of American Family Physicians* (1999).

Aging, viral infections, blood diseases, and a variety of drugs, as well as cancer chemotherapy and radiation therapy, can cause deficits in red blood cells, white blood cells, and blood platelet production (*Annu. Rev. Nutr.*, 1999; 19:357–77).

Dietary anemia is caused by not consuming enough nutrients, losing needed nutrients, or the inability to absorb enough required nutrients. Anemia can sometimes be caused by a hormone deficiency.

Symptoms of Anemia

- ▼ Weakness and faintness
- ▼ Shortness of breath
- ▼ Increased heart rate
- ▼ Headaches
- ▼ Sore tongue
- ▼ Nausea and loss of appetite
- ▼ Dizziness
- ▼ Bleeding gums
- ▼ Confusion and dementia
- ▼ Severe cases may cause heart failure.

Common Dietary Anemias

Pernicious Anemia (Lack of Vitamin B_{12})

Pernicious anemia occurs when the body does not have enough vitamin B_{12}. Pernicious anemia usually means the person can't absorb the vitamin, rather than lack of the vitamin in the diet.

> Vitamin B_{12} deficiency is estimated to affect 10 to 15% of people over the age of 60, and the laboratory diagnosis is usually based on low serum vitamin B_{12} levels or elevated serum methylmalonic acid and homocysteine levels (*Annu. Rev. Nutr.*, 1999; 19:357–77).

Vitamin B_{12} is important and is used by our bodies in the bone marrow to make red blood cells. Interestingly, this disease is more common in the people of northern Europe.

The risks of getting pernicious anemia are increased by eating only a vegetarian diet, having stomach surgery (removing a part of the stomach which makes intrinsic factors needed to absorb vitamin B_{12}), thyroid disease, diabetes mellitus, or family history of the disease.

There is a special test for vitamin B_{12} called the Schilling Test in which a doctor gives an injection of radioactive vitamin B_{12}. By measuring how much of it comes out in the urine, the doctor can tell whether a lack of vitamin B_{12} is causing the anemia. Your physician may also look at your bone marrow to see whether there is a problem in red blood cell production.

If untreated, pernicious anemia can lead to serious health problems such as congestive heart failure, neurological problems, increased incidences of infections, and even impotence in males. Those with coronary artery or pulmonary disease are especially vulnerable to the oxygen deprivation that can be caused by anemia.

Folic-Acid-Deficiency Anemia

Folate deficiency is generally found in malnourished individuals, especially alcoholics, infants fed solely on cows' milk, and pregnant women. Malabsorption syndromes often produce folate deficiency, and certain drugs (e.g., phenytoin, phenobarbital, primidone, isoniazid, and cycloserine) are associated with attenuation of folate absorption and metabolism.

Folic acid is a vitamin found in many foods, especially asparagus, broccoli, endive, spinach, and lima beans. Folic acid is metabolically inactive until it is converted into tetrahydrofolic acid (THF).

Tetrahydrofolic acid is important to general health as it produces thymidylate, which acts as a courier of "genetic messages" to cell DNA. Additionally, folate has been shown to play a role in no fewer than six biochemical reactions, including synthesis of methionine, synthesis of purines (thymine is a pyrimidine), and catabolism of histidine. Failure of folate to break down histidine results in accumulation of an intermediary metabolite, formiminoglutamic acid (FIGlu), which can be measured clinically and is a clinical marker for folate deficiency.

Iron-Deficiency Anemia

When there is insufficient iron available for the normal production of hemoglobin, iron-deficiency anemia results.

According to the World Health Organization, iron-deficiency anemia (IDA) has not been responsive to prevention and control efforts.

> Subclinical consequences of micronutrient deficiencies, i.e., "hidden hunger," include compromised immune functions that increase the risk of morbidity and mortality, impaired cognitive development and growth, and reduced reproductive and work capacity and performance (*Bull. World Health Org.*, 1998; 76 Suppl. 2:34–7).

Iron-deficiency anemia, the most common type of anemia, strikes 20% of all premenopausal women in the United States. The primary cause is loss of blood through menstruation. This type of anemia also commonly occurs during pregnancy.

The body's iron stores can be depleted either through insufficient intakes or excessive loss. In America, dietary insufficiency is a very rare condition, thanks to the combination of our meat-rich diet and the iron fortification of our food staples. The one notable exception to this is the case with milk-fed infants and their mothers. Bovine milk has almost no iron. An iron-deficient state in babies may begin in the antenatal life of the mother who may be overtly or borderline iron-deficient (iron requirements are markedly increased in pregnancy due to the demands of developing the fetal tissues). Fortunately most infant formulas are now fortified with iron. Still, nutritional cases of IDA do occur. Although dietary deficiency of iron is rare, individuals with gastrointestinal lesions (scarring) that cause poor absorption may fail to assimilate sufficient iron.

As mentioned above, the more important cause of iron depletion is chronic blood loss. In females, this is usually due to menstruation. Other underlying causes of blood loss include chronically bleeding lesions of the gastrointestinal tract, reflux esophagitis, peptic ulcers, or gastric or colorectal adenocarcinomas.

Because these diseases may be undetected, all cases of iron-deficiency anemia should be thoroughly investigated for the presence of hidden bleeding sites. This is especially true in cases involving females who are not of reproductive age and in all males. Patients should insist on clinical testing to determine the source of any suspected bleeding.

The Anti-Anemia Drug

When the drug Epogen was approved, it provided physicians with a relatively safe method of treating anemias caused by defective red blood cell production. Epogen is a recombinant human erythropoietin that stimulates the division and differentiation of red blood cell progenitors in the bone marrow. Epogen is prescribed to treat anemias caused by cancer chemotherapy drugs, certain anti-HIV drugs, testosterone deficiency, and chronic kidney failure (erythropoietin is naturally produced in the kidneys). Epogen is administered by injection by a physician experienced in using this drug.

It should be noted that a clinically significant resolution to an anemic condition may require 2 to 6 weeks of Epogen therapy. This means that Epogen is not intended for patients who require immediate correction of a life-threatening anemic condition. Despite Epogen being approved by the FDA several years ago, most conventional doctors are still not familiar with it and often fail to prescribe it appropriately.

Acute anemia therapy usually requires blood transfusions. The goal of therapy in acute anemia is to restore the hemodynamics of the vascular systems and replace lost red blood cells. To achieve this, the practitioner may use mineral and vitamin supplements, blood transfusions, vasopressors, histamine antagonists, and glucocorticosteroids.

Treatment of Pernicious Anemia

Doctors have long prescribed vitamin B_{12} injections, though recent studies show that orally ingested vitamin B_{12} works as well as B_{12} shots (*Life Extension Magazine;* 1999, August, pp. 34–40).

Treatment of Folic-Acid-Deficiency Anemia

Oral supplementation with folic acid and vitamin B_{12} is a common treatment of folic-acid deficiency.

Treatment of Iron-Deficiency Anemia

Oral iron preparations are available for treatment of these cases. The least expensive and typically the best absorbed is a noncoated ferrous sulfate ($FeSO_4$). It is important to specify on the prescription that nonenteric, coated preparations are used, so as to maximize iron availability for absorption. Since acute iron overdoses are potentially fatal, iron tablets should be kept out of reach of children.

In certain cases, such as in gastrointestinal malabsorption syndromes, it may be necessary to give parenteral iron. This preparation, iron dextran (Imferon7), may be given intramuscularly or intravenously. Since it may produce anaphylactic shock, it needs to be given under direct physician supervision. Transfusion, which immediately restores all iron stores, is very dangerous in chronically anemic patients because of the demand this new blood volume puts upon the already taxed heart. This is rarely indicated for iron-deficiency anemia.

Since excess iron in the body can generate massive free-radical reactions, supplemental iron to correct an iron deficiency should be used sparingly. Some people mistakenly continue taking iron supplements long after a deficient state is corrected. The penalty for overloading the body with too much iron is dramatically increased risks of cancer, heart disease, and neurological degeneration.

Other Nutritional Approaches

Anemia and associated diseases compromise the oxygen-transport capabilities of red blood cells and the normal immune function of both red and white blood cells due to increased adhesion, reduction, or malfunction. Scientific study strongly suggests that trace minerals may act as an adjunctive preventive therapy and/or reduce the effect of anemia on normal blood cell function.

Researchers at the Nichols Institute in San Juan Capistrano, California, reported the importance of trace minerals in a 1998 study quoted below:

> Copper, zinc, selenium, and molybdenum are involved in many biochemical processes supporting life. The most important of these processes are cellular respiration, cellular utilization of oxygen, DNA and RNA reproduction, maintenance of cell membrane integrity, and sequestration of free radicals (*Clin. Lab. Med.*, 1998 Dec; 18 [4]:673–85).

We recommend the consumption of trace minerals such as 2 to 3 mg daily of copper, 30 to 60 mg of zinc, and 200 to 600 mcg daily of selenium, as an adjunctive therapy for anemia and associated disease.

Preventing and Treating Anemia Caused by HIV Antiviral Drugs

Infection by the human immunodeficiency virus (HIV) is commonly associated with hematologic abnormalities (anemia, leukopenia, and thrombocytopenia). A 1998 study by The National Center for HIV states that "the 1-year incidence of anemia was 36.9% for persons with acquired immunodeficiency syndrome (AIDS)." Several causes have been identified, including direct HIV injury on bone marrow (as mentioned above), anti-HIV drugs such as AZT, opportunistic infections in bone marrow, vitamin B_{12} and folate deficiency, radiation therapy, and hemophagocytic syndrome. Patients have an increased risk of infection, since the neutrophils play an important role in the defense against bacterial and certain fungal infections.

Treatment strategies may include reducing or eliminating anti-HIV drugs and other conventional therapies that suppress bone marrow production of blood cells. Supplementation with 2000 mcg of vitamin B_{12} sublingual or oral tablets and 1600 mcg of folic acid is strongly suggested because deficiencies of these vitamins can cause numerous AIDS-related complications. The drug Epogen would be an appropriate conventional therapy.

THROMBOCYTOPENIA

Thrombocytopenia is a multisystem, life-threatening disorder of unknown cause, first observed and described in 1924. Thrombocytopenia is characterized by microvascular leakage with platelet aggregation. The disease is most common in adults and is associated with pregnancy and diseases such as HIV, cancer, bacterial infection, vasculitis, bone marrow transplantation, and drugs.

Many drugs can induce thrombocytopenia mediated by drug-dependent antiplatelet antibodies. Management of patients with unexpected thrombocytopenia who are taking multiple drugs remains a difficult clinical problem (*Curr. Opin. Hematol.,* 1999 Sept; 6 [5]:349–53).

Platelet damage generally accompanies thrombocytopenia, releasing a substance into the bloodstream, which dramatically increases platelet adhesiveness and causes further complications.

In some cases of megaloblastic anemia (anemia conditions that have a common failure mechanism in which the body is unable to synthesize adequate amounts of normal DNA), there is concomitant leukopenia and thrombocytopenia, reflecting the abnormal development of white blood cells and platelets (*Int. J. Clin. Pract.,* 1999 March; 53 [2]:104–6).

Anemia Chronic Disease (ACD) often accompanies or can cause thrombocytopenia and leukopenia. This is a condition found in patients suffering from chronic infections, noninfectious inflammatory diseases (such as rheumatoid arthritis), and neoplasms. The following characterize this type of anemia:

- Decreased red blood cell (RBC) life span. The cause is completely unknown.
- Impaired iron metabolism. Iron accumulates in the body, but its absorption by red blood cells is impaired.

This disease contributes to the further reduction of red and white blood cells, causing the disease or complicating the treatment of anemia and anemia-associated diseases.

A specific natural therapy to restore healthy platelet production is 5 capsules a day of standardized shark liver oil, containing 200 mg of alkylglycerols per capsule. Studies have shown that shark liver oil can boost the production of blood platelets. Studies have also shown the immune enhancement capabilities of shark liver oil (*J. Alt. Compl. Med.,* 1998 Spring; 4 [1]:87–99). As will be discussed later, melatonin may be an especially effective and safe therapy to treat thrombocytopenia.

CAUTION: Shark oil capsules should be taken in high doses for a maximum period of only 30 days, because otherwise too many blood platelets might be produced.

LEUKOPENIA

Preventing and Treating Chemotherapy-Induced Leukopenia

Studies have shown that supplemental melatonin in doses of 10 to 40 mg a night can protect and restore normal blood cell production caused by the toxicity of chemotherapy. A study was performed in 80 patients with metastatic solid tumors to evaluate the benefits of melatonin. Patients received either chemotherapy alone or chemotherapy plus 20 mg each night of melatonin. Thrombocytopenia was significantly less frequent in patients receiving melatonin.

Other common side effects of cancer chemotherapy, such as malaise, asthenia, stomatitis, and neuropathy, occurred less frequently in patients receiving melatonin. This corroborated previous studies showing that the administration of melatonin during chemotherapy can prevent some side effects, especially myelosuppression (blood cell production suppression) and neuropathy.

The Life Extension Foundation recommends that cancer patients using cytotoxic chemotherapy drugs be placed on FDA-approved immune-protective drugs a week before the first chemotherapy drug is administered. Depending on the type of cancer and the chemotherapy regimen that will be used, some of these FDA-approved drugs may include

- Neupogen, a granulocyte-colony stimulating factor drug (G-CSF).

- Leukine, a granulocyte macrophage–colony stimulating factor (GM-CSF).

  These FDA-approved drugs stimulate the production of T-lymphocytes, macrophages, and other immune cells that are valuable in preventing the toxic effects on the bone marrow during chemotherapy. These immune-protecting drugs enable chemotherapy to be given at a higher dose that may make it effective. Stimulated macrophages are powerful tumor killers, as has been demonstrated by clinical studies using interleukin-2 and (GM)-CSF, or G-CSF. In addition, colony growth factors are able to accelerate regeneration of blood cells following chemotherapy. Initial clinical experience with GM-CS and G-CSF has shown that severe neutropenia (immune impairment) due to chemotherapy drugs may be prevented or at least decelerated, thus reducing the number of severe infections.
- Immune cytokines such as alpha-interferon and interleukin-2. Interferon directly inhibits cancer cell proliferation and has already been used in the therapy of hairy cell leukemia, Kaposi's sarcoma, and malignant melanoma. Interleukin-2 allows for an increase in the cytotoxic activity of natural killer (NK) cells.
- Retinoic acid (vitamin A) analog drugs enhance the efficacy of some chemotherapy regimens and reduce the risk of secondary cancers.
- T-cell suppressor inhibiting agents, such as cimetidine, prevent cancer cells from prematurely shutting down the immune system.

The proper administration of these drugs—1 week prior to the initiation of chemotherapy—can dramatically reduce the immune damage that chemotherapy inflicts on the body and increase the cancer-cell killing efficacy of conventional chemotherapy drugs. Please remember that we are talking about drugs that require physician administration. The patient can self-administer melatonin, CoQ_{10}, tocopherol succinate, and many other nutrients that have been shown to protect immune function and improve chemotherapy efficacy. These nutrients have saved the lives of numerous cancer patients in clinical trials. The administration of the FDA-approved drugs, however, is still important to the cancer patient, even though nutrients such as melatonin have similar mechanisms of action. There are too many published studies about the prophylactic benefits of these FDA-approved drugs for them not to be used prior to the administration of chemotherapy.

To treat low white blood cell counts, the FDA-approved drug Neupogen or Leukine may be considered by your immunologist or hematologist. Drugs such as Neupogen, Leukine, and Intron A (alpha-interferon) can restore immune function debilitated by toxic cancer chemotherapy drugs. In one study, patients with refractory (resistant to treatment) solid tumors treated with standard chemotherapy and GM-CSF had a 33.3% objective response rate, versus 15% with chemotherapy alone. If you are on chemotherapy, and your blood tests show immune suppression you should demand that your oncologist use the appropriate immune restoration drug(s).

Summary

The following steps are important in preventing and treating anemia.

1. Vitamin B_{12}, 2000 to 4000 mcg a day orally or sublingually.
2. Folic acid, 1600 to 5000 mcg a day.
3. Iron, the minimum amount needed to correct an iron deficient state; 30 to 200 mg a day should be taken until blood parameters return to normal.
4. Zinc, 30 to 60 mg daily.
5. Selenium, 200 to 600 mcg daily.
6. Copper, 2 to 3 mg daily.
7. Melatonin, 3 to 10 mg at bedtime.
8. A multivitamin supplement that provides a potent B-complex and vitamin E.
9. Coenzyme Q_{10}, 100 mg a day.
10. If nutrients don't work, ask your doctor to administer the drug Epogen.

The following steps are important to prevent or treat thrombocytopenia:

1. Melatonin, 10 to 40 mg a night (some people may only be able to tolerate 3 mg a night of melatonin).
2. Standardized shark oil capsules, 5 capsules daily, containing 200 mg of alkylglycerols.

CAUTION: Limit consumption to 30 days to avoid overproduction of platelets.

3. Take a potent multinutrient supplement like Life Extension Mix (3 tablets, 3 times a day) to guard against a nutritional deficiency.

The following steps are important to prevent and treat leukopenia:

1. Melatonin, 10 to 40 mg a night (some people may be able to tolerate only 3 mg a night of melatonin).
2. Take a potent multinutrient supplement like Life Extension Mix (3 tablets, 3 times a day) to guard against a nutritional deficiency.
3. Ask your doctor to consider prescribing immune-cell boosting drugs like Neupogen, Leukine, alpha-interferon, and interleukin-2 *before* leukopenia develops. These drugs are not totally free of side effects and have to be carefully monitored for safety and efficacy.

Regular blood testing should be done to monitor the effectiveness of any blood-cell boosting therapy you are taking.

For more information. Contact the National Heart, Lung, and Blood Institute Information Center, (301) 251-1222.

Product availability. Standardized shark liver oil capsules, vitamin B_{12}, folic acid, copper, zinc, selenium, and pharmaceutical grade melatonin can be obtained by phoning (800) 544-4440, or order on-line at www.lef.org.

ANESTHESIA AND SURGICAL PRECAUTIONS

Anesthesia and surgery, though often necessary to preserve life or repair damage to the human body, can have unfortunate side effects. Some anesthesia and surgery have even resulted in temporary or permanent brain damage. Other undesirable complications can be induced by free radicals that occur during anesthesia or during the surgical process.

Risks from Surgery and Anesthesia

Risks to the body from free radicals may be substantially increased during and after anesthesia and surgery. Several free radicals have been implicated as primary culprits in interfering with the re-establishment of a regular heart rhythm following surgery, and in contributing to the common complication of pancreatitis. Some of the mechanisms of neurological injury following anesthesia and surgical procedures have also been identified in the scientific literature.

Benefits of Antioxidants

There are specific nutrients and drugs that, when taken in advance of surgery, can help protect against the more common forms of neurological injury that may occur during anesthesia and surgery. Because of the energy released by their inherent instability, free radicals can interfere with the ability of body cells to function normally. Antioxidants can reduce the energy of free radicals in several ways. Their presence in a cell can prevent the free radical from forming, or they can minimize damage by interrupting an oxidizing chain reaction.

The body also produces its own antioxidant defenses. These include several enzymes, such as catalase, superoxide dismutase (SOD), and glutathione peroxidase, that neutralize many kinds of free radicals. These compounds can be taken as supplements, but taking supplements containing the building blocks of these enzymes may actually be more helpful. Some nutrients containing such building blocks are copper, manganese, selenium, and zinc.

Many vitamins, minerals, and herbs also act as antioxidants. Among these are beta carotene (a source of vitamin A), bilberry (anthocyanoside), vitamin C, Coenzyme Q_{10} (CoQ_{10}), cysteine (an amino acid), ginkgo biloba (flavone glycosides), grape seed (bioflavonoid) or pine bark extract, vitamin E, and turmeric (curcumin). A combination of these substances may provide the best protection against free-radical damage.

Clinical Research

A study conducted on 30 patients undergoing vascular surgery for abdominal aortic aneurysm or obstructive aortoiliac disease yielded the following results. Patients in the first group were treated with CoQ_{10} at a rate of 150 mg per day for 7 days before surgery, while patients in the second group were given a placebo. Group 1 patients (Coenzyme Q_{10}) showed significantly lower markers of free-radical activity and tissue damage (malondialdehyde, conjugated dienes, creatine kinase, and lactate dehydrogenase) than did patients from group 2. Pretreatment with CoQ_{10} may play a protective role during routine vascular procedures by attenuating the degree of peroxidative free-radical damage.

Significant free-radical damage to cells can result from the administration of some forms of anesthesia used during surgical procedures. This is especially true of anesthetics that cause temporarily reduced blood flow. One study assessed the effect of vitamin E administered during prolonged anesthesia. The vitamin E produced a statistically significant decrease in the amount of peroxidation products in the blood.

There is a growing body of evidence to support the role free radicals play in delaying functional and metabolic myocardial recovery following cardiopulmonary bypass surgery in humans. A clinical study evaluated the extent to which ginkgo extract inhibited reperfusion-induced lipid peroxidation, ascorbate depletion, tissue necrosis, and cardiac dysfunction. Patients received either ginkgo extract (320 mg a day) or a placebo before surgical intervention. Plasma samples were collected before incision, during ischemia, and within the first 30 minutes after unclamping. Samples were also collected up to 8 days after surgery from the peripheral circulation and the coronary sinus.

Ginkgo extract inhibited the formation of free radicals on aortic "unclamping" and significantly reduced delayed leakage of myoglobin. Ginkgo also preserved the ascorbic acid pool and had a very slight effect on ventricular myosin leakage. Surgeons concluded that adjuvant (assisting) ginkgo extract therapy was useful in limiting oxidative stress in cardiovascular surgery. Discussion also considered the possible role of highly bio-available terpene constituents of the extract.

Adjuvant Therapies

The best way to obtain high-potency antioxidants to protect against the free radicals induced by anesthesia and surgery is to take—starting at least a week before surgery—3 tablets, 3 times a day, of Life Extension Mix, along with 200 mg a day of CoQ_{10}, and 120 mg a day of ginkgo extract. In addition, at least 3 to 10 mg of melatonin should be taken every night for a week before surgery. Another 3 to 10 mg of melatonin may be taken just prior to anesthesia to provide further protection against anesthesia- and surgery-induced complications. Research funded by the Life Extension Foundation has shown that melatonin given prior to anesthesia protects cells throughout an animal's body (but especially in the brain) against ischemic injury caused by the lack of blood flow.

Some surgeons request their presurgical patients to avoid nutrients that may promote excessive bleeding during surgery. Ginkgo biloba and some of the nutrients in Life Extension Mix (such as vitamin E) may inhibit abnormal blood clotting and cause excessive bleeding during and after surgery. For some surgical procedures, excessive bleeding can be a problem, but experienced surgeons should be able to deal successfully with it.

Conversely, a significant risk factor during and after surgical procedures and long hospital stays is the development of abnormal blood clots (thrombosis). This development can cause stroke, heart attack, or lethal pulmonary embolism (a thrombosis that has traveled to the lung). The platelet aggregation-inhibiting effect of vitamin E, ginkgo, and other nutrients in Life Extension Mix could prevent surgery-induced blood clots from forming.

A recent study published in the British journal *Lancet* showed that low doses of aspirin are effective in preventing post-operative side effects following certain surgical procedures. Physicians from 74 hospitals worldwide evaluated low-dose aspirin (81 or 325 mg) versus high-dose aspirin (650 or 1300 mg) taken daily by more than 2800 patients undergoing endarterectomy to remove fatty plaque from carotid arteries in the neck. Patients receiving low doses of aspirin had fewer strokes (18 versus 38) and heart attacks (5 versus 18) than high-dose patients 3 months following surgery. Overall, 9 patients taking low-dose aspirin died compared with 12 taking high-dose aspirin. The authors cautioned that different doses of aspirin may be required to prevent strokes for patients not undergoing surgery. In describing the effectiveness of lower-dose aspirin, Dr. John Marler of the National Institute of Neurological Disorders and Stroke stated, "This is good news because lower doses are easier to take and better tolerated, so more people can get the full benefit of aspirin."

Some published studies have demonstrated that fewer complications result when open-heart surgery patients take antioxidants before surgery. The scientific literature contains contradictions on the subject of whether or not vitamin E and other antioxidants cause enough excessive bleeding to create a problem during or following surgery. Neurological benefits, protection against damage by free radicals, protection against abnormal blood clot formation, and overall health benefits provided by these nutrients may lead physicians and their patients to decide to include them in their presurgery medication.

Neuroprotection

The brain is especially vulnerable to oxidative stress because of its rich oxygen supply and high fatty acid content. Unfortunately, the brain is relatively underdefended against this stress, and its vulnerability increases with age. In a series of studies by neurologist M. Flint Beal and colleagues at the Massachusetts General Hospital and Harvard Medical School, it was found that the neurotoxins malonate, 3-NP, and MTPT inflicted significantly less brain damage on animals treated with CoQ_{10}. Beal's studies provided the first demonstration that oral CoQ_{10} supplements exert neuroprotective effects in the living brain and significantly raise CoQ_{10} levels in brain tissue and brain mitochondria. Studies also demonstrated that CoQ_{10} protects the brain by raising neuronal energy levels.

In addition to such antioxidants as CoQ_{10}, the patient should consider taking at least 5 mg a day of Hydergine and 2400 mg daily of piracetam for a week before surgery to protect brain cells against the effects of erratic blood flow that may occur during the procedure.

Surgical Wound Healing

A variety of nutrients can be taken after surgery to accelerate the healing process. Refer to the *Wound Healing protocol* for complete information.

Summary

1. It is possible to reduce exposure to free radicals by avoiding ionizing radiation (from x-rays and the sun), exposure to heavy metals, and cigarette smoke.
2. Specific nutrients, taken before surgery, can help protect against some of the most common forms of neurological injury that can occur during anesthesia and surgery.
3. Antioxidants can reduce the energy and harmful effects of free radicals. Antioxidants include beta carotene, bilberry, vitamin C, CoQ_{10}, cysteine (an amino acid), ginkgo biloba, grape seed and pine bark extract, vitamin E, and turmeric (curcumin).

4. It is often helpful to take supplements containing the building blocks of naturally produced antioxidant enzymes: copper, manganese, selenium, and zinc all provide such building blocks.
5. A combination of antioxidants may provide the best protection against free-radical damage.
6. Life Extension Mix and melatonin may provide protection against anesthesia- and surgery-induced complications. The best way to obtain high-potency antioxidants is to take—starting at least a week before surgery—3 tablets, 3 times a day, of Life Extension Mix, along with 200 mg a day of CoQ_{10}, and 120 mg a day of ginkgo extract. In addition, at least 3 to 10 mg of melatonin should be taken every night for a week before surgery, and another 3 to 10 mg of melatonin may be taken just prior to anesthesia.
7. Other agents deemed beneficial are 5 mg daily of Hydergine and 2400 mg daily of piracetam for a week before surgery to protect brain cells.
8. The platelet aggregation-inhibiting effect of vitamin E, ginkgo, and other nutrients in Life Extension Mix could prevent surgery-induced blood clots. Although substances such as aspirin, ginkgo biloba, and some nutrients contained in Life Extension Mix (such as vitamin E) may cause excessive bleeding during or after surgery, the scientific literature contains contradictions on whether or not they and other antioxidants cause enough excessive bleeding to create problems during and after surgery.
9. Oral CoQ_{10} supplements exert neuroprotective effects in the human brain and help to protect it from injury during surgery.

Product availability. Life Extension Mix, ginkgo biloba, CoQ_{10} (Coenzyme Q10), low-dose Healthprin aspirin, and melatonin can be ordered by calling (800) 544-4440, or order on-line at www.lef.org. Hydergine can be obtained with a medical doctor's prescription. Ask the Foundation for a list of offshore pharmacies which carry piracetam.

ANXIETY AND STRESS

Anxiety and stress are two of the most common types of mental disorders in the United States. The National Institute of Mental Health reports that 19 million Americans per year are afflicted by these illnesses. In 1990, the direct and indirect costs of these debilitating conditions to the American economy were more than $46 billion. In Britain, the Office of National Statistics reported that approximately one in seven adults has some form of diagnosable mental disorder, with anxiety being the most commonly reported complaint. Conditions associated with anxiety and stress include depression, phobias, and chronic fatigue. Furthermore, accumulated stress and anxiety can predispose patients to medical conditions such as chronic headaches, hypertension, ulcers, and heart disease. Some physicians estimate that stress and anxiety may be a contributing factor in 90% of all illnesses.

Anxiety Disorders

Anxiety disorders are illnesses that cause people to feel frightened and apprehensive for no apparent reason. These conditions are often related to the biological and psychological makeup of the individual and may be familial in nature. If untreated, these illnesses can significantly reduce productivity and inhibit a person's ability to function in daily life. There are five types of anxiety disorders.

Panic disorder is characterized by repeated episodes of intense fear of sudden onset, often occurring without warning and with varying frequency. Symptoms of panic disorder include chest pains, heart palpitations, sweating palms, dizziness, shortness of breath, a sense of unreality, or an uncontrollable fear of death. Panic disorder affects between three and six million Americans and is twice as likely to occur in women. Onset may occur at any age but generally begins in early adulthood.

Obsessive-Compulsive Disorder (OCD) is characterized by anxious thoughts and uncontrollable ritualistic behavior: obsessions are the anxious thoughts, and compulsions are the rituals used to dispel those thoughts. No pleasure is derived from performing the rituals; rather, the rituals provide only temporary relief. OCD appears to afflict men and women equally, and approximately 1 in 50 people may experience some sort of obsessive-compulsive behavior. Onset is typically in early adulthood, although it may occur in childhood or adolescence.

Post-Traumatic Stress Disorder (PTSD) is a debilitating illness that can result from a traumatic event. Originally defined as battle fatigue or shell shock, this disorder can be precipitated by any traumatic life event such as a serious accident, crime victimization, and natural disasters. People diagnosed with PTSD may relive the event in nightmares or have disturbing recollections of it during waking hours. Ordinary events can trigger flashbacks that may result in a loss of reality, causing the person to believe the event is happening again. PTSD may occur at any age, and although the course of the illness is variable, it can become chronic.

Phobias may be either specific or social in nature. Specific phobias are irrational fears of certain things or situations such as heights, elevators, or closed-in places. This type of phobia may affect 1 in 10 people. Currently, there are no medications for specific phobias. Social phobias are an intense fear of humiliation in a public situation and may be characterized by a feeling of dread beginning weeks in advance of a social event.

Generalized Anxiety Disorder (GAD) is much more serious than the daily anxiety most people feel. It is chronic, excessive worrying about health, personal finances, work, and family. GAD is characterized by difficulty sleeping, trembling or twitching, lightheadedness, irritability, muscle tension, and headaches, among other symptoms. Depression may accompany the anxiety. The onset of GAD is gradual, generally occurring in childhood or adolescence, although adult onset is not uncommon. GAD occurs more frequently in women and may be familial in nature.

Stress

Stress is a psychological and physical response to the demands of daily life that exceed a person's ability to cope successfully. Stress is often characterized by fatigue, sleep disorders, irritability, and constant worrying. Depression often accompanies stress. The accumulated effects of stress may lead to more serious medical problems. Stress may be work-related, or it may stem from personal problems such as divorce, family conflict, or financial concerns. Most often, stress results from a combination of these pressures. Stress may also be a factor in critical illnesses, and the use of specific therapies in these instances is a topic of current research.

Conventional Treatments for Anxiety and Stress

Conventional treatments for anxiety and stress include psychotherapy and medication. There are two types of psychotherapy: behavioral therapy and cognitive-behavioral therapy. Behavioral therapy uses several techniques such as diaphragmatic breathing and exposure therapy. Diaphragmatic breathing teaches people how to control anxiety by taking slow, deep breaths. Exposure therapy gradually exposes people to whatever frightens them to help them cope with their fears. Two new behavioral techniques, "cut-thru" and "heart lock-in," are designed to teach the elimination of negative thoughts and to promote a sense of well-being. Research suggests that these behavioral modification techniques may have significant value in the treatment of stress and anxiety. Cognitive-behavioral therapy teaches people to react differently to the bodily sensations and situations that trigger anxiety and stress. Modification of thinking patterns that control the thoughts and sensations accompanying anxiety is an integral part of this form of therapy. Often, psychotherapy is used in combination with medication.

Antidepressants are frequently used in combination with behavioral therapy to mitigate anxiety and stress. The two major classes of antidepressants are selective serotonin reuptake inhibitors (SSRIs), such as Zoloft and Prozac, and tricyclic antidepressants (TCAs), such as Elavil and Tofranil. These medications work by inhibiting the reuptake of neurotransmitters, such as dopamine and serotonin, resulting in the accumulation of these neurotransmitters. Monoamine oxidase (MAO) inhibitors are also used to treat anxiety and function much the same as SSRIs and TCAs. Antidepressants are among the most widely prescribed medications in the United States.

Less frequently, benzodiazepines, such as Valium, may be used in the treatment of anxiety, but these are highly addictive agents that often cause depression. Worse than addiction is the tolerance effect that causes the patient to take increasing quantities of the benzodiazepine until the drug stops working altogether. Tolerance to benzodiazepines can occur in as little as a few weeks. Withdrawal symptoms can include hyperanxiety, confusion, anorexia, shaking, memory loss, and a re-emergence of the original symptoms. There are alternatives to these medications.

Moderate Exercise

Regular exercise such as running, walking, and strength training three times a week for 20 to 60 minutes has been shown to have a positive effect on mental health. In a recent issue of the journal *Professional Psychology: Research and Practice,* Canadian researchers report that individuals suffering from depression, anxiety, panic disorder, substance abuse, and even schizophrenia have shown improvement after following a regular exercise program for 5 to 10 weeks. In a study of 46 people with moderate to severe panic disorder, those who ran three times a week for 10 weeks and took antianxiety medication felt better than those on placebo. The same researchers note that treatment with the drug chlomipramine was faster and more effective than exercise in treating these patients. In the treatment of depression, a combination of factors that includes the release of the brain chemicals endorphins is most likely involved. Endorphins are known to produce a calm, soothing effect upon release. The researchers conclude that exercise is a viable, low-cost intervention therapy that should be recognized by the healthcare community.

Adapton

Adapton is widely used in Europe and Japan for the treatment of stress, anxiety, and depression. Some physicians in the United States are now prescribing its use in lieu of antidepressants. An extract of a deep sea fish, the garum, Adapton is a naturally occurring substance. It functions at the cellular level to increase energy efficiency, resulting in improved concentration, mood, and sleep while promoting a general sense of well-being. A number of European clinical trials document the beneficial effects of Adapton:

> Twenty patients with chronic, stress-related fatigue participated in a study in which they were given a placebo for 2 weeks, followed by a 2-week trial usage of Adapton. Patients reported a 14% reduction in fatigue and a 4% reduction in the symptoms of anxiety and insomnia following the placebo trial period. After using Adapton for 2 weeks, patients reported a 51% decrease in fatigue, and the symptoms of anxiety improved by 65%. The results of the study indicated that Adapton was effective in the treatment of patients with chronic stress and fatigue.
>
> In a study of 40 patients with chronic fatigue syndrome, Adapton was prescribed for a 2-week period. Using the Fatigue Study Group's criteria for the 10 functions that most accurately measure fatigue and depression, the results of the study showed that 50% of the participants reported beneficial effects from Adapton.
>
> A study of 60 patients using garum extract reported three cases of mild side effects, including nervous irritation, heartburn, and diarrhea. No emotional stress or fatigue was reported, leading researchers to conclude that garum was a safe and effective treatment of anxiety and stress. Other beneficial effects included improved learning and enhanced electroencephalograph (EEG) readings.

> Overall, Adapton benefits 90% of patients suffering from chronic stress and fatigue as compared with a 30% improvement rate in patients using placebos.
>
> In Europe, hyperactive children with attention deficit disorder are being treated with Adapton rather than Ritalin, with positive results.

Overall, researchers in these European clinical trials reported that Adapton was well-tolerated, produced no major side effects, and had no apparent contraindications.

Adapton consists of a standardized dosage of polypeptides, which act as precursors to neurotransmitters and exert a regulatory effect on the nervous system, thereby improving the body's ability to adapt to mental and physical stress. Adapton contains an omega-3 essential fatty acid that enhances certain prostaglandins and prostacyclin, the chemical mediators that regulate major biological functions. These polypeptides are believed to contribute to the stress-relieving effects of Adapton. Adapton is a safe, effective, low-cost alternative to traditional antidepressant medications and may provide substantial beneficial effects to people suffering from chronic, stress-induced anxiety, fatigue, or depression. The recommended dosage of Adapton is 4 capsules taken in the morning on an empty stomach for 15 days. Thereafter, the dose is reduced to 2 capsules each morning. If complete relief of the symptoms occurs, Adapton may be discontinued and restarted if the symptoms return. There is no toxicity involved in the daily use of Adapton. Some patients use 2 to 3 capsules of Adapton every other day and still report relief of their symptoms.

For people who suffer from panic attacks, the addition of a 10-mg dose of the cardiovascular medication propranolol can produce immediate results. Propranolol is a beta-adrenergic blocker that inhibits the overproduction of adrenaline during a panic attack. The low dose of propranolol required to produce this effect is well-tolerated by the majority of patients.

Other Beneficial Treatments for Anxiety and Stress

In addition to Adapton, there are a number of other stress-reducing treatments currently available. One of these treatments is KH3, a European medication. KH3 mitigates the effects of the overproduction of cortisol, the adrenal hormone that can occur with anxiety and stress. The overproduction of cortisol has been shown to damage the immune system, arteries, and brain cells, and it may cause premature aging. The recommended dosage of KH3 is 1 to 2 tablets taken on an empty stomach in the morning and afternoon. KH3 should not be taken by people allergic to procaine (the active ingredient in the medication), is contraindicated for patients taking sulfa drugs, and should not be used by children or pregnant or lactating women. In addition to KH3, the hormones melatonin and dehydroepiandrosterone (DHEA) may also reduce and protect against the effects of cortisol. The recommended dose range of melatonin is from 500 mcg to 3 mg taken approximately one half hour before bedtime. DHEA should be taken in a dose of 25 to 50 mg a day.

CAUTION: Prior to taking DHEA, refer to the *DHEA Replacement Therapy protocol*.

Summary

Prescription antidepressants and other prescription medications for the treatment of anxiety-related disorders often produce unwanted side effects, have more contraindications, and may become habit forming in some cases. Alternatives to these treatments, such as Adapton, have proven to be safe and effective in the treatment of stress, anxiety, and fatigue. There are fewer reported side effects in those patients using natural substances such as Adapton, KH3, DHEA, and melatonin, and there may be greater long-term benefits involved. As with any medication, it is advisable to consult your physician prior to any treatment program.

1. Reduce environmental causes of stress as much as possible.
2. Behavioral modification techniques such as diaphragmatic breathing and exposure therapy may be beneficial.
3. Moderate, regular exercise can reduce symptoms of stress and anxiety.

4. Adapton, 4 capsules in a.m. on an empty stomach for 15 days; reduce to 2 capsules in a.m. after 2 weeks.
5. For patients with panic attacks, the addition of 10 mg of propranolol in combination with Adapton may be highly effective.
6. KH3, 1 to 2 capsules in a.m. taken on an empty stomach.

CAUTION: Patients allergic to procaine should not use KH3.

7. Melatonin, 500 mcg to 10 mg in p.m., one half hour prior to bedtime.
8. DHEA, 25 to 50 mg a day. (*Refer to DHEA Replacement Therapy protocol.*)
9. Consider conventional medications such as SSRI and tricyclic antidepressants.

Product availability. Adapton, DHEA, and melatonin are available by calling (800) 544-4440, or order on-line at www.lef.org. Ask for a listing of offshore companies that sell KH3 to American citizens by mail for personal use. Propranolol must be prescribed by a physician.

ARRHYTHMIA (CARDIAC)

Palpitations are a symptom described as the sensation of having an irregular heart beat. This is a fairly common symptom that just about everyone experiences at one time or another. Palpitations occur when the heart beats irregularly. Whether or not palpitations are of medical concern is ultimately determined by medical history, physical exam findings, and testing. Most people know when it's time to go to see their physician because the palpitations have become sustained and very uncomfortable, or they are associated with another symptom such as shortness of breath.

Heart rhythm is controlled by factors both intrinsic and extrinsic to the heart itself. The most common damage to the heart's "wiring" comes from damage caused by decreased blood flow from clogged coronary arteries, or from muscle death caused by a heart attack. Additionally, certain drugs and toxins can affect heart rhythm as well.

The classification of abnormal heart rhythm, or dysrhythmia, is too complex to describe here. However, despite this complexity, some basic information can be given. The heart has an amazing ability to tolerate markedly abnormal rhythms. In fact, a double-blind study had to be discontinued because it was found that the group taking the antiarrhythmic drug was experiencing more deaths than the group taking the placebo. The majority of antiarrhythmic drugs have proarrhythmic effects; that is to say they can themselves cause arrhythmias.

Anyone who experiences sustained palpitations for the first time should see a physician before taking any medications and should follow these suggestions: no matter what the cause of a dysrhythmia, ensuring that the heart gets enough blood is essential. (*Patients with a family or personal history of coronary heart disease should consult the Atherosclerosis protocol and follow the suggestions given there.*) A course of chelation therapy should be considered as well.

Acute Myocardial Infarction (Heart Attack)

The development of potentially life-threatening dysrhythmias during the immediate period following an MI (myocardial infarction) is the reason that heart-attack patients are monitored very closely in a CCU (coronary care unit). One therapy which can increase the risk of dysrhythmia is thrombolytic treatment of the clogged coronary artery. When this is successful, there is a sudden influx of blood into the blood-starved area. This often results in dysrhythmia, which can be fatal. The culprit is in part a free-radical reaction. Therefore, any therapy directed at this free-radical burden could be potentially helpful.

In fact, recent studies have shown that such treatment is important in this setting. A 1998 study looked at patients with a recent AMI (acute myocardial infarction). For 28 days one group received oral treatment with Coenzyme Q_{10} (CoQ_{10}, 120 mg a day), and the other group received a placebo. After treatment, total arrhythmias were 9.5% in the CoQ_{10} group, compared to 25.3% in the placebo group. When measuring angina pectoris, only 9.5% of CoQ_{10}-supplemented patients were symptomatic compared to 28.1% on placebo, while poor left ventricular function was observed in 8.2% of those patients taking CoQ_{10} compared to 22.5% on placebo.

Total cardiac events, including cardiac deaths and nonfatal infarction, were also significantly reduced in the CoQ_{10} group compared with the placebo group (15.0% vs. 30.9%). Other recent studies have demonstrated that giving patients who have recently suffered an AMI omega-3 fatty acids protects them from the development of dysrhythmias in the immediate post-AMI period. Omega-3 fatty acids may be found in flaxseed, perilla, and fish oils.

Based upon clinical findings, the intravenous administration of vitamin C 3 times a week for the 4 weeks immediately following an AMI is recommended. It is hoped that future studies will demonstrate this to be an efficacious treatment. Those interested in this type of therapy should find a physician who practices complementary medicine.

Other antiarrhythmia nutrients include the minerals magnesium (500 to 2000 mg a day), potassium (200 to 500 mg a day), and selenium (300 to 600 micrograms a day). CoQ_{10} is used at 100 to 300 mg a day in Japan as a treatment for cardiac arrhythmia. Acetyl-*L*-carnitine is used at 1000 to 2000 mg a day in Europe to treat cardiac arrhythmia.

Vitamin D_3 enhances calcium metabolism in the sinoatrial node of the heart when given at 1000 IU a day. Vitamin E (at 400 to 800 IU a day) is used to treat coronary artery disease, but also helps establish normal heart rhythms. Five to eight capsules a day of fish-oil concentrates have been shown in several published studies to regulate cardiac arrhythmias. Studies on perilla oil show that it works as well as fish oil, without the unpleasant gastrointestinal side effects.

The use of any of these natural therapies should be with the full cooperation of a trained physician, since any errors could result in sudden death from a heart attack. Those with cardiac arrhythmias should avoid caffeine, heavy alcohol intake, and saturated fats.

Summary

1. Do not utilize any of these suggestions without being under the care of a physician.
2. If you have a personal or family history of myocardial infarction, follow the suggestions of the *Atherosclerosis protocol*.
3. Consider chelation therapy.
4. CoQ_{10}, 100 to 300 mg a day.
5. Perilla oil, six 1000-mg capsules a day; flax oil, 1 tablespoon a day; or highly concentrated fish oil, 5 to 8 capsules (minimum 400 mg EPA/300 mg DHA a day).
6. Magnesium citrate, 500 to 2000 mg a day.
7. Potassium, 200 to 500 mg a day.
8. Selenium, 300 to 600 mcg a day.
9. Acetyl-*L*-carnitine, 1000 to 2000 mg a day.
10. Vitamin D_3, 1000 IU a day.
11. Vitamin E, 400 to 800 mg a day.
12. Avoid caffeine-containing beverages, excessive alcohol, and saturated fats.

WARNING: Do not take ephedra-containing herbs such as Ma Huang.

For more information. Contact the American College for the Advancement of Medicine, (800) 532-3688 for the location and phone number of a physician in your area who specializes in complementary medicine.

Product availability. Magnesium, potassium, acetyl-*L*-carnitine, Coenzyme Q10, taurine, Mega EPA, selenium, and vitamin D_3, can be obtained by calling (800) 544-4440, or order on-line at www.lef.org.

ARTHRITIS

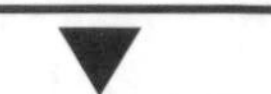

OSTEOARTHRITIS & RHEUMATOID ARTHRITIS

What's the difference? Can arthritis be prevented or cured? New research is shedding light on old natural remedies and opening up new treatment possibilities.

By Karin Granstrom Jordan, M.D.

Arthritis is all too well-known by most of us as a source of discomfort and pain. There are different forms of arthritis, however, with distinctive symptoms and prognosis.

Osteoarthritis is the most common form. It is the kind that seems to come with the wear-and-tear process of aging, affecting approximately 70 to 80% of the population over age 50. The onset is marked by morning stiffness, crackling joints, and perhaps some pain. As it gets worse it causes discomfort, pain, and disability in varying degrees for millions of people. It also causes an enormous consumption of painkillers and anti-inflammatory drugs that many times have undesirable long-term effects. Does it have to be this bad?

Modern medicine does not have much to offer for these chronic conditions, only symptomatic, temporary relief. Painkillers and the so-called NSAIDs, non-steroidal anti-inflammatory drugs, are effective in reducing symptoms quickly but often cause serious side effects such as ulcers and gastrointestinal bleeding, and they do not stop the progression of the disease. In the long run they have actually proven to worsen the condition by accelerating joint destruction.

The last few years of research, however, have brought some hope to this dismal picture. Old herbal remedies such as ginger, nettle, and willow bark, as well as fish oils and the already well-known cartilage constituents glucosamine sulfate and chondroitin sulfate, are about to revolutionize the treatment of arthritis. These substances not only give symptomatic relief but actually intervene at the root of the problem and help the body to rebuild functioning joints.

The Normal Joint

To understand the pathological processes in the joint, we need to take a look at the normal healthy joint. Joints are held together by a joint capsule and designed to allow smooth movement between adjacent bones. In the type of joint commonly affected by arthritic diseases, the highly movable joints, we find the bone ends covered by articular cartilage and the joint space enclosed by a synovial membrane. This thin membrane secretes synovial fluid that lubricates the space between the cartilage-covered joint-forming bones. The cartilage contains no blood vessels or nerves and receives its nutrients by diffusion from the synovial fluid and from the bone.

Joint function depends on the health of the cartilage in the joint. Cartilage is a gel-like substance that acts as a shock absorber, essential for smooth and easy movement in the joint. Cartilage gets its elasticity from collagen fibers and its sponge-like quality from water, held by a structure of big molecules called proteoglycans. Collagen and proteoglycans are produced by special cells, called chondrocytes, in the cartilage. Joints can withstand enormous pressure by slowly releasing water from the cartilage.

As we age, the ability to restore and maintain a normal cartilage structure seems to decrease. The activity of important repair enzymes is reduced, the water content diminished, and the joints become more prone to damage. But the full pathological mechanism for arthritis development is not yet known.

Osteoarthritis (OA)

Osteoarthritis/arthrosis is a disease mainly characterized by degenerative processes of the articular cartilage, but changes also involve the synovial membrane and the bone next to the cartilage. It is a gradual decay that most often affects the weight-bearing joints (knees, hips, and spinal joints) and the joints of the hand. A breakdown of the cartilage matrix leads to cracks and ulcers and a thinning of the cartilage with a loss of shock absorption. The underlying bone starts to thicken as a response to the increasing stress, and bone spurs are formed. In the advanced phases of osteoarthritis, an inflammatory reaction in the synovial membrane can be seen. This severe degeneration causes pain, swelling, deformation, and reduced range of motion.

Traditionally, osteoarthritis has been connected to aging, obesity, and repeated mechanical joint stress. Predisposing factors such as trauma or inherited abnormalities are also known to trigger degenerative changes and cause secondary osteoarthritis at even younger ages. New research is beginning to shed light on how osteoarthritis develops at the cellular and molecular levels.

Evidence is accumulating that the culprits may be factors called cytokines together with enzymes that break down the collagen matrix. Cytokines are proteins that carry messages between cells and regulate immunity and inflammation. Two cytokines, tumor necrosis factor alpha (TNF-a) and interleukin one beta (IL-1B), play an essential role in the cartilage destruction and inflammation process (Feldman et al., 1996). They have been found in elevated levels in the synovial membrane, the synovial fluid, and the cartilage of osteoarthritis patients. In animal models it was shown that inhibition of TNF-a results in decreased inflammation, while inhibition of IL-1B effectively prevents cartilage destruction (Plows et al., 1995).

TNF-a has proven to be an even more important factor in rheumatoid arthritis (RA), where it is a key factor in promoting inflammation and damage to cartilage and bone (Bertolini et al., 1986; Saklatvala, J., 1986).

Rheumatoid Arthritis (RA)

Unlike osteoarthritis, rheumatoid arthritis is a so-called autoimmune disease, characterized by chronic inflammation and thickening of the synovial lining in addition to cartilage destruction. In autoimmune diseases the immune system attacks body tissues as if they were foreign invaders. As in most other chronic inflammatory diseases, the etiology and pathogenesis of RA is poorly understood. Contributing factors are thought to include food allergies, leaky gut syndrome, hereditary factors, and microbes.

RA affects approximately 3% of the population, striking women three times as often as men. The typical onset is at 20 to 40 years of age. The clinical picture varies from mild chronic joint inflammation with occasional flare-ups to painfully deformed joints. The disease is often accompanied by low-grade fever, weight loss, and a general feeling of sickness and soreness.

Biochemical Mechanisms

The destruction of cartilage and bone in both OA and RA is currently believed to be due mainly to the action of matrix enzymes (metalloproteinases), which include collagenases and stromelysins (Birkedal-Hansen et al., 1993; Hill et al., 1994). These enzymes are under the control of cytokines, such as IL-1 and TNF-a, which are highly activated in rheumatoid arthritis. Some of the enzymes have pro-inflammatory characteristics and some have anti-inflammatory properties. The varying balance between these forces probably accounts for the variation in disease activity as it flares up and subsides.

Inflammation is a living tissue response to mechanical, chemical, and immunological challenge. It is characterized by high levels of arachidonic acid metabolites, which are metabolized along two different enzymatic pathways: cyclooxygenase and lipoxygenase, leading to prostaglandin PGE-2 and leukotriene LTB4, which are the most prominent metabolites and important mediators of inflammation (Srivastava et al., 1992). They play a crucial role in arthritis by causing resorption of bone, stimulating the secretion of collagenase and inhibiting the formation of proteoglycans.

Data from many studies confirm the important role of TNF-a in regulating production of both inflammatory and anti-inflammatory mediators in RA. Because of the demonstrated excess of pro-inflammatory cytokines, such as TNF-a, it was hypothesized that a blockade of TNF-a should be beneficial. Several experimental as well as clinical studies have been conducted with anti-TNF-a antibody (Paulus et al., 1990). The results have confirmed that TNF-a is a good therapeutic target in RA.

A placebo-controlled trial by Feldman et al. (1997) provided the first convincing evidence that blockade of a specific cytokine could be effective treatment in human autoimmune or inflammatory diseases. Interesting results with TNF-a blockade have also been achieved in trials conducted on Crohn's disease, sepsis, and HIV/AIDS.

The effectiveness and reproducibility of short-term anti-TNF-a antibody therapy, which has severe limitations, has stimulated the development of more convenient and practical alternatives to this kind of therapy. Interestingly enough, the leaves of the common nettle plant have recently been shown to lower TNF-a levels.

Current Medical Treatment

The basic conventional treatment for both osteoarthritis and rheumatoid arthritis consists of NSAIDs, including aspirin. Even "stronger" drugs such as corticosteroids, gold salts, and methotrexate are often prescribed for RA in an aggressive attempt to stop the development of the disease. These drugs are all aimed at alleviating pain and reducing inflammation. They can sometimes be effective, but more often, however, they prove unsatisfactory and many times intolerable due to toxicity. Aspirin, for example, which is the most commonly used, is quite effective, but it often causes gastric irritation and tinnitus (ringing in the ears) with the high dosages needed. Other NSAIDs may be somewhat better tolerated but have an even greater risk for serious side effects, which limits their use. These treatments are only symptomatic, because they do not act on the causes of arthritis and do not stop the progression of the disease. In fact, the opposite has proven to be true. It has been demonstrated in many studies that NSAIDs actually have an inhibitory effect on cartilage repair and accelerate cartilage destruction (Brooks et al., 1982; Shield, M.J., 1993; Newman et al., 1985; Solomon, L., 1973; Ronningen et al., 1979). How can it be that NSAIDs help and destroy at the same time?

NSAIDs exert their analgesic and anti-inflammatory effects through the inhibition of the enzyme cyclooxygenase (COX). The discovery (Needleman et al., 1979) that two forms of COX exist, COX-1 and COX-2, have clarified the dual nature of NSAIDs. While relieving pain and inflammation through COX-2 blockade, they also block, via COX-1, the biotransformation of arachidonic acid to substances that carry out various homeostatic (balancing) physiological functions, one of which is to protect the gastrointestinal mucosa and limit gastric acid output. While NSAIDs inhibit prostaglandin and leukotriene synthesis through COX-2 blockade, they fail to influence the TNF-a and IL-1B activation of cartilage-destroying enzymes.

With this enhanced understanding of the underlying mechanisms for current medical treatment, researchers are now looking for new compounds that will relieve pain and inflammation and enhance the repair process in the joints, without inhibiting important physiological functions. A COX-2-specific inhibitor has recently come out on the pharmaceutical market, and other products are underway.

There are many anti-inflammatory drugs approved by the FDA to treat arthritis. The problem is that anti-inflammatory drugs kill about 7000 Americans every year, despite the fact that they can be obtained only by prescription from an attending physician. We are intentionally not discussing these drugs in detail because of their extreme toxicity. The newer COX-2 inhibiting drugs are ostensibly safer, yet side effects have been reported.

Nettle Leaf (*Urtica dioica*)

Nettle leaf is an herb that has a long tradition of use as an adjuvant remedy in the treatment of arthritis in Germany. Nettle leaf extract has recently been found to contain a variety of active compounds, such as cyclooxygenase and lipoxygenase inhibitors and substances that affect cytokine secretion (Obertreis et al., 1996; Teucher et al., 1996).

Not only does nettle leaf reduce TNF-a levels, as mentioned above, but it has recently been demonstrated that it does so by potently inhibiting the genetic transcription factor that activates TNF-a and IL-1B in synovial tissue (Riehemann et al., 1999). This proinflammatory transcription factor, known as nuclear factor kappa beta (NF-KB), is known to be elevated in chronic inflammatory diseases and is essential to activation of TNF-a. Nettle is thought to work by preventing degradation of the natural inhibitor of NF-KB in the body. It has also been shown that TNF-a activates NF-KB in synovial cells, leading to the suggestion that a cycle of cross-activation between TNF-a and NF-KB may sustain and amplify the disease process in rheumatoid arthritis (Jue et al., 1999).

A study on healthy volunteers showed the anti-inflammatory potential of nettle (Obertreis, B., 1998). Lipopolysaccaride was used to stimulate and increase the secretion of proinflammatory cytokines. When nettle extract was given simultaneously in a dose-dependent manner, TNF-a and IL-1B concentration was significantly reduced.

Another study conducted on 40 patients suffering from acute arthritis compared the effects of 200 mg of a NSAID (diclofenac) with 50 mg of the NSAID in combination with 50 g of stewed nettle leaf per day (Chrubasik et al., 1997). Total joint scores improved significantly in both groups by approximately 70%. The nettle leaf extract clearly enhanced the anti-inflammatory effect of the NSAID. The addition of nettle extract made possible a 75% dose reduction of the NSAID, while still retaining the same anti-inflammatory effect with reduced side effects.

Ginger

Ginger (*Zingiber officinale*) is mostly known to us in the West as a spice and a flavor. In China, however, it has been used for thousands of years for medicinal purposes, such as nausea, stomachache, rheumatism, and toothache. Modern research has found ginger to be a powerful anti-oxidant and to have strong anti-inflammatory effects.

The pharmacologically active components of the ginger root are thought to be aromatic ketones known as gingerols. These have been shown in experimental studies to inhibit both the cyclooxygenase and lipoxygenase pathways and the production of prostaglandins, thromboxane, and leukotrienes (Kiuchi et al., 1992; Srivastava, K.C., 1986; Flynn, D.L. et al., 1986), just as the NSAIDs do. No significant side effects have been reported.

Ginger oil is obtained by steam distillation of dried ginger root. In an experimental study on rats (Sharma et al., 1997), arthritis was induced in the knee and paw by injection of bacilli, leading to inflammation. One group of rats was also given ginger oil by mouth for 28 days starting the day before the injection. The rats given ginger oil had less than half the knee and paw inflammation compared to the controls.

Glucosamine Sulfate

Among the natural therapies for osteoarthritis, glucosamine sulfate is probably the best known. It is extensively used as a drug for osteoarthritis in Europe, and it has been readily available in health food stores in the United States in recent years.

Glucosamine is a naturally occurring substance in the body, synthesized in the chondrocytes. In osteoarthritis this synthesis is defective and insufficient, and the supplementation with glucosamine has proven to be useful. The body uses supplemented glucosamine to synthesize the proteoglycans and the water-binding glycosaminoglycans (GAGs) in the cartilage matrix. In addition to providing raw material, the presence of glucosamine seems to stimulate the chondrocytes in their production of these substances. Glucosamine also inhibits certain enzymes, which destroy the cartilage, e.g., collagenase and phospholipase. By blocking pathogenic mechanisms that lead to articular degeneration, glucosamine delays the progression of the disease and relieves symptoms even for weeks after termination of the treatment (Qiu et al., 1998).

There are many studies confirming the excellent effect and safety of glucosamine sulfate. In one well-designed study of 178 patients suffering from osteoarthritis of the knee (Qiu et al., 1998), one group was treated for 4 weeks with glucosamine sulfate, 1500 mg daily, and the other group with ibuprofen at 1200 mg per day. Glucosamine relieved the symptoms as effectively as ibuprofen, and was significantly better tolerated than ibuprofen. The safety and tolerability of glucosamine can easily be explained by the fact that it is a physiological substance normally used by the body.

As with most natural remedies, the therapeutic effect of glucosamine does not come immediately, and usually takes some weeks to appear (1 to 8 weeks). Once achieved, it tends to persist for a notable time even after discontinuation of the treatment.

Chondroitin Sulfate

Chondroitin sulfate is a major component of cartilage. It is a very large molecule, composed of repeated units of glucosamine sulfate. Like glucosamine, chondroitin sulfate attracts water into the cartilage matrix and stimulates the production of cartilage. Likewise it has the ability to prevent enzymes from dissolving cartilage. Although the absorption of chondroitin sulfate is much lower than that of glucosamine (10 to 15% versus 90 to 98%), a few recent studies have shown very good results from long-term treatment with chondroitin sulfate, reducing pain and increasing range of motion.

A one-year long, double-blind clinical study including 42 patients with osteoarthritis showed that chondroitin sulfate was well tolerated and significantly reduced pain and increased joint mobility. The patients were given 800 mg chondroitin sulfate per day or placebo (Uebelhart et al., 1998).

In another double-blind study 119 patients with finger-joint osteoarthritis were followed for 3 years. The chondroitin dosage was 400 mg three times daily. X-rays of the finger joints were carried out at the start and at yearly intervals. The number of patients that developed progression of the disease was significantly less in the group treated with chondroitin sulfate (Verbruggen et al., 1998).

The improvement in walking time was studied in 80 patients with osteoarthritis in the knee. In this double-blind study the treatment period was 6 months and the chondroitin sulfate dosage 400 mg twice daily. The minimum time to perform a 20-meter walk showed a constant reduction of time only in the chondroitin group. Lower consumption of pain-killing drugs and excellent tolerability was also observed (Bucsi et al., 1998).

Glucosamine alone or in combination with chondroitin sulfate is more and more becoming recognized as the treatment of choice for osteoarthritis even in the United States. Its ability to actually repair and improve joint function in addition to providing pain relief gives it a significant advantage compared to conventional treatment.

Willow Bark

Salicylic acid, the basis of aspirin, was first prepared from willow bark by an Italian chemist in 1838. The name of the compound is derived from *Salix,* the Latin name for the willow genus. Aspirin, or acetylsalicylic acid, is a synthetic form of salicylic acid. Willow bark is rich in salicin and related salicylates that metabolize into salicylic acid. Many plants, such as meadowsweet and wintergreen, also contain these compounds. They have a long tradition of use in Europe, and far fewer side effects than aspirin.

While aspirin/salicin has been shown to have a lowering effect on some of the pro-inflammatory factors, it can also increase leukotriene LTB4, which is a major inflammation-promoting mediator. An interesting study (Engstrom et al., 1997) compared the effect on pro-inflammatory substances of aspirin alone with a combination of low-dose aspirin and fish oil. The results showed that the combination of fish oil and low-dose aspirin has significantly more favorable effects on the pattern of pro- and anti-inflammatory factors than the aspirin alone. LTB4 increased 19% when aspirin was taken by itself, but decreased 69% after intake of aspirin and fish oil together.

Fish Oil

It is established that dietary fatty acids determine the composition of lipids in the cell membranes, which influences the production of prostaglandins and leukotrienes that regulate inflammation, a fact that has given rise to interest in the potential of these dietary substances.

Omega-3 oils, such as fish oil (EPA and DHA) and flaxseed oil, have the ability to suppress the production of inflammatory mediators and thereby influence the course of chronic inflammatory diseases such as RA (Kremer et al., 1985 and 1992).

A new enteric-coated fish-oil preparation was used in a 1-year, double-blind study of 78 patients with inflammatory bowel disease. The absorption rate and tolerability was high with this preparation, and after 1 year 59% of the fish-oil group remained in remission compared to 36% in the placebo group, indicating a significant anti-inflammatory effect (Belluzzi et al., 1996)

In recent studies, dietary omega-3 oils have shown a suppressive effect on the production of the cytokines IL-1B and TNF-a, which stimulate the production of collagenase and pro-inflammatory prostaglandins (PGE2) (James et al., 1997; Caugey et al., 1996). When fish oil supplementation was given to rheumatoid arthritis patients, arachidonic acid levels were reduced by 33% compared to pre-supplement values (Sperling et al., 1987), suggesting that increase of dietary omega-3 oils can be complementary in treating rheumatoid arthritis.

A large number of publications from around the world have confirmed the usefulness of dietary supplementation with omega-3 oils in relieving tender joints and morning stiffness in patients with RA, in some cases eliminating the need for NSAID medication (Kremer et al., 1995). Skoldstam et al. (1992) and Lau et al. (1993) found that patients consuming fish oil were able to significantly reduce their NSAID dose compared with a control group.

Of 12 published double-blind and placebo-controlled studies with a duration of 12 to 52 weeks, decreased joint tenderness was the most common favorable outcome reported. Fish-oil supplementation significantly decreased the use of NSAIDs in the three studies in which NSAIDs was used. Unlike NSAID use, fish-oil consumption is not associated with gastrointestinal toxicity. The results of the studies suggest that the effective dose of fish oil is approximately 3 to 6 grams a day. Higher dosages did not give better results. There are indications that the combination of EPA and DHA, as it is found in fish oil, has a synergistic effect (Robinson et al., 1989).

A study by James et al. (1997) emphasizes the potential for increased efficacy of anti-inflammatory drugs when using omega-3 oils in the diet. It was observed that diets rich in omega-3 oils and low in omega-6 fats had a drug-sparing effect with decreased side effects. Drug toxicity is estimated to contribute 60% of the total cost of treating RA patients in the United States (Prashker et al., 1995). Use of omega-3 oils in the diet would appear to offer a simple, safe, and inexpensive way to reduce toxicity and side effects from RA medications.

Oxidative Damage

Food is not conventionally accepted as influential in the course of inflammatory or degenerative diseases (in contrast to diabetes and vascular heart disease). We know, however, that oxidative stress or free-radical damage is a factor of importance in the development of osteoarthritis, just as it is a major cause of most chronic degenerative diseases as well as aging. There is also strong evidence that oxidative damage occurs in RA patients. Increased oxidation of lipids (peroxidation) as well as depletion of ascorbate in serum and synovial fluid has been observed. High doses of vitamin E, which is a powerful antioxidant, are reported to diminish pain. Most importantly, tumor necrosis factor alpha (TNF-a), which plays a key role in RA, is well known to cause oxidative stress.

In order to counteract free-radical damage, antioxidants are needed. A diet rich in vegetables and fruits is likely to add important antioxidants to the body. This may not always be enough, however. Vitamin C and vitamin E supplements have been studied and found to be important in the treatment of osteoarthritis. Deficient vitamin C intake, which is common with elderly people, impairs the synthesis of collagen, the main protein of cartilage (Bates, C.J., 1977). Studies on vitamin E have shown its ability to stimulate the production of cartilage components, such as glycosaminoglycans, as well as to inhibit the breakdown of cartilage.

Healthy food and a minimum of toxins may be more important for our health than we want to believe. The body strives to heal itself, whether it is a cut finger, a cold, or a damaged or inflamed joint. It makes sense to find ways to support the body with natural substances that the body can use in the healing process.

Recent research has provided us with new insights into the mechanisms of arthritis, and left us with a scientific understanding of how natural remedies work in harmony with the body rather than against it.

Natural Therapies

New factors have been identified in the pathology of both common forms of arthritis C osteoarthritis and rheumatoid arthritis. This research has enabled scientists to develop novel natural therapies that work along multiple pathways not taken into account by FDA-approved drugs. These botanical extracts and natural agents have an extraordinary safety profile and a long track record of clinical success in Europe.

Glucosamine is extensively used as a drug for osteoarthritis in Europe, and it has been readily available in health food stores in the United States for many years. Chondroitin sulfate is often combined with glucosamine because of the synergistic effects these two cartilage-protecting nutrients have shown. Fish-oil supplements are popular to prevent cardiovascular disease, but some arthritis patients find it difficult to use fish oil because of gastric upset. Pharmaceutical nettle leaf, salicin and gingerol extracts are not widely sold in the United States.

A product called ArthroPro combines all this technology into one formulation, including enteric-coated fish oil capsules, that provide the nutrients shown to alleviate arthritis via the following mechanisms:

Suppressing Tumor Necrosis Factor (TNF-a)

Tumor necrosis factor (TNF-a) and another inflammatory cytokine called *interleukin-1B* (IL-1B) have been identified as factors in the destruction of cartilage in both osteo- and rheumatoid arthritis. Studies show that the blockade of these aberrant immune factors can produce therapeutic results.

Nettle leaf has been shown to reduce TNF-a levels and IL-1B. Nettle also inhibits the genetic transcription factor that activates TNF-a in synovial tissue.

A placebo-controlled human trial showed that leaves of the nettle exhibited a potent effect in lowering TNF-a levels in arthritis patients. Another study compared the effects of 200 mg of a NSAID drug with 50 mg of the NSAID in combination with nettle leaf on arthritis patients. Total joint scores improved in both groups by approximately 70%. The addition of nettle extract made possible a 75% dose reduction of the toxic NSAID, while still retaining the same anti-inflammatory effect with reduced side effects.

Anti-arthritic drugs are being developed to suppress TNF-a, but similar effects can be obtained today using the safe nettle leaf. Please note that nettle *leaf* extract contains different phyto-chemicals than the nettle *root* extract used to treat benign prostate disease.

Inhibiting COX-2

The most popular prescription drug in the United States works by suppressing the pro-inflammatory enzyme cyclooxygenase-2 **(COX-2)**. Cyclooxygenase and lipoxygenase cause the formation of prostaglandin E2 and leukotriene B4, two pro-inflammatory agents that stimulate other enzymes to degrade cartilage in the joint. **Nettle leaf** extract contains a variety of natural cyclooxygenase and lipoxygenase inhibitors. While COX-2 inhibition can be obtained from either nettle leaf extract or FDA-approved drugs, only nettle has been shown to *also* interfere with the TNF-a and IL-1B activation of cartilage destroying enzymes. Nettle leaf has a long tradition of use as a safe adjuvant remedy in the treatment of arthritis in Germany.

The pharmacologically active components of the **ginger root** have also been shown to inhibit the cyclooxygenase and lipoxygenase pathways. This results in a suppression of the production of pro-inflammatory prostaglandins, thromboxane and leukotrienes, just as the NSAIDs do, but without the side effects. In one experimental arthritis study, rats given ginger oil had less than half the inflammation that the controls had.

Suppressing Leukotrienes

Aspirin has been shown to have a lowering effect on some pro-inflammatory factors, but it can also increase the joint-destroying **leukotriene** (LTB4) cytokine, which is a major inflammation promoting agent. A study compared the effect on pro-inflammatory substances of aspirin alone with a combination of *low-dose aspirin* and *fish oil*. The results showed that the combination of fish oil and low-dose aspirin has significantly more favorable effects than the aspirin alone. The pro-inflammatory LTB4 increased 19% when aspirin was taken by itself, but decreased 69% after intake of aspirin and fish oil together. The combination of low-dose aspirin and moderate intake of fish oil is thus a potent weapon in the regulation of pro-inflammatory leukotrienes.

Preventing the Formation of Prostaglandin E2

Omega-3 oils have been shown to suppress the production of prostaglandin E2 (PGE2), which contributes to arthritis by degrading collagen needed for the cartilage that lines the joints. PGE2 is also a pro-inflammatory prostaglandin that contributes to the arthritis inflammatory cascade. A large number of studies have confirmed the usefulness of omega-3 oils in relieving tender joints and morning stiffness, in some cases eliminating the need for NSAID medication. One study found that patients consuming fish oil were able to significantly reduce their NSAID dose compared with a control group. Of 12 published placebo-controlled studies using fish oil to treat arthritis, a decrease in joint tenderness is the most common outcome reported.

Protecting the Cartilage Matrix

Glucosamine is a naturally occurring substance in the body, synthesized by chondrocytes for the purpose of producing joint cartilage. In osteoarthritis this synthesis is defective, and supplementation with glucosamine has proven to be useful. The body uses supplemented glucosamine to synthesize the proteoglycans and the water-binding glycosaminoglycans in the cartilage matrix. In addition to providing raw material, the presence of glucosamine seems to stimulate the chondrocytes in their production of these substances. Glucosamine also inhibits certain enzymes which destroy the cartilage, e.g., collagenase and phospholipase. By blocking pathogenic mechanisms that lead to articular degeneration, glucosamine delays the progression of the disease and relieves symptoms even for weeks after termination of the treatment.

Many studies confirm the efficacy of glucosamine. One study showed that glucosamine relieved the symptoms as effectively as ibuprofen, and was significantly better tolerated than ibuprofen. The safety of glucosamine can easily be explained by the fact that it is a substance normally used by the body. As with most natural remedies, the therapeutic effect of glucosamine does not come immediately and usually takes some weeks to appear (1 to 8 weeks). Once achieved, it tends to persist for a notable time even after discontinuation of the treatment.

Chondroitin sulfate is a major component of cartilage. Like glucosamine, chondroitin sulfate attracts water into the cartilage matrix and stimulates the production of cartilage. Likewise it has the ability to prevent enzymes from dissolving cartilage. Although the absorption of chondroitin sulfate is much lower than that of glucosamine (10 to 15% versus 90 to 98%), recent studies have shown very good results from long-term treatment with chondroitin sulfate, reducing pain and increasing range of motion. Glucosamine alone or in combination with chondroitin sulfate has the ability to repair and improve joint function in addition to providing pain relief.

All of the cartilage-protecting and anti-inflammatory agents listed in this section, including endemically coated fish-oil capsules, have been put together in one convenient formula called ArthroPro. Suggested dose is one packet of 4 capsules, twice a day.

Gamma-Linolenic Acid (GLA)

GLA (gamma-linolenic acid) is a fatty acid found in evening primrose oil, borage oil, and black currant seed oil that has been used to suppress chronic inflammation.

In the *Annals of Internal Medicine* (1993, 119/9), the findings of a 24-week, double-blind, placebo-controlled trial with GLA derived from borage oil was reported. The patients receiving the borage oil experienced a 36% reduction in the number of tender joints, a 45% reduction in the tender joint score, a 41% reduction in the swollen joint score, and a 28% reduction in the swollen joint count. The placebo group showed no benefits.

A paper in the *British Journal of Rheumatology* (1994, 33/9) reports the findings of a 24-week, double-blind, placebo-controlled trial in rheumatoid arthritis patients treated with black currant seed oil rich in GLA and alpha-linolenic acid. Patients receiving black currant seed oil showed reductions in the signs and symptoms of the disease. The placebo group showed no change in disease status. According to the researchers, the study showed that black currant seed oil is a potentially effective treatment for active rheumatoid arthritis. No adverse reactions were observed, although some people dropped out of the trial because of the size and number of capsules they were required to take.

In *Seminars in Arthritis and Rheumatism* (1995, 25/2), there was a review of all the published literature on the use of GLA for the treatment of rheumatoid arthritis. GLA reduced the effects of autoimmune disease on joint linings, though more research was needed to determine the ideal dose of GLA for arthritis. Suggested dose is 4 to 5 borage oil (1400 mg) capsules per day. Those taking Arthro Pro may not need borage oil.

Summary

Unlike toxic FDA-approved drugs, natural therapies safely provide relief from chronic inflammation and pain. While FDA-approved drugs can cause cartilage destruction, natural therapies correct the underlying factors involved in arthritic cartilage degeneration.

To attack the multiple causes of joint cartilage destruction while reducing chronic inflammation and pain, natural therapies have been shown to work by the following mechanisms:

1. Inhibiting cyclooxygenase-2 (COX-2).
2. Suppressing tumor necrosis factor (TNF-a) and interleukin-1B.
3. Suppressing leukotriene B4.
4. Inhibiting the formation of prostaglandin E2.
5. Promoting the synthesis of proteoglycans and glycosaminoglycans in the joint.
6. Suppressing cartilage-destroying enzymes collagenase and phospholipase.
7. Attracting water to the cartilage to enhance synovial lubrication.

Combined Natural Therapies

Arthritis patients have enjoyed considerable success using one or more of the natural approaches discussed in this protocol. The ArthroPro formula was designed to provide all effective natural therapies (except borage oil) in one convenient package. ArthroPro comes in boxes containing 60 cellophane packettes. Each packette consists of two enterically coated softgel caps and two dry powder capsules. The softgels provide the proper portion of fish and ginger oils while the dry powder capsules deliver the precise glucosamine sulfate, chondroitin sulfate, and *N*-acetyl-glucosamine. The suggested dose for the first three months is one packette twice a day, with or without food. After three to six months, some people may be able to reduce the dose to just one packette a day. The ingredients in ArthroPro should provide the same effects as the GLA found in borage, primrose, and black currant seed oils.

Each packette of ArthroPro contains the following:

- ▼ Two enterically coated oil capsules that provide

EPA	720 mg
DHA	500 mg
Ginger oil (rhizome)	120 mg
Vitamin E	20 IU

Enteric coating prevents the gastric upset complications some people experience with fish oil capsules.

▼ Two dry-powder capsules that provide

Nettle Leaf Extract	750 mg
Glucosamine (in sulfate and *N*-acetyl forms)	500 mg
Chondroitin sulfate	400 mg
Salicin combination	120 mg

Salicin contains 25% salicylic derivatives obtained from Windergreen, Purple willow bark, and Meadowsweet (contains no methyl salicylate).

Caution: Those who are allergic to aspirin may not be able to use ArthroPro because of the small amount of naturally derived aspirin contained in willow bark extract.

For more information. Contact the Arthritis Foundation, (800) 283-7800.

Product availability. The ArthroPro formula, borage oil, and antioxidant supplements can be purchased by calling (800) 544-4440, or order online at www.lef.org.

ASTHMA

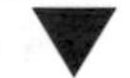

Asthma, a chronic obstructive pulmonary disease, is a reversible airway obstruction not caused by any other disease. It is characterized by an increased responsiveness of the airways (i.e., the bronchial tubes close). With proper care, there is no need for asthma to become a permanent debilitating condition.

Description

The common symptoms of asthma include difficulty in breathing, coughing, wheezing, and the use of accessory muscles to facilitate breathing; apprehension; fast heart rate (up to 120 beats a minute); flared nostrils and increased symptoms of respiratory distress. Serious attacks include a feeling of tightness in the chest with thick and tenacious production of mucus. The underlying mechanisms, which bring about the sudden attacks of wheezing, are not fully understood.

Asthma affects approximately 4% of the American population (about 9 million people) with up to 7% of Americans experiencing asthma at one time or another during their lifetimes. Asthma occurs most frequently in children and young adults, and fortunately, 50 to 70% of children outgrow the disease. Asthma is the most common cause of school absence and hospital admission in children.

Factors that have been confirmed to contribute to asthma are genetic predisposition, viral respiratory infection, emotional upset, inhalation of cold air, fumes from fresh paint, tobacco smoke, chemicals, and other airborne irritants. The exposure to specific allergens (foods, liquids, or fabrics), and such nonspecific factors as change in temperature can also cause symptoms. A family history of asthma or allergies, such as eczema, appears in about half of all asthmatics.

Asthma is divided into two broad categories:

Extrinsic or allergic asthma is brought on when the person comes in contact with allergens—airborne pollens and molds, animal danders, foods, drugs, and house dust. These symptoms are IgE mediated: IgE or immunoglobulin E is an antibody produced by the cells lining the respiratory and intestinal tracts. In asthmatics, when an allergen enters the respiratory tract, an allergen–IgE antibody reaction takes place. This leads to the allergic reaction. As a result, mast cells will secrete "slow-releasing anaphylaxis substance" (SRS-A) and other inflammatory compounds. SRS-A causes spasms of bronchiole tubes. From 10 to 20% of the adult asthmatic population is affected by this category of asthma.

Intrinsic asthma. This type of asthma occurs in people who have not been identified by medical history or by tests as having and suffering from allergies. The precipitating causes may be, for example, infections, irritants, or emotional factors.

Status asthma describes a prolonged and potentially dangerous attack of very severe asthma.

Biological Overview

Asthma usually produces three sets of physical changes:

1. Bronchial spasms may develop to the point where considerable obstruction occurs in the airway.
2. Irritated bronchial walls become inflamed and swell, causing the airway to narrow further.
3. The mucus glands of the patient produce a thick, tenacious mucus.

These physical changes can lead to hyperinflation of the lungs simply because inhaling is easier than exhaling. For most patients, the short period of time necessary for air exchange problems and increasingly labored respiration to develop is offset by a short and spontaneous recovery as symptoms disappear in a matter of minutes.

Asthma seems to be created by an imbalance in the relative functions of the sympathetic and parasympathetic nervous systems as they relate to the lungs. The sympathetic nervous system is stimulated by two important adrenal-gland secretions, epinephrine and norepinephrine. The adrenal system is often deficient in asthma patients. Normally, these hormones calm mast cell inflammatory response and relax bronchial muscles. In this case, however, the parasympathetic nervous system, via the vagus nerve, has an opposite action. The parasympathetic nervous system, often overactive in asthma patients, stimulates inflammation and bronchial constriction, thereby aggravating this condition.

Balance must be restored by means of proper adrenal-gland functioning. Subclinical adrenal-gland deficiency generally is not recognized by the medical profession. Yet this is frequently an underlying cause of asthma.

Therapeutic Recommendations

Foods

Certain foods can trigger an asthmatic attack, particularly in children. Cow's milk, yeast, cheese, fish, nuts, chocolate, wheat, eggs, shellfish, tomatoes, and other foods of the nightshade family (for example, eggplants and potatoes) are potential offenders. High-salicylate foods can aggravate 10 to 20% of asthmatics. Aspirin, food colorings, and monosodium glutamate (MSG) can also initiate an episode. Avoid processed and salted foods as much as possible.

Flaxseed and linseed oils, and salmon, if tolerated, are rich in essential fatty acids. These can be useful long-term promoters of bronchial relaxation. Red meat can have the opposite effect, stimulating constriction. Therefore it should be eaten no more than once or twice a week.

For children and adults using steroids recently or for a period of time, there are special nutritional considerations. In particular, these patients will need to balance their blood sugar, keep their potassium levels up, and reduce their salt intake. Small frequent meals and protein snacks (beans, chicken, turkey) can be helpful. Most fruits, vegetables, and whole grains are high-potassium foods, especially avocados, carrots (best taken in the high-potency form of carrot juice), and bananas. Mineral repletion may be necessary, as corticosteroids deplete the body of calcium, magnesium, and zinc.

Vitamin-Mineral-Amino Acid Therapeutics

Most asthmatics are not aware of the many published studies showing that high-potency vitamin supplements induce a reduction in the incidence and severity of asthmatic attacks. These studies also show that high dietary magnesium intake is associated with improvement in lung function, less wheezing, and fewer asthma attacks. Asthmatics should consider taking an additional 1000 mg a day or more of elemental magnesium. Histamine is a major factor in asthmatic attacks, and vitamin C is involved in the natural destruction of excess histamine. Asthmatics should take at least two 600-mg capsules of *N*-acetylcysteine (NAC) a day, along with 2 grams or more of vitamin C, to break up mucus that could worsen an asthma attack. Buffered vitamin C, 500 to 1000 mg taken at bedtime, seems to lessen or prevent the asthma attacks that occur around 4 a.m., according to Carmen Fusco. Sublingual DMG before vigorous activity, vitamins B_6 and B_{12}, and citrus bioflavonoids also prove helpful, she adds.

In addition to C.O.P.D. recommendations, take the following:

Vitamin B_6 is specifically helpful for asthma, presumably by catalyzing neurohormonal mediator response in lung tissues, and also useful in counteracting MSG poisoning.

Pantothenic acid is an excellent promoter of adrenal hormone production—epinephrine and norepinephrine. Pantothenic acid strengthens the sinus tissues and has an antihistaminic action.

Vitamin C stimulates antihistamine response. When used with B-complex, the balanced production of epinephrine and norepinephrine will reduce bronchial constriction. Vitamin C strengthens the adrenals and therefore is essential, especially if steroids have been or are in use by the patient.

Folic acid works with tyrosine to reduce bronchial constriction through activation of norepinephrine and epinephrine.

L-tyrosine stimulates production of epinephrine and norepinephrine, thereby helping to prevent bronchial constriction.

Perilla or flaxseed oils stimulate production of prostaglandin E1, which dilates the bronchioles and calms inflammation. These oils may also stabilize the mast cells.

Hydrochloric acid and/or pancreatin are most useful if asthma attacks are related to food sensitivity. These help break down food proteins most completely, thereby minimizing allergic reactions.

Bioflavonoids are potent antihistamines.

An Alternative Drug Therapy

Asthmatics also should consider taking the drug Hydergine to safely boost intracellular levels of the messenger molecule cyclic adenosine monophosphate (cAMP). Higher levels of cAMP often reduce bronchial constriction. The recommended dose of Hydergine is 5 to 10 mg a day with food. The FDA-approved drug theophylline is used to treat asthma because it boosts cAMP levels. (*For more information about the multi-faceted benefits of the drug Hydergine, refer to the Age-Associated Mental Impairment protocol.*)

Prevention and Healing

Stress is a fact of life, and it is impractical to attempt to eliminate all stress, but for the asthmatic, one of the keys to the restoration of free breathing is stress management. Mental and emotional tolerance of daily stress can be strengthened through avoidance of troublesome stimuli and by using stress management training, including meditation and setting aside a time and place for "emotional space."

Enhancing tolerance means raising the distress threshold so that stress does not immediately precipitate an asthma attack. For this reason asthmatics need to adopt an environmental awareness of such substances as chemicals, fumes, dust, molds, pet dander, and allergenic foods. Many sufferers from childhood asthma find that their asthma clears when they leave home. In many such cases, it is likely that changing the home environment removes such irritating substances as pet dander, tobacco smoke, mold, etc. from the child's environment. Such environmental changes can benefit adults in exactly the same way.

Tolerance to asthma stimuli can also be dramatically improved by changing diet through the elimination of problem foods and substituting recommended foods, herbs, and nutritional supplements. The asthmatic needs to support the adrenals, minimize allergen and chemical exposure, enhance tolerance and strength, and create enough "space to breathe."

Withdrawing from the use of inhalers and other medications is a challenge for many asthmatics, but it can be done with careful nutritional planning using both elimination and supplementation and with attention to stress management. Most asthmatics are much improved by carefully defining their own physical (environment and nutrition) and emotional (stress) limitations.

CAUTION: Do not try this alone. Before beginning a program to reduce reliance on inhaler-type medications, seek the guidance and support of a qualified physician who is willing to monitor a gradual reduction of the amounts and frequency of use of your medication. Under the supervision of such a physician, the following general guidelines may be used.

1. Begin elimination or reduction of one medicine at a time by gradually reducing the dosage. Reduce the prescription amount as recommended by a medical professional or by the smallest practical amount. This may require breaking tablets into halves or quarters, or receiving a reduced prescription dosage.
2. Stabilize the prescription amount for one week at the adjusted level before reducing further.
3. Eliminate prescription drugs under controlled conditions; i.e., completely eliminate one drug through gradual steps before beginning to withdraw from any other medications.
4. If asthma symptoms develop or worsen, return to the previous dosage level(s) until symptoms clear. Stabilize for one week as before and continue the reduction process as outlined above.

If you are cutting down on antihistamines, increasing your intake of vitamin C, bioflavonoids, and pantothenic acid will be helpful. These act as natural antihistamines, stimulating your cells' ability to process and reduce the inflammatory histamines.

As you cut down on cromolyn and other inhalers, coltsfoot (5 times a day) and *L*-cysteine (3 times a day) may be used to help keep your lungs clear and breathing freely. You also may find it helpful during this process to gradually increase the distance between the inhaler spray and your mouth. Passion flower can be especially useful in calming tension related to changing medicinal schedules. These herbs and nutrients strengthen the tissues as they provide support. They can be discontinued gradually within 3 months to 2 years after you have successfully withdrawn the medications.

Visualization (Meditation Technique Application)

Imagine that you are in a large, clear, and open space. You have all the room that you need. You can invite anyone into your space, and you can ask anyone to leave your space. Feel the peace and strength of "your space" inside you.

Summary

Asthmatics can improve their health and suppress their asthma by careful elimination testing to learn their asthma "triggers," by improving their surroundings (home and work environment), and by applying this information to adopt a different lifestyle to minimize the potential for asthma attacks. Particular care should be taken to avoid any foods that are known to cause an allergic reaction possibly triggering an asthma attack. A goal of reducing the need for prescription drugs by developing a plan to substitute nutritional supplements should be undertaken with the assistance of a qualified physician. Meditation techniques offer a simple, effective method of circumventing an asthma attack before it begins or reducing symptoms during an asthmatic episode.

With careful elimination testing under the care of a physician, a workable combination of botanicals and nutritional supplements can be developed that will support a better control of asthma. A physician must carefully monitor any prescription-drug elimination technique.

Some dosing recommendations include

1. Elemental magnesium, 1000 mg a day.
2. NAC, 600 mg, twice a day.
3. Vitamin C, 2000 mg 3 times a day.
4. Sublingual DMG (100–200 mg) before strenuous exercise.
5. *L*-tyrosine, 250 to 500 mg, twice a day before meals.
6. Perilla or flaxseed oil, 1000 to 5000 mg, once a day with meals.
7. Digestive enzymes after large meals.
8. Bioflavonoids, 1000 mg, 1 to 3 times a day.
9. Hydergine, 5 to 10 mg a day with food.
10. Life Extension Mix, 3 tablets 3 times a day.

Note: Children should take the lowest recommended dose, unless otherwise recommended by a qualified health practitioner.

For more information. Contact the National Jewish Center for Immunology and Respiratory Medicine, (800) 822-5864.

Product availability. Magnesium, NAC, *L*-tyrosine, perilla oil, and Life Extension Mix are available by calling (800) 544-4440, or order on-line at www.lef.org. Hydergine is available from overseas companies for personal use only. For a list of companies offering Hydergine call (800) 544-4440.

ATHEROSCLEROSIS (CORONARY ARTERY DISEASE)

Atherosclerosis is a leading cause of death and impairment in America today. It is estimated that 1,100,000 new or recurrent coronary attacks occur per year in America. It affects close to 60 million Americans. To better place this disease in perspective, every 20 seconds a person in the United States has a heart attack, and one third of these attacks lead to death. Moreover, 50% of Americans have levels of cholesterol that place them at high risk of coronary artery disease, and cholesterol is only one factor that causes the occlusion of arteries that is technically known as atherosclerosis.

The high mortality of the disease, widespread suffering, and huge economic impact demand an integrated medical approach and therapies. This protocol reflects that meticulous approach.

The most common form of heart disease is caused by atherosclerosis, generally known as coronary heart disease, hardening and/or thickening of the arteries. It involves the slow buildup of deposits of fatty substances, cholesterol, body cellular waste products, calcium, and fibrin (a clotting material in the blood) in the inside lining of an artery. The buildup that results, called plaque, may partially or totally block the blood's flow through the artery. This can lead to the formation of a blood clot (thrombus) on the plaque's surface. If either of these occurs and blocks the entire artery, a heart attack or stroke may result.

One researcher reported that otherwise-healthy soldiers examined after returning from World War II had arteries already occluded 22%, even though they were only 20 years old. Sometimes referred to as the "silent killer," atherosclerosis and cardiovascular disease can progress for years undetected by an individual who may have, or be at great risk from, the disease.

Generally few symptoms arise with the early, and in some cases later, stages of the disease. An elevated or high blood pressure for an individual with normal blood pressure may be an indication of disease presence; however, blood pressure increases generally occur over a long period of time, as the disease slowly advances. A study reported in *Circulation* (March 4, 1997) confirmed that even borderline blood pressure readings (140/90) represent a risk factor for atherosclerosis and stroke. However, blood-pressure is associated with many other factors such as being overweight, lack of exercise, higher blood sugar, and cholesterol.

Atherosclerosis is a slow, progressive disease that may start in childhood. In some people, this disease progresses rapidly in their 30s and early 40s—in others it doesn't become threatening until later in life.

Exactly how atherosclerosis begins or what causes it isn't known, but some theories have been proposed. Many scientists think atherosclerosis begins because the innermost layer of the artery, called the endothelium, becomes damaged. Possible causes of damage to the arterial wall are free-radical reactions, elevated levels of oxidated serum cholesterol, triglycerides, fibrinogen and homocysteine, high blood pressure, obesity, lifestyle issues, cigarette smoke, and environmental pollutants.

Specific diseases caused by atherosclerosis include coronary artery disease, angina pectoris, cerebral vascular disease, thrombotic stroke, transient ischemic attacks, and diabetic vascular complications.

Three mechanisms that have been identified as the most probable causative factors in the development of atherosclerosis include the following:

1. LDL cholesterol oxidation. LDL stands for *low-density lipoprotein* and is often referred to as "bad cholesterol." Oxidation of LDL renders it "sticky" and facilitates its deposition on the internal lining of blood vessel walls. The oxidation of LDL cholesterol, other blood fats, and homocysteine can initiate and significantly contribute to the development of atherosclerosis.

2. Homocysteine overload. There is growing consensus that homocysteine may be a major contributor to degenerative diseases such as atherosclerosis. Detoxification of excess homocysteine requires "methylating factors" such as folic acid, vitamin B_{12}, and trimethylglycine (TMG). Methylation factors function to convert (remethylate) homocysteine back into the nontoxic amino acid methionine. Some individuals with elevated serum homocysteine also require higher amounts of vitamin B_6, which converts homocysteine to safer substances via a different (trans-sulfuration) metabolic pathway.

Homocysteine often causes the initial lesions on arterial walls that enable LDL cholesterol and fibrinogen to accumulate and eventually to obstruct blood flow. Homocysteine also contributes to the oxidation of LDL cholesterol and the accumulation of arterial plaque and subsequent vascular blockage. Homocysteine damages cells directly by promoting oxidative stress. Homocysteine also can cause abnormal arterial blood clots (thrombosis) that can completely block an artery. Homocysteine alone has been demonstrated to promote atherosclerosis and thrombosis, even if cholesterol and triglyceride levels are not significantly elevated. That is why homocysteine blood testing is strongly recommended (*see Medical Testing protocol*).

3. Abnormal platelet aggregation (clotting inside an artery). Fibrinogen, platelets, and other clotting factors aggregate with LDL cholesterol, triglycerides, and calcium on the arterial wall to further promote the development of atherosclerotic plaques. Abnormal platelet aggregation can lead to the development of a blood clot (thrombus) on the arterial walls inside the heart, brain, or any other organ, resulting in ischemia (reduced blood flow) and/or infarction (cell death). Abnormal platelet aggregation can cause an acute arterial blood clot that can lead to a suddenly fatal heart attack or stoke.

Integrated and alternative therapies.

There now exists a massive body of evidence that supplementation, combined with appropriate lifestyle, diet, and exercise can prevent and even help reverse cardiovascular disease, evidenced by an April 1998 recommendation by the *New England Journal of Medicine* titled, "Eat Right and Take a Multivitamin." The conventional medical establishment has long ridiculed vitamin supplementation, but for the first time, a 1998 editorial in the *New England Journal of Medicine* encouraged the use of homocysteine-lowering vitamin supplements to reduce the risks of cardiovascular disease.

Homocysteine Testing: Measuring Your Risk of Atherosclerosis and Cardiovascular Diseases

The dangers of homocysteine were first recognized and reported in the early 1950s. Numerous studies since then have substantiated the role that homocysteine plays in the development of atherosclerosis. In 1995, Dr. Harpel reported that the levels of homocysteine directly correlated with the risk and incidence cardiovascular disease based on the Hordaland Homocysteine Study, a long-term study of over 10,000 patients in Norway.

Since then, conventional doctors have begun recognizing the role that homocysteine plays in causing heart attacks and strokes. With recommendations for lowering homocysteine levels published in the *Journal of the American Medical Association (JAMA)* (Dec. 18, 1996) and the *New England Journal of Medicine* (April 9, 1998), more doctors are recommending folic acid to their coronary artery disease patients. As you will soon read, it takes a lot more than just folic acid to adequately suppress homocysteine concentrations in the blood.

A large multicenter European trial published in the June 11, 1997, issue of *JAMA* found that among men and women younger than age 60, the overall risk of coronary and other vascular disease was 2.2 times higher in those with plasma total homocysteine levels in the top fifth of the normal range compared with those in the bottom four fifths. This risk was independent of other risk factors, but was notably higher in smokers and persons with high blood pressure.

A Norwegian study, published in the July 24, 1997, issue of the *New England Journal of Medicine* found that among 587 patients with coronary heart disease, the risk of death after 4 to 5 years was proportional to plasma total homocysteine levels. The risk rose from 3.8% in those with the lowest levels (below 9 µmol per liter) to 24.7% in those with the highest levels (greater than 15 µmol per liter).

More recently, in March of 1999 the Life Extension Foundation reported a flaw in conventional homocysteine-reduction therapy. The Foundation showed that although folic acid, vitamin B_{12}, vitamin B_6, and trimethylglycine (TMG) all lower homocysteine levels, it is impossible for any individual to know if they are taking the proper amount of nutrients to attain safe levels of homocysteine unless they have a homocysteine blood test to establish their individual homocysteine level.

Based on recent scientific findings, the clear message is that there is *no* safe "normal range" for homocysteine. While commercial laboratories state that normal homocysteine can range from 5 to 15 µmol per liter of blood, epidemiological data reveal that homocysteine levels above 6.3 cause a steep progressive risk of heart attack (see the American Heart Association's journal *Circulation,* Nov. 15, 1995, pp. 2825–2830). One study found each 3-unit increase in homocysteine caused a 35% increase in heart-attack risk (see the *American Journal of Epidemiology* 1996, 143[9]:845–59).

People taking vitamin supplements may presume they are being protected against the lethal effects of homocysteine, when in actuality, even supplement users can have homocysteine levels far above the accepted safe level of 6.3 to 7.0.

Recommendation. For that reason the Life Extension Foundation now recommends that individuals consider homocysteine blood testing as an indicator of present disease risk, to establish a baseline which can be used to monitor the successful effects and appropriate dosages of homocysteine-lowering supplements throughout one's lifetime. (*See Medical Testing protocol for information about homocysteine blood testing.*)

The Life Extension Foundation's long-time position (first published in 1981) about the role that homocysteine plays in cardiovascular disease is being confirmed by new studies showing that homocysteine, like cholesterol, is strongly associated with risk of heart disease.

A study conducted at the Agricultural University in Wageningen, Netherlands, 1999, has identified homocysteine levels as a "new risk factor" for atherosclerosis. In fact, this study has implicated this risk factor as second only to cholesterol in predicting the onset of heart disease. As published in the *Journal of Atherosclerosis, Thrombosis, and Vascular Biology,* every 10% increase in homocysteine levels carries with it about a 10% increase in the risk of developing heart disease. A similar percentage increase in cholesterol levels would imply about a 20% increased risk for heart disease. This study is important, because it is the first of its size to show a positive correlation with risk of atherosclerosis of both "fasting" plasma homocysteine levels and "postload" homocysteine levels (the "postload" blood levels are measured after giving a "load" of oral methionine, the precursor of homocysteine).

From the data, Dr. Verhoef, the study director, found that there was a linear relationship between the number of blocked arteries and homocysteine levels (both fasting and postload), regardless of sex, age, or any other risk variables. Therefore, the study found that the more severe the blockages in the coronary arteries, the higher the homocysteine levels. Researchers concluded that an elevated plasma homocysteine level is an independent risk for severe coronary atherosclerosis.

Dr.Verhoef especially recommends that those people with a family history of heart disease should have their homocysteine levels checked. Finally, Dr.Verhoef believes that the study's findings have implications for the importance of controlling homocysteine levels and testing in the general population, and not just for those people with clearly abnormal levels.

Homocysteine and Degenerative Diseases Such as Atherosclerosis

Elevated homocysteine can be a sign of a methylation deficiency throughout the body. Methylation is fundamental to the body's ability to repair DNA. If DNA is not adequately repaired, mutations and gene strand breaks may result. This may lead to disease and accelerated aging, as greater amounts of faulty proteins are synthesized from the damaged DNA. The liver depends on methylation to perform the numerous enzymatic reactions required to detoxify every drug and foreign substance that the body is exposed to. Methylation is required for the growth of new cells. Without it, new cells cannot be made.

A study published in the 1998 journal *Medical Hypothesis* (vol. 51), provides evidence that aging may be exclusively a result of cellular "demethylation," or said differently, the aging process is caused by the depletion of enzymatic "remethylation" activity that is required to maintain and repair cellular DNA. This study suggests that aging may be reversible if aged cells could be programmed to remethylate rather than demethylate.

Homocysteine induces cellular damage by interfering with the methylation process. Methylation will be compromised if homocysteine is elevated, and elevated homocysteine is a warning sign that the methylation cycle is not functioning properly. Homocysteine may also damage cells directly by promoting oxidative stress.

There is a growing consensus that deficient methylation is the major cause of the degenerative diseases of aging such as atherosclerosis and cancer. The consumption of methylation-enhancing nutrients such as TMG, choline, folic acid, and vitamin B_{12} may be one of the most readily available and effective anti-aging therapies presently known. However, it is important to tailor the intake of methylation-enhancing nutrients to one's individual biochemistry. The best way of assessing your body's rate of methylation is to measure blood levels of homocysteine. Elevated serum homocysteine is the classic sign of a methylation deficiency (or demethylation) that is correctable with the proper intake of methylation-enhancing nutrients such as TMG, folic acid, and vitamin B_{12}.

Homocysteine Detox Mechanisms: How Do the Right Supplements and Dosages Neutralize the Adverse Effects of Homocysteine?

Elevated homocysteine can be reduced (or detoxified) in two ways. The most common pathway is via the remethylation process, where "methyl groups" are donated to homocysteine to convert it into methionine and *S*-adenosylmethionine (SAMe).

A potent remethylation agent is TMG, which stands for tri-methyl-glycine. The "tri" means there are three "methyl" groups on each "glycine" molecule that can be transferred to homocysteine to convert (remethylate) it into methionine and SAMe. The remethylation (or detoxification) of homocysteine requires the following minimum factors: folic acid, vitamin B_{12}, zinc, and TMG. All of these factors (supplements) are included in our recommendations for atherosclerosis treatment.

Choline is another "methyl donor" that helps to reduce elevated homocysteine levels, and this conversion doesn't require co-factors. However, choline only enhances remethylation in the liver and kidney, which is why it is so important to take adequate amounts of remethylating factors such as folic acid and vitamin B_{12} to protect the brain and the heart. The published literature emphasizes that folic acid and vitamin B_{12} are critical nutrients in the remethylation (detoxification) pathway of homocysteine.

The other pathway whereby elevated homocysteine is diminished is by its conversion into cysteine and eventually glutathione via the "trans-sulfuration" pathway. This pathway is dependent on vitamin B_6. The amount of vitamin B_6 required to lower homocysteine has considerable individual variability.

Methionine is the only amino acid that creates homocysteine. People who eat foods that are high in methionine, such as red meat and chicken, may need more vitamin B_6. Elevated homocysteine can occur when there are insufficient vitamin co-factors (such as folate and vitamin B_6) to detoxify the amount of methionine being ingested in the diet.

Elevated homocysteine can also be caused by a genetic defect that blocks the trans-sulfuration pathway by inducing a deficiency of the B_6-

dependent enzyme, cystathione-*B*-synthase. In this case, high doses of vitamin B_6 are required to suppress excessive homocysteine accumulation. Since one would not want to take excessive doses of vitamin B_6 (greater than 300 to 500 mg a day for a long period of time), a homocysteine blood test can help determine whether you are taking enough B_6 to keep homocysteine levels in a safe range. There are some people who lack an enzyme to convert vitamin B_6 into its biologically active form, pyridoxal-5-phosphate. In this case, if low-cost vitamin B_6 supplements do not sufficiently lower homocysteine levels, then a high-cost pyridoxal-5-phosphate supplement may be required. (*See Atherosclerosis supplement recommendations at the end of this protocol*).

Benefits of Vitamin Supplementation

Vitamin C

One of the most significant reports regarding the benefits of vitamin supplementation originated from UCLA in 1992, where it was reported that men who took 800 mg a day of vitamin C lived 6 years longer than those who consumed the FDA's recommended daily allowance of 60 mg a day. The study, which evaluated 11,348 participants over a 10-year period of time, showed that high vitamin C intake prolonged average lifespan and reduced mortality from cardiovascular disease by 42%. This study was published in the journal *Epidemiology* (1992, 3/3:194–202).

High-potency antioxidant supplements can reduce atherosclerosis in humans. This compelling discovery was published in the August 1996 issue of the *American Journal of Clinical Nutrition*. This study involved 11,178 elderly people, who participated in a trial to establish the effects of vitamin supplements on mortality from 1984 to 1993. The results showed that the use of vitamin E reduced the risk of death from all causes by 34%. Effects were strongest for coronary artery disease, where vitamin E resulted in a 63% reduction in death from heart attack. In addition, the use of vitamin E resulted in a 59% reduction in cancer mortality. When the effects of vitamin C and E were compared, overall mortality was reduced by 42% (compared to 34% for vitamin E alone).

These results reported in the prestigious *American Journal of Clinical Nutrition* are the most significant evidence yet presented about the value of vitamin supplementation.Another study published in the *Journal of Clinical Investigation* (1998; July 1) looked at the effects of nitrate drug therapy on human patients. Tolerance development was monitored by changes in arterial pressure, pulse pressure, heart rate, and activity of isolated patients. All patients experienced the deleterious effects of nitrate tolerance. However, when vitamin C was co-administered with the nitrate drugs, the adverse effects of nitrate tolerance were virtually eliminated. The most significant improvement was a 310% improvement in the arterial conductivity test.

Additionally, nitrate drugs sometimes induced dangerous up-regulated activity of platelets; this activity was reversed with vitamin C supplementation. The doctors who conducted this study indicated that vitamin C may be of benefit during long-term, nonintermittent administration of nitrate drugs in humans.

A double-blind study published in the *Journal of the American College of Cardiology* (1998, 31:6, 1323–29) compared the effects of nitrate drugs in people receiving vitamin C to a placebo group not receiving vitamin C. The doctors administered nitrate drugs to both healthy people and patients with coronary artery disease and then measured vasodilation response and cellular levels of cyclic guanasine monophosphate (cGMP), an energy substrate that is depleted by nitrate drugs. At day zero, all participants were measured to establish a baseline. After 3 days of vitamin C administration (2 grams, 3 times daily), there was no change in either group.

After 6 days of vitamin C therapy, an impressive 42% improvement in vasodilation response was observed, and a 60% improvement in cellular cGMP levels was measured in coronary artery disease patients receiving vitamin C compared to placebo. A similar improvement occurred in the healthy subjects taking vitamin C compared to the placebo group. The doctors concluded the study by stating, "These results indicate that combination therapy with vitamin C is potentially useful for preventing the development of nitrate tolerance."

Vitamin supplementation has also been shown to be effective relative to chronic heart failure (CHF). CHF is associated with reduced dilating "stretch" capacity of the endothelial lining of the arterial system. In a February 1998 issue of the *Journal of Circulation,* scientists tested heart failure patients by high-resolution ultrasound and Doppler to measure radial artery diameter and blood flow. They reported vitamin C restored arterial dilation "stretch" response and blood flow velocity in patients with heart failure.

Additionally, another positive aspect of vitamin C's effect on coronary artery disease was recently discovered. A study published in the *Journal of the American College of Cardiology* (1998, 41/5:980-86) showed that low plasma ascorbic acid levels independently predict the presence of an unstable coronary syndrome in heart disease patients. According to the doctors, the study's results showed that the beneficial effects of vitamin C in treating coronary artery disease may result, in part, from an influence on arterial wall lesion activity, rather than a reduction in the overall extent of fixed disease.

Benefits of CoQ_{10}

Coenzyme Q_{10}, also known as ubiquinone, is a fat-soluble vitamin-like substance. It is involved in several key steps in the production of energy within a cell, and it also functions as an antioxidant, a feature that explains its clinical advantages. It has no known toxicity or side effects.

There have now been numerous studies in various countries detailing the use of Coenzyme Q_{10} as a treatment in heart disease. The efficacy and safety of the treatment has been well established, including in large trials. One study, by Baggio et al., which took place in Italy, involved almost 2664 patients with heart failure.

A study by Greenberg and Frishman found that 150 mg of CoQ_{10} reduced the frequency of angina attacks by up to 46%, while improving the capacity for physical activity in those patients. That work was published in the *Journal of Clinical Pharmacology* in 1990.

A study by Sunamori et al., published in 1991, reported that pretreatment with Coenzyme Q_{10} minimized the myocardial injury caused by cardiac bypass surgery and improved heart function compared with patients not pretreated with CoQ_{10} (*Cardiovascular Drugs and Therapy*).

More recently, R.B. Singh, from the Heart Research Laboratory at the Medical Hospital and Research Center in Moradabad, India, told the inaugural conference of the International Coenzyme Q10 Association that, in a randomized double-blind trial of 144 patients with acute myocardial infarction, Coenzyme Q_{10} was seen to be associated with a significant reduction in angina pectoris, arrhythmias, and left ventricular dysfunction. Nonfatal infarction and cardiac deaths also were significantly lower in the Coenzyme Q_{10} group than in the control group.

Early in 1999, as part of a double-blind study, scientists in Melbourne, Australia, gave Coenzyme Q_{10} to elderly people about to undergo cardiac surgery in a bid to make their old hearts young again. (A double-blind study is one in which neither the subjects nor the persons administering the treatment knows which treatment a subject is receiving.)

Dr. Franklin Rosenfeldt, head of cardiac surgical research at the Baker Institute, says he expects the treatment will make the hearts of people over the age of 70 perform as well as those of 30 year-olds. Rosenfeldt believes CoQ_{10} will improve heart function in two ways. The antioxidant fights free radicals released at times of stress, such as during cardiac interventions (including angioplasty, thrombolysis, and surgery). It also improves the way cells convert oxygen and food to energy, strengthening the heart and making it beat more strongly. "We are giving the patients CoQ_{10} for a week before surgery to build up the energy levels in their cells, and we are testing to see whether their recovery after surgery is better, whether their heart shows less damage, and whether cardiac tissue removed at the time has greater energy capacity and also can stand up to stress better," Rosenfeldt says.

Benefits of Artichoke Extract

As early as 1939 scientists discovered that artichoke may have favorable effects on arteriosclerosis and heart disease in general. Subsequent studies in the 50s, 60s, 70s, and 80s supported the possible benefits of artichoke extract. In a 1996 double-blind study conducted by Petrowicz, the cholesterol-lowering effect of artichoke leaf extract was studied on 44 healthy individuals under strictly controlled conditions, resulting in a significant decrease in cholesterol levels in those individuals who had the highest starting levels of cholesterol, further documenting the potential benefits of artichoke extract relative to lowering of cholesterol.

Benefits of B Vitamins

In a landmark study, researchers at the USDA Human Nutrition Research Center on Aging at Tufts University used ultrasonography methods to further explore the relationship between plasma homocysteine and stenosis (narrowing) of the carotid arteries. Study participants were 1041 men and women, aged 67 to 96 years, who were part of the Framingham Heart Study, a large, on-going population-based trial, begun in 1948 and designed to assess cardiac risk factors over time. Dietary intake of folic acid, vitamin B_{12}, and vitamin B_6 was assessed, and blood samples were analyzed to obtain plasma levels of these vitamins. Plasma concentrations of homocysteine also were determined. Ultrasonography was used to estimate vascular stenosis in both the left and right carotid arteries, and the results were analyzed in a blinded fashion by a single examiner. The doctors who conducted this study conclusion stated,

> The study findings indicate that high plasma levels of homocysteine and low levels of folic acid and vitamin B_6 are associated with increased narrowing of the carotid arteries (*New England Journal of Medicine,* 1995, 332:286–91).

The results of other studies using B vitamins are summarized below:

> Subclinical deficiencies of vitamins B_6, B_{12}, and folic acid may be common in men with hyperhomocysteinemia. Moreover, homocysteine levels can be normalized by supplementation with moderate doses of these vitamins (*American Journal of Clinical Nutrition,* 1993, 57:47–53).
>
> Recently, elevated homocysteine blood concentrations have been identified as an independent risk factor for the development of atherosclerotic lesions. The amino acid homocysteine is metabolized in the human body involving the vitamins folic acid, B_{12}, and B_6 as essential cofactors and coenzymes, respectively. There is an inverse relationship between the status of the relevant B vitamins and the homocysteine blood concentration. Supplementation of these vitamins results in a significant reduction of the homocysteine level (*Arch. Latinoam. Nutr.* (Venezuela), June 1997).
>
> Deficiencies of vitamins B_6 and B_{12} also can contribute to hyperhomocyst(e)inemia. Successful treatment of hyperhomocyst(e)inemia usually is accomplished by increasing intake of folic acid above 400 to 800 micrograms daily, with the addition of vitamins B_6 and B_{12} if indicated (*Endocrinologist* (United States), 1998).
>
> Combined vitamin supplementation reduces homocysteine levels effectively in patients with venous thrombosis and in healthy volunteers, either with or without hyperhomocysteinemia. Even supplementation with 0.5 mg of folic acid led to a substantial reduction of blood homocysteine levels (*Arteriosclerosis, Thrombosis, and Vascular Biology* (United States), 1998).
>
> Numerous epidemiological studies have shown the relationship between moderate hyperhomocysteinemia and the occurrence of vascular diseases, cerebral, coronary, peripheral artery diseases, (*and*) venous thrombosis. In addition, hyperhomocysteinemia is a predictive risk factor of vascular diseases or even of mortality. There is a relation between plasma homocysteine levels and folate, vitamin B_6, and B_{12} levels (*Hematologie* (France), 1998).
>
> Low vitamin B_{12} concentrations were associated with an increased risk of coronary atherosclerosis, partly independently of homocysteine. Although low folate status was a strong determinant of elevated homocysteine concentrations, it was not associated with increased risk of coronary atherosclerosis (*Journal of the American College of Nutrition* (United States), 1998).

Benefits of Niacin

The B vitamin niacin, also known as nicotinic acid, has been used for many years in relatively high doses (e.g., 1 to 4.5 grams/day) as an inexpensive treatment for hyperlipidemia, a condition characterized by elevated blood levels of cholesterol and/or triglycerides (fats). High concentrations of these fatty compounds are associated with increased risk of coronary heart disease (CHD).

Recent research indicates that, in addition to reducing cholesterol and triglyceride levels, nicotinic acid treatment also significantly increases the concentration of high-density lipoproteins (HDL), the "good" form of cholesterol associated with reduced risk of CHD.

Despite its advantages, high-dose nicotinic acid treatment also produces undesirable side effects, including flushing, itching, gastrointestinal upset, and at higher dosages possible liver abnormalities. Although these side effects appear to be dose-related, few studies have attempted to clarify the optimal dose of nicotinic acid needed to alter lipid levels while producing the fewest side effects.

To determine whether lower doses of nicotinic acid are as effective and better tolerated than the typical regimen currently used, researchers at the University of Texas Southwestern Medical Center in Dallas (*Arch. Intern. Med.* 1996, 156:1081–88) conducted a trial using two different doses of nicotinic acid. The study participants were 44 middle-aged men, 24 with normal blood lipid levels and 20 with moderately elevated triglyceride levels and low levels of HDL. Although the subjects were taking various cardiac medications, none were taking drugs to alter lipid levels. The trial was divided into three 8-week phases consisting of either diet alone (30% fat) or diet plus 1.5 or 3.0 grams/day of nicotinic acid daily. The results showed that low-dose nicotinic acid treatment significantly lowered triglyceride levels, raised HDL concentrations by approximately 22%, and favorably altered the ratio of total cholesterol to HDL-cholesterol in both normal patients and those with abnormal lipid levels at baseline. Further improvement in lipid levels was also observed in those patients who tolerated the higher dose of nicotinic acid. In this study, significant improvement in blood lipid levels was observed among the 75% of patients who tolerated low-dose nicotinic acid therapy. The authors conclude that use of nicotinic acid in lower doses than traditionally prescribed is both well-tolerated and effective in altering blood lipid levels. In addition, they suggest that this vitamin may be particularly worthwhile when combined with other lipid-lowering medications.

"Niacin is a useful lipid-modifying drug because it (1) decreases low-density lipoprotein (LDL) cholesterol, total cholesterol, triglycerides, and lipoprotein(s), and (2) raises high-density lipoprotein (HDL) cholesterol" as reported in the *American Journal of Cardiology,* December 1998.

The *Journal of Cardiovascular Risk* (June 1997, 4/3:165–71) concluded a report by stating, "This study of hypertriglyceridemic men has shown that long-term treatment with nicotinic acid not only corrects serum lipoprotein abnormalities, but also reduces the fibrinogen concentration in plasma and stimulates fibrinolysis."

A 1998 study reported in the *Journal of Cardiology* indicates niacin increased "good" HDL by almost 30% in a study of patients over a 5-year period. The study also reported that the presence of low HDL was an independent predictor of coronary artery disease.

Many people have not been able to use high-dose niacin because of the unpleasant "flushing" effects. However, given the results of the studies above and other studies recently completed, we are now suggesting the approach using the low dosages used in the study discussed above.

CAUTION: Some side effects from niacin consumption may be encountered such as flushing, itching, and minor gastrointestinal upset. Measurement of liver enzyme levels every 3 to 6 months via a blood test is mandatory because niacin can cause liver damage in a minority of people. Those with liver disease such as hepatitis C cannot use niacin.

Benefits of Vitamin E

Vitamin E was advocated as an effective treatment for heart disease by Dr. Even Shute of London, Ontario, more than 50 years ago. His pioneering claims, which were unacceptable to the medical community at large, have been confirmed by recent findings from epidemiologic studies and clinical trials. Evidence is presented that vitamin E protects against the development of atherosclerosis. Vitamin E enrichment has been shown to retard LDL oxidation, inhibit the proliferation of smooth muscle cells, inhibit platelet adhesion and aggregation, inhibit the expression and function of adhesion molecules, attenuate the synthesis of leukotrienes, and potentiate the release of prostacyclin through up-regulating the expression of cytosolic phospholipase A2. Collectively, these biological functions of vitamin E may account for its protection against the development of atherosclerosis. (*Journal of Nutrition,* 1998 [Oct], pp. 1593–96).

Some other studies about vitamin E and cardiovascular disease have been summarized as follows:

> Vitamin E acts as an important antioxidant against oxidative modification of low-density lipoprotein (LDL), which is accepted as an initial event in the pathogenesis of atherosclerosis (*Free Radical Research* (United Kingdom), 1998, 28/6:561–72).
>
> Epidemiologic studies have suggested that vitamin E (alpha-tocopherol) may play a preventive role in reducing the incidence of atherosclerosis. Our economic evaluation indicates that vitamin E therapy in patients with angiographically proven atherosclerosis is cost-effective in the Australian and US settings (*American Journal of Cardiology,* 1998, 82/4:414–17).
>
> There is growing evidence that supplementation with vitamin E in higher doses has a protective role in prevention of atherosclerosis (*Medizinische Welt* (Germany), 1998, 49/5:250–55).
>
> Evidence indicates that antioxidant supplements, particularly vitamin E, can reduce oxidation of LDLs (*American Journal of Epidemiology,* 1994, 139:1180–89).
>
> There is increasing evidence that free radical reactions are involved in the early stages, or sometimes later on, in the development of human diseases. Put simply, the proposition is that by improving human diets by increasing the quantity in them of antioxidants, it might be possible to reduce the incidence of a number of degenerative diseases. Of particular significance to these considerations is the likely role of the primary fat-soluble dietary antioxidant vitamin E in the prevention of degenerative diseases such as arteriosclerosis, which is frequently the cause of consequent heart attacks or stroke, and prevention of certain forms of cancer, as well as several other diseases. Substantial evidence for this proposition now exists, and this review is an attempt to give a brief account of the present position. Two kinds of evidence exist: on the one hand there is very substantial basic science evidence which indicates an involvement of free radical events, and a preventive role for vitamin E, in the development of human disease processes. On the other hand, there is also a large body of human epidemiological evidence which suggests that incidence of these diseases is lowered in populations having a high level of antioxidants, such as vitamin E, in their diet, or who have taken steps to enhance their level of intake of the vitamin by taking dietary supplements. There is also some evidence which suggests that intervention with dietary supplements of vitamin E can result in a lowered risk of disease, in particular of cardiovascular disease, which is a major killer disease among the developed nations of the world. The intense interest in this subject recently has as its objective the possibility that, by making some simple alterations to dietary lifestyle, or by enhancing the intake of vitamin E by fortification of foods, or by dietary supplements, it may be possible to reduce substantially the risk of a large amount of common, highly disabling human disease. By this simple means, therefore, it may be possible to improve substantially the quality of human life, in particular for people of advancing years (*Free Radical Research,* June 1997).
>
> Dose-response studies in humans have reported that 400 IU/day vitamin E increased its levels in plasma two-fold and prolonged the lag time before LDL oxidation. It has been reported that oxidizability of LDL was correlated to the atherosclerotic score of coronary angiography in CHD patients. About 400 IU/day vitamin E, which increases its levels two-fold and prolongs sufficiently the lag time before LDL oxidation, might be beneficial in decreasing the individual risk of CHD (*Biofactors Journal*, 1998).

As mentioned earlier, the August 1996 issue of the *American Journal of Clinical Nutrition* showed that the use of vitamin E resulted in a 63% reduction in death from heart attack. Vitamin E has clearly established itself as a front-line preventative and treatment for coronary artery disease.

Benefits of Omega-3 Oils

The healthy body requires large amounts of the fatty acids EPA and DHA, which are found in or are made from omega-3 (fish, flax, or perilla) oils. Regrettably, the typical Western diet provides large amounts of linoleic acid (omega-6) that in high amounts contribute to most forms of degenerative disease. The bad saturated fatty acids and their metabolites compete with the beneficial fatty acids EPA and DHA and their metabolites.

Scientific studies have demonstrated that alpha-linoleic acid (from flax or perilla oil) reduces the incidence of atherosclerosis, stroke, and second heart attacks. One study showed a 70% reduction in second heart attacks in those consuming this type of fatty acid.

Results of a 1998 25-year follow-up study on plasma cholesterol and coronary heart disease mortality in seven countries indicated there was an eightfold difference in coronary heart disease mortality between West Scotland and Catalonia in Spain, without significant differences in blood cholesterol concentration. These observations clearly indicate that, while plasma cholesterol is one of the risk factors for coronary heart disease, other factors can be more important. It is now becoming obvious that Western diets contain too many of the artery-clogging saturated fats, and not enough friendly fats that provide the body with EPA and DHA omega-3 oils.

Experimental studies suggest that an intake of 3 to 4 grams per day of alpha-linoleic acid is necessary to obtain the protective effect against coronary heart disease.

However, may people suffer stomach upset when taking fish oil, which is a direct source of EPA and DHA. Perilla oil, on the other hand, provides a high concentration of the beneficial alpha-linoleic acid (that converts to EPA and DHA in the body). New studies are showing significant health benefits without gastrointestinal side effects. A review of the scientific literature indicates that perilla oil—which comes from the beefsteak plant (*Perilla frutescens*) and is relatively common in East Asian countries—may be superior to other oils and is tolerable by virtually everyone.

Perilla oil inhibits abnormal blood clotting, alleviates chronic inflammation, prevents certain types of arrhythmia, maintains cardiac cell energy output, and preserves youthful cell membrane structure.

Platelet-activating factor (PAF) is a major cause of arterial blood clots that cause heart attacks and strokes, and are the leading cause of death in the West. Perilla oil was shown to decrease PAF by 50% in rats, compared with the administration of safflower oil. (*Journal of Lipid Mediators and Cell Signaling* (Netherlands) 1997, 17/3:207–20)

The effects of perilla oil on nutritional status and the production of thromboxane A2, a significant cause of abnormal blood-clot formation, were compared with those of soybean oil in diabetic rats. After only 7 days, perilla oil improved body-weight gain and nitrogen balance and reduced inflammatory cytokine formation and thromboxane A2 production by platelets. Perilla oil improved the overall nutritional state of these diabetic rats (*Nutrition* (USA), 1995, 11/5:450–55).

Benefits of Folic Acid

Folic acid is now being prescribed by conventional medical doctors to lower homocysteine. As discussed already in this protocol, it takes more than just folic acid to optimally suppress serum homocysteine to safe levels. Here are some studies that relate what the doctors are saying about the importance of folic-acid supplementation:

> Supplementation with B vitamins, in particular with folic acid, is an efficient, safe, and inexpensive means to reduce an elevated homocysteine level. Studies are now in progress to establish whether such therapy will reduce cardiovascular risk. The basis for these conclusions is data from about 80 clinical and epidemiological studies including more than 10,000 patients (*Annual Review of Medicine* (United States), 1998, 49:31–62).
>
> Since atherosclerosis risk may increase continuously with decreasing plasma homocysteine, it may be wise to keep plasma homocysteine levels as low

as possible. To reach this goal, the recommended dietary allowance of folic acid may have to be increased (*Tijdschrift voor Geneeskunde* (Netherlands), 1998, 142/14:782–86).

Plasma levels of folic acid, on the other hand, appeared protective, with more than a 60 percent reduction in risk of heart attack (*American Journal of Epidemiology,* 1996, 143:845–59).

The results of this study demonstrate that supplements containing modest levels of folic acid or a combination of folic acid, vitamin B_6, and vitamin B_{12} are effective in lowering plasma levels of homocysteine (*Journal of Nutrition,* 1994, 124:1927–33).

The results of this study provide further evidence that homocysteine is an independent risk factor for cardiovascular disease. These findings also suggest that adequate folic acid intake from diet or supplements may help to normalize plasma homocysteine levels (*American Journal of Epidemiology,* 1996, 143:845–59).

Benefits of Herbals

Herbal extracts are among the world's best-studied medicines. Almost all of what we know as modern-day medicine has been derived either directly or indirectly from folk medicine, which relies on herbal treatments. Even today, 80% of the world (4 billion people) use herbal treatments as part of their primary health care. Many of the drugs that are commonly used today are herbal in origin. In fact, the Office of Alternative Medicine of the National Institutes of Health reports that about one fourth of the prescription drugs dispensed in the United States have at least one active ingredient derived from plant material.

Green Tea Extract

Some studies suggest that green tea extract may inhibit the oxidation of LDL, so-called "bad" cholesterol, and thereby prevent heart disease. Moreover, tea, especially green tea, provides antioxidants and flavonoids which have been shown to inhibit abnormal platelet aggregation that can result in an arterial blood clot (thrombus) that can cause an acute heart attack or stroke.

Ginkgo Biloba Extract

The following excerpts from leading journals describe the indications for gingko biloba in the treatment of vascular disease:

> Ginkgo biloba is one of the oldest, still-existing plants. Extracts from its leaves were already used in ancient China, whereas in the western world, they have been utilized only since the sixties when it became technically possible and feasible to isolate the essential substances of ginkgo biloba. Pharmacologically, there are two groups of substances which are of some significance: the flavonoids, effective as oxygen-free radical scavengers, and the terpenes with their highly specific action as platelet activating factor (PAF) inhibitors. Clinically important indications for ginkgo biloba extracts are cerebral insufficiency and atherosclerotic disease of peripheral arteries of intermediate severity. In several placebo-controlled clinical studies, symptoms of cerebral insufficiency and vascular disease have been effectively and significantly influenced (As reported in *Rundsch. Med. Prax.* (Switzerland), 1995, 84/1:1–6).

Gingko biloba was used with heart patients in a treadmill test in France:

> In a comparison of the differences before and after treatment, the areas of ischemia decreased by 38% after its use (*Angiology* (USA), 1994, 45/6:413–17).

A German 1994 technical journal *Therapiewoche* article describes the therapeutic value of hawthorn, ginkgo, and garlic. "Circulatory effective herbs such as hawthorn, ginkgo and garlic have a very important share in the entire phytotherapy. Due to their good tolerance, they are used in less severe classes of the frequent circulatory system's diseases as such arteriosclerosis and consequent symptoms, heart failure, and orthostatic dysfunction."

Garlic

The mechanisms by which garlic has been shown to protect against cardiovascular disease include preventing abnormal blood-clot formation inside of blood vessels, protecting LDL cholesterol against oxidation, and protecting the endothelial lining of the arterial system against oxidation.

A mechanism by which atherosclerotic plaque accumulates on the walls of arteries is the oxidation of LDL cholesterol. Garlic has been shown in repeated studies to protect against LDL cholesterol oxidation and oxidation in the linings of the arteries themselves.

A study published in the journal *Nutrition Research* (1987, 7:139–49) showed that a liquid garlic extract made by Kyolic caused a 12 to 31% reduction in cholesterol levels in the majority of test subjects after 6 months. The study showed that 73% of the subjects given the Kyolic garlic experienced greater than 10% reduction in cholesterol, compared with only 17% in the placebo group showing the same improvement.

If you have high LDL cholesterol levels, garlic supplementation is especially important because LDL cholesterol oxidation causes atherosclerosis, and garlic specifically inhibits LDL oxidation. And, as noted, garlic helps protect the arterial lining against oxidation. Most importantly, garlic prevents abnormal platelet aggregation (thrombosis) via several different mechanisms.

The formation of arterial blood clots is the primary cause of most heart attacks and strokes.

In a study published in the *American Journal of Clinical Nutrition* (1996, 64:866–70), the daily administration of 7.2 grams of Kyolic garlic powder for 6 months produced a modest reduction (of between 6.1 and 7%) in total cholesterol, compared with the placebo group. The more dangerous LDL cholesterol was reduced 4 to 4.6% in the Kyolic group.

The heart-healthy benefits of garlic include protecting the endothelial lining of the arterial system against oxidative damage. A study published in *Atherosclerosis* (1999, 144:237–49) shows an actual reduction in build-up of fatty plaque in arteries in garlic supplement users. Fatty plaque is comprised of many substances, including cholesterol. When plaque accumulates in the coronary arteries, the condition can lead to heart attack.

In a study of 280 adults, German researchers report that participants who took 900 mg of garlic powder per day had up to 18% less plaque in their arteries than those who took a placebo or "dummy" powder. Male study participants who took placebo had a 5.5% increase in plaque volume, while those who took the garlic powder experienced just a 1.1% increase in plaque build-up during the 4-year study period. By comparison, women who took the garlic showed a 4.6% decrease in plaque volume, while those who took the placebo powder had a 5.3% increase. Garlic may affect plaque build-up by reducing blood platelet stickiness (aggregation) and specifically preventing the oxidation of LDL cholesterol onto the lining of the arteries. Platelet aggregation helps plaque cling to the arteries.

Bromelain

Bromelain is a mixture of sulfur-containing proteolytic enzymes obtained from the stem of the pineapple plant. Bromelain breaks down fibrinogen and has been shown to be useful in treating cardiovascular disease. Cardiovascular disease patients should test their fibrinogen levels to see if bromelain can lower serum fibrinogen to a safe level.

Curcumin

Curcumin is the yellow pigment of tumeric. When rats were fed small doses of curcumin, their cholesterol levels fell to one half those in rats not receiving curcumin (*Journal of Nutrition*, 1970, 100:1307–16).

Curcumin reduces cholesterol by interfering with intestinal cholesterol uptake, increasing the conversion of cholesterol into bile acids, and increasing the excretion of bile acids (*International Journal of Vitamin Nutritional Research*, 1991, 61:364–69).

Curcumin prevents abnormal blood-clot formation by interfering with the formation of thromboxanes, the promoters of platelet aggregation. Curcumin increases levels of prostacyclin, the body's natural inhibitor of abnormal platelet aggregation (*Arzneim. Forsh.*, 1986, 36:715–17).

When 500 mg per day of curcumin was given to ten volunteers, there was a 29% increase in beneficial HDL cholesterol after only 7 days. Total cholesterol was reduced by 11.6% and lipid peroxidation was reduced by 33% (*Indian Journal of Physiology,* 1992, 36(4):273–75). While FDA-approved cholesterol-lowering drugs can cause liver damage, curcumin's ability to help prevent cancer and inhibit dangerous viruses is well documented. Curcumin also has anti-inflammatory effects.

Curcumin neutralizes dietary carcinogens and has been shown to inhibit cancer at the initiation, promotion, and progression stages of development.

Curcumin is a potent antioxidant and has been shown to be an inhibitor of HIV replication via several different mechanisms. Unlike FDA-approved drugs, curcumin may protect against liver damage caused by viral hepatitis.

CAUTION: Do not use curcumin if you have a biliary tract obstruction because curcumin increases the excretion of cholesterol-bile acids through the bile duct. High doses of curcumin on an empty stomach may cause stomach ulcers.

Gugulipid

Gugulipid extract produces a blood-fat lowering effect with no side effects. In a study in the *Journal of Associated Physicians—India* (1989, 37/5:323–28), 125 patients who received gugulipid experienced an 11% decrease in total cholesterol and a 16.8% decrease in triglyceride levels within 3 to 4 weeks. Patients with elevated cholesterol responded better than patients with normal cholesterol. HDL cholesterol increased in 60% of the patients receiving gugulipid.

In a placebo-controlled study conducted by the same researchers, 205 patients received gugulipid (25 mg 3 times a day). Of the gugulipid-treated patients, 70 to 80% showed cholesterol reduction compared to virtually none in the placebo group.

In another placebo-controlled trial in 40 patients with high blood fat levels, serum cholesterol declined by 21.75% and triglycerides by 27.1% after 3 weeks of administration of gugulipid. After 16 weeks, HDL cholesterol increased by 35.8%. The placebo group did not achieve statistically significant results (*Indian Journal of Medical Research,* 1988, 87:356–60).

Ginger

Thromboxane A2 initiates a cascade of events that can result in the formation of abnormal blood clots. Ginger is a potent inhibitor of thromboxane synthesis, just like aspirin is. Unlike aspirin, however, ginger also raises prostacyclin, which inhibits abnormal platelet aggregation (clotting). Thus, ginger inhibits abnormal platelet aggregation by at least two mechanisms of action (*Medical Hypothesis,* 1986, 20:271).

In a study in *Prostaglandins Medicine* (1984, 13:277), ginger inhibited platelet aggregation *in vitro* more effectively than onion or garlic.

In the *New England Journal of Medicine* (1980, 303:756–7), it was reported that ginger completely inhibited arachidonate-induced platelet aggregation in platelet-rich plasma that had been incubated for 1 to 60 minutes. Ethanol showed no effect.

Ginger also increases the contractile strength of the heart. Scientists call ginger a "cardiotonic agent" because of its ability to increase ATP energy production in the heart and to enhance calcium pumping within heart cells that is required for optimal cardiac output.

The Need for Trace Minerals

A recent 1998 study in the *Annales Pharmaceutiques Francaises* suggests the need for and synergistic effect of trace minerals relative to the antioxidant action of supplements.

> Epidemiological studies suggest a negative correlation between the occurrence of cardiovascular diseases and blood concentrations of lipophilic antioxidants such as vitamin A and E and beta-carotene. Trace elements such as selenium, zinc and copper are involved in the activity of antioxidant enzymes.

The study further pointed out the need for adequate trace elements to fuel the activity of antioxidants.

> Our results showed that, as compared with normocholesterolemic subjects, patients treated by LDL-apheresis were not deficient in vitamin E, beta-carotene and copper but had low plasma levels

> of selenium, zinc and vitamin A. The low selenium and vitamin A levels were due to the treatment by LDL-apheresis by itself, while the hypercholesterolemia of these patients might have provoked the low plasma levels of zinc. This study pointed out the interest of a supplement of selenium, zinc and vitamin A in patients treated by LDL-apheresis.

Research conducted in 1986 by the U.S. Department of Agriculture and published in *Acta Pharmacol. Toxicol.* (Denmark, 1986) first suggested the importance of adequate mineral supplementation and its effect on cardiovascular disease as follows:

> Evidence linking marginal intakes of the trace elements chromium, copper, zinc and selenium with abnormal lipid metabolism and ultimately cardiovascular diseases is accumulating from both animal and human studies. Chromium supplementation of normal adult men, as well as diabetics, has been reported to increase high-density lipoprotein cholesterol and decrease triglycerides and total cholesterol. Subjects with the highest total cholesterol and triglycerides usually respond the most to supplemental chromium. Selenium may also affect cardiovascular diseases since selenium is postulated to be involved in platelet aggregation. These data demonstrate that the trace elements chromium, copper, and selenium have beneficial effects on risk factors associated with cardiovascular diseases suggesting that a decreased risk of cardiovascular disease may be achieved by adequate intake of trace elements.

A 1997 study in the *Journal of the American Dietetic Association* by Kwiterovich, Jr., also documents and discusses the possible benefits of trace-mineral (selenium) activity and its synergetic effect on antioxidants, vitamin E, beta-carotene, and vitamin C.

A 1997 study entitled "Erythrocyte Selenium-Glutathione Peroxidase Activity is Lower in Patients with Coronary Atherosclerosis" was conducted in Europe and reported in November of 1997 in the *Japan Heart Journal*. Researchers confirmed that selenium levels decreased as severity of atherosclerosis increased, further suggesting the linkage between heart disease and "subclinical" levels of minerals, "and further...the need for adequate mineral supplementation as part of any preventive or restorative vascular disease therapy."

Benefits of Aspirin

Aspirin has an immediate and 2-day lasting effect on blood platelets, making them less likely to clump together and form a catastrophic clot in arteries. A low dose of aspirin (81 mg) has been shown to be beneficial in the prevention of heart attacks, strokes, and transient ischemic attacks (little strokes).

More than 50 randomized clinical trials have documented the safety and effectiveness of aspirin as a cardiovascular drug. Low-dose aspirin is advised by legions of physicians as well as a 70-member panel convened by the American College of Chest Physicians, which recommended aspirin for all people over 50 with one risk factor and no conditions that make aspirin use inadvisable. This translates into the majority of people over 50, since risk factors for heart disease include male gender, high blood pressure, elevated cholesterol, diabetes, cigarette smoking, lack of exercise, and family history of heart attack or stroke.

While many of the nutrients included in the *Prevention protocols* will reduce the risk of an abnormal blood clot forming inside a blood vessel, it is still beneficial for most older people to take aspirin in the low dose provided by the Healthprin tablet, which minimizes stomach irritation.

We also recommend that it be taken with a heavy meal to further decrease the possibility of stomach irritation.

Benefits of TMG

TMG's (Tri-Methyl-Glycine) unique biological effect makes it a critical component of a disease-prevention program: it is the most effective facilitator known of youthful methylation metabolism. Published research shows that methylation is related to a variety of diseases, including cardiovascular disease, cancer, liver disease, and neurological disorders. Enhancing methylation improves health and slows premature and, perhaps, normal aging. Methylation lowers dangerous homocysteine levels, thus lowering the risk of heart disease and stroke.

TMG is extracted from sugar beets. It has a distinctive taste that is mildly sweet with a mild aftertaste. TMG is also known as glycine betaine. Don't confuse "betaine hydrochloride" with glycine betaine (TMG). Betaine HCL does not provide the methylation enhancement of TMG and could elevate stomach acidity in some people.

There are no reports of side effects with TMG other than brief muscle tension headaches if it is taken in large quantities without food. TMG should be taken with co-factors vitamin B_{12} and folic acid.

Benefits of Dietary Soy

Soy made headlines in late 1998 and early 1999 when the Food and Drug Administration said studies showed that soy protein, in combination with a diet low in saturated fat and cholesterol, can reduce heart disease, the number one cause of death in the United States. The FDA also said that soy protein, when part of a low-fat, low-cholesterol diet, can lower total blood cholesterol and reduce low-density lipoprotein (LDL), the "bad" cholesterol.

In its report, the FDA said soy protein differs from other vegetable proteins because it changes the way the liver processes cholesterol. According to the agency, the benefit to the heart comes from consuming a minimum of 25 grams of soy protein a day.

Soybeans are the source of soy protein, a major protein source worldwide. It is used in making soy noodles and tofu, as well as meat substitutes such as tempeh and soy burgers. It is also available as a dietary supplement.

Accumulating evidence from molecular and cellular biology experiments, animal studies, and, to a limited extent, human clinical trials suggests that phytoestrogens may potentially confer health benefits related to cardiovascular diseases, cancer, osteoporosis, and menopausal symptoms. These potential health benefits are consistent with the epidemiological evidence that rates of heart disease, various cancers, osteoporotic fractures, and menopausal symptoms are more favorable among populations that consume plant-based diets, particularly among cultures with diets that are traditionally high in soy products (*Journal of Clinical Endocrinology Metabolism,* 1998 [July], 83/7:2223–35).

"It has long been recognized that coronary heart disease rates are lower in Japan, where soy consumption is common, than in Western countries. Potential mechanisms by which soy isoflavones might prevent atherosclerosis include a beneficial effect on plasma lipid concentrations, antioxidant effects, antiproliferative and antimigratory effects on smooth muscle cells, effects on thrombus formation, and maintenance of normal vascular reactivity" (*American Journal of Clinical Nutrition,* 1998 [Dec], 68/6 Suppl.:1390S–93S).

Conventional Therapies

Drugs. Various medications constitute the first-line treatment of coronary artery disease. These include the following:

Beta-blocking drugs. These agents act by blocking the effect of the sympathetic nervous system on the heart, slowing heart rate, decreasing blood pressure, and thereby reducing the oxygen demand of the heart. Studies have found that these drugs also can reduce the chances of dying or suffering a recurrent heart attack if they are started shortly after suffering a heart attack and continued for 2 years. Commonly prescribed beta-adrenergic blockers drugs are atenolol (Tenoretic, Tenormin), metoprolol (Lopressor, Toprol XL), nadolol (Corgard, Corzide), and propranolol (Inderol).

Calcium-channel-blocking drugs. All muscles need varying amounts of calcium in order to contract. By reducing the amount of calcium that enters the muscle cells in the coronary artery walls, spasms can be prevented. Some calcium-channel-blocking drugs also decrease the work load of the heart and some lower the heart rate as well. Commonly prescribed calcium-channel blockers are diltiazem (Cardizem CD, Cardizem SR, Dilacor XR), nifedipine (Procardia XL), verapamil (Calan, Calan SR, Isoptin, Isoptin SR, Verelan).

Centrally acting drugs. These agents decrease the heart rate and lower the amount of blood pumped with each beat by decreasing sympathetic nervous system activity, which controls involuntary muscle action. They are usually taken with the thiazide class of diuretic drug. Commonly prescribed central alpha-adrenergic agonist and blockers are guanfacine (Tenex) and terazosin (Hytrin).

Angiotensin-Converting Enzyme (ACE) inhibitors. These drugs block the formation of angiotensin, a naturally occurring substance that constricts blood vessels. They also decrease the body's ability to retain salt and water. ACE inhibitors are used to treat a number of conditions in addition to high blood pressure. Some commonly prescribed ACE inhibitors are captopril (Capoten, Capozide), enalapril (Vasotec), and lisinopril (Prinivil, Zestril).

Vasodilators. These drugs relax the muscles in the blood vessel walls, causing them to enlarge or widen. There are four types of drugs that could be classified as indirect or direct vasodilators: (1) beta blockers such as propranolol (Inderal) and metoprolol (Lopressor); (2) direct-acting vasodilators such as Hydralazine and Minoxidil that directly cause the muscle in the walls of the blood vessels to relax; (3) angiotensin-converting enzyme (ACE) inhibitors such as captopril (Capoten), enalapril (Vasotec), lisinopril (Zestril, Prinivil), benazepril (Lotensin), and fosinopril (Monopril). The angiotensin enzyme makes the arteries constrict or narrow. These drugs don't allow angiotensin to be made, and so the arteries dilate, or open up, lowering the blood pressure; (4) calcium channel blockers such as felodipine (Plendil) and bepridil (Vascor). These drugs block calcium from getting into the muscle, so the muscles can't contract (Source: Boston University Medical Center, 1999).

Cardiac glycoside/anti-arrhythmic drugs. Prescribed to control arrhythmia or abnormal heart rates: digoxin (Lanoxicaps, Lanoxin).

Diuretics. Commonly called "water pills," these drugs lower blood pressure by reducing the body's sodium and water volume. The most commonly used diuretics in treating hypertension are the thiazides; if these fail to lower the blood pressure adequately, a different diuretic or other drugs to take with a thiazide may be prescribed. Commonly prescribed drugs are loop diuretics: bumetanide (Bumex), furosemide (Lasix); thiazide diuretics: hydrochlorothiazide (Aldactazide, Aldoril, Esidrix, HydroDIURIL, Moduretic, Oretic, Thiuretic); potassium supplements: potassium chloride (K-Dur, K-Lor, K-Norm, K-Tab, Kaochlor, Kaon-Cl, Kay Ciel, Klotrix, Klorvess, Micro-K, Slow-K, Ten-K).

Nitroglycerin and nitrates. Nitrate-type medications may be prescribed to both treat and prevent attacks of angina. This drug dilates the large coronary arteries, thereby increasing the flow of blood to heart muscle. Commonly prescribed drugs are nitroglycerins (Deponit, Minitran, Nitro-Bid, Nitro-Dur, Nitrodisc, Nitrogard, Nitroglyn, Nitrol, Nitrolingual, Nitrostat, Tridil).

Anti-anginal drugs. Drugs commonly prescribed to suppress the occurrence of angina are isosorbide dinitrate (Dilatrate-SR, ISMO, Iso-Bid, Isordil, Sorbitrate, Sorbitrate-SA).

Surgical treatment. An estimated 200,000 Americans undergo coronary artery bypass surgery each year. This operation, once considered difficult, is now almost routine in many medical centers. There is a good deal of controversy over whether it is being used unnecessarily to treat coronary disease that could be controlled just as effectively by more conservative, less costly medical therapies.

There remains some disagreement among doctors as to the indications for coronary bypass surgery. Studies have conclusively demonstrated that the operation prolongs life in patients who have a severely blocked left main coronary artery. It is also indicated in most cases in which three major arteries are diseased. There is less agreement about when it is appropriate for other patients. In general, it is recommended for people with disabling angina that cannot be controlled by conventional therapy who are also good candidates for surgery.

The operation itself is relatively simple. A segment of healthy blood vessel, usually an artery from the chest (mammary artery) or vein from one of the legs (saphenous vein), is interposed between the aorta and the blocked coronary arteries. During the operation, which takes about 2 hours, circulation is maintained by a heart-lung machine.

Coronary bypass patients usually spend 2 or 3 days in an intensive care recovery unit following the operation, and another week in the hospital. Costs of the operation vary depending on the individual's condition and geographic locale, but the average cost is $32,000 to $35,000. (Refer to the *Anesthesia and Surgical Precautions protocol* to learn what can be done to reduce the risk of surgically induced complications.)

Caution: Although bypass surgery greatly improves the way most patients feel, it is not a cure for heart disease. Unless other preventive steps are taken, the processes that caused the artery disease will continue. In fact, the grafts seem to become diseased even faster than the natural coronary arteries. Therefore, it is particularly important for bypass patients to follow a prudent lifestyle following the operation.

Angioplasty. A relatively recent—and increasingly popular—treatment for atherosclerotic arterial diseases is transluminal angioplasty, also referred to as balloon angioplasty. Used to treat severely blocked coronary arteries as well as arteries diseased with atherosclerotic plaque in other parts of the body, this technique involves threading a catheter with an inflatable balloon-like tip through the artery to the area of blockage. The balloon is inflated, flattening the fatty deposits and widening the arterial channel, allowing more blood to reach the heart muscle.

Angioplasty offers several obvious advantages. (1) The operation is performed under local anesthesia. (2) Although invasive, it does not involve surgery or the use of a heart-lung machine. (3) It is not as costly as coronary bypass surgery, nor does it involve more than 1 or 2 days of hospitalization under ordinary circumstances.

Unfortunately, it is not appropriate for all types of coronary artery disease, nor does it work in all people. Several recent studies show that women are not as likely as men to benefit from the operation; they also have a higher mortality rate from the procedure. Some studies have put the success rate at about 60%; people who undergo an unsuccessful angioplasty still may require coronary bypass surgery. As technology advances, the applicability and success rates of angioplasty may improve. It also should be noted that it is not a cure for the disease. In a significant number of patients, the occlusions recur, and a repeat angioplasty may be required after 2 or 3 years.

Angioplasty is also being used to treat blockages in the arteries of the legs and the carotid artery, the major vessel carrying blood to the brain.

A variation of balloon angioplasty uses a tiny drill-like device to shave away fatty deposits, similar to a Roto-Rooter. Another still-experimental variation, called laser ablation, is performed through a special viewing tube (fiber-optic catheter) that is inserted into the clogged artery. A laser is used to vaporize the plaque (Source: Columbia University, 1999).

Estrogen Drugs May Not Provide Significant Protection

Heart disease is a serious problem for women. It kills more women over the age of 60 than any other disease. At half a million deaths, it dwarfs breast cancer, which will claim about 43,000 lives this year.

In 1994, a large-scale study called the Heart and Estrogen/Progestin Replacement Study (HERS) was begun at 20 medical centers across the United States. It was the second largest study of its type ever attempted. Funded by pharmaceutical giant Wyeth-Ayerst, every expectation was that HERS would prove that synthetic hormones would prevent heart attacks in postmenopausal women. Two thousand women with heart disease were put on "Prempro," a combination of Premarin and medroxyprogesterone acetate (a synthetic progestin). By 1998, the results were in: Prempro substantially increased heart attacks the first year and had no effect on heart attacks in subsequent years. Blood clots were 3 times higher in the group that took Prempro, and gall bladder disease was also increased.

A Nutritional Approach to Prevent and Treat Atherosclerosis

To prevent the known atherogenic factors from causing a heart attack, stroke, or other arterial occlusive disease, the following protocols should be followed:

To inhibit the oxidation of serum cholesterol, we suggest

- Life Extension Mix: 3 tablets, 3 times a day, preferably with meals. Life Extension Mix contains a potent spectrum of such antioxidants as vitamin E, vitamin C, folic acid, and B vitamins that have been shown to inhibit the oxidation of cholesterol. Life Extension Mix also contains trace minerals that have been shown to increase "good" cholesterol and decrease triglycerides and total cholesterol. Additionally, trace elements such as zinc and selenium are involved in the activity of antioxidant enzymes and may have a positive impact on those with severe hypercholesterolemia, according to a 1998 French study and a USDA study report in 1996.
- Coenzyme Q_{10}: 100 to 200 mg a day. CoQ_{10} works synergistically with vitamin E to prevent LDL cholesterol oxidation. CoQ_{10} also enhances heart cell energy function. CoQ_{10} in a base of rice bran oil should be used, based on studies showing superior assimilation and cardiac benefits.
- Life Extension Herbal Mix: 1 tablespoon early in the day. This formula contains plant extracts that have been documented to maintain the health of the vascular system and reduce the incidence of cardiovascular disease. Life Extension Herbal Mix contains pharmaceutical doses of such premium-grade herbal extracts as green tea, ginkgo biloba, ginseng, bilberry, and grape seed-skin extract. The suggested dose is one tablespoon mixed with water or juice early in the day.

To inhibit the formation of atherogenic homocysteine, we suggest

- Folic acid: 800 mcg with every meal. Folic acid has been shown to significantly lower blood levels of artery-clogging homocysteine. Use a folic acid supplement that also contains at least 1000 micrograms of vitamin B_{12}. Folic acid works synergistically with vitamin B_{12} to lower homocysteine levels.
- Vitamin B_6: 100 to 200 mg a day. Vitamin B_6 reduces homocysteine using a different mechanism than folic acid. There is enough vitamin B_6 in Life Extension Mix to keep homocysteine levels under control in most people. In the case of the disease called familial homocysteinemia, however, folate will not reduce homocysteine levels adequately, but doses of vitamin B_6 in excess of 250 to 500 mg daily can do so.

CAUTION: Since chronic high doses of vitamin B_6 can cause peripheral nerve toxicity, high doses (500 mg a day and higher) should only be used when a blood test documents the failure of folic acid to lower homocysteine levels.

- Trimethylglycine (TMG): 500 to 1500 mg a day with meals. TMG is the most effective homocysteine-lowering substance known. If homocysteine levels are too high, then up to 9000 mg of TMG may be needed along with higher amounts of other remethylation cofactors.

To inhibit the formation of blood clots inside arteries, we suggest

- Low-dose aspirin: take 1/4 aspirin tablet every day with the heaviest meal of the day.
- Perilla oil: take six 1000-mg capsules of perilla oil a day (provides 3300 mg of alpha-linoleic acid). (Fish or flax oils may work as well as perilla oil).
- Garlic: take 900 to 6000 mg a day.

- Trace minerals such as selenium (minimum 200 mcg per day), zinc (minimum 30 mg per day), chromium (200 mcg per day), and copper (1.5 mg a day—only if copper deficient).

To lower cholesterol levels, we suggest

- Artichoke extract: take 300 mg of a 15% chlorogenic acid artichoke extract, 3 times a day.
- Niacin: 1.5 to 3 grams a day (if tolerable).

Herbal Cardiovascular Formula contains potent extracts of ginger and curcumin. These extracts produce anti-inflammatory effects that may slow the progression of aortic stenosis. Ginger also inhibits abnormal platelet aggregation.

- Herbal Cardiovascular Formula: take 1 capsule in the morning and 1 in the evening. If your cholesterol levels are not significantly lower in 30 days, double or triple this dose.
- Soy protein concentrate: take 1 heaping tablespoon (10 to 20 grams) of soy protein powder containing a standardized amount of soy isoflavones such as genistein and daidzein. A product called Mega Soy Extract provides in two small capsules the amount of genistein and other isoflavones found in 10 to 20 grams of soy protein powder. It is not yet known if these two capsules of genistein extract will lower cholesterol levels. The Mega Soy Extract supplement is used primarily for cancer and osteoporosis risk reduction.

In addition to reducing cholesterol levels, soy protein has been shown to induce a significant improvement in insulin sensitivity, glucose effectiveness, fasting insulin levels, and insulin-to-glucose ratios. In female monkeys, soy genistein has been shown to enhance the dilator response to acetylcholine in atherosclerotic arteries. This means that the daily ingestion of soy could prevent sudden heart attack or stroke by processes other than its known cholesterol-lowering effect.

- Fiber: take 10 to 30 grams of soluble fibers, including pectins, guar, and psyllium. You can take fiber powder along with soy protein powder.

It should be recognized that there is an overlapping beneficial effect in the above recommendations. For instance, the homocysteine-reducing effect of folic acid can inhibit the progression of atherosclerosis and also reduce the risk of abnormal blood clots forming inside arteries. Folic acid, therefore, protects against heart attack and stroke via two well-documented mechanisms of action. Also, fish oil has been shown in published studies to reduce triglyceride levels by about 35% on average. Thus, fish oil may prevent abnormal arterial clotting and reduce triglyceride-induced arterial clogging.

(For information on aortic valve stenosis, refer to the Valvular Insufficiency / Heart Valve Defects protocol.)

Summary

The nutritional supplements discussed in this protocol are designed to prevent the development of atherosclerosis and arterial blockage by

1. Lowering and inhibiting the oxidation of LDL cholesterol.
2. Elevating beneficial HDL cholesterol.
3. Lowering serum triglycerides, fibrinogen, glucose, homocysteine, and iron levels.
4. Inhibiting blood clotting within blood vessels.

Please note that cholesterol levels below 180 mg/dL increase the risk of hemorrhagic stroke and premature death. Ideal cholesterol levels therefore may be between 180 and 200 mg/dL.

Following this protocol involves a lot of pill-taking. There are many factors that can cause atherosclerosis and abnormal blood clotting that can lead to a heart attack, stroke, and even diminished mental capacity. Failure to use the known "integrated therapies" could increase your disease risk to cardiovascular disease, or risk of a life-threatening cardiovascular event.

Many Foundation members already are following our atherosclerosis protocols because the same antioxidant nutrients used to prevent cardiovascular disease may also help to prevent cancer, cataract, Alzheimer's disease, and a host of other aging-related illnesses.

For more information. Contact the American Heart Association, Dallas, TX, (214) 373-6300.

Product availability. You can obtain Life Extension Mix, Coenzyme Q_{10}, Life Extension Herbal Mix, folic acid, vitamin B_6, fish oils, Herbal Cardiovascular Formula, garlic, fiber food, Artichoke extract, Healthprin (aspirin), perilla oil, TMG, niacin (vitamin B3), Super Soy Extract, and other supplements by calling (800) 544-4440 or order on-line at www.lef.org.

Blood testing availability. Homocysteine testing information and costs are available by calling (800) 208-3444, or review testing information and order on-line at www.lef.org/bloodtest.htm.

ATTENTION DEFICIT DISORDER

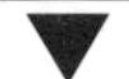

Attention Deficit Disorder (ADD) is characterized by a poor or short attention span and an impulsiveness that is inappropriate for a child's age. When children with symptoms of ADD are also hyperactive, the disorder is called attention deficit hyperactivity disorder (ADHD). Although ADD is commonly diagnosed in children, adults can suffer from it as well. The disorder is usually inherited and is often caused by abnormalities in neurotransmitters. There are three types of disorders: ADD without hyperactivity, ADD with hyperactivity, and ADD residual type. The latter applies when ADD persists into adulthood.

In Children

ADD affects 5 to 20% of school-aged children, with boys being diagnosed 10 times more often than girls. However, more conservative estimates put the figure at 3 to 5% as refinements have been made in diagnosing ADD. Signs of ADD can be noticed in children under the age of 4, but it is not until middle school that it can seriously interfere with performance. Symptoms of the disorder include a lack of sustained concentration, attention, and task completion. Impulsiveness and overactivity may also be present. Preschool-aged children with ADD may have difficulty communicating and interacting, and they may have associated behavior problems. Older children may constantly fidget and move hands and legs, talk impulsively, and forget easily.

About 20% of children with ADD also have learning disabilities and a full 90% have academic problems. Although typically not aggressive, children with the disorder may demonstrate conduct and behavioral problems. By adolescence, about 40% of young sufferers will be depressed, anxious, and confrontational. They will also display a low tolerance for frustration. It is important to note that other childhood problems can trigger what appear to be symptoms of ADD. These include physical and sexual abuse, family violence, tension, depression, and stress. Food allergies and sensitivities may also play a role in ADD-type symptoms, as discussed below. In addition, in recent years, many children have been labeled with ADD when their behavior is actually normal for their age or situation.

Diagnosis and Treatment

A child with suspected ADD must first be examined for the presence of physical disorders. Next, a battery of neuropsychiatric testing should be done by a clinician who has experience with the disorder. This is extremely important since ADD and ADHD have become "fad" diagnoses and are therefore easily overdiagnosed.

Traditional treatment is to manage ADD with medication, primarily the psychostimulant methylphenidate (Ritalin). The drug may improve attention and concentration in some children; however, many experts believe that Ritalin is overprescribed. Common side effects are sleep disturbances, insomnia, decreased appetite, depression, headaches, stomachaches, and high blood pressure. The drug therapy is usually combined with behavior therapy conducted by a psychologist, and parenting techniques that include providing a routine and structured environment.

Other stimulants such as dexadrine and cylert have been used. Since these drugs may decrease appetite, the child's weight and growth development should be followed closely.

Newly published research in the journal *Pediatric Neurology* indicates that antithyroid medications may be an effective treatment in some children. Researchers detected higher than normal thyroid hormone levels in three children aged 2 to 7 years exhibiting varying degrees of learning disabilities and diagnosed with ADHD. The children did not demonstrate physical signs of hyperthyroidism. After treatment with the anti-thyroid medication neomercazole, a decrease in hyperkinetic behavior and an increase in attention span was noted in all three children. When medication was stopped in one child, the hyperactive behavior returned, and again diminished upon reinstatement of medication. Due to the improvement in behavior, all three were able to participate in speech therapy. Although screening for elevated thyroid hormone levels may seem cost prohibitive, the researchers suggest that ". . . selective screening of children with familial attention deficit-hyperactivity disorder and those with ADHD in association with developmental learning disabilities and pervasive development disorders appears to be justified."

Nutrition and Food Allergies

Benjamin Feingold, M.D., was the first person to promote the idea that food additives might be responsible for causing the problem. Food additives are essentially anything that nature did not put in your food. Examples are food colorings, preservatives, bleaching agents, thickeners, and anti-caking agents. It is estimated that 8 to 10 pounds of food additives are consumed by each American every year. Feingold's work has created tremendous controversy in the past because many studies failed to support his observations. However, under closer scrutiny, these studies were faulty in terms of their design. As an example, one study compared a control group using chocolate cookies as a placebo. This was hardly an appropriate choice considering the fact that chocolate causes reactions in 30 to 60% of children depending upon the study. Additionally, cookies have ingredients and additives which may cause reactions according to Feingold's work. Therefore, the Feingold diet described below should be considered a place to start in treating both ADHD and ADD.

Studies done in the past 5 years have shown that the effects of diet, including adverse reactions to certain food products and additives, can play a significant role in triggering the symptoms of ADHD in children. A study on preschool-aged boys diagnosed with hyperactivity showed that elimination of food products containing substances such as artificial colors and flavors, monosodium glutamate, preservatives, chocolate, and caffeine produced reliable improvements in at least half the sample group studied. The 10-week study diet was also low in simple sugars and dairy free if a family history showed a possible reaction to cow's milk. In the study, other nonbehavior variables that improved included halitosis, night awakenings, and latency to sleep onset.

According to one study, sucrose, or table sugar, and artificial food dyes may play a role in the disorder. A study by Langseth and Dowd demonstrated abnormal glucose metabolism in 74% of the 261 hyperactive children he studied. The abnormality was reactive hypoglycemia, occurring when the child ate refined sugar, causing a large burst of insulin. This caused the glucose level (sucrose turns into glucose) to crash to low levels. This resulted in a burst of adrenaline, the fight-or-flight hormone.

Magnesium deficiency may also play a role in children with ADHD. In a study by English researchers, 50 hyperactive children, 7 to 12 years of age with recognized magnesium deficiency, were assessed after the addition of 200 mg a day of supplemental magnesium. The control group consisted of 25 children with diagnosed ADHD given no supplemental magnesium. In the group of children given magnesium independently of other mental disorders coexisting with hyperactivity, a significant decrease in hyperactivity was achieved compared to their clinical state before supplementation and compared with the control group that was not treated with magnesium.

Another 6-week study reported the effects of two nutritional products on the severity of symptoms in children with diagnosed ADHD. The dietary substances tested were a glyconutritional product containing saccharides that are known to be important to healthy functioning, and a phytonutritional product containing flash-dried fruits and vegetables. The test group consisted of 17 children: five were not taking methylphenidate, six were on full doses of methylphenidate, and six had their dosage cut in half 2 weeks into the study. The glyconutrition supplement decreased the number and severity of ADHD and associated Conduct Disorder (CD) and Oppositional Deficit Disorder (ODD) and side effects in all groups during the first 2 weeks of the study. There was little further improvement with the addition of the phytonutrient product. The results of the study suggest that symptoms of ADHD may be reduced by the addition to the diet of saccharides used by the body in glycoconjugate synthesis.

The first step is to determine if the child has allergies and/or sensitivities to certain foods or food additives. Dietary allergies cause more than skin rashes, asthma attacks, and intestinal disruptions. Studies have proven that many foods and food additives cause brain-wave disruptions so severe that a child cannot process in-coming information, exercise behavior self-control, or demonstrate emotion-based reasoning. The elimination diet that identifies foods or additives that may be causing neurological disruption is a simple method to follow. The Feingold Foundation suggests a very comprehensive elimination diet, but users must be aware that bovine dairy products are allowed on this diet. Since many children have mild to severe reactions to bovine dairy products, they may have to be eliminated at the very beginning of the diet to get accurate results. Once the child's diet is clear of all offenders, the body will be able to heal itself when given the proper supplemental nutrients.

For more information on the Feingold Foundation, write to P.O. Box 6550, Alexandria, VA, 22306, or call (800) 321-3287.

Once dietary problems have been identified and eliminated, the nutrients used by the body to increase memory and concentration, and to assist in emotional maturation, will need to be boosted. The most difficult aspect of using supplements is getting children to take them. The following is a list of supplements used by the body to increase neurotransmitters and memory function.

Life Extension Mix. Vitamin deficiency is common in children with learning difficulties. Unfortunately, most children do not like chewable vitamins. If you have a problem getting your child to take vitamins, try using 1 teaspoon of the Life Extension Mix powder with juice in a blender.

Choline Cooler. A product used to increase choline in the brain. Mixed with juice or water, Choline Cooler contains a synergistic blend of acetylcholine precursors that are ideal to boost memory and concentration.

Twin Lab Amino Fuel. 2 to 3 tablespoons before breakfast. Neurotransmitters are made from protein; protein is made from amino acids. It has been proven that children with no learning problems increase their concentration and memory skills with amino-acid supplementation. Amino acids also work on the nervous system to calm the body.

Cognitex. A formulation of memory-enhancing, brain-boosting nutrients. Be sure to get Cognitex *without* pregnenolone for children. If able to swallow capsules, the child should take 4 capsules before breakfast.

Udo's Choice Oil Blend. Essential fatty acids are necessary for proper growth and help to make prostaglandins that are essential for brain function. Essential fatty acids are a structural component of all brain cells, the blood-brain barrier, the myelin sheath that wraps around nerves, and cellular walls. Essential fatty acids comprise more than 50% of the brain itself, and help with nerve transmission.

Adapton. Most children with ADD/ADHD problems are under a tremendous amount of self-imposed stress. Adapton will calm the nervous system without sedation and works very well. A loading dose of 2 pills before breakfast and 2 pills after school for 14 days, followed by 2 pills before breakfast 3 days a week, is all that is necessary. Adapton works very well when combined with behavior training and diet.

Behavior Modification and Biofeedback

In addition to diet, behavior training is essential for successful treatment. ADD and ADHD children need structured daily routines. When the child is spoken to, he/she must look at the person speaking, and acknowledge what was said. Daily schedule and time limits must be set and adhered to for television, playtime, and bath time, so that the child becomes accustomed to following a set order of activities such as school, playtime, dinner, homework, bath, and bed. His/her school day is structured and home time should be as well. Most ADD/ADHD children are "creatures of habit," and a set routine is vital to their emotional and mental security.

A very exciting, promising form of treatment that is showing success in the treatment of ADD/ADHD is electroencephalograph (EEG) biofeedback based on the work of Dr. Eugene Pennisten. Children with ADD/ADHD are taught how to enter a very specific brainwave state called alpha/theta that is a rate of 4 to 6 cyavioles per second. This is a very specialized state and has dramatic effects on behavior. Dr. Pennestin has been successful in treating alcoholism with this modality. While relatively new to ADD/ADHD treatment, it has been used in several inner-city schools with astounding success. The teachers and special education counselors are reporting students are more emotionally centered and focused on school work with little to no teacher intervention to complete assignments. Parents are reporting that children formerly on drug therapy no longer need the drug to function. In one school district, neurofeedback has kept 20 out of 60 students treated with EEG out of expensive special education classrooms. Remember that food allergies and diet must go hand in hand with any outside treatment to obtain optimal results.

For more information on EEG biofeedback, contact EEG Spectrum, 16100 Ventura Blvd, Suite #3, Encino, California, 91436-2505; phone (818) 789-349; fax: (818) 788-6137.

ADD in Adults

The focus of this protocol has been aimed at children with ADD. However, many experts believe that some form of the disorder will continue into adulthood. Adults with ADD may be highly disorganized, prone to outbursts of temper, and feel they are not able to adequately cope with the stresses of life. Other problems may surface that include low self-esteem, anxiety, depression, and inappropriate behavior in social situations. Left untreated, difficulties may also be manifested in drug or alcohol problems and personal relationships. Although academic failure may persist throughout adulthood, individuals with ADD seem to function better in work than in school situations. An adult that exhibits symptoms of ADD that interferes with work or daily life should consult a mental health professional.

The following recommended reading is available from the Life Extension Foundation:

What's Food Got To Do with It?, Hills, Wyman
No More Ritalin, Dr. Mary A. Block
Nutrition and Behavior, Keats Publishing

Summary

ADD affects 3 to 5% of school-aged children and can seriously affect behavior and academic achievement. The disorder is treated primarily with the psychostimulants Ritalin, amphetamine, and cylert, combined with behavior modification and establishing a routine structured environment. Food allergies and nutritional deficiencies are shown to trigger symptoms of ADD and hyperactivity in some children, indicating that a change in diet may be the more appropriate treatment in these cases.

1. Life Extension Mix, 1 tsp. mixed with juice.
2. Choline Cooler, 1 tablespoon mixed with water or juice.
3. Twin Lab Amino Fuel, 2 to 3 tablespoons.
4. Cognitex, 4 capsules before breakfast.
5. Udo's Choice Oil Blend, 1 tablespoon of oil or 12 capsules.
6. Adapton, a loading dose of 2 pills before breakfast and 2 pills after school for 14 days, followed by 2 pills before breakfast 3 days a week.
7. No sugar.

8. Consider allergy testing.
9. Feingold-type elimination diet.
10. Consider alpha/theta biofeedback training.

For more information. Contact Children and Adults with Attention Deficit Disorder (CHADD), (800) 233-4050.

Product availability. Cognitex, Udo's Choice Oil Blend, Choline Cooler, and Life Extension Mix are available by calling (800) 544-4440, or order on-line at www.lef.org. Ask for a list of offshore pharmacies that sell piracetam to Americans for personal use.

AUTISM

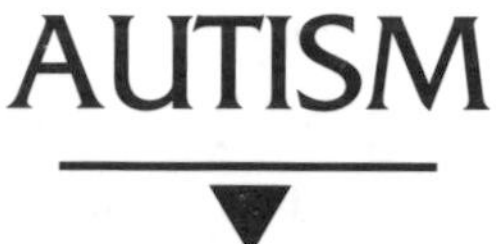

Autism is a genetic mental ailment or syndrome that manifests during the first 2 years of life. Persons afflicted with autism are found to be chronically deficient in neurons in an area in the brain. This characterizes a developmental disability resulting in a neurological disorder that affects functioning of the brain. However, recent biochemical and genetic studies have led to the hypothesis that the disorder is due to an organic defect in brain development. Autism is thought to be a result of abnormal serotonin metabolism in the brain. Autism has been estimated to occur in as many as 1 in 500 births, and 80% of autistic children born with this syndrome are males with low body weight implications at birth; the lower the birth weight the higher the risk of autism.

Diagnostic Summary

A syndrome of early childhood (first diagnosed no later than 30 months) autism is characterized by (1) failure to develop social relationships, (2) language disorder with impaired understanding, (3) compulsive phenomena, and (4) retardation in intellectual development.

The male to female ratio of children born with autism is 4 to 1. There are other ailments that resemble autism such as Rett's syndrome, a rare neurological disorder that affects only girls.

Demographics

Over one half million people in the United States today have some form of autism. It's the third most common developmental disability and is more common than Down's syndrome.

Professionals in the medical, educational, and vocational fields remain unaware of how autism affects people and how to work effectively with individuals with autism. Phenothiazines are used to control severe forms of aggressive and self-destructive behavior, but they do not abort the psychosis. Although not effective for all autistic children, vitamin B_6 and magnesium, when used in combination, have been shown in a number of studies to greatly help a significant portion of autistic individuals.

Social Impact

Autism affects the normal development of the brain in the areas of social interaction and communication skills. Autistic individuals have difficulty with verbal and nonverbal communication, social interactions, and leisure activities. In some cases, aggressive and/or self-injurious behavior may be present.

Causes and Prevention

Although researchers are unsure of what causes autism, studies suggest that autism might be caused by biological factors that include metabolic disorders, infant vaccinations, food allergies, viral infections, fetal alcohol syndrome, lead poisoning, decreased brain stem size, defective nerve fibers, parasite infestation, and yeast infections.

Scientists believe they may have found the genes that are responsible for autism; knowledge of these genes might help doctors diagnose the disorder in other children in the near future. Other research studies have found that people with autism have problems in several parts of their brain. These studies indicate that autism may be caused by abnormal brain development before birth or trauma during birth delivery.

Researchers also are learning how certain physical factors may affect later behavior. For example, poor dietary management affects the way that autistic children process information, thus preventing them from normal social interactions and the ability to pay attention to other people. This in turn may cause poor development of social skills, knowledge, and awareness.

Scientists have also identified chemicals in the brain and the immune system that may be involved in autistic syndrome. During normal development of the brain, the level of the chemical serotonin declines. In some children with autistic disorder, however, the serotonin levels do not decline. Researchers are now trying to determine whether this only happens to children with autism, why, and other factors that may be involved.

Therapeutic Considerations

Abnormalities in serotonin metabolism that have been documented in autistic individuals include abnormal release and uptake of serotonin by platelets, abnormal kynurenine metabolism, increased serum serotonin and free tryptophan levels, abnormal urinary 5-hydroxyindolacetic acid (5-HIAA) levels, and abnormal urinary serotonin metabolites. The basic defect appears to be a decrease in central nervous system (CNS) serotonin activity despite elevated free tryptophan levels in the serum.

The following are possible mechanisms of action that have been suggested to explain the brain-serotonin hypoactivity seen in autism:

- Reduced tryptophan hydroxylase or *L*-aromatic amino acid decarboxylase activity results in impaired serotonin synthesis and, via feedback control, leads to increased serum free tryptophan levels.
- Increased tryptophan oxygenase activity results in high levels of kynurenine, which reduces the available tryptophan for serotonin synthesis and inhibits tryptophan transport across the blood-brain barrier. In turn, increased free tryptophan levels result in increased tryptophan oxygenase activity, thus setting up a positive feedback cycle.

These two theories are the most plausible and the most supported in the scientific literature. They are discussed below in conjunction with the therapeutic approaches that have been shown to normalize the aberrations. The metabolic pathways of tryptophan, serotonin, and their metabolites are too complex to be discussed in this protocol.

Vitamin B_{12}, Folic Acid, and Vitamin C

If the metabolic defect is due to a decrease in tryptophan hydroxylase metabolic activity (a tetrahydrobiopterin-[BH4] dependent enzyme), supplementation with folic acid, ascorbic acid, and B_{12} may increase the activity of tryptophan hydroxylase by increasing BH4. Although no studies have been done with autistic children, increasing CNS BH4 levels has offered some benefit in patients with affective disorders and Parkinson's disease.

Pyridoxine Paradox

If the metabolic defect is in the decarboxylation or the abnormal kynurenine metabolism, pyridoxine supplementation is indicated. Pyridoxine supplementation of autistic children has been investigated in several double-blind clinical studies. The results indicate that there is a subgroup that improves with B_6 supplementation and shows significantly reduced levels of urinary HVA. About 20% of autistics will show moderate improvement in symptom scores, while about 10% will demonstrate dramatic clinical improvement. It has also been observed that B_6 supplementation has a greater effect when used in combination with magnesium.

A 1985 study of 60 autistic children used four crossed-sequential, double-blind therapeutic trials. The children were divided into two groups and given various combinations of vitamin B_6, magnesium, and placebo. Therapeutic effects were measured using behavioral rating scales, urinary excretion of homovanillic acid (HVA), and evoked potential recordings (EP). The combination of B_6 and magnesium resulted in significant improvement in behavior that was closely associated with decreases in HVA excretion and a normalized EP amplitude and morphology. However, magnesium and vitamin B_6 were not significantly effective when used alone.

The tryptophan load test may be indicated as a screening test for B_6-responsive patients and as a monitor of B_6 dosage. Although B_6 may not result in a cure of autism, sufficient evidence exists to support a clinical trial in which improvement may be noted. Rimland pioneered the use of pyridoxine in treating autistic children. His findings show that a quarter to half of the children were significantly helped, and about 20% showed dramatic improvement.

Allergy-Induced Autism

In allergy-induced autism, the symptoms become apparent during early infant life. The children have several almost unnoticeable physical problems, including excessive thirst, excessive sweating (especially at night), low blood sugar, diarrhea, bloating, rhinitis, inability to control temperature, red face and/or ears, and dark circles under the eyes.

Some children have autism that has been triggered by intolerance to foods and/or chemicals, the main offenders being wheat, dairy products, corn, sugar, and citrus fruits, although each child's allergies may be affected by different substances.

Vitamin Therapy

Dimethylglycine (DMG) is a food substance and is most often used for the nutritional deficiencies of autistic individuals as part of their vitamin/mineral therapy. DMG is found in small amounts in brown rice and liver. Its chemical make-up resembles that of water-soluble vitamins, specifically vitamin B_{15}. DMG does not require a prescription, and it is available through the Life Extension Foundation. There are no apparent side effects.

For the autistic child, one-half of a 125-mg tablet at breakfast should be administered for a few days. It may be advisable to increase to 1 to 4 tablets a day if the results are positive. Reports from parents giving their children DMG indicate improvements in the areas of speech, eye contact, social behavior, and attention span. Two weeks after starting on the DMG, B_6 and magnesium can be added. Studies have shown that vitamin B_6 may help control hyperactivity and improve overall behavior. Although improvements vary considerably among individuals, other possible improvements are speech improvements, improved sleeping patterns, lessened irritability, increased attention span, decrease in self-stimulation, and overall improvement in general health. The information for developing an effective therapy for autism is incomplete at best. Tremendous amounts of research need to be done. Despite these limitations, the following suggestions may offer some improvement in the condition.

Diet

Eliminate those factors that play a role in aggravating CNS dysfunction in autistic children. Remember that the autistic child has a weak stomach. The permeability of the lining of their digestive system allows for food to enter into the bloodstream, thus causing brain allergies, the primary cause of autism.

Supplements

The doses given below are general levels suitable for children ages 2 and 6.

- Vitamin C, 1 gram a day
- Pyridoxal phosphate, 5 to 20 mg a day
- Pyridoxine (vitamin B_6), 25 to 100 mg a day
- Folic acid, 400 mcg a day
- Vitamin B_{12}, 500 mcg a day
- Magnesium, 75 to100 mg a day

Anti-Yeast Therapy

There is some evidence that *Candida albicans* may exacerbate behavior and cause health problems in autistic individuals. An overgrowth of *Candida albicans* causes toxins to be released into the body that are known to impair the central nervous system and the immune system. Some of the behaviors related to this are confusion, hyperactivity, short attention span, lethargy, irritability, and aggression. Reported health problems can include headaches, intestinal problems (constipation, diarrhea, flatulence), distended stomach, and cravings for carbohydrates, fruits, and sweets. Unpleasant odor of hair and feet, acetone smell from mouth, and skin rashes may also be present. Candida overgrowth is often attributed to long-term antibiotic treatments. These clinical observations suggest an association between gastrointestinal and brain function in patients with autistic behavior.

Secretin: "The New Hope"

At the department of pediatrics of the University of Maryland School of Medicine, three children with autistic spectrum disorders underwent upper gastrointestinal endoscopy and intravenous administration of secretin to stimulate pancreaticobiliary secretion. All three had an increased pancreaticobiliary secretory response when compared with nonautistic patients (7.5 to 10 mL/min versus 1 to 2 mL/min). Within 5 weeks of the secretin infusion, a significant amelioration of the children's gastrointestinal symptoms was observed, as was a dramatic improvement in their behavior, manifested by improved eye contact, alertness, and expansion of expressive language.

Secretin is a polypeptide neurotransmitter involved in digestion. This agent has been approved by the Food and Drug Administration for use in the diagnosis of gastrointestinal problems in adults; repeated use has not been approved by the FDA. Several anecdotal reports have suggested that secretin may ameliorate some of the symptoms of autism, and one open study of three children has been reported. The mechanism of action is unclear; there are not yet appropriate controlled studies that support the use of this agent, nor has it been determined that it is safe for repeated administration. Accordingly, the use of this agent should be considered unproven and experimental.

Summary

1. Dimethylglycine (DMG), one half of a 125 mg tablet at breakfast to be increased to up to 4 tablets a day if improvements are seen.
2. Vitamin C, 1 gram a day.
3. Pyridoxal phosphate, 5 to 20 mg a day.
4. Pyridoxine (vitamin B_6), 25 to 100 mg a day.
5. Folic acid, 500 mcg a day.
6. Vitamin B_{12}, 500 mcg a day.
7. Magnesium, 75 to 100 mg a day.
8. Allergies may play a significant role in autistic behavior. Testing and the elimination of potentially harmful food products is recommended.
9. The presence of elevated levels of the yeast, *Candida* may exacerbate health and behavior problems in autistic children. Testing is recommended.

For more information. Contact the Autism Society of America, (800) 328-8476.

Product availability. DMG; vitamins B_6, B_{12}, and C; folic acid; and magnesium are available by phoning (800) 544-4440, or order on-line at www.lef.org.

AUTOIMMUNE DISEASES

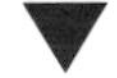

Autoimmune diseases are characterized by the body's immune responses being directed against its own tissues, resulting in inflammation and destruction. A wide range of degenerative diseases are caused as a result. Immune dysfunction can cause immune responsive cells to attack the linings of the joints, resulting in rheumatoid arthritis, or prompt defectively functioning immune cells to attack the insulin-producing islet cells of the pancreas, resulting in insulin-dependent diabetes.

A healthy immune system first recognizes bacteria, viruses, and cancer cells that are not normally present in the body and then attacks and destroys the foreign agents using a variety of mechanisms, such as engulfing. A defective immune system, on the other hand, wreaks havoc throughout the body.

There is a whole class of degenerative diseases that are caused by changes in the immune system that result in the immune system attacking normal cells in the body. Any disease is considered autoimmune if antibodies of cytotoxic cells are directed against self-antigens in the body's own tissues. Diseases such as lupus erythematosus, autoimmune hepatitis, diabetes, pancreatitis, and rheumatoid arthritis can develop and become dangerous diseases requiring drastic measures to control and correct. Allergy is also the result of disordered immune function. Additionally, there are other diseases that may be the result of autoimmune dysfunction, such as multiple sclerosis.

Aging

Age is an important factor in the appearance of autoimmune diseases. However, some people experience these types of diseases very early in life. The immune system may also be suppressed or weakened as a result of factors not associated with a degenerative disease but due to the intake of alcohol, caffeine, tobacco, drugs, sugar, and of course poor diet and lack of sleep. These lifestyle factors can have a substantial effect on the trends of autoimmune diseases.

As we age, our autoimmune system declines in its effectiveness due in large part to oxidative damage caused by the recurrent presence of significant amounts of free radicals. This kind of oxidative damage has been implicated in such autoimmune diseases as rheumatoid arthritis, autoimmune hepatitis, and lupus.

Basic Pathways of Autoimmune Dysfunction

Autoimmune diseases tend to be viewed as separate entities. A broader perspective, however, may reveal shared mechanisms that are the cause of disease, rather than just its by-product. If this perspective were applied, patients would benefit from improved therapies and early intervention, before the development of irreversible tissue damage. As reported in the journal *Hospital Practice,* Dr. Majid Ali has long considered that there must be a single initial common pathway to all disease, including immune dysfunction.

Of concern is the fact that our environment—our air, water and food in particular—is full of toxic substances. There is no doubt that these toxins play a role in immune dysfunction. Even substances considered by most people as safe to eat actually impair immune function. Glucose, fructose, and sucrose are all forms of sugar. Eating 100 grams will impair the ability of white cells to destroy biological agents. The effect begins within a half hour and lasts for 5 hours. After 2 hours, there is a 50% reduction in immune function. Other factors that decrease immune function are obesity, eating excess fats and alcohol, and stress and fatigue.

The Effect of Natural Supplements on the Autoimmune System

The autoimmune system needs a good nutritional foundation over a long period of time to alleviate or reverse lifestyle autoimmune dysfunction and to assist with combating fully developed autoimmune diseases. The fundamental causal basis for autoimmune system boosting was shown in a study that was designed to measure the serum concentrations of vitamin E, beta-carotene, and vitamin A in patients prior to developing rheumatoid arthritis or systemic lupus erythematosus. Two to fifteen years after the volunteer patients had originally donated their blood to the serum bank (1974), the serum samples were assayed for vitamin E, beta-carotene, and vitamin A. Those patients who developed rheumatoid arthritis or lupus showed lower serum concentrations of vitamin E, beta-carotene, and vitamin A in their serum from 1974. Those who had the lowest serum level of beta-carotene in 1974 were the most likely to develop rheumatoid arthritis later in life. This indicates the long-term importance of maintaining adequate vitamin status for the prevention of autoimmune diseases.

Vitamin C also plays an important role in immune function; intravenous administration of large doses of vitamin C can stimulate healthy immune function in patients.

In a study conducted at the University of Texas Health Sciences Center (*Lipids,* 1994), it was found that fish oil containing vitamin E delayed the onset of autoimmune diseases in autoimmune-prone mice. Another study on the effects of vitamin E deficiency was conducted in the United Kingdom and published in *Inflammation Research* (1995). It was found that dietary components that alter the antioxidant/oxidant status may contribute to the treatment of inflammatory/autoimmune diseases.

Supplementation with omega-3 essential fatty acids from fish, flax, or perilla oils—along with borage oil, evening primrose oil, or black currant seed oil, which contain the essential omega-6 fatty acid gamma-linoleic acid (GLA)—can alleviate many symptoms of autoimmune disease through their anti-inflammatory activity.

One protocol used with a great deal of success involves daily supplementation with 4 capsules a day of a concentrated fish oil encapsulated supplement called Mega EPA, along with 5 capsules a day of a borage oil preparation called Mega GLA. These two oils provide the essential fatty acids that have been shown to favorably modulate immune function and help correct autoimmune disease. For those who don't like fish oil supplements, flax or perilla oils can be substituted. When consuming supplemental oils, it is especially important to protect the body from excessive oxidation that would normally occur in response to ingestion of these fatty acids. Most members of The Life Extension Foundation take 3 tablets, 3 times a day of an antioxidant preparation called Life Extension Mix that provides ideal doses of free-radical-suppressing nutrients, including vitamin E, beta-carotene, and selenium. In general, a good ratio for essential fatty acid supplementation is two parts of an omega-3 rich essential fatty acid supplement to one part of a supplement rich in omega-6 essential fatty acid. Omega-6 essential fatty acid taken alone can follow a pro-inflammatory pathway that is blocked by the omega-3 essential fatty acids by inhibiting the delta-5 desaturation enzyme system.

L-carnitine has been shown to reduce the impairment of immune function caused by the dangerous fats found in the typical American diet. This is probably due to *L*-carnitine's ability to lower serum lipids (fats) by enhancing the transport of fatty acids into the cell's mitochondria, where they are used to produce energy. Acetyl-*L*-carnitine is the most effective form of *L*-carnitine.

The trace element selenium showed promise according to a study conducted in Würzburg, Germany, and cited in *Medizinische Klinik* (Germany), 1997. Selenoproteins (such as selenomethionine) were shown to block cell damage caused by environmental peroxides, and these selenium compounds were found to aid in the "prevention and therapy of metabolic bone disease as well as chronic (autoimmune) inflammation."

Those with existing autoimmune diseases may need more than essential fatty acids and antioxidant supplements to gain control over their disease. The hormone DHEA can suppress certain unwanted immune-system reactions in patients with autoimmune diseases by blocking the action of a cytokine called interleukin-6.

Intestinal dysbiosis, or leaky gut syndrome with increased intestinal permeability, is thought to play a role in some autoimmune diseases (by allowing bacterial and other antigens similar to self-antigens in some tissues to penetrate and simulate an autoimmune response). Eating a healthy diet, the use of a probiotic such as Life Flora, and nutritional support for friendly bacteria such as NutraFlora are desirable, as is avoidance of excessive exposure to antibiotics, alcohol, aspirin, nonsteroidal anti-inflammatory drugs, and other agents which may alter intestinal-wall permeability and the normal ecology of the bowel bacterial flora.

Other Considerations

To prevent and treat immune dysfunction it is important to get regular exercise; even walking will do. Sleep is also very important. One of the major contributors to immune dysfunction is stress. The mechanism is simple. Prolonged, even low-level stress stimulates the adrenal glands to produce cortisol, which in excess impairs immune function. Depression and emotional distress are also contributors to immune dysfunction. There is a connection between the limbic system and the part of the brain from which emotions arise. Limbic function affects immune function. One of the ways to deal with stress and directly with immune function is guided imagery and biofeedback. Therefore, stress reduction is a must for treating immune dysfunction. Poor thyroid function can also contribute to impaired immune function since many autoimmune processes are involved in many thyroid diseases.

Summary

Autoimmune diseases may be prevented by adopting a healthy lifestyle, a nutritional diet, and by boosting the strength of the autoimmune system with supplements. Those with developed autoimmune diseases such as lupus, pancreatitis, and rheumatoid arthritis—or those whose autoimmune systems are degraded because of toxic substances such as tobacco and alcohol—can also use supplements to suppress autoimmune diseases. The protocols needed may include the supplements listed below as well as prescription drugs.

1. To decrease oxidative damage associated with autoimmune dysfunction, dietary supplements of vitamins A, C, E, and beta-carotene should be taken daily.
2. Life Extension Mix containing the above vitamins along with the trace element selenium should help favorably modulate immune function.
3. Mega EPA (4 capsules daily) and Mega GLA (5 capsules daily), which contain the essential fatty acids, will alleviate symptoms of immune dysfunction.
4. DHEA, 25 to 50 mg a day (*refer to DHEA Replacement Therapy protocol for precautions*).

Product availability. Mega EPA, Mega GLA, DHEA, and Life Extension Mix can be obtained by calling (800) 540-4440, or order on-line at www.lef.org.

BACTERIAL INFECTIONS

Bacterial infections are caused by the presence and growth of microorganisms that damage host tissue. The extent of infection is generally determined by how many organisms are present and how virulent (toxic) they are. Worldwide, bacterial infections are responsible for more deaths than any other cause. Symptoms can include inflammation and swelling, pain, heat, redness, and loss of function. The most important risk factors are burns, severe trauma, low white blood cell counts, very old or young patients, patients on immunotherapy treatment, and anyone suffering from malnutrition or vitamin deficiency.

Bacteria are generally spread from an already infected person to the newly infected person. The most common invasion routes are inhalation of airborne bacteria, ingestion into the stomach from dirty hands or utensils or through contaminated food or water, direct contact with an infected area of another person's body, contaminated blood, and by insect bite.

The first of the body's three primary lines of defense includes naturally occurring chemicals such as the lysozymes found in tears, gastric acid of the stomach, pancreatic enzymes of the bowel, and fatty acids in the skin. The body's immune response becomes involved only if the infective organism manages to invade the body. Nonspecific immune response (the body's second line of defense) consists primarily of inflammation, whereas specific immune response (the third line of defense) relies on the activation of lymphocytes, which send T- and B-cells to try to recognize the specific type of organism involved. T-cells marshal cytotoxic cells, which are sent to destroy the organism, and B-cells produce the antibodies (immunoglobulins) that can destroy specific types of bacteria. (*For more information about preventing infections in general, please refer to the Foundation's Immune Enhancement protocols.*)

Acute bacterial infections require immediate conventional medical care. If FDA-approved antibiotics fail to work, European antibiotics, which are several years more advanced than American antibiotics, may be effective.

Limitations of Modern Antibiotics

When antibiotics were discovered in the 1940s, they were incredibly effective in the treatment of many bacterial infections. Over time many antibiotics have lost their effectiveness against certain strains of bacteria, as resistant strains have developed, mostly through the use of "resistance genes." In 1998 a potentially deadly bacterium, *Staphylococcus aureus* ("staph"), which causes widespread nosocomial (infections contracted in a hospital or clinic) infections, failed to respond to the most potent antibiotic vancomycin. The most troubling aspect was that this failure occurred in three patients in widely separated geographic areas.

There are several ways in which bacteria are becoming resistant to antibiotic therapy. One is that some bacteria have now developed "efflux" pumps. When the bacterium recognizes invasion by an antibiotic, the efflux pump simply pumps the antibiotic out of its cells. Resistance genes code for more than pumps, though. Some lead to the manufacture of enzymes that degrade or chemically alter (and therefore inactivate) the antibiotic. Where do these resistance genes come from? Usually, bacteria actually get them from other bacteria. In some cases they pick up a gene containing plasmid from a "donor" cell. Also, viruses have been shown to extract a resistance gene from one bacterium and inject it into a different one. Furthermore, some bacteria "scavenge" DNA from dead cells around them, and occasionally, scavenged genes are incorporated in a stable manner into the recipient cell's chromosome or into a plasmid and become a part of the recipient bacterium. A few resistance genes develop through random mutations in the bacterium's DNA.

Recent research shows great promise for a novel concept: the introduction of susceptible strains of bacteria following treatment by antibiotics. The idea is for the susceptible strain to colonize the resistant strain. The resulting colony is then antibiotic sensitive.

New Wonder Drugs?

As the problems of antibiotic resistance become ever more global, scientists see an increasing role for aminoglycosides in clinical practice. Aminoglycosides are chemical compounds that are present in a variety of antibiotics. Some are derived naturally from microorganisms, while others are synthesized. Their broad antimicrobial spectrum and ability to act synergistically with other drugs make them very useful in treating serious nosocomial infections. Though aminoglycosides show great promise, more research is needed before they will become widely available.

The Last Line of Antibiotic Defense

When a patient is faced with a life-threatening staph or other bacterial infection that is resistant to all other known antibiotics, the last drug of choice is called Vancocin (vancomycin). This potentially lethal drug must be administered by a bolus injection in a hospital setting because it has so many side effects. Vancocin is not systemically effective when administered orally. Vancocin is the drug to ask your doctor for when all else fails.

Herbal and Natural Alternatives

Researchers around the world are taking another look at folk medicine, herbal remedies, and other alternatives to pharmacological drugs. Recent research has confirmed the antibacteriological value of herbal extracts from many parts of the world. Examples of useful herbal remedies abound. Herbal extracts from goldenseal and echinacea may be effective natural antibiotics. Raw garlic has potent antibacterial effects. Kyolic, an aged garlic product, does not kill bacteria directly but does boost immune function, enabling the body to fight off some chronic bacterial infections.

Alkylglycerols

Alkylglycerols, or AKGs, are a family of compounds that have been found to play a crucial role in the production and stimulation of white blood cells. They occur in freshwater fish and in cow, sheep, and mother's milk. AKGs help give nursing mammals, including breast-fed babies, protection against infection until their own immune systems can develop fully. Alkylglycerols are thought to act as immune boosters against infectious diseases. No side effects have been seen in patients taking 100 mg 3 times a day. Shark liver oil capsules containing a minimum of 200 mg of alkylglycerols per capsule, at the dose of 5 capsules a day, can have a direct antibiotic effect.

CAUTION: Do not take shark liver oil for more than 30 days because it may cause overproduction of blood platelets.

Enzymes

Bromelain, a proteolytic digestive enzyme, can potentiate (augment or strengthen) the effects of conventional antibiotics, making them more effective in killing bacteria. (Proteolytic substances contribute to the hydrolysis of proteins or peptides and help form simpler, soluble products.) It should be taken with meals. The suggested dose is 2000 mg a day of a highly concentrated bromelain.

Amino Acids

Arginine, a crystalline basic amino acid derived from guanidine, can stimulate antibacterial components of the immune system when taken in doses ranging from 6 to 20 grams per day. Arginine promotes the synthesis of nitric oxide, which is believed to help protect against bacterial infections. The role of nitric oxide was studied in host defense against *Klebsiella pneumoniae* infection of the lung. The results suggested that nitric oxide plays a critical role in antibacterial host defense against *Klebsiella pneumoniae,* in part by regulating macrophage phagocytic and microbicidal activity.

Fruit Juice

Cranberry juice has proven to be an effective nondrug therapy against urinary tract infections. The active ingredients of the juice keep bacteria from attaching to the walls of the bladder and urinary tract. Recent research concludes that cranberry juice also helps to prevent the formation of dental plaque, which can eventually lead to tooth decay. Because the recommended daily intake of juice is so great, the Life Extension Foundation suggests a dietary supplement called Cran-Max Cranberry Juice Concentrate that provides the equivalent of sixteen 8-ounce glasses of cranberry juice in just 1 capsule. One capsule a day provides the equivalent of the recommended amount of cranberry juice for proven results in fighting urinary tract infections.

Honey and Bee Propolis

Before the discovery of antibiotics, honey was known to have antibacterial properties. Recent research has confirmed those earlier findings. In addition, recent electron microscope studies show that bee propolis has a potent antibacterial effect by preventing cell division and inhibiting protein synthesis.

CAUTION: Bee products should not be administered to children under the age of three.

Trace Elements

Zinc has been found to potentiate antiseptic agents. A South African study concluded that zinc is also critical in the maintenance of a healthy immune system. Life Extension Mix contains zinc as well as other supplements needed to maintain immunity.

Conclusion

Ironically, the advent of the new "miracle drugs," the antibiotics developed in the 1940s and since, also set the stage for drug-resistant bacteria that do not respond to antibiotics. Avoiding or neutralizing bacterial infections requires a strong, effective immune response. Research demonstrates preventive benefits from herbal and natural alternatives. These include alkylglycerols, enzymes, amino acids, the active ingredients in fruit juice, honey and bee propolis, and trace elements. Advanced European antibiotics and natural and herbal remedies can provide effective treatment when FDA-approved American antibiotics fail.

Summary

1. The primary symptom of bacterial infection is inflammation. Other symptoms are swelling, fever, pain, heat, redness, and loss of function.
2. Positive diagnosis of an infection (such as strep throat) often requires a culture or blood workup.
3. With the arrival of drug-resistant bacteria, prevention becomes more important than ever. The body's immune system can be strengthened by vitamin and trace-element supplementation. Three Life Extension Mix tablets 3 times a day (at meal times) provide all essential vitamins and trace elements for basic immune-system health.
4. Life Extension Herbal Mix incorporates 27 different herbs with demonstrated therapeutic value into a powder designed to make one daily drink. One teaspoon a day mixed in fruit juice supplies immune-enhancing nutrients.
5. Shark liver oil contains alkylglycerols, a family of compounds proven beneficial to the production and stimulation of white blood cells; 1000 mg a day of shark liver oil capsules can have a direct antibiotic effect.
6. Bromelain, a proteolytic digestive enzyme, augments conventional antibiotics and makes them more effective in killing bacteria. The suggested dose is 2000 mg a day with meals.
7. Arginine, an amino acid, stimulates the immune system's antibacterial components when taken at the rate of 6 to 20 grams per day.
8. The active ingredients of cranberry juice, fructose, and an unidentified polymer, simply prevent harmful bacteria from adhering to the walls of the urinary tract, preventing and actually helping to cure urinary tract infections. These ingredients have also been found to help prevent dental cavities. Cranex, a purified extract of cranberry juice, contains the equivalent of eight glasses of juice in each capsule. The recommended dose is two capsules a day.
9. Both honey and bee propolis are known to have antibacteriological properties. They work by preventing bacterial cell division and inhibiting protein synthesis.

CAUTION: Do not administer bee products to children under the age of three.

10. Zinc potentiates antiseptic agents and is critical to the maintenance of a healthy immune system. When treating a bacterial infection, 90 to 120 mg a day of zinc is suggested.

Product availability. Life Extension Mix, Life Extension Herbal Mix, Kyolic garlic, Norwegian shark liver oil, bromelain, echinacea, arginine, Cran-Max Cranberry Juice Concentrate, and bee propolis can be obtained by calling (800) 544-4440, or by ordering online at www.lef.org. Ask for a listing of offshore companies that sell European antibiotics.

BALDNESS

Description

Baldness, the loss of hair, is in most cases a cosmetic problem. It is more common in men than women. There are different forms of baldness: male-pattern baldness, female-pattern baldness, toxic baldness, alopecia areata, alopecia universalis, alopecia totalis, trichotillomania, and scarring alopecia. There is no known cure for baldness. Hair loss can be responsible for depression, feelings of inadequacy, and low self-esteem.

Types of Hair Loss

Baldness is usually the result of genetic factors, aging, local skin conditions, diseases, and the taking of certain medicines. Balding is always symmetrical in both male- and female-pattern baldness. If hair loss is nonsymmetrical, e.g., hair loss on only one side of the head, there more than likely is another reason and a biopsy may have to be performed.

Male-Pattern Baldness

Male-pattern baldness, the most common type of balding in men, is controlled by a single dominant autosomal gene. This type of balding usually starts at the temples, then will gradually recede to form an "M" shape on the head. The hair on the top of the head will start to thin out. Over time, the male is left with a horseshoe-shaped pattern of hair around his head. Some males will have only a receding hairlines or bald spots on the crowns of their heads. The hair that remains in the balding areas starts out as long, thick, and pigmented and changes into fine, unpigmented sprouts that grow at a slower rate. If a man begins losing his hair during his mid-teen years, there is a good chance he will go completely bald on top of his head.

Androgenic alopecia is another factor that can cause male-pattern baldness. Androgenic alopecia is caused by three factors: advanced age, an inherited tendency to bald early, and an overabundance of dihydrotestosterone (DHT), a highly active form of testosterone within the hair follicle. DHT influences male behavior, from the sex drive to aggression. Testosterone converts to DHT by 5-alpha reductase, an enzyme produced in the prostate, various adrenal glands, and the scalp. What appears to happen is that DHT (and perhaps other androgenic hormones) causes the immune system to react to the hair follicles in the affected areas as foreign bodies. This is suggested by the presence of hair-follicle antibodies, as well as by the infiltration of immune system cells around the hair follicles of balding men (as well as women).

Female-Pattern Baldness

Female-pattern baldness is caused by aging, genetic susceptibility, and levels of endocrine hormones known as androgens. This type of balding usually begins around the age of 30 and becomes more noticeable at age 40; it can be more evident after menopause. Female-pattern baldness usually causes the hair to thin out all over the head, but rarely progresses to total or near baldness as it does in men. This type of hair loss is permanent.

Females may also suffer hair loss because of temporary shedding, known as telogen effluvium; breaking of the hair due to styling treatments and the twisting or pulling of the hair; alopecia areata, an immune disorder temporarily causing patchy areas of total hair loss; oral medications; and certain skin diseases.

Toxic Baldness

Toxic baldness occurs in males as well as females. Hair may fall out for as long as 3 or 4 months before it grows back. Many cancer chemotherapy medications, as well as certain cholesterol-lowering drugs, Parkinson's medications, ulcer drugs, anticoagulants, antiarthritics, drugs derived from vitamin A, anticonvulsants for epilepsy, antidepressants, beta blocker drugs for high blood pressure, antithyroid agents, blood thinners, and anabolic steroids can cause baldness. When a doctor prescribes any drug, he should be asked if it causes hair loss. If he doesn't know, have him look it up in the *Physicians' Desk Reference,* which lists the side effects of all prescription drugs. A pharmacist can also be asked.

Alopecia Areata, Universalis, and Totalis

Sudden hair loss in a certain area, such as the scalp or beard, is called alopecia areata and is sometimes caused by an autoimmune illness. Alopecia universalis is a condition in which all body hair may be lost. The total loss of all body hair—including eyebrows, eye lashes, facial and body hair, and hair loss on top of the head—is known as alopecia totalis. Unless hair loss is widespread, new hair may grow back within a few months, but with no color.

Trichotillomania and Scarring Alopecia

Trichotillomania, known as hair pulling, is found mostly in children, although it can prevail throughout a person's lifetime. Children with trichotillomania suffer from chronic scratching or will brush their hair for no apparent reason.

Scarring alopecia describes skin that is scarred because of burns, x-ray therapy, skin cancer, or a severe injury that produces hair loss.

Treatment

A doctor may need to perform a biopsy to determine what type of baldness a person is suffering from. The biopsy will ascertain whether the follicles are normal. There are basically four choices a person has in regard to treating hair loss: do nothing, begin to take better care of the scalp and use products such as minoxidil (Rogaine), get a hair transplant or a scalp reduction, or have the hair replaced nonsurgically.

Successful prevention and treatment of accelerated hair loss necessitates dealing with some, if not all, of the factors involved in the process, except for the genetic component of baldness, which is still in the research phase.

Since the male hormone dihydrotestosterone is involved in premature hair loss, scientists have experimented with a wide variety of anti-androgens in an attempt to prevent or reverse the process. Among the anti-androgens that have been used to treat hair loss are progesterone, spironolactone (Aldactone), flutamide (Eulexin), finasteride (Proscar), cimetidine (Tagamet), serenoa repens (Permixon), and cyproterone acetate (Androcur/Diane). Of these anti-androgens, the most effective have proven to be oral finasteride (Proscar) and topical spironolactone, both of which have been able to grow hair to some degree with minimal side effects.

In the hair-loss process, it is the immune reaction caused by male hormones such as DHT that plays, perhaps, the most significant role. Stimulated by androgens, the immune system targets hair follicles in genetically susceptible areas to cause the premature loss of hair that is characteristic of male-pattern baldness.

Among the most potent hair-growth stimulators are topical oxygen-radical scavengers such as the superoxide dismutases (SODs), enzymes that play a critical role in countering excessive free-radical activity throughout the body.

SODs not only inhibit oxygen radicals, but also may inhibit the localized immune response implicated in so much hair loss, and may offset some of the damage and inflammation already incurred. Unless the immunologic factors involved in the hair-loss process are dealt with effectively, the potential for significant hair regrowth may be very limited.

There are many available agents (such as Rogaine) that can stimulate some degree of hair growth in some people, but cannot by themselves produce the kind of health and cosmetic benefits that balding people desire. What's needed is a multimodal approach that combines anti-androgens with autoimmune protective agents, oxygen free-radical inhibitors, and other hair-growth stimulators to halt hair loss and generate hair regrowth to a degree well beyond the abilities of single compounds.

Dr. Proctor's Hair Regrowth Formulas

Dr. Peter Proctor is the only hair-treatment practitioner in the world who has developed unique, patented, multi-ingredient hair formulas that address all the known factors in the balding process. He is the author of more than 30 scientific articles and book chapters, and holds several broad patents for hair-loss treatment.

Dr. Proctor offers both prescription and nonprescription hair-treatment formulas that vary both in potency and cost. However, even the least-potent of Dr. Proctor's formulas has proven to be superior to Rogaine, the only FDA-approved hair-treatment product on the market.

The least expensive of Dr. Proctor's hair-growth formulas is sold under the name Dr. Proctor's Hair Regrowth Shampoo. This formula includes an abundant supply of the most potent natural hair-growth stimulator available, NANO (3-carboxylic acid pyridine-N-oxide), which is known as "natural" minoxidil.

Dr. Proctor's Hair Regrowth Shampoo has been shown to work effectively for many people who did not respond to Rogaine. It may be all you need if you have experienced only small to moderate hair loss, or if your primary need is for a prophylactic program that will prevent hair loss in the future. Dr. Proctor's Hair Regrowth Shampoo should be used whenever you shower or wash your hair (at least 3 times a week). It should be used just like any other shampoo.

The second formula developed by Dr. Proctor, which is sold under the name Dr. Proctor's Advanced Hair Regrowth Formula, includes a potent dose of "natural" minoxidil (NANO) combined with the following natural hair-protection and hair-growth agents: EDRF enhancers, SODs, and various free-radical scavengers.

This multi-agent natural formula is the most potent natural hair-growth formula you can buy. It includes every type of natural hair-treatment agent available to counter the DHT, autoimmune, and inflammatory effects that are at the root of hair loss and baldness. Dr. Proctor's Advanced Hair Regrowth Formula is a liquid that is applied to the scalp.

Dr. Proctor's Advanced Hair Regrowth Formula should be applied 8 to 10 drops once or twice a day to the thinning areas. Its side effects include contact dermatitis, an itchy, scaly rash at the site of application.

If you have a really serious hair-loss problem, you may need to try Dr. Proctor's most potent hair-growth formula—Dr. Proctor's European Prescription Hair Regrowth Formula—that uses an array of natural hair-growth protectors combined with several drugs compounded into a cream base. Natural agents in Dr. Proctor's European Prescription Hair Regrowth Formula include topical anti-androgens, which increase EDRF levels and oxygen free-radical scavengers. These agents are combined with the following drugs: minoxidil, phenytoin (Dilantin), tretinoin (Retin-A), and spironolactone.

The protocol for using Dr. Proctor's European Prescription Hair Regrowth Formula is as follows: apply one tenth of a teaspoon (a dab on the end of your finger) once a day for 8 to 12 months, then every other day for maintenance. Its side effects include contact dermatitis.

Summary

Baldness is in most cases a cosmetic problem and usually the result of genetic influences, aging, skin conditions, or the ingesting of certain medications. The most common form of balding is male- and female-pattern baldness. At this time there is no known cure for baldness, and there are limited choices on how to cope with it: do nothing; start taking better care of your scalp and use minoxidil; get a hair transplant or a scalp reduction; or have hair replaced by a nonsurgical procedure, e.g., a toupee.

Dr. Peter Proctor has developed unique, patented multi-ingredient hair formulas that address all the known factors in the balding process:

1. For natural hair-growth stimulation, Dr. Proctor's Hair Regrowth Shampoo, used like any other shampoo.
2. For the benefits of "natural" minoxidil, Dr. Proctor's Advanced Hair Regrowth Formula, 8 to 10 drops applied once or twice a day to the thinning areas.
3. For serious hair-loss problems, Dr. Proctor's European Prescription Hair Regrowth Formula, one tenth of a teaspoon (a dab on the end of your finger) applied once a day for 8 to 12 months, then every other day for maintenance.

For more information. Contact the National Alopecia Areata Foundation, P.O. Box 150760, San Rafael, CA, 94915, phone (415) 456-4644; the American Hair Loss Council, 401 North Michigan Avenue, Chicago, IL, 60611, phone (312) 321-5158.

Product availability. You can order Dr. Proctor's Hair Regrowth Shampoo and Advanced Hair Regrowth Formula by calling (800) 544-4440, or order online at www.lef.org. European Prescription Hair Regrowth Formula is available by prescription from his office. For further information, call (800) 544-4440.

BELL'S PALSY

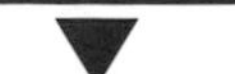

by Ben Best

Incidence, Symptoms, and Causes

Bell's palsy is a paralysis of the facial muscle, usually only on one side of the face. Approximately one person of every 4000 contracts the disease in any given year. It is more common among diabetics with high blood pressure and among pregnant women in the last third of their pregnancy.

The facial nerve passes through a narrow channel of bone in the face, so when the nerve swells due to inflammation, the result may be nerve compression and degeneration. The resulting lack of nerve function mainly prevents facial movement, but salivation, tear production, and facial sensation may also be reduced.

Recovery from Bell's palsy typically begins 3 weeks after onset of symptoms for 85% of patients, who fully recover within 6 months. About 5% experience permanent deformity. Younger patients have a better recovery rate than older ones. About 10% of patients will experience a recurrence of the disease some time after recovery.

Traditionally, Bell's palsy was defined as facial paralysis of unknown cause, but that definition has become controversial. It is now widely believed that as many as 80% of cases are due to herpes simplex virus, with the remainder largely due to infectious agents such as influenza virus, HIV, Lyme disease, herpes zoster, and tuberculosis. Facial paralysis can also be due to cancer or facial trauma (frequently seen in infants delivered by forceps).

There are two herpes simplex viruses which are similar in genetic composition, designated HSV-1 (oral) and HSV-2 (genital). In both diseases the virus enters the body though a mucous membrane or skin abrasion and is transported to nerve cell bodies in nerve ganglia where it "hides". Various stress conditions can cause the disease to manifest as cold sores (HSV-1) or genital sores (HSV-2). These stresses include menstruation, dental extraction, coldness, or exposure to other infectious agents, particularly upper respiratory tract infection—and these same stresses are associated with Bell's palsy. The evidence has become strong that Bell's palsy is usually the only manifestation of a herpes reactivation. In the great majority of cases, HSV-1 is the causative agent, but there is a well-documented case of a 24-year old man who developed paralysis on both sides of his face within 2 weeks of performing oral sex on a female partner who had active genital herpes blisters.

Therapy

In addition to the risk of permanent nerve damage, Bell's palsy patients can experience serious eye damage. Artificial tears, ophthalmic ointments, and protective goggles may be required, under the guidance of a physician. In some cases, physical therapy is required to strengthen facial muscles.

In most clinical trials the proven therapies for speeding recovery and reducing the risk of permanent damage have been combinations of the anti-inflammatory drug prednisone (steroid) with the herpes-suppressive drug acyclovir. In one clinical trial (not including acyclovir), intramuscular injections of 500 mcg of the methylcobalamin form of vitamin B_{12} 3 times weekly resulted in faster recovery than treatment with steroid.

The value of methylcobalamin for Bell's palsy is supported by the fact that methylcobalamin is also used in therapy for diabetic neuropathy and a number of other neurological diseases. Methylcobalamin is known to promote synthesis of DNA and myelin proteins, facilitate regeneration of crushed nerves in animal experiments, and protect cultured neurons from glutamate toxicity. Methylcobalamin can be taken as sublingual tablets in the dose of 40 mg a day, or by intramuscular injection (500 mcg, 3 times a week) administered by a physician.

Another clinical trial has shown that 1 gram 3 times daily of acetyl-*L*-carnitine in combination with steroid resulted in earlier functional improvement in Bell's palsy over steroid alone. Although this experiment has not yet been repeated by other researchers, acetyl-*L*-carnitine has also been shown to promote nerve regeneration in animal experiments, to improve nerve function in diabetic neuropathy, and to be of proven value in a number of other neurological diseases.

Summary

1. Eye protection as directed by a physician.
2. Steroid and/or antiviral (such as acyclovir) or other appropriate treatment if another infectious organism has been demonstrated.
3. Physical therapy if advised by a physician.
4. Methylcobalamin, 500 mcg 3 times weekly by intramuscular injection by a physician. Alternatively, the Life Extension Foundation provides 5 mg sublingual lozenges which bypass digestion.
5. Acetyl-*L*-carnitine, 1 gram, 3 times daily.

Product availability. Acetyl-*L*-carnitine and sublingual vitamin B_{12} can be ordered by calling (800) 544-4444 or order online at www.lef.org.

BLOOD TESTING

(See Medical Testing)

BREAST CANCER

by Andy Baer, M.D.

The very words strike fear into any woman. With one in eight women developing the disease, most women know either a friend or a relative who has or had breast cancer. The impact on women in light of the potential for disfiguring surgery and the possibility for metastatic spread and death cannot be understated.

According to the American Cancer Society, 173,000 women will be diagnosed with breast cancer in the coming year, and about 43,000 women will die from it. Breast cancer has become the second largest cause of cancer death in women, after lung cancer, and the leading cause of death for women between the ages of 35 and 54. This protocol will deal with the treatment of breast cancer and will also contain information for preventing the disease.

Introduction

Like most other cancers, once breast cancer has been detected there is already the chance that the disease has spread. Once a lump has been discovered on the breast or even discovered early on a mammogram, there may already be an average of 45 billion cancer cells present, and some of these malignant cells may have metastasized to other parts of the body. As in other types of cancer, conventional medicine stages the disease based on certain factors including tumor size, presence of lymph node involvement, or distal spread. Depending on the stage, the oncologist may recommend a number of options and combinations ranging from simple lumpectomy to complete mastectomy, radiation, and chemotherapy.

As discussed in the *Cancer protocols*, most physicians practicing complementary medicine believe the net effect of radiation and chemotherapy weakens the very system that protects us from cancer in the first place—the immune system. This leaves the cancer patient more vulnerable to the development of metastatic lesions in critical organs of the body. Despite this, studies demonstrate that radiation and chemotherapy can improve survival in certain breast cancer patients when appropriately used. The Life Extension Foundation cannot overemphasize the need for the breast cancer patient to become as well informed as possible regarding the disease and to be under the care of an oncologist who specializes in the treatment of the disease. Only then can a patient make informed decisions regarding the appropriate therapies to utilize.

Hormonal Manipulation

Although the cause of breast cancer has not been found, it has become clear that hormonal manipulation may have a therapeutic impact on the course of the disease. This is why the tumors, when removed during surgery, are studied to find whether or not they are so-called estrogen-receptor positive or negative. If the cancer is estrogen-receptor positive, theoretically there should be a response to manipulation of estrogen. This is exactly the role tamoxifen has played as an adjuvant drug therapy in the treatment of the disease. However, studies have demonstrated that after 2 years, tamoxifen can cause an increase of estrogen in the blood. This is one reason that breast cancer cells may become resistant to tamoxifen treatment. Another reason tamoxifen fails to control cell proliferation is that estrogen-receptor-positive cells often mutate into a cancer cell type that does not need estrogen to proliferate. Tamoxifen can cause serious side effects after 2 years, and for this reason it has been suggested that tamoxifen treatment not go beyond a 2-year time period. Those using tamoxifen should also follow the *Thrombosis Prevention protocol* because tamoxifen and cancer itself can increase the risk of abnormal blood clots.

Melatonin and vitamin D_3 have been shown to synergistically enhance the beneficial effects of tamoxifen, and for this reason, women taking tamoxifen should also take 4000 to 6000 IU of vitamin D_3 and 3 to 50 mg of melatonin nightly. While tamoxifen's side effects may limit its use to 2 years, most people can take melatonin and moderate doses of vitamin D_3 indefinitely. A few people experience kidney toxicity and abnormal calcium metabolism when taking high doses of vitamin D_3, and breast cancer patients are also at a high risk for developing blood calcium disorders. For all these reasons, breast cancer patients who use therapeutic doses of vitamin D_3 (4000 to 6000 IU a day) should have a regular blood chemistry panel that will reveal kidney toxicity and calcium imbalances while these problems are still reversible. The importance of melatonin and vitamin D_3 will be discussed later in this protocol.

What You Should Know about Tamoxifen

The most well-publicized aspect of tamoxifen's mode of action against breast cancer is that it occupies the estrogen receptor and blocks the "grow" signal. However, what's not usually appreciated is that tamoxifen has other modes of action besides blocking estrogen. The other actions are just as important, or in some cases more important, than the estrogen-blocking effect, and they are not unique to tamoxifen. Tamoxifen also works in estrogen-receptor-negative breast cancers and progesterone-receptor-positive breast cancers. This is because tamoxifen not only blocks the estrogen "grow" signal, but also blocks another type of "grow" signal known as protein kinase C (PKC). PKC is another one of those contact points inside the door jamb, and blocking this signal stops oncogenes (cancer genes) from activating. PKC also controls other signals that could lead to runaway growth and transformation of cells.

Another aspect of tamoxifen's anti-cancer action is its ability to interfere with the cell cycle. The cell cycle is a predetermined program a cell goes through to divide. In a healthy state, certain processes occur, then the cell moves on to the next step, finally creating a new cell. At points during the cell cycle, everything stops at predetermined points so that checks can be made to ensure that abnormal cells don't replicate. Cancer cells have abnormal cell cycles because they have lost those checkpoints. Cancer cells proceed through cell division at break-neck speed. One of the ways traditional chemotherapy works is to restore a checkpoint and stop the cell cycle. Tamoxifen is used as a chemotherapeutic agent because it stops the cell cycle.

While some studies show that tamoxifen works better at 5 years than at 2 years, other research has confirmed that tamoxifen may "turn" on its user in months to years, and begins feeding new, tamoxifen-dependent cancer. A new drug is being tested to combat this "problem," but the new drug may create problems of its own.

Meanwhile, there are hints that tamoxifen "resistance," as it's known, is the result of permanent damage caused by the drug. One area that might be damaged is tumor-suppressor gene p53. Gene p53 is a player in the process that stops the cell cycle and makes sure cancer cells don't replicate. In a healthy person, p53 sends signals that stop the cell cycle when abnormal cells are involved and cause them to self-destruct. Using human breast cancer cells, researchers in France showed that tamoxifen stops p53 from working. While this may sensitize cancer cells to the effects of chemotherapy, the same phenomenon in a healthy person would cripple p53's ability to stop cancer.

Natural Estrogen Manipulation

In 1991 researchers at the Institute for Hormone Research announced that they had been able to induce the body to convert the stronger form of estrogen (estradiol) into the weaker form (estriol) without using drugs. Estriol is considered to be a more desirable form of estrogen. It is less active than estradiol, so when it occupies the estrogen receptor, it effectively blocks estradiol's strong "grow" signals.

It took only 1 week to prove that the conversion of estradiol to estriol can be accomplished without drugs. Using a natural substance, researchers were able to increase the conversion of estradiol to estriol by 50% in 12 healthy people. Next, they tested the natural substance in female mice prone to developing breast cancer. The incidence of cancer and the number of tumors fell significantly. What was the substance? Indole-3-carbinol (IC3), a phytochemical isolated from cruciferous vegetables (broccoli, cauliflower, Brussels sprouts, turnips, kale, green cabbage, mustard seed, etc.).

I3C was then given to 17 men and women for 2 months. Again, levels of strong estrogen declined, and levels of weak estrogen increased. But more importantly, the level of an estrogen metabolite associated with breast and endometrial cancer (16-alpha-hydroxyestrone) fell.

In 1997, researchers at Strang Cancer Research Laboratory at Rockefeller University discovered that when I3C changes "strong" estrogen to "weak" estrogen, stops human cancer cells from growing (54–61%) and provokes the cells to self-destruct (apoptosis). Subsequent studies done at the University of California at Berkeley, show that I3C inhibits MCF7 human breast cancer cells from growing by as much as 90% in culture. Growth arrest does not depend on estrogen receptors.

I3C does more than just turn strong estrogen to weak estrogen. 16-alpha-hydroxyestrone (16OHE) and 2-hydroxyestrone (2OHE) are metabolites of estrogen in addition to estriol and estradiol. 2OHE is biologically inactive, while 16OHE is biologically active—i.e., like estradiol, it can send those "grow" signals. In breast cancer, the bad 16OHE is elevated, and the good 2OHE is decreased. Interestingly, cancer-causing chemicals change the metabolism of estrogen so that 16OHE is elevated. Studies show that people who take I3C not only have beneficial increases in estriol, they also have beneficial increases in 2OHE.

In an experiment at New York University, researchers gave African-American women I3C, 400 mg for 5 days. Most of them experienced an increase in the "good" 2OHE and a decrease of the "bad" 16OHE. However, some did not. It turns out that those who did not have a mutation in a gene that helps metabolize estrogen to the 2OHE version. These women have an 8 times higher risk of breast cancer.

I3C Stops Cancer Cells from Growing

I3C has other modes of action similar to tamoxifen. I3C also interrupts the cell cycle. In studies from the University of California mentioned above, I3C inhibited the growth of estrogen-receptor-positive breast cancer cells by 90% compared to tamoxifen's 60% by stopping the cell cycle. Adding tamoxifen to I3C gave a 5% boost (95% inhibition). In estrogen-receptor-negative cells, I3C stopped the synthesis of DNA for new cells by about 50% whereas tamoxifen had no significant effect. I3C also restores p21 and other proteins that act as checkpoints during the synthesis of a new cell. Tamoxifen has no effect on p21. Restoration of these growth regulators is extremely important. Tumor suppressor p53, for example, works through the p21 that I3C restores. I3C also inhibits cancers caused by other types of chemicals. If animals are fed I3C before exposure to cancer-causing chemicals, DNA damage and cancer is virtually eliminated. A study on rodents shows that damaged DNA in breast cells is reduced 91% by I3C. Similar results happen in the liver. And in a study from New York University Medical Center, female smokers taking 400 mg of I3C significantly reduced their levels of a major lung carcinogen. Cigarette chemicals are known to adversely affect estrogen metabolism.

There is no proven breast cancer prevention. The best and most comprehensive scientific evidence so far stands behind phytochemicals such as I3C. I3C beat out more than 80 other substances, including tamoxifen, for anticancer potential in one assay. Recently, researchers at the Hoechst Marrion Roussel drug company staked their claim to dozens of indole-3 look-alikes. They claim that the indoles, which down-regulate estrogen receptors, can be used to treat and prevent cancer and autoimmune diseases such as multiple sclerosis, arthritis, and lupus. They hope to replace all the chemically altered estrogen drugs such as tamoxifen with a new generation of chemically altered indole drugs that fit in the Ah receptor and regulate estrogen indirectly.

How to Use I3C

While the evidence is compelling, it is too premature to know exactly how effective I3C will be as an adjuvant breast cancer therapy. (*See the Breast Cancer Reference List for citations pertaining specifically to I3C.*)

The suggested dose is one 200-mg capsule, twice a day for those under 120 pounds. For those who weigh over 120, three 200 mg capsules a day may be needed. ***Take Note****: A little is good; a lot is not necessarily better. As with certain antioxidants that can actually promote oxidation at high levels, too much I3C can have the opposite effect of what you want. Therefore, don't exceed the dosage.*

CAUTION: Pregnant women should not take I3C because of its modulation of estrogen. The reported aversion to cruciferous vegetables by pregnant women may be associated with their ability to change estrogen metabolism. Estrogen is a growth factor for the fetus.

I3C Summary

A summary of recent studies shows that this vegetable extract (indole 3 carbinol) can

- Increase the conversion of estradiol to the safer estriol by 50% in 12 healthy people in just 1 week.
- Prevent the formation of the carcinogenic estrogen metabolite 16-alpha-hydroxyestrone in 2 months in 17 men and women.
- Stop human cancer cells from growing (54 to 61%) and provoke the cells to self-destruct (apoptosis).
- Inhibit MCF7 human breast cancer cells from growing by as much as 90% in culture.
- Inhibit an estrogen metabolite (16-alpha-hydroxyestrone) that prompts breast cancer cells to grow.
- Compete with dioxin for the Ah receptor to help keep dioxin out of cells. In breast cancer cells with I3C and dioxin at the same time, dioxin's adverse effects were reduced 90% by I3C.
- Prevent chemically induced breast cancer in rodents by 70 to 96%. Prevent other types of cancer, including aflatoxin-induced liver cancer, leukemia, and colon cancer.
- Inhibit free radicals, particularly those that cause the oxidation of fat.
- Inhibit the growth of estrogen-receptor-positive breast cancer cells by 90%, compared to tamoxifen's 60%, by stopping the cell cycle.
- Stop the synthesis of DNA for new cells by about 50% in estrogen-receptor-negative cells, whereas tamoxifen had no significant effect.
- Restore p21 and other proteins that act as checkpoints during the synthesis of a new cancer cell. Tamoxifen has no effect on p21.
- Virtually eliminate DNA damage and cancer if animals are fed it before exposure to cancer-causing chemicals.
- Reduce DNA damage in breast cells by 91%. Similar results happen in the liver.
- Reduce levels of a major carcinogen in female smokers.

Flavonoids

Soy contains genistein, which belongs to a group of substances called flavonoids. Studies have demonstrated that genistein has certain anti-estrogenic properties and can inhibit the development of breast cancer cells. Soy can also inhibit the tendency for cancerous tissue to create new capillaries to supply it with blood. Indeed, substances that demonstrate anti-angiogenesis properties have recently been a hot topic in the war against cancer. The theory is that if you can prevent the tumor from developing new blood vessels, you can starve and ultimately kill it. Genistein has been demonstrated to affect the ability of cancer cells to stick to one another. Cancer-cell adhesiveness is part of the process by which metastatic colonies of breast cancer cells form tumors in other parts of the body. Another study suggests that genistein may enhance the benefits of certain chemotherapeutic regimens.

There have been a number of studies conducted on genistein to determine its effect on the proliferation and maturation of breast cancer cells. In one, genistein inhibited growth but not maturation in both estrogen-positive and -negative cell lines. This would suggest that the inhibition of cell growth is not dependent on genistein's inhibition of estrogen. Genistein was tested with a number of other naturally occurring flavonoids and was found to inhibit cell proliferation in estrogen-receptor-positive breast cancer cells. This inhibition was reversed when excess competing estrogen was added. Interestingly, the other flavonoids inhibited cell proliferation even when high levels of estrogen were added suggesting that they work by a different mechanism than genistein. One of those flavonoids is quercetin. This suggests that taking supplemental quercetin might be useful in treating breast cancer. Quercetin is effective only in a water-soluble form, and it is difficult to find water-soluble quercetin in the United States. It is expected that this form will soon be available as a dietary supplement. Water-soluble quercetin supplementation should be considered in treating and perhaps preventing breast cancer.

Another study was done in which both genistein and supplemental curcumin were tested to evaluate their ability to inhibit the growth of estrogen-receptor-positive breast cancer cells that were induced by pesticides. Pesticides and other petrochemicals have estrogenic effects. One theory regarding the increased incidence of breast cancer is the proliferation of these types of chemicals in our environment. The study demonstrated a synergistic effect resulting in the total inhibition of cancer cell growth. Though more studies are needed, curcumin should be considered, along with genistein, water-soluble quercetin, and green tea (that will be described later).

CAUTION: Breast cancer patients about to undergo radiation therapy should stop using soy products 1 week before, during, and after being treated. The therapeutic effects of radiation therapy are dependent on the activity of an enzyme called protein kinase C. Soy inhibits this activity and therefore could theoretically undermine the radiation therapy. The most potent soy extract on the market is called Mega Soy Extract. It contains more than 40% pure soy isoflavones . . . much higher than previous soy products. The suggested dose for nonestrogen-receptor-positive breast cancer patients is five 700-mg capsules of Mega Soy Extract 4 times a day. This provides the optimal daily dose of approximately 2800 mg of standardized genistein. Genistein is rapidly metabolized within the body, which makes it necessary for cancer patients to take Mega Soy Extract in 4 divided doses spaced evenly throughout the day.

CAUTION: Women with any type of breast cancer should test their serum estrogen levels to make sure that too much estrogen is not present if they are taking high doses of soy. Estrogen can combine with the genistein to cause some breast cancer cells to grow faster. Other studies show that genistein blocks certain types of estrogen-receptor sites, thus inhibiting the proliferation of these types of breast cancer cells.

Melatonin

One of the most important supplements for the breast cancer patient is the hormone melatonin. High doses of the hormone should be taken at bedtime. Melatonin blocks estrogen receptors somewhat similarly to the drug tamoxifen without the long-term side effects of tamoxifen. Furthermore, when melatonin and tamoxifen are combined, synergistic benefits occur. Melatonin can be safely taken for an indefinite period of time. The suggested dose of melatonin for breast cancer patients is 3 to 50 mg at bedtime. Melatonin not only blocks estrogen-receptor sites on breast cancer cells, but directly inhibits breast cancer cell proliferation and boosts the production of immune components that kill metastasized cancer cells.

There have been some studies demonstrating changes in melatonin and other hormone levels in breast cancer patients. In one study, breast cancer patients demonstrated lower melatonin levels than women without breast cancer. Normally, we undergo a seasonal variation in the production of certain hormones like melatonin. A study comparing healthy women to women with a history of breast cancer demonstrated that the women with breast cancer did not have a seasonal variation in melatonin levels as did the healthy women. Of course this begs the question: are these findings a contribution to the cause of breast cancer or a result of the disease?

Vitamins A, D, and E and Selenium

Vitamin A and vitamin D_3 inhibit breast cancer cell division and can induce cancer cells to differentiate into mature, noncancer cells. Vitamin D_3 works synergistically with tamoxifen (and melatonin) to inhibit breast cancer cell proliferation. Breast cancer patients should take 4000 to 6000 IU of vitamin D_3 every day on an empty stomach. Water-soluble vitamin A can be taken in doses of 100,000 to 300,000 IU every day. Monthly blood tests are needed to make sure toxicity does not occur in response to these relatively high daily doses of vitamin A and vitamin D_3. After 4 to 6 months, the doses of vitamin D_3 and vitamin A can be reduced.

Vitamin E succinate has been shown to inhibit tumor cell growth *in vitro* and *in vivo*. In a recently published study, vitamin E succinate, a derivative of fat-soluble vitamin E, inhibited growth and induced apoptic cell death in estrogen-receptor-negative human breast cancer cell lines. The study concluded that vitamin E succinate may be of clinical use in the treatment of aggressive human breast cancers, particularly those that are resistant to anti-estrogen therapy. Those with estrogen-receptor-negative breast cancers should consider taking 1200 IU of vitamin E succinate a day. In breast cancer cells of the mouse, selenium has been shown to directly induce growth arrest and cell death. Although no human studies have been done, it is suggested that patients with breast cancer take 200 mcg of organic selenium (selenomethionine) 2 to 3 times a day.

CAUTION: Refer to the symptoms of vitamin A toxicity in *Appendix A: Avoiding Vitamin A Toxicity*. When taking doses of vitamin D_3 in excess of 1100 IU a day, regular blood chemistry tests should be taken to monitor kidney function and serum calcium metabolism.

DHEA and Pregnenolone

Dehydroepiandrosterone (DHEA) and pregnenolone may be thought of as steroid precursors whose exact function is unclear. They are both present in the body at any given time and are part of the synthetic pathway that many of the adrenal steroids take. At the present time, existing studies make it unclear whether or not these hormones should be taken by breast cancer patients. Some studies have demonstrated a positive impact while others have shown a negative one. From the standpoint of preventing breast cancer, the preponderance of scientific literature indicates that maintaining youthful levels of DHEA is beneficial. The Life Extension Foundation, however, cannot support the use of pregnenolone or DHEA by breast cancer patients at this time and recommends that they not be used.

CoQ_{10}

CoQ_{10} (Coenzyme Q_{10}) has demonstrated promise in treating breast cancer. Although there are only a few studies, the safe nature of CoQ_{10} coupled with this promising research suggests that breast cancer patients should take 100 mg 3 times a day. It is important to take CoQ_{10} with some kind of oil such as fish or flax since dry powder CoQ_{10} is not readily absorbed without it.

CAUTION: Some studies indicate that Coenzyme Q_{10} should not be taken at the same time as chemotherapy. If this is true, it would be disappointing, since CoQ_{10} is so effective in protecting against adriamycin-induced cardiomyopathy. Adriamycin is a chemotherapy drug sometimes used as part of a chemotherapy cocktail. Until more research is known, it is not possible to make a definitive recommendation whether to take CoQ_{10} during chemotherapy.

Green Tea

The most current research shows that some of the ingredients in green tea may have a beneficial effect in treating cancer. While drinking green tea is a well-documented method of preventing cancer, it is difficult for the cancer patient to obtain a sufficient quantity of anti-cancer components in that form. We suggest that a person with breast cancer take 4 to 10 decaffeinated green tea extract capsules every day. These capsules contain a standardized extract of epigallocatechin gallate, which is the component of green tea that makes it a potentially effective adjunct therapy in the treatment of breast cancer.

A Novel Herbal Preparation

The September 17, 1998, issue of the *New England Journal of Medicine* published a study on a product called *PC Spes* that was 100% effective in reducing PSA levels in advanced prostate cancer patients. The company that makes *PC Spes* also makes another herbal preparation called *Spes* to treat breast and certain other cancers. The *Spes* preparation has been shown effective in the 2 years that Foundation members have been using it. The studies show that *Spes* works best against cancers with a mutated p53 oncogene and an over-expressed N-RAS gene. Cancer patients have been getting good results when combining *Spes* with high-dose genistein, soy extract, curcumin, and 95% green tea extract. What follows is a highly technical description of the molecular mechanisms of action of *Spes*. Please don't be intimidated if you can't understand all of this; it is written to inform the oncologist as well as the layperson.

Spes has been shown to inhibit prostaglandin E2 (PGE2) by about 50%. Cancer patients often develop high concentrations of PGE2 that can promote the proliferation of some cancer cell lines and also damage immune function. PGE2 inhibits the T cell response, causes a decrease in natural killer (NK) cells, and inhibits lymphokine production. PGE2 enhances tumor survival by blocking the natural destruction via the lysis process of tumor cells. In addition, PGE2 promotes abnormal platelet aggregation, a common feature that enables cancer cells to enter the interstitial tissue through a blood vessel wall to establish metastatic sites. PGE2-induced endothelial cell damage attracts metastatic cancer cell colony formation. Many cancer patients succumb to acute death when an abnormal blood clot (thrombus) causes a heart attack or stroke. It is clearly desirable to suppress PGE2, and *Spes* does this by about 50%. The suppression of PGE2 by *Spes* has resulted in a dramatic increase in NK activity. While cancer drugs are in development that work by suppressing PGE2 formation, *Spes* is available as a dietary supplement for use today.

Nearly all cancer cells secrete a peptide hormone called substance P that promotes tumor growth. Substance P also functions as a neurotransmitter involved in pain pulse transmission through the nerves. *Spes* appears to lower the levels of Substance P, thus potentially slowing tumor growth and alleviating pain.

Spes increases enkephalin production. Enkephalins are peptides produced in the brain that act as opiates, binding to receptor sites involved in pain perception. This could be a mechanism by which *Spes* alleviates pain. *Spes* may increase enkephalins between 30 to 50% in about 1 hour.

Beta-endorphin levels are markedly depressed in the cerebrospinal fluid of cancer patients. Endorphins are polypeptides produced in the brain that also act as opiates, producing an analgesic effect by binding to opiate receptor sites. The most active of the endorphins is beta-endorphin. *Spes* has been shown to normalize beta-endorphin levels. Another mechanism by which *Spes* provides analgesic action is by lowering norepinephrine in relation to serotonin. *Spes* raises acetylcholine levels in the brain by an average of 60.4%. This also has a positive effect on pain reduction.

Spes reduces the afferent peripheral pain signals and increases the central pain-modulating function. This is a fancy way of saying *Spes* causes a reduction in internal organ pain or bone pain.

In the animal model, *Spes* was directly injected into the tumor site and caused an inhibition rate of 133% in tumor weight or volume. On hepatocarcinoma cell lines, *Spes* markedly reduced the number of survived cells in a total unit area, reversed the self-keeping system of the cancer cells and causing the differentiation of the cancer cells to normal cells. By causing the cancer cells to differentiate normally, *Spes* may markedly inhibit the advancement of the tumor.

Alpha-Fetoprotein (AFP) is a specific marker for gene expression in hepatocellular carcinoma. AFP is a serum protein produced by the fetal liver and yolk sac during prenatal development and reaches its full expression at 15 weeks of gestation, falling rapidly thereafter until normal adult levels are reached. High levels in an adult are an indication of hepatocellular carcinoma. *Spes* was shown to block expression of AFP by 83.5%.

N-RAS gene is a "transforming" gene whose overexpression is required for the activation of hepatocellular carcinoma and approximately 30% of all other cancers. A mutation in the N-RAS gene tends to turn off the switch for cell cycle progression. N-RAS thus interacts with other proteins and simulates cell growth. *Spes* was shown to block the overexpression of the N-RAS gene.

Ribosomal RNA instructs specific ribosomes to join into a group called ribosomal complex. This is the production facility for making protein. A ribosome is a cell organelle. It is the site of amino acid assembly in the exact sequence ordered by messenger RNA (mRNA). mRNA receives instructions (the genetic code) in the nucleus for the exact sequence of the 22 different amino acids necessary to make a specific protein. This process is called transcription. It is at this point that overexpression often occurs and the cell turns cancerous. IGF-II has a growth-promoting effect on cells, and *Spes* blocks the overexpression of mRNA for IGF-II synthesis.

Finally, *Spes* increases SOD production in the blood serum by 50% and suppresses free-radical generation.

Dosage recommendations are based on body weight. Patients who weigh under 150 lbs. should take 2 capsules 2 hours prior to breakfast on an empty stomach and again 2 capsules 2 hours prior to dinner on an empty stomach. Patients who weigh over 150 lbs. should take 3 capsules 2 hours prior to breakfast on an empty stomach and again 3 capsules 2 hours prior to dinner on an empty stomach. An empty stomach means no food or any other medication or supplement during the 2-hour period. *Spes* requires a noncompetitive stomach environment for proper absorption.

The pain-relieving effect should be felt within 2 hours. Also, mood and appetite should improve as well. Botaniclab, the manufacture of the product, claims that *Spes* works as well as hydrazine sulfate in countering the cachexia that occurs in late-stage cancer. Testing for blood tumor markers and tumor volume should be done regularly to determine if *Spes* is effective against the individual's cancer.

Preventing Breast Cancer Cell Metastasis

Breast cancer cells frequently metastasize to the bone, where they cause severe degradation of bone tissue.

The bisphosphonates are a class of drugs that protect against the degradation of bone, primarily by inhibiting excess activity of osteoclasts. The osteoclasts are bone cells that absorb and remove bone tissue so that the osteoblasts can bring together the minerals calcium, magnesium, and phosphorus to form new healthy bone. When osteoclasts become overactive, they break down too much bone, which can result in a pathological reduction of bone density.

Among the known inhibitors of osteoclast activity, the bisphosphonates are the most promising drugs. Clodronate, one of the most investigated bisphosphonates, has been clinically utilized for over 15 years in treating malignant diseases. It is the most-used, most effective, and safest drug in the treatment of hypercalcemia (too much calcium in the blood). It inhibits bone destruction, prevents bone fractures, relieves bone pain, and prevents the development of new bone lesions. Clodronate may even reduce mortality.

Bisphosphonates such as clodronate are potent osteoclast inhibitors that have opened the way for a nontoxic medical treatment of bone metastasis. Large-scale studies in humans with breast cancer indicate the benefits of prolonged administration of clodronate to reduce the frequency of pathological skeletal events and also the need for radiation therapy.

A *New England Journal of Medicine* study (Aug. 6, 1998) confirmed many previous studies showing that breast cancer patients receiving clodronate experienced about half the number of metastatic lesions to the bone compared to the placebo group. What was remarkable about the *New England Journal of Medicine* study was that it showed that clodronate also prevented metastasis to the visceral organs and that it significantly improved patient survival over a 36-month time period.

Another study showing improved survival was conducted in Finland, where breast cancer patients were treated with clodronate or placebo. Bone pain, extension of bone metastasis, and formation of new bony metastatic lesions were reduced by clodronate, and development of severe hypercalcemia was prevented during the first 12-month period. The patients were then withdrawn from clodronate treatment and were followed up for at least 12 months. There were fewer fractures and less hypercalcemia (too much calcium in the blood) in the patients previously treated with clodronate than in the placebo group. The survival rate was higher in the clodronate group compared to the placebo group. No side effects were observed in either group. While clodronate has been investigated as a therapy for advanced metastatic bone cancer in dozens of human studies, only two studies show that clodronate improved breast cancer patient survival. It would appear that if clodronate were administered earlier in the disease state, it could significantly prolong survival, as was demonstrated in the *New England Journal of Medicine* study.

Since 1980, the Europeans have been studying the effects of clodronate in the management of hypercalcemia, bone pain, and skeletal complications in patients with bone metastasis. Controlled studies show that bone metastasis can be prevented or delayed in patients receiving clodronate. The bisphosphonate drug clodronate is now the standard therapy (after hydration) that German doctors use to treat malignant states of hypercalcemia.

As was previously stated, tumor-induced hypercalcemia is essentially due to an increase in osteoclast-induced breakdown of the bone into the blood. During this process of bone destruction, substances such as growth factors are released that promote tumor-cell growth. Since the bisphosphonates are potent inhibitors of osteoclast activity, they represent an effective method of safely treating hypercalcemic events that frequently occur in patients with breast cancer and other diseases.

In a double-blind multicenter study, the effect of intravenous clodronate plus hydration was compared with placebo plus hydration in the treatment of hypercalcemia in breast cancer patients with bone metastases. A significant difference in favor of clodronate was observed in the time to reach normal blood calcium. A total of 17 patients of 21 patients on clodronate achieved normal blood levels of calcium compared with only 4 of 19 patients on placebo. The only adverse event associated with clodronate was symptomatic hypocalcemia (too little calcium in the bone) in one patient.

The reason hypocalcemia is such a rare event is that patients having a good response to clodronate normally show an increase in calcium-regulating hormones such as parathyroid hormone. This homeostatic response probably explains why hypocalcemia occurs rarely in clodronate-treated patients. In 1991, Italian scientists reviewed 126 publications on clinical studies concerning the use of clodronate in the therapy of bone disease. These studies evaluated a total of 1930 patients in order to ascertain the effects following the short- and long-term administration of clodronate. The results of the large number of studies indicate that clodronate therapy does not have any clinically significant side effects and confirm its tolerability and safety. It is still, however, advisable to have a blood test within 10 days of initiating clodronate therapy, just to make sure that clodronate is not removing too much calcium from the blood.

Bisphosphonate drugs like clodronate exert their analgesic effect by several mechanisms. The long-term effects are probably due to osteoclast inhibition. The acute pain-relieving effect, which occurs within days or a week, is likely to be associated with the reduction of various potentially pain-producing substances. In a controlled trial using clodronate in patients with metastatic bone disease and pain, 57% of patients in pain chose clodronate, while 26% chose placebo, and eight (17%) had no preference. For the investigators who also made a blinded selection, clodronate was chosen in 65% of patients compared to placebo in 22% patients, and no difference was apparent in 13%.

In an observational study involving 398 tumor patients with bone metastases or related hypercalcemia, the effect of treatment with clodronate over a period of 12 months was investigated. Bone pain, analgesic requirements, quality of life, and laboratory parameters were recorded at monthly intervals. The results showed that some 71.4% of all patients indicated an improvement in quality of life. In another study, 20 postmenopausal women (between 46 and 67 years old) with skeletal metastases from breast cancer were treated with clodronate for 15 days. All patients received standard hormonal therapy (tamoxifen). These results showed that clodronate provided pain relief in 75% of treated patients, and serum bone-marker levels indicated stabilization of skeletal metastatic lesions.

In a randomized, double-blind, placebo-controlled trial of oral clodronate, 173 breast cancer patients with bone metastasis were treated with clodronate or an identical placebo. In patients who received clodronate, there was a 47% reduction in the number of episodes of hypercalcemia, a 32% reduction in the incidence of vertebral fractures, and a 43% reduction in the rate of vertebral deformity. Trends were seen in favor of clodronate for nonvertebral fracture rates and bone pain. In patients who receive clodronate before developing bone metastasis, the results are more dramatic, showing consistent 50% reductions in skeletal metastasis and fractures. An inevitable conclusion may be that all breast cancer patients should consider supplementing with an 800-mg clodronate supplement twice a day for prophylactic purposes.

Women with primary breast cancer who receive chemotherapy may experience ovarian failure or early menopause, leading to a loss of bone-mineral density. A double-blind trial was conducted to evaluate women with breast cancer who were given clodronate or placebo for 2 years. Those who received oral clodronate showed reduced bone-density loss compared to placebo. All of the patients in the trial received conventional treatment for breast cancer. In another study, the effect of clodronate on bone-mineral density was studied in 121 postmenopausal breast cancer patients without skeletal metastases. At 2 years, clodronate combined with the anti-estrogen drugs tamoxifen or toremifene markedly increased bone-mineral density in the lumbar spine and femoral neck by 2.9 and 3.7%. There were no significant changes in the patients given anti-estrogen drugs only. Doctors often advise cancer patients using clodronate to take plenty of calcium, magnesium, and even phosphorus to enable the bone to regenerate.

The molecular mechanisms by which tumor cells degrade bone involve tumor cell adhesion to bone as well as the release of toxic chemicals from tumor cells that stimulate osteoclast-induced bone degradation. Bisphosphonates inhibit cancer cell adhesion to the bone matrix and inhibit osteoclast activity. By preventing tumor cell adhesion, bisphosphonates are useful agents for the prophylactic treatment of patients with cancer that is known to preferentially metastasize to bone.

There is evidence that growth factors such as insulin-like growth factor and transforming growth factor are released when the bone matrix is degraded. These growth factors could stimulate tumor cell proliferation throughout the body, which may be a reason that early use of clodronate significantly improved survival.

In a study to determine the effects of clodronate in women with advanced breast cancer, 133 patients with recurrent breast cancer—but no evidence of skeletal metastases—were randomly allocated to receive clodronate by mouth or an identical placebo for 3 years under double-blind conditions at two clinical oncology centers in the United Kingdom and Canada. The number of skeletal metastases was significantly lower with clodronate treatment than with placebo. The complications of skeletal disease were fewer by 26% in clodronate-treated patients compared to controls. Compared to placebo, significant effects in favor of clodronate were observed for vertebral deformities and nonvertebral fractures. The doctors concluded that oral clodronate significantly decreases the number and complications of skeletal metastasis in women with advanced breast cancer.

The reported studies of clodronate in the management of bone metastasis suggest a significant palliative role for this drug in those with advanced disease. An analysis of the hospital costs associated with the management of metastatic disease suggested that there are significant savings to be gained from the use of clodronate if only a 20% reduction occurs in the incidence of fractures, hypercalcemia, and hospital-based treatment for pain control (via radiation therapy).

Of the many compounds belonging to the bisphosphonate family, clodronate has been the most widely used in treating hypercalcemia and metastatic malignancy to the bone. All published reports indicate that clodronate can normalize plasma calcium in the majority of cancer patients. A large number of clinical studies indicate that clodronate is a safe and efficacious drug.

Some Published Studies on Clodronate

A study published in 1988 concluded

> Breast-cancer patients with multiple bone metastasis were treated with clodronate (1600 mg/day) or placebo for 12 months. After withdrawal of treatment, the patients were followed up for at least 12 months. There were fewer fractures and less hypercalcemia in the clodronate group than in the placebo group. The survival rate was higher in the clodronate group than in the placebo group. No side-effects were observed in the clodronate group (*Biomed. Pharmacother.* (France), 1988, 42/2:111–116).

Two studies published in 1987 state

> The possibility of reducing symptomatic hypercalcemia and of maintaining total serum calcium concentrations with clodronate was evaluated in 28 patients with various types of malignant tumors. Oral clodronate successfully reduced a mean serum calcium concentration in 22 out of 25 patients after 3 to12 days (800 to 3200 mg/day). It is concluded that clodronate is a valuable clinical tool in the management of patients with malignancy-associated hypercalcemia (*Acta Med. Scand.* (Sweden), 1987, 221/5:489–494)
>
> We investigated the acute effect of hydration plus intravenously administered clodronate By the third day of observation, the clodronate produced a significant reduction in serum calcium levels compared to the placebo patients who received hydration only. There were no toxicities observed. Intravenously administered clodronate appears to be an excellent agent for the acute treatment of malignancy-associated hypercalcemia (*Arch. Intern. Med.* (United States), 1987, 147/5:937–939).

A study published in 1985 states

> We have assessed the effects of clodronate daily by mouth for up to 3 months in 17 episodes of hypercalcaemia and osteolysis due to carcinoma. Clodronate reduced serum calcium in 14 episodes and bone resorption in all patients. These remained suppressed for the duration of treatment, but recurred promptly when treatment was stopped. Clodronate may be a useful measure for controlling hypercalcaemia and osteolysis in patients with carcinoma (*Br. J. Cancer* (England), 1985, 51/5:665–669).

A study published in 1984 states

> Clodronate is very effective against osteoclasts. We studied its effects on calcium balance in patients with malignant osteolytic lesions. Ten normocalcemic patients with advanced metastatic bone disease or myeloma were randomized to a clodronate or placebo regimen. The results show that both calcium balance and calcium absorption increased from base

line in the clodronate group and that these changes were significantly different from those in the placebo group. Our results suggest that clodronate may be a useful adjuvant in managing metastatic bone disease (*Presse Med.* (France), 1984, 13/8:479–482; also published in the *N. Engl. J. Med.*, 1983, 308/25:1499–1501).

A study published in 1981 states

Clodronate and etidronate were injected in various doses in 6 patients with one or multiple episodes of malignant hypercalcemia. All patients responded well to the drugs after a delay period of 2 to 7 days. The tolerance of the drugs was excellent. Etidronate, and especially clodronate, are promising agents for treating hypercalcemia and inhibiting bone resorption in malignant disorders (*Cancer* (Philadelphia), 1981, 48/8:1922–1925).

A study published in 1980 states:

[Thirty] patients with disorders of calcium metabolism were treated with clodronate by mouth (1.6 g/day). Serum-alkaline-phosphatase and urinary hydroxyproline fell to normal or near-normal within 3 to 7 months, and there was a clinical improvement in all but 1 patient. Clodronate also reduced plasma-calcium and urinary calcium in 17 patients with hypercalcaemia due to primary hyperparathyroidism or secondary to malignant disease. Clodronate seems to be an effective oral drug for inhibiting excessive bone resorption in man (Douglas, D.L., Duckworth, T., Russell, R.G. et al., Dept. Hum. Metab., Univ. Sheffield Med. Sch., Sheffield, United Kingdom; *Lancet* (England), 1980, 1/8177:1043–1047).

As mentioned earlier, clodronate is not approved in the United States, but the FDA did approve some expensive bisphosphonate drugs a few years ago. These drugs may not work as well as clodronate, and they produce side effects that could keep some breast cancer patients from using them for 3 to 5 continuous years. One FDA-approved bisphosphonate drug is called pamidronate and is sold under the trade name Aredia. The problem with Aredia is that it costs about $2,000 a month and must be administered in a medical setting via intravenous infusion.

The high cost of Aredia has caused HMOs and other insurance companies to refuse to pay for it in early-stage breast cancer. What's worse, many physicians are not even familiar with bisphosphonate drug therapy, and therefore won't prescribe it to their patients.

One reason insurance companies can avoid paying for Aredia in early-stage breast cancer is that the FDA has approved it for the treatment of "moderate to severe hypercalcemia associated with malignancy." Women with metastatic breast cancer often do not manifest serious hypercalcemia until the disease has significantly progressed. The FDA has thus restricted the use of Aredia in a way that makes it more of a palliative therapy in advanced disease rather than a potential lifesaving therapy.

Out of concern for toxicity, the FDA cautions against immediate retreatment with Aredia if the initial dose fails. Cancer patients are advised to undergo intravenous infusions of Aredia every 3 to 4 weeks. At $2,000 per infusion, few people can afford it.

Clodronate, on the other hand, is so safe that cancer patients can start taking two 800-mg capsules a day as soon as they are diagnosed. The fact that clodronate is nontoxic, is not terribly expensive, and has been shown to improve survival would make it the drug of choice in a free market. Americans, however, are not free to make their own choices about medicines. The FDA does this for us.

A review of the published literature provides conflicting results as to whether clodronate or Aredia is the better drug. Proponents of Aredia state it provides a longer period of remission from hypercalcemia. One study compared single infusions of either Aredia or clodronate at the highest doses commonly used. A total of 100% of patients in the Aredia group achieved normal serum calcium following infusion of Aredia, compared to 80% receiving clodronate. The median time to achieve normal serum calcium was a range of 4 days for Aredia and 3 days for clodronate. The median duration of normalized serum calcium was 28 days after Aredia and 14 days after clodronate. Two patients who failed to respond to clodronate were successfully treated with Aredia. Another two patients experienced fever after Aredia, but no significant toxicity was observed with either treatment. The doctors concluded by stating, "Both agents are effective in the management of hypercalcaemia of malignancy. At the doses studied, the effects of Aredia are more complete and longer lasting than those of clodronate."

What the study did not mention is that clodronate can be taken orally every day, while Aredia administration is restricted to intravenous infusion. The fact that the calcium-normalizing effects of a single dose of Aredia lasted twice as long as a single dose of clodronate does not reveal much since it was already known that clodronate should be taken every day by mouth to maintain its effects.

The major unpleasant side effect to Aredia is a transient fever, sometimes accompanied by flu-like symptoms such as myalgias and lymphopenia. These effects occur commonly after the first infusion of Aredia. Other reported adverse events include transient neutropenia, mild thrombophlebitis, asymptomatic hypocalcemia, and, rarely, ocular complications (uveitis and scleritis) and irritation at the site of infusion. Clodronate, on the other hand, appears to be free of unpleasant side effects other than the very rare case of it causing too little calcium in the blood (hypocalcemia).

There is no evidence to show that Aredia increases survival or prevents the development of metastasis in breast cancer, while there are two studies that show clodronate can improve survival. The greatest concern to cancer patients, however, may be that Aredia has been consistently shown to significantly elevate blood levels of the cytokines tumor necrosis factor (TNF) and interleukin-6 (IL-6). Clodronate does not increase these cytokines. TNF and IL-6 have differing effects on various cancer cell lines.

One study to compare the effects of Aredia and clodronate on cancer patients showed a significant decrease in lymphocyte and leukocyte count in the Aredia group. In the same group, seven patients (24%) showed a transient increase of body temperature. These changes were not found in the patients treated with clodronate. Plasma IL-6 and TNF levels increased significantly after Aredia treatment, whereas no change was seen after clodronate infusion.

Breast cancer patients already have elevated levels of TNF and IL-6. Elevation of these two cytokines reflects an advanced disease state and impending death. TNF is also involved in inducing autoimmune inflammatory disease. A study evaluated the possible anti-inflammatory action of Aredia and clodronate and found that low concentrations of Aredia induced the IL-6 secretion while higher levels of Aredia were toxic. The induction of IL-6 or toxic effects were not observed with clodronate.

A study was undertaken to evaluate the relationship between serum TNF and cachexia (wasting syndrome) in patients with prostate cancer. Serum TNF activity was positive in 76% of the patients with relapsed disease, whereas only 11% of the untreated patients and 0% of the patients in remission as a result of endocrine therapy were positive. The serum total protein and albumin levels, hemoglobin levels, and body mass index of the patients with elevated serum TNF levels were significantly lower than the corresponding values in patients with undetectable serum TNF levels. There was a significant correlation between the detectability of serum TNF and performance status. Patients with elevated serum TNF levels had a significantly higher mortality rate than those with undetectable serum TNF levels. These findings suggest that TNF may be one of the factors contributing to cachexia in patients with prostate cancer. This study clearly shows that prostate cancer patients do not want to elevate TNF. Aredia elevates serum TNF, but clodronate does not. When it comes to prostate cancer, clodronate appears to be a lot safer.

A high serum level of IL-6 is regarded as a predictor of poor prognosis in multiple myeloma. A 3-year study evaluated the effect of IL-6 on a large group of multiple myeloma patients. The patients with high levels of IL-6 were at very high risk of dying within 3 years from diagnosis. The doctors concluded that serum IL-6 is a significant marker of disease progression in multiple myeloma. A study on serum in human breast cancer patients revealed levels of serum IL-6 correlated with the stage of progression and with axillary lymph node involvement. The doctors concluded that high levels of IL-6 indicates more advanced disease. Aredia increases IL-6 levels, and is also used frequently by doctors in the United States to treat multiple myeloma. However, in the United States, doctors cannot treat patients with clodronate, even though it does not boost toxic IL-6, because the FDA will not allow it to be sold to American citizens.

Angiogenesis (the formation of new blood vessels) is an essential requirement for tumor growth and metastasis. TNF is a factor known to promote tumor angiogenesis in breast cancers. Scientists are looking at therapies to lower TNF as a way of inhibiting tumor angiogenesis. It would appear that most cancer patients would not want to increase their TNF level because the resulting formation of new blood vessels would enable their tumor to grow and develop metastatic colonies. Aredia causes TNF to elevate, whereas clodronate does not affect TNF levels.

The oncologist should be encouraged to prescribe 1.25 to 2.5 mg of the drug Parlodel, also known as bromocriptine. Parlodel must be taken after meals because severe nausea can occur when it is taken on an empty stomach. A better way to suppress prolactin is with Dostinex. Twice a week dosing of 0.25 to 0.50 mg is all that is needed, and side effects are rare. Breast cancer patients should endeavor to keep their prolactin to under 3 nanograms per milliliter on a standard prolactin blood test, and Dostinex will accomplish this in most people.

Diet

Although there has been some controversy regarding the association between types of dietary fat and the development of breast cancer, some suggestions can be made. The American diet, particularly in the last 15 years with the push for higher consumption of carbohydrates and the robust incorporation of fat, is likely associated with the development of breast cancer. One reason may be that the high fat and carbohydrate diet increases the development of so-called free radicals, which cause DNA damage and can affect cell development, the immune system, and hence lead to the propensity to develop cancer in general. Additionally, carbohydrates with a high glycemic index (meaning they are quickly converted to glucose) cause the release of insulin, resulting in rapid fluctuations in the glucose level, which may have an impact on the development of breast cancer. Therefore, breast cancer patients should markedly decrease their intake of both saturated and unsaturated fats and simple carbohydrates containing a high glycemic index. Additionally, patients should follow a diet as recommended in the *Cancer protocols*.

Other Treatment

(*See the Cancer protocols for other alternative cancer treatments that may help breast cancer.*)

Laboratory Testing

Breast cancer patients whose tumor cells have a mutant p53 oncogene are far more likely to benefit from soy extract supplementation. Only a pathology examination of the actual cancer cells can determine p53 status. An immunohistochemistry test can help to determine the p53 status of tumor cells. The following laboratory can perform this new test:

IMPATH Laboratories
1010 Third Avenue, Suite 203
New York, N.Y. 10021
Phone: 1-800-447-5816

IMPATH Laboratories measures the presence of mutant p53 oncogene. If the test is positive, you have mutant p53 and are more likely to benefit from soy extracts. If the test is negative, it indicates that you have functional p53 and are less likely to benefit from soy extracts. The Foundation realizes that many cancer patients seeking to use soy supplements may find it difficult to have an immunohistochemistry test performed to ascertain p53 status. Monthly blood testing for breast cancer patients is mandatory. Every patient responds differently to both conventional and alternative cancer therapies. The results of blood tests provide critically important data to evaluate the effectiveness of whatever therapies are being used. The blood tests commonly used by doctors to evaluate progression or regression of breast cancer are CA 27.29, CEA, prolactin, GGTP, and alkaline phosphatase. If, for instance, the CA 27.29 tumor marker were to continue to elevate 30 to 60 days after initiating soy-extract supplementation, discontinue its use and seek another therapy immediately.

Monthly blood tests should include a complete blood chemistry with tests for liver function and serum calcium levels, prolactin levels, parathyroid hormone levels, and the tumor marker CA 27.29 as well as cancer profile tests (CA Profile) that include the CEA and GGTP tests. These tests monitor the progress or failure of whatever therapies are being used, and also are able to detect toxicity from high doses of vitamin A and vitamin D_3. The patient should insist on obtaining a copy of her blood workups every month. (*Please refer to the Cancer protocols for additional suggestions.*)

Conventional Therapies

Surgery, radiation, and cytotoxic chemotherapy are conventional treatments for breast cancer that have statistically increased survival rates in published studies. Despite the known short- and long-term toxicities of chemotherapy, it is difficult to argue against it since breast cancer cells have such an exceptional propensity to metastasize. The high failure rates associated with conventional breast cancer therapy has motivated most educated women to integrate alternative therapies into their treatment program. Few conventional oncologists, however, have sufficient knowledge of these alternative therapies, and it is often up to the patient to stay fully informed.

A nontoxic conventional drug called Arimidex (anastrozole) may be prescribed to suppress estrogen synthesis in the body. Arimidex works by inhibiting the aromatase enzyme that is responsible for the conversion of androstenedione to estrone in the peripheral tissues (such as adipose tissue). Estrone further converts to estradiol, the more potent form of estrogen that patients with estrogen-receptor positive cancer cells want to suppress.

Summary

1. Take 3–50 mg of melatonin at bedtime.
2. Take indole-3-carbinol. Take one 200-mg capsule twice a day if you weigh under 120 pounds. Take three 200-mg capsules a day in two divided doses if you weigh over 120 pounds.
3. Vitamin D_3, 4000 to 6000 IU taken daily on an empty stomach with monthly blood testing to monitor for toxicity. Reduce dosage at 6 months.
4. Take water-soluble vitamin A, 100,000 to 300,000 IU daily with monthly blood testing to monitor for toxicity. Reduce dosage at 6 months. (*Refer to vitamin A precautions.*)
5. Take vitamin E succinate, 1200 IU daily.
6. Take quercetin, 400 mg 3 times a day. (Water-soluble form will have a different dosage.)
7. Take curcumin, 900 to 2700 mg daily.
8. Take dostinex, 0.25 to 0.50 mg twice a week to suppress serum prolactin to under 3 nanograms a milliliter, if elevated.
9. Mega Soy, five 700-mg capsule taken 4 times a day. Note cautions stated in this protocol.

CAUTION: Pregnant women should not take indole-3-carbinol because of its modulation of estrogen.

10. Take CoQ_{10}, 100 mg 3 times a day. Note cautions stated in this protocol.
11. Take decaffeinated green tea extract, 4 to 10 capsules daily.
12. Take organic selenium (selenomethionine), 200 mcg 2 to 3 times a day.
13. Take conjugated linolenic acid, ten 50-mg capsules a day.
14. Take flax B—The Missing Link For Humans—2 to 5 tablespoons a day.
15. Take Garlic Caps, 900 mg 5 times a day.
16. Consider 1 to 2 tablespoons of Phyl-Food vegetable complex each day.
17. Consider whey protein, 20 to 30 grams taken a day.
18. Consider *Spes,* 2 to 3 capsules, twice a day, 2 hours before meals. Individuals over 150 pounds should take 3 capsules and those under 150 pounds should take 2 capsules.

(*See general guidelines for cancer treatment in the Cancer Protocols.*)

19. Consider conventional therapies such as tamoxifen and Arimidex. Surgery, chemotherapy, and radiation therapy have been proven effective in improving survival.

(*For a basic introduction to the nature of cancer, please see the Cancer protocols.*)

For information about clinical research studies. Contact the American Cancer Society, (800) ACS-2345.

Product availability. Melatonin, Phyto-Food, Mega Soy Extract, Coenzyme Q_{10}, green tea, water-soluble vitamin A, vitamin D_3 caps, conjugated linolenic acid, indole-3-carbinol, and The Missing Link For Humans can be ordered by calling (800) 544-4440, or order online at www.lef.org. Ask for a listing of innovative physicians in your area who may be able to help you implement an alternative-therapy cancer program. For information about how to obtain clodronate, call (800) 226-2370.

BURSITIS

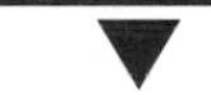

(See Arthritis)

CANCER (ADJUVANT) TREATMENT

More than 4 million Americans are currently being treated for cancer. Each year, 1.3 million Americans are newly diagnosed with cancer. For the past four decades, both the incidence and age-adjusted death rate from cancer in America have been climbing steadily.

Cancer is an abnormal growth, caused by underlying disease involving the whole body. It is not just limited to a lump or bump. The successful treatment of cancer is best accomplished by the precise administration of multiple therapies. Neither conventional nor alternative medicine recognizes the importance of multimodality treatment, and the end result is that too many cancer patients needlessly die.

Although the mainstream therapies of chemotherapy, radiation, and surgery often do reduce tumor burden, these therapies do not change the underlying causes of the disease. Given the blatant failures of conventional cancer therapies, it is imperative that we examine optional and complementary therapies to assist the swelling ranks of American cancer patients. These therapies need to be considered earlier, rather than as a last resort by cancer patients.

The purpose of this protocol is to help cancer patients bridge critical gaps in their treatment programs so they can increase the odds of long-term disease remission. The information provided is based solely on peer-reviewed studies published in respected medical journals throughout the world. It is important for the reader to know that this protocol is based on the results of published research, as there are many fraudulent "cancer cures" that are not substantiated in the medical literature.

We call these "adjuvant" treatment recommendations because the primary therapy will inevitably be administered by the attending physician. The problem is that even the best oncologist may not be able to keep up with the latest findings because of the sheer volume of new treatment data. Our mission, therefore, is to provide insightful cancer-treatment information that is too often overlooked by practicing oncologists.

The Importance of "Measuring" Success or Failure

It is of critical importance in any cancer treatment program to measure success or failure. This can be accomplished in most cancers by evaluating tumor markers in the blood and/or by looking at the actual tumor(s) via medical imagery. When using any kind of cancer therapy, it is crucial that blood tumor marker tests be performed every 30 to 45 days. If the tumor markers reveal regression of the cancer, then existing therapy may be continued. If tumor markers indicate disease progression, then a different treatment approach should be implemented immediately. At the end of this protocol, we provide a listing of blood tumor marker tests as they relate to specific types of cancer.

An Overlooked Therapy

Many types of cancer cells use an enzyme called cyclooxygenase-2 (COX-2) to propagate. This includes cancers of the colon, pancreas, breast, prostate, bladder, lung, head and neck, to name a few. The good news is that COX-2 is also involved in the rheumatoid arthritis process, so there are drugs that are already approved to treat arthritis that may also be prescribed for cancer patients.

Drugs that inhibit the cyclooxygenase enzyme are known as COX-2 inhibitors. The two newest COX-2 inhibitors are Celebrex and Vioxx, but we suggest that cancer patients consider older drugs that have a more predictable safety history. One drug that oncologists may consider prescribing is *Lodine XL,* a drug used to treat arthritis that also interferes with COX-2 activity. A safer COX-2 inhibiting drug called *nimesulide* is sold in Europe but is not yet approved by the FDA.

Cancer cells often produce large amounts of COX-2 and use it as a biological fuel to cause rapid proliferation of cell division. An article in the journal *Cancer Research* (1999 March 1; 59 [5]:987–90) shows that COX-2 levels in pancreatic cancer cells are 60 times greater than in adjacent normal tissue. A handful of physicians knowledgeable about COX-2 and cancer are prescribing COX-2 inhibitors to their patients. It was back in 1997 that the Life Extension Foundation recommended the European drug nimesulide to cancer patients. The FDA has aggressively blocked the personal-use importation of this potential life-saving medication to cancer patients.

Scientists are now actively investigating COX-2 inhibitors as drugs that would be effective in both the prevention and treatment of many cancers. When COX-2 drugs are given to patients with colon polyps (precancerous lesions), the lesions completely disappear. When a group of rats were given a potent carcinogen, there was a 90% reduction in those who developed cancer if they were on COX-2 inhibition therapy. In the few rats that did develop the tumors while taking COX-2 inhibition therapy, the tumors were 80% smaller and less numerous than in the group not on COX-2 inhibition (*Wall Street Journal,* Sept. 7, 1999).

We predict that COX-2 inhibiting drugs will eventually be approved to treat cancer, but in the meantime, cancer patients should ask their doctors to consider prescribing a COX-2 inhibiting drug as an adjuvant therapy.

Drugs that Inhibit COX-2

Lodine XL is an arthritis drug approved by the FDA that interferes with COX-2 metabolic processes. The maximum dosage for Lodine is 1000 mg daily. Everyone now appears to be using Lodine XL extended-release tablets for convenient once-a-day dosing. The Lodine XL 500-mg tablet enables physicians to prescribe the maximum dosage of Lodine XL—1000 mg per day—as two tablets in a single daily dose. As with any nonsteroidal anti-inflammatory drug (NSAID), extreme caution and physician supervision are a must.

The most common complaints associated with Lodine XL use relate to the gastrointestinal tract. Serious GI toxicity such as perforation, ulceration, and bleeding can occur in patients treated long term with NSAID therapy. Serious renal and hepatic reactions have been reported only rarely. Lodine XL should not be given to patients who have previously shown hypersensitivity to it or in whom aspirin or other NSAIDs induce asthma, rhinitis, urticaria, or other allergic reactions. Fatal asthmatic reactions have been reported in such patients receiving NSAIDs.

Nimesulide is a safer COX-2 inhibitor, but is not approved by the FDA. It is available from Mexican pharmacies or can be ordered by mail from European pharmacies. The suggested dose for nimesulide is two 100-mg tablets a day. It is important that your physician know you are taking nimesulide as an adjuvant cancer therapy.

Please refer to the "molecular oncology" section of this protocol for a detailed description of the connection between COX-2 and cancer.

Why Many Cancer Patients Need Cholesterol-Lowering Drugs

The regulation of cancer cell growth is often governed by a family of proteins known as RAS oncogenes. The RAS family is responsible for modulating the regulatory signals that govern the cancer cell cycle and proliferation. Mutations in genes encoding RAS proteins have been intimately associated with unregulated cell proliferation (i.e., cancer).

There is a class of cholesterol-lowering drugs known as the "statins" that have been shown to inhibit the activity of RAS oncogenes. Some of these cholesterol-lowering "statin" drugs are lovastatin, simvastatin, and pravastatin.

The highest incidences of RAS mutations are found in cancers of the pancreas (90%), the colon (50%) and the lung; in thyroid tumors (50%), in liver tumors (30%), and in myeloid leukemia (30%). If you have one of these cancers, you should consider requesting an immunohistochemistry for the mutated RAS oncogene or a biopsied specimen in order to ascertain whether the combination of chemotherapy and a statin drug may be effective. (Information about obtaining RAS testing appears later in this protocol.)

As far as dosing is concerned, if the drug lovastatin (Mevacor) were chosen, a cancer patient with a mutated RAS oncogene should take as high as 80 mg a day for several months. Another approach is to take 80 mg a day of lovastatin for 3 weeks, take 2 weeks off, and then resume. It may be especially important to use a statin drug during chemotherapy. Statin drugs given with cytotoxic chemotherapy could provide the necessary one-two punch to kill a sufficient number of tumor cells for the patient to enter a period of long-term remission. Careful monitoring of liver enzymes is needed to guard against liver toxicity of the statin drugs. There are other potential side effects to watch out for, but in many cancers, statin drugs appear to be a powerful inhibitor of cancer cell proliferation. The "molecular oncology" section of this protocol provides more details about the use of statin drugs as an adjuvant cancer therapy.

Combining a COX-2 Inhibitor with a Statin

A novel approach would be to combine a "statin" drug such as lovastatin with a COX-2 inhibitor.

A study published in the journal *Gastroenterology* (1999, Vol. 116, No. 4, Suppl. A369) showed that lovastatin augmented by up to fivefold the cancer cell killing effect of a drug with COX-2 inhibiting properties (Sulindac). In this study, three different colon cancer cell lines were killed (made to undergo programmed cell death) by depriving them of COX-2. When lovastatin was added to the COX-2 inhibitor, the kill rate increased by up to fivefold.

Thus, those with certain cancers might benefit if their oncologists prescribed for several months 80 mg a day of Mevacor (lovastatin) and 1000 mg a day of Lodine XL.

Physician involvement is crucial to help protect against potential side effects of these drugs. Those who are concerned about potential toxicity should take into account the fact that the types of cancers these drugs might be effective against have extremely high mortality rates.

The Importance of Nutritional Support

Nutrition therapy helps to change the conditions in the body that favor tumor growth and return the cancer patient to a healthier status. More wellness in the body means less illness. Fungus grows on the bark of a tree due to the underlying conditions of heat, moisture, and darkness. One could "cut, burn, and poison" this fungus, but as long as the prevailing conditions of heat, moisture, and darkness were present, the fungal growth would return until the host was consumed. Similarly, a patient develops cancer due to a collection of conditions that compromise the host.

Nutrition is a low-cost, nontoxic, and scientifically validated adjuvant modality in the treatment of cancer. Adjuvant (helpful) nutrition and traditional oncology are synergistic, not antagonistic. Some reasons and rationale for using an aggressive nutrition program in comprehensive cancer treatment include

- Avoiding malnutrition.
- Reducing the toxicity of medical therapy, making chemotherapy and radiation therapy more selectively toxic to the tumor cells.
- Stimulating immune function.
- Selectively starving the tumor.
- Providing biological response modifiers to assist mechanisms and improve outcomes in cancer therapy.

A complete nutritional support plan of action will be provided later in this protocol.

A Promising New Therapy

Angiogenesis (new blood vessel growth) is a key step in tumor growth, invasion, and metastasis. A substance that cuts the supply of blood to cancer cells can stop the primary tumor and its spread throughout the body. A new anti-angiogenesis cancer drug will enter human clinical trials in the United States at the end of 1999. The scientific literature shows that this drug induces a consistent and significant reduction in tumor growth in laboratory animals. In many cases the primary and metastatic cancer lesions are put into a dormant state and no longer propagate.

To date, a number of anti-angiogenesis agents have been identified. In animal models, treatment with angiogenesis inhibitors has proven antitumor effects. Early clinical experience with angiogenesis inhibitors indicates that optimal anti-angiogenesis therapy will likely be based on their long-term administration to cancer patients in adjunct to other therapies.

The published evidence indicates that the new angiogenesis-inhibitors offer great promise to cancer patients. The therapy is nontoxic and has shown efficacy against every type of cancer it has been tested against. One study showed that it suppressed metastatic tumor growth rates by 90%. Another study showed primary tumors regressing to become "dormant microscopic lesions."

Before raising any premature hope, we want to state that this new anticancer therapy consists of two drugs, *endostatin* and *angiostatin*. The FDA, however, is only permitting one of these two drugs (endostatin) to be used in the initial clinical trials. In other words, the FDA is not allowing terminally ill humans to use the two drugs that worked so remarkably well together in the animal studies. There is still reason to believe, however, that just one half of this drug combination (the endostatin) could save the lives of human cancer victims who have been sentenced to death by the medical establishment.

Those suffering from a nontreatable form of cancer should consider entering those clinical trials where endostatin, a potent angiogenesis-inhibiting drug, will be tested in humans. It is hoped that the other angiogenesis-inhibiting drug, angiostatin, will soon be added to endostatin in order to replicate the successful two-drug combo that so effectively treated cancer in the laboratory studies.

Primary and metastatic tumors require ongoing angiogenesis (new blood vessel formation) to support their growth. This is an undisputed fact based on today's understanding of oncological processes. Weak angiogenesis-inhibiting agents such as shark cartilage have not shown adequate efficacy. Angiostatin and endostatin are naturally produced proteins that shut off new blood vessel formation to tumors.

Angiostatin and/or endostatin have produced dramatic remissions in animal studies. Human cancer patients can access endostatin in FDA-sanctioned human clinical trials. The drug endostatin is derived from a protein found in the human body. In animal trials, the protein drug wiped out several forms of cancer by choking off the blood supply to tumors.

Although many cancer patients develop a resistance to conventional drugs, they aren't likely to do so with endostatin. What's more, the new natural treatment appears to stop cancer from spreading to other parts of the body.

So far, endostatin has worked only in mice. Now the National Cancer Institute in Frederick, MD, wants to find out whether the drug can starve human tumors. The initial trials are scheduled to begin at the University of Texas, M.D. Anderson Cancer Institute in Houston, and the University of Wisconsin's Comprehensive Cancer Center in

Madison. The "molecular oncology" section of this protocol provides more detailed information about endostatin and angiostatin.

(To find out specific information about entering these clinical trials, refer to the Life Extension Foundation's Web site at www.lef.org or call (800) 544-4440).

Protecting against Chemotherapy Toxicity

Cancer patients using cytotoxic chemotherapy drugs should ask their oncologists to place them on FDA-approved immunoprotective drugs 1 week before the first chemotherapy drug is administered. Depending on the type of cancer and the chemotherapy regimen that will be used, two of the most important FDA-approved drugs to consider are *Neupogen,* a granulocyte-colony stimulating factor drug (G-CSF) and *Leukine,* a granulocyte-macrophage-colony stimulating factor (GM-CSF).

Neupogen and Leukine stimulate the production of T-lymphocytes, macrophages, and other immune cells which are valuable in preventing the toxic effects on the bone marrow during chemotherapy. These immune-protecting drugs enable chemotherapy to be given at a higher dose that may make it effective. Stimulated macrophages are powerful tumor killers, as has been demonstrated by clinical studies using interleukin-2 and GM-CSF, or G-CSF. In addition, colony growth factors are able to accelerate regeneration of blood cells following chemotherapy. Initial clinical experience with GM-CSF and G-CSF has shown that severe neutropenia (immune impairment) due to chemotherapy drugs may be prevented or at least decelerated, reducing the number of severe infections.

Alpha-interferon and interleukin-2 are immune cytokines (regulators) that should also be considered by cancer patients. Interferon directly inhibits cancer cell proliferation and has already been used in the therapy of hairy cell leukemia, Kaposi's sarcoma, and malignant melanoma. Interleukin-2 allows for an increase in the cytotoxic activity of Natural Killer (NK) cells. These drugs must be carefully administered by an oncologist, as they can produce temporary side effects.

Retinoic acid (vitamin A) analog drugs enhance the efficacy of some chemotherapy regimens and reduce the risk of secondary cancers. Ask your oncologist to consider prescribing vitamin A analog drugs such as Accutane. Again, the use and dosage of potentially toxic drugs such as Accutane must be carefully prescribed by your attending oncologist.

Some cancer patients produce too many T-suppressor cells that shut down optimal immune function. The administration of drugs such as cimetidine prevent cancer cells from prematurely shutting down the immune system. An *immune cell subset* blood test will reveal the status of your T-helper cells, T-suppressor cells, and natural killer cell count and activity.

The proper administration of Neupogen or Leukine prior to the initiation of chemotherapy can dramatically reduce the immune damage that chemotherapy inflicts on the body and increase the cancer cell killing efficacy of conventional chemotherapy drugs. Please remember that, so far, we have only talked about drugs that require physician administration. There are safe nutrients that can be self-administered that also protect against chemotherapy toxicity and immune impairment.

Some of these nutrients include Coenzyme Q_{10}, which has been shown in several studies to protect against chemotherapy damage to the heart. CoQ_{10} was highlighted as the topic of professional medical discussion as a complementary treatment for cancer at a recent meeting (*Oncology Hunting*) 1999 Feb; 13 [2]:166). Natural vitamin E succinate has also been shown to protect organs throughout the body from the damaging effects of cytotoxic chemotherapy.

CAUTION: Some studies indicate that Coenzyme Q_{10} should not be taken at the same time as chemotherapy. If this is true, it would be disappointing, since CoQ_{10} is so effective in protecting against adriamycin-induced cardiomyopathy. Adriamycin is a chemotherapy drug sometimes used as part of a chemotherapy cocktail. Until more research is known, it is not possible to make a definitive recommendation whether to take CoQ_{10} during chemotherapy.

Supplemental melatonin in doses of 10 to 40 mg a night can protect and restore normal blood-cell production caused by the toxicity of chemotherapy. A study was performed in 80 patients with metastatic solid tumors to evaluate the benefits of melatonin. Patients received either chemotherapy alone or chemotherapy plus 20 mg each night of melatonin. Thrombocytopenia was significantly less frequent in patients receiving melatonin. Other common side effects of cancer chemotherapy—such as malaise, asthenia, stomatitis, and neuropathy—occurred less frequently in patients receiving melatonin. This corroborated previous studies showing that the administration of melatonin during chemotherapy can prevent some side effects, especially myelosuppression (blood-cell production suppression) and neuropathy.

The administration of FDA-approved drugs such as Neupogen or Leukine are important to cancer patients, even though melatonin has similar mechanisms of action. There are too many published studies about the prophylactic benefits of these FDA-approved drugs for them not to be used prior to the administration of chemotherapy.

To treat low white blood cell counts, the FDA-approved drug Neupogen or Leukine may be considered by your immunologist or hematologist. Drugs such as Neupogen, Leukine, and Intron A alpha-interferon (an immune-modulating cytokine) can restore immune function debilitated by toxic cancer chemotherapy drugs. In one study, patients with refractory (resistant to treatment) solid tumors treated with standard chemotherapy and GM-CSF had a 33.3% objective response rate, versus 15% with chemotherapy alone. If you are on chemotherapy and your blood tests show immune suppression, you should demand that your oncologist use the appropriate immune restoration drug(s).

(Please refer to the *Cancer Chemotherapy protocol* for additional suggestions on protecting against the multiple toxicities these drugs can cause.)

Immunohistochemistry Testing

Cancer patients whose tumor cells have a mutant p53 oncogene are far more likely to benefit from certain therapies than are others. Only a pathology examination of the actual cancer cells can determine p53 status. An immunohistochemistry test can help to determine the p53 and RAS oncogene status of tumor cells. The following laboratory can perform this test:

IMPATH Laboratories
1010 Third Avenue, Suite 203
New York, N.Y. 10021
Phone: (800) 447-5816

IMPATH Laboratories measures mutant p53. If the test is positive, you have mutant p53 and are *more* likely to benefit from products such as soy genistein. If the test is negative, it indicates that you have functional p53 and are *less* likely to benefit from soy extracts.

The Life Extension Foundation first recommended immunohistochemistry testing in 1997. An article that appeared in a September 1999 issue of the *Lancet* (1999; 354:896–900) showed that immunohistochemical detection aids in the diagnosis and staging of breast cancer and should become "a standard method of node examination in postmenopausal patients." While the *Lancet* study looked only at breast cancer cells, the Foundation continues to recommend that all cancer patients consider immunohistochemical testing of their tumor cells to determine p53, RAS, and other oncogene status.

Integrated Cancer Therapy

With one in three Americans now using alternative medicine therapies regularly, many conventional oncologists are still not incorporating the published findings of nutritional science that benefit their patients' fight against cancer.

The Life Extension Foundation has researched an impressive collection of published studies showing that the disease process can be favorably mitigated with nutritional factors. These adjuvant treatments present approaches to boost immune system function, inhibit cancer cell division, induce cancer cells to differentiate back into mature cells, inhibit cancer cell metastases, prevent angiogenesis, and modulate the effect of hormones on cancer cell growth. These studies also reveal complementary methods for reducing the toxicity and the suppression of the immune system for both chemotherapy and radiation therapy.

It is impossible to completely describe all the mechanisms of action for the nutrients and hormones recommended in this Cancer Treatment protocol. What follows are discussion and studies that substantiate key recommendations of the protocol. The inclusion of certain nutrients in the following descriptions does not mean that they are more important than nutrients such as vitamin C and selenium, which are not discussed because of lack of space.

Many cancers require aggressive conventional therapies. The Life Extension Foundation has not found an effective alternative therapy that is sufficiently potent to shrink large primary or widely disseminated cancer. Treatment of such advanced tumors may yet require conventional therapies such as chemotherapy, radiation therapy, and surgery. The conventional approach to cancer using one or more of the big three can leave the patient's immune system suppressed and can induce a catabolic (or wasting) state with rapid weight loss. Cancer patients should insist that their oncologists accept their desire to support their immune systems with nutritional therapies and the benefits of using such protocols to assist the conventional medicine.

Continued Testing and Monitoring Is Crucial

The Foundation emphasizes the importance of regular tumor marker testing to measure and monitor cancer status and therapy. Patients should establish with their doctors a planned schedule for cancer testing to monitor their progress during treatment. Modern testing is one of the most important tools for combating cancer, and both the patient and the doctor should be cognizant of the latest testing methods and should establish a monthly or regular testing schedule. Some cancers will require x-ray, MRI, or CAT scans to be detected and/or monitored, while other cancers can be monitored using blood tumor markers. For cancers that do not have an established blood tumor marker test, patients should use MRI, CAT scans, and other imaging diagnostics every 30 to 60 days to determine whether tumor shrinking is actually occurring and to measure the progress of any remissions seen.

Nutritional Therapies

Patients who have been diagnosed with large primary tumors may have to rely on conventional cancer therapy to treat the primary tumor, however, the nutrient and hormone adjuvant therapies presented in this book may help control metastasized cancer cells and reduce the toxicity of chemotherapy and radiation therapy. It should be noted that nutritional therapy is a long-term therapy requiring consistent and proper use of nutritional supplements and the measuring of cancer status (via regular blood testing) to determine the patient's response. The use of nutritional support is gaining in popularity because of high public demand and scientific findings.

Chemotherapy has a poor overall record of success over the past 30 years, but the Life Extension Foundation has identified adjuvant therapies to augment chemotherapies by making these drugs less toxic to healthy cells and more toxic to cancer cells, and by reducing the suppression of the immune system.

It should be noted that many cancer patients turn to alternative therapy fairly late in the course of the disease. Under such circumstances, and after the failure of conventional medicine, the prognosis for a cure is poor and the best many patients can hope for is an increased survival rate and reduced pain. In many cases, the failure of alternative medicine at the latest stages of cancer is used as a political statement by the medical establishment on the general topic of alternative therapies for cancer therapy. Keep in mind that conventional medicine has, in most cases, failed to offer any improvement or hope for the majority of desperate patients with advanced-stage cancers.

The Science behind Cancer Nutrition Therapies

Finnish oncologists used high doses of nutrients along with chemotherapy and radiation for lung cancer patients. Normally, lung cancer is a "poor prognostic" malignancy advanced with a 1%-2%

expected survival at 30 months under normal treatment. In this study, however, 8 of 18 patients (44%) were still alive 6 years after therapy.

Oncologists at West Virginia Medical School randomized 65 patients with transitional cell carcinoma of the bladder into either the "one-per-day" vitamin supplement providing the RDA, or a group which received the RDA supplement plus 40,000 IU of vitamin A, 100 mg of B_6, 2000 mg of vitamin C, 400 IU of vitamin E, and 90 mg of zinc. At 10 months, tumor recurrence was 80% in the control group (RDA supplement) and 40% in the experimental "megavitamin" group. Five-year projected tumor recurrences were 91% for controls and 41% for "megavitamin" patents. Essentially, high-dose nutrients cut tumor recurrence in half.

In a nonrandomized clinical trial, Drs. Hoffer and Pauling instructed patients to follow a reasonable cancer diet (unprocessed food low in fat, dairy, and sugar), coupled with therapeutic doses of vitamins and minerals. All 129 patients in this study received concomitant oncology care. The control group of 31 patients who did not receive nutrition support lived an average of less than 6 months. The group of 98 cancer patients who did receive the diet and a supplement program was categorized into three groups:

- Group 1. Poor responders or approximately 20% of treated group. These had an average lifespan of 10 months or a 75% improvement over the control group.
- Group 2. Good responders, or approximately 47%, who had various cancers including leukemia, lung, liver, and pancreas; this group had an average lifespan of 72 months (6 years).
- Group 3. Good female responders or approximately 32% with involvement of reproductive areas (breast, cervix, ovary, uterus); group 3 had an average lifespan of over 10 years. Many were still alive at the end of the study.

In examining the diet and lifespan of 675 lung cancer patients over the course of 6 years, researchers found that the more vegetables consumed, the longer the lung cancer patient lived.

In 200 cancer patients studied who experienced "spontaneous regression," 87% made a major change in diet, mostly vegetarian in nature, 55% used some form of detoxification, and 65% used nutritional supplements.

Researchers at Tulane University compared survival in patients who used the macrobiotic diet versus patients who continued with their standard western lifestyle. Of 1467 pancreatic patients who made no changes in diet, 146 (10%) were alive after one year, while 12 of the 23 matched pancreatic patients (52%) consuming macrobiotic foods were still alive after one year.

Benefits of Genistein

Genistein has shown significant cell-inhibiting effects in many different types of cancer. A study was conducted to examine the role genistein played in growth factors'—such as protein tyrosine kinase and in thymidine incorporation into cancer cells. Genistein suppressed protein tyrosine kinase activity and the subsequent growth stimulatory incorporation of thymidine into cancer cells. The scientists speculated that genistein has potential value in the prevention and treatment of some tumors *in vivo*.

In other studies, genistein has shown anti-angiogenesis properties, cancer cell adhesion-inhibition properties, estrogen-receptor blocking properties, and apoptosis-inducing effects. An investigation into the effect of soy genistein on the growth and differentiation of human melanoma cells showed that genistein significantly inhibited cell growth. Some studies suggest that genistein may enhance the efficacy of certain chemotherapy regimens.

Soy protein contains several anticancer agents including genistein and other isoflavones. In one study, a lower incidence of prostate cancer was shown in Chinese men who had higher amounts isoflavonoid phytoestrogens, daidzein, and equol within their prostatic fluids and in their blood plasma. The study concluded that the high concentrations of isoflavones present in the prostatic fluid of Asian men may protect them from prostate disease.

A study in a 1999 issue of the *Journal of Nutrition* reported that "dietary soy products may inhibit prostate tumor growth through a combination of direct effects on tumor cells and indirect effects on tumor neovasculature." Earlier in 1999, a study in the *British Journal of Cancer* reported an inhibitory effect of genistein and quercetin on the growth of tumors.

Curcumin and genistein have both been shown to inhibit the growth of estrogen-positive human breast cancer cells induced by pesticides. When curcumin and genistein were added to breast cancer cells, a synergistic effect resulted in a total inhibition of cancer cell growth caused by pesticide-induced estrogenic activity. This study suggested that the combination of curcumin and genistein in the diet has the potential to reduce the proliferation of estrogen-positive cells induced by mixtures of pesticides or estrogen. Since it is difficult to remove pesticides completely from the diet, and since neither curcumin nor soy genistein is toxic to humans, their inclusion in the diet in order to prevent hormone-related cancers deserves consideration. Curcumin appears to function via several different mechanisms to inhibit cancer cell proliferation.

Differentiation-inducing agents such as genistein, retinoids, and vitamin D analogs inhibited tumor cell–induced angiogenesis *in vitro* and *in vivo*. Simultaneous administration of retinoids and 1,25-dihydroxy vitamin D_3 led to a synergistic inhibition of tumors associated with angiogenesis in mice. Recently, these compounds have been shown to induce and act in concert with natural angiogenic inhibitors such as interferons.

A study was conducted to determine whether genistein could induce human breast adenocarcinoma cell maturation and differentiation. Treating these cells with genistein resulted in growth inhibition accompanied by increased cell maturation. These maturation markers were optimally expressed after 9 days of treatment with genistein. Both estrogen-receptor-positive and estrogen-receptor-negative cells became differentiated in response to genistein, which is a crucial step in inducing cancer cell apoptosis (programmed cell death). Despite this study, we do not recommend that women with estrogen-receptor-positive breast cancer use soy genistein because of the following evidence.

Genistein appears to be especially effective against prostate cancers. One study showed that genistein inhibited the proliferation and expression of the *in vitro* invasive capacity of tumoral prostatic cells. In a cell culture system, genistein appeared to be cytotoxic and inhibitory to PC-3 cells. The more aggressive the prostate cancer cell culture studies, the more effective was the genistein, both with respect to proliferation rate and inhibition of growth factors.

More recently, the *Japanese Journal of Cancer Research* (1999 April; 90 [4]:393–98) reported results of a comprehensive rat study which provides further evidence that soybean isoflavones have a potential as chemopreventive agents against carcinogenesis in the prostate.

Other investigators have reported anticancer effects of genistein on lung cancer in the 1999 *Journal of Nutritional Cancer,* where researchers reported a specific effect on lung cancer cells.

Breast cancer and genistein

One study tested the effects of naturally occurring flavonoids on the proliferation of an estrogen-receptor-positive human breast cancer cell line. Genistein inhibited cell proliferation, but this effect was reversed when estrogen was added. The flavonoids hesperidin, naringenin, and quercetin inhibited breast cancer cell proliferation even in the presence of high levels of estrogen. These flavonoids apparently exert their antiproliferative activity via a mechanism that is different from that of genistein. Women with any type of breast cancer should test their serum estrogen levels to make sure that too much estrogen is not present if they are taking high doses of soy. Estrogen can combine with the phytoestrogen genistein to cause some breast cancer cells to grow faster. Other studies, however, show that genistein blocks certain types of estrogen receptor sites, thus inhibiting the proliferation of these types of breast cancer cells.

CAUTION: The Foundation has made a preliminary determination that women with estrogen-receptor-positive breast cancer should not take soy supplements based on evidence that an estrogenic growth effect could occur in some forms of estrogen-receptor-positive breast cancer. Until more is known about the effects of soy phytoestrogens in this type of cancer, compounds such as genistein should be avoided in those with estrogen-receptor- positive breast cancer.

Summing up the possible benefits of genistein and other natural therapies is a May 1999 study in the *North American Urological Clinical Journal* regarding findings of new nontoxic cancer therapies. Researchers reported, "Other agents that promise low toxicity include vitamin D and its analogs, genistein and related isoflavones, green tea polyphenols, and retinoic acid analogs."

Information on how cancer patients should use soy genistein appears at the end of this protocol. The Foundation reiterates that regular testing is recommended for all cancer patients to measure the status and progression of the cancer and the trend of any protocol used; i.e., if tumor markers elevate for 30 to 60 days after beginning soy extract supplementation, discontinue use and seek another therapy immediately.

Benefits of Green Tea

Green tea is the staple beverage of the Japanese and Chinese cultures. It contains a chemical known as epigallocatechin gallate, which is one of the polyphenolic catechins, a family of chemicals many times more potent against free radicals than vitamin E. In a study to measure the effect of green tea consumption in Japanese populations, it was found that green tea had a "preventative effect against cancer among humans." This study surveyed 8552 people over a 9-year period (71,248 person years) and found that cancer incidence was low for those people who consumed green tea regularly. The study also found that the more green tea was consumed, the lower the risk of cancer. Many women interviewed for the study consumed more than 10 cups of green tea daily, and their cancer incidence was the lowest in the study. The overall consumption of green tea correlated with both men and women.

University Hospitals of Cleveland researchers reported in the May 1999 *Journal of Urological Oncology* that prostate cancer (PC) is the second leading cause of cancer-related deaths among males in the United States. According to an estimate, 1 of every 11 American men will eventually develop PC. Researchers suggested that one way to reduce the occurrence of cancer is through natural chemoprevention. PC represents an excellent candidate disease for chemoprevention because it is typically diagnosed in men over 50 years of age, and therefore even a modest delay in neoplastic development achieved through pharmacological or nutritional intervention could result in a substantial reduction in the incidence of clinically detectable disease. The ideal agent(s) suitable for chemoprevention of PC should be the one(s) with proven efficacy in the laboratory experiments on one hand, and with proven epidemiological basis on the other hand. This review attempts to address the issue of possible uses of tea, especially green tea, for the prevention of PC.

The researchers provided an experimental as well as an epidemiological basis for this possibility. They also pointed out that many laboratory experiments conducted in cell culture systems and in animal models have shown the usefulness of green tea—and the polyphenols present in it—against PC.

The epidemiological basis for this possibility is twofold. First, some epidemiological observations have suggested that people who consume tea regularly have a lower risk of PC-related deaths. Second, the incidence of PC in China, a population that consumes green tea on a regular basis, is the lowest in the world (*Semin. Urol. Oncol.,* 1999 May; 17 [2]:70–76).

Another study reported in the July 1999 *Japanese Journal of Cancer Research* further substantiated the benefits of green tea against specific cancer cells. Researchers emphasized its role in the prevention and treatment of cancers such as stomach cancer.

Investigators reported in the September 1999 *American Journal of Clinical Nutrition* that "herbal teas inhibit mevalonate synthesis and thereby suppress cholesterol synthesis and tumor growth," further supporting the section in this protocol which discusses the reduction of cholesterol in the fight against cancer (*Am. J. Clin. Nutr.,* 1999 Sept; 70 [3 Suppl]:491S–99S).

A study found that apoptosis occurred in prostate cancer cell lines LNCaP, PC-3, and DU125 in response to green tea extract. The cancer cell morphology and DNA fragmentation were induced by the most active constituent of green tea, epigallocatechin gallate (EGCG). The study concluded that EGCG triggered apoptosis (programmed cell death) in human prostate cancer cells.

Another study found that two phenols contained in green tea extract had inhibitory effects on several cancer cell lines including lung, stomach, and mammary cancers. It was found that the phenols, epigallocatechin (EGC), and epicatechin gallate (ECG) inhibited the growth of human lung cancer cell PC-9.

Collectively, the results indicate that tea possesses anticarcinogenic activity in the colon, and this most likely involves multiple inhibitory mechanisms (*Proc. Soc. Exp. Biol. Med.,* 1999 April; 220 [4]:239–43).

A review published in a 1999 issue of *Experimental Biological Medicine* summarizes the mechanisms of action of green teas as follows:

- ▼ Tea polyphenols are powerful antioxidants that may play a role in lowering the oxidation of LDL-cholesterol, with a consequent decreased risk of heart disease, and may also diminish the formation of oxidized metabolites of DNA, with an associated lower risk of specific types of cancer.
- ▼ Tea and tea polyphenols selectively induce Phase I and Phase II metabolic enzymes that increase the formation and excretion of detoxified metabolites of carcinogens.
- ▼ Tea lowers the rate of cell replication and thus the growth and development of neoplasms.
- ▼ Tea modifies the intestinal microflora, reducing undesirable bacteria and increasing beneficial bacteria. The accumulated knowledge suggests that regular tea intake by humans might provide an approach to decreasing the incidence of and mortality from major chronic diseases.

Benefits of Garlic

Epidemiological studies in China have provided reasons to suspect that a rich garlic content in the diet might reduce the proliferation of tumors in humans. Researchers reported in the March 1999 issue of *Phytomedicine* relative to experiments conducted on human tumor cell lines to determined the influence of garlic to inhibit the growth of human liver or colon cancer cell lines. Results suggest a strong antiproliferative effect of garlic on human cancer cells (*Phytomedicine,* 1999 Mar; 6 [1]:7–11).

Although the herb garlic by itself possesses these medical properties, aged garlic extract (AGE) has additional benefits due to tightly controlled manufacturing. The process of cold-aging garlic may enhance its medicinal factors, and the aging process also reduces the tendency of garlic to irritate the digestive tract.

A study investigated aged garlic extract in an effort to determine whether it could inhibit proliferation of cancer cells. The proliferation and viability of erythroleukemia and hormone-responsive breast and prostate cancer cell lines were evaluated. The erythroleukemia cells were not significantly affected by the garlic extract, but the breast and prostate cancer cell lines clearly were susceptible to the growth-inhibitory influence of aged garlic extract. The antiproliferative effect of aged garlic extract was limited to actively growing cells. This study provided evidence that garlic can exert a direct effect on established cancer cells.

A Chinese study revealed that garlic effectively prevented oral precancer and oral cancer cell proliferation (*Hunan I Ko Ta Hsueh Hsueh Pao,* 1997; 22 [3]:246–48).

There is a debate among alternative doctors as to whether aged "odorless" garlic is better than high-allicin garlic supplements. For those fighting cancer on an acute basis, perhaps both forms of garlic should be considered. Specific garlic dosing suggestions are provided at the end of this protocol.

Benefits of Vitamins A and D

Nutrients with an inhibitory effect on cancer-cell proliferation include vitamin A (and synthetic vitamin A analogs). The best example of the effectiveness of vitamin A and beta-carotene in inhibiting cell proliferation is with patients who suffer from cancer of the mouth. Vitamin A or beta-carotene supplementation may induce a remission in early stage I mouth cancer as long as these nutrients continue to be consumed. A similar study of 44 patients with mouth lesions caused by chewing tobacco found that spirulina's (chlorella) high concentration of beta-carotene also proved effective for 20 patients after one year.

Vitamin D_3 and its analogs may inhibit cancer cell growth and induce cancer cells to differentiate back into normal cells. An experimental study was performed on a prostate cancer cell line, PC-3, to measure the effect of a vitamin D analogue. A control medium was conducted in parallel. Cell proliferation was measured at 7 and 12 days, and it was found that results "were dose dependent varying from 40 to 70% of controls." The maximum inhibitory effect was at 0.1 micromol/L; however, the study found that "longer incubation times" were more effective than high concentrations of the vitamin D analog. The study concluded that vitamin D deficiency increased the risk of prostate cancer.

The vitamin D analog was used in another study of MCF-7 breast cancer cells grafted into nude mice to determine whether vitamin D could mediate apoptosis of breast cancer *in vivo*. Two delivery methods were used to administer the vitamin D time release pellets and daily injections. At 4 weeks the volume of tumors was reduced fourfold versus the control group. Characteristic "apoptotic morphology" was observed at 5 weeks with MCF-7 tumor cells showing a sixfold increase in DNA fragmentation measured by in situ labeling. The study found that vitamin D demonstrated apoptotic morphology and regression of human breast tumors and that the study "supported the concept that vitamin D compounds can effectively target human breast cancer."

CAUTION: Both vitamin A and vitamin D can have toxic effects in high doses. Consult with health care professionals before increasing doses of either vitamin to high levels.

Benefits of EPA Fish Oil

Fish oil may enhance the effectiveness of cancer chemotherapy drugs. A study compared different fatty acids on colon cancer cells to see whether they could enhance mitomycin C, a chemotherapy drug. The fish oil containing high amounts of eicosapentaenoic acid (EPA) was shown to sensitize colon cancer cells to mitomycin C. Fish oil has been shown to specifically induce apoptosis of pancreatic cancer cells and to inhibit metastasis of breast and lung cancer cells.

A June 1999 study demonstrated the benefits of EPA in reducing acute protein phase response which leads to wasting in cancer patients. Researchers indicated that "the presence of an acute-phase protein response has been suggested to shorten survival and contribute to weight loss in patients with pancreatic cancer. The acute-phase protein response tends to progress in untreated patients but may be stabilized by the administration of a fish oil–enriched nutritional supplement. This may have implications for reducing wasting in such patients" (*Journal of Nutrition,* 1999 June; 129(6):1120–25).

Other studies have found that EPA induced alternations of the fatty-acid composition of cancer cells, which made them more vulnerable to the chemotherapy effects. Although preliminary, these findings imply that EPA specifically enhances the chemosensitivity of malignant cells.

Conjugated Linoleic Acid (CLA)

CLA has been shown both *in vitro* and in animal models to have strong antitumor activity. An early protective effect was noted in one study that focused on the maturation of mammary cells, and the study concluded that "exposure to CLA during Y-maturation may modify the development of Y-target cells that are normally susceptible to carcinogen-induced transformation."

Investigators at Roswell Park Cancer Institute in Buffalo, New York, conducted rat studies and reported inhibited breast cancer cell outgrowth using CLA *(Exp. Cell. Res.,* 1999 July 10; 250 [1]:22–34).

Another study investigated the effect of dietary CLA on the growth of human breast adenocarcinoma cells in immunodeficient mice. Similarly it was found that CLA inhibited the development and growth of mammary tumors. Moreover, CLA completely abrogated the spread of breast cancer cells to lungs, peripheral blood, and bone marrow. These results indicate the ability of dietary CLA to block both the local growth and systemic spread of human breast cancer via mechanisms independent of the host immune system.

CLA has been shown to inhibit initiation and promotion stages of carcinogenesis in several experimental animal models. A study of mice with skin tumors showed that CLA inhibited tumor yield. This study confirmed previous studies showing that CLA inhibits tumor promotion in a manner that is independent of its cancer-prevention effects.

Benefits of Echinacea

The popularity of echinacea has grown during the last couple of years because of its ability to enhance the immune system, especially during the cold and flu season. However, echinacea also has profound anticancer effects related to its ability to increase NK cell activity, which was improved by 221% in one study of patients suffering from metastasized cancers of the colon and esophagus. Another naturally occurring chemical found in echinacea (arabinogalactan) is known to stimulate macrophages' B tumor killing cells.

Benefits of Whey Protein

Whey protein concentrate has been studied for cancer prevention and treatment. When different groups of rats were given a powerful carcinogen, those fed whey protein concentrate showed fewer tumors and a reduced pooled area of tumors. The researchers found that whey protein offered "considerable protection to the host" over that of other proteins, including soy.

At low concentrations, whey appears to inhibit the growth of breast cancer cells. One clinical study with cancer patients showed a regression in some patients' tumors when they were fed whey protein concentrate at 30 grams per day. As noted in a related protocol (but worth repeating in this context), this discovery led researchers to discover a relationship between cancerous cells, whey protein concentrate, and glutathione. Glutathione is an antioxidant that protects the body against harmful compounds. It was found that whey protein concentrate selectively depletes cancer cells of their glutathione, thus making them more susceptible to cancer treatments such as radiation and chemotherapy.

It has been found that cancer cells and normal cells will respond differently to nutrients and drugs that affect glutathione status. What is most interesting is that the concentration of glutathione in tumor cells is higher than that of the normal cells that surround it. This difference in glutathione status between normal cells and cancer cells is believed to be an important factor in cancer cells' resistance to chemotherapy. As the researchers put it, "Tumor cell glutathione concentration may be among the determinants of the cytotoxicity of many chemotherapeutic agents and of radiation, and an increase in glutathione concentration in cancer cells appears to be at least one of the mechanisms of acquired drug resistance to chemotherapy."

They further state, "It is well known that rapid glutathione synthesis in tumor cells is associated with high rates of cellular proliferation. Depletion of cancer cell glutathione *in vivo* decreases the rate of cellular proliferation and inhibits cancer growth." The problem is, it's difficult to reduce glutathione sufficiently in tumor cells without placing healthy tissue at risk and putting the cancer patient in a worse condition. What is needed is a compound that can selectively deplete the cancer cells of their glutathione while increasing, or at least maintaining, the levels of glutathione in healthy cells. This is exactly what whey protein appears to do.

This research found that cancer cells subjected to whey proteins were depleted of their glutathione, and their growth was inhibited, while normal cells had an increase in glutathione and increased cellular growth. These effects were not seen with other proteins. Not surprisingly, the researchers concluded, "Selective depletion of tumor cell glutathione may in fact render cancer cells more vulnerable to the action of chemotherapy and eventually protect normal tissue against the deleterious effects of chemotherapy." The exact mechanism by which whey protein achieves this is not fully understood, but it appears that it interferes with the normal feedback mechanism and regulation of glutathione in cancer cells. It is known that glutathione production is negatively inhibited by its own synthesis. Since baseline glutathione levels in cancer cells are higher than those of normal cells, it is probably easier to reach the level of negative-feedback inhibition in the cancer cells' glutathione levels than in the normal cells' glutathione levels.

(See the Benefits of Whey Protein section of the Cancer Chemotherapy protocol.)

Benefits of Melatonin

The evidence continues to mount that melatonin may be an effective adjuvant cancer therapy because melatonin boosts immune system function, suppresses free radicals, inhibits cell proliferation, and helps to change cancer cells back into normal cells.

A randomized study of 70 patients with advanced nonsmall lung cancer was conducted using chemotherapy (cisplatin) and melatonin support to measure immune system improvement during chemotherapy. The study was conducted using the World Health Organization specifications for clinical response and toxicity, and it was found that "chemotherapy was well tolerated in patients receiving melatonin and, in particular, the frequency of myelosuppression, neuropathy, and cachexia was significantly reduced in the melatonin group." The study concluded that chemotherapy with 20 mg daily of melatonin may improve the chemotherapy particularly with respect to the patient's survival time and the mitigating effect of "chemotherapeutic toxicity" for patients with advanced nonsmall cell lung cancer. This same hospital facility conducted a melatonin survey (several different but related cancer studies using the same dosage of melatonin = 20 mg/daily) that found similar results for patients being treated with the chemotherapy drugs mitoxantrone, cisplatin, etoposide, and 5-fluorouracil.

A 1999 Slovak research study regarding the use of melatonin in the treatment of tumors reported that "melatonin has potentially important influence on the neoplastic growth and direct and indirect oncostatic effect in some forms of neoplasia. The beneficial influence of melatonin alone or its combination with immunotherapy, radiotherapy, or chemotherapy in many clinical studies in patients with tumors was demonstrated" (*Cesk. Fysiol.,* 1999 Feb; 48 [1]:27–40).

Another 1999 study in the *Mutagenesis Cancer Journal* (1999 Jan; 14 [1]:107–12) confirmed that melatonin is able to modulate and reduce chromosome damage by its involvement in regulating adverse oxidative stress and processes, thereby reducing DNA damage. In particular, researchers reported that melatonin is able to decrease damage at the chromosomal level.

Combining Melatonin with Interleukin-2

Melatonin has been seen to enhance the anticancer action of interleukin-2 (IL-2) and to reduce IL-2 toxicity. Melatonin use in association with IL-2 cancer immunotherapy has been shown to have the following actions:

- Amplification of IL-2 biological activity by enhancing lymphocyte response and by antagonizing macrophage-mediated suppressive events.
- Inhibition of production of tumor growth factors, which stimulate cancer cell proliferation by counteracting lymphocyte-mediated tumor cell destruction.
- Maintenance of a circadian rhythm of melatonin, which is often altered in human neoplasms and influenced by cytokine exogenous injection.

The subcutaneous administration of 3 million IU a day of interleukin-2 (IL-2) and high doses of melatonin (40 mg a day orally) in the evening has appeared to be effective in tumors resistant either to IL-2 alone or to chemotherapy. The dose of 3 million IU a day of interleukin-2 is a low dose, while serious toxicity normally begins at 15 million IU a day. At present, 230 patients with advanced solid tumors and life expectancy less than 6 months have been treated with this melatonin/IL-2 combination. Objective tumor regressions were experienced in 44 patients (18%), mainly in patients with lung cancer, hepatocarcinoma, cancer of the pancreas, gastric cancer, and colon cancer. A survival longer than one year was achieved in 41% of the patients. The preliminary data show that melatonin synergizes with tumor necrosis factor (TNF) and alpha-interferon by reducing their toxicity.

Importance of Vegetables

Indole-3-carbinol (I3C), isothiocyanate, and sulforaphane are *phytochemicals* found in cruciferous vegetables. They have an inhibitory effect on cancer cell proliferation. Sprague-Dawley rats were subjected to 7,12-dimethylbenzanthracene-(DMBA) induced mammary tumors in a study to report on antitumorigenic activity of di-indolylmethane (DIM), an acid B catalyzed metabolite of I3C that is formed in the intestines. The study found that DIM inhibited the proliferation of MCF-7 cells and that DIM (at 5 mg/kg every other day) inhibited the mammary tumor growth induced by DMBA. The study concluded that DIM metabolized from the phytochemicals of cruciferous vegetables presents a new class of relatively nontoxic Y antiestrogens that inhibit E2-dependence without affecting normal cells.

Can Nutrition Help the Malnourished Cancer Patient?

A position paper from the American College of Physicians published in 1989 basically stated that total parenteral nutrition (TPN) had no benefit on the outcome of cancer patients. Unfortunately, this article excluded malnourished patients, which is bizarre, since TPN only treats malnutrition, not cancer. Most of the scientific literature shows that weight loss drastically increases the mortality rate of most types of cancer, while also lowering the response to chemotherapy. Chemotherapy and radiation therapy are sufficient biological stressors to induce malnutrition by themselves.

In the early years of oncology, it was thought that one could starve the tumor out of the host. Pure malnutrition (cachexia) is responsible for at least 22% and up to 67% of all cancer deaths. Up to 80% of all cancer patients have reduced levels of serum albumin, which is a leading indicator of protein and calorie malnutrition. Dietary protein restriction in the cancer patient does not affect the composition or growth rate of the tumor, but does restrict the patient's well being.

Parenteral feeding improves tolerance to chemotherapeutic agents and immune responses. One study indicated that malnourished cancer patients who were provided TPN had a mortality rate of 11%, while the group without TPN feeding had a 100% mortality rate. Preoperative TPN in patients undergoing surgery for GI cancer provided general reduction in the incidence of wound infection, pneumonia, major complications, and mortality. Patients who were the most malnourished experienced a 33% mortality and 46% morbidity rate, while those patients who were properly nourished had a 3% mortality rate with an 8% morbidity rate.

In 20 adult hospitalized patients on TPN, the mean daily vitamin C needs were 975 mg/day, which is over 16 times the RDA. Of the 139 lung cancer patients studied, most tested deficient or scorbutic (clinically vitamin-C deficient). Another study of cancer patients found that 46% tested scorbutic while 76% were below acceptable levels for serum ascorbate. Experts now recommend the value of nutritional supplements, especially in patients who require prolonged TPN support. Remember that 40% or more of cancer patients actually die of malnutrition, not from the cancer, according to medical experts. Nutrition therapy is the only treatment for malnutrition.

Properly nourished patients experience less nausea, malaise, immune suppression, hair loss, and organ toxicity than patients on routine oncology programs. Antioxidants such as beta-carotene, vitamin C, vitamin E, and selenium appear to enhance the effectiveness of chemotherapy, radiation, and hyperthermia while minimizing damage to the patient's normal cells. Protecting healthy cells thus makes these conventional therapies more of a "selective toxin."

An optimally nourished cancer patient can better tolerate the rigors of cytotoxic therapy. While, in simplistic theory, vitamin K might inhibit the effectiveness of anticoagulant therapy (Coumadin), vitamin K actually seems to augment the antineoplastic activity of Coumadin. In a study with human rheumatoid arthritis patients being given methotrexate, folic acid supplements did not reduce the antiproliferative therapeutic value of methotrexate. Tumor-bearing mice fed high doses of vitamin C (antioxidant), along with the pro-oxidant chemotherapy drug adriamycin, had a prolonged life and no reduction in the tumor-killing capacity of adriamycin. Lung cancer patients who were provided antioxidant nutrients prior to, during, and after radiation and chemotherapy had enhanced tumor destruction and significantly longer lifespan. Some of the benefits of complimentary nutrition therapy include the following:

Improved tolerance to radiation therapy. Tumor-bearing mice fed high doses of vitamin C experienced an increased tolerance to radiation therapy without reduction in the tumor-killing capacity of the radiation.

Improved tolerance to cytotoxic chemotherapies. In both human and animal studies, nutrients improve the host tolerance to cytotoxic medical therapies while allowing for unobstructed death of tumor cells. Nutrition therapy makes medical therapy more of a selective toxin on the tumor issue.

Bolstering immune functions. We must rely on the capabilities of the 20 trillion cells that make up an intact immune system to find and destroy the undetectable cancer cells that inevitably remain after medical therapy. There is an abundance of data linking nutrient intakes to the quality and quantity of immune factors that fight cancer.

Selectively starve the tumor. Tumors are primarily obligate glucose metabolizers, meaning "sugar feeders." Americans not only consume about 20% of their calories from refined sucrose, but often manifest poor glucose tolerance curves due to stress, obesity, low chromium and fiber intake, and sedentary lifestyles. Since this topic is of crucial importance, further information on how the cancer patient should properly regulate glucose will follow.

Providing antiproliferative factors. Certain nutrients such as selenium, vitamin K, vitamin E, the fatty acid EPA, melatonin, and CoQ_{10} appear to have the ability to slow down the unregulated growth of cancer. Various nutritional factors—including vitamins A, D, and E; folic acid; bioflavonoids; and soybeans—have been shown to alter the genetic expression of tumors.

Cancer Is a "Sugar Feeder"

Nobel laureate Otto Warburg, Ph.D., discovered in 1955 that cancer cells primarily use glucose for fuel, with lactic acid being an anaerobic by-product. Lactic acid buildup then generates a lower pH, fatigue, and enlarged liver (where lactic acid is converted back to pyruvate in the Cori cycle). Cancer causes a breakdown in normal energy metabolism, which is one of the reasons why so many cancer patients die of malnutrition or cachexia.

Since Warburg's pivotal study was published in a 1956 issue of the journal *Science,* other research has shown that the glucose utilization rate is high in neoplastic tissues. Glucose is, in fact, the preferred energy substrate for cancer cells, utilized mainly via the anaerobic glycolytic pathway. The large amount of lactates produced by this process is then transported to the liver where it is converted to glucose, thus contributing to further increase the host's energy wasting.

Interfering with carbohydrate and/or energy metabolisms could preferentially impair the malignant cells. Studies show that *in vivo* consumption of glucose by neoplastic tissues is very high. It is well known that the brain is one of the highest consumers of glucose among the normal tissues. Hepatomas and fibrosarcomas have been shown to consume roughly as much glucose as the brain does, and more prevalent carcinomas consume about twice as much.

One study showed lactate levels to be 27 to 83% higher in cancer patients than in related controls. If cancer cells use glucose through anaerobic fermentation, then lactic acid must accumulate as the inefficient by-product of energy metabolism. Hence, cancer therapies need to take into consideration the importance of regulating blood glucose levels.

Another study on ten healthy human volunteers assessed fasting blood glucose levels and the phagocytic index of neutrophils. Glucose, fructose, sucrose, honey, and orange juice all significantly decreased the capacity of neutrophils to engulf bacteria as measured by the slide technique. Starch ingestion did not have this effect. One epidemiological study showed that the risk associated with the intake of sugars, independent of other energy sources, more than doubled for biliary tract cancer in older women. Other studies show a correlation between breast cancer mortality and sugar consumption.

Starving Cancer

In his book *Beating Cancer with Nutrition,* Dr. Patrick Quillin makes specific recommendations about how glucose modulation can be utilized to help the cancer patient. Some of his recommendations include

- Diets designed to lower glycemic index to regulate rises in blood glucose, hence selectively starving the cancer cells.
- Low glucose total parenteral nutrition (TPN) solution.
- Avocado extract (mannoheptulose), which inhibits glucose uptake in cancer cells.
- Systemic Cancer Multistep Therapy, which injects glucose into the cancer patient to induce rapid malignancy growth and then uses hyperthermia to selectively destroy the rapidly dividing cells.

Dr. Quillin provides a compelling case for the role of glucose in the growth and metastasis of cancer cells. According to Dr. Quillin, a frequent characteristic of many tumors is a high rate of glucose consumption along with an increase in anaerobic glycolysis (the conversion of glucose to lactase). By manipulating glucose levels, cancer cells can be starved over an extended time, or, conversely, glucose can be injected into the patient when a therapy is being utilized that targets rapidly dividing cells.

Glucose modulation therapy is an underutilized component in the treatment of cancer. There is not sufficient space in the protocol to discuss the complete aspects of glucose modulation therapy, but this is described in detail in Dr. Quillin's book, *Beating Cancer with Nutrition*. You can order it directly from the publisher by calling (918) 495-1137. (The cover price is $14.95.)

The Foundation's Adjuvant Cancer Treatment Protocol

The Foundation's Adjuvant Cancer Treatment Protocol is for most forms of cancer. This protocol assumes that the patient's primary tumor has been eradicated, at least partially, by surgery or by some other treatment. However, it may be followed even if the primary tumor has not yet been eradicated. The following is a step-by-step treatment plan.

Step One—Arrange for monthly blood tests, including

- Tumor marker tests. The type of cancer dictates the type of test used. Some cancers do not have a specific tumor marker test available.
- Immune cell subset test. (This is an expensive test.)
- Complete blood chemistry. To include all standard liver, thyroid, heart, and kidney function tests. (This is a low-cost test.)

These blood tests must be taken on a regular basis under the supervision of a physician in order to follow scientifically the Foundation's Cancer Treatment Protocol. It's the best way of knowing whether what you are taking is working and/or whether significant toxicity is developing. This is no time to guess! Since you will be having these tests performed monthly, you should price-shop for the best deal. The Life Extension Foundation offers these tests at discount prices, but if you have health insurance, it would save you money in the long run to have these tests performed by your physician.

Here are some accepted blood tumor markers for common cancers:

Type of Cancer	Tumor Marker Blood Test
Ovarian cancer	CA 125
Prostate cancer	PSA and prolactin
Breast cancer	CA 27.29, CEA, alkaline, phosphatase, and prolactin (some doctors use the CA 15-3 in place of the CA 27.29)

Type of Cancer	Tumor Marker Blood Test
Colon, rectum, liver, stomach, and other organ cancers	CEA, GGTP
Pancreatic	CA 19.9, CEA, GGTP
Leukemia, lymphoma, and Hodgkin's disease	CBC with differential, immune cell differentiation and leukemia profile
Lung cancer	CEA, CA 125, alkaline phosphatase PT, PTT, and D-Dimer of fibrin

Step Two—Nutritional support

- Life Extension Mix (high-potency multinutrient supplement): the standard daily dose involves 3 tablets, 3 times a day. It is also available in powder or capsule form to be taken in 3 divided doses.
- Life Extension Herbal Mix—powder only. Take 1 tablespoon early in the day.
- Super Selenium Complex: take 1 tablet, 2 times a day.
- Green Tea capsules (decaffeinated): take 4 to 10 capsules a day in divided doses.
- Coenzyme Q_{10} (oil-filled capsules): take 200 to 400 mg early in the morning.
- Garlic–Kyolic Garlic Formula 105: take 4 capsules a day; and PureGar (high allicin garlic): take four 900-mg capsules a day with meals.
- Essential fatty acids. Mega EPA fish oil or Udo's Choice Ultimate Oil: take the highest tolerable dose. The suggested dose is 8 to 12 Mega EPA caps along with 4 MEGA GLA capsules to balance the high amount of omega-3 being consumed in the fish oil. (Some studies suggest not taking these oils if you have prostate cancer.)
- Vitamin C capsules or powder: take the highest tolerable dose (4000 to 12,000 mg) of pharmaceutical grade vitamin C (to be taken throughout the day).
- Phyto-Food powder: take 1 to 2 tablespoons daily. Juicing organic vegetables is an alternative to Phyto-Food powder.
- Curcumin: take four 500-mg capsules daily.
- Conjugated linoleic acid (CLA): Take four 1000-mg capsules in two divided doses.

Step Three—Boosting immune function

If the immune system is weakened enough, cancer cells can survive and multiply. The most critical part of the immune system is the thymus gland, a small organ just below the breast bone that governs the entire system. There are several products that promote healthy thymic activity.

Thymex is a product used by alternative physicians to stimulate immune function. It provides extracts of fresh, healthy tissue from the thymus and other glands that produce the disease-fighting cells of our immune system. The primary ingredient in Thymex is immunologic tissue from the thymus gland. Also included in Thymex is tissue from the lymph nodes and spleen that produces the white blood cells that engage in life-or-death combat with invading organisms in our bloodstream under the "instruction" of the thymus gland. Thymex is a synergistic formula that contains herbal activators and a full complement of natural homeopathic nutrients, in addition to fresh, healthy thymus, lymph, and spleen tissues. Thymex is a professional formula normally dispensed through doctor's offices. Thymex has been used extensively to amplify the immune potentiating effect of DHEA replacement therapy. According to a physician most familiar with DHEA, thymus extract is required to obtain the immune system–boosting benefit of DHEA.

KH3. Cancer patients usually have elevated cortisol levels that can suppress immune function. Take 1 to 2 tablets of KH3 daily on an empty stomach first thing in the morning and 1 or 2 KH3 tablets in the mid-afternoon on an empty stomach to suppress the damaging effects of cortisol.

DHEA can also suppress dangerously high cortisol levels while boosting immune function via other mechanisms. Doctors usually prescribe at least 25 mg per day of DHEA for their male cancer patients and a minimum of 15 mg a day of DHEA for females. Your monthly or bimonthly DHEA-S and immune cell subset tests and tumor marker tests will determine whether DHEA is producing a beneficial effect. Do not use DHEA if you have prostate cancer or estrogen-sensitive breast cancer.

Melatonin boosts immune function via several mechanisms of action. It also exerts an inhibitory effect on cancer cell proliferation and induces the differentiation of cancer cells into normal cells. Melatonin should be taken every night in doses ranging from 3 to 40 mg.

CAUTION: Some doctors are under the impression that leukemia, Hodgkin's disease, and lymphoma patients should avoid melatonin until more is known about its effects on these forms of cancer. If melatonin is tried in these types of cancer, tumor blood markers should be watched closely for any sign that melatonin is promoting tumor growth.

Show your oncologist the information in this book regarding the use of the FDA-approved drugs interleukin-2 or interferon and melatonin. Studies document that low doses of interleukin-2 or alpha-interferon combined with high doses of melatonin (10 to 50 mg nightly) are effective against advanced, normally untreatable cancers. Ask your doctor to prescribe these agents:

- ▼ Interleukin-2 at a dose of 3 million units injected subcutaneously six out of every seven days for 6 weeks.
- ▼ (One month later) Alpha-interferon at a dose of 100,000 to 300,000 units injected subcutaneously six out of seven days for six weeks. Subcutaneous injections can be self-administered at home.

This immune-boosting program should be adjusted if the immune cell subset test or tumor marker tests fail to show marked improvement in the patient's immune function. For example, if there are too many T-suppressor cells, 800 mg a day of the drug Tagamet (now available over the counter) can lower the T-suppressor cell activity. T-suppressor cells often are elevated in cancer patients, which prevents them from mounting a strong immune response to the cancer.

Step Four—Inhibiting cancer cell proliferation

- ▼ Water-soluble vitamin-A liquid in doses of 100,000 to 300,000 IU a day should be used for several months. In lieu of high-dose vitamin A supplementation, it would be better to have a physician prescribe a vitamin A analog drug such as Accutane.

CAUTION: Monthly blood tests can help ascertain whether toxicity is occurring in response to these high doses of vitamin A. Do not take vitamin A if you have thyroid cancer or suffer severe thyroid deficiency. (*Refer to the Vitamin A Precautions in Appendix A.*)

- ▼ Melatonin (taken to boost immune function) also inhibits cancer cell proliferation.
- ▼ Mega Soy Extract: take five 700-mg capsules 4 times a day. Soy may be effective in treating certain cancers. Genistein is the most substantiated soy isoflavone that produces multiple cancer-inhibiting effects. Genistein has been shown to work especially well against certain leukemias and cancers of the skin, prostate, and brain.

CAUTION: For most cancers, the determining factor of whether soy may work is whether your cancer cells carry a mutated p53 tumor suppressor gene, or whether they carry functional p53. If functional p53 is present, then soy genistein will probably not work. In small-cell lung cancer, however, it was recently determined that genistein's growth-inhibiting effects were independent of p53 function. Only specialized tumor cell tests (immunohistochemistry) can determine the p53 status of your particular cancer. Estrogen-receptor-positive breast cancer patients should avoid high doses of genistein.

- ▼ Take whey protein concentrate powder, 30 to 60 grams a day (1 to 2 scoops). Whey protein concentrate inhibits cancer cell glutathione levels, making cancer cells more vulnerable to free-radical destruction than normal cells.

Step Five—Inducing cancer cell differentiation

Cancer cells are aberrant, transformed cells that proliferate (divide) more rapidly than normal cells until they kill the patient. Inducing cancer cells to "differentiate" back into normal cells is a primary objective of cancer researchers.

- Vitamin D_3 and its analogs may be the most effective therapies to induce cancer cell differentiation. Vitamin D_3 can cause too much calcium to be absorbed into the bloodstream, so the monthly blood chemistry test, which includes serum calcium levels and kidney and liver function tests, is crucial to guard against vitamin D_3 overdose. A daily dose of 2000 to 3000 IU of vitamin D_3 is suggested. Increase vitamin D_3 if blood tests show blood calcium levels are not being affected and if parathyroid hormone (PTH) levels are not suppressed. Decrease or eliminate vitamin D_3 supplementation if hypercalcemia occurs. Underlying kidney disease precludes high-dose vitamin D_3 supplementation. Note the importance of competent, professional guidance by a physician.

CAUTION: Monthly blood testing is mandatory when taking high doses of vitamin A or vitamin D_3.

- The Nutritional Support protocol supplies nutrients such as beta-carotene and the phytochemicals found in fresh fruits and vegetables that induce cancer cell differentiation into normal cells and inhibit cancer cell proliferation.
- Melatonin, which boosts immune function and inhibits cancer cell proliferation, also induces cancer cell differentiation.

Step Six—Adjuvant Drug Therapies

There are drugs approved by the FDA that may be of enormous benefit to certain cancer patients. These drugs include COX-2 inhibitors, the "statins," retinoid analogs, the interferons, interleukin-2, and immune-protecting drugs such as Leukine. These drugs are described throughout this protocol and require a prescription from a knowledgeable and cooperative oncologist for safe administration.

There are also drugs approved in other countries that may be effective against certain cancers. These drugs are not discussed because the FDA routinely seizes these life-saving medicines, thus making consistent administration virtually impossible.

Step Seven—Diet

For the malnourished patient, low-glucose, total parental nutrition is a must from the beginning of therapy. Reducing intake of sugars appears to be especially important, because cancer cells use glucose as a primary substrate.

Step Eight—Call the Life Extension Foundation

If following the above protocols does not result in significant immune enhancement, improvements in blood tumor markers, tumor shrinkage, weight stabilization, and an overall improvement in well being within two months, please call the Life Extension Foundation at (800) 544-4440 or refer to the Web site at www.lef.org for other, more aggressive options. Life Extension Foundation can also provide the latest in cancer testing services.

The Science behind Life Extension's Cancer Protocol

The recommendations made in this protocol are based exclusively on published scientific studies. The Foundation continues to research new therapies to provide the most comprehensive database of information to support this cancer treatment protocol. For the latest findings about cancer treatment and the actual abstracts that substantiate these recommendations, please refer to our Web site www.lef.org

Specific Cancer Protocols

The Life Extension Foundation currently publishes separate protocols for the more common forms of cancers. The cancer protocols are available on the Foundation's Web site www.lef.org and are contained in this book.

MOLECULAR ONCOLOGY

CAUTION: The following information is extremely technical. The cooperation of your oncologist is vital to most cancer patients who seek to use the following information in an attempt to save their lives.

Determining RAS Mutations

The family of RAS proteins plays a central role in the regulation of cell growth and integration of regulatory signals that govern the cell cycle and proliferation. Mutant RAS genes were among the first oncogenes described for their ability to transform cells to a cancerous phenotype. Mutations in one of three genes (H, N, or K-RAS) encoding RAS proteins have been intimately associated with unregulated cell proliferation and are found in an estimated 30% of all human cancers. The frequency of RAS mutations appears to depend upon the specific tumor type analyzed. For example, 90% of pancreatic carcinomas contain a mutated oncogenic RAS protein, whereas RAS mutations are rarely found in breast carcinomas.

Approximately one third of liver cancers harbor a mutated RAS oncogene. Pravastatin, an inhibitor of the rate-limiting enzyme of cholesterol synthesis, inhibits growth of liver cancer cells. One of the possible mechanisms of pravastatin inhibition of cell growth is that pravastatin may inhibit the activity of RAS proteins. In a recently published study, patients with primary liver cancer were treated either with the chemotherapeutic drug 5-FU or with a combination of 5-FU and 40 mg per day of pravastatin. Median survival was 26 months in the combination therapy group, versus 10 months in the monotherapy (5-FU) group.

The highest incidences of RAS mutations are found in adenocarcinomas of the pancreas (90%), the colon (50%), and the lung; in thyroid tumors (50%); in liver tumors (30%); and in myeloid leukemia (30%). If you have one of these cancers, you should consider requesting an immunohistochemistry for the mutated RAS oncogene or a biopsied specimen in order to ascertain whether the combination of chemotherapy and a statin drug may be effective.

Determining p53 Oncogene Status

Cancer patients whose tumor cells have a mutant p53 oncogene are far more likely to benefit from soy extract supplementation. Only a pathology examination of the actual cancer cells can determine p53 status. An immunohistochemistry test can help to determine the p53 status of tumor cells. The following laboratory can perform this new test:

IMPATH Laboratories
1010 Third Avenue, Suite 203
New York, N.Y. 10021
Phone: (800) 447-5816

IMPATH Laboratories measures mutant p53. If the test is positive, you have mutant p53 and are more likely to benefit from soy extracts. If the test is negative, it indicates that you have functional p53 and are less likely to benefit from soy extracts. The Foundation realizes that many cancer patients seeking to use soy supplements may find it difficult to have an immunohistochemistry test performed to ascertain p53 status. In order to find out whether you have p53, please contact your oncologist and ask him to request this test from IMPATH. IMPATH is unable to provide information about the likelihood of p53 expression on an individual basis without samples and test requests from your treating oncologist.

Another of the most widely studied molecular changes in epithelial malignancies is mutation in the p53 tumor suppressor gene. A p53 mutation has been found in approximately 50% of solid tumors.

The p53 gene product is regarded as a cell-cycle checkpoint, arresting progression through the G phase of the mitotic cycle in response to cellular injury and allowing time for repair of replication errors. Mutant p53 allows tumor cells to bypass the cell cycle constraints that facilitate repair or promote apoptosis (programmed cell death).

In addition, p53 dysfunction promotes the spontaneous emergence of mutant cells and encourages the progression of cancer. Mutant p53 might restrict therapeutic efficacy, since many cancer drugs and radiotherapy operate via the induction of DNA damage and p53-dependent apoptosis.

Clinically, the presence of p53 mutations is indeed associated with intransigence to treatment, and both *in vitro* and *in vivo* studies with human cell lines and transplantable tumors have demonstrated enhanced survival of p53 mutant or null cells in the face of normally lethal concentrations of cytotoxic drugs and ionizing radiation. A determination of p53 status by immunohistochemistry can help to ascertain whether genotoxic chemotherapy and/or radiotherapy are likely to work, and can even help determine whether natural therapies such as soy genistein will be effective.

In a recently published study, genistein was shown to inhibit growth and induce differentiation in human melanoma cells *in vitro*. The effects of genistein were regulated by cellular p53. Functional p53-containing cells were not suppressed by genistein. However, mutant p53-containing cells were significantly more sensitive to genistein's inhibitory and cell-differentiating effects.

IMPATH Laboratories, cited earlier in this protocol, can ascertain immunohistochemistries, which will determine RAS and p53 status.

Determining Thrombotic Risk Factors

In patients affected with different tumors, blood clotting disorders are frequently observed. The biological processes leading to coagulation are probably involved in the mechanisms of metastasis. About 50% of all cancer patients, and up to 95% of those with metastatic disease, show some abnormalities, a prethrombic state, in the coagulation-fibrinolytic system. Thromboembolic complications are seen in up to 11% of cancer patients, and hemorrhage occurs in about 10%. Thromboembolism and hemorrhage, taken as a whole, are the second most common cause of death after infection.

In a recently published study, subclinical changes in the coagulation-fibrinolytic system were frequently detected in lung cancer patients. Five conventional tests and one new test of blood coagulation—that is, platelet count (P), prothrombin time (PT), partial thromboplastin time (PTT), fibrinogen (F), and D-Dimer of fibrin (DD)—were prospectively recorded in a series of 286 patients with new primary lung cancer. A prethrombotic state (depicted by a prolongation of PT, PTT, and increase of D-Dimer of fibrin) was significantly associated with an adverse outcome.

Anticoagulant treatment of cancer patients, particularly those with lung cancer, has been reported to improve survival. These interesting, though preliminary, results of controlled trials lend some support to the argument that activation of blood coagulation plays a role in the natural history of tumor growth. Two recent studies compared the effectiveness of standard heparin with low molecular weight heparin (LMWH) in the treatment of deep vein thrombosis (DVT). In both studies, mortality rates were lower in the patients randomized to LMWH. The analysis of these deaths reveals a striking difference in cancer-related mortality.

Cancer-related mortality of patients treated with standard heparin was 31%, versus only 11% among those treated with low molecular weight heparin. This difference cannot be attributed solely to thrombotic or bleeding events. Because large numbers of cancer patients were included in the studies, it seems unlikely that patients with more advanced tumors were present in the standard heparin group. Although it is also possible that standard heparin increases cancer mortality, such an adverse effect has not been reported. These considerations suggest that low molecular weight heparin might exert an inhibitory effect on tumor growth that is not apparent with standard heparin. The evidence of lowered cancer mortality in patients on LMWH has occasioned renewed interest in these agents as antineoplastic drugs. If your oncologist will not test for thrombotic risk factors, contact the Life Extension Foundation at (800) 544-4440 or online at www.lef.org.

Assessing Immune Function

In order to assess the effectiveness of immune-boosting therapies, a complete immune cell subset test could be performed bimonthly in order to measure CD4 (T-helper) total count, CD4/CD8 (T-helper to T-suppressor) ratio, and NK (natural killer) cell activity.

CD4 T-cells have been shown to differentiate into TH1 or TH2 cells, with different cytokine profiles and functions. TH1 cells produce interleukin-2 and gamma interferon, activate macrophages, and cause delayed hypersensitivity reactions, whereas TH2 cells produce interluken-4, interleukin-5, and interleukin-10, cause eosinophilia, and are more specialized in providing B cell (antibody) help for immunoglobulin production. The differential development of these immune system subjects is a major determinant of the outcome of physiological as well as pathological immune responses to cancer.

One of the soluble factors secreted by monocytes, interleukin-12, is a major cause of differentiation of T-cells toward the TH1 type, while suppressing TH2 cytokine development. The capacity of interleukin-12 to stimulate growth and gamma interferon production in T-cells and NK cells is probably the main reason for its TH1-inducing capacity.

Another product of activated monocytes, prostaglandin E2, has been shown to be an important regulatory factor in inducing TH2 responses. PGE2 affects T-helper responses opposite to interleukin-12: the synthesis of TH1 cytokines (interleukin-2 and gamma interferon) is much more sensitive to inhibition by PGE2 than is TH2 cytokine production (IL-4, IL-5, IL-10). Because TH1 and TH2 cytokines negatively cross-regulate each other's production, the selective inhibition of TH1 cytokines by PGE2 could result in dominant TH2 responses. These findings provide opportunities to treat patients with dominant TH2 responses by selectively inhibiting synthesis of PGE2 during therapy, as this would increase interleukin-12 production and cause a shift toward TH1 cytokine production.

Many human tumors—including gastric, colon, estrogen-receptor-negative breast, prostate, and lung tumors—produce more prostaglandin E2 than their associated normal tissues. The mechanisms and implications are not fully understood, but PGE2 may act as a tumor promoter in tumor angiogenesis, in cachexia (wasting syndrome), and in the suppression of immune function.

Prostaglandins are synthesized from arachidonic acid by the enzyme cyclooxygenase. There are two isoforms of cyclooxygenases: COX-1 is expressed constitutively in most tissues and helps maintain gastric mucosal integrity; COX-2 is inducible and is associated with cellular growth and differentiation.

In a recently published study, PGE2 was shown, for the first time, to upregulate the MRNA levels of its own synthesizing enzyme, COX-2, in four lines of human cells. In this regard, it is conceivable that cells continuously sustain their growth, in part, by using extracellular PGE2 that they themselves produce and release to up regulate the expressions of COX-2 (and possibly other growth-related genes). Elevated COX-2 expression may make cancer cells resistant to apoptosis. Inhibition of excess activity with COX-2 specific nonsteroidal anti-inflammatory drugs might restore the cell's ability to die by apoptosis and so cause tumor regression.

Super Aspirins

Super aspirins that selectively inhibit COX-2 are being developed by several drug companies for the purpose of avoiding the side effects of NSAIDS. The currently commercially available NSAIDS are nonselective COX inhibitors and are associated with peptic ulceration in the stomach. Nimesulide is a novel NSAID that is 100 times more selective for COX-2 than for COX-1. In a recently published study, patients received either nimesulide or aspirin for 14 days. PGE2 formation fell markedly in the nimesulide treated patients, whereas aspirin had no effect. In contrast, nimesulide had no significant effect on thromboxane B2, which was suppressed by aspirin. Nimesulide suppressed COX-2 *in vivo* with no detectable effect on platelet COX-1.

Nimesulide has been commercially available throughout most of the rest of the world for more than 10 years. It has not been licensed by the FDA for use in the United States. The Life Extension Foundation has identified sources that will ship nimesulide to Americans for personal use. There are also COX-2 inhibiting drugs approved by the FDA, such as Lodine XL, Celebrex, and Vioxx.

Lodine is an FDA-approved arthritis drug that interferes with COX-2's metabolic processes. The maximum dosage for Lodine is 1000 mg daily. Everyone now appears to be using Lodine XL extended-release tablets for convenient once-a-day dosing. The Lodine XL 500-mg tablet enables physicians to prescribe the maximum dosage of Lodine XL—1000 mg per day—as 2 tablets in a single daily dose. As with any NSAID, extreme caution and physician supervision is a must. The most common complaints associated with Lodine XL use relate to the gastrointestinal tract. Serious GI toxicity such as perforation, ulceration, and bleeding can occur in patients treated long term with NSAID therapy. Serious renal and hepatic reactions have been reported rarely. Lodine XL should not be given to patients who have previously shown hypersensitivity to it or in whom aspirin or other NSAIDs induce asthma, rhinitis, urticaria, or other allergic reactions. Fatal asthmatic reactions have been reported in such patients receiving NSAIDs.

Nimesulide is a safer COX-2 inhibitor but is not approved by the FDA. It is available from Mexican pharmacies or can be ordered by mail from European pharmacies. The suggested dose for nimesulide is two 100-mg tablets a day. It is important that your physician know you are taking nimesulide as an adjuvant cancer therapy.

Cancer and Angiogenesis

Cancer has long baffled medical science. The debilitating, frequently fatal disease often spreads throughout the body at an alarming rate. Until recently, scientists did not fully understand why. Dr. Judah Folkman, a professor of surgery at Children's Hospital in Boston, an affiliate of Harvard Medical School, has spent the last 30 years championing a controversial theory.

Almost every tissue in the body derives blood from the thinner-than-hair capillaries that lace our tissues. Through capillaries, nutrients, oxygen, and various signaling molecules diffuse into cells. Tumors start out without circulation. In early stages, they are limited to a trickle of nutrients that can diffuse from the nearest capillary. Then, somehow, tumors begin to stimulate healthy tissue to make thousands of new blood vessels to supply the cancerous growth. Without this ability to nourish itself and grow, a tumor cannot enlarge.

At the same time, a primary tumor also sends chemical signals that prevent other tumors from growing in other parts of the body. When the tumor is removed, there is nothing to stop other tumors from growing elsewhere. That's why some people become riddled with cancer after undergoing tumor removal.

In recent years, several drugs—including interferons, steroids, and certain hormonal agents—have been developed to stop or slow angiogenesis. In fact, at least 11 anti-angiogenic drugs are in clinical trials now, and three have proved effective enough to make it to the final phase. Some of the drugs, such as endostatin, are derived from proteins; others are based on smaller molecules. Ironically, one promising drug now on trial is thalidomide, which at one time was sold as a sedative, causing notorious birth defects in the children of women who took it.

Another drug, 2-methoxyestradiol (2-ME), is a natural estrogen metabolite believed to be an inhibitor of angiogenesis and also an antitumor agent. Dr. Robert D. Amato and colleagues at Children's Hospital discovered in preclinical studies that 2-ME inhibited the growth of breast cancer cells and stopped tumors from sprouting new blood vessels.

In March of 1999, researchers reported that 2-methoxyestradiol (2-ME) inhibited growth and tumorigenesis in human pancreatic cancer cells. They reported that 2-ME inhibited the growth of these cell lines 50 to 90% (*Clin. Cancer Res.,* 1999 March; 5[3]:493–99).

In addition, the NCI is investigating a drug called Col-3 and negotiating with several biotechnology companies to examine other anticancer compounds. But of all the anti-angiogenic drugs, endostatin and angiostatin appear to hold the greatest potential for saving lives.

The Premise behind Anti-Angiogenesis

Angiostatin and endostatin drugs were discovered by Dr. Michael O'Reilly, a research fellow at Children's Hospital who has worked closely with Folkman. (O'Reilly discovered angiostatin first.) The cancer-preventing chemical turned up in the urine of mice afflicted by large tumors. Angiostatin, O'Reilly later determined, is used by the human body as part of a blood-clotting mechanism.

Endostatin appears to be produced by tumors to stop other tumors from developing throughout the body. O'Reilly and Folkman found that the drugs could eradicate several forms of cancer in mice by starving tumors of nutrient-rich blood. In fact, the drugs were so powerful that they shriveled tumors in mice that would have weighed several pounds in a human being. Unlike some anticancer drugs, though, endostatin and angiostatin do not harm normal cells. In addition, the new drugs suppress metastasis, the process by which tumor cells spread to other sites in the body.

Folkman called the protein combination "very promising" when he announced the discovered in May of 1998, but added, "We have to be careful with expectations. You always have the risk that something will fail. But if [the drugs] work in patients as well as they work in laboratories—and that's a big if—then one might hope that they improve our ability to treat cancer."

How the Drugs Work

Scientists are excited about the new drugs because cancer is a difficult disease to treat with existing medicines. Tumor cells can do things with their genes that are amazing. They can shuffle their genetic information. They can amplify certain genes. They can turn off some genes and mutate others. Because you're dealing with a moving target, cancer can be hard to hit with a killing drug.

In addition, conventional cancer therapies often cause severe side effects. That's because the drugs slow down cell division, particularly in the gut and bone marrow, where cells divide rapidly. Angiostatin and endostatin, however, slow cell growth only in blood vessels and in the heart, where cells divide much less frequently. Thus, although the new drugs don't appear to cause side effects such as the nausea often produced by chemotherapy, they could cause bleeding and difficulty with wound healing, two potential problems that doctors will be monitoring closely.

Another problem with existing cancer drugs is that they sometimes stop working after patients develop a resistance to them. Of the more than 500,000 annual deaths from cancer in the United States, many follow the development of resistance to chemotherapy.

Drugs that work at first often lose effectiveness over time because cancer cells divide rapidly and sloppily, forming thousands of mutant cells. If any of these mutant cells resists the anticancer drugs, it divides and forms a drug-resistant line of cancer cells. That's what happened after scientists gave a conventional anticancer drug to mice with aggressive lung cancer. The drug controlled the tumors for 13 days, but the cancer in the mice soon developed a resistance to the drug, and the tumors resumed growing.

To find out whether tumors would develop resistance to angiostatin and endostatin, researchers gave the new drugs to mice in an on-off cycle. In other words, they attempted to stimulate any drug resistance the mice might develop for the new medicines. Remarkably, there was no resistance, no matter how many times the scientists gave the drugs to the mice. Every time the mice received the blood-vessel inhibitors, their tumors shrank as rapidly as they had the first time they were exposed to the drugs.

What accounts for the lack of resistance to the new drugs? Angiogenesis occurs when genetically stable endothelial cells in blood vessels divide to build new blood vessels. It is those cells that the inhibitor drugs affect.

The tumor cells could mutate and develop resistance, but it will be more difficult for the endothelial cells to do so, explains James Mixson, a research assistant professor at the University of Maryland School of Medicine who also studies angiogenesis in mice. "Endostatin and angiostatin are not directed at the actual tumor cell, but rather at the blood vessels that feed it," says Dr. John W. Holaday, chairman, president, and chief executive officer of EntreMed, a small biotech company in Rockville, MD, that produces endostatin. Thus, Holaday says, the drugs retain their tumor-shrinking abilities.

Even more important is the fact that the new drugs appear to keep on working even after therapy is discontinued. After mice stopped taking the drugs, for example, tumors remained dormant for up to 165 days. That's the human equivalent of 16 years. All endostatin-treated mice remained healthy and gained weight normally, according to studies completed thus far.

How is it that tumors remain dormant after the drug therapy is stopped? Perhaps, researchers speculate, the drugs leave a residual "capsule" of angiogenesis inhibitors around the tumor. Or they may initiate a sort of programmed cell death in tumors.

Tests in Mice

In trials with mice, endostatin and angiostatin worked remarkably well to kill cancers in the colon, prostate, breast, and brain. Twenty mice had large cancerous growths, which researchers removed. Ten mice were given salt water and ten were given angiostatin. There was no recurrence of cancer in any of the ten mice treated with angiostatin, but all of the water-treated mice developed new cancers.

Endostatin was given to mice in cycles. Small amounts of the protein caused tumors to shrink until they were barely visible. Treatment then was stopped and did not begin again until tumors had grown to more than 1% of body size in the mice. Miraculously, endostatin not only shrank the tumors, but caused them to become dormant so that they remained inactive even after the treatment had ended.

Initial Problems with Replication

Scientists from the NCI were unable to reproduce some initial study results involving endostatin and angiostatin. Researchers attributed the failure to technical problems, including possible trouble in transporting the fragile proteins, or improperly injecting them in the mice. There are often many problems which must be overcome in transferring a new technique from one lab to another, explained study scientists, adding that it usually takes at least 2 years for other scientists to repeat an experiment and publish results.

Eventually, other scientific teams, including one from the NCI, succeeded in independently testing endostatin and angiostatin. The two new drugs, which block the tumor blood vessels, were independently demonstrated to be incredibly effective at preventing the growth of cancers in mice, even in those with large tumors.

Human Trials

But several steps had to be taken before human trials could begin. First, scientists had to figure out a way to get adequate supplies of endostatin for preclinical and initial human clinical trials. So far it has been difficult to produce the large quantities needed for human tests. To overcome the problem, the NCI is working closely with EntreMed. Researchers are developing bacterial, mammalian-cell, or yeast "factories" that produce the proteins.

Scientists must also ensure that drugs produced for the trials are free of any impurities that might cause side effects in people. In recent months, researchers have developed a drug-production process that ensures purity. As part of the preclinical development process, researchers must perform necessary toxicologic and pharmacologic studies of the new drug. Scientists have been developing tests that measure the drug's action on body chemistry and organ systems. Required safety testing will follow.

Although endostatin and angiostatin have been used in combination to treat mice, the human trials will involve only endostatin. Presumably, angiostatin will be tested later in humans. During the first phase of the endostatin trials, scientists will test for adverse side effects and will also look for signs that the drug is halting the growth of tumors. If the drug is found to be safe, it will be tested for effectiveness.

The first phase will begin at Dana-Farber Cancer Institute, Brigham and Women's Hospital, and Massachusetts General Hospital in Boston. Candidates will have tumors caused by lymphoma or cancers of the colon, breast, or other organs. Additional, similar phase I tests will begin after the Boston trials. These will be done at the University of Texas, M.D. Anderson Cancer Institute in Houston and at the University of Wisconsin's Comprehensive Cancer Center in Madison. Both sites will conduct trials on 15 to 25 patients with solid tumors caused by lung cancer, lymphoma, breast cancer, colon cancer, and prostate cancer.

Some Concerns

NCI investigators hope that the new drugs will work in humans as well as it has worked in mice, but there are several variables to consider. So far, scientists have been treating tumors that were transplanted in mice. The biology of transplanted tumors is different from that of naturally occurring tumors. Often transplanted tumors are not accurate predictors of what will happen with natural human cancers.

Laboratory animals such as mice don't metabolize drugs the same way that humans do. This can affect the success of treatments with proteins. Because humans are much larger than mice, they will require much larger quantities of the drug. Scientists don't know what effect large amounts of endostatin might have on humans. Other anti-angiogenesis drugs have shown promise in the laboratory and then performed poorly in human tests. Interleukin-2, for example, was very successful in treating tumors in mice. But subsequent studies in people showed that it caused significant side effects such as a severe drop in blood pressure and leaking of fluid from blood vessels.

What the Future Holds

Human trials of endostatin will enable researchers to learn much more than they now know about cancer and how it kills. In fact, scientists may be able to learn more about every stage of cancer development, and that knowledge could help them to devise more innovative treatments.

If the new drug works in humans, it eventually will become available for consumption by patients. Medications in late-phase clinical trials may be approved by the U.S. Food and Drug Administration for general use as cancer treatments within 2 to 5 years. Some anti-angiogenesis drugs are already at that stage. These include Marimastat, a matric metalloproteinase inhibitor, and thalidomide, a drug with multiple mechanisms that has shown some evidence of biologic activity in gliomas (brain tumors) and Kaposi's sarcoma.

If all goes well, endostatin may become available early in the next century. But some patients may be able to get it sooner. The FDA sometimes approves "compassionate use" for promising drugs that have not been fully approved. The compassionate-use mechanism allows patients to receive such drugs if no other satisfactory options exist.

But, at this point, no one knows how costly the drug might be—or whether it will have unforeseen long-term side effects. It is likely that scientists will discover that endostatin is effective against some tumors at a particular stage in the disease process. As such, the drug could be valuable in treating cancer as a chronic disease, enabling patients to live longer, healthier lives.

Summary

Treating cancer is a lifetime commitment. The good news is that scientists are developing new cancer therapies at the fastest pace in medical history. The bad news is that all this science still requires FDA approval, which means millions of cancer patients will die in the FDA's "waiting room."

Medical oncologists do not require FDA approval to prescribe drugs like COX-2 inhibitors and the "statins" to the cancer patient. Cancer patients, however, require a continuous flow of new information to make sure they are getting the best therapies science has to offer. Much of this new information can be found on the Life Extension Foundation's Web site www.lef.org

Members of the Life Extension Foundation receive a 96-page monthly magazine that carries exclusive and timely articles about potential cancer treatment breakthroughs from around the world. To inquire about joining the Life Extension Foundation, call (800) 544-4440.

Alternative Therapy Books on Cancer Available from LEF

Call (800) 544-4440 to order the following:

1. *Beating Cancer with Nutrition,* Dr. Patrick Quillin with Noreen Quillin.
2. *An Alternative Medicine Definitive Guide to Cancer,* W. John Diamond, M.D., and W. Lee Cowden, M.D., with Burton Goldberg.
3. *Cancer Therapy, The Independent Consumer's Guide to Non-toxic Treatment and Prevention,* Ralph W. Moss, Ph.D. (also the author of *The Cancer Industry*).

Please refer to the References section at the end of this book for additional studies.

For some forms of cancer, you may be able to get into a free program utilizing experimental cancer therapies sponsored by the National Cancer Institute. For information about experimental cancer therapies, call (800) 4-CANCER. Make sure you do not enroll in a study where you may be part of a placebo group or where the toxicity of the drug may potentially kill you before the cancer does.

Product availability. You can order Life Extension Mix, Life Extension Herbal Mix, selenium complex, Thymex, DHEA, melatonin, vitamin A emulsified drops, vitamin D_3, Mega Soy Extract, Green Tea capsules, Coenzyme Q_{10}, garlic (Aged Garlic Extract), vitamin C, Phyto-Food, and conjugated linoleic acid (CLA) by calling (800) 544-4440, or order online at www.lef.org. Ask for the names of companies that will ship nimesulide and other cancer drugs to Americans for personal use.

CANCER CHEMOTHERAPY

Respected cancer journals are publishing articles that identify safer and more effective chemotherapy drug regimens, yet only a few medical institutions in the United States are incorporating these synergistic methods into clinical practice. Cancer patients, for the most part, are suffering through brutal chemotherapy regimens that have long ago proven themselves to be ineffective.

The Foundation's chemotherapy protocol provides concise information about reducing some of the side effects of cytotoxic chemotherapy and utilizing other drugs to enhance the cancer cell–killing effects of these drugs.

(After reading this protocol, it is important that chemotherapy patients refer to the Cancer (Adjuvant) Treatment protocol for additional information about enhancing the efficacy of chemotherapy drug therapies).

How Does Chemotherapy Work?

According to the National Cancer Institute, normal cells grow and die in a controlled way through a process called apoptosis. Cancer cells keep dividing and forming more cells without a control mechanism. Anticancer drugs destroy cancer cells by stopping them from growing or multiplying at one or more points in their growth cycle. Chemotherapy may consist of one or several cytotoxic drugs, depending on the type of cancer being treated.

In addition to chemotherapy, other methods are sometimes used to treat cancer. For example, your doctor may recommend that you have surgery to remove a tumor or to relieve certain symptoms that may be caused by your cancer. You also may receive radiation therapy to treat your cancer or its symptoms. Sometimes your doctor may suggest a combination of chemotherapy, surgery, and/or radiation therapy.

The goal of chemotherapy is to shrink primary tumors, slow the tumor growth, and to kill cancer cells that may have spread (metastasized) to other parts of the body from the original tumor. Chemotherapy kills both cancer and healthy cells. The goal is to minimize damage to normal cells and to enhance the cytotoxic effect to cancer cells.

An Integrated Approach

Nutrients and hormone therapies can be used to mitigate the toxicity of chemotherapy. The use of chemotherapy can cause health problems over and above those of the cancer itself such as severe heart muscle damage, gastrointestinal damage, anemia, nausea, and lethal suppression of immune function.

Bolstering the immune system may help alleviate or lower the severity of the complications associated with chemotherapy. If possible, these methods should be undertaken several days or even weeks before any planned chemotherapy is begun and should be continued well after the chemotherapy has completed.

Benefits of Vitamins E and C and *N*-Acetyl-Cysteine

Vitamins E and C, and *N*-acetyl-cysteine (NAC), may protect against heart muscle toxicity for cancer patients undergoing high doses of chemotherapy. A controlled study examined the effects of these nutrients on cardiac function on a group of chemotherapy and radiation patients. One group was given vitamins C and E supplements and NAC supplements while the other group was not supplemented. In the group not supplemented, left ventricle function was reduced in 46% of the chemotherapy patients compared to those who took the supplements. Furthermore, none of the patients from the supplement group showed a significant fall in overall ejection fraction, but 29% of the nonsupplement group showed reduced ejection fraction.

Vitamin C may be used to potentiate the effects of chemotherapy. Patients report improved appetite while taking vitamin C, as well as a reduced need for pain killers.

Vitamin E has been shown to protect against cardiomyopathies induced by chemotherapy. Vitamin E has also been used in combination with vitamin A and Coenzyme Q_{10} to reduce the side effects of the chemotherapy drug Adriamycin. Vitamin E is also complementary to chemotherapy in that it boosts the effectiveness of the drugs. The dry powder succinate form of vitamin E appears to be most beneficial to cancer patients. The more common acetate form has proven ineffective in slowing cancer cell growth in some studies, whereas natural dry powder vitamin E succinate has shown efficacy.

Benefits of Coenzyme Q_{10}

Coenzyme Q_{10} is used with vitamin E to protect patients from chemotherapy-induced cardiomyopathies. Coenzyme Q_{10} is nontoxic even at high dosages and has been shown to prevent liver damage from the drugs Mitomycin C and 5-FU (5-fluorouracil). Adriamycin-induced cardiomyopathies have been prevented by concomitant supplementation with CoQ_{10}.

CAUTION: Some studies indicate that Coenzyme Q_{10} should not be taken at the same time as chemotherapy. If this is true, it would be disappointing, since CoQ_{10} is so effective in protecting against adriamycin-induced cardiomyopathy. Adriamycin is a chemotherapy drug sometimes used as part of a chemotherapy cocktail. Until more research is known, it is not possible to make a definitive recommendation whether to take CoQ_{10} during chemotherapy.

Benefits of Selenium

Selenium has been used in combination with vitamin A and vitamin E to reduce the toxicity of chemotherapy drugs, particularly Adriamycin. The synergistic effect of vitamin E and selenium together to enhance the immune system is greater than either alone.

Benefits of Whey Protein

Glutathione balance is very important for the cancer patient. Glutathione is an antioxidant that protects cells from toxic compounds. Unfortunately, it is believed that glutathione actually benefits cancer cells at the expense of normal adjacent cells. A group of researchers showed that "tumor cell glutathione concentration may be among the determinants of the cytotoxicity of many chemotherapeutic agents and of radiation, and an increase in glutathione concentration in cancer cells appears to be at least one of the mechanisms of acquired drug resistance to chemotherapy."

Whey proteins used in combination with glutathione appear to reduce the concentrations of glutathione in cancer cells, thereby making them more vulnerable to chemotherapy while maintaining or even increasing glutathione levels in normal healthy cells. Researchers found that cancer cells had reduced glutathione levels in the presence of whey protein while at the same time normal cells had increased levels of glutathione levels with increased cellular growth of healthy cells. The study concluded, "Selective depletion of tumor cell glutathione may, in fact, render cancer cells more vulnerable to the action of chemotherapy and eventually protect normal tissue against the deleterious effects of chemotherapy."

Glutathione production in cancer and healthy cells is negatively inhibited by its own synthesis. Since glutathione levels are higher in cancer cells, it is believed that cancer cells would reach a level of negative-feedback inhibition for glutathione production more easily than normal cells. Chemotherapy patients should consider taking 30 to 60 grams a day of whey protein concentrate 10 days before initiation of chemotherapy, during the chemotherapy, and at least 10 days after the chemotherapy session is completed.

Note: If blood testing shows that chemotherapy has suppressed the immune system, patients should insist that their oncologists use the appropriate immune restoration drug(s), as outlined in the *Cancer (Adjuvant) Treatment protocol*.

Research using whey protein concentrate has led researchers to a discovery regarding the relationship between cancerous cells, glutathione, and whey protein concentrate. As mentioned above, it was found that whey protein concentrate selectively depletes cancer cells of their glutathione, making them more susceptible to cancer treatments such as radiation and chemotherapy.

This difference in glutathione status between normal cells and cancer cells is believed to be an important factor in cancer cells' resistance to chemotherapy.

Benefits of EPA Fish Oil (Omega-3 d-Alpha Tocopherol)

Fish oil may enhance the effectiveness of cancer chemotherapy drugs. A study compared different fatty acids on colon cancer cells to see if they could enhance Mitomycin C, a chemotherapy drug. Eicosapentaenoic acid (EPA) concentrated from fish oil was shown to sensitize colon cancer cells to Mitomycin C. It should be noted that fish oil also suppresses the formation of prostaglandin E2, which is involved in the synthesis of COX-2. Colon cancer cells use COX-2 to stimulate propagation.

Anti-Nausea Drugs for Chemotherapy Patients

Nausea is one of the most common and difficult aspects of chemotherapy for cancer patients. Nausea can have secondary effects on cancer patients by interfering with their eating habits during and immediately after chemotherapy.

Drugs to mitigate chemotherapy-induced nausea include Megace and Zofran. The high cost of Zofran has kept many cancer patients not covered by insurance from obtaining this potentially beneficial drug. If you are receiving chemotherapy and are suffering from nausea, you should be able to demand that any HMO, PPO, or insurance carrier pay for this drug. Zofran can enable a cancer patient to tolerate chemotherapy long enough for it to be possibly effective.

Medical marijuana was approved by referendum in California and Arizona, primarily for the beneficial medical use by cancer patients to alleviate nausea following chemotherapy. It is interesting to observe the objections of the federal government regarding the concept of medical marijuana as their "war on drugs" is brought to bear on an herb. Life Extension Foundation has provided financial help for the legal battle on behalf of the medical rights of those cancer patients in California and Arizona.

Researchers have embarked on evaluating the medical benefits of marijuana, and we will follow these studies and report the results to you. One study evaluated glutathione and vitamins C and E for their antivomiting properties. Cisplatin-induced vomiting in dogs was significantly reduced by glutathione and vitamins C and E. The anti-vomiting activity of antioxidants was attributed to their ability to react with free radicals generated by cisplatin. Ginger extract has also been shown effective in reducing nausea symptoms.

Benefits of Melatonin

Melatonin has been shown to protect against chemotherapy-induced immune depression. One study specifically suggested that cancer patients treated with Adriamycin, a toxic chemotherapy drug, should supplement with vitamins A and E and selenium to reduce its side effects.

Melatonin mediates the toxicity of chemotherapy and inhibits free-radical production. In a randomized study to evaluate the effect of melatonin on the toxicity of chemotherapy drugs, the patients receiving melatonin with chemotherapy had lower incidences of neuropathies, thrombocytopenia, stomatitis, alopecia, malaise, and vomiting.

The study suggests that adding melatonin to a chemotherapy regimen may prevent some toxic effects of the chemotherapy drugs, especially myelosuppression and neuropathies.

A study was performed to evaluate the influence of melatonin on chemotherapy toxicity. Patients randomly received chemotherapy alone or chemotherapy plus melatonin (20 mg each evening). Thrombocytopenia, a decrease in the number of blood platelets, was significantly less frequent in patients treated with melatonin. Malaise and lack of strength also were significantly less frequent in patients receiving melatonin.

Finally, stomatitis (inflammation of the mouth area) and neuropathy were less frequent in the melatonin group. Alopecia and vomiting were not influenced. This pilot study seems to suggest that administration of melatonin during chemotherapy may prevent some chemotherapy-induced side effects, particularly myelosuppression and neuropathy.

Expensive drugs like Neupogen (granulocyte-colony stimulating factor: GC-SF), granulocyte-macrophage-colony (white blood cells) stimulating factor (GM-CSF), and interferon-alpha (an immune modulating cytokine) can restore immune function debilitated by toxic cancer-chemotherapy drugs. If you are on chemotherapy and your blood tests show immune suppression, you should request the appropriate immune restoration drug(s) from your medical oncologist.

Studies have shown that melatonin specifically exerts colony-stimulating activity and rescues bone marrow cells from apoptosis (programmed cell death) induced by cancer chemotherapy compounds. Melatonin has been reported to "rescue" bone marrow cells from cancer chemotherapy-induced death. The number of granulocyte-macrophage colony-forming units has been shown to be higher in the presence of melatonin.

Combining Melatonin with Interleukin-2

Melatonin has been seen to enhance the anti-cancer action of interleukin-2 (IL-2) and to reduce IL-2 toxicity. Melatonin use in association with IL-2 cancer immunotherapy has been shown to have the following actions:

1. Amplification of IL-2 biological activity by enhancing lymphocyte response and by antagonizing macrophage-mediated suppressive events.
2. Inhibition of production of tumor growth factors, which stimulate cancer cell proliferation by counteracting lymphocyte-mediated tumor cell destruction.
3. Maintenance of a circadian rhythm of melatonin, which is often altered in human neoplasms and influenced by cytokine exogenous injection.

The subcutaneous administration of 3 million IU a day of interleukin-2 (IL-2) and high doses of melatonin (40 mg each evening orally) has appeared to be effective in tumors resistant either to IL-2 alone or to chemotherapy. The dose of 3 million IU a day of interleukin-2 is a low dose, while serious toxicity normally begins at 15 million IU a day. At present, 230 patients with advanced solid tumors and life expectancy less than 6 months have been treated with this melatonin/IL-2 combination.

Objective tumor regressions were experienced in 44 patients (18%), mainly in patients with lung cancer, hepatocarcinoma, cancer of the pancreas, gastric cancer, and colon cancer. A survival longer than one year was achieved in 41% of the patients. The preliminary data show that melatonin synergizes with tumor necrosis factor (TNF) and alpha-interferon by reducing their toxicity.

Melatonin Precautions

The Life Extension Foundation introduced the world to melatonin in 1992. And it was the Life Extension Foundation that issued the original warnings about who should not take melatonin. These warnings were based on preliminary findings, and in two instances the Foundation was overly cautious.

First, we suggested that prostate cancer patients might want to avoid high doses of melatonin. However, subsequent studies indicated that prostate cancer patients could benefit from moderate doses of melatonin, though the Foundation still advises prostate cancer patients to have their blood tested for prolactin. Melatonin could possibly elevate prolactin secretion, and if this were to happen in a prostate-cancer patient, the drug Dostinex could be used to suppress prolactin so that the melatonin could continue to be taken (in moderate doses of 1 to 6 mg each night).

Some doctors initially thought that melatonin should not be taken by ovarian cancer patients, but a study published in *Oncology Reports* ((Greece), 1996; 3[5] 947–49), indicates that high doses of melatonin may be beneficial in treating ovarian cancer. In this study, 40 mg of melatonin were given nightly, along with low doses of interleukin-2, to 12 advanced ovarian cancer patients who had failed chemotherapy. While no complete response was seen, a partial response was achieved in 16% of patients, and a stable disease was obtained in 41% of the cases. This preliminary study suggests that melatonin is not contraindicated in advanced ovarian cancer patients. It is still not known what the effects of melatonin are in leukemia, so leukemia patients should use melatonin with caution.

Drugs That Protect against Chemotherapy Toxicity

Cancer patients using cytotoxic chemotherapy drugs should ask their oncologist to place them on FDA-approved immune-protective drugs 1 week before the first chemotherapy drug is administered. Depending on the type of cancer and the chemotherapy regimen that will be used, two of the most important FDA-approved drugs to consider are *Neupogen,* a granulocyte-colony stimulating factor drug (G-CSF) or *Leukine,* a granulocyte-macrophage-colony stimulating factor (GM-CSF).

Neupogen or Leukine stimulates the production of T-lymphocytes, macrophages, and other immune cells which are valuable in preventing the toxic effects on the bone marrow during chemotherapy. These immune-protecting drugs enable chemotherapy to be given at a higher dose that may make it effective. Stimulated macrophages are powerful tumor killers, as has been demonstrated by clinical studies using interleukin-2 and GM-CSF, or G-CSF. In addition, colony growth factors are able to accelerate regeneration of blood cells following chemotherapy. Initial clinical experience with GM-CSF and G-CSF has shown that severe neutropenia (immune impairment) due to chemotherapy drugs may be prevented or at least decelerated, thus reducing the number of severe infections.

Alpha-interferon and/or interleukin-2 are immune cytokines (regulators) that should also be considered by cancer patients. Interferon directly inhibits cancer cell proliferation and has already been used in the therapy of hairy cell leukemia, Kaposi's sarcoma, and malignant melanoma. Interleukin-2 allows for an increase in the cytotoxic activity of natural killer (NK) cells. These drugs must be carefully administered by an oncologist as they can produce temporary side effects.

Retinoic acid (vitamin A) analog drugs enhance the efficacy of some chemotherapy regimens and reduce the risk of secondary cancers. Ask your oncologist to consider prescribing vitamin A analog drugs like Accutane. Again, the use and dosage of potentially toxic drugs like Accutane must be carefully prescribed by your attending oncologist.

Some cancer patients produce too many T-suppressor cells that shut down optimal immune function. The administration of drugs such as cimetidine helps to prevent cancer cells from prematurely shutting down the immune system. An *immune cell subset* blood test will reveal the status of your T-helper cells, T-suppressor cells, and NK cell count and activity.

The proper administration of Neupogen or Leukine prior to the initiation of chemotherapy can dramatically reduce the immune damage that chemotherapy inflicts on the body and increase the cancer cell–killing efficacy of conventional chemotherapy drugs. Please remember that so far we have only talked about drugs that require physician administration. There are safe nutrients that can be self-administered that also protect against chemotherapy toxicity and immune impairment.

To treat low white blood cell counts, the FDA-approved drug Neupogen or Leukine may be considered by your immunologist or hematologist. Drugs such as Neupogen, Leukine, and Intron A alpha-interferon (an immune-modulating cytokine) can restore immune function debilitated by toxic cancer chemotherapy drugs. In one study, patients with refractory (resistant to treatment) solid tumors treated with standard chemotherapy and GM-CSF had a 33.3% objective response rate, versus 15% with chemotherapy alone. If you are on chemotherapy and your blood tests show immune suppression, you should demand that your oncologist use the appropriate immune restoration drug(s).

Additional Information on Cancer Treatment

Cancer patients may want to refer to the other protocols in this edition or visit our web site at www.lef.org

General information sources. U.S. Department of Health and Human Services, Public Health Service, National Institutes of Health National Cancer Institute, Bethesda, Maryland 20892, and NIH Publication No. 94-1136

Summary

The following natural supplements may reduce side effects and damage caused by chemotherapy:

1. Vitamin E, 800 IU a day of vitamin E succinate (dry powder natural vitamin E).
2. Vitamin C, 4000 to 12,000 mg throughout the day.
3. Coenzyme Q_{10}, 200 to 300 mg daily in a softgel oil capsule for maximum absorption. (Refer to cautions about CoQ_{10} and chemotherapy.)
4. EPA fish oil, 8 to 12 Mega EPA caps throughout the day. This should be balanced with at least one capsule a day of MEGA GLA (gamma-linolenic acid) CAUTION: Some studies suggest not taking these oils if you have prostate cancer.
5. Melatonin: 20 mg at bedtime. Dose may be reduced after chemotherapy ends if too much morning drowsiness occurs. After several months, most cancer patients take 3 to 10 mg of melatonin at bedtime.
6. Selenium: 200 to 600 mcg of selenium daily.
7. Whey protein concentrate-isolate: 30 to 60 grams daily. Note: Cancer patients undergoing chemotherapy should consider taking whey protein concentrate at least 10 days before beginning therapy and during therapy, and then continuing with the whey protein for at least 30 days after completion of the therapy.
8. Ask your oncologist to consider prescribing drugs suggested in this protocol, such as Neupogen, Leukine, and alpha interferon.

(*For more complete information, refer to the Cancer (Adjuvant) Treatment protocol*). We suggest you check www.lef.org regularly for the latest information regarding cancer chemotherapy and related subjects.

Product availability. Coenzyme Q_{10}, whey protein concentrate, vitamin A, vitamin C, vitamin D, vitamin E, selenium, melatonin, and EPA fish oil Mega GLA can be obtained by calling (800) 544-4440, or order online at www.lef.org.

CANCER RADIATION THERAPY

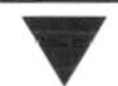

Radiation therapy is given to about 60% of all cancer patients, but may inflict tremendous tissue damage to healthy cells. Radiotherapy can also cause secondary cancers after the primary cancer has been treated, leading to secondary diseases such as pneumonitis and radiation fibrosis. Radiation therapy is associated with both acute and late disease conditions that affect a patient's nutritional status.

Radiation therapy relies on the local destruction of cancer cells through ionizing radiation that disrupts cellular DNA. Radiation therapy can be externally or internally originated, high or low dose, and delivered with computer-assisted accuracy to the site of the tumor. Brachytherapy, or interstitial radiation therapy, places the source of radiation directly into the tumor as implanted "seeds."

Newer radiotherapy technologies such as stereotactic radiosurgery, which uses tightly focused x-rays or gamma rays to target tumors without widespread irradiation of surrounding tissues, may improve radiotherapy results; these approaches, however, are limited to certain types of cancers.

Complications Caused by Radiation Therapy

Radiation Pneumonitis

Radiation-induced pneumonitis can be treated with antioxidants; however, the exact cause of pneumonitis is not known. It is thought to occur as a result of excessive free radicals generated following radiotherapy.

In vitro studies have shown that large doses of radiation can cause membrane lipid peroxidation and the oxidation of protein groups. Radiation-induced pneumonitis was studied using 25 patients who underwent radiotherapy for non-small cell lung cancer (inoperable). Blood samples were taken over a 3-month period, and it was found that 40% (10 out of 25) of the patients developed pneumonitis and that these patients had significantly higher levels of free radicals and iron in their blood. Iron is a catalyst for free-radical reactions.

Benefits of Antioxidants

The risk of pneumonitis may be reduced by antioxidant therapy. There are several specific nutrients that can be taken to improve the immune system after radiotherapy. General supplementation with antioxidants such as vitamins A, C, and E, and with the sulfur amino acids cysteine and glutathione, are known to reduce free-radical damage caused by radiation therapy. For these nutrients to be effective, the nutrients or their precursors must be consumed before the radiotherapy treatment.

Radiation Fibrosis

Radiation fibrosis is an extreme complication, without effective treatments, after radiation therapy. Surgical removal and healing of a radiation-induced fibrosis is rarely successful.

One published case involved a 58-year-old woman who developed a radiation fibrosis in the irradiated area of a squamous cell carcinoma. Following the surgery the woman was treated with a combination of pentoxifylline tablets (400 mcg 3 times daily) and vitamin E (one 400-mg capsule each day). The woman tolerated the treatment well and a noted improvement in the condition of the affected skin was seen, beginning at 4 months. A decrease in skin thickness could be demonstrated from the 6th month on, with the patient experiencing no side effects from this protocol. The data indicates a therapeutic effect on radiation-induced fibrosis by the synergistic administration of pentoxifylline and vitamin E. Pentoxifylline is a prescription drug that inhibits abnormal platelet aggregation and which may allow more blood flow to the irradiated area.

Another study published in the August 1998 issue of the *British Journal of Radiology* reported a "striking regression of radiation-induced fibrosis by a combination of pentoxifylline and tocopherol." Researchers reported a 50% regression of superficial radiation-induced fibrosis regression after a 6-month administration of pentoxifylline and tocopherol (vitamin E) in half of the patients studied.

The British journal study also reported on a 67-year-old woman with a bulky radiation-induced fibrosis who, 10 years previously, had received radiochemotherapy for a small cell thyroid carcinoma with severe acute radiation side effects. She had palpable cervico-sternal fibrosis measuring 10 × 8 cm, with local inflammatory signs and functional consequences (cough, restricted cervical movement, dyspnea, and bronchitis). A CAT scan revealed deep radiation-induced fibrosis extending from the vocal cords to the carina, with laryngotracheal compression but without cancer recurrence. The patient received pentoxifylline (800 mg/day) and vitamin E (1000 IU/day), orally administered daily for 18 months. The patient exhibited clinical regression and functional improvement at 6 months and complete response with no measurable fibrosis at 18 months.

The combination of pentoxifylline and vitamin E seems to promote a significant antifibrotic effect by reversing deep radiation-induced fibrosis.

Sexual Dysfunction after Radiotherapy—New Therapy Now Available

One of the unpublicized side effects of radiotherapy is male impotency, especially in those being treated for prostrate cancer, as reflected in a study published in the July 1999 issue of the journal *Urology*. This study reported that a high percentage of men suffer this dysfunction after radiotherapy with little hope for recovery.

However, treatment of erectile dysfunction with the drug Viagra after radiation therapy for prostate cancer was reported a success just 1 month later (August 1999) in that same urological journal. Researchers reported the success based on research conducted by the Department of Urology at the Cleveland Clinic Foundation in Cleveland, Ohio.

The study was conducted to determine the response to Viagra in patients with erectile dysfunction after radiation therapy for localized prostate cancer. Twenty-one patients presenting with erectile dysfunction after radiation treatment for clinical T1-2 prostate cancer were studied. Two patients had undergone iodine-125 seed implantation, and the remaining 19 had undergone conformal external beam irradiation.

All 21 patients were considered to have erectile dysfunction as assessed by the International Index of Erectile Function and were prescribed sildenafil at a dosage of 50 mg, with a titration to 100 mg if needed.

Seventy-one percent of patients had a positive response, with a corresponding spousal satisfaction rate of 71%. No patient discontinued the drug because of side effects. On the global efficacy question (ability to achieve firm erections), 71% of the patients responded positively.

If you are experiencing impotency you may consider consulting your physician and having him or her prescribe 50 to 100 mg of Viagra daily to correct this sometimes overlooked adverse side effect of radiotherapy. Viagra is not without side effects, but, for otherwise healthy people, it appears safe.

Vitamin A May Improve the Tolerance and Effectiveness of Radiation Therapy

Radiation-induced lung injury frequently limits the total dose of thoracic radiotherapy that can be delivered to a patient undergoing radiation therapy, limiting its effectiveness.

Several small animal studies including a study reported in the October 1998 issue of the *Journal of Nutrition* suggest that supplemental vitamin A may reduce lung inflammation after thoracic radiation and be an important modifiable radioprotective agent in the lung (*J. Nutr.,* 1998 Oct; 128 [10]:1661–64).

Researchers have also reported the radioprotective effect of beta-carotene from a study conducted on over 700 children exposed to radiation by the Chernobyl nuclear accident. The results showed that natural beta-carotene protected against the susceptibility of lipids to oxidation and may act as an *in vivo* lipophilic antioxidant or radioprotector.

Patients undergoing radiotherapy should be taking 25,000 IU of vitamin A a day.

CAUTION: Refer to vitamin A precautions in *Appendix A: Avoiding Vitamin A Toxicity* to avoid toxic overdose.

Radiation Therapy Reduces Taurine

The amino acid taurine is severely depleted when people undergo radiation therapy. The March 1992 issue of the *American Journal of Clinical Nutrition* suggested a possible therapeutic effect of taurine supplementation relative to radiation therapy. Supplementation with 2000 mg a day of taurine is, therefore, recommended to people undergoing cancer radiation therapy.

Benefits of Melatonin

The possible benefits of melatonin were reported in a preliminary study in the February 1996 issue of the journal *Oncology* (1996 Jan–Feb;53 [1]:43–46) in which researchers suggested that radiotherapy plus melatonin may prolong the survival time and improve the quality of life of patients affected by glioblastoma.

More recently, an issue of *Mutation Research* (1999, March:10; 425 [1]:21–27) reported that "high doses of melatonin are effective in protecting mice from lethal effects of acute whole-body irradiation."

Patients with brain glioblastoma generally experience a poor survival rate, which is typically less than 6 months. However, when 20 mg of melatonin were given to patients treated with radical or adjuvant radiotherapy, both the mean survival rates and the percentage of survivors after one year were significantly higher among patients treated with melatonin therapy compared with patients who did not receive melatonin. Researchers also reported that patients had reduced radiation and steroid-related toxicities when melatonin was consumed nightly.

Avoid Soy Extracts

Soy extracts have a strong impact on protecting both healthy and cancerous cells and are strongly recommended as an adjuvant cancer therapy. However researchers have documented that soy extracts may reduce the effectiveness of radiotherapy. Based on these preliminary results, cancer patients undergoing radiation therapy should avoid soy or genistein extracts 1 week before, during, and 1 week after radiation therapy, because soy may prevent radiation from killing cancer cells.

Reducing Tumor Cell Glutathione Levels

It has been found that cancer cells and normal cells will respond differently to nutrients and drugs that affect glutathione status. Some studies show that the concentration of glutathione in tumor cells is higher than that of the normal cells that surround them. This difference in glutathione status between normal cells and cancer cells is believed to be an important factor in cancer cells' resistance to chemotherapy. Whey protein concentrate has been shown to selectively deplete cancer cells of their glutathione, thus making them more susceptible to cancer treatments such as radiation and chemotherapy.

As the researchers put it, "Tumor cell glutathione concentration may be among the determinants of the cytotoxicity of many chemotherapeutic agents and of radiation, and an increase in glutathione concentration in cancer cells appears to be at least one of the mechanisms of acquired drug resistance to chemotherapy." They further state, "It is well-known that rapid glutathione synthesis in tumor cells is associated with high rates of cellular proliferation. Depletion of cancer cell glutathione *in vivo* decreases the rate of cellular proliferation and inhibits cancer growth."

It's difficult to reduce glutathione sufficiently in tumor cells without placing healthy tissue at risk and putting the cancer patient in a worse condition. What is needed is a compound that can selectively deplete the cancer cells of their glutathione, while increasing or at least maintaining the levels of glutathione in healthy cells. This is what whey protein appears to do.

Scientists have found that cancer cells subjected to whey proteins are depleted of their glutathione, and their growth is inhibited, while normal cells have an increase in glutathione and increased cellular growth. These effects were not seen with other proteins. Not surprisingly, the researchers concluded, "Selective depletion of tumor cell glutathione may in fact render cancer cells more vulnerable to the action of chemotherapy and eventually protect normal tissue against the deleterious effects of chemotherapy."

The exact mechanism by which whey protein achieves this is not fully understood, but it appears that it interferes with the normal feedback mechanism and regulation of glutathione in cancer cells. It is known that glutathione production is negatively inhibited by its own synthesis. Since baseline glutathione levels in cancer cells are higher than those of normal cells, it is probably easier to reach the level of negative-feedback inhibition in the cancer cells' glutathione levels than in the normal cells' glutathione levels.

Cancer patients undergoing radiation therapy may consider taking 30 to 60 grams a day of whey protein concentrate, starting at least 10 days before beginning therapy, during therapy, and then continuing for at least 10 days after completion of the therapy.

Benefits of Alpha-Interferon/Retinoic Acid and Accutane

It is well established that solid tumors contain oxygen deficient (hypoxic) areas, and that cells in such areas will cause tumors to be resistant to ionizing radiation. Inoperable cervical cancer is normally treated with radiotherapy. Several previous *in vivo* and *in vitro* trials suggest an improvement of radiosensitivity by adding retinoids and alpha-interferon in squamous cell cervical cancer.

In an early pilot trial, 33 women with squamous cell cervical cancer were treated with 6 million units of alpha-interferon a day and 1 mg per kilogram of body weight of the retinoid drug Accutane a day for 12 days prior to radiotherapy. During radiotherapy, all dosages were reduced to prevent toxic side effects: 3 million units of alpha-interferon 3 times a week and 0.5 mg per kilogram of body weight of Accutane daily were administered until the maximum dosage of radiation was reached. Twenty-nine patients were totally evaluated and four patients were still under treatment.

Complete response occurred in 26 patients, partial response in three patients, and almost all patients tolerated treatment well while toxicity was mild. Treatment with alpha-interferon and Accutane improved oxygenation of squamous cell cancers and may enhance the efficacy of radiotherapy.

In a 1998 study, German researchers conducted a 2-week pretreatment with retinoic acid plus interferon-alpha-2a prior to definitive radiation therapy in cervical cancer patients. Investigators reported a complete clinical remission of the local tumor in 19 of 22 patients after radiotherapy and additional retinoic acid plus interferon-alpha-2a treatment. In primarily hypoxic tumors, four out of five achieved complete remission (*Strahlenther Onkol.* 1998 [Nov]; 174[11]:571–74).

A 1999 study published in the *International Journal of Radiation Oncology Biological Physics* (1999, Jan 15; 43[2]:367–73) confirmed the German study regarding the oxygenation of cervical cancers during radiotherapy using radiotherapy plus cis-retinoic acid/interferon. Researchers found that in patients with well-oxygenated tumors, 87% (20 out of 23) achieved a clinically complete response. In patients with primarily hypoxic tumors, 6 out of 6 patients whose primarily hypoxic tumors showed an increase of the median oxygen levels achieved a complete remission. In contrast, only 4 out of 7 patients with a low pretreatment and persisting low median O2 achieved a complete remission. Researchers concluded there are evident changes in the oxygenation of cervical cancers during a course of fractionated radiotherapy. In primarily hypoxic tumors, a significant increase of the median oxygen was found. An additional treatment with cis-retinoic acid and interferon further improved the oxygenation.

If you (or a member of your family) are undergoing radiotherapy, this new information should be brought to your physician's attention.

Possible Benefit to Ginseng

In animal studies, when ginseng was administered along with radiation therapies, a far greater percentage of the animals survived in the ginseng-supplemented group, compared with the group administered radiation without ginseng. Cancer patients should consider taking 2 to 4 capsules daily of Sports Ginseng by Nature's Herbs, which combines Korean and Siberian ginseng.

Shark Liver Oil for 30 Days

Shark liver oil containing standardized alkylglycerols can prevent immune impairment and irradiation injury to healthy tissues. Cancer patients should take six 200-mg standardized shark liver oil capsules a day for 30 days. Shark liver oil can cause an overproduction of blood platelets, so high doses of shark liver oil should not be taken for more than 30 days.

Hyperthermia and Microwave Hyperthermia Therapy—New Emerging Cancer Therapies

Worth mentioning are several other emerging cancer therapies including hyperthermia and microwave hyperthermia. Hyperthermia therapy has been used to fight metastatic cancer and is usually combined with immune therapy treatment. Microwave hyperthermia is generally used to treat a specific region or tumor. This therapy is generally combined with radiation therapy.

Millennium Health Care in Atlanta, Georgia, is considered one of the leading organizations for this emerging therapy and can be contacted at (770) 390-0012, or information can be obtained online at www.millennium-healthcare.com.

Summary

The following natural supplements may reduce side effects and damage caused by radiotherapy. In addition, they may aid in the selective destruction of cancer cells and protection of healthy body tissue.

1. Melatonin, 20 mg nightly. Dose may be reduced to 3 to 10 mg each night after 30 days if too much morning drowsiness occurs.
2. Taurine, 2000 mg daily for those patients undergoing radiotherapy.
3. Ginseng, two to four 200-mg standard dosage Ginseng Sport capsules daily.
4. Shark liver oil, six 200-mg standardized shark liver oil capsules a day for 30 days prior to radiation therapy.

CAUTION: Shark liver oil can cause an overproduction of blood platelets, so high doses of shark liver oil should not be taken for more than 30 days.

5. Pentoxifylline and vitamin E, three 400-mg pentoxifylline tablets daily with two 400-IU capsules of vitamin E.
6. Vitamin A, 25,000 IU a day (*refer to Vitamin A Precautions in the Appendix to avoid toxic overdose*).
7. Vitamin C, 4,000 to 12,000 mg a day.
8. *N*-acetyl-cysteine (NAC), 600 mg, 3 times a day.
9. Whey protein concentrate-isolate, 30 to 60 grams a day at least 10 days before beginning therapy and during therapy, and then continuing with the whey protein for at least 30 days after completion of the therapy.
10. Alpha-interferon and Accutane. Consult your physician. A recent study reports on dosages of 6 million units of alpha-interferon and 1 mg per kilogram body weight of the retinoid drug Accutane daily for 12 days prior to radiation therapy. (During the radiation therapy sessions, the dosages were reduced to 3 million units of alpha-interferon 3 times a week and 0.5 mg per kilogram of body weight of Accutane until the maximum dosage of radiation was achieved).

Product availability. Vitamins A, C, D, and E; selenium; shark liver oil capsules; whey protein concentrate; taurine; ginseng; and melatonin can be obtained by calling (800) 544-4440, or order online at www.lef.org.

CANCER SURGERY

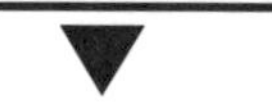

Surgery poses many risks to a cancer patient. The known side effects associated with the surgical removal of tumors include anesthesia complications, infections, and immune suppression.

A newly discovered surgery side effect of concern to cancer patients is that the removal of the primary tumor may directly stimulate the propagation of metastatic lesions. The theory is that an intact primary tumor regulates the growth of metastatic lesions by naturally secreting anti-angiogenesis agents such as endostatin and angiostatin. Metastatic tumors require the formation of new blood vessels (called angiogenesis) in order to grow. Once the primary tumor has been surgically removed, the amount of endostatin and angiostatin to control new blood vessel growth is drastically reduced, and metastasized lesions begin proliferating out of control. If the immune depression that surgery induces is factored in, the failure of surgery to meaningfully prolong the life of cancer patients becomes quite understandable. Surgery takes away growth control factors (endostatin and angiostatin) while simultaneously weakening the immune surveillance that might be keeping metastatic lesions under some degree of control.

Cancer has long baffled medical science. Until recently, scientists did not fully understand why the disease so often begins rapidly spreading throughout the body after surgery. The good news is that the drugs endostatin and angiostatin are finally entering clinical trials. If the FDA ever gets around to approving these drugs, the surgical removal of a large primary tumor might actually "cure" a lot more cancer patients. In the meantime, there are other anti-angiogenesis drugs that may help prevent the rapid growth of metastatic lesions after the primary tumor is removed.

How Tumors Grow

Almost every tissue in the body derives blood from the thinner-than-a-hair capillaries that lace our tissues. Through capillaries, nutrients, oxygen and various signaling molecules diffuse into cells. These mechanisms maintain health, fight disease, and allow the body to flourish and grow.

Scientists have found that tumors start out without circulation. In the early stages of tumor development, they are limited to a trickle of nutrients that can diffuse from the nearest capillaries. Then, somehow, tumors begin to stimulate healthy tissue to make thousands of new blood vessels to supply the cancerous growth—a process called angiogenesis. Without this ability to nourish itself and grow, a tumor cannot enlarge. If the blood supply can be reduced or cut off, the tumor will shrink or die.

Removing One Tumor May Stimulate the Growth of Many More

Scientists believe that a primary tumor sends chemicals to signal new blood vessels to grow into itself, but at the same time also sends a chemical signal that prevents other tumors from growing in other parts of the body. Advanced biomedical technology has now pinpointed those signals, and most scientists accept that the angiogenesis process (stimulation of new blood vessel growth) regulates the growth of metastatic tumors.

Once the primary tumor is removed, there is nothing to stop other tumors from growing elsewhere. That's why some cancer patients often get worse after undergoing tumor removal.

In recent years, several drugs—including interferons, steroids, and certain hormonal agents—have been developed to stop or slow angiogenesis. In fact, at least 11 anti-angiogenic drugs are now in clinical trials and three have proved effective enough to make it to final phase.

Some of the drugs, like endostatin, are derived from natural proteins, while others are based on smaller molecules. Ironically, one promising drug on trial now is thalidomide, which once was sold as a sedative which caused notorious birth defects in the children of women who took it.

Another drug, 2-methoxyestradiol (2-ME), is a natural estrogen metabolite believed to be an inhibitor of angiogenesis and also an antitumor agent.

In addition, researchers are investigating a drug called Col-3 and are negotiating with several biotechnology companies to examine other anticancer compounds.

Of all the anti-angiogenic drugs, endostatin and angiostatin appear to hold the greatest potential for saving lives. These drugs are nontoxic and have shown efficacy against every type of cancer they have been tested against. One study showed that these drugs suppressed metastatic tumor growth rates by 90%. Another study showed primary tumors regressing to become dormant microscopic lesions.

Based on this new information, angiostatin and endostatin may greatly increase the number of cancer patients who become disease free after surgery.

How to Enter Clinical Trials

Endostatin will be entered into clinical trials before the end of 1999. It is hoped that angiostatin human trials will soon follow.

For more information about human trials of endostatin, call The University of Wisconsin Cancer Connect Line, (800) 622-8922 or (608) 262-5223. Or call the M.D. Anderson Information Line, (800) 392-1611 and select option 3. For more information on current clinical trials from PDQ, the National Cancer Institute's database, call the Cancer Information Service, (800) 4-CANCER.

Physicians may request information about trials from the PDG Search Service by calling (800) 345-3300, faxing (800) 380-1575, or e-mailing [pdqsearch@icicc.nci.nih.gov].

There are many anti-angiogenesis drugs in clinical studies. In some cases, the FDA may allow an unapproved drug to be released before it is officially approved. Here are some of the anti-angiogenesis drugs being tested and the sponsoring companies:

Drug	Phase	Sponsor
TNP-40	II	TAP Pharmaceuticals Inc., Deerfield, Wisc.
Squalamine		Magainin Pharmaceuticals Inc., Plymouth Meeting, Pa.
Vitaxin	I	Ixsys Inc., San Diego, Calif.
Thalidomide	II	ExtreMed Inc., Rockville, Md.
RhuMab, VEGF	II	Genentech Inc., South San Francisco, Calif.
SU5416	II	Sugen Inc., Redwood City, Calif.
Marimastat	III	British Biotech Inc., Annapolis, Md.
Bay 12-9566	III	Bayer Corp., West Haven, Conn.
AG3340	III	Agouron Pharmaceuticals Inc., La Jolla, Calif.
Col-3	I	CollaGenex Pharmaceuticals, Inc.
CM101	I	Carbomed, Brentwood, Tenn.

Summary

A study conducted several years ago in Germany showed that, for most forms of cancer, surgical removal of the primary tumor did not result in prolonged survival compared with patients with similar cancers who refused surgery. For many forms of cancer, however, the surgical removal of the primary tumor is crucial if long-term remission is to occur. Anti-angiogenesis drugs given prior to cancer surgery may improve the chances of a long-term remission.

(For cancer patients undergoing surgery, or any other type of cancer therapy, it is important to review the new information that appears in the Cancer (Adjuvant) Treatment protocol. There are therapies discussed in the general Cancer protocol that are available now which can help protect against surgically induced immune depression, thus improving the odds of long-term survival.)

For the latest information about how cancer surgery can be made safer and more effective, check out the Foundation's Web site at www.lef.org and enter "cancer surgery" in the disease treatment search engine.

CANDIDA (FUNGAL, YEAST) INFECTIONS

Candidiasis is an infection caused by strains of the yeast, Candida, the most common being *Candida albicans*. Candida is normally present in the digestive tract and the vagina. During certain favorable conditions such as warm, humid weather or when an individual's immune system is impaired, the yeast can infect the skin. Mucous membranes in the mouth and vagina are commonly infected. In rare instances, Candida can invade blood and deeper tissues causing life-threatening infection.

People may sometimes develop a Candida infection after taking antibiotics. The antibiotics kill the bacteria that normally keep the Candida under control, allowing the Candida organism to grow unchecked. Pregnant women, diabetics, and obese people are also prone to Candida infections. Corticosteroids, given after organ transplantation, can also promote growth of Candida.

Commonly Infected Areas

- Skinfolds, including the navel and anus. Symptoms include a red rash with patchy areas oozing whitish fluid. Pus may also appear. The area will itch or burn. Perlèche is a Candida infection at the corners of the mouth, creating cracks and tiny cuts. It is often caused by ill-fitting dentures.
- Vagina (vulvovaginitis), occurring most often in pregnant women, those taking antibiotics, or those with diabetes. Symptoms include a white or yellow discharge, with burning, itching, and redness on the walls and the external areas of the vagina.
- Penis, occurring mostly to men having diabetes or whose sexual partner has a vaginal Candida infection. A red, scaly, often painful rash appears on the underside of the penis. However, an infection of the penis (or vagina) will not always cause discernible symptoms.
- Thrush, caused by a Candida infection of the mouth. Creamy white patches will appear on the tongue or sides of the mouth. Thrush can appear in a healthy child; however, in an adult it may be a symptom of a more serious disorder such as diabetes or AIDS. The use of antibiotics can also cause thrush.
- Paronychia is caused from Candida growing in the nail beds resulting in a painful swelling and secretion of pus. Infected nails may turn white or yellow and separate from the surrounding skin.

Candidiasis and the Yeast Syndrome

Most conventional physicians restrict a diagnosis of candidial infection to the previously mentioned conditions. When there is doubt, cultures may be obtained to prove the diagnosis and check for susceptibility to antifungal agents. Conventional physicians may also encounter the particularly vexing problem of women who have multiple vaginal yeast infections that are difficult to control. Many of these women are treated with multiple courses of potent antifungal drugs, often without relief.

Another, more controversial perspective is that which was popularized by Crook in *The Yeast Connection*. Dr. Crook used the term candidiasis to mean something different from what conventional medicine has described. What Crook and others refer to is a syndrome in which the predominant features are fatigue, a generalized malaise, gastrointestinal complaints, recurrent chronic infections, allergies, skin problems, decreased concentration, depression, irritability, and craving for sweets or carbohydrates. The mechanism is purported to be an overabundance of yeast in the bowel and perhaps elsewhere. While this has not been investigated and subjected to the rigors of peer review scrutiny, there is certainly substantial clinical and anecdotal evidence that this syndrome exists and appears to be connected with the overuse of antibiotics. Many patients who have been diagnosed with yeast syndrome do get better when they follow a diet essentially devoid of sugar, yeast-containing substances, and wheat.

If you utilize the questionnaire following this protocol which comes from Dr. Crook's book, you may better understand the problem. Physicians experienced with this condition can also look for Candida antibody levels in the blood and do an ELISA-ACT test for T-cell mediated allergy. (*See the Allergies protocol for a discussion of this very useful test.*) It is also useful to check the acidity of the stomach and the alkalinity of the first part of the duodenum with a Heidelburg test. This is a noninvasive test utilizing a small capsule with a sensitive pH probe and radio transmitter that is swallowed by the patient. A radio receiver picks up the signals and measures the perspective values. The capsule passes harmlessly into the test probe afterlife! Abnormalities of stomach and pancreatic secretions can be corrected with the proper supplements.

Treatment

Treatment of Candida depends upon the location of the infection. Infection of the skin is easily treated with medicated creams and lotions often containing nystatin. Suppositories may be used for vaginal and anal infection. Thrush medications may be taken as a liquid swished around the mouth or as a slowly dissolving lozenge. Along with an antifungal cream, hydrocortisone for skin infection may be used to relieve pain and itching. Keeping the skin dry will help to clear up the infection and prevent its return.

Treatment with Natural Agents

Most people have an occasional bout with a candidial infection at one time or another in their lives. This discussion is directed to the patients that either have recurrent infections or suffer from yeast syndrome. It is very important to screen for the more obvious and common predisposing things like diabetes or chronic steroid use. The challenge is to look for more subtle problems that impair immunity. One must realize that especially in yeast syndrome, there is a vicious circle. A person may become predisposed because of antibiotic overuse. Then when the syndrome takes hold, immune function is further impaired, making it all the more difficult to treat. Therefore, based on the clinical experience of many physicians, it is fair to say that anyone suffering from either recurrent yeast infections or the yeast syndrome should adhere to most of the suggestions that follow, especially with respect to dietary changes.

The importance of the removal of sugar from the diet cannot be overemphasized. For reasons that are not entirely clear, many patients suffering from this problem have serious sugar and carbohydrate cravings that are of an addictive nature. There is no magic bullet. Failure to change the diet will result in failure to recover from the problem. Anyone who tells you that you can merely take an antifungal drug to cure the problem is mistaken! If ELISA-ACT testing reveals food allergies, those foods need to be avoided during the recovery period.

Some authorities suggest that decreasing honey and fruit juice during the period of recovery is sufficient. Many physicians feel that people may need to eliminate these foods entirely during the recovery period and reintroduce them slowly following recovery. The same may be said for dairy products. Yeast-containing products are a definite no. The reader is referred to Dr. Crook's book for an exhaustive description of the proper diet. In addition, as mentioned, consideration should be given to supplemental hydrochloric acid and pancreatic enzymes if indicated.

Many readers are probably thinking "how long must I stay on this diet?" The truth is that as far as sugar is concerned, one should never resume its use. The other foods may often be reintroduced slowly. Again, it is wise to work with a physician experienced with recurrent yeast infections. It may also be said that as a person gets more attuned to their body's health a certain sensitivity develops letting one know that eating certain things leaves one feeling "not right." This question is the same as when a patient asks how long they should avoid using an injured limb. The answer, of course, is "when it no longer hurts!" Your body knows what is right and wrong for it. It always knew. One just has to relearn by self-observation.

Often a person will report that after following this diet for 2 to 4 weeks they begin to feel worse. This is most probably a result of the yeast dying off and releasing toxins. It is for this reason that the diet should include plenty of fiber to ensure proper elimination. Additionally, 2 to 4 weeks of a proper diet should be undertaken before initiating treatment with antifungal agents, natural or otherwise.

Natural agents are frequently neglected for the treatment and prevention of selected intestinal and vaginal infections. Placebo-controlled studies demonstrated that natural agents have been used successfully to prevent antibiotic-associated bacterial infections and Candida vaginitis. Few adverse effects have been reported. There is now significant evidence that administration of selected microorganisms is beneficial in the prevention and treatment of certain intestinal infections, and possibly in the treatment of vaginal infections. These are called probiotics and are particularly useful in treating yeast syndrome.

The intake of bifido bacteria concentrate capsules every day can dramatically increase the quantity of beneficial bacteria in the gut to help fight Candida infections. Acidophilus bacteria also can help to fight Candida in the upper intestinal tract. Bifido bacteria feed on a special sugar trademarked under the name Nutraflora. One teaspoon a day of Nutraflora promotes the proliferation of friendly bifido bacteria in the gut.

Garlic (not Kyolic garlic), biotin, and caprylic acid have a direct yeast-killing effect in the intestine. Fiber in the diet also can help remove yeast and fungus from the intestines. A product called Yeast Fighters capsules contains an odorless garlic concentrate, caprylic acid, biotin, acidophilus, and a fiber blend to control Candida overgrowth in the intestine before it spreads to other parts of the body.

Other things to consider are goldenseal (*Hydrastis canadensis*) and volatile oil from oregano. Both have antifungal properties. Goldenseal is probably best taken as an infusion such as a tea bag or about 4 grams, 3 times a day in capsule form. Oregano oil comes in an enteric-coated capsule to protect you from a bad bout of dyspepsia (heartburn.) Take one capsule on an empty stomach 3 times a day.

Although research has not yet proven orthomolecular therapies to be useful for this, some physicians who practice complementary therapies administer nutritional intravenous vitamins, particularly vitamin C, during the recovery period. Clinically, patients seem to feel stronger more quickly when this is done.

When diet and "natural" therapies fail, a number of antifungal drugs can be considered. One is nystatin, which works only in the bowel and is not absorbed systemically. The dosage is variable and is usually given mixed in water. The other is the most potent FDA-approved drug available: Diflucan. One month's treatment with Diflucan can temporarily eradicate a systemic Candida infection so that anti-Candida nutritional supplements like Yeast Fighters, bifido bacteria, and Nutraflora can prevent a new Candida infection from occurring.

Shark liver oil has demonstrated an antifungal effect in laboratory studies. Shark liver oil capsules, containing 200 mg of alkyl glycerol, can be taken in doses of five capsules a day for up to 30 days. As for dietary modifications, sucrose and fructose should be avoided, since these types of sugars can cause yeast overgrowth.

Studies have shown that the daily ingestion of 150 mL of yogurt enriched with live Lacto acidophilus is associated with an increased colonization of friendly bacteria in the rectum and vagina. This results in reduced episodes of bacterial vaginitis. Yogurt is often used by women with chronic vaginal Candida infections. This should not be used for treating yeast syndrome or for those with known milk sensitivity.

Recent studies have demonstrated the antifungal properties of tea tree oil (*Melaleuca alternifolia*) against a wide range of fungal isolates including species of Candida. Studies indicate that controlled doses of tea tree oil may be used as an effective topical treatment for dermatologic Candida infection and paronychia.

Summary

1. Investigate carefully for underlying problems.
2. For one-time infection, use traditional local treatment with a topical antifungal.
3. Follow the yeast syndrome diet for 2 to 4 weeks prior to initiating antifungal therapy, but probiotics (#4) may be initiated during this time.
4. Take probiotics with *Lactobacillus acidophilus* and *Lactobacillus bifidum* such as Nutraflora, 1 teaspoon a day up to 3 times a day.
5. Consider ELISA-ACT allergy testing.
6. Consider Heidelburg testing for gastrointestinal secretions.
7. Use HCl and/or pancreatic enzymes if indicated.
8. Consider garlic, biotin, and caprylic acid.
9. Consider goldenseal infusion or about 4 grams, 3 times a day in capsule form.
10. Consider oregano oil, enterically coated, one capsule 3 times a day on an empty stomach.
11. Consider shark oil, up to 5 capsules a day for no more than 30 consecutive days.
12. If above remedies fail consider a course of oral nystatin or Diflucan.
13. Consider orthomolecular therapy with intravenous vitamins, in particular vitamin C, 50 grams I.V., 1 to 3 times a week.

Please note that studies have not been done to ascertain exact dosing. Additionally, whether to combine the antifungals or use them one at a time is unclear as well. It is probably best to begin with single agents and add others if necessary.

For more information. Contact the National Women's Health Network, (202)-628-7814. A staffer will answer questions on vaginitis and yeast infections. An information packet costs $6 for members, $8 for nonmembers. Refer to *The Yeast Connection* by W. G. Crook.

Product availability. Yeast Fighters capsules (combination anti-fungal nutrients), bifido bacteria, standardized shark liver oil capsules, and Nutraflora can be ordered by calling (800)-544-4440, or order online at www.lef.org. Diflucan is an expensive prescription drug that needs to be prescribed by your physician.

Candida Questionnaire

History	Point	Score
1. Have you taken tetracycline or other antibiotics for acne for 1 month or longer?	25	______
2. Have you at any time in your life taken other "broad-spectrum" antibiotics for respiratory, urinary, or other infections for 2 months or longer, or in short courses 4 or more times in a 1-year period?	20	______
3. Have you ever taken a broad-spectrum antibiotic (even a single course)?	6	______
4. Have you at any time in your life been bothered by persistent prostatitis, vaginitis, or other problems affecting your reproductive organs?	25	______
5. Have you been pregnant. . .		
One time?	3	______
Two or more times?	5	______
6. Have you taken birth-control pills . . .		
For 6 months to 2 years?	8	______
For more than 2 years?	15	______
7. Have you taken prednisone or other cortisone-type drugs . . .		
For 2 weeks or less?	6	______
For more than 2 weeks?	15	______
8. Does exposure to perfumes, insecticides, fabric shop odors, and other chemicals provoke. . .		
Mild symptoms?	5	______
Moderate to severe symptoms?	20	______
9. Are your symptoms worse on damp, muggy days or in moldy places?	20	______
10. Have you had athlete's foot, ringworm, "jock itch," or other chronic infections of the skin or nails?		
Mild to moderate	10	______
Severe or persistent	20	______
11. Do you crave sugar?	10	______
12. Do you crave breads?	10	______
13. Do you crave alcoholic beverages?	10	______
14. Does tobacco smoke really bother you?	10	______
Total Score for This Section		______

Major Symptoms

For each of your symptoms, enter the appropriate figure in the Point Score column

If a symptom is occasional or mild	score 3 points
If a symptom is frequent and/or moderately severe	score 6 points
If a symptom is severe and/or disabling	score 9 points

1. Fatigue or lethargy ______
2. Feeling of being "drained" ______
3. Poor memory ______
4. Feeling "spacey" or "unreal" ______
5. Depression ______
6. Numbness, burning, or tingling ______
7. Muscle aches ______
8. Muscle weakness or paralysis ______
9. Pain and/or swelling in joints ______
10. Abdominal pain ______
11. Constipation ______
12. Diarrhea ______
13. Bloating ______
14. Persistent vaginal itch ______
15. Persistent vaginal burning ______
16. Prostatitis ______
17. Impotence ______
18. Loss of sexual desire ______
19. Endometriosis ______
20. Cramps and/or other menstrual irregularities ______
21. Premenstrual tension ______
22. Spots in front of eyes ______
23. Erratic vision ______

Total Score for This Section ______

Other Symptoms

For each of your symptoms, enter the appropriate figure in the Point Score column

If a symptom is occasional or mild	score 3 points
If a symptom is frequent and/or moderately severe	score 6 points
If a symptom is severe and/or disabling	score 9 points

1. Drowsiness ______
2. Irritability ______
3. Lack of coordination ______

4. Inability to concentrate
5. Frequent mood swings
6. Headache
7. Dizziness/loss of balance
8. Pressure above ears, feeling of head swelling and tingling
9. Itching
10. Other rashes
11. Heartburn
12. Indigestion
13. Belching and intestinal gas
14. Mucus in stools
15. Hemorrhoids
16. Dry mouth
17. Rash or blisters in mouth
18. Bad breath
19. Joint swelling or arthritis
20. Nasal congestion or discharge
21. Postnasal drip
22. Nasal itching
23. Sore or dry throat
24. Cough
25. Pain or tightness in chest
26. Wheezing or shortness of breath
27. Urinary urgency or frequency
28. Burning on urination
29. Failing vision
30. Burning or tearing of eyes
31. Recurrent infections or fluid in ears
32. Ear pain or deafness

Total Score for This Section

Interpretation

	Women	Men
Yeast-connected health problems are almost certainly present	>180	>140
Yeast-connected health problems are probably present	120–180	90–140
Yeast-connected health problems are possibly present	60–119	40–89
Yeast-connected health problems are less likely to be present	<60	<40

(Taken from W. G. Crook, ***The Yeast Connection.***)

CARDIOVASCULAR DISEASE

(See Fibrinogen and Cardiovascular Disease protocols)

CATABOLIC WASTING

Catabolic wasting or cachexia is a clinical wasting syndrome that is characterized by unintended and progressive weight loss, weakness, and low body fat and muscle. At least 5% of body weight is lost. Cachexia is not caused by poor appetite and nutritional intake but rather by a metabolic state in which a "breaking down" rather than a "building up" occurs in bodily tissues no matter how much nutritional intake occurs. Additionally, whether a patient receives nutrition orally or intravenously makes no difference. The patient simply cannot gain weight, so eating more is not an answer.

It is estimated that one half of all cancer patients experience catabolic wasting, with a higher occurrence seen in cases of malignancies of the lung, pancreas, and gastrointestinal tract. The syndrome is equally common in AIDS patients and can also be present in bacterial and parasitic diseases, rheumatoid arthritis, and chronic diseases of the bowel, liver, lungs, and heart. It is usually associated with anorexia and can manifest as a condition in aging or as a result of physical trauma. Catabolic wasting is a symptom that diminishes the quality of life, worsens the underlying condition, and is a major cause of death.

Cachexia and Cancer

Researchers previously believed that cancer increased metabolic demand (stolen protein), produced toxins, and suppressed appetite, resulting in malnutrition. New research, however, shows that although cancer may raise resting metabolic rate, improved nutrition does not alleviate the symptoms of anorexia, chronic nausea, early satiety, and changes in taste that make even favorite foods unpalatable to some cancer patients. The view of clinicians is that bodily wasting is the result of a combined action of tumor products and host immune factors—in particular— cytokines, that lead to poor appetite, muscle wasting, and an altered metabolism. The cytokines interleukin-1 (IL-1), IL-6, interferon-gamma, tumor necrosis factor-alpha (TNFa), and brain-derived neurotrophic factor appear to increase and play a role in the progression of cachexia in cancer as well as in other diseases associated with bodily wasting.

Other metabolic alterations associated with the syndrome are hyperglyceridemia, lipolysis, and accelerated protein turnover, all leading to a loss of fat mass and body protein. The dysregulation of metabolic processes produces a negative energy balance.

Clinicians are currently treating cancer-related catabolic wasting with a variety of interventions, including nutritional supplementation, administration of cytokine inhibitors, steroids, hormones, cannabinoids, and thalidomide. Gemcitabine, a chemotherapeutic drug, has shown clinical benefits in treating cachexia. Newer nutritional intervention with megestrol acetate derivatives, gamma-receptor agonists, amino acid manipulations, myostatin inhibitors, and uncoupling protein modifiers is currently being explored. Further research must be done to investigate gender differences in relation to pathophysiology and therapy.

There is some evidence that the drug hydrazine sulfate may help cancer patients gain weight and improve the cachectic state. The drug is by prescription and should be given by a complementary physician familiar with its use. The dose is usually 60 mg a day. Narcotic painkillers or benzodiazepine anxiety-reducing agents cannot be given concomitantly. Unfortunately, the FDA has recently prevented compounding pharmacists from dispensing it. Patients may need to import it from European sources.

Cachexia and HIV

Bodily wasting is a common manifestation of HIV, occurring at any state of infection and indicative of disease progression. Malnutrition, a result of appetite loss, is commonly due to nausea and vomiting. Weakness and diarrhea are often present as well. HIV sufferers may also experience malabsorption of nutrients due to enteric infections associated with the disease, even if they consume sufficient calories.

The effects of malnutrition are thought to contribute to increased immune suppression including a reduction in T-lymphocyte helper and suppressor cells, altered phagocytic functions, and decreased killer-cell activity, leading to opportunistic infections and cancers. Pro-inflammatory cytokines IL-1, IL-6, and TNF have been cited in many studies as potential causes of wasting. Most people with advanced HIV and AIDS suffer some degree of wasting.

To reverse weight loss, appetite stimulants, anabolic agents (such as growth hormone or testosterone), cytokine inhibitors, and hormones are often prescribed. Megestrol acetate and dronabinol (which contains the active ingredient in marijuana) are approved for the treatment of wasting. Thalidomide, which aids in the healing of aphthous ulcers of the mouth and esophagus, is now available.

Diagnosis

Sadly, the cachectic state is all too apparent to any observer. In severe chronic disease with the development of multiple organ failure, some degree of malabsorption of nutrients probably contributes to the cachectic state. The entire picture is reflected in a continuing decline of the serum albumin as the illness progresses. Conversely, an increase in serum albumin suggests an improvement in the nutritional state. As long as a patient is maintained on nutrition by the normal route (by mouth), optimizing the state of digestive secretions is probably advisable although there may not be clinical studies demonstrating this. The Heidelburg test reflects this environment and can be used to ascertain the need for either hydrochloric acid or pancreatic enzyme supplementation.

Fish Oil Studies

Depletion of muscle and adipose tissue in cancer cachexia appears to arise not only from decreased food intake but also from the production of catabolic factors secreted by certain tumors such as tumor necrosis factor and other autoimmune cytokines. Experiments with a cachexia-inducing tumor in mice showed that, when part of the carbohydrate calories in their diet was replaced by fish oil, host body weight loss was inhibited. The catabolic-inhibiting effect occurred without an alteration of either the total calorie consumption or nitrogen intake.

Fish oil that is high in EPA (the fatty acid eicosapentaenoic acid) was found to inhibit tumor-induced lipolysis directly. The catabolic fat loss-preventing effect of EPA arose from an inhibition of the elevation of cyclic AMP (adenosine monophosphate, a nucleotide involved in energy metabolism) in fat cells. The increased protein degradation in the skeletal muscle of catabolic animals was also inhibited by EPA; this effect was due to the inhibition of muscle prostaglandin E_2 production in response to a tumor-produced proteolytic factor by EPA. Thus, reversal of cachexia by EPA in this mouse model results from its capacity to interfere with tumor-produced catabolic factors. Similar factors have been detected in human cancer cachexia. Catabolic wasting patients should consider taking five capsules a day of the Mega EPA fish oil concentrate.

Beneficial Effects of Glutamine

Glutamine has been one of the most intensively studied nutrients in the field of nutrition support in recent years. Animal studies show that glutamine is effective against catabolic stress. Glutamine supplementation was shown to improve organ function, survival, or both in most published studies. These studies also have supported the concept that glutamine is a critical nutrient for the gut mucosa and immune cells.

Recent molecular and protein chemistry studies are beginning to define the basic mechanism involved in glutamine action in the gut, liver, and other cells and organs. Double-blind prospective clinical investigations to date suggest that glutamine-enriched diets are generally safe and effective in catabolic patients. Intravenous glutamine has been shown to increase plasma glutamine levels; exert protein anabolic effects; improve gut structure and function; and reduce important indices of disease, including infection rates and length of hospital stay in selected patient subgroups.

Glutamine is the most abundant free amino acid in the human body. In catabolic stress situations, such as after surgical operations or trauma and during sepsis, glutamine is rapidly transported to organs and to blood cells. This results in an intracellular *depletion* of glutamine in the muscles and the ensuing catabolic wasting effect. Increasing evidence suggests that glutamine is a crucial substrate for immunocompetent cells. Glutamine depletion decreases the proliferation of lymphocytes, possibly by arresting a critical phase of the cells' growth cycle.

Glutamine is a precursor for the synthesis of glutathione and stimulates the formation of heat-shock proteins. Moreover, there are suggestions that glutamine plays a crucial role in the stimulation of intracellular protein synthesis. Experimental studies revealed that glutamine deficiency causes a necrotizing enterocolitis—an inflammation of the small intestine and colon, leading to cell death—and increases the mortality of animals subjected to bacterial stress.

A clinical human study involving bone-marrow transplant patients demonstrated, after supplementation with glutamine, a decrease in the incidence of infections and a shortening of hospital stay. In critically ill patients, parenteral glutamine reduced nitrogen loss and caused a reduction of the mortality rate. In surgical patients, glutamine evoked an improvement of several immunological parameters. Moreover, glutamine exerted a nutritional (tropic) effect on the intestinal mucosa, decreased the intestinal permeability, and thus may prevent the translocation of bacteria.

In conclusion, glutamine is an important metabolic substrate of rapidly proliferating cells. It influences the cellular hydration (molecular water content) state and has multiple effects on the immune system, intestinal function, and protein metabolism. In several disease states, glutamine may become an indispensable nutrient supplement. Catabolic wasting patients should consider supplementing with 2000 mg of glutamine a day.

Whey Protein

Scientists have examined the impact of whey protein concentrate on preventing or treating catabolic wasting, immune dysfunction, and cancer. A study involving HIV-positive men fed whey protein concentrate found dramatic increases in glutathione levels, with most men reaching their ideal body weight. In another study, when different groups of rats were given a powerful carcinogen, those fed whey protein concentrate showed fewer tumors and reduced tumor masses. Whey appears to inhibit the growth of breast cancer cells at low concentrations. In one clinical study, when cancer patients were fed whey protein concentrate at 30 grams a day, some patients' tumors showed a regression.

The research using whey protein concentrate has led researchers to a discovery regarding the relationships between cancerous cells, whey protein concentrate, and glutathione. Glutathione is an antioxidant that protects the body against harmful compounds. It was found that whey protein concentrate selectively depletes cancer cells of their glutathione, thus making them more susceptible to such cancer treatments as radiation and chemotherapy. It has been found that cancer cells and normal cells will respond differently to nutrients and drugs that affect glutathione status.

The concentration of glutathione in tumor cells is higher than that in the normal cells that surround the tumor. This difference in glutathione status between normal cells and cancer cells is believed to be an important factor in cancer cells' resistance to chemotherapy. Research has shown that cancer cells subjected to whey proteins were depleted of their glutathione, and their growth was inhibited, while normal cells had an increase in glutathione and increased cellular growth. These effects were not seen with other proteins.

Not surprisingly, the researchers concluded, "Selective depletion of tumor glutathione may, in fact, render cancer cells more vulnerable to the action of chemotherapy and eventually protect normal tissue against the deleterious effects of chemotherapy."

Whey protein also appears to play a direct role in bone growth. Researchers found that rats fed whey protein concentrate showed increases in bone strength as well as such bone protein as collagen. Whey protein was found to stimulate total protein synthesis, DNA content, and increased hydroxyproline content of bone cells in a dose-dependent manner.

It should be noted that not all whey protein concentrates are created equal. Processing whey protein to remove the lactose and fats, but without losing its biological activity, takes special care by the manufacturer. The protein must be processed under low-temperature and low-acid conditions so as not to denature it. Maintaining the natural state of the protein is essential to its biological activity.

Whey protein has the highest biological value rating of any protein. When the biological value is high, that means protein is absorbed, used, and retained better in the body. High biological values also are associated with tissue sparing. Thus, whey protein concentrate can be beneficial for people suffering from wasting catabolic diseases.

Other Nutritional Supplementation

Conjugated linoleic acid (CLA), a fatty acid, has anticatabolic properties. This has been demonstrated in laboratory mice injected with endotoxin to produce catabolic response. By 72 hours after feeding them with linoleic acid, the mice presented body weights similar to controls. The researchers concluded that conjugated linoleic acid prevented anorexia in endotoxin-injected test subjects. The suggested dose of CLA for a person in a catabolic state is two 1000-mg capsules taken twice a day. Cancer patients taking CLA also should take a soy supplement that provides at least 800 mg a day of genistein.

The amino acid arginine can help to generate anabolic cell replacement throughout the body, and can suppress excess levels of ammonia in the body, a common problem associated with catabolic breakdown. The suggested dose for arginine to counteract catabolism is 5 to 20 grams a day. Additional amino acid supplementation should include 2400 mg of *L*-carnitine and four capsules a day of the standard branched-chain amino acid complex, which includes leucine, isoleucine, and valine.

WARNING: Some nutritionists are concerned about the use of high doses of glutamine or arginine in cancer patients. Glutamine and arginine promote cellular growth, and the concern is that these amino acids could cause cancer cells to grow faster. Scientific studies, however, show that glutamine and arginine provide beneficial effects to cancer patients. Only one study on breast cancer patients hinted at a risk for arginine supplementation.

Resistance Training

Resistance or strength training is defined by resisting, lifting, and lowering weights. Resistance exercise training for a period of 8 to 12 weeks results in significant increases in muscle mass, muscle strength, and muscle function. Even in cases where dietary intake of protein falls below recommended daily allowances, the anabolic effect of resistance training appears to improve energy intake and protein use, allowing nitrogen retention. The benefits of resistance training have been shown to improve muscle strength and functioning in people suffering from disease-causing muscle wasting and in healthy but frail elderly people. Resistance exercise training should be considered as an adjunct treatment modality that is cost-effective, noninvasive, and a means to improve the quality of life.

Potential Considerations

WARNING: The possibilities discussed below have not been thoroughly studied with respect to potentially worsening cancer (if this is the source of the cachectic state). It is suggested that you discuss a potential treatment with a physician practicing complementary medicine prior to initiating therapy.

Testosterone is a natural anabolic steroid and can help place patients in a positive nitrogen balance. Dosages of 100 to 200 mg a week can be given to both men and women without androgenizing effects. Consideration can be given to DHEA (*see DHEA Replacement Therapy*) and pregnenolone as well. The intravenous administration of vitamins—in particular, vitamin C, 25 to 50 grams 2 to 3 times a week—may be helpful.

Consideration should be given to "adrenal support." Patients suffering from catabolic wasting should be assumed to have some degree of adrenal fatigue from the stress of chronic disease (*please see Adrenal Disease).*

Summary

Catabolic wasting can be counteracted by proper nutrient supplementation. A daily dose of 2000 mg of glutamine is suggested. Fish oil supplementation, in the dose of five Mega EPA fish oil capsules a day, should be considered. Two 1000-mg CLA capsules should be taken twice a day to facilitate the transport of glucose into muscle cells. The intake of 30 grams a day of biologically active whey protein concentrate, 10 to 20 grams of arginine, 2400 mg of *L*-carnitine, and a branched-chain amino acid complex may produce a dramatic anticatabolic tissue-sparing effect and regulate immune system cytokines that are thought to cause cachexia.

The standard dose of Life Extension Mix should be given to all people suffering from catabolic breakdown to provide the nutrient building blocks the body needs to start rebuilding.

1. Supplementation with glutamine, 2000 mg a day.
2. Mega EPA fish oil, five capsules a day.
3. Conjugated linoleic acid (CLA), 2000 mg 2 times a day to improve glucose utilization.
4. Biologically active whey protein concentrate, 30 grams a day.
5. Arginine, 10 to 20 grams a day in divided doses.
6. *L*-carnitine, 2400 mg a day in divided doses.
7. Life Extension Mix, the standard dose daily.
8. Consider hydrazine sulfate, 60 mg a day. Must not be taking narcotic painkillers or benzodiazepine anxiety-reducing agents.
9. Consider growth hormone, DHEA, and/or testosterone replacement therapy.

Product availability. Glutamine, specially designed whey protein, arginine, Life Extension Mix, CLA, Mega EPA, *L*-carnitine, and the branched-chain amino acid formula can be ordered by calling (800) 544-4440 or order online at www.lef.org. Ask about hydrazine sulfate, imported from European sources. Growth hormone and testosterone are prescription drugs.

CATARACT

Few people know that poor vision from cataracts affects 80% of people 75 years of age and older. Cataract surgery costs Medicare more money than any other medical procedure, with 60% of those who initially qualify for Medicare already having cataracts. For most people, the question is not whether you ever will suffer from cataracts, but when? We may all suffer from cataracts at some time in our lives, so taking steps to prevent the disease early in life may mean you are one of those 20% of people who enjoy good eye health and never suffer from cataracts.

A cataract is the clouding of the lens of the eye, which reduces the amount of incoming light and results in deteriorating vision. The condition is often described as similar to looking through a waterfall or a piece of waxed paper. Daily functions such as reading or driving a car may become difficult or impossible. Sufferers may need to change eyeglass prescriptions frequently. It is estimated that 20 million people worldwide suffer from cataracts. More than 350,000 cataract operations are performed in the United States yearly.

Many people are born with minor lens opacities that never progress, while others progress to the point of blindness or surgery. Many factors influence vision and cataract development such as age, nutrition, heredity, medications, toxins, health habits, sunlight exposure, and head trauma. Cataracts can also be caused by high blood pressure, kidney disease, diabetes, or direct trauma to the eye.

The good news is that a lot of published research exists showing that the cataract progression can be slowed or prevented by the use of natural therapies and minor lifestyle changes.

The Stages of Cataract Development

The first stage of cataract development occurs when there is a separation of laminated lens (cartilage-like) protein fibers, appearing as water and/or debris in eye vacuoles (spaces) in the eye.

The second or middle stage of the disease presents with an increase in the size of the vacuole (space) area within the eye. This is when people can noticeably see a halo around lights at night, or may have an increase in visual glare, increase in nearsightedness, and decrease in farsightedness.

In the third, or maturing stage, there is a large increase in vacuole space located in the lens, taking in water and distending protein fibers. These factors in turn cause a decrease in water in the aqueous humor, increasing disintegration of the cortex and calcification of the lens capsule and the lens.

The release of lens proteins into the aqueous and vitreous humor may cause inflammation leading to the development of glaucoma. The lens is drying out at this stage. In the last stage, the disintegration causes byproducts to escape the lens capsule, leaving a shrunken, dried, yellow or brown lens.

Types of Cataracts

There are three main types of cataracts. The first, most common type, is a *nuclear cataract* that occurs when the proteins of the nucleus (center) degenerate and darken, causing light to scatter. The second most common type of cataract occurs in the cortex (periphery) of the lens and is termed a *cortical cataract*. This forms when the regular order of fibers in the cortex is disturbed and the gaps in fibers fill with water and debris, thus altering light by scattering and/or absorbing it. The third and least common type affects the back of the lens, called a *posterior subcapsular cataract* (behind the lens).

Common Symptoms of a Cataract

Here are some signs of a cataract:

- Cloudy, fuzzy, foggy, or filmy vision.
- Changes in the way you see colors.
- Problems driving at night because headlights seem too bright.
- Problems with a glare from lamps or the sun.
- Frequent changes in your eyeglass prescription.
- Double vision.
- Better near vision for a while only in farsighted people.

Note: These symptoms also can be signs of other eye problems.

Diagnosis of Cataracts

A regular eye exam is all that is needed to find a cataract. Your eye physician will ask you to read a letter chart to see how sharp your sight is. You probably will get eye drops to enlarge your pupils (the round black centers of your eyes). This helps the doctor to see inside of your eyes. The doctor will use a bright light to see whether your lenses are clear and to check for other problems in the back of your eyes.

Other eye tests may also be used occasionally to show how poorly you see with a cataract or how well you might see after surgery. Only a few people need these tests:

- Glare tests.
- Contrast sensitivity tests.
- Potential vision tests.
- Specular photographic microscopy.

Source: American Society Cataract Refractory Surgery, 1999.

Conventional Medical Treatment

A change in your glasses, stronger bifocals, or the use of magnifying lenses may help improve your vision and be treatment enough. The way to surgically treat a cataract is to remove all or part of the lens and replace it with an artificial lens.

Just because you have a cataract does not mean it must be removed immediately. Cataract surgery can almost always be put off until you are unhappy with the way you see.

Your eye physician will tell you whether you are one of a small number of people who must have surgery. For example, your doctor may need to see or treat an eye problem that is behind the cataract. Or surgery may be required because a cataract is so large it could cause blindness.

Ninety-eight percent of cataract problems can be improved after surgery and cataracts will not grow back once they are surgically removed.

Free-Radical Damage to the Aging Eye

Researchers at Brigham and Women's Hospital, Harvard Medical School, stated in a scientific research report published in the January–February 1999 issue of *Journal of Association American Physicians* that

> Basic research studies suggest that oxidative mechanisms may play an important role in the pathogenesis of cataract and age-related macular degeneration, the two most important causes of visual impairment in older adults.

The researchers recommended that additional research be conducted in the promising area of preventive therapy and treatment.

The aging lens suffers metabolic changes that may predispose it to cataract development. Some of this occurs due to low supply of oxygen and nutrients, which leaves the eye open for free radical damage. According to a 1983 report from the National Academy of Science, cataracts are initiated by free-radical hydrogen peroxide found in the aqueous humor. Free radicals such as hydrogen peroxide oxidize glutathione and destroy the energy-producing system of the eye and allow leakage of sodium into the lens. Water follows the sodium, and the edema phase of the cataract begins. Then, body heat in the lens of the eye oxidizes (cooks) lens protein, and it becomes opaque and insoluble (similar to egg protein).

Free radicals reside in the aqueous fluid and bathe the lens of the eye, destroying enzymes that produce energy and maintain cellular metabolism. Free radicals also break down fatty molecules in membranes and lens fibers, generating more free radicals and creating a cross-linking (denaturing or breakdown) of the laminated-like structural proteins inside the lens capsule. The lens capsule has the ability to swell or dehydrate. In doing so the increase and/or decrease in pressure can cause breaks in the lens fiber membranes, resulting in microscopic spaces in the eye in which water and debris can reside.

Integrated and Alternative Medical Therapies

Supplements Protect Against Free Radicals

Prevention and treatment of cataracts are probably one of the more scientifically documented and beneficial uses of dietary supplements. Free-radical action has been directly linked to and accepted as one of the major causes of cataracts and damage to the healthy eye. Numerous well conceived, scientific studies have been conducted to test and document the possible effect of supplements due to their capability to reduce free-radical damage, and in some cases allow the body to reverse the damage done by free radicals.

Although it is difficult to treat cataracts with oral antioxidants since there is only minimal blood circulation within the eye compared to other parts of the body, nutritional supplements have been shown to reduce the risks of cataracts as well as slow or reverse their progression.

Benefits of Glutathione

The eye consists of 65% water and 35% protein (the highest protein content in the body). The eye also contains the highest percentage of potassium in the body, along with a high percentage of vitamin C and glutathione.

If glutathione levels are abnormal, they can affect the health of the eye in a major way. Glutathione helps maintain the water balance in the lens. It also is synthesized within the lens and is made of three amino acids: glycine, cysteine, and glutamic acid. Glutathione can affect the function of the lens and is essential to its normal metabolism in the following ways:

1. Preserving the physicochemical balance of proteins within the lens.
2. Maintaining the action of the sodium–potassium transport pump and the molecular integrity of lens fiber (protein) membranes.
3. Maintaining molecular integrity of lens fiber membranes and acting as a free-radical scavenger to protect membranes and enzymes from oxidation (cooking).
4. Maintaining an affect on proper energy production (glutathione indirectly preserves the glycolysis pathway for energy production within the lens).

Higher levels of glutathione are present in the cortex (edge) of the lens, preventing free radical–induced photochemical generation of harmful by-products. Oxyradicals (free radicals) generate cataracts, and experiments demonstrate that glutathione reactivates oxidized vitamin C, which in turn improves antioxidant potential within the lens.

Bioflavonoids

Bioflavonoids are powerful inhibitors of the enzyme, aldose reductase. Accordingly, if aldose reductase is decreased, then sorbitol will not form, reducing the danger of water accumulating in the lens. The bioflavonoids quercetin, myrcetin, and kaempferol (found in limes) are specifically noted in inhibiting diabetic cataracts. Ginkgo is a widely used flavonoid in maintaining microcirculation to the eye and inhibiting free radicals.

Vitamin C

Vitamin C is crucial for normal ocular metabolism. Vitamin C occurs in the lens concentration and is 30 to 50 times higher than that found in circulating blood. This concentration is second only to the nervous system and the adrenal cortex. Vitamin C is found in high concentrations in the eyes of animals that are active during the daylight hours and in low concentrations in the eyes of animals that are nocturnal. Vitamin C acts to

1. Protect delicate lens-protein sulfa-hydroxyl groups from oxidation in the eyes of nocturnal animals.
2. Ensure proper formation of collagen and many other structures.
3. Stimulate the immune system.
4. Play a major role in protecting the lens from photochemical oxidation.
5. Feed the delicate membranes that regulate the transport of nutrients and ions (minerals/electrolytes) into the lens.

Because the pupillary part of the eye is transparent (where the iris cannot shield and protect it), UV radiation and light can more easily generate the superoxide radical O_2, which is known to be extremely destructive in every cell of the body, including the lens. The superoxide radical can self-mutate into hydrogen peroxide and hydroxide radicals. Just prior to cataract formation, researchers have reported a significant drop of vitamin C concentrations in the eye.

B Vitamins

Vitamin B_2 (riboflavin) is necessary for the production of glutathione reductase. This enzyme is utilized within the lens to activate glutathione and glutathione–selenium peroxidase. These two glutathione forms are crucial in the protective mechanism for operation of the glutathione system.

Light, especially ultraviolet light, destroys B_2. B vitamins are not stored, so they must be replaced on a daily basis. Riboflavin deficiency is the prime cause of photosensitivity, making eyes more sensitive to damage; 50 to 150 mg a day of riboflavin can help reduce photosensitivity.

Vitamin B_6 (pyridoxine) is essential for protein metabolism, for absorption of vitamin B_{12}, and for proper synthesis of antiaging nucleic acids. Its coenzyme is necessary for many protein reactions and metabolic functions. Vitamin B_6 is suggested for nutritional support for cataract patients.

N-Acetyl-Cysteine and Garlic

A 1998 study in the *Journal of Ocular Pharmacology and Therapeutics* tested the treatment effects of diallyl disulfide (DADS) and *N*-acetyl-cysteine (NAC) using acetaminophen (the active ingredient in Tylenol) to induce rapid cataract formation. Acetaminophen is a potent generator of free radicals. Injection of acetaminophen (350 mg/kg body weight) produced acute cataract and other ocular tissue damage. However, treatment with DADS (200 mg/kg body weight), one of the major organosulfides in garlic oil, prevented cataract development and prolonged survival time. *N*-acetyl-cysteine also prolonged survival time but was only weakly effective in preventing cataract formation. *The remarkable finding was that a combination of DADS and NAC completely prevented cataractogenesis, and that all of the treated animals survived the acetaminophen toxicity.*

Melatonin

Melatonin is a potent antioxidant that may be especially effective in preventing and treating cataracts. A compelling study published in the *Journal of Pineal Research* (1994 [Sept]; 17[2]:94–100) showed a potent inhibitory effect of melatonin on cataract formation in newborn rats. By administering a drug that inhibited glutathione synthesis, scientists were able to induce cataracts in rats. The glutathione-depleted rats all developed cataracts, but only 6.2% of the rats given melatonin acquired them. When glutathione levels in the eye lens were measured, the melatonin group had more glutathione than the group not receiving melatonin. The scientists concluded that the inhibitory effects of melatonin on cataract formation could be due to melatonin's free-radical scavenging activity or due to its stimulatory effect on glutathione production.

Melatonin production slows down in people over the age of 40, and by age 60 there is virtually no melatonin being naturally produced. It is over the age of 60 when most cataracts develop. The suggested dose for melatonin is 500 mcg to 3 mg taken at bedtime.

Other Supplements for Healthy Eyes

Eye lenses afflicted with cataracts have decreased concentrations of potassium and magnesium. Supplementation with 400 mg of elemental potassium and 800 mg of elemental magnesium would theoretically increase the availability of these minerals to the eye lens. Potassium and magnesium are often deficient in aging humans, and supplementation with these low-cost minerals helps protect the arterial system.

Selenium and vitamin E may work synergistically in protecting against cataracts and these two nutrients have been shown to reduce the risk of cancer and cardiovascular disease. Therefore, 400 to 800 IU a day of vitamin E and 200 to 600 mcg a day of selenium would appear to be prudent methods of protecting against cataract formation and maintaining good overall health. Selenium works with alpha-lipoic acid to increase cellular concentrations of glutathione. As previously discussed, glutathione is a critical antioxidant in protecting against free radicals in the eye lens.

Ginkgo biloba extract should be taken at a dose of 120 mg a day by anyone suffering from cataracts. Bilberry extract should be taken at a dose of 150 mg a day by cataract patients. These two flavonoid nutrients may help to restore microcapillary circulation to the eye.

After taking ginkgo and bilberry for a month, add 600 mcg of the mineral selenium, 500 mg of the amino acid glutathione, and 500 mg of alpha-lipoic acid every day.

Inositol occurs in high concentrations within the lens. Inositol is indispensable for intercellular transport of amino acids in the lens metabolism and speeds the ATP energy to pump inositol into the lens itself. Inositol performs best when taken in combination with the B complex vitamins.

Inhibiting Glycation

Glycation (glycosylation) of proteins has been shown to play a prominent role in the development of diabetic cataract formation and retinopathy. The glycosylation process also occurs as a result of general aging.

Acetyl-*L*-carnitine was recently shown effective in reducing glycation protein damage leading to cataract formation. Scientists who were published in the July 1999 *Journal of Experimental Eye Research* stated

> This *in vitro* study shows, for the first time, that acetyl-*L*-carnitine could acetylate potential glycation sites of lens crystallins, and protect them from glycation-mediated protein damage.

Investigations have been conducted to explore the possibility of preventing glycation through the use of pyruvate and alpha-ketoglutarate. The results demonstrate that both these compounds are effective in preventing the initial glycation reaction, as well as the formation of eye disease.

Both pyruvate and alpha-keto glutarate also inhibit the generation of high molecular weight aggregates associated with cataract formation. The preventive effects appear to be due to competitive inhibition of glycation by the keto acids and the antioxidant properties of these compounds. These agents might be useful in preventing glycation-related protein changes and consequent tissue pathological manifestations associated with cataract, diabetes, and normal aging. The best form of pyruvate is calcium pyruvate. A 500-mg capsule of calcium pyruvate provides 405 mg of elemental pyruvic acid. Those with cataract should consider taking 500 mg of calcium pyruvate along with 650 mg of ornithine alpha-ketoglutarate 3 times a day.

The most potent drug to inhibit glycosylation is called aminoguanidine and is sold in Europe. In a study published in *Experimental Eye Research* (1996 [May]; 62 [5]:505–10), aminoguanidine was shown to inhibit cataracts in moderately diabetic rats. Aminoguanidine functioned as an inhibitor of advanced glycation on the development of cataracts in diabetic rats. The scientists showed that aminoguanidine treatment inhibited the formation of damaging advanced glycated endproducts by about 56 to 75% in moderately diabetic rats and by 19 to 52% in severely diabetic rats. The formation of cataracts, however, was only observed in the moderately diabetic rats, showing that a diabetic must maintain some degree of control over blood sugar levels if they can expect antiglycating agents like aminoguanidine to be effective in protecting against cataract.

Aminoguanidine may also help save the vision of patients with hard-to-treat glaucoma, according to the August 17, 1999 issue of the *Proceedings of the National Academy of Sciences* (1999; 96:9944–9948). This study showed that only 10% of crucial vision cells in the retina were lost in a group of aminoguanidine-supplemented rats compared to a 36% loss of retinal cells in the group not receiving aminoguanidine. The study was funded by the National Eye Institute and the Glaucoma Foundation. Dr. Robert Ritch, chair of the Foundation's scientific advisory board, said, "Although the current investigations do not yet translate into clinical use, this [study] is the sort of breakthrough research that could eventually lead to a stemming of vision loss from glaucoma."

The recommended safe dose of aminoguanidine is 300 mg a day. Aminoguanidine is especially important for diabetics, who suffer from greatly accelerated glycosylation throughout their body.

Glaucoma is the second leading cause of vision loss in the United States and it appears that the glycosylation mechanism of damage is responsible for vision problems caused by cataract and glaucoma.

Avoid Arginine for Now

Arginine facilitates the natural synthesis of nitric oxide and this has been shown to enhance arterial elasticity in the diabetic patient. Nitric oxide enables arteries to easily expand and contract with each heartbeat. While most people benefit from increased nitric oxide production, a new study in rats suggests that nitric oxide might contribute to cataract. Until this issue is resolved, those with cataract might want to avoid taking large amounts of arginine since arginine promotes nitric oxide synthesis. It has long been known that nitric oxide is damaging if other antioxidants are not present. Most people who take supplemental arginine also take large amounts of antioxidant supplements like selenium and vitamin E and are probably protected against any oxidizing effects that could occur in response to elevated synthesis of nitric oxide.

Further Recommendations for Care of the Eye

Protection from Ultraviolet (UV) Sunlight

It is crucial for cataract patients to wear protective eyeglasses to shield against free-radical damage induced by ultraviolet (UV) sunlight. If UV-blocking sunglasses were to be worn throughout life, the risk of cataract would be reduced greatly. Exposure to sunlight is a major risk factor in the development and progression of cataract disease. Low-cost, wrap-around sunglasses called Sun-Shields are available; they fit over regular glasses to provide almost 100% protection against UV penetration to the eye.

Additional Antioxidant Protection

Some cataract patients apply vitamin drops, called Viva Drops, to their eyes every day. While there is no published data on whether vitamin drops can slow the cataract disease process, these vitamin drops do provide antioxidant protection directly to the lens of the eye.

Conclusion

Metabolic changes in the aging lens may predispose it to cataract formation. Free-radical damage due to oxygen and nutrient deficiencies in the eye can create a denaturing effect causing damage to the lens membranes. Supplements, as a preventive approach or as an adjunctive therapy, have been well documented in the scientific literature.

Summary

Cataract surgery costs Medicare more money than any other medical procedure. Cataract is epidemic among the aged and its incidence is often linked to controllable lifestyle factors such as cigarette smoking, unprotected sun exposure, and poor dietary practices. The following integrated therapy may be beneficial to the prevention and/or treatment of cataracts.

1. Alpha-lipoic acid, 250 mg, 2 times a day (to boost glutathione production).
2. Melatonin, 500 mcg to 3 mg each night.
3. Aminoguanidine, 300 mg a day (available only from European pharmacies).
4. Glutathione, 500 mg a day.
5. *N*-acetyl-cysteine (NAC), 600 to 1200 mg a day (to boost glutathione levels).
6. Life Extension Mix, three tablets, 3 times a day to obtain NAC, selenium, inositol, vitamins B_2, B_6, C, and E, bioflavonoids, and many other antioxidant and antiglycating nutrients such as calcium pyruvate and ornithine alpha-ketoglutarate.
7. Potassium, 300 mg a day.
8. Ginkgo extract, 120 mg a day.
9. Bilberry extract, 150 mg a day.
10. High-allicin garlic powder, 1800 mg a day; or garlic oil extract, 10 mg a day; or Kyolic Garlic Formula 105, 4 capsules a day.

The Life Extension Mix is a full-spectrum vitamin and mineral concentrate, balanced and coordinated to offer cellular nutrition as well as antioxidant protection.

For more information. Contact the National Eye Health Education Program of the National Institutes of Health, (301) 496-5248 or the American Society of Cataract Surgery, (703) 591-2220.

Product availability. Viva Drops, bilberry, Sun-Shields, glutathione, vitamin C, cysteine, Life Extension Mix, ginkgo and bilberry extracts, garlic, alpha-lipoic acid, potassium, melatonin, garlic, NAC, and selenium can be ordered by calling (800) 544-4440 or order online at www.lef.org.

CEREBRAL VASCULAR DISEASE

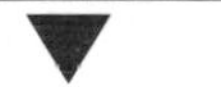

For those suffering from hemorrhagic cerebral vascular disease, such as cerebral aneurysm or cerebral hemorrhage, it is suggested that nutrients that help build collagen and elastin be taken, to help rebuild the endothelial lining of the cardiovascular arterial system. Nutrient supplements have also been reported to help reduce the risk of or damage caused by aneurysm or hemorrhage.

Fifty percent of all patients diagnosed with an aneurysm or cerebral hemorrhage have hypertension. Cerebral atherosclerosis is also an underlying risk factor for cerebral vascular disease.

Cerebral artery aneurysm, one of the cerebral vascular diseases, can be fatal. An aneurysm is a weakened portion of the heart or a blood vessel, usually an artery, that fills up with blood under pressure, causing it to balloon outward. Aneurysm can be caused by a hereditary weakness in the vessel wall, high blood pressure, atherosclerosis, direct injury, infection, and other diseases.

Approximately 30,000 people a year in the United States suffer an aneurysm rupture, causing cerebral hemorrhage. It has been estimated that if five people suffer a cerebral hemorrhage today, in 1 year, only one of those people will be alive and well, one will be disabled, and the other three will be dead.

Cerebral vascular hemorrhage may also produce delayed problems such as water on the brain (hydrocephalus) and narrowing of the blood vessels because of the irritation of the blood on the blood vessels, known as vasospasm. Rebleeding, hydrocephalus, and vasospasm can happen days to weeks after the initial bleed. Aneurysms can and do grow. If they reach a certain size, usually more than 25 mm (1 inch), they may start applying pressure on the surrounding brain tissue and cause additional problems.

Cerebral aneurysm is very uncommon in patients below 20 years of age and is increasingly common in older patients. In people over 65, they may be found in as high as 5% of the population. It appears they are related to an absence of a muscular layer that makes up part of the blood vessels; over time, it stretches and thins and creates the aneurysm. Smoking appears to markedly increase the chance that one will develop a cerebral aneurysm.

Indications of the presence of an aneurysm depend on the location of the aneurysm. Aneurysm generally exhibits few symptoms and is discovered by accident on x-ray films or imaging scans performed for some other reason.

The rupture or hemorrhage of an aneurysm usually produces severe pain. The location of the aneurysm usually determines the amount of bleeding, shock, loss of consciousness, or if death will occur. In some cases, the aneurysm may leak blood, causing warning pain without the rapid deterioration and damage characteristic of a rupture. The threat of aneurysm goes beyond the immediate site damage it can cause. Blood clots often form in an aneurysm, creating a danger of embolisms and clotting in distant organs or vessels.

Cerebral hemorrhagic problems occur when an aneurysm ruptures, causing internal bleeding. For example, aneurysm affecting the arteries supplying the brain can occur at any age, but more often in people more than 60 years of age with a history of hypertension. The aneurysm may rupture, causing hemorrhage and blood leakage into the membrane surrounding the brain. A cerebral artery aneurysm is particularly important, because it can lead to fatal subarachnoid hemorrhage, which occurs underneath one of the layers of tissue lining the brain. This aneurysm frequently occurs from inherited vascular defects, at the branch points of cerebral arteries.

If your physician suspects an aneurysm or the possibility of hemorrhage, he or she will probably recommend an ultrasound test, computed tomography scanning (CT scan), magnetic resonance imaging (MRI), or angiography of the area to determine the size, severity, and to predict the possibility of rupture and subsequent hemorrhage.

Conventional Treatment

If an aneurysm is large and the risk of rupture is significant, surgery may be necessary.

When an aneurysm ruptures, emergency surgery is necessary to stop the bleeding. Surgical intervention into cerebral aneurysm or hemorrhage may be difficult or impossible, given the constraints of access to the damaged or threatened areas of the brain.

Hypertensive drugs may also be prescribed in an attempt to lower blood pressure and reduce the chances of additional aneurysm or cerebral hemorrhage. (*See the Hypertension protocol for more information on natural ways to reduce blood pressure.*)

Integrated or Alternative Therapies

Researchers have speculated in a 1998 issue of *Life Sciences Journal* that "an acute systemic oxidative stress condition might influence the rupture of intracranial aneurysm." Vitamin E was specifically identified by investigators to act as an antioxidant by scavenging free radicals and thus reducing the conditions that precipitate these cerebral vascular ruptures. We recommend taking 400 to 800 IU of vitamin E daily to reduce the risk of aneurysm ruptures. Vitamin C at 2000 to 5000 mg a day is suggested, along with 300 mg a day of the flavonoid proanthocyanidin (from grape seed or pine bark) for further protection against underlying factors that cause cerebral vascular disease.

Magnesium is crucial for arterial structure, and it is suggested that 1500 mg a day of elemental magnesium be taken along with 1000 mg a day of calcium and 500 mg a day of potassium.

Mechanisms that regulate cerebral circulation have been intensively investigated in recent years, and this research is increasingly focused on the effects of nitric oxide. Nitric oxide is an important regulator of cerebral vascular tone. Nitric oxide maintains the cerebral vasculature in a dilated state. Arginine, a natural supplement, specifically enhances nitric oxide synthesis. Those with cerebral vascular disease may consider taking 4 to 5 grams of arginine 3 times a day to better maintain the health of vessels.

Activation of potassium channels appears to be a major mechanism for *dilatation* of cerebral arteries. Agents that increase the intracellular concentration of cyclic adenosine monophosphate (cAMP) produce vasodilatation. Supplementation with 500 mg a day of potassium and 5 to 20 mg a day of Hydergine may enhance vasodilatation in cerebral vascular disease, helping to restore vessels to a healthier state.

Additionally, alcohol consumption poses a risk for development of hypertension (high blood pressure), strokes, and sudden death through the depletion of magnesium from the body. The dietary intake of magnesium modulates the hypertensive actions of alcohol. Experiments indicate that chronic ethanol ingestion results in the contraction of the cerebral arteries and capillaries, a contraction that causes increased cerebral vascular resistance. Chronic ethanol ingestion increases the reactivity of intact microvessels to vasoconstrictors and results in decreased reactivity to vasodilators. However, pretreatment of animals with magnesium prevents ethanol from inducing a stroke, and prevents the adverse cerebral vascular changes from taking place. Magnesium influences the response of cerebral arteries to several other natural or synthetic stimulators (agonists), and has been shown to decrease cerebral vascular resistance. Contractility of cerebral arteries is dependent upon the actions and interactions of calcium and magnesium.

It is clear from published studies that magnesium can induce healthy vascular tone in all types of vascular smooth muscle. Magnesium appears to act on voltage-, receptor-, and leak-operated membrane channels in vascular smooth muscle. Standard channel blocker drugs do not have this uniform capability. Calcium channel–blocking drugs, however, can block calcium infiltration into brain cells, lower cerebral vascular resistance, relieve cerebral vasospasm, and lower arterial blood pressure.

Magnesium can also cause significant vasodilatation of intact cerebral arteries. Although magnesium is 3 to 5 orders of magnitude less potent than the standard calcium channel–blocking drugs, it possesses unique and potentially useful effects in maintaining healthy cerebral vascular circulation. Those with cerebral vascular disease, and especially those who consume alcohol, should take 1500 mg a day of elemental magnesium.

Essential fatty acids in the form of flax, perilla, or fish oil concentrates also should be considered. Mega EPA enables a person to get pharmacologic doses of fish oils by taking only five capsules a day. Extreme caution should be exercised when taking these supplements because they inhibit blood clotting. There is a chance that a cerebral hemorrhage could occur because of the blood-thinning effects these nutrients can produce. Blood tests that measure clotting time can be used to make sure these nutrients are not reducing the clotting factors in your blood too much.

Nimotop (nimodipine) is an FDA-approved calcium channel–blocking drug specific to cerebral circulation and brain-cell activity. It has been shown to work better in the restoration of cerebral circulation than any other calcium channel–blocking drug yet tested. The normal dose is 30 mg of Nimotop, taken 3 times a day.

New Medical Device Advances The Treatment of an Aneurysm

By using the device known as the Guglielmi coil, physicians can now correct an aneurysm that is not approachable surgically, either because of its position in the brain or other factors that present a high risk.

The coil is an extremely fine wire made from platinum—one of the softest metals—at the end of a longer stainless steel wire. Several coils, depending on the size of the aneurysm, are inserted inside the bubble-like aneurysm through a catheter (a long, narrow tube) threaded through the patient's blood vessels. When the coil is in the correct position—verified by a blood vessel x-ray called an angiogram—it is given a positive electric charge. The charge causes the steel wire to dissolve at the point of a junction with the platinum coil, and the positively charged coil attracts blood cells to form a clot within the aneurysm.

The coils and resulting blood clot fill up the aneurysm, essentially sealing it off. Eventually, the lining of the blood vessel grows over the aneurysm's neck and the aneurysm is essentially healed.

Conclusion

Cerebral vascular disease can be life threatening. Aneurysm and the subsequent rupture-causing hemorrhage are caused by inherited vascular defects and may be unavoidable. Aneurysm is often precipitated by atherosclerosis and hypertension. High blood pressure increases your risk of aneurysm. Reduction of high blood pressure is imperative in reducing the risk of cerebral vascular disease. Natural supplements combined with lowered blood pressure can reduce the risk and/or damage caused by cerebral vascular disease.

(Refer to the Age-Associated Mental Impairment and Stroke protocols for additional suggestions about restoring cerebral circulation. See Hypertension, Cholesterol Reduction, and Atherosclerosis protocols for more information on prevention and treatment of cerebral vascular disease.)

Summary

The following are most important in preventing cerebral vascular disease.

1. Arginine, 4 to 5 grams daily.
2. Calcium, 1000 mg daily.
3. Flavonoid proanthocyanidin (grape seed-skin extract), 300 mg daily.
4. Hydergine, 5 to 20 mg daily.
5. Magnesium, 1500 mg daily.
6. Potassium, 500 mg daily.
7. Vitamin C, 2000 to 5000 mg daily.
8. Vitamin E, 400 to 800 IU daily.
9. Mega EPA, 6 to 9 grams a day (6 to 8 Mega EPA capsules.)

For more information. Contact the National Institute of Neurological Disorders and Stroke, (800) 352-9424.

Product availability. Mega EPA, proanthocyanidins (grape seed-skin extract), vitamin C, vitamin E, magnesium, calcium, arginine, and potassium are available by calling (800) 544-4440, or order on-line at www.lef.org.

CERVICAL DYSPLASIA

Cervical dysplasia is a premalignant or precancerous change that occurs in the cells of a woman's cervix.

Cervical dysplasia is the third leading cause of cancer deaths in women in the United States, second in China, and first in developing countries. Smoking, oral contraception, a poor diet, nutritional vitamin and mineral deficiencies, and stress have been implicated as the primary causes of the disease.

Some experts have estimated that as high as 70% of women have had or are currently infected by human papilloma virus (HPV), the most frequent cause of cervical dysplasia. HPV is commonly called the wart virus. More than 60 types of HPV have been identified. Generally, types 1, 3, and 5 can cause warts on the hands and feet of children. Types 6 and 11 can cause warts on men's and women's bottoms (genital warts). Other types, such as 16, 18, 31, 33, and 35 may not cause warts but can cause changes to the cells of your vagina or cervix, such as dysplasia.

There are three types of cervical dysplasia: mild, moderate, and severe. Mild dysplasia is by far the most common, and is not considered a true premalignant disease by many experts. Mild dysplasia represents a tissue response to the HPV virus.

Up to 70% of women with mild dysplasia will have abnormal cervical cells return to normal over time without any medical treatment. However, even mild dysplasia can advance to a more serious disease. Moderate and severe dysplasia should be treated immediately when discovered, as left untreated they can lead to cervical cancer.

Detection of the Disease

Many women do not know they have been in contact with or have the disease. A pap smear often detects abnormal cervical cells caused by HPV, as only 1 person in 100 with HPV will exhibit any symptoms such as warts. Even if HPV is not noted on the pap smear, there is an 80 to 90% chance that you have the HPV virus if you have been diagnosed by a physician with any type of cervical dysplasia.

As routine testing for the presence of HPV varies across the United States, the Foundation strongly recommends that you request testing for the virus to facilitate early HPV detection along with your routine pap smear testing.

Additionally, if you have been diagnosed with abnormal cells (cervical dysplasia) you should request testing to specifically determine from which HPV virus you are suffering. This will ensure that the best information possible regarding your disease is available to aid you and your physician in determining the best course of treatment for your specific disease condition.

Protecting yourself from HPV is difficult. Generally, you acquire the virus through sexual contact. Condoms can prevent the spread of many diseases, but not HPV. HPV is found on all the genital tissues, and a condom on the penis usually will not prevent transmission of HPV. The virus can lie dormant on your cervix for 20 years before it causes warts or changes to the cells. If your physician has just discovered an abnormal Pap smear, you may not have recently acquired the virus.

Disease Risks

Smoking

Cigarette smoking has been implicated as a cause of dysplasia. More than 53% of women with cervical dysplasia were smokers. Women who smoke concentrate the chemicals ingested by smoking (nicotine and cotinine) into their cervix. These chemicals have been shown to damage cervical cells.

Interestingly, smoking men also concentrate these chemicals into their genital secretions, and can bathe the cervix with these chemicals during intercourse. Partners who smoke may want to consider the use of condoms as a preventive approach to reduce the risk or progression of the disease.

A number of studies link smoking directly to cervical dysplasia and neoplasia. Several studies indicate that smoking at a younger age increases risk factors for cervical intra-epithelial neoplasia and squamous cell intra-epithelial lesions.

Smoking has also been shown to lower plasma vitamin C and beta-carotene levels, which adversely affect the pathology and increase the risks of contracting cervical intra-epithelial neoplasia.

Smoking can cause low-grade squamous cell intra-epithelial lesions (SIL) to develop into a high-grade lesion and possibly progress to cancer. One study observed changes in and compared smokers to nonsmokers. The authors concluded that the mutagenic effect of cigarette smoking on cervical cells has an effect on chromosomal damage of the tissue, which means smoking increases the risk of dysplasia's progression toward cancer.

Additionally, vitamin C status in cervical tissue and leukocytes in the blood has been examined to compare smokers to nonsmokers. The findings show that nonsmokers have 4 times as much vitamin C as leukocytes, while smokers had lower levels of vitamin C and higher levels of leukocytes in their cervical tissue. This reversal of normal levels of vitamin C and leukocytes further illustrates the ongoing damage of smoking. The study further discusses the free-radical–induced cellular damage due to smoking and the possible benefits of antioxidants.

Oral Contraceptive Use

Oral contraceptive use and duration appear to increase the risk and subsequent development of cervical dysplasia and neoplasia. Studies indicate low levels of folic acid in the blood of oral contraceptive users have a positive correlation with development of cervical dysplasia and neoplasia. Researchers have demonstrated that oral contraceptives can cause an imbalance in the nutrient status of folic acid, B_6, zinc, and vitamin A, thereby leaving the tissue void of the nutrients that would otherwise protect it.

Studies have reported that women with mild to moderate cervical dysplasia who were using oral contraceptives have experienced improvement when they received folic acid supplementation.

Another group of investigators studied the long-term effects of oral contraceptives by following 195 women for more than 12 years. They found those women were twice as likely to have adenocarcinoma of the cervix.

Another study screened 726 subjects for possible factors leading to dysplasia. They identified 294 cases of dysplasia (with 170 controls) as defined by coexistent cytologic and colposcopic evidence. The results indicated that the key risk factors leading to dysplasia and cancer were the use of oral contraceptives, number of sexual partners, and the presence of HPV-16 infection. The presence of all or one of these factors increased the risk of cervical dysplasia.

CAUTION: Both vitamins E and B_6 should be supplemented in women who are taking oral contraceptives. However, those supplements need to be taken at different times, since B_6 can nullify the effects of vitamin E on blood hematocrit.

Exposure to HPV

Unprotected, and even protected, sex with a male with genital warts carries risks. Warts are lower grades of HPV that are believed to mutate sometimes to cancer-causing HPVs. Research has revealed that the earlier the age an individual first contracts genital warts, the more likely they are to contract cervical neoplasia later on in life.

Multiple Sex Partners

Multiple studies indicate that the number of sexual partners is a risk factor. Often this number is taken into consideration along with other factors, such as the lack of condom use, smoking, low levels of vitamin C, beta-carotene, vitamin A, or folic acid, and oral contraceptive use. These factors seem to play a very large role in development of cervical dysplasia. Risks have been reported to be as much as 72% greater with all of these risk factors present.

Diet and Dietary Risk Factors

For those with a high risk of dysplasia, or who already have dysplasia, diets high in fruits and vegetables, as well as foods which are high in carotenoids may be beneficial. A healthy diet would also include raw nuts, complex carbohydrates, and foods high in essential fatty acids but low in animal fat.

A high-quality, easily digestible protein is also beneficial. Protein is extremely important for a strong immune system and tissue repair. Many women are "on the go" and suffer from a low protein intake. It would be advisable for these women to consume protein. One easy approach used by many smart women is to make a protein shake in the blender each morning. Since it is convenient, fast, and easy, it can make an ideal breakfast. Whey or soy proteins would be excellent choices as a breakfast shake, along with some frozen fruit, banana, Udo's Multi-Blend Oil, vitamin B_{12}, and folic acid mixed in a blender.

There are studies indicating that a diet higher in fruits and vegetables, especially those higher in beta-carotene and vitamin C, has a direct effect on the development of cervical dysplasia into the more dangerous cervical neoplasia. Several studies show a positive correlation between risk factors for cervical dysplasia and consumption of fruits and vegetables, yet the risk factors for squamous cell carcinoma of the cervix were not positive in this area. It would seem diet might be better as a preventive mechanism for cervical dysplasia. Once cervical dysplasia continues to develop into a neoplasia, diet alone may not be a significant factor in stopping the progression, but should be maintained to support recovery and future prevention.

There is a relationship between several nutrients and the severity of cervical dysplasia. A study in *Cancer and Nutrition 1984* revealed that

> There is approximately a 3-fold greater risk for severe dysplasia or CIS in women with lowered vitamin A or beta-carotene intake.

Stress is a Risk Factor

Stress and a feeling of hopelessness have been implicated as having an adverse effect on immunity. Clinical researchers reported that stress contributed to the promotion of CIN and squamous cell cervical cancer. If you have been diagnosed with cervical dysplasia you should take steps to reduce your daily stress as part of an integrated therapeutic approach for the disease.

Other risk factors are

- Intercourse before the age of 18,
- Having an immune deficiency disorder, and
- Giving birth before the age of 22.

Traditional Medical Treatment

Getting rid of the HPV virus is difficult. Even if your entire cervix is burned or frozen, the virus generally still remains. The goal of treatment today is not elimination of the virus, but for the body's immune system to control the virus.

Cervical dysplasia can be removed by many techniques such as LEEP conization (Loop Electrosurgical Excisional Procedure) or cryosurgery. The purpose of LEEP and cryosurgery is to remove or kill abnormal cells on or around the cervix before they can turn into cancer. These procedures are aimed at getting rid of the unhealthy infected tissue. Your physician can discuss these treatments with you if they are needed.

Generally, women with normal immune system function can limit the progression or be cured of mild to moderate cervical dysplasia without surgery. See the integrated therapies suggested below.

Integrated and Alternative Medical Therapy

Supplements taken orally, as well as delivered topically, have been shown to be an effective integrated treatment approach for cervical dysplasia.

Benefits of Vitamin A

In one study where 34 women were biopsied, the researchers concluded that supplementation of vitamin A may help prevent cervical neoplasia. Another case-control study of 87 cases and 82 controls showed that with all factors considered, about a threefold greater risk for severe dysplasia or carcinoma was found in women with lowered vitamin A or beta-carotene intake and nutritional status.

CAUTION: Please refer to Appendix A before supplementing with high doses of vitamin A.

Topical Vitamin A

Topical vitamin A in the form of various retinoids has been studied and showed positive results for cervical dysplasia and cervical cancers. Retinoids are regulators of epithelial differentiation and necessary for maintenance, which is the basis for study of their chemopreventive effects on cervical tissues.

Several studies using topical vitamin A applied directly to cervical tissue using a cervical cap sponge have been completed. Investigators reported a successful and complete response rate in 50% of those suffering mild to moderate forms of dysplasia. Patients with severe dysplasia did not benefit from the therapy. Topical application of vitamin A appears only to be effective in mild to moderate cases of dysplasia.

A large Latin American study of 387 women reported a decrease in disease risk associated with higher levels of beta-carotene consumption. Additionally, after supplementation with beta-carotene, normal cervicovaginal cells (a positive indicator) were significantly increased in 79% of the patients, as compared to baseline levels.

Benefits of Vitamin B_6

Oral contraceptives deplete vitamin B_6, which increases the risk of dysplasia. If a woman has diabetes or is overweight and taking oral contraceptives, her need for vitamin B_6 is increased. Vitamin B_6 plays an important role in protein synthesis, carbohydrate metabolism, and glucose tolerance. We recommend taking 50 to 250 mg of vitamin B_6 daily if you are using oral contraceptives.

Benefits of Vitamin C

Vitamin C has been reported as an independent risk factor for dysplasia. Nutritional levels that are less than recommended daily allowance (RDA) levels have been shown to increase the odds of dysplasia. Of United States women who are of reproductive age, a dietary survey estimated that 68% of women receive inadequate levels of vitamin C.

Demonstrating the need for adequate vitamin C levels, another controlled case study looked at vitamin C's impact on the risk of contracting dysplasia. The study examined women with completely normal pap smears and no gynecological problems as well as women who had two consecutive abnormal pap smears. These test subjects were evaluated for vitamin C blood plasma levels. Those women with normal pap smears had twice the vitamin C blood plasma levels than those with abnormal smears.

Benefits of Vitamin E

Oral contraceptive use can also deplete vitamin E levels, increasing the risk of dysplasia. There have been a number of studies where low levels of tocopherols (vitamin E) were noted in women with cervical dysplasia and cancer. Investigators have reported an inverse relationship between vitamin E levels and increased risk and severity of the disorder.

Benefits of Folic Acid and Lycopene

Folic acid has also been reported to play a therapeutic role in preventing cervical dysplasia and reducing the risks of neoplasia in ulcerative colitis.

Folic acid is involved in red blood cell health, as well as other functions in maintaining healthy tissues. Folic acid has been shown to prevent neural tube defects, both indirectly, in the synthesis of transfer RNA, and through its function as a methyl donor to create methylcobalamin, which is used in the remethylation of homocysteine to methionine.

Folic acid is also important to healthy cervical tissue. In a number of studies on oral contraceptive users, it has been shown that folate levels are decreased by oral contraceptives. Oral ontraceptives appear to have a role in disrupting normal folate metabolisms, and supplementation with folic acid can reverse this problem. It would appear extremely prudent for oral contraceptive users to be on folic acid daily.

Additional studies have demonstrated that folic acid supplementation in oral contraceptive users with mild to moderate dysplasia has arrested progression of the disease. In some cases, folic acid supplementation was reported to have reversed dysplasia.

Several studies have reported the importance of lycopene relative to the risk and treatment of cervical dysplasia. A 1990 study titled "Nutritional Factors and the Risk of Cervical Dysplasia" reported in *Dissertation Abstracts International* stated that "there appeared to be an inverse association between the presence of cervical dysplasia and intakes of lycopene and folacin (folic acid)."

Benefits of Selenium

Numerous studies on cervical uterine cancers have found that low selenium levels are associated with risk and treatment. These studies show that patients who do not have dysplasia (controls) have higher levels of tissue selenium compared to patients who suffer cervical dysplasia. Low selenium intakes and levels increase the risk of cervical and uterine neoplasia.

Benefits of Zinc

Zinc is well known for its function of enhancing immunity. Though not studied conclusively for its independent effects on cervical dysplasia, it should be included in a woman's supplement program to improve general health and reduce the risk of disease.

Worth mentioning is a study in which high levels of retinol were related to regression of cervical dysplasia and the protective effect of zinc was noted by the researchers.

A Topical Therapeutic Approach for Cervical Dysplasia

A phase-one pilot study investigation has reported positive results in 50% of those treated with a vitamin A analog therapy. The approach delivered all-trans-retinoic acid (RA) directly to the cervix using a collagen sponge, called a Vag-Pack.

Researchers have demonstrated that retinoic acid, a topical form of vitamin A, can reverse or suppress the epithelial preneoplasia factor of cervical dysplasia. Similar results were found in another study, where total regression of the disease was again found in 50% of the patients treated.

Based on the scientific literature reported thus far, retinoic acid appears effective for mild to moderate dysplasia, but not for severe dysplasia. This topical application of retinoic acid further supports the possibility that prevention of human cancer may be feasible.

Vag-Pack is available from the Bezwecken company. Several different types of vaginal inserts for the treatment of different types of cervical dysplasia are available and must be ordered by your physician. Refer to the order information that follows for your physician.

The Vag-Pak may be a good treatment option if your dysplasia is mild to moderate, rather than conventional therapies such as LEEP conization or cryosurgery which may cause adverse side effects. You should discuss your best option with your physician.

If You Have Been Diagnosed

Communicate with your physician. Help him or her to understand your desire for a long-term positive outcome, with as little surgical intervention as possible.

Conclusion

Integrated medicine works best when one focuses on all the cofactors of the disease.

1. Do not smoke.
2. Using a condom has been shown to somewhat lower the risk of contracting the HPV virus, which is associated with almost all dysplasia, even though HPV virus can be transmitted between sexual partners even when condoms are being used.
3. Eat a well-balanced diet, including an adequate protein intake and fruits and vegetables.
4. Take a multiple supplement high in the B vitamins, zinc, selenium, beta-carotene, lycopene, vitamin E, vitamin C, and additional folic acid and vitamin A. (If you might become pregnant, do not take extra vitamin A, as it can cause birth defects.)
5. If you are taking oral contraceptives, an extra B-complex vitamin that is high in B_6 would be wise.
6. If you do smoke, all vitamins need to be taken in the higher optimal dose range.
7. Find a physician willing to treat you with a Vag-Pak. Have the physician's office contact the Life Extension Foundation for the phone number and additional information.

Summary

The following nutrients are important in the prevention and treatment of cervical dysplasia.

1. Vitamin A, 5000 to 25,000 IU daily.
2. Beta-carotene, 25,000 IU daily.

3. Vitamin B_6, 50 to 250 mg daily.
4. Vitamin C, 2000 to 6000 mg daily.
5. Vitamin E, 400 to 800 IU daily.
6. Folic acid, 800 to 10,000 mcg daily.
7. Selenium, 200 to 400 mcg daily.
8. Zinc, 15 to 50 mg daily.
9. Lycopene, 10 to 30 mg daily.

For more information. To find out more about the effects of drug-induced vitamin depletion, read a new book on the subject called *The Drug-Induced Nutrient Depletion Handbook* by Dr. Ross Pelton, Dr. Jim LaValle, Ernest Hawkins, R.Ph., M.S., and Dan Krinsky, R.Ph., M.S.

If you are currently diagnosed and would like to contact A Woman's Time, the phone number is (503) 222-2322. A Woman's Time specializes in women's ailments and provides information on the Vag-Paks by Bezwecken (which include topical vitamin A, proteolytic enzymes with zinc, and other nutrient-based treatments for cervical dysplasia). A Woman's Time also provides phone consulting ranging in price from 40 to $80 an hour.

Product availability. Life Extension Mix (a multi-nutrient formula), vitamin A, beta-carotene, vitamin B_6, folic acid, vitamin C, vitamin E, lycopene extract, selenium, zinc, and whey protein can be ordered by phoning (800) 544-4440 or order online at www.lef.org.

CHOLESTEROL REDUCTION

Elevated cholesterol is associated with a greater-than-normal risk of atherosclerosis and cardiovascular disease. While antioxidants can inhibit cholesterol from oxidizing onto the linings of the arteries, knowing and controlling your cholesterol levels is still an important step in preventing cardiovascular disease.

Estimates are that 52% of the total population have cholesterol levels of 200 mg/dL, and about 21% have levels of 240 or above. In adults, total cholesterol levels from 200 to 239 mg/dL are considered borderline-high, while levels above 240 are considered dangerously high. Knowing cholesterol numbers can allow a person to manage "fat intake," which has other benefits, such as lowering one's risk of various cancers caused by fat-soluble toxins.

During the past 20 years, deaths from heart disease have gone down 33% in the United States saving as many as 250,000 lives each year! This is because people are beginning to learn about and take the proper precautions to prevent and treat heart problems. Keeping cholesterol levels in the safest range (between 180 and 200 mg/dL) is one way of statistically reducing your risk of suffering a heart attack or stroke.

Types of Cholesterol, and the Impact on Your Health

Low Density Lipoprotein (LDL)

Low density lipoprotein (LDL) is called the "bad" form of cholesterol. LDL carries most of the cholesterol in the blood, and the cholesterol from LDLs is the main source of damaging accumulation and blockage in the arteries. Thus, the more LDL-cholesterol you have in your blood, the greater your risk of disease. If you have coronary heart disease (CHD) and your LDL is higher than 100 mg/dL, your cholesterol may well be too high for you.

High Density Lipoprotein (HDL)

High density lipoprotein (HDL) is called the "good" form of cholesterol. HDL picks up and transports cholesterol in the blood back to the liver, which leads to its elimination from the body. HDL can help keep LDL cholesterol from building up in the walls of the arteries. If your level of HDL cholesterol is below 35 mg/dL, you are at substantially higher risk for CHD. The higher your HDL cholesterol level, the better. The average HDL-cholesterol for men is about 45 mg/dL, and for women it is about 55 mg/dL.

Triglycerides

Triglycerides are a form of fat carried through the bloodstream. Most of your body's fat is in the form of triglycerides stored in fat tissue. Only a small portion of your triglycerides are found in the bloodstream. High blood triglyceride levels alone do not cause atherosclerosis. But lipoproteins that are rich in triglycerides also contain cholesterol, which causes atherosclerosis in many people with high triglycerides. So high triglycerides may be a sign of a lipoprotein problem that contributes to CHD.

Serum (blood) cholesterol levels are affected not only by what you eat, but also by how quickly your body creates LDL cholesterol and eliminates it. Most people manufacture all the cholesterol they need in their liver, and it is not necessary to obtain any surplus cholesterol from food.

Patients with coronary artery disease typically have too high a level of LDL cholesterol in their blood. Multiple factors help determine whether your LDL cholesterol level is high or low. The factors discussed next are the most important:

Heredity

Your genes control how high your LDL cholesterol is by affecting how fast LDL is made and removed from the blood. One specific form of inherited high cholesterol is familial hypercholesterolemia, which often leads to early CHD. Even if you do not have a specific genetic form of high cholesterol, genes play a role in affecting your LDL cholesterol level.

What You Eat

Saturated fat, found mostly in foods that come from animals, increases your LDL cholesterol level more than anything else in your diet. Dietary cholesterol also plays a part. The average American man consumes about 360 mg of cholesterol a day; the average woman, between 220 and 260 mg. Eating too much saturated fat and cholesterol-rich foods such as eggs is the main reason for high levels of cholesterol and a high rate of heart attacks in the United States according to the Centers for Disease Control. Reducing the amount of saturated fat and cholesterol you eat is a very significant step in reducing blood cholesterol levels.

Here are the 1999 dietary recommendations from the American Heart Association:

"Cholesterol is found in meat, poultry, seafood and dairy products. Foods from plants—such as fruits, vegetables, vegetable oils, grains, cereals, nuts, and seeds—don't contain cholesterol. Egg yolks and organ meats are high in cholesterol. Shrimp and crayfish are somewhat high in cholesterol. Chicken, turkey, and fish contain about the same amount of cholesterol as do lean beef, lamb and pork."

As can be seen from the above recommendations, it is hard to avoid consuming foods that cause cholesterol to build up in the blood.

Weight

Excess weight tends to increase LDL cholesterol level. If you are overweight and have a high LDL cholesterol level, losing weight may help lower it. Weight loss also helps to lower triglycerides and raise HDL. Conversely, it is now accepted that even small increases in weight may increase cholesterol and the general risk of cardiovascular disease.

Physical Activity/Exercise

Frequent physical activity may lower LDL-cholesterol and raise HDL-cholesterol levels.

Age and Sex

Before menopause, women usually have total cholesterol levels that are lower than those of men the same age. As women and men get older, their blood cholesterol levels rise until about 60 to 65 years of age. In women, menopause often causes an increase in LDL cholesterol and a decrease in HDL cholesterol level, and after the age of 50, women often have higher total cholesterol levels than men of the same age.

Alcohol

Alcohol intake increases HDL cholesterol but does not lower LDL cholesterol. Drinking too much alcohol can damage the liver and heart muscle, lead to high blood pressure, and raise triglycerides. Because of the risks, doctors don't recommend alcoholic beverages as a way to prevent CHD, yet the consumption of just one glass of red wine or other alcoholic beverage statistically reduces the risk of heart attack and stroke without causing other health problems for most people.

Stress

Stress over the long term has been shown in several studies to raise blood cholesterol levels. One way that stress may do this is by affecting your habits. For example, when some people are under stress, they console themselves by eating fatty foods. The saturated fat and cholesterol in these foods contribute to higher levels of blood cholesterol.

Who's at Risk?

"At risk" cholesterol numbers are considered to be anything above 200 mg/dL for total serum cholesterol with the caveat that the dangerous LDL cholesterol (low density lipoprotein) number be less than 100 mg/dL. HDL cholesterol (high density lipoprotein), the aptly named "good" cholesterol, can be increased using specific nutrient supplements and by limiting total serum cholesterol intake. If your HDL is less than 35 mg/dL, your physician will try to help you increase it, while lowering LDL cholesterol.

Here's a fact for you to consider! A person with a total serum cholesterol number of 260 mg/dL increases his or her chance of a heart attack by 500% (*Annals of Internal Medicine* (United States), 1979).

Cholesterol is a vital substance that is synthesized by the liver and other bodily tissues. The body uses cholesterol as a building block for essential organic molecules such as steroid hormones, cell membranes, and bile acids. Our bodies produce between 500 to 1000 mg total serum cholesterol each day, and this amount is added to the typical American's diet, which may contain an additional 500 to 1000 mg a day of additional cholesterol—half of which is absorbed into the body. Therefore, the total elimination of all cholesterol from dietary sources may not be enough for some people, and over time they may face elevated cholesterol levels and require additional measures to control or reduce cholesterol (*Heart Disease, Preventive Medicine,* 1992).

Source of risk factors: Columbia and Boston Universities, 1999.

Cholesterol and the Threat of Unstable Plaque

Cholesterol is a major ingredient of the plaque that collects in the coronary arteries and causes CHD, so it is important to understand how plaques develop. Excess cholesterol is deposited in the artery walls as it travels through the bloodstream. Then special cells in the artery wall gobble up this excess cholesterol, creating a "lump" in the artery wall. This cholesterol-rich "lump" then is covered by a scar that produces a hard coat or shell over the cholesterol and cell mixture. It is this collection of cholesterol covered by a scar that is called plaque.

The plaque buildup narrows the space in the coronary arteries through which blood can flow, decreasing the supply of oxygen and nutrients to the heart. If not enough oxygen-carrying blood can pass through the narrowed arteries to reach the heart muscle, the heart may respond with a pain called angina. The pain usually happens with exercise when the heart needs more oxygen. It is typically felt in the chest or sometimes in other places like the left arm and shoulder. However, this same inadequate blood supply may cause no symptoms. Cardiovascular disease is often a "silent" disease, until something happens.

Plaques come in various sizes and shapes. Throughout the coronary arteries many small plaques build themselves into the walls of the arteries, blocking less than half of the artery opening. These small plaques are often invisible on many of the tests doctors use to identify coronary heart disease. It used to be thought that the most dangerous plaques and the ones most likely to cause total blockage of coronary arteries were the largest ones. The largest plaques are in fact the ones most likely to cause angina. However, small plaques that are full of cholesterol but not completely covered by scar are now thought to be very unstable and more likely to rupture or burst, releasing their cholesterol contents into the bloodstream.

When this happens, it precipitates blood clotting inside the artery. If the blood clot totally blocks the artery, it reduces or stops blood flow, and a heart attack occurs. The muscle on the far side of the blood clot does not get enough oxygen and begins to die. The damage can be permanent.

Lowering your blood cholesterol level can slow, stop, or even reverse the buildup of plaque. Cholesterol lowering can reduce your risk of a heart attack by lowering the cholesterol content in unstable plaques to make them more stable and less prone to rupture. This is why lowering your LDL cholesterol is such an important way to reduce your risk for having a heart attack. Even in people who have had one heart attack, the chances of having future attacks can be substantially reduced by cholesterol reduction.

One of the best methods of reducing cholesterol is through dietary modification (*see Dash Diet in Hypertension protocol*). Supplements offer excellent synergistic benefits to augment dietary measures.

The Benefits of Lowering Cholesterol

A 5-year clinical trial with over 4400 patients with heart disease found that lowering cholesterol can prevent heart attacks and reduce death in men and women who already have heart disease and high cholesterol. Researchers say that the following benefits could be expected if physicians were to treat their heart disease patients for the same 5-year period and lower cholesterol to the same extent.

For every 1000 patients,

- Forty people would be saved out of the 90 who would otherwise die from heart disease.
- Seventy of the expected 210 nonfatal heart attacks would be avoided.
- Heart procedures such as bypass surgery would be avoided in 60 of the 210 patients who would be expected to need these procedures.

The most recent report of the *National Cholesterol Education Program* identified low HDL cholesterol as a coronary artery disease risk factor and recommended that "all healthy adults be screened for both total cholesterol and HDL cholesterol levels" (*Am. J. Cardiol.,* Nov. 1998, 82:9A, 13Q–21Q).

Landmark clinical studies in the past several years have demonstrated diminished mortality and first coronary events following lowering of low density lipoprotein (LDL) cholesterol. The *Framingham Heart Study* (a long-term research study) produced compelling evidence indicating that a low level of HDL cholesterol was an independent "predictor" of coronary artery disease (CAD).

Many community health organizations, local drug stores, and health food stores regularly provide low-cost or free cholesterol screening for those interested in monitoring their serum cholesterol. Seek the advice of a competent physician experienced in cholesterol management using dietary modification and nutritional supplements. A physician with this kind of background can also help with the substitution of nutrient-based cholesterol-reduction plans which may allow the reduction or elimination of prescription drugs.

If you already have high blood pressure as well as high blood cholesterol (and many people do), your physician may also tell you to cut down on sodium or salt. As long as you are working on getting your blood cholesterol number down, this is a good time to work on your blood pressure, too.

Traditional Therapies

HMG-CoA Reductase Inhibitors

Drugs that inhibit the enzyme HMG-CoA reductase are referred to as "statins." These drugs lower cholesterol by slowing down the production of cholesterol and by increasing the liver's ability to remove the LDL cholesterol already in the blood.

The latest introduction to the powerful group of lipid-lowering drugs known as statins, or HMG reductase inhibitors, is atorvastatin (Lipitor). It is the only statin approved for the reduction of triglycerides as well as total and LDL cholesterol. It reduces LDL by 40 to 60%, triglycerides by 20 to 40%, and raises HDL cholesterol by 5 to 10%, changes which may be bigger than those produced by other statins. It can be taken once a day, at any time of day, and the recommended dose range is from 10 to 80 mg a day. Atorvastatin provides the lowest cost per percentage of LDL cholesterol reduction of available statins. Other available statins which primarily reduce LDL cholesterols are cerivastatin (Baychol), fluvastatin (Lescol), lovastatin (Mevacor), pravastatin (Pravachol), and simvastatin (Zocor).

Additional drugs that are commonly prescribed and approved for lowering elevated triglyceride levels are gemfibrozil and clofibrate. These drugs may be prescribed alone or in combination with other drugs. These triglyceride-lowering drugs have toxic side effects that cause many people to avoid them.

Integrated and Alternative Medical Approaches

Some people with high cholesterol are able to reduce to safe levels by using combinations of dietary supplements that have been shown to lower serum cholesterol, protect against LDL cholesterol oxidation, and reduce the risk of an abnormal arterial blood clot formation.

Benefits of Curcumin

Curcumin, also known as turmeric root, an ancient spice in the ginger family, is gaining attention for its positive impact on a number of diseases, including cholesterol reduction. Scientific evidence has been building since the mid-1980s of curcumin's potential cholesterol-lowering capabilities.

For example, animals fed small doses of curcumin had their cholesterol levels drop by one half (50%) over those that did not receive curcumin. Curcumin reduces cholesterol by interfering with intestinal cholesterol uptake, increasing the conversion of cholesterol into bile acids, and increasing the excretion of bile acids, according to the *International Journal of Vitamin Nutritional Research* (1991, 61:364–69).

The 1992 *Indian Journal of Physiology* reported that ten human volunteers taking curcumin showed a 29% increase in beneficial HDL cholesterol in only 7 days. Total cholesterol also fell 11.6% and lipid peroxidation was reduced by 33%.

In January of 1997, the *Journal of Molecular Cell Biochemistry* reported curcumin has demonstrated, *in vivo,* the ability to decrease total cholesterol and LDL cholesterol levels in serum and to increase the beneficial HDL cholesterol. "Blood cholesterol was lowered significantly by dietary curcumin in these diabetic animals. Significant decrease in blood triglyceride and phospholipids was also brought about by dietary curcumin in diabetic rats."

The research has continued and curcumin's ability to lower blood cholesterol levels was reported in the April 1998 issue of *Molecular Cell Biochemistry,* and again, later that year, researchers in *Biofactors* (1998, 8:1–2, 51–57) reported that "curcumin extract may be protective in preventing lipoperoxidation of subcellular membranes."

Curcumin also provides an additional benefit by potentially reducing the risk of cardiovascular-related disease as it inhibits platelet aggregation and significantly decreases the level of lipid (LDL) peroxidation. "Observation of curcumin's mechanism of action shows that it blocks the formation of thromboxane A2, a promoter of platelet aggregation, thereby inhibiting abnormal blood clot formation. Curcumin also increases a prostacyclin, a natural inhibitor of platelet aggregation" (*Arzneim. Forsch.,* 1986, 36:715–17).

Benefits of Gugulipid (*Commiphora mukul*)

This powerful ancient remedy has been rediscovered by Western culture. Gugulipid is made from the resin of the commiphora mukul tree of north central India. Gugulipid (gugulestones) has been used for thousands of years to alleviate problems associated with obesity, acne, viral infections, and other ailments.

In a study published in 1989 by the *Journal of Associated Physicians—India,* 125 patients receiving gugulipid showed an 11% decrease in total serum cholesterol, a drop of 16.8% in triglycerides, and a 60% increase in HDL cholesterol within 3 to 4 weeks. Patients with elevated cholesterol levels showed much greater improvement than normal patients.

The study quoted a second trial (included in the article noted above) where 205 patients receiving gugulipid at a dose rate of 25 mg administered 3 times daily showed a 70 to 80% reduction of serum cholesterol, whereas no response was found in the placebo group (*Journal of Associated Physicians—India,* 1989, 37[5]:328).

A placebo-controlled trial of 40 patients with high blood-fat levels showed a serum cholesterol reduction of 21.75%, with triglycerides being reduced by 27.1% in only 3 weeks, and after continuing the study for 16 weeks it was learned that HDL cholesterol was increased by 35.8% (*Journal of Associated Physicians—India,* 1989, 37[5]:328).

Benefits of Garlic

A study published in the *Journal Nutrition Research* (1987, 7:139–49) showed that a liquid garlic extract made by Kyolic caused a 12 to 31% reduction in cholesterol levels in the majority of test subjects after 6 months. The study showed that 73% of the subjects given the Kyolic garlic experienced a greater than 10% reduction in cholesterol, compared with only 17% of the subjects in the placebo group showing the same improvement.

If you have high LDL cholesterol levels, garlic supplementation is especially important because LDL cholesterol oxidation causes atherosclerosis, and garlic specifically inhibits LDL oxidation. And garlic helps protect the arterial lining against oxidation. Most importantly, garlic prevents abnormal platelet aggregation (thrombosis) via several different mechanisms. The formation of arterial blood clots is the primary cause of most heart attacks and strokes.

Investigators reported in a study published in the *American Journal of Clinical Nutrition* (1996, 64:866–70) that the daily administration of 7.2 grams of Kyolic garlic powder for 6 months produced a modest reduction (of between 6.1 and 7%) in total cholesterol, compared with the placebo group. The more dangerous LDL cholesterol was reduced 4 to 4.6% in the Kyolic group.

The heart-healthy benefits of garlic include protecting the endothelial lining of the arterial system against oxidative damage. A study published in *Atherosclerosis* (1999, 144:237–49) shows an actual reduction in buildup of fatty plaque in arteries in garlic-supplement users. Fatty plaque is comprised of many substances, including cholesterol. When plaque accumulates in the coronary arteries, the condition can lead to heart attack. In a study of 280 adults, German researchers reported that participants who took 900 mg of garlic powder a day had up to 18% less plaque in their arteries than those who took a placebo, or "dummy," powder. Male study participants who took a placebo had a 5.5% increase in plaque volume, while those who took the garlic powder experienced just a 1.1% increase in plaque buildup during the 4-year study period. By comparison, women who took the garlic showed a 4.6% decrease in plaque volume, while those who took the placebo powder had a 5.3% increase. Garlic may affect plaque buildup by reducing blood platelet stickiness (aggregation) and specifically preventing the oxidation of LDL cholesterol onto the lining of the arteries. Platelet aggregation helps plaque cling to the arteries.

An April 1998 study reported on the effect of garlic on blood lipids, blood sugar fibrogen, and fibrinogenic activity of 30 patients who received 4 grams of garlic daily for 3 months. The patients were monitored at 1.5 and 3 months when it was determined that garlic had "significantly reduced total serum cholesterol and triglycerides, and significantly increased HDL cholesterol." With regard to fibrinogenic activity, it was determined that the garlic inhibited platelet aggregation (*Prostagland. Leuk. Essent. Fatty Acids,* April 1998, 58[4]:257–63).

An earlier study in June 1994, the University of Massachusetts Medical School published a report that found that those U.S. adults who consumed one-half to one clove of garlic each day showed cholesterol levels that were reduced by 9% (*JAMA,* June 1, 1994, 271[21]:1660–61). A survey of 7 out of 8 studies on garlic showed that dosages of between 600 to 900 mg of garlic powder (*Allium sativum L.*) produced a 5 to 20% reduction in cholesterol and triglycerides. (*Fortschr. Med.* (Germany) 1990, 108[36]:49–54). Other studies have shown that much higher doses of garlic were required for cholesterol reduction.

Human patients fed a daily dose of Kyolic ("Aged Garlic Extract") over a 10-month study showed that "adhesion to fibrinogen was reduced by 30%—compared to placebo . . . and that . . . the beneficial effect of garlic preparations on lipids and blood pressure extends also to platelet function" (*Journal of Cardiovascular Pharmacology* [United States], 1998, 31[6]:904–8).

Note: Overall studies seem to indicate that dosages of garlic may be a factor in its efficacy. The suggested dose of high allicin garlic extract should be between 6000 mg and 8000 mg daily taken with meals. Since large amounts of garlic may cause stomach upset, we recommend that garlic be taken with the largest meal of the day.

In summary, the mechanisms by which garlic have shown to protect against cardiovascular disease include the following: cholesterol reduction, preventing abnormal blood clot formation inside of blood vessels; protecting against LDL cholesterol oxidation; and protecting the endothelial lining of the arterial system against oxidation. A review of all the studies on garlic indicates that high doses are required for effective cholesterol reduction. If you were to use garlic alone to lower serum cholesterol, you should take 6000 to 8000 mg a day. When used in combination with other cholesterol-lowering nutrients, lower doses of garlic may be effective.

Benefits of Vitamin E

To say that vitamin E is very important to our health is an understatement: it is protective against approximately 80 diseases.

The National Institute of Aging, Tufts University, and the University of Arizona, College of Medicine have found that vitamin E may help inhibit and slow the development of LDL oxidation, the progression of cardiovascular-related diseases, and possibly slow aging.

Oxidation of low density lipoprotein is involved in the development of atherosclerotic disease. An extensive study by the National Institute of Aging of 11,178 seniors aged 67 to 109 found that seniors who supplement with vitamin E are less likely to die prematurely. The research, reported in the *American Journal of Clinical Nutrition* late in 1997, discovered that vitamin E has the ability to stabilize free radicals. Free radicals are unstable oxygen molecules that can break down and degenerate cells, much as oxygen causes rust on iron. Partly caused by increased LDL cholesterol oxidation, free radicals result in increased plaque deposits and restricted blood flow, making them extremely dangerous to the interior of arteries.

A study by the National Institute of Aging found that people who took vitamin E supplementation over a 9-year period (1984 to 1993) had a 27% lower risk of all-cause mortality, a 41% reduction in heart disease risk!

Similarly, Dr. Jeffrey Blumberg, professor of nutrition at Tufts University in Boston, who heads the Antioxidant Research NIH Laboratories found that vitamin E helped prevent exercise-induced muscular damage based on many of the same mechanisms mentioned above, in the publication *Advanced Nutrition,* 1997. "The potential benefit is great, data are consistent and compelling, and the risk of side effects is essentially nil. It makes a clear case for recommending supplements," Dr. Blumberg said.

Increased blood cell adhesion to human aortic endothelial cells (ECs) lining veins and arteries is one of the early events in the development of atherogenesis. Investigators in 1997, in the *Journal of Thrombosis and Vascular Biology* (United States), indicate that vitamin E has an "inhibitory effect" on LDL-induced production of adhesion molecules and adhesion of blood cell to ECs via its antioxidant function and/or its direct regulatory effect on cell adhesion and arteriosclerosis.

The elderly may receive extra value from vitamin E supplementation, as supplementation with 100 IU vitamin E in the elderly has been reported as beneficial in lowering the rate of oxidation of LDL, slowing the progression of atherosclerosis (*Atherosclerosis*, Sept. 1997, 133[2]:255–63).

Smokers may benefit from long-term vitamin E supplementation, as it has been reported to improve endothelium-dependent relaxation in forearm resistance in vessels of hypercholesterolemic smokers which are characterized by increased levels of auto-antibodies against oxidized LDL. These findings suggest the beneficial effect of vitamin E for subjects with increased exposure to oxidized LDL such as smokers (*J. Am. Coll. Cardiol.,* Feb., 1999, 33[2]:499–505).

Vitamin E may even work as well as some hypocholesterolemic drugs. Results of a study in the *Journal of Circulation Research,* August 1998, suggest that vitamin E and selenium inhibited atherosclerosis as effectively as an equally hypocholesterolemic dose of the drug probucol.

The recommended dose of vitamin E ranges from 400 to 800 IU a day. Minimum effective dose for selenium supplementation is 200 mcg a day. Selenium works with vitamin E to protect against LDL oxidation.

Benefits of Soy

The FDA has approved soy as a method of lowering the risk of coronary heart disease. For this dietary supplement, one research abstract says it all:

> Soy has been a staple part of the Southeastern diet for nearly 5,000 years and is associated with a reduction in the rates of cardiovascular disease, and certain types of cancer. The research is now showing that phyto-chemicals in soy are the mechanism of action responsible (*Society for Experimental Biology and Medicine* [United States], 1998, 217[3]:386–92).

Diets rich in soy protein can protect against the development of atherosclerosis. The mechanisms of action of soy protein include cholesterol lowering, inhibition of LDL oxidation, protection against the development of atherosclerosis, and reduction in risk of thrombosis. The active constituents in soy responsible for these benefits are the isoflavones genistein, daidzein, and glycitein. In a study to determine whether soy isoflavones would protect against atherosclerosis in mice, it was reported that mice fed a soy diet averaged 30% lower cholesterol (*J. Nutr.* [United States], June 1998, 128[6]:954–59).

In a study in *Metabolism,* June 1997, investigations suggest that dietary soybean protein has a beneficial effect on cardiovascular risk factors. According to another study completed at about the same time, "Potential mechanisms by which soy isoflavones might prevent atherosclerosis include a beneficial effect on plasma lipid concentrations, antioxidant effects, antiproliferative and antimigratory effects on smooth muscle cells, effects on thrombus formation, and maintenance of normal vascular reactivity" (*American Journal of Clinical Nutrition,* Dec. 1988, 68[6] Suppl., 1390S–93S).

Postmenopausal women may also benefit from intake of soy protein, and it is suggested to be beneficial by researchers in a 1998 issue of *American Journal of Clinical Nutrition* for diseases and the risk factors (cholesterol) associated with cardiovascular disease.

Adding to the evidence that soy is beneficial, conclusions of a September 1998 *Journal of Nutrition* study are that "the efficacy of the American Hospital Association Step I cholesterol-lowering diet can be improved with the addition of soy protein." If you want to reduce your disease risk to heart disease and avoid elevated cholesterol levels, it is recommended that you take soy.

Benefits of Niacin

Niacin (vitamin B_3) improves cholesterol profiles when given in doses well above the vitamin requirement. Nicotinic acid lowers total cholesterol, LDL-cholesterol, and triglyceride levels, while raising HDL-cholesterol levels. Most people cannot use the high doses (1000 to 3000 mg a day) of niacin required to suppress cholesterol levels. Niacin causes a flushing effect, resembling an acute allergic reaction that many people find intolerable. While niacin is considered relatively safe, like other cholesterol-lowering drugs, it can cause liver toxicity when taken in high doses. Monitoring liver enzymes every 6 months is important when taking more than 1000 mg of niacin a day. Those with hepatitis should avoid niacin.

Flush-free niacin may lower cholesterol while boosting the beneficial HDL fraction. In a report on the antiatherogenic role of HDL (high density lipoprotein) cholesterol, flush-free niacin (inositol hexanicotinate) "appears to have the greatest potential to increase HDL cholesterol [by] 30%."

This study was made over a 5-year period and focused on the effect of high LDL numbers exhibited before a patient's first coronary event(s).

As reported in a November 1998 *American Journal of Cardiology* research study, "Nicotinic acid (niacin) has been shown to decrease triglyceride, increase HDL cholesterol, lower LDL cholesterol, and decrease lipoprotein (a); it also decreases fibrinogen," an additional benefit that reduces the risk of related cardiovascular disease.

To determine whether lower doses of nicotinic acid are as effective and better-tolerated than the typical regimen currently used, researchers at the University of Texas Southwestern Medical Center in Dallas, as reported and described in the *Archives of Internal Medicine,* 1996, conducted a trial using two different doses of nicotinic acid.

The results showed that low-dose (1.5 mg to 3 mg) nicotinic acid treatment significantly lowered triglyceride levels, raised HDL concentrations by approximately 22%, and favorably altered the ratio of total cholesterol: HDL cholesterol in both normal patients and those with abnormal lipid levels at baseline. Further improvement in lipid levels was also observed in those patients who tolerated the higher dose of nicotinic acid.

> In this study, significant improvement in blood lipids levels was observed among the 75% of patients who tolerated low-dose nicotinic acid therapy. The authors conclude that use of nicotinic acid in lower doses than traditionally prescribed is both well-tolerated and effective in altering blood lipid levels. In addition, they suggest that this vitamin may be particularly worthwhile when combined with other lipid-lowering medications.

(Nicotinamide, another form of the vitamin B_3, does not lower cholesterol levels and should not be used in the place of niacin.)

Benefits of Fiber

High intake of soluble fiber is a very effective way of lowering serum cholesterol. Most people, however, find that high amounts of fiber produce gastrointestinal upset, and therefore do not consistently take enough fiber to lower cholesterol levels.

In populations with reported higher incidence of elevated cholesterol, fiber may be of benefit as found in a 1998 study conducted in Mexico City.

> Psyllium and oat bran have been shown to lower plasma LDL cholesterol levels in different populations. Hypercholesterolemia is prevalent in the Northern part of Mexico and might be associated to dietary habits and sedentary lifestyle. These results indicate that psyllium and oat bran are efficacious in lowering plasma LDL cholesterol in both normal and hypercholesterolemic individuals from this population (*Journal of the American College of Nutrition,* Dec. 1998, 17(6):601–8).

Another study contradicts this as follows:

> Various soluble fibers reduce total and LDL cholesterol by similar amounts. The effect is small within the practical range of intake. For example, 3 grams soluble fiber from oats (3 servings of oatmeal, 28 grams each) can decrease total and LDL cholesterol by approximately 0.13 mmol/L. Increasing soluble fiber can make only a small contribution to dietary therapy to lower cholesterol (*Am. J. Clin. Nutr.,* (United States), Jan. 1999, 69(1):30–42).

CAUTION: DO NOT take psyllium if you are presently taking the prescription drugs digitalis or nitrofurantoin.

Chitosan is a fiber composed of chitin, which is a component of the shell of shellfish. Scientists in Norway have processed chitin to provide a magnetic binding affinity for fat and cholesterol in the digestive tract. Chitosan can absorb as much as seven to eight times its weight of fat and bile in the digestive tract. The fat and cholesterol are then excreted through the bowel, thereby improving bowel function and reducing cholesterol levels in the body.

One of the first studies to show a direct correlation between lowering of serum cholesterol with chitosan—suggesting that the agent could be used to inhibit the development of atherosclerosis in individuals with hypercholesterolemia—appeared in the June 1998 issue of *Atherosclerosis Journal*. Researchers at the Department of Medicine, University of Auckland, New Zealand, found that animals fed for 20 weeks on a diet containing 5% chitosan or on a control diet attained blood cholesterol levels significantly lower in the chitosan-fed animals throughout the study and at 20 weeks were 64% below that of control animals. That's right, 64%!

Additionally, when the area of aortic plaque in the two groups of animals were compared, a highly significant inhibition of plaque deposits was observed in the chitosan-fed animals—42% and 50%, compared to 42% in the control animals.

Earlier in the August–October 1994 issue of the journal *ARM Medicina,* Helsinki, clinical studies with chitosan demonstrated that in 5 weeks total cholesterol (LDL) was reduced by 32%, HDL increased by 7.5%, and triglycerides were lowered by 18%.

Another study done almost 20 years ago in the April 1980 *Journal of American Clinical Nutrition* reported a 25 to 30% reduction in cholesterol over a several-month period, initially documenting chitosan's potential cholesterol-lowering effectiveness.

Because of chitosan's ability to bind fat, chitosan is also an excellent aid in weight loss as well as normalization of cholesterol levels in the body.

CAUTION: Chitosan, like other fibers, can reduce absorption of trace minerals as well as dietary fat. For that reason, it is recommended that trace minerals be taken at a separate time than when the fiber is consumed.

Benefits of Fish Oil (Omega-3)

Fish oil has been shown to reduce high levels of triglycerides by an average of 35%. Fish oil does not appear to reduce cholesterol to that extent, but does offer benefits when consumed as part of an integrated therapy.

A study conducted in The Netherlands on mice and published in June 1998 stated, "Triglyceride turnover studies revealed that fish oil significantly decreased the hepatic VLDL-triglyceride production rate (down 60%)" (*Journal of Lipid Research* (United States), June 1998, 39(6):1181–88).

Another study indicates, "Our results suggest that fish oil lowers plasma lipid levels significantly" (*J. Formos. Med. Assoc.,* Sept. 1997, 96(9):718–26). Investigations published in the *American Journal of Clinical Nutrition* in 1997 examined the effects of *n*-3 fatty acids on serum lipid and lipoprotein concentrations in seven species of experimental animals. *n*-3 Fatty acids consistently lower serum triglyceride concentrations in humans, but not in most animals. These differences between animals and humans may arise from underlying species differences in lipoprotein metabolism.

Scientific studies have demonstrated that alpha-linolenic acid (from flax or perilla oil) reduces the incidence of atherosclerosis, stroke, and second heart attacks. One study showed a 70% reduction in second heart attacks in those consuming this type of fatty acid. Additionally, perilla oil suppresses platelet-activating factor (PAF), a major cause of arterial blood clots that cause heart attacks and strokes. Perilla oil was shown to decrease PAF by 50% in rats, compared with the administration of safflower oil (*Journal of Lipid Mediators and Cell Signaling* (Netherlands), 1997, 17/3:207–20).

Fish oil and garlic is a beneficial combination: Forty subjects, all with cholesterol over 200 mg/dL, were enrolled in a single-blind, placebo-controlled crossover study to evaluate both fish oil and garlic extract used in a synergistic regimen. Each patient received 1800 mg of fish oil plus 1200 mg of garlic for 1 month. Crossovers were then made to placebos for 1 month. This study found an 11% decrease in cholesterol, a 34% decrease in triglycerides, and a 10% decrease in LDL levels as well as a 19% decrease in HDL risk. Although not significant, there was a trend toward increase in HDL. The doctors concluded by stating

> These results suggest that in addition to the known anticoagulant and antioxidant properties of both fish oil and garlic, the combination causes favorable shifts in the lipid subfractions within 1 month. Triglycerides are affected to the largest extent. The cholesterol lowering and improvement in lipid/HDL risk ratios suggests that these combinations may have antiatherosclerotic properties and may protect against the development of coronary artery disease (*J. Natl. Med. Assoc.,* [United States], Oct. 1997, 89[10]:673–78).

Although fish oil appears to be beneficial for cholesterol reduction, there is a remaining problem: fish and flax oil, traditional sources of omega-3 fatty acids, can cause gastrointestinal side effects as well a stomach upset. There is good news in this regard; a new source of essential fatty acids, perilla oil, is showing superior health benefits without adverse gastrointestinal side effects. For cardiovascular disease risk reduction, we recommend 6000 mg of perilla oil a day.

Benefits of Green Tea

Green tea has been shown to lower "bad" LDL cholesterol and serum triglyceride levels. Further, green tea's potent antioxidant effects inhibit the oxidation of LDL cholesterol in the arteries, which plays a major contributory role in the formation of atherosclerosis. "There is considerable epidemiological evidence that tea drinking lowers the risk of heart disease" (*FEBS Lett.*, Aug. 1998, 433(1–2):44–46).

The cholesterol-lowering (hypocholesterolemic) effects of green tea (as well as black tea) have been confirmed by both animal and human epidemiological studies. High consumption of green tea by humans, especially more than 10 cups a day, was found to be associated with higher HDLs and lower LDL and VLDL cholesterol, as well as with various biomarkers indicating better liver health. Lower levels of lipid peroxides in the liver are one well-confirmed benefit of green-tea supplementation found in study after study.

A Japanese study relates, "Green tea catechin acts to limit the excessive rise in blood cholesterol" based on a series of studies reported in 1996 *(Journal Nutritional Science Vitaminol.*, 32:613).

Additionally, some very exciting results were found when rats were fed 2.5% green tea leaves in their diet. The experimental group showed a drop in total cholesterol, low-density cholesterol, and triglycerides. The body weight of green tea–fed rats was 10 to 18% lower than that of rats not consuming green tea. In addition, the activity of antioxidant enzymes superoxide dismutase (SOD) and catalase, and of anticarcinogenic phase-II enzyme glutathione S-transferase (GST), were significantly higher in the green tea group, as was the glutathione level in the liver. There was no liver or kidney toxicity. Thus, the study demonstrated combined cardiovascular and anticancer effects of green tea.

The relation between green tea consumption and serum lipid concentrations were examined using cross-sectional data on 1306 males in Japan. Results indicated that total cholesterol levels were found to be inversely related to the consumption of green tea. "Adjusted mean concentrations of total cholesterol were significantly lower in men drinking nine cups or more a day than in those consuming zero to two cups a day" (*Prev. Med.* July 1992, 21(4):526–31). No wonder the Japanese people have the longest life span. Most Japanese sip tea all day long.

Green tea also has been shown to elevate levels of HDL, the good cholesterol that helps remove atherosclerotic plaque from arterial walls. Green tea is a natural ACE inhibitor. This is an extra benefit for those with high cholesterol and blood pressure, as published studies show lowered blood pressure in animals and humans given green tea extracts. We recommend one capsule (350 mg) of green tea 95% extract daily, or drinking one to ten cups of green or black tea a day.

Benefits of Artichoke

The discovery that artichoke leaf extract reduces elevated cholesterol levels opens up exciting perspectives in the prevention and treatment of arteriosclerosis and coronary heart disease.

It was as early as the 1930s that scientists first discovered that artichoke extract had a favorable effect on atherosclerotic plaques in the arteries (Tixier, 1939). Later animal studies, in which rats were fed a high-fat diet, also showed that artichoke extract prevented a rise in serum cholesterol levels and the manifestation of atherosclerotic plaque (Samochowiec, 1959 and 1962).

In addition to findings in animal experiments (Samochowiec et al., 1971; Frohlich and Ziegler, 1973; Wojcicki 1976; Lietti 1977 and 1978), a study by Fintelmann in 1996 of 553 outpatients demonstrated a significant effect of the extract on fat (lipid) metabolism. The researchers found a significant decline in both the cholesterol and triglyceride levels in the blood, which confirmed a discovery made as early as the 1930s.

Recent research confirms these earlier findings. The study by Fintelmann demonstrated a significant reduction in cholesterol and triglyceride levels in spite of the relatively short duration of the study (6 weeks). On an average, there was an 11.5% reduction in serum cholesterol from 264 mg/dL initially to 234 mg/dL. Serum triglycerides were similarly reduced from 215 mg/dL initially to 188 mg/dL, corresponding to a decrease of 12.5%. Although this was an open study, its reliability is buttressed by the relatively large number of patients (302) and the very high level of statistical significance attained for the main results.

Very fascinating results came out of an excellent double-blind clinical trial conducted by Petrowicz in 1996. He studied the cholesterol-lowering effect of artichoke leaf extract on 44 healthy individuals under strictly controlled conditions over a 12-week period. There was a significant decrease of cholesterol levels in the volunteers who had high initial levels (greater than 220 mg/dL). In fact, the higher the initial cholesterol value, the more significant was the reduction in cholesterol levels. It was moreover observed that the protective HDL cholesterol levels showed a tendency to increase.

The restricting effect of artichoke leaf extract on cholesterol synthesis was demonstrated in some very interesting studies by Gebhardt (1995, 1996, and 1997) on rat hepatocytes (liver cells). A highly significant concentration-dependent inhibition of cholesterol synthesis was found. The 1997 study indicates that artichoke leaf extract reduces the formation of cholesterol in a physiologically favorable, long-lasting manner. This reduction of cholesterol synthesis persisted for hours following the period of exposure.

The study further indicates that

> artichoke extract may work through indirect inhibition of the enzyme HMGCoA-reductase, which might avoid problems known to occur with strong direct inhibitors of HMGCoA-reductase during long-term treatment. The indirect inhibition was supported by the fact that artichoke leaf extract effectively blocked insulin-dependent stimulation of HMGCoA-reductase without affecting insulin in general. HMGCoA-reductase is a key enzyme in cholesterol synthesis, and HMGCoA-reductase inhibitors generally reduce total cholesterol, LDL cholesterol and triglyceride levels

The International Antioxidant Research Centre, UMDS-Guy's Hospital, London, UK, published its research in September 1998 in *Free-Radical Research,* in which investigators stated, "Artichoke extract retarded LDL oxidation. . . and . . . overall, the results demonstrate the antioxidant activity of the artichoke extract."

Summary

Diseases associated with high cholesterol (and fats) are the number one killer. Fats also play a key role in the incidence of cancers and many other degenerative diseases. Cholesterol exists only in animal tissues, therefore, one's diet is an important first step in its control. For some people, however, limiting fat and cholesterol intake alone is not enough to reduce serum cholesterol to safe levels because of their own liver's production of excess cholesterol. The use of supplements to augment dietary modification can help reduce cholesterol without the side effects of many drugs.

The effectiveness of any cholesterol-reduction therapy varies considerably between individuals. The nutrients we recommend have not only been shown to lower cholesterol, but also protect against cardiovascular disease by other mechanisms such as inhibition of cholesterol-oxidizing free radicals and abnormal blood clots inside arteries (thrombosis).

The following nutritional supplements offer synergistic benefits to assist dietary modification to reduce total serum cholesterol and elevate HDL cholesterol:

1. Garlic, 900 to 8000 mg a day.
2. Curcumin, 900 to 1800 mg a day.
3. Gugulipid, 140 mg 1 to 2 times a day.
4. Artichoke extract, 300 mg, 3 times a day.
5. Chitosan, three to six 500-mg chitosan capsules and one 1000-mg ascorbic acid capsule right before a high-fat meal.
6. Soluble fiber (psyllium, guar gum, and/or pectin), 4 to 6 grams before any high-fat meal.
7. Green tea, 350 mg a day of green tea, 95% polyphenol extract.

8. Niacin, 1500 to 3000 mg a day (if tolerable). Consider flush-free niacin (inositol hexanicotinate) to avoid a "red face."
9. Perilla oil, 6000 mg a day. We suggest taking six 1000-mg gel caps daily. If triglycerides are high, take 6000 mg of fish oil instead.
10. Soy protein extract, 2 heaping teaspoons (5 to 6 grams) of soy powder daily. Soy powder can be easily dispersed and has a light peanut butter taste. For those who want to avoid powders, one capsule of Mega Soy Extract (135 mg/40% extract) twice a day may work as well.
11. Vitamin E, 400 to 800 IU daily.
12. Selenium, 200 to 600 mcg daily.

CAUTION: Anyone who is seeking to use dietary supplements to lower high cholesterol must verify efficacy by having a cholesterol blood test 45 to 60 days after initiating a nutritional regimen. If supplements fail to work, cholesterol-lowering drugs should be considered. While blood testing is not mandatory for healthy people seeking to reduce their risk of heart attack or stroke, it is recommended that everyone have an annual blood test to establish a benchmark giving you the ability to monitor and optimize your life extension program.

For more information. Contact the National Heart, Lung, & Blood Institute (301) 251-1222.

Blood testing availability. Cholesterol testing information and costs can be obtained by calling (800) 208-3444, or review information testing and order online at www.lef.org/bloodtest.htm.

Product availability. Herbal Cardiovascular Formula (containing curcumin and gugulipid, flush- free niacin, super soy extract, mega soy extract) and soy power, garlic powder extract, vitamin E, garlic, niacin, perilla oil, fiber food, chitosan, and artichoke extract are available by phoning (800) 544-4440, or order online at www.lef.org.

CHRONIC FATIGUE SYNDROME

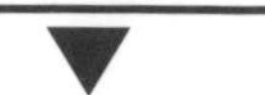

Definition

Chronic Fatigue Syndrome (CFS) is defined as debilitating fatigue and associated symptoms lasting at least 6 months and primarily affecting women. Although there is no known cure for this illness, prognosis for patients is usually good through the treatment of symptoms. Preliminary studies also indicate that there may be a genetic predisposition to CFS.

Chronic Fatigue Syndrome is a controversial issue. Some physicians believe the illness to be psychosomatic, while others remain open-minded. Most are determined to help their patients who are suffering from the debilitating symptoms of this illness.

Some experts believe CFS to be closely related to another chronic condition, fibromyalgia (FMS). A preliminary follow-up study by the Centers for Disease Control reveals that, for those individuals whose chronic fatigue does not significantly improve after a 5-year duration, the most prominent symptom changes from fatigue to muscle pain. This muscle pain is the prominent symptom of fibromyalgia. Doctors usually perform a complete blood count (CBC) and urinalysis when attempting to diagnose a patient with CFS.

Symptoms

Clinically evaluated, unexplained chronic fatigue can be classified as Chronic Fatigue Syndrome if the following criteria are met:

- Unexplained, persistent, or relapsing fatigue that is not a result of ongoing exertion, is new (not lifelong), is not alleviated by rest, and results in a substantial reduction in previous levels of occupational, social, or personal activity.

- The concurrence of four or more of the following symptoms that have persisted or recurred for 6 or more consecutive months and that do not predate the fatigue:
  - Substantial impairment in short-term memory or concentration
  - Sore throat
  - Tender lymph nodes
  - Muscle pain
  - Multijoint pain without swelling or redness
  - Headaches of a new type, pattern, or severity
  - Unrefreshing and/or interrupted sleep
  - Post-exertional malaise lasting more than 24 hours
  - Sensitivity to odors, noise, bright lights, medications, and various foods

Possible Causes

The causes of CFS are as yet undetermined, but studies have shown that multiple nutrient deficiencies, food intolerance, or extreme physical or mental stress may trigger chronic fatigue. Studies have also indicated that CFS may be activated by the immune system, various abnormalities of the hypothalamic-pituitary axes, or by the reactivation of certain infectious agents in the body. Some CFS patients were found to have low levels of PBMC beta-endorphin and other neurotransmitters. Thyroid deficiency may also be a contributing factor in chronic fatigue syndrome. (*Refer to the Thyroid Deficiency protocol to find out how you can determine whether you are deficient in thyroid hormone production.*)

Virus and CFS

Symptoms of CFS resemble a post-viral state and, for this reason, chronic viral conditions have been thought to contribute to CFS in some patients. Medical tests for herpes, Epstein-Barr virus, and cytomegalovirus antibody activity are recommended. (*For those with a viral-induced chronic fatigue syndrome, refer to the Foundation's protocol on Immune Enhancement.*) If you are infected with a chronic, energy-depleting virus, there are conventional and alternative therapies that may be of help. It should be noted that most individuals have been exposed to pathogenic viruses that can be reactivated by adverse environmental conditions and cause chronic fatigue and other diseases. Studies indicate that the Epstein-Barr virus may be suppressed with bilberry extract (anthocyanins), curcumin, carotenoids, and chlorophylls. The exact doses of these natural plant extracts that might be effective against Epstein-Barr have yet to be determined.

Patient Management of CFS

Physicians advise patients to pace themselves carefully and to avoid unusual emotional or physical stress. Follow a regular and manageable daily routine and take modest regular exercise supervised by a physician or physical therapist. In some instances, acupuncture, aquatic therapy, chiropractic, massage, self-hypnosis, stretching, tai chi, therapeutic touch, and yoga have proven helpful in managing CFS. Certain psychotherapies such as family therapy have shown promise in the development of coping skills necessary to counter the adverse effects of chronic illness on the family or patient caregiver.

Energy-Boosting Therapies and Antioxidant Supplementation

A recent report in the *Annual Review of Medicine* stated that CFS "is an illness characterized by activation of the immune system, various abnormalities of several hypothalamic-pituitary axes, and reactivation of certain infectious agents." This suggests that the sufferer of CFS should follow a regimen that involves protecting and enhancing the immune system with proper nutritional supplements, proteins, and hormones. Free radicals play a role in causing damage to the immune system. Alpha-lipoic acid, a potent antioxidant, has improved energy levels in some people on doses of 500 to 800 mg a day. Two multinutrient formulas that contain nutrients shown to maintain healthy immune function and also fight free-radical activity are Life Extension Mix and Life Extension Booster.

Boosting energy levels is necessary for people suffering from CFS. Coenzyme Q_{10}, 100 mg taken 3 times a day, often helps victims of severe chronic fatigue syndrome. Another energy-boosting therapy involves taking 5 mg of NADH 2 times a day. The amino acid *L*-carnitine is known to boost energy levels. Taking 1000 to 2000 mg a day of acetyl-*L*-carnitine has helped people with low energy.

Deficiencies in brain hormones and neurotransmitters are also known to cause low levels of energy. The amino acids phenylalanine or tyrosine, taken in daily doses of 1500 mg, can boost epinephrine and norepinephrine levels. (*Refer to Phenylalanine and Tyrosine—Dosing and Precautions protocol before taking phenylalanine or tyrosine products.*) Phenylalanine and tyrosine are available in capsule and powder forms. The European anti-anxiety medication, Adapton, has been shown to alleviate chronic fatigue symptoms when 2 to 4 capsules a day are taken. DHEA has been reported to improve energy levels in chronic fatigue patients. One study showed the value of DHEA and vitamin C infusion treatment in the control of chronic fatigue syndrome. (*Refer to the DHEA Replacement Therapy protocol before embarking on this therapy.*)

Summary

Chronic Fatigue Syndrome is debilitating fatigue and associated symptoms lasting at least 6 months. The cause of CFS is as yet undetermined, but it may be triggered by infectious agents, stress, vitamin deficiencies, immunologic dysfunction, or thyroid deficiency. There may be a genetic predisposition to Chronic Fatigue Syndrome. Although there is no known cure, energy-boosting treatments and proper management of stress levels and physical activity can significantly reduce the effects of CFS.

1. Alpha-lipoic acid to fight free radicals and improve energy levels, 500 to 800 mg a day.
2. Life Extension Mix and Life Extension Booster, as directed, to provide the nutrients needed to maintain a healthy immune system.
3. Coenzyme Q_{10}, 100 mg 3 times a day, for increased energy.
4. NADH, 5 mg 2 times a day, for increased energy.
5. Acetyl-*L*-carnitine, 1000 to 2000 mg a day, for increased energy.
6. The amino acids phenylalanine or tyrosine, taken in daily doses of 1500 mg, to boost levels of brain hormones and neurotransmitters (*refer to Phenylalanine and Tyrosine—Dosing and Precautions protocol*).
7. Consider DHEA and vitamin C-infusion treatment to control CFS (*refer to the DHEA Replacement Therapy protocol*).

For more information. Contact the American Association for Chronic Fatigue Syndrome, c/o Harborview Medical Center, 325 Ninth Avenue, Box 359780, Seattle, WA, 98104.

Product availability. Alpha-lipoic acid, acetyl-*L*-carnitine, NADH, Coenzyme Q_{10}, Adapton, DHEA, phenylalanine, and tyrosine are available by phoning (800) 544-4440, or order online at www.lef.org. Ask for availability of Adapton from offshore pharmacies.

CIRRHOSIS

(See Liver Cirrhosis)

COGNITIVE ENHANCEMENT

(See Age-Associated Mental Impairment)

COLITIS (ULCERATIVE)

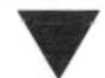

Ulcerative colitis is a chronic disease in which the large intestine becomes inflamed and ulcerated, leading to episodes of bloody diarrhea, abdominal cramps, and fever. Unlike Crohn's disease, ulcerative colitis usually doesn't affect the full thickness of the intestine and never affects the small intestine. The disease usually begins in the rectum or sigmoid colon and spreads partially or completely through the large intestine. The cause of ulcerative colitis is not known, but heredity and an overactive immune response are suspected factors.

Conventional treatment aims to reduce inflammation, reduce symptoms, and replace any lost fluid or nutrients. While symptoms can be alleviated by dietary changes and drug therapies, there are specific nutritional therapies that have been shown to be effective without inducing side effects.

The first part of this protocol is a succinct description of the various conventional and alternative therapies that have been shown in published studies to be useful. At the end, a specific supplement menu is provided that reveals the actual doses required to obtain the beneficial effects.

Fish Oil Studies

Fish oil may be a useful therapeutic agent in the management of colitis. Studies on the use of dietary supplements of fish-oil-derived fatty acids have indicated a beneficial effect on inflammatory bowel disease. Recent studies suggest that marine fish-oil supplements, which are rich in omega-3 fatty acids, may reduce the inflammation associated with ulcerative colitis. Fish oils may exert their anti-inflammatory effects by modulating tissue levels of certain immune factors that promote inflammation. In prospective, randomized, and controlled studies, omega-3 fatty acids have been shown to be therapeutically useful. These studies also show that fish oil reduces the doses needed of toxic steroid drugs.

Butyrate and Mucin Synthesis

Butyrate is the major fatty acid fuel source for the epithelial cells lining the colon, and there is evidence to suggest that butyrate metabolism is impaired in ulcerative colitis. The human *in vitro* model system suggests that topical treatment using sodium butyrate may reverse symptoms in ulcerative colitis. Several reports on the use of butyrate enemas for the treatment of distal ulcerative colitis have appeared. One study showed a striking increase in colon cell mucin synthesis in response to butyrate added to standard nutrient medium. Boosting the rate of mucin synthesis and restoring the colon's mucous lining may explain the therapeutic effect of butyrate in colitis. Butyrate enemas are prescribed by alternative doctors for the treatment of Crohn's disease and colitis.

Butyrate enemas can be ordered from the following pharmacies:

Lloyd Center Pharmacy

(800) 358-8974

The Butyrate Enema Kit includes 2 reusable enema bottles, with 200 ml of concentrated Butyrate, which makes 2800 ml of reconstituted Butyrate (this is a 2-week supply). The patient supplies distilled water. The kit also includes directions.

Key Pharmacy

(800) 878-1322

The Butyrate Enema Kit includes 28 disposable single-use enema bottles with tops, 12 oz of concentrated Butyrate (which when reconstituted is a 2-week supply) a funnel, and a measuring cup. The patient must supply the distilled water. The kit also includes complete directions. Please call for prices.

A prescription from your doctor is needed when ordering butyrate enemas.

Glutamine and Endotoxin Levels

Colitis can enable toxins to be absorbed into the blood from the intestines. The effect of oral glutamine was studied in a guinea pig model of experimentally induced colitis. The mean endotoxin level in the blood of guinea pigs fed a glutamine-enriched elemental diet was 64% lower compared with animals given a standard elemental diet. The scientists concluded that a glutamine-enriched diet may be therapeutically beneficial in patients with inflammatory bowel disease.

The Effects of RNA and Arginine on Ulcerative Ileitis

A study showed that dietary supplementation of RNA and arginine promoted healing of small-bowel ulcers in experimental ulcerative ileitis. Rats with experimental ileitis who received yeast RNA and/or arginine showed a significant decrease in ulcer number compared to controls. The scientists concluded that yeast RNA and/or arginine-supplemented diets accelerated ulcer healing by promoting increased cell proliferation. Additional research has shown that arginine suppresses the growth of some strains of unfavorable bacteria and inhibits bacterial toxin release, a common problem in those suffering from chronic colitis. Other studies, however, contraindicate the use of arginine for some models of colitis. Arginine promotes nitric oxide synthesis, and several studies have found excess nitric oxide production to be detrimental to colitis patients. Most people benefit from the healthy effects of arginine-induced nitric oxide synthesis, but some colitis patients may not.

Soluble Fiber and Colonic Microflora

Fiber is an important physiologic component of the diet. Dietary fiber contains soluble and insoluble substrates. Soluble fiber components are fermented by colonic micro flora, with the resultant production of short-chain fatty acids and gas. Short-chain fatty acids (such as butyric acid) are important fuels not only for colonic mucosa, but also for the small intestine through secondary metabolism to glutamine and ketone bodies. The clinical importance of dietary fiber and its metabolic products on gastrointestinal and nongastrointestinal functions have yet to be fully realized. During the past decade it has become evident that colonic mucosal metabolism is more complex than previously suspected. Luminal short-chain fatty acids are recognized as an essential fuel source for colonocytes, particularly in the distal colon. The histologic, endoscopic, and metabolic observations of ulcerative colitis suggest that a nutritional short-chain fatty acid deficiency (such as butyric acid) may play a role in the pathogenesis of this disorder. This can be confirmed by observations in experimental models of enterocolitis demonstrating enhancement of gut growth and function in response to intestinal nutrients such as glutamine for the small intestine and short-chain fatty acids for the colon.

Since exacerbation of colitis seems to be associated with stress, scientists evaluated the influence of stress on experimental colitis in rats. The results showed that stress may exacerbate experimental colitis in rats. (*Refer to the Anxiety and Stress protocol for information about alleviating the physiological effects of stress.*)

Colitis and Bone Loss

Osteoporosis is a serious complication of inflammatory bowel disease that has not received adequate recognition despite its high prevalence and potentially devastating clinical effects. Data derived from a retrospective survey of 245 patients with inflammatory bowel disease suggest that the prevalence of bone fractures is unexpectedly high, particularly in patients with a long duration of disease, frequent active phases, and high cumulative doses of corticosteroid intake. Recent advances in the diagnosis and management of osteoporosis have facilitated early detection of bone loss and identified means by which this may be prevented. Bone-density measurements to predict fracture risk and define thresholds for prevention and treatment should be performed routinely in patients with inflammatory disease. Those with colitis should consider reducing the risk of incurring a bone fracture. (*See the Osteoporosis protocol.*)

Long-Term Nutritional Deficiencies

Colitis patients often suffer from multiple nutrient deficiencies. Supplementation with a multinutrient formula such as Life Extension Mix could prevent complications of long-term nutritional deficiencies. Studies have shown potential lethal effects caused by colitis-induced nutritional deficiencies. Free radicals have been implicated in the colitis inflammatory process. Vitamin E and selenium are two nutrients that appear to be especially effective in suppressing free radical–generated inflammation.

Folate and Colon Cancer

Two case-control studies have shown that folate may protect against the development of colon cancer caused by ulcerative colitis. The most recent study showed that folate use for at least 6 months reduced the risk of colon cancer by 28% in 98 patients who had ulcerative colitis for at least 8 years. Of the ulcerative colitis patients, 29.6% developed cancerous lesions, indicating the high risk for colon cancer in colitis patients. The greater the dose of supplemental folate consumed, the lower the rate of colon cancer. The scientists concluded that "daily folate supplementation may protect against the development of neoplasia in ulcerative colitis."

Dietary Intake

Colitis patients should avoid raw fruits and vegetables to reduce physical injury to the inflamed lining of the large intestine. A diet free of dairy products may decrease symptoms and is worth trying.

The chief purpose of the gut is to digest and absorb nutrients in order to maintain life. Studies have shown that colitis is often associated with a reduction in pancreatic enzyme secretion. Supplementation with pancreatic enzymes could enable better absorption of many critical nutrients.

Drug Therapy

Successful conventional drug treatments for inflammatory bowel disease include topically active or rapidly metabolized steroids that have fewer long-term side effects than the standard steroid drugs. The cancer chemotherapy drug methotrexate can promote remission in approximately 50% of patients, but is less effective in maintaining remission. Cyclosporin is valuable for treating patients with severe ulcerative colitis but is less valuable for patients with Crohn's disease. In patients with distal colitis, lignocaine appears to be effective.

Nutritional Therapies and Dosage

The major news over the past year, however, is the effect of nutrients, particularly fish oils and glutamine, on gut inflammation and permeability, bacterial translocation, and immune cell profiles. The major nutrients for the large bowel and small bowel mucosa are, respectively, butyrate and glutamine. The use of butyrate enemas, along with yeast-derived RNA, the amino acid glutamine, and fish oil capsules, represent novel nutritional therapies for patients suffering with chronic inflammatory bowel disease.

Here is a protocol of nutritional therapies for the ulcerative colitis patient to consider:

1. Glutamine, four to six 500-mg capsules a day
2. RNA, four to six 500-mg capsules a day
3. Fish Oil, 8 to 10 capsules a day of the MEGA EPA* supplement
4. Life Extension Mix, 3 tablets, 3 times a day (basic multinutrient formula)
5. Life Extension Booster, 1 capsule a day (for extra folate, selenium, and vitamin E)
6. Butyrate enemas, 2 a day are suggested
7. Soluble fiber, 1 to 3 tablespoons a day of the Fiber Food powder supplement
8. Pancreatin, one to two 500-mg capsules right before each meal
9. Follow the recommendations in the *Osteoporosis and the Anxiety and Stress protocols*

*MEGA EPA is a free fatty-acid form of fish oil that is able to be absorbed better than standard MAX EPA supplements. Each MEGA EPA capsule equals more than 2 standard MAX EPA capsules. This is important because some people experience digestive problems with fish oil and are unable to take the dose required to achieve therapeutic results.

For more information. Contact the Crohn's and Colitis Foundation of America (800) 343-3637.

Product availability. Glutamine, RNA, MEGA EPA, butyrate enemas, and the other suggested supplements are available by calling (800) 544-4440, or order online at www.lef.org.

COMMON COLD

Modern medicine can probe the depths of the human brain and successfully transplant limbs, but for the most part, conventional physicians have been hard-pressed to cure the common cold or find a vaccine to prevent it. Why is this the case? The common cold is caused by over 300 serologically distinct viruses belonging to many groups such as rhinoviruses and adenoviruses. Since there are so many different types, it is impossible to develop a single vaccine effective against them all. The influenza vaccine represents a guess on the part of the Centers for Disease Control as to which strain or strains of flu virus will probably be present for the coming season. Usually three are chosen. If the CDC picks the wrong ones, the vaccine will not be effective. One can see the problem for dealing with over 300 potential viruses responsible for the common cold. Additionally, unlike bacteria, which to date still have many antibiotics that are effective against them, the very nature of the biology of viruses has made antiviral agents difficult to produce.

The common cold is spread by airborne droplets from an infected person breathing, coughing, or sneezing. Viruses will generally not stay alive on inanimate objects long enough to be a problem, as on a phone for instance. The droplets must be inhaled. However, when considering any infection, one must keep in mind a number of things. Infection is by no means automatic. Just because a person is exposed to an infection does not mean that an infection will ensue. Infection is dependent on three important aspects; virulence of the organism, inoculation size of the organism, and host resistance.

Virulence refers to the inherent ability of a particular organism to cause infection. Some strains may have a low infectivity rate while others have a higher one. Inoculation size refers to the number of biological agents the host (the person exposed) is exposed to. Host resistance refers to the immunological state of the person exposed. What this means is that if two people are standing side by side when an infected person sneezes directly into their faces and we assume that they both receive the same number of organisms into their airways, it is possible that one or both of them may not get sick. How can this be? One or both of the two people may have a weakened immune system as a result of stress or recent illness, making them more susceptible.

Sadly, most of us are all too familiar with the most common symptoms of the common cold: headache, nasal congestion, watery rhinorrhea (runny nose), sneezing, and a scratchy throat accompanied by general malaise (body aches).

One of the things that physicians find most frustrating in treating patients is the continual demand by patients for antibiotics to treat the common cold. Simply put, viruses do not respond to antibiotics. Taking antibiotics inappropriately only contributes to antibiotic resistance and placing patients at risk for serious disease. The majority of the infections adults have throughout the healthy time of their lives are viral in origin. Having a common cold with congested sinuses is *not* sinusitis. Patients may even have greenish nasal discharge with sinus congestion due to a common cold. Sinusitis is a *bacterial* infection of the sinuses that is very painful and is associated with fever, moderate sinus pressure, and nausea. Only with bacterial sinusitis is an antibiotic necessary.

The same can also be said for a cold associated with a bad cough producing sputum. Usually, this represents a viral infection for which antibiotics are of no use. The only caveat from a clinical perspective is that many physicians will give antibiotics prophylactically to smokers and patients whose immune function may be impaired by other illnesses such as diabetes or asthma.

Treatment

Stress is a factor that can increase susceptibility to the common cold. This was shown in a recent study conducted at Carnegie Mellon University in Pittsburgh and reported in the *Journal of Psychosomatic Medicine*. Researchers measured the severity of respiratory symptoms, mucus production, and interleukin-6 in test subjects injected with influenza A virus. Volunteers who reported greater psychological stress before inoculation, reacted to infection with more intense symptoms, increased mucus production, and higher concentrations of interleukin-6. The same researchers further believe that interleukin-6, a protein produced in the body, may be a biological link between psychological stress and the severity of upper respiratory infections such as cold and flu.

Rest and relaxation while recovering enables the individual to strengthen immune function and enhance detoxification. Avoiding contact with others will help to prevent spreading the infection. While there is no cure for the common cold, there are certain steps that can be taken to relieve symptoms and discomfort.

- ▼ Eating properly may help to shorten duration or make the symptoms less severe.
- ▼ Drink a minimum of eight to ten glasses of fluids a day to avoid dehydration, keep mucous membranes moist, and loosen phlegm.
- ▼ Abstain from alcohol as it reduces the body's ability to fight infection.
- ▼ Avoid smoking and smoky places.
- ▼ To relieve aches and fever, take an aspirin substitute.
- ▼ Use saline-based over-the-counter nose drops to relieve a stuffy nose.
- ▼ To keep nasal passages moist, use a cool-mist humidifier.
- ▼ Certain dietary supplements as described below have been shown to lessen the discomfort and duration of a cold.

Patients often wonder if they should go to work while they are sick. The answer is simple—do what your body tells you to do. If you are sick, tired, and feel that you would be more comfortable at home under the covers resting, that is exactly what you should do. You do not need a doctor to tell you that. Your body communicates exactly what it needs. It is when you resist what your body is telling you and push yourself to work when you should rest that you get into trouble. You can't "catch" a cold from being out in the cold. However, if your body is already under stress, being out in the cold may be the additional stress that lowers your immune threshold to the point that you become ill.

Many over-the-counter cold medications provide far more ingredients than are needed to ease symptoms of the common cold. Physicians generally recommend one-ingredient generic brands over expensive mega formulas that attempt to treat several symptoms at once. A simple cough suppressant or oral decongestant should provide satisfactory relief. If a cold formula is necessary, read packaging information carefully for drug interactions to avoid.

A unique therapy to treat the common cold involves the one-time injection of 500,000 to 3 million IU of interferon (alpha-interferon-2a), combined with 40 mg of melatonin every night. Studies document the ability of interferon to kill many common-cold viruses. Interferon is a component of the immune system that kills viruses (and cancer cells). Since it is a prescription drug, a doctor must prescribe and inject the one-time dose of interferon. (*For additional suggestions, refer to the Immune Enhancement protocol.*) Getting the average family physician to prescribe alpha-interferon for a cold may be difficult. Most physicians are not familiar with it. It is generally used to treat leukemia and hepatitis C among other diseases. Long-term use carries with it certain side effects. However, using alpha-interferon for a few days is generally safe. Those interested in this type of therapy should find a physician who practices complementary medicine. Presenting him or her with this book may make them more open to the idea.

Ribavirin is a broad-spectrum antiviral-approved drug for hepatitis C in the United States. There is evidence that some cold virus strains can be stopped from replicating with ribavirin at a dose of 800 mg a day. It is difficult to purchase because of severe FDA restrictions on its use, even though it is a safe drug to use in the short term.

Vitamin C

Vitamin C in doses of 5,000 to 20,000 mg has been used by many people as a natural antihistamine and antiviral therapy to treat common colds. In 1971, Linus Pauling carried out a meta-analysis of four placebo-controlled trials, concluding that it was highly unlikely that the decrease of common cold symptoms in vitamin C groups was caused by chance alone. Studies carried out since then have found that high doses of vitamin C alleviate common cold symptoms, indicating that the vitamin does indeed have physiologic effects on colds. However, despite the large number of placebo-controlled studies showing that vitamin C supplementation alleviates the symptoms of the common cold, widespread skepticism about vitamin C persists. A cup of hot tea taken one hour before consuming vitamin C and an immune-boosting formula containing thymus may help at the very first sign of a cold.

In a review of six large studies on vitamin C supplementation of 1000 mg a day or less, it was shown that common-cold incidence is not reduced in the low-dose vitamin C-supplemented groups. A further analysis of these studies, however, reveals that some groups do benefit from low-dose vitamin C supplementation. In four studies with British male schoolchildren, a statistically significant reduction in common-cold incidence was found in groups supplemented with low-dose vitamin C. One study showed that those who engaged in heavy exercise were 50% less likely to get a common cold if they took only 600 to 1000 mg a day of vitamin C.

As vitamin C has an individually based maximum dose prior to the development of diarrhea, some complementary physicians give patients with bad colds 50 grams of intravenous vitamin C every other day for 3 treatments. While there may be few studies to date proving efficacy for this treatment, anecdotal clinical experience suggests that it is indeed helpful.

In addition to vitamin C, oxidative therapy with intravenous hydrogen peroxide 0.03%, popularized by Dr. Charles Farr, may be helpful. Ultraviolet blood irradiation may also be helpful as well.

Zinc Gluconate

A randomized, double-blind, placebo-controlled clinical trial has shown that zinc gluconate lozenges produce a significant reduction in the duration of cold symptoms. In this study, patients received zinc lozenges or placebo lozenges every 2 hours for the duration of cold symptoms. The median time to complete resolution of cold symptoms was 4.4 days in the zinc group, compared with 7.6 days in the placebo group.

Another study to test the benefits of zinc gluconate lozenges showed that the time to complete resolution of symptoms was significantly shorter in the zinc group than in the placebo group. The zinc group had significantly fewer days with coughing, headache, hoarseness, nasal congestion, nasal drainage, and sore throat. By dissolving 2 zinc lozenges in the mouth every few hours, the zinc will help inactivate cold viruses multiplying in the throat.

Echinacea

In the past 50 years echinacea has achieved worldwide fame for its antiviral, antifungal, and antibacterial properties. Four to six standardized capsules should be taken at onset and then two capsules every 4 hours thereafter, until symptoms are gone for more than 2 days. Standardized liquid herbal extract is effective at a dose of 6 full droppers followed by 2 full droppers every 2 waking hours until the 2-ounce bottle is empty.

Astragalus

This herb brings support to all deep immune functions and activates cellular immunity. Astragalus herbal extract at 300 mg a day can boost immune function and produce direct antiviral effects.

N-Acetyl-Cysteine (NAC)

The amino acid *N*-acetyl-cysteine (NAC) helps to break up excessive mucus and can have a direct antiviral effect. If you get a cold, it is suggested that 600 mg of *N*-acetyl cysteine be taken with at least 2000 mg of vitamin C 3 times a day.

Sambucol

Sambucol, a standardized elderberry extract, is used as an herbal remedy for colds and flu. Sambucol should be taken in doses of 1 tablespoon 4 times a day.

Ganmaoling

Some physicians have limited clinical experience with a Chinese proprietary drug called Ganmaoling, which is a mixture of the Chinese herbs honeysuckle flower, flower of Indian Dendranthema, leaf of Negundo chostetree, leaf and twig of thin evodia, root of rough-haired holly, menthol, and root of indigowood. The recommendation is to take 4 tablets 3 times daily. For "severe" cases, 8 tablets 3 times daily for 3 to 7 days should be taken.

Can Infection Be Prevented?

As mentioned earlier, the best way to avoid becoming sick is to maintain baseline health. Remember, the one factor that you can control is host (this means you!) immunity. Ganmaoling may help prevent a cold. The recommendation is to take 2 tablets twice daily for 3 days when exposed to someone who has a cold. The immediate use of zinc gluconate lozenges as soon as cold symptoms appear can stop some cold viruses dead in their tracks. Zinc lozenges are cheap and can be kept in the medicine cabinet for easy access.

Signs of a More Serious Infection

Most common colds do not require a visit to the doctor or a prescription medication. However, certain symptoms may indicate that a more serious infection is present. Consult a physician if you experience one or more of the following:

- A sustained fever of 100 degrees or higher for more than 4 days
- Chills and rigors (shakes)
- Facial swelling and/or pain in the ears
- A severe sore throat with a white or yellow coating
- A severe cough with thick discolored mucus; a cough that lasts more than 10 days
- Headache with pain in the face, sensitivity in the upper jaw, yellow or green mucus being expelled from the nose or throat

Summary

1. The best offense is a good defense. Maintain good health, take basic supplementation, and avoid stress.
2. Zinc gluconate lozenges every 2 hours.
3. If a cold has you down—rest, drink fluids, and stay home if that is what your body tells you to do.
4. Vitamin C, as much as can be tolerated every 2 hours daily without causing diarrhea.
5. Echinacea, standardized capsules, 2 to 4 capsules at onset and 1 to 2 capsules every 4 hours; an echinacea tea can be made 4 times a day until symptoms are gone. Echinacea is not for chronic use.
6. Astragalus, 300 mg a day of the standard extract. Some people who are under stress take this indefinitely. Long-term use has not been subjected to study. A tea can be made once a day.
7. If exposed to a cold, consider Ganmaoling, 2 tablets twice a day. If you have a cold, consider Ganmaoling, 4 to 8 tablets, 3 times a day for 5 to 7 days.
8. Consider taking *N*-acetyl-cysteine, 600 mg with 2000 mg vitamin C, 3 times a day.
9. Consider Sambucol, 1 tablespoon 4 times a day.
10. For refractory cold, consider one-half million to 3 million IU of alpha-interferon for 3 days. Those interested in this type of therapy should find a physician who practices complementary medicine.
11. For refractory cold, consider 800 mg of ribavirin a day.
12. For refractory cold or "I don't have the time for this," consider i.v. vitamin C, 50 grams 3 times a week for 1 week. Those interested in this

type of therapy should find a physician who practices complementary medicine.

13. For refractory cold or "I don't have the time for this," consider oxidative therapy. Those interested in this type of therapy should find a physician who practices complementary medicine.
14. For refractory cold or "I don't have the time for this," consider ultraviolet blood irradiation. Those interested in this type of therapy should find a physician who practices complementary medicine.

For more information. For the location and phone number of a physician in your area who specializes in complementary medicine, call the American College for the Advancement of Medicine, (800) 532-3688.

Product availability. Zinc lozenges, NAC, echinacea, astragalus, vitamin C, and melatonin are available by calling (800) 544-4440, or order online at www.lef.org. Ask for a listing of offshore companies that sell ribavirin to Americans by mail. If you live close to the Mexican border, you can buy ribavirin in a Mexican pharmacy and bring it back into the United States under the FDA's personal-use provision. Ganmaoling is available at Chinese and Vietnamese herb shops.

CONGESTIVE HEART FAILURE AND CARDIOMYOPATHY

The American Heart Association estimates that 4.7 million Americans have congestive heart failure (CHF) and that 400,000 new cases will be diagnosed in the coming year. Heart failure is the leading cause for hospitalization in people over the age of 65, and the risk for developing the disease increases with age. The risk for developing heart failure is slightly greater in men than in women. African-Americans are twice as likely to acquire the disease as Caucasians, and mortality from the disease is also twice as great in this group. Since the 1970s, heart failure has been on the increase because the number of people aged 65 or older has grown. Approximately 20% of CHF patients will die within 1 year of diagnosis, and 50% will die within 5 years.

Congestive heart failure occurs when the heart is unable to pump blood throughout the body (but not all patients with heart failure have congestion). There are two categories of congestive heart failure: systolic and diastolic. In the systolic type of the disease, blood coming into the heart from the lungs may be regurgitated so that fluid accumulates in the lungs (*pulmonary congestion*). In the diastolic type, the heart muscle becomes stiff and cannot relax, leading to an accumulation of fluid in the feet, ankles, legs, and abdomen.

Congestive heart failure is in itself not a diagnosis. Rather it is the physiological result of damage to the heart caused by some underlying condition. Therefore, it is not enough to say that a person has congestive heart failure. The CHF has to be due to some underlying process, and that diagnosis is important in terms of treatment and prognosis.

Cardiomyopathy is a condition in which the heart muscle is damaged and no longer functions properly. It is divided into three categories: dilated, hypertrophic, and restricted. Dilated cardiomyopathy, where the heart muscle becomes thin and stretched, may be caused for unknown reasons (idiopathic), by alcoholism, and by endocrine or genetic diseases. Restrictive cardiomyopathy results when some disease process restricts the movement of the heart. This may be caused by amyloidosis, prior heart surgery, and diabetes, for example. Hypertrophic cardiomyopathy, where the heart muscle becomes enlarged and thickened, is due to high blood pressure and failure of the heart's valves.

Risk Factors for Congestive Heart Failure

The most common underlying cause for congestive heart failure is *hypertension* (high blood pressure). The Framingham Heart Study recently reported that high blood pressure increased the risk of developing heart failure about 2 times for men and 3 times for women. A second important risk factor for the disease is diabetes mellitus. The incidence of heart failure among diabetics is three to eight times greater than in the normal population. Other forms of cardiac disease, such as myocardial infarction, valve disease, rheumatic heart disease, and certain types of congenital conditions, also increase the potential for developing heart failure. Secondary risk factors include smoking, obesity, and high cholesterol.

Signs and Symptoms

A number of generalized symptoms are associated with heart failure; they include fatigue, fluid accumulation (*edema*), and persistent coughing. The symptom most associated with the disease is *dyspnea,* or shortness of breath. In particular, the patient may develop orthopnea or cardiac asthma. This is the case when a patient needs several pillows to sleep on to prevent shortness of breath. Another way orthopnea manifests is that the patient may awaken short of breath and go stand up by a window to breathe better. The shortness of breath is positional, caused by positional changes in blood flow. Heart failure generally develops slowly, and the patient is often unaware of the condition until symptoms appear.

Diagnosis of Congestive Heart Failure and Cardiomyopathy

In many cases, the diagnosis of congestive heart failure is made on physical examination. The patient may present with edema, shortness of breath, and fatigue and orthopnea as described above. Risk factors (e.g., hypertension, diabetes etc.) for the disease are evaluated during the examination. A relatively simple procedure for determining the presence of heart failure is the electrocardiogram (ECG). Echocardiograms, which evaluate heart function, may also be ordered by the physician. Chest x-rays can reveal the size and shape of the heart and rule out other causes of the patient's symptoms.

Conventional Treatments for CHF

Although CHF can be treated and improved by therapy, it is important to treat the underlying cause to prevent progression and worsening of symptoms leading to death. The protocols dealing with specific problems such as high blood pressure or vascular disease should be consulted.

Various types of medications are used in the treatment of CHF, each of which has a different function. ACE (angiotensin-converting enzyme) inhibitors and vasodilators expand blood vessels, thereby allowing the heart to function more efficiently. Beta-blockers reduce oxygen demand in the left ventricle, which is often damaged in patients with CHF. Digitalis increases the pumping action of the heart, and diuretics eliminate fluid accumulation. In some cases, successful control of hypertension can eliminate CHF.

One new medication recently approved by the FDA, Carvedilol, was found to be of significant value to patients with mild to moderate CHF when used in conjunction with diuretics, ACE inhibitors, and digoxin. Clinical trials of this medication indicate that hospitalization time for CHF, as well as morbidity and mortality from the disease, was considerably reduced. In the most severe cases of CHF, cardiac transplant may be necessary. A study of conventional medications for the treatment of CHF reported the following percentages of use:

Diuretics, 82%
ACE inhibitors, 53%
Nitrates, 49%
Digoxin, 46%
Potassium, 40%
Aspirin, 36%
Calcium antagonists, 20%
Coumadin (Warfarin), 17%
Beta-blockers, 15%
Magnesium, 10%

CAUTION: Diuretics deplete the body of potassium and magnesium. Patients who are taking diuretics should consult with their physician regarding supplementation of these electrolytes.

In a clinical trial of 111 CHF patients, a left ventricular assist device (LVAD) was implanted in the patients while they awaited transplantation. Five patients implanted with the LVAD prior to transplant were successfully weaned from the device and were no longer in need of the transplant. More importantly, the study indicated that LVADs worked to modify cardiac function and could potentially benefit patients with cardiomyopathy as well. A surgical strategy for congestive heart failure, mitral valve repair, may offer another alternative to transplantation. In this procedure, the mitral valve is strengthened by surgically implanting a small, flexible ring at the valve opening, thereby preventing regurgitation. The results of the study indicated that the procedure could improve exercise tolerance and cardiac function, and decrease heart enlargement.

Natural Treatments for Congestive Heart Failure

Coenzyme Q_{10} is a naturally occurring substance that may have considerable value as an adjunct therapy for the treatment of CHF. Clinical studies indicate that Coenzyme Q_{10} can improve the quality of life, allow for a reduction of other pharmacological agents, and decrease the incidence of cardiac complications from CHF. In those patients who receive little benefit from conventional medications, Coenzyme Q_{10} may be a highly effective form of therapy. One study evaluated the cardiac parameters of 17 CHF patients after a 4-month trial period of Coenzyme Q_{10}. The following results were reported:

- Heart function improved by 20%, and the mean CHF score increased significantly.
- Left ventricular ejection fraction (a measure of the heart's capacity to pump efficiently) improved nearly 35%.
- Cardiac output improved by 15.7%.
- Stroke volume index improved nearly 19%.
- Systolic blood pressure decreased by 4.4%.
- End-diastolic volume area decreased by 8.4%.
- Mean exercise duration improved by 25.4%.
- Cardiac workload improved by 14.3%.

The researchers concluded that Coenzyme Q_{10} was associated with significant functional, clinical, and hemodynamic improvements and that the risk-to-benefit ratio was extremely favorable. Coenzyme Q_{10} exerted a positive influence on the muscular contractility of the myocardium while enhancing vasodilation. Additional clinical trials of Coenzyme Q_{10} conducted in the United States, Great Britain, and Denmark had similar results; there was notable improvement in several cardiac parameters when Coenzyme Q_{10} was used in conjunction with conventional therapies.

Because low magnesium levels are associated with frequent arrhythmias and higher mortality in patients with CHF, patients may benefit from magnesium therapy, which improves hemodynamic function and controls arrhythmias. There is little clinical evidence that magnesium therapy alone will provide substantial improvement in the overall condition of patients with CHF. However, in a recent study at the Arizona Heart Institute, patients with CHF who received oral magnesium oxide showed significant improvement in heart rate, mean arterial pressure, and exercise tolerance.

The use of human growth hormone may be of significant value in the treatment of idiopathic dilated cardiomyopathy (IDC) and CHF. A recent study of seven patients with IDC and moderate to severe CHF evaluated the effects of human growth hormone. The patients were given 14 international units (IU) of growth hormone in conjunction with conventional treatments for 3 months. Use of the hormone was discontinued for an additional 3 months. The results of the study indicated that growth hormone improved cardiac output and clinical symptoms, doubled ventricular mechanical function, and increased exercise capacity. After discontinuation of growth hormone, many of the beneficial effects were partially reversed. A second study had similar results; the researchers concluded that growth hormone, used in addition to conventional therapies, reduced the workload of the myocardium and deactivated the levels of the neurohormone aldosterone. The drawback to the use of human growth hormone in the treatment of CHF and IDC is its cost. For patients who cannot afford this therapy, 6 to 10 grams daily of arginine, an amino acid, may help to improve cardiac output.

The amino acid carnitine may be used in the treatment of IDC. In one study of children with IDC, supplemental doses of *L*-carnitine produced favorable results, in particular, improved left ventricular ejection fraction. There is some indication that *L*-carnitine, used in conjunction with taurine (a derivative of cysteine, an amino acid), Coenzyme Q_{10}, magnesium, chromium, and potassium, may be beneficial in patients with CHF. High intakes of fish oil may also provide some improvement of myocardial workload while reducing blood viscosity and the risk of arrhythmias. Prior to using any adjunctive therapies, patients should consult with their cardiologist regarding potential benefits and risks derived from the use of these therapies.

Chelation therapy may also be beneficial in treating CHF. Chelation increases blood flow, particularly to tiny arterioles.

Summary

Congestive heart failure is a debilitating disease that is the most common cause for hospitalization in patients 65 or older. The risk factors for developing CHF are hypertension, diabetes, and other types of cardiac disease. Cardiomyopathy is a related condition in which the heart muscle is weakened or damaged. CHF and cardiomyopathy cause the heart to work much harder than normal. The goal of the various therapies used in the treatment of these diseases is to decrease the cardiac workload, reduce the risk of arrhythmias, increase cardiac function and hemodynamics, and improve the overall quality of life. Conventional medications used in the treatment of these diseases include diuretics, beta-blockers, antihypertensives, ACE inhibitors, and digoxin, among other medications. Recent studies indicate that Coenzyme Q_{10}, human growth hormone, taurine, magnesium, and *L*-carnitine can be of substantial benefit in the treatment of CHF and IDC when used as adjunctive therapies. Chelation therapy may be beneficial. Patients who do not respond well to medication may benefit from other types of therapy such as LVAD devices and mitral valve surgery. Organ transplantation may be the last option for a number of patients with CHF or cardiomyopathy. Prior to considering any adjunctive therapy, consult with your cardiologist. Here is a review of the treatment options:

1. Coenzyme Q_{10} has proven to be an effective treatment for patients with CHF and cardiomyopathy by improving cardiac workload and contractility of the heart muscle and increasing exercise tolerance. The recommended dosage of Coenzyme Q_{10} is 100 mg, 3 times daily.
2. Carnitine has been shown to benefit patients with IDC (particularly children) by increasing left ventricular function. The recommended dose is 2000 mg a day.
3. Taurine, when used in combination with other therapies, may benefit CHF patients. The daily dosage of taurine is 2000 mg.
4. Growth hormone, when used in conjunction with conventional medications, was proven to increase cardiac output, particularly left ventricular function. The recommended dosage for growth hormone is 1 to 2 IU daily, or as recommended by a cardiologist.
5. In lieu of growth hormone, arginine may provide the same benefits. Daily dosage of arginine is 6 to 10 grams.
6. When used in conjunction with other therapies, magnesium can improve cardiac hemodynamics and reduce the risk of arrhythmia in patients with CHF. The daily dose of magnesium is 1000 mg. Patients may want to consider taking magnesium-rich Life Extension Mix. The recommended dose is 3 tablets, 3 times daily.
7. Fish oil may increase cardiac output and reduce the risk of arrhythmia. The recommended dosage is 5 to 8 capsules a day containing at least 400 mg of EPA and 300 mg of DHA.
8. Consult the protocols relating to the underlying causes of CHF (*e.g. the Hypertension, Diabetes, Atherosclerosis protocols*).
9. Conventional medications for the treatment of CHF and cardiomyopathy include diuretics,

antihypertensive agents, digoxin, ACE inhibitors, beta-blockers, aspirin, and calcium antagonists, among other medications.

10. Cardiac transplantation may be necessary for patients who do not respond to medications.
11. New treatment options include the use of LVAD devices and mitral valve repair.

For more information. Contact the National Heart, Lung, & Blood Institute, (301) 251-1222.

Product availability. Coenzyme Q_{10}, *L*-carnitine, taurine, magnesium, potassium, and high-potency fish oil capsules are available by calling (800) 544-4440, or order online at www.lef.org. Growth hormone must be prescribed by a knowledgeable physician. Contact the American College for the Advancement of Medicine for a physician knowledgeable about chelation and growth hormone at (800) 532-3688.

CONSTIPATION

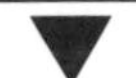

Chronic constipation is the number one gastrointestinal complaint in the United States, particularly among the elderly. Constipation accounts for more than 2.5 million physician visits a year and is among the most frequent reasons for patient self-medication.

The *American Family Physician* journal reported in 1998 that constipation affects as many as 26% of elderly men and 34% of elderly women. Constipation is one of those health problems that has been related to diminished perception of quality of life. The good news is that there are conventional and alternative treatments that can provide immediate relief.

Common Symptoms

Most individuals with uncontrolled constipation develop a variety of symptoms, ranging from large bowel pain, rectal discomfort, abdominal fullness, nausea, anorexia, and a general feeling of malaise. These people feel like they never completely evacuate their bowels. Severe chronic constipation may be accompanied by fecal impaction resulting in severe diarrhea, ulceration of the colon, and intestinal obstruction.

Fiber Is Not the Solution for Most People

Conventional and alternative physicians often recommend fiber supplements to prevent constipation. Yet published studies show that a significant number of chronically constipated people do not find relief from fiber supplements.

An example of fiber not working was a trial that showed that 80% of patients with slow transit and 63% of patients with a disorder of defecation did not respond to dietary fiber treatment. In 85% of patients *without* these disorders, fiber was effective. This study showed that slow gastrointestinal transit and/or a disorder of defecation may explain a poor outcome of dietary fiber therapy in some patients with chronic constipation and why nutritional laxative therapy may be important.

Another example of fiber not working was a trial with 73 consecutive constipated children whose mean fiber intake was the same as in healthy controls, although energy and fluid intakes were lower. The conclusion was that the amount of dietary fibers played no role in chronic constipation. Dietary advice did not change the mean fiber content of the diet. In addition, changes in fiber intakes had no effect on colonic transit time or cure.

Still another study evaluated whether laxatives and fiber therapies improve symptoms and bowel movement frequency in adults with chronic constipation. Fiber and laxatives decreased abdominal pain and improved stool consistency compared with a placebo. The conclusions were that both fiber and laxatives modestly improved bowel movement frequency in adults with chronic constipation. The results of this study showed that there was inadequate evidence to establish whether fiber was superior to laxatives, or if one laxative class was superior to another. Clearly, fiber is not the solution to chronic constipation for many people, despite endless TV commercials and physician recommendations that tout the benefits of fiber.

Aggressive Alternative Therapies

Dietary modifications can help some people, but many people's constipation is caused by insufficient peristalsis, which means there is not enough colon contractile activity to completely evacuate the bowel. However, there are specific nutrients that, if taken at the right time, can induce healthy colon peristaltic action without producing side effects. While pharmaceutical laxatives have been linked to the development of cancer, nutritional laxatives have many health benefits.

Nutrients that induce healthy colon peristalsis work best when taken on an empty stomach. One combination is 4 to 8 grams of vitamin C powder and 1500 mg of magnesium oxide powder taken with the juice of a freshly squeezed grapefruit. A convenient product sold by several vitamin companies is a buffered vitamin C powder product that contains magnesium and potassium salts mixed with ascorbic acid. Depending on the individual, a few teaspoons, or in some cases, 1 to 2 tablespoons of this buffered vitamin C powder produces a powerful but safe laxative effect within 45 minutes. This therapy has to be carefully individually adjusted so it will not cause day-long diarrhea.

Most Americans suffer from a deficiency of magnesium, and the use of a magnesium laxative several times a week could prove beneficial for cardiovascular health. However, chronic use of very high doses (over 3000 mg every day) of magnesium could allow excessive magnesium into the bloodstream, and this could affect kidney function.

Vitamin B_5 (pantothenic acid) in a dose of 2000 to 3000 mg on an empty stomach will produce a rapid evacuation of bowel contents. Vitamin B_5 powder tastes terrible, but there are many health benefits attributed to this vitamin in addition to its ability to stimulate peristalsis.

One way of taking vitamin B_5 and other peristalsis-inducing nutrients is to use a multi-nutrient formula called Powermaker II developed by Durk Pearson and Sandy Shaw and sold by many supplement companies. This decent-tasting powder contains vitamin B_5, vitamin C, choline, and arginine, all of which induce significant peristaltic action when 1 to 2 tablespoons are taken on an empty stomach.

Nutritional laxatives such as magnesium, ascorbic acid, and pantothenic acid are becoming more popular in those afflicted with constipation that is resistant to fiber therapies.

Some Lifestyle Changes That May Help

There are number of factors that can contribute to constipation, including not eating enough fiber, not drinking enough water, not getting enough exercise, improper laxative use, hypercalcemia, inflammatory bowel disorders, neuromuscular disorders (e.g., scleroderma, dermatoamyocytes), and acute diverticulitis. Additionally, taking antacids containing aluminum or calcium as well reactions to taking medications (e.g., painkillers containing codeine, antidepressants, antiparkinsonism drugs, and diuretics) may cause constipation. In many people, anxiety, depression, and grief may also precipitate constipation. Even pregnancy can cause constipation.

Aging itself may increase the incidence of constipation. As a person ages, the colon wall thickens. When this thickening is combined with a lifetime diet low in fiber, constipation can result.

Constipation can also contribute to loss of bladder control by weakening the pelvic floor muscles due to straining. A full bowel pressing on the bladder and causing it to empty prematurely or blocking the outflow of urine is another common effect of constipation. People with bladder control problems often don't drink enough for fear of wetting, which can result in constipation, causing further discomfort and anxiety.

Diet can have a significant effect on constipation. People may become constipated if they start eating fewer vegetables, fruits, and whole grains. Eating more high-fat meats, dairy products, and eggs can be another cause of constipation. So can eating more rich desserts and other sweets high in refined sugars.

Unfortunately, many elderly people who live alone may lose interest in cooking and eating. As a result they start using a lot of convenience foods. These foods tend to be low in fiber, so they may contribute to constipation. In addition, bad teeth may cause older people to choose soft, processed foods that contain little, if any, fiber.

People sometimes do not drink enough fluids, especially if they are not eating regular meals. Water and other liquids add bulk to stools, making bowel movements easier.

Despite all of the above known causes, many people suffer chronic constipation because of a sluggish bowel (insufficient peristalsis) and need to follow aggressive interventions to properly evacuate their colon on a regular basis.

What the Europeans Are Doing

The most popular digestive aid sold in Europe is called Digest RC. This product was introduced in Europe over 45 years ago, and today over 100 million doses of the product are sold annually, primarily in Eastern Europe.

The mechanism of action of the formula is to stimulate peristalsis of the intestines, speed digestion of fats, and prevent stagnation of food in the digestive tract. The benefits the user finds are a reduction in esophageal acid reflux, alleviation of the feeling of fullness and bloating after eating, decreased digestive tract tension, alkalinization of the gastric content, constipation relief, and normalized elimination.

Black radish juice extract is the primary active ingredient in Digest RC. Virtually unknown in the United States, the radish contains a variety of chemicals that increase the flow of digestive juices. The most important function of black radish extract is that it encourages the liver to produce fat- and protein-digesting bile and lowers the tension of the bile ducts. It also improves peristaltic movement. Constipation is another problem to benefit from radish consumption. Rich in fiber and digestive stimulants, regular consumption of radishes helps regulate the bowels. Since dehydration is a major cause of constipation, radishes help hydrate and lubricate the intestines and encourage relaxed bowel movements. The root juice extract of the black radish used in Digest RC is the most potent part of the plant.

The charcoal in Digest RC is particularly useful in absorbing toxins. It is used in emergency departments to treat drug overdoses. It also calms a stressed digestive system, allowing digestive enzymes to be produced and released. Indigestion and nervous vomiting are also treated with this ingredient. The charcoal in Digest RC is actually a special herbal preparation of linden tree bark, traditionally used in Europe as a digestive aid. This special preparation has antibacterial properties, which when used as directed helps balance the digestive tract and supports the creation of the proper intestinal flora. At the same time, it creates an inhospitable environment for parasitic infestation.

Another key ingredient in Digest RC is cholic acid, or pure processed ox bile, a liver enzyme used for digestion. It is particularly helpful in digesting fats and meat protein.

Independent clinical research was conducted on Digest RC to analyze the therapeutic effectiveness of the product among patients with chronic digestive problems. Results showed statistically significant improvement in patients' symptoms during treatment. Digest RC was most successful in eliminating the most frequently occurring symptoms, such as gas, in over 95% of the cases. Symptoms such as constipation, intestinal pains and cramps, heartburn (reflux), and stomach pains and cramps, were helped or completely eliminated in over 90% of the cases. Bloating ceased in over 80%, diarrhea in about 75%, and nausea and vomiting in approximately 65% of the cases. Digest RC was found to minimize the assimilation of undigested toxic products, which often stay in the gut for a prolonged period of time. Due to its cholepoietic and cholagogic abilities, Digest RC was particularly effective in preventing stagnasis of food and bloating in those patients whose diet was rich in animal protein and fat. As there are no specific contraindications, Digest RC can be taken together with any medication and can be taken by patients suffering from different respiratory, cardiovascular, and musculoskeletal disorders. The only people who should avoid Digest RC are those with biliary tract obstruction or gall bladder disease because of the bile-stimulating effects of the black radish and artichoke extracts. It is not known how this product would affect those who have had their gall bladder removed. The suggested dose is 2 to 3 tablets of Digest RC with every heavy meal for the first 2 to 3 weeks. The dose may then be reduced as symptoms of digestion discomfort are alleviated.

Additional Suggestions

As previously discussed, fiber supplements frequently fail to correct chronic constipation. However, one fiber that may work when all others fail is chitosan. Chitosan is a fiber composed of chitin, which is a component of the shell of shellfish and is used for weight and cholesterol reduction. Chitosan has been reported in research conducted in Helsinki, Finland, "to make the feces softer and smoother, which made defecation easier" (*ARS Medicina,* (Helsinki), 1994 Aug.–Oct.). If you're not getting results with other commonly used fiber, we suggest you try six 500-mg capsules of chitosan along with 1000 mg of vitamin C before each meal. Chitosan requires ascorbic acid to become soluble in the gut.

A trial on functional constipation in children showed that most children with fecal incontinence benefit from a strict treatment plan that includes defecation trials, a fiber-rich diet, and laxative medications. Surgery followed by medical treatment was required in patients with Hirschsprung's disease (congenital colon defect) and in some patients with anal stenosis (narrowing).

Chronic constipation can be a disabling condition that may require removal of part or all of the colon (colectomy). However, one study showed fiber, cathartic laxatives, or biofeedback therapy to be successful in 65% of patients. Among the remaining patients, two thirds underwent surgery, of which 83% were successful.

Laxative use was significantly reduced in a long-term care facility when an interdisciplinary program based on a philosophy of prevention and health promotion was implemented. Specifically, increased fluid and fiber intake, timely toileting habits, and regular activity or exercise led to a 50% reduction in the number of patients receiving laxatives as required, relative to preprogram levels and a control unit not receiving the program.

Constipation is a problem frequently encountered during pregnancy, as is excessive weight gain. Treatments commonly used to control constipation are endowed with some drawbacks and often do not help control weight. However, a preparation of lactulose and glucomannan was shown to be effective and well-tolerated in patients with constipation and was also shown to be effective in controlling excessive food intakes. Fifty pregnant females with constipation were treated with a preparation of glucomannan (3 to 6 grams) and lactulose (8 to 16 grams) twice a day for 1 to 3 months. This preparation resulted in a return to normal frequency of weekly number of evacuations and a parallel control of weight gain.

It is common for constipation to occur following severe spinal cord injury. One study suggested that increasing dietary fiber in spinal cord injury patients does not have the same effect on bowel function as has been previously demonstrated in individuals with "normally functioning" bowels. Indeed, the effect may be the opposite to that desired. As had been seen in previous studies, fiber will work only in certain people suffering from constipation.

Drug Therapies

Some constipated people benefit from prescription drugs. A drug called Propulsid promotes upper gastrointestinal peristalsis that often results in quicker lower bowel evacuation. Recent reports of deaths occurring when Propulsid was combined with certain cardiovascular drugs make the use of this medicine risky.

A new drug called Procalopride was shown to help relieve chronic constipation. A report of a clinical study using Procalopride was published in the June 1999 *Digestive Diseases Journal.* Researchers reported on a 253-patient double-blind, placebo-controlled evaluation of Procalopride that showed that over a 12-week period, patients treated with Procalopride had more frequent stools of improved consistency and less severity of constipation versus placebo. A majority of the patients in the study were women with chronic constipation that didn't improve with fiber or laxatives. Side effects from long-term use of this drug are not known.

Some Conventional Therapies

Doctors often recommend fiber supplements (bulk producers) to prevent constipation. Also recommended are more fresh fruits and vegetables, either cooked or raw, and more whole grain cereals and breads. Dried fruit such as apricots, prunes, and figs are especially high in fiber. Drink plenty of liquids (1 to 2 quarts daily), unless you have heart, blood vessel, or kidney problems. Be aware that some people become constipated from drinking large amounts of milk.

Some doctors suggest adding small amounts of unprocessed bran ("miller's bran") to baked goods, cereals, and fruit. Some people suffer from bloating and gas for several weeks after adding bran to their diets. Make diet changes slowly to allow the digestive system to adapt. Remember, if your diet is well balanced and contains a variety of foods high in natural fiber, it may not be necessary to add bran to other foods.

Other therapies may include

- **Bulk producers**—As mentioned above, bulk producers are natural or semisynthetic polysaccharide and cellulose, which hold water, soften the stool, and increase the occurrence of the passage of a stool. They are the most physiologic of the laxatives. Generally recommended for managing irritable bowel syndrome. Results occur within 12 to 24 hours (may be delayed up to 72 hours).
- **Saline laxatives**—These compounds attract water into the lumen of the intestines. The fluid buildup alters the stool consistency, expands the bowel, and encourages peristaltic movement. Used mostly as a bowel preparation to clear the bowels for rectal or bowel examinations. Results occur rapidly (within 0.5 to 3 hours).
- **Stimulant laxatives**—These increase motor activity of the bowels by direct action on the intestines. Used to evacuate the bowel for rectal or bowel examinations. Most of these laxatives act on the colon, but castor oil acts on the small intestine. Results occur in 6 to 10 hours.
- **Lubricant laxatives**—These lubricate intestinal mucosa and soften stools. Used prophylactically to prevent straining in patients for whom it would be dangerous to strain. Generally, mineral oil is recommended: 5 to 30 cc at bedtime—results vary.
- **Fecal softeners**—These promote water retention in the fecal mass, thus softening the stool. Generally used to prevent straining. Most beneficial when stool is hard. However, it may require 3 days before results are experienced. Stool softeners and emollient laxatives have limited use because of their resorption of water from the forming stool. Fecal softeners should not be used exclusively, but may be useful given in combination with stimulant laxatives.
- **Lactulose**—This synthetic material passes to the colon undigested. Used to clear the bowel with minimal water and sodium loss or gain. When it is broken down in the colon, it produces lactic acid, formic acid, acetic acid, and carbon dioxide. These products increase the amount of water in the stool, which softens the stool and increases the frequency. Results generally occur in 24 to 48 hours.
- **Golytely**—This electrolyte solution used to clear the bowel with minimal water and sodium loss or gain. Good for elderly patients with congestive heart failure or renal disease.

Source for these conventional therapies: National Cancer Institute, 1999.

Summary

Constipation is a universal affliction of Western civilization. Americans spend more than $725 million annually on over-the-counter (OTC) laxatives in an attempt to self-treat the most common gastrointestinal complaint in the country. There are alternative therapies that are safer and more effective than conventional laxatives and work better for more people than fiber supplements.

For relieving *acute* constipation, *one* of the following techniques may be tried to induce peristaltic action within 45 to 60 minutes:

1. Mix 4000 to 8000 mg of ascorbic acid powder with 1500 mg of magnesium oxide powder and take with juice of fresh squeezed grapefruit or orange juice. Should be taken on an empty stomach.
2. Mix 1 to 6 teaspoons of a "buffered vitamin C powder" that contains magnesium and potassium salts along with ascorbic acid (vitamin C). This should be taken on an empty stomach using room-temperature water.

3. Mix 1 to 2 tablespoons of Power Maker II Sugar-Free Powder in water or juice and take on an empty stomach.
4. Take 2000 to 3000 mg of pantothenic acid (vitamin B_5) powder on an empty stomach. Pantothenic acid powder does not taste good.

Note that drinking several cups of green tea will enhance the bowel evacuating effects of any one of the above four suggestions. Drinking green tea late in the day may cause insomnia. Those with gastritis or stomach ulcers may not be able to tolerate these aggressive peristalsis-inducing approaches.

For relieving *chronic* constipation, one or all of the following may be used:

1. Chitosan: take six 1000-mg capsules of chitosan before each meal with one 1000-mg capsule of vitamin C.
2. Digest RC: take 2 to 3 tablets with every meal that contains fat or protein for 3 weeks. Dosage may be reduced after symptomatic relief occurs.
3. Soluble fibers: take 6 to 15 grams of a soluble fiber blend that contains guar gum, apple and/or citrus pectin, and psyllium seed husk.
4. Follow the diet and lifestyle changes discussed in this protocol.

Refer to the *Digestive Disorders protocol* for additional information.

For more information. Contact the Consumer Nutrition Hotline of the National Center for Nutrition and Dietetics, (800) 366-1655.

Product availability. You can order pure ascorbic acid powder, magnesium oxide powder, buffered vitamin C or vitamin B_5 powder, Power Maker II Sugar-Free Powder, chitosan capsules, Digest RC, or soluble fiber blends by calling (800) 544-4440, or order online at www.lef.org.

CROHN'S DISEASE

Crohn's disease is a chronic disorder of the intestines. Of unknown etiology, the gastrointestinal tract in persons suffering from this disease becomes inflamed and weak, making digestion difficult and leading to general physical debility. It is a relatively rare disease, occurring in approximately 1 to 5 people out of every 10,000. The symptoms are similar to ulcerative colitis, and they are both categorized as inflammatory bowel diseases; to distinguish between them, your doctor may need to examine a sample of intestinal tissue.

Crohn's disease can attack any part of your intestines from the mouth to the anus, but most commonly it strikes the ileum (lower portion of the small intestine) or the colon (large intestine). Ulcers form on the inner intestinal lining and eventually spread through the intestinal wall. As the affected part of the intestine becomes scarred and thick, the passage narrows, disrupting nutrient absorption and normal bowel function.

Symptoms and Diagnosis

Crohn's disease is typically diagnosed among people in their 20s and 30s, but the disease can also occur in infants and children. More common in women than in men, it is rare in people of Asian or African descent who live outside the United States. The disease is a lifelong ailment that can be controlled, but at present there is no cure or even a definitive cause. Crohn's patients usually experience excruciatingly painful attacks of abdominal pain and diarrhea followed by weeks, months, or years of remission.

A common complication of Crohn's disease is the development of abscesses or fistulas, which are tubes that form a connection between two organs and allow passage of fluid and stool. This can happen between the intestinal loops, the intestines, and the bladder or the intestines and the skin. They often occur near the anus. Surgery may be required to close the fistulas. Some Crohn's patients have a tendency to also manifest nonintestinal disorders, such as inflammation of the eye; skin eruptions or rashes; kidney stones; or arthritis in the knees, ankles, and wrists. People who have had Crohn's for 10 years or more are at risk of developing colorectal cancer. Therefore, if you have Crohn's disease and are over 30, you should get regular checkups.

The following are the most prevalent symptoms of this difficult disease:

- Severe abdominal pain and diarrhea that is occasionally mixed with blood. Unlike ulcerative colitis, in which patients may have episodes of diarrhea as often as 10 to 15 times a day, people with Crohn's may have fewer episodes, though each episode may be extraordinarily painful. However, as with many other elements of this disease, it is difficult to make sweeping generalizations.
- Cramps or pain after eating, especially in the lower right side of the abdomen.
- Chronic low-grade fever, loss of appetite, fatigue or weight loss, especially if accompanied by persistent nausea and vomiting.
- Arthritis flareups in the arms or legs, with the symptoms above.
- In young children, any of the symptoms above, plus failure to thrive; in older children, failure to grow at a normal rate.
- Anemia.

The actual cause of Crohn's disease is unknown, but it may be an autoimmune disorder. The inflammation apparently occurs when the body's own immune system—for reasons not yet understood—attacks a part of the intestine. Some scientists are studying whether a virus causes Crohn's, but no specific viral agent has been identified.

Crohn's disease can usually be diagnosed from a variety of methods. It is difficult, in some cases, to distinguish this disease from ulcerative colitis; therefore doctors may employ more than one diagnostic method. Common diagnostic tools include:

- X-rays of the large and small intestines.
- Sigmoidoscopy.
- Colonoscopy, which will usually include tissue biopsy.
- Barium enema.

Once diagnosed, routine tests of liver function, blood iron levels, and other blood work may be ordered, depending also on treatment being offered, in order to ensure other problems are not interfering with the healing process.

Conventional Treatments

At present, Crohn's disease is not curable. Medical treatment typically involves a three-pronged approach to controlling the disease—depending on the severity of the symptoms. Drug therapy and a restricted diet are first explored, then hospital treatment if necessary. The last resort is surgery.

Because there is no cure for this disorder, Crohn's patients and their doctors try to keep patients free from attacks for as long as possible. If that is not possible in cases of active disease, remission is sought as quickly as possible. Some patients take maintenance medications even when the symptoms are not present. Children with Crohn's disease may need high-protein, high-calorie liquid supplements to keep their growth on track, as this is a particularly devastating disease in youths.

Aminosalicylates, such as sulfasalazine, mesalamine, Asacol, Pentasa, and Rowasa, are intestinal anti-inflammatory agents that are the cornerstone of conventional medical treatment. They may be prescribed for years at a stretch and are given in varying dosages depending on the severity of the symptoms. Many people find they have an allergy to the aminosalicylates, sometimes manifested as vomiting and headaches or even more severe symptoms. If, when a patient starts taking these medications, new symptoms of this sort appear, it is important to keep the doctor advised.

In cases of active disease, steroids such as prednisone are often prescribed with aminosalicylates or alone to reduce the inflammation of the intestines. This represents its own difficulties because of potentially severe side effects. These side effects can include

- Cushing's syndrome.
- Steroid myopathy.
- Hair loss.
- Weight gain.
- Suppressed immune system and the accompanying risks.

Steroids are often used during the acute stage to help get symptoms under control. Then they are slowly tapered, leaving the aminosalicylates for maintenance therapy. Tapering represents a critical time during disease treatment as many patients find themselves precariously trying to keep themselves in remission while weaning from the steroids.

To reduce the need for steroids, an immunosuppressant such as azathioprine, 6-mercaptopurine, or cyclosporine may be substituted. Chemotherapy agents and organ transplant antirejection drugs are sometimes used. Again, all these medications contain their own dangerous side effects, and treatment coordinated with the patient's doctor must be well thought out and communicated effectively. Patients may also take an antidiarrheal agent for mild bouts of diarrhea, as well as antispasmodics for cramping. In cases where patients suffer from arthritis-like symptoms, anti-arthritis medications may also be taken. In cases of severe disease, patients are often put on a bland, well-balanced diet.

If patients become severely ill with diarrhea and weight loss, intravenous (i.v.) feedings in a hospital can allow the intestines to rest. Total parenteral nutrition (TPN) is also used. After stabilization, some patients may need i.v. feedings at home with the help of a visiting nurse.

If the disease does not respond to drugs and diet, doctors may recommend surgery. Because Crohn's disease can affect the entire intestinal tract from the mouth to the anus, surgery only removes the severely inflamed part of the intestine. The goal of surgery is to preserve as much of the intestine as possible. This commonly involves the colon or small intestine. Occasionally, the end of the intestine left in place needs to be brought to the skin's surface. If it is the small intestine that's involved, it is called an ileostomy. If it involves the colon, it's called a colostomy. Although the disease may recur after surgery, the symptoms are likely to be less severe and less debilitating than before. However, when the disease does recur, it usually does so at the area where the last surgery was done.

Nutrition, Diet, and Vitamin Supplementation

Because most medications for Crohn's disease have an abundance of side effects, many patients understandably focus on nutrition and diet as a means of staving off active disease or helping to induce remission. To that end, omega-3 fatty acids from fish and flaxseed oils are said to help reduce inflammation. Flavonoids such as quercetin may also reduce inflammation.

Once active disease states occur, patients must carefully guard against dehydration and vitamin and mineral deficiency. For instance, a recent Scandinavian study noted selenium deficiency in inflammatory bowel patients. Selenium supplements might therefore be beneficial in correcting this deficiency.

A 1998 German study examined deficiencies of vitamins and trace elements in patients with inflammatory bowel disease. The records from 392 outpatients—279 with Crohn's disease and 113 with ulcerative colitis—were analyzed. Deficiencies were found in 85% of patients with Crohn's disease, predominantly deficiencies of iron and calcium. Less frequently, deficiencies of zinc, protein, cyanocobalamin, and folic acid were found. Given this broad cross section of deficiencies, a basic multivitamin nutrient supplement may be helpful to stave off secondary weakness and complications from such deficiencies. Note that calcium deficiency, in particular, carries with it a risk of osteoporosis.

Men with Crohn's disease are at risk of osteoporosis, but the factors contributing to low bone-mineral density and its optimum treatment have not been established. Researchers in Britain investigated levels of sex hormones on men with Crohn's disease to determine their influence on bone metabolism. Bone density was measured by dual energy x-ray absorptiometry at the hip and lumbar spine in 48 men with Crohn's disease.

Total serum testosterone and gonadotrophins were measured in all subjects, and the free androgen index was calculated in men with low or borderline total testosterone. Serum osteocalcin, procollagen carboxy-terminal peptide, bone-specific alkaline-phosphatase, and urinary deoxypyridinoline were measured as markers of bone turnover. The results showed that 8 (17%) men had osteoporosis, and a further 14 (29%) had osteopenia. Three (6%) men had a low free-androgen index and normal gonadotrophins consistent with secondary hypogonadism, and two of these had osteopenia of the hip and spine. Age ($p = 0.002$) and small-bowel Crohn's disease ($p = 0.02$) were the only independent predictors of serum testosterone. There was a significant association between total testosterone and osteocalcin ($r = 0.53$, 95% CT: 0.290.71, $p = 0.0001$) which was independent of age and current steroid use ($p = 0.0001$). The researchers concluded that undiagnosed hypogonadism is an uncommon cause of low bone density in men with Crohn's disease. The independent association between testosterone and the bone-formation marker osteocalcin suggests sex-hormone status influences bone metabolism in men with Crohn's disease. The results further suggest that testosterone replacement might be effective treatment for some men with osteoporosis and Crohn's disease.

A 1998 *Japanese Pharmacology and Therapeutics* study examined the use of barley foodstuff (GBF) derived from the aleurone layer, scutellum, and germ of germinated barley, containing a large quantity of glutamine-rich protein and fermentable dietary fibers, especially hemicellulose. The study sought to verify the effect of GBF on diarrhea in humans and animals and concluded that GBF did increase stool bulk, thereby reducing frequency and quantity of diarrhea. This would point to the use of fiber supplements, particularly barley.

Another study, published in *Digestive Diseases and Sciences,* concluded that rats who followed a diet supplemented with yeast-RNA and arginine showed a significant improvement in ulcer healing.

There is no evidence that food allergies cause Crohn's, but food sensitivities may add to the irritation of the colon. To check for sensitivities, avoid a suspected food for 10 to 30 days, then reintroduce it into the diet. If a reaction occurs, eliminate the food from your diet. Common allergens are dairy products, eggs, and wheat. Nutrition and intestinal function are, by their very relationship, intimately connected. A published Scandinavian study suggests that fiber, starches, glutamine, and fish oils may all help Crohn's patients with issues of malnutrition.

Butyrate

A recent Irish study published in Diseases of the Colon and Rectum examined mucosal metabolism of butyrate impaired in ulcerative colitis. The study sought to confirm if a similar change occurs in Crohn's colitis and to establish whether a panenteric disorder of butyrate metabolism exists in either condition. The results indicated that in the colon, the mucosal metabolic fluxes of both butyrate and glutamine are reduced in both ulcerative colitis and Crohn's colitis compared with healthy controls. Therefore some patients may want to try butyrate enemas as an alternative treatment.

Summary

Crohn's disease is a debilitating disease of unknown etiology that attacks the gastrointestinal tract, making digestion difficult and leading to a wide variety of physical problems. It is a lifelong, incurable disease that may move in and out of remission in patients. It presents with multiple complications, both from the disease process itself and the medications taken for it, which do not cure the disease, but may induce remission.

Some Crohn's patients have a tendency to also manifest nonintestinal disorders, such as inflammation of the eye, skin eruptions or rashes, kidney stones, or arthritis in the knees, ankles, and wrists. People who have had Crohn's for 10 years or more are at risk of developing colorectal cancer. The most prevalent symptoms of this difficult disease include weight loss, severe abdominal pain, diarrhea, bleeding, anemia, low-grade fever, cramping, fatigue, arthritis, and failure to thrive in children.

The following is a nutritional protocol for Crohn's disease patients to consider:

1. Glutamine, four to six 500-mg capsules a day.
2. RNA, four to six 500-mg capsules a day.
3. Fish oil, 8 to 10 capsules of the Mega EPA supplement.
4. Life Extension Mix, 3 tablets, 3 times a day to restore depleted vitamins and trace minerals.
5. Life Extension Booster, 1 capsule a day (for extra selenium, folate, and vitamin E).
6. Butyrate enemas, 2 a day.
7. Soluble fiber, 2 to 3 tablespoons a day of Fiber Food supplement.
8. Barley foodstuffs to increase stool bulk.

(Refer to the Colitis (Ulcerative) protocol for additional information.)

For more information. Contact the Crohn's and Colitis Foundation of America, (800) 343-3637.

Product availability. *L*-glutamine, RNA, Mega EPA, Life Extension Mix, Life Extension Booster, and Fiber Food can be obtained by phoning (800) 544-4444, or order online at www.lef.org.

DEAFNESS

▼

(See Hearing Loss protocol.)

DEPRESSION

▼

Depression is a serious problem with a biochemical basis. It results from an upset in the delicate balance of brain chemicals that regulate mood. Depression is a "whole body" disease that skews the way we think and behave, often damaging our physical health as well as our emotional state. It's a powerful disease that can leave us debilitated, unable to work, maintain relationships, or deal with other responsibilities.

Who is Affected?

Depression is an "equal opportunity" disease, striking all ages and races, both sexes, and people in all socioeconomic groups:

- Each year more than 10 million Americans are hit by depression.
- One in five women will suffer from major depression at some time in her life, as will 1 in 15 men.
- If you have just one episode of major depression, there's a 50/50 chance you'll have more, perhaps as many as one or two a year.
- Millions of depression cases are never diagnosed or treated.
- Untreated, major depression may last for 6 months to a year, becoming more frequent and severe.
- Depression costs our society an estimated $44 billion a year, including
- $24.2 billion for lowered productivity and absenteeism at work and $12.3 billion for medical and psychiatric care.
- More than 18,000 people commit suicide each year, partly or completely as a result of depression, costing us $7.5 billion.

Depression is one of the most commonly misdiagnosed problems. Many doctors treat the obvious symptoms of depression, such as poor appetite, insomnia, and headaches, but overlook the real problem. Untreated, depression can become more frequent and severe, leading to physical and emotional suffering, loss of job and relationships, even to suicide.

What is Depression?

Medical textbooks describe depression as a mood disorder, lasting at least 2 weeks, that produces exaggerated, inappropriate feelings of sadness, worthlessness, emptiness, and dejection.

"Exaggerated" and "inappropriate" are two important words to keep in mind. To feel upset because of a job layoff, a broken marriage, a bankruptcy, or the loss of a loved one is a perfectly normal response to an unhappy event. Generally, our upset feelings are proportional to our loss, and this "reactive depression," as doctors call it, goes away with time.

But endogenous, or major depression often strikes for no apparent reason. It doesn't seem to be caused by outside events, such as the loss of a job. Instead, the black mood grows and grips from within. This crippling darkness can last for weeks, months, or years, and may make it impossible for us to carry on our normal lives. The many and varied symptoms of endogenous depression may include:

- ▼ Profound, persistent sadness.
- ▼ Profound, persistent irritability.
- ▼ Unexplained crying.
- ▼ Loss of self-esteem.
- ▼ Feelings of hopelessness.
- ▼ Feelings of pessimism.
- ▼ Feelings of helplessness.
- ▼ Feelings of worthlessness.
- ▼ Feelings of guilt.
- ▼ Feelings of emptiness.
- ▼ Continually mulling over the past, reviewing the errors you've made.
- ▼ Changes in sleeping patterns.
- ▼ Changes in eating habits.
- ▼ Unexplained weight gain or loss.
- ▼ Restlessness.
- ▼ Fatigue.
- ▼ A "slow down" in physical movements.
- ▼ Inability to concentrate.
- ▼ Memory difficulties.
- ▼ Difficulty making decisions.
- ▼ Loss of interest in usually pleasurable activities.
- ▼ Loss of interest in sex.
- ▼ Unexplained headaches, stomach upset, or other physical problems that are not helped with standard treatment.
- ▼ Thoughts of suicide or death.
- ▼ Suicide attempts.

The symptoms may come in any combination. They can build gradually or strike hard and fast. Some of the symptoms may manifest as either too much or too little of the same thing. Mildly depressed people, for example, may gain weight as they seek comfort in favorite foods, and those suffering from more profound depression may lose weight as their appetites are deadened by sadness. Sleep patterns also may be affected this way. Some depressed people have difficulty falling or staying asleep, while others sleep more than usual but awaken feeling tired.

What Causes Depression?

Although we're only beginning to pull back the curtains that hide the inner workings of the human brain, we do know that several neurotransmitters (chemical messengers), including norepinephrine and serotonin, help to regulate our moods and keep us happy. Depressed people tend to have lower levels of norepinephrine and serotonin. If, for any reason, the amounts of these key neurotransmitters drop below critical levels, the result may be an endogenous depression that seems to come from nowhere, linger forever, sap our energy, and ruin our lives.

Why do brain levels of mood regulators fall in some people but not in others? We can't fully answer that question, although we know that genetics plays a major role. Depression, like other mood disorders, tends to run in families. Depression is even more likely to be shared by identical twins: if one is depressed, there's a better than 50% chance that the other will be, too.

A great deal of research has looked into possible environmental or psychological causes of depression. Some investigators believe that people who are pessimistic, often feel overwhelmed by life, or have low self-esteem are more likely to suffer from depression. It may be that some of us are lucky enough to have large reserves of "happy" neurotransmitters in our brains, but others have just enough to barely keep a smile on their faces.

Although biochemistry is the biggest factor in major depression, we're also affected by what happens to us in our lives. We're all hit by unpleasant events that may cause brain levels of norepinephrine and dopamine to fall temporarily. People with naturally large reserves usually get through the troubling times with minimal difficulties, but those with low chemical levels to begin with are more likely to fall into a depression.

Women, moreover, seem to suffer more from depression than men. Some researchers argue that this disparity is caused by gender hormonal differences; others suggest that the difference is due to socialization. Girls in our society are taught to monitor their feelings and to ask for help when they are troubled. Boys, on the other hand, are encouraged to ignore their feelings. It may be that men and women are equally likely to become depressed, but that men are more reluctant to admit that they are down. In any case, it seems clear that biochemistry is the major cause of endogenous depression, with psychology and hormones playing supporting roles.

How Doctors Treat Depression

Depression is a big business, supporting legions of physicians, psychiatrists, psychologists, social workers, and other health professionals. The therapies they offer are numerous, but basically boil down to three types: electroconvulsive shock therapy, "talking therapy," and drugs, administered individually or in combination.

Although not as gruesome as it is has seemed in movies, electroconvulsive therapy (ECT) is not a pleasant experience. Electricity shot though the brain can sideline a bout of depression, but it is only a temporary measure. It does not cure the disease, and often it destroys parts of the memory.

Also ineffective at curing the underlying biochemical upset that causes endogenous depression are various forms of talking therapy, including behavioral therapy, cognitive therapy, and psychodynamic therapy. Psychologists have not been able to determine which therapy works best for which patients, or why. Such therapies are wonderful tools that have helped many people, but they are not the answer to achieving a cure. Perhaps that's why so many depression victims turn to pills.

In the 1950s, doctors used stimulants, such as amphetamines, to treat depression. But side effects of those drugs include nervousness, increased blood pressure, rapid heartbeat, and irregular heart rhythms. Sometimes sedative antidepressant drugs were used to put patients to sleep for days at a time.

In the 1960s, doctors started using lithium to treat manic depression. The 1960s also marked the advent of iproniazide, the first really effective antidepressant. The drug's antidepressant actions were discovered accidentally after doctors noted that tuberculosis patients taking a similar drug (isoniazide) seemed to become happier.

Commonly Used Prescription Medications

Today, physicians and psychiatrists have numerous drugs at their disposal. Tricyclic antidepressants (TCAs) include Tofranil (imipramine) and Elavil (amitriptyline). Called tricyclics because of their three-ringed chemical structure, they work by altering the way the brain responds to norepinephrine and serotonin. Hundreds of clinical studies involving tricyclic antidepressants have produced only moderate results. In only about 60% of these tests have the tricyclics proved to be more effective than placebos such as sugar pills.

Monoamine oxidase inhibitors (MAOIs), such as Nardil (phenelzine) and Parnate (tranylcypromine), act as "shields" to norepinephrine and dopamine, preventing their breakdown by enzymes. But MAOIs can have serious side effects if mixed with certain foods.

Selective serotonin reuptake inhibitors (SSRIs) include Zoloft (sertraline), Paxil (paroxetine), and Prozac (fluoxetine), one of the most widely prescribed of all drugs today. SSRIs enhance or increase serotonin levels by preventing the hormone from being reabsorbed and "taken out of circulation."

These powerful medications have helped many people to regain their sense of equilibrium. But they have potentially serious side effects and must be used with caution. Many patients on these drugs suffer problems ranging from minor sleep difficulties to life-threatening allergic reactions.

Prozac, for example, may cause diarrhea, nervousness, sleepiness, inability to sleep, headaches, chills, fever, chest pain, nightmares, decreased sexual drive, menstrual difficulties, tremors, nausea, vomiting, increased appetite, rapid heart action, abdominal pain, and difficulty in breathing.

Zoloft's side effects include weight loss, insomnia, heart palpitations, dizziness, chest pain, mania, dry mouth, headaches, and sweating. Tofranil may elevate or lower blood pressure and cause strokes, irregular heartbeat, anxiety, delusions, insomnia, seizures, nausea, vomiting, abdominal cramps, impotence, and altered liver function.

Parnate may cause anxiety, weakness, dizziness, nausea, abdominal pain, anorexia, chills, blurred vision, and impotence. Patients, moreover, must be especially careful when taking Parnate, Nardil, or other MAOIs, because they can cause or worsen high blood pressure and other problems if consumed with aged cheese, wine, beer, pickled herring, chocolate, yogurt, liver, or other foods containing tyramine.

Paxil, a brand name for paroxetine, can cause problems with erections and ejaculation, as well as weakness, sleepiness, dry mouth, dizziness, inability to sleep, sweating, anxiety, decreased appetite, and nervousness.

Potential side effects of lithium—marketed as Carbolith, Euralith, Lithane, and Lithonate—include dizziness, dry mouth, increased urination, lack of appetite, vomiting, diarrhea, stomach pain, irregular heartbeat, shortness of breath, swelling of hands and feet, slurred speech, headaches and muscle aches, weakness, sleepiness, and confusion.

In addition, countless cases of depression are actually caused by medicines. Medicines that may cause or worsen depression include ibuprofen, Benadryl, Xanax, Valium, Librium, Klonopin, Butisol, Fiorinal, Inderal, Lopressor, Seconal, Halcion, Compazine, Thorazine, Percodan, Darvocet, Percocet, and Dalmane. If you are taking any of these medicines, ask your physician to review with you all of the potential side effects before taking any drug. And if you or anyone in your family has or has had problems with depression, make sure your doctor knows about this before he or she writes you a prescription.

Pills are not the panaceas we've been led to believe they are. Studies have shown that drugs are of no value in treating about 33% of depression cases. In another 33% of cases, the drugs were only a little more effective than placebos.

Meanwhile, we must remember that all drugs have potentially serious side effects, and must be used cautiously.

Natural Supplements to Fight Depression

It is possible to treat the underlying causes of depression without taking synthetic drugs. Several natural remedies have brought relief to many people who suffer from depression. Unless otherwise noted, follow dosing information on labels. Helpful supplements include

SAMe. The safest and most effective antidepressant in the world is the European drug S-adenosylmethionine (SAMe). SAMe is a simple natural metabolite produced from the essential amino acid methionine and adenosine triphosphate (ATP) by an enzyme known as MAT (methionine adenosyl transferase). It is found in every cell within the body and plays an important role in critical biochemical processes. For one thing, it serves as a precursor for glutathione, Coenzyme A, cysteine, taurine, and other essential compounds.

When compared with other antidepressants, SAMe works faster and more effectively, with virtually no adverse side effects. In fact, unlike FDA-approved antidepressants that have both lethal and nonlethal side effects, SAMe produces side benefits, such as improved cognitive function, protection of liver function, and a potential slowing of the aging process. Some people take SAMe for its antiaging properties alone.

The major drawback of SAMe is that it is a difficult-to-produce natural substance with high manufacturing and packaging costs. At this time, the retail price of using SAMe to treat depression is more than the price of Prozac. The suggested dose of SAMe to treat depression ranges from 400 to 1600 mg a day. In one study, as little as 35 mg a day was used to treat depression, but most people have used 800 to 1600 mg a day.

A lack of SAMe is associated with an increase in clinical depression, and supplying the missing SAMe can relieve the problem. Used in Germany and Italy to treat osteoarthritis, SAMe also proved itself to be a powerful weapon against depression in 1973, during the first SAMe depression trial. By 1986 doctors knew that SAMe was helpful with endogenous depression caused by chemical imbalances in the brain.

SAMe gets to "where the action is," because clinical measurements have shown a significant rise in SAMe in the cerebral spinal fluid of treated patients. SAMe has been shown to be is as good as conventional antidepressant drugs, because it has been compared with tricyclic and other medications in single- and double-blind randomized trials, with doses ranging from 75 to 400 mg a day. The results, including scores on the Hamilton rating used to gauge depression, show that SAMe is as effective as tricyclic drugs.

As the clinical and scientific information on the benefits of SAMe mounted, scientists and physicians from around the world came together at an international symposium called "A New Treatment for Depression," held in Trieste, Italy, in June 1987. Here is some of the exciting information from the studies reported at the conference:

- ▼ Researchers from the University of Alabama at Birmingham found that depressed patients were not making enough SAMe in their brains. After checking the red blood cells from patients suffering from depression and schizophrenia, they discovered a decreased amount of methionine adenosyl transferase (MAT), an enzyme necessary for the formation of SAMe. (It was, however, higher in people with mania.)
- ▼ In a double-blind, randomized study, 14 women suffering from bipolar, unipolar, reactive or neurotic depression were given 45 mg of SAMe a day, and 5 women with reactive or neurotic depression received a placebo. Treatment ranged from 5 to 11 days. There was a "significant improvement" in the SAMe patients compared with those on the placebo.
- ▼ Forty-nine people suffering from moderate to severe depression, as well as rheumatoid arthritis, were observed in a double-blind, randomized study. Over 21 days, 25 of the patients were given 200 mg of SAMe a day, and 24 received a placebo. The patients who were treated with SAMe showed larger drops in depression, as measured by the Hamilton Depression system, than the placebo group.
- ▼ In a 1986 double-blind, randomized study, 32 severely depressed patients were divided into two groups. One group received 200 mg of SAMe for 14 days and the other was given a placebo. SAMe reduced depression by 50% on the Hamilton or Beck scale, and was more effective in counteracting endogenous than neurotic depression. There were no side effects except a possible increase in agitation.
- ▼ Twenty-two women and 18 men suffering from dysthymic disorder, atypical depression, or major depression were enlisted in a 1987 study of SAMe. The volunteers, with an average age of about 44, were divided into two groups of 20 each. The first group received 200 mg of SAMe for 30 days; the second, a placebo. SAMe was found to be superior to the placebo.
- ▼ A 1990 study examined SAMe and the depression often associated with Parkinson's disease. Twenty-one patients participated in this double-blind, crossover study with SAMe and a placebo. The patients' depression was rated using various scales; then they were given either SAMe for a while and then the placebo, or the placebo first and then SAMe. Neither the doctors nor the patients knew who was receiving what, or when. The researchers concluded that SAMe was a useful treatment for the depression associated with Parkinson's disease (72% of the patients said they had improved), and that it had few side effects. That's significant, when you consider that many Parkinson's patients are routinely turned into "zombies" by the side effects of the powerful medicines they take.

These studies clearly showed that SAMe was an effective antidepressant. But how would SAMe fare when pitted against conventional antidepressant drugs with a proven track record? The results speak well for SAMe:

- A 1975 study compared SAMe to imipramine, a standard medicine for depression. The double-blind, random study involved 31 patients, who ranged in age from 28 to 82, and suffered from endogenous, involutional, neurotic, and endoreactive depression. Sixteen of the volunteers were given 25 mg of SAMe 3 times a day, and the other 15 received 25 mg of imipramine 3 times a day. Researchers concluded that SAMe was just as effective as the drug, with slight differences favoring the natural substance.
- Eighteen men and women ranging from 20 to 65 years old participated in a 14-day double-blind study comparing intravenous SAMe to oral imipramine. The researchers found that SAMe produced "superior results" by the end of the first week of treatment. By the end of the second week, 66% of SAMe patients enjoyed a clinically significant improvement in depressive symptoms, compared with 22% of imipramine patients. The researchers also noted that SAMe is "rapid, effective, and has few side effects."
- In the opening discussion of a 1988 study on SAMe, Jerrold Rosenbaum, M.D., Associate Professor of Psychiatry at Harvard Medical School, reported that double-blind studies showed that SAMe was "equally more effective" than tricyclic antidepressants, including clomipramine, amitriptyline, and imipramine. Rosenbaum and colleagues also noted that SAMe produced an earlier response (3 to 7 days) and had fewer side effects.
- SAMe was compared with desipramine in a 1994 study headed by a researcher from the University of California. In this 4-week, double-blind, randomized study of 26 patients, 62% given SAMe showed significant improvement, compared with only 50% given the drug. Moreover, plasma levels of SAMe rose in patients reporting a 50% or better improvement, suggesting that SAMe plays a major role in depression.
- A 1994 meta analysis was performed on the SAMe studies, comparing it with placebo and standard antidepressants. The analysis, which looked at many studies already conducted on a large number of patients in a variety of conditions, found that SAMe was superior to placebo and just as good as the tricyclic medications. But because it is a naturally occurring compound, SAMe had relatively few of the side effects of standard drugs.

SAMe's benefits are numerous. In addition to relieving depression, it

- Protects against aging by maintaining cellular "energy factories" called mitochondria.
- Prevents DNA mutations.
- Restores cellular membrane fluidity.
- Guards against hepatitis and liver disease caused by toxins and drugs.
- Protects against neuronal death caused by lack of oxygen.
- May confer protection against heart disease.
- Regenerates nerves and helps nerve fibers "re-shield" themselves.
- May help in treating Alzheimer's disease. Brain levels of SAMe are low in Alzheimer's patients. Restoring them to normal levels may help the problem.

Adrafinil. This is another European antidepressant drug that is being successfully used by Europeans and Americans who import it for personal use. The dose is usually two tablets twice a day.

DHEA. Also known as dehydroepiandrosterone, this hormone is produced in the ovaries, and in the glands of women and men. It's important for good brain function; the brain contains six and a half times more DHEA than any other organ. From puberty, DHEA levels rise steadily, peaking at about the age of 25. By age 70 or 80, there is only about 10% of that peak amount left. Thus, it may be helpful for many people to take supplemental DHEA. Among other things, DHEA

- Relieves depression by improving psychological well-being.

- ▼ Enhances memory.
- ▼ Improves general physical condition.
- ▼ Strengthens the immune system.
- ▼ Reduces body fat and increases lean body mass.
- ▼ Makes it easier to handle stress.
- ▼ Helps to lower blood pressure.
- ▼ Reduces the risk of heart disease.
- ▼ Helps to reduce the need for insulin in diabetes.

Pregnenolone. This is another hormone produced by the ovaries and by adrenal glands in men and women, and it can be very useful for treating depression. Some studies have shown that depressed people have less-than-normal amounts of pregnenolone in their spinal fluid. Pregnenolone likely works by preventing the brain from being overwhelmed by GABA (gamma-aminobutyric acid) and other hormones that slow its activity.

Although pregnenolone helps to relieve depression, it may earn its greatest accolades through its beneficial effect upon the mind, especially the memory. Studies have shown that giving this hormone to older men and women improves their performance on tests of memory and concentration. Research, moreover, indicates that pregnenolone

- ▼ Improves the ability to remember and retrieve information.
- ▼ Increases the ability to handle stress.
- ▼ Has a beneficial effect on the myelin sheath membranes, which protect the brain and nervous system.
- ▼ Helps to keep the nervous system on an even keel.

DLPA. The 50/50 mixture of the "*d*" and "*l*" forms of the amino acid phenylalanine works well against depression, and also chronic pain. Soon after phenylalanine's endorphin-protecting abilities were discovered, it was tested against depression. From the very first study, the results have been impressive.

DLPA, when taken with the nutrients in the Life Extension Mix, can boost endorphin levels in the brain to help lift a person out of a depressed state. The suggested dose is two 500-mg capsules of *dl*-phenylalanine in the morning on an empty stomach and one 500-mg capsule in midafternoon on an empty stomach.

In addition, some people use the powder formula Rise & Shine, designed by Durk Pearson and Sandy Shaw, which provides phenylalanine and cofactors. The suggested dose is 1 tablespoon in the morning and 1 tablespoon in midafternoon. If phenylalanine does not work after several weeks, then the amino acid tyrosine should be tried at the same dose. (See below for more information on tyrosine.)

There are some people who are genetically sensitive to phenylalanine and cannot take it. Avoid the supplement if you are pregnant or lactating. Neither should anyone suffering from the genetic disease called phenylketonuria (PKU) take DLPA, because they cannot metabolize phenylalanine normally. This also applies to those on a phenylalanine-restricted diet. Children should not take DLPA. And DLPA can elevate blood pressure in people who already have hypertension. Cancer patients should avoid taking extra phenylalanine and tyrosine, because the amino acids can contribute to cancer cell proliferation.

But other people with depression may want to consider this supplement. The research backing it up is significant.

Fifteen people suffering from endogenous depression were studied at the North Nassau Mental Health Center in New York in the early 1970s. They were suffering from pervasive feelings of helplessness and hopelessness, disturbed sleep, lack of drive, and other symptoms of serious depression. They were given either DLPA or DPA, twice a day. Within 5 days, the symptoms were substantially better in 10 of the 15, and they required no other treatment.

Phenylalanine did not by itself cure the other five, but it did work with their antidepressant drugs, making them more powerful. No side effects were noted in this early, very successful test of the new, natural treatment for depression.

Even better results were chalked up in a 1975 study, when 23 patients suffering from endogenous depression were given either DLPA or DPA. Two weeks later, the depression had been lifted in 17 of the 23—and these were "tough customers" who had not been helped by previous therapy with antidepressants.

A 1978 study involved more than 400 patients suffering from various types of depression. It was the largest study pitting DLPA against depression to date. The patients were physically examined once a week, evaluated by psychiatrists every 5 days, and were subjected to numerous tests measuring their responses to the DLPA.

By day 15 of the study, all depressive symptoms had vanished in 73% of those suffering from endogenous depression, and most of the symptoms had cleared up in another 23%. By day 60, a full 80% were enjoying complete relief, while most of the symptoms were gone in another 15% of the participants. Here was compelling evidence of DLPA's ability to combat depression without the strong side effects seen with drug therapy.

In a separate, double-blind portion of the same study, researchers compared phenylalanine with a tricyclic antidepressant called Tofranil (imipramine), a commonly prescribed medication. Two groups of 30 depressed patients each were studied. For the first 15 days, one group took phenylalanine, the other Tofranil. For the next 5 days, each group received a placebo. For the final 10 days, each group went back to its original medication. Neither the doctors nor the participants knew whether they were getting phenylalanine or the drug. Throughout the 30-day period, phenylalanine was at least as effective as the medicine, without the side effects. In another double-blind study testing DLPA against imipramine, the amino acid was found to be just as effective as the drug, again without the side effects.

The studies show that DLPA is a powerful, safe, and natural antidepressant. (Some people may have trouble falling asleep if they take their DLPA too late in the afternoon.)

DMAE (dimethylaminoethanol). A naturally occurring nutrient found in sardines and other foods, DMAE is a remarkably powerful tool for relieving depression and/or fatigue. A brain stimulant, DMAE passes through the blood-brain barrier into the brain, where it helps increase the levels of acetylcholine (a neurotransmitter that plays an important role in both mood and energy levels).

DMAE has been shown to elevate mood, improve memory and learning, and increase intelligence, and is even more effective when taken with vitamin B_5 (pantothenate). DMAE has also been used with great success in the treatment of ADD (attention deficit disorder) in children and adults.

Depression often manifests itself as fatigue. By directly increasing energy levels and through its ability to alleviate depression, DMAE attacks fatigue on two levels. In summary, this nutrient

- Increases physical energy.
- Decreases daytime fatigue and allows for more natural sleep at night.
- Is a safe antidepressant that elevates the mood.
- Increases the ability to learn (it can raise IQ while you're taking it).
- Helps reduce "brain debris" called lipofuscin, thereby improving brain function.
- Increases longevity as measured in laboratory animals.

Tyrosine. A nonessential amino acid that can either be manufactured by the body or absorbed from our food, the body uses tyrosine to make the neurotransmitters dopamine, norepinephrine, and epinephrine, all of which play a role in elevating mood and keeping us alert. The amino acid is found in fish, poultry, and other foods. Some people find that 500 to 1500 mg a day of tyrosine works better than phenylalanine.

KH3. Is a European drug that inhibits the enzyme monoamine oxidase (MAO). Inhibiting this enzyme has helped many people to overcome depression, but many standard MAO-inhibitors can have several side effects. KH3 works without producing negative side effects. It is mild and very inexpensive.

L-carnitine. Another amino acid, it has been reported to safely alleviate depression in some people in doses of 1000 mg twice a day. Acetyl-*L*-carnitine has cognitive-enhancing and antiaging effects.

NADH (nicotinamide-adenine dinucleotide). Enhances brain cell energy and has alleviated depression in studies of people who took 5 to 10 mg a day.

Vitamins and Minerals to Fight Depression

Just as they help the body to heal physical wounds, vitamins and minerals can aid in the recovery from emotional ailments. Here are some you may want to consider.

Vitamin B_1, also know as thiamin, was the first of the B-family of vitamins to be discovered. A severe lack of this vitamin leads to beriberi, which causes confusion, high blood pressure, problems with the heart, and other symptoms. But a more subtle deficiency leads to depression and fatigue, as well as constipation and numbness or a "pins-and-needles" sensation in the legs. Some patients given powerful antidepressant drugs by physicians have suffered side effects including dry mouth, insomnia, and stomach upset. Taking B_1 supplements, or in some cases simply eating lots of foods containing good amounts of this vitamin, quickly solved the problem—inexpensively and with no side effects. Begin with 50 mg a day of vitamin B_1. And eat plenty of foods containing B_1, including kale, spinach, turnip greens, green peas, lettuce, cabbage, and many other vegetables.

Vitamin B_2, also known as riboflavin, has been linked to happiness for many years. In 1973, researchers discovered that if normal, healthy men were given diets almost completely devoid of the vitamin, they would soon score higher ratings on tests designed to detect depression. Take 50 mg of B_2 twice a day. Because it's also a good idea to eat foods containing this vitamin, add asparagus, broccoli, spinach, and whole wheat bread to your diet.

Vitamin B_3, also known as niacin or niacinamide, helps to beat the bad blues. The body needs B_3 in order to convert the amino acid tryptophan into serotonin, a neurotransmitter that plays an important role in keeping us happy. Not enough B_3 means not enough serotonin, leading to depression, worry, and fear. In fact, the newest drugs for depression (the SSRIs) work by increasing brain levels of this neurotransmitter.

The vitamin B_3 story began in the early part of the 20th century, when a disease called pellagra burst onto the scene in the southern part of the United States. Pellagra, which had been known about for some time but was a relatively minor problem, caused the "4Ds": diarrhea, dermatitis, dementia, and death. The rapid rise in the number of pellagra cases was caused by refined corn meal.

You see, many Southerners lived on the "3M Diet," which consisted of meat (mostly fatback), molasses, and meal (cornmeal). But improvements in food refining and railroad transportation led to many Southerners dropping "whole" corn meal in favor of the refined version. Unfortunately, the outer husk of the corn is discarded in the refining process, along with vitamin B_3.

Lacking sufficient B_3, the victim's bodies could not convert tryptophan into serotonin, and their mental/emotional balance was upset. Many victims wound up in the hospital; others ended up in the cemetery. But significant numbers of pellagra victims responded well to doses of B_3. And when the U.S. government ordered that certain vitamins be added back into refined flour and other foods, the pellagra problem receded.

In 1950, the famous physician Abram Hoffer followed up on the B_3–pellagra connection by treating schizophrenia patients with a nutritional program featuring B_3. Many of the patients improved immediately, and were still doing fine when rechecked 15 years later. These were not pellagra patients. Instead, they were suffering from "vitamin dependency," a condition in which they need larger amounts of a vitamin or vitamins than do the rest of us.

You may want to start with a single dose of 25 mg on day one. Some people may notice a red flushing of the skin of the face or neck. Gradually increase the dose incrementally to 100 mg 3 or 4 times a day, for a total of 300 to 400 mg a day. The flush may be avoided by using niacin in combination with the nutrient inositol. There are also "non-flush" combinations available.

Vitamin B_5, also known as pantothenate, helps the body convert dietary choline into the neurotransmitter acetylcholine. By "pushing" more choline in the brain, it may lighten depression. This vitamin is very important in Alzheimer's disease, in which there is a progressive loss of neurons that use acetylcholine. Note, however, that some depressed people get worse when acetylcholine levels are elevated. You may want to start out with 250 mg of vitamin B_5 in divided doses.

Vitamin B_6, also known as pyridoxine, is needed for conversion of the amino acid tryptophan to serotonin. This member of the B-family of vitamins is found in brewer's yeast, sunflower seeds, soybeans, walnuts, lentils, lima beans, hazelnuts, brown rice, avocados, and many other foods.

It is particularly helpful for women who develop depression as a result of taking oral contraceptive pills. The vitamin has been quite helpful in ameliorating the emotional difficulties sometimes associated with premenstrual syndrome and as part of the treatment for depression in postmenopausal women, which is often related to low levels of the neurotransmitter serotonin.

Serious deficiencies of B_6 are not common, but minor deficiencies, which are common, can cause depression, convulsions, and other problems. Alcoholics are more likely to be lacking this vitamin, as are those who have heart disease, liver disease, diarrhea, or other illnesses or injuries. Pregnant and lactating women may also be at risk for B_6 deficiency. Start out with 20 mg of supplemental B_6 in divided doses.

Vitamin B_{12}, also called cobalamin, is needed by the body only in very small quantities. A major deficiency causes a serious disease called pernicious anemia. Lesser deficiencies, which are common among the elderly, can produce depression, confusion, and other symptoms. B_{12} may help to fight depression by inhibiting monoamine oxidase (MAO), an enzyme that "attacks" and destroys certain neurotransmitters that help to elevate mood. In that sense, B_{12} works like the MAOI (monoamine oxidase inhibitors) drugs prescribed for depression. The vitamin is not as strong as the drugs, but being natural, it hasn't the side effects of the drugs.

We know that perhaps 20% of senior citizens have difficulty absorbing B_{12} from food, which means that they can suffer a deficiency even if there is plenty of the vitamin in their food. This may help to explain why depression is more common among the elderly—and point the way to a simple, inexpensive, and safe treatment for selected cases of depression.

You'll find good amounts of this vitamin in beef liver, chicken liver, clams, oysters and sardines, with smaller amounts in eggs, many fish, and cheeses. Vegetarians who eat no foods coming from animals should scrutinize their diets and consider taking supplements to make sure they're getting enough of this vital vitamin. If you take supplements, try 500 mcg of sublingual B_{12} twice a day.

Choline, a member of the B-family of vitamins, is converted by the body into the important neurotransmitter acetylcholine, which plays an important role in learning and memory. Choline is more effective when taken with vitamin B_5, which helps to "push" it into the brain. Some depressed people get worse when they take choline, however. You may find that 2000 mg a day, taken in divided doses, is a good starting point. Also eat plenty of choline-containing foods, including eggs, brewer's yeast, soybeans, peanuts, green peas, and peanuts.

Folic acid, another member of the B-family of vitamins, has been linked to depression in a number of studies, and depression is a common problem among those who are deficient in this vitamin. In fact, folic acid deficiency is common in a number of psychiatric disorders, not just depression.

Many studies have examined folic acid's ability to fight depression, including one in which 36 patients with either endogenous depression or schizophrenia had low levels of folic acid. Thirteen of them were given standard treatment plus folic acid, while the remaining 26, acting as the control group, received only the standard treatment. The results? Ninety-two percent of the folic acid group made a full recovery, compared with only 70% of the control group. Folic acid was especially helpful to those suffering from endogenous depression. Those who received the vitamin spent only 23.3 days in the hospital, while those in the control group averaged 32.9 days.

The RDA for folic acid is 400 mcg a day. People who are depressed may want to take 1000 mcg (1 mg) of folic acid. You also may want to eat bananas, green leafy vegetables, whole wheat bread, wheat germ, and other foods containing this member of the B-family of vitamins. Spinach is a good source of folic acid.

Vitamin C, also known as ascorbic acid, is a powerful antioxidant that helps to strengthen the immune system, guard against cancer and heart disease, reduce the risk of cataracts, and otherwise help us to lead long and healthy lives. We know that a deficiency of vitamin C can lead to depression and mental confusion, among other problems. In fact, depression is the first clinical symptom detected when humans are deliberately deprived of vitamin C for purposes of study.

How strong is the relationship between vitamin C and depression? It varies from person to person, but studies can give us clues. In one study, the diets of 12 women who attempted suicide were compared with 12 women who were not depressed and had not attempted suicide. The diets of the "suicide" and "happy" groups were very similar, except that the "suicide" group was taking in much less vitamin C.

And when researchers compared the amount of vitamin C in the blood of 885 psychiatric patients and 110 healthy controls, the mentally ailing were found to have significantly less of the vitamin in their blood.

A lack of vitamin C does not cause all cases of depression, so not all patients would be expected to recover if given the vitamin. However, supplemental doses of vitamin C have helped depressed patients of all ages, suggesting that a deficiency is implicated in an unknown number of cases. Start with 1 gram (1000 mg) of vitamin C twice a day. Then gradually increase the dosage until you are taking at least 3000 mg twice a day. This vitamin also is found in red chili peppers, guavas, parsley, green and sweet red peppers, broccoli, strawberries, oranges, mangoes, cantaloupe, and many other foods.

Potassium, a mineral that helps to keep the heart beating regularly, has also been linked to depression. Mood upsets, fatigue, and weakness, all symptoms of depression, have been associated with low levels of the mineral. These problems can occur if there isn't enough of the mineral inside the cells, even if there is enough potassium in the body fluids (outside the cells). Lower levels of potassium in the brain have been found in suicide victims. Replenishing potassium stores helps to reverse the fatigue and muscle weakness that may be associated with depression—or may be present on its own.

Unless potassium levels are dangerously low, it is probably best to get more of the mineral by increasing your intake of foods high in potassium, such as bananas, nonfat milk, oranges, and fresh peas. Enjoying four to five servings of fresh vegetables and fruit a day is usually enough to ensure that you are getting enough of this mineral.

Herbs to Fight Depression

Many herbs as well as vitamins have been used for centuries to treat depression. An affordable herbal antidepressant long used in Europe and now available in the United States is hypericum, an extract from the herb St. John's wort.

Hypericum (St. John's wort). In Germany, where it is covered by health insurance as a prescription drug, some 20 million people take hypericum for depression.

For treating depression we suggest 300 mg of hypericum 3 times a day (with a standardized concentration of 0.3% hypericin, the primary active ingredient of hypericum). Take the first 300-mg dose in capsule form on awakening, the second late in the morning, and the final dose no later than early afternoon. Or you may take two of the 300-mg doses on arising and a third in mid-day. Some people find that hypericum is an effective sleep aid. If you do, take the first dose in the morning, the second one around lunchtime, and the third dose late in the evening or just before bedtime.

Small children should be limited to 300 mg a day; larger children may take 600 mg a day; adolescents may take the full adult dose.

As with all antidepressants, it takes a while for the effects of hypericum to be felt. Many patients will notice a change in 2 to 3 weeks, although it may take as long as 4 to 6 weeks.

Hypericum's side effects are very mild, and may include slight gastrointestinal irritation and fatigue. In one study involving more than 1000 patients, hypericum produced fewer side effects than a placebo.

However, there are certain light-skinned sheep in Australia that become more sensitive to the sun and may suffer from serious sunburns after grazing on large amounts of the hypericum leaf. This is not a problem with people taking the recommended doses of hypericum for depression, but you should be aware of the potential problem. Those rare individuals who are hypersensitive to the sun, and/or those taking medications such as Terramycin, which can increase sun sensitivity, should be cautious about taking hypericum, and discuss its use with their physicians.

Also, the herb is not recommended for people who are taking monoamine oxidase (MAO) inhibitors such as Parnate and Nardil. If you are taking such drugs, wait at least a month after discontinuing the MAO inhibitors before starting hypericum.

And some types of depression, such as severe, debilitating depression and bipolar depression (also known as manic-depressive illness), do not respond to hypericum. Indeed, these are very difficult problems to treat even with standard antidepressants.

The research on St. John's wort is impressive. A meta-analysis and review of 23 randomized clinical trials involving 1757 people with mild or moderately severe depressive disorders showed that St. John's wort was 2.67 times superior to a placebo in relieving depressive symptoms, and was as effective as standard antidepressant drugs. Side effects occurred in 19.8% of patients on St. John's wort, compared with 52.8% of those taking standard antidepressant drugs. The conclusion of the researchers was that St. John's wort is more effective than a placebo for treatment of mild to moderately severe depressive disorders.

Hypericum was compared to the antidepression drug imipramine in a double-blind, randomized study involving 135 outpatients. The 71 men and 64 women, ranging in age from 18 to 75, were suffering from typical depression, neurotic depression, and adjustment disorder with depressed mood. After being medically and psychologically examined, they were given either 0.9 mg of hypericum extract LI 160 3 times a day, or 25 mg of imipramine 3 times a day for 6 weeks. The results of the study showed that "Hypericum was clearly superior to imipramine in terms of patient tolerance and fewer side effects."

In an observation group study, 72 volunteers ranging in age from 18 to 70, and all suffering from major depression, were given either a hypericum preparation or a placebo for 4 weeks. For the next 2 weeks, everyone was given hypericum. After 4 weeks on hypericum, the volunteers getting the real thing saw their depression scores drop to normal values. The placebo group also enjoyed improvement during the last 2 weeks (while taking hypericum). The researchers concluded that, "Most of the patients benefited from taking hypericum extract. Because of its potent and specific efficacy, with few or no side effects, hypericum extract LI 160 can be recommended as an antidepressant."

Other herbs as well have been used with success in treating depression. These include the following.

Ginseng. An ancient remedy long prized in the Orient as an overall tonic and rejuvenator. A great deal of anecdotal and scientific evidence has been amassed, suggesting that the herb is a stimulant and also has antioxidant and anticancer properties. Some scientists also believe that ginseng is an adaptogen, a substance which helps the body adapt to stress by keeping body chemistry within normal limits when stressful situations threaten to upset our internal balance.

Many depression patients have found that drinking one cup of ginseng tea a day gives them a "lift." There are three types of ginseng; the stronger Chinese ginseng (also known as *Panax ginseng*), the milder American ginseng (also known as *Panax quinquefolius*), and Siberian ginseng (also known as *Eleutherococcus senticosus*), which is actually a relative of ginseng.

CAUTION: Ginseng has mild estrogenic effects. That is, it can "mimic" some of the effects of the female hormone. In rare cases, it may cause vaginal bleeding in women. If you have vaginal bleeding, see your doctor immediately, and be sure to tell him or her that you are taking ginseng. Also, you should avoid ginseng if you have heart irregularities, high blood pressure, or a family history of high blood pressure.

Ginkgo biloba. From the leaf of the ginkgo tree, this extract is used to increase the flow of blood to the head and other parts of the body. It also has beneficial effects on thinking. It has been used to treat depression by itself, or in combination with DMAE and/or tyrosine. Studies have shown that ginkgo biloba can improve cognition and increase both vigor and lifespan in animals. Try 50 to 100 mg a day, in divided doses.

Nutrition and Depression

Hippocrates, the great Greek physician and Father of Medicine, said: "From the brain, and from the brain only, arise our pleasures, joys, laughter, and jests, as well as our sorrows, pains, griefs, and tears."

It's startling to learn that there are 15 thousand million nerve cells called neurons in the human brain. And there are far more glial cells (neuroglia) that fill the spaces between the neurons, Schwann cells, and miles and miles of blood vessels to nourish the 3 or so pounds of brain tissue in the average head.

Three pounds isn't much, only 2% of the body weight of a person weighing 150 pounds. But brain cells are hungry cells, demanding nourishment from as much as 30% of circulating blood. We used to think that the brain could somehow protect itself from nutrient deficiencies, but today we know that the brain requires specific nutrients. If the brain doesn't get them, its biochemistry changes, resulting in fatigue, depression, irritability, and other symptoms.

For example, the brain needs a good supply of B vitamins to act as coenzymes (catalysts) for many functions, including converting nutrients from food to fuel that our bodies can use. Glucose is the brain's primary fuel. If glucose levels fall, we may feel depressed, tired, or unable to think clearly.

B vitamins also are needed to help the brain make neurotransmitters, the "messengers" that enable brain cells to communicate with each other. Vitamin B_6 is needed to manufacture serotonin, a neurotransmitter that produces feelings of well-being. Without proper supplies of vitamin B_{12}, the brain could not make acetylcholine, an important neurotransmitter involved in learning and memory. The B vitamin known as folate (folic acid) is needed to make an important group of mood-regulating chemicals called catecholamines, including dopamine, norepinephrine, and epinephrine.

In many cases, depressed people with blood levels indicating that they lacked key nutrients respond quite well to supplements. Unfortunately, most physicians do not prescribe natural supplements to treat depression.

In general, people who are depressed should follow these dietary guidelines:

Avoid alcohol. It may make us feel giddy at first, but that's only because it's dulling our inhibitions. In the long run, alcohol is a depressant, which is the last thing depressed people need. If you must drink, limit yourself to one drink a day. (One drink means a single serving of a single alcoholic beverage a day, either 1 ounce of hard liquor, straight or mixed, 4 ounces of wine, or 12 ounces of beer.

Quit caffeine. Although it promises energy forever, caffeine is a liar. It can leave you mentally and physically drained. Avoid the caffeine in coffee, tea, soft drinks, chocolate, and cocoa, as well as the "hidden" caffeine in Excedrin, Midol, Anacin, and many other medicines. (Ask your doctor or pharmacist if the medicines you are taking contain caffeine. If they do, talk to your physician about switching to other medications.)

Shun sugar. Sugar jolts us with a sudden burst of energy, which can make us feel excited, talkative, and ready to take on the world. But when the body responds by snatching the excess sugar out of circulation, it often takes too much, leaving us tired and depressed. Many depressed patients suffer from nothing more than wild, sugar-induced gyrations in their moods. Convincing them to stay away from cakes, candy, soda, refined and processed foods solves the problem.

Consider the benefits of fish oil. Researchers have found that the fatty oil in salmon, cod, and other types of fish may alleviate symptoms of manic depression. We already know that certain fish oils can help to prevent and treat heart disease and arthritis. Now scientists are learning that this dietary ingredient can affect the brain as well.

In a recent landmark study, patients suffering from manic depression were given capsules containing fish oil. Over 4 months, they experienced a dramatic improvement in their symptoms.

The study, published in the American Medical Association's *Archives of General Psychiatry*, involved 30 patients diagnosed with bipolar disorders, characterized by chronic bouts of mania and depression.

Half of the subjects received fish oil supplements and half got capsules containing olive oil, a placebo. They underwent psychological testing at 2-week intervals.

The chemicals in the fish oil that seemed to help the patients were omega-3 fatty acids, found in many types of fatty fish, as well as in canola and flaxseed oils. Omega-3 fatty acids have many health benefits, including helping blood to flow through the constricted arteries of heart-disease patients, lubricating painful joints in rheumatoid arthritis sufferers, cutting women's risk of breast cancer, preventing an intestinal inflammation known as Crohn's disease, and even ridding the body of cellulite.

But there have been few studies looking at the effect of omega-3 fatty acids on the brain. Scientists now think that omega-3 fatty acids boost levels of the neurotransmitter serotonin in the brain, just like antidepressants such as Prozac. But they're not sure how the fish oils accomplish this.

Nonetheless, the discovery could help many people suffering from manic depression. Patients in the study received up to seven capsules daily with concentrated fish oil from menhaden, a type of Atlantic herring, containing nearly 10 grams of fatty acids.

Manic-depressive patients might want to take omega-3 fatty acids in supplemental form as an adjunct to antidepressant drugs or lithium, which is commonly prescribed to treat bipolar disorders.

A Missing Link In Depression Therapy

As men enter their fourth decade of life, hormonal changes occur that often produce a noticeable effect on physical, sexual, and cognitive energy levels, as well as a loss of feeling of well being. Until recently, these changes were attributed to "growing old," and men were expected to accept the fact that their body was entering into a long degenerative process that would some day result in death.

A remarkable amount of data has been gathered over the last 3 years that indicates that many of the diseases that men begin experiencing over age 40, including depression, abdominal weight gain, prostate, and heart disease, are directly related to hormone imbalances that are correctable with currently available drug and nutrient therapies. To the patient's detriment, conventional doctors are increasingly prescribing antidepressant, cholesterol-lowering, and other drugs to correct symptoms of a possible hormone imbalance. If doctors checked their male patient's blood levels of estrogen, progesterone, testosterone, prolactin, thyroid, and DHEA (instead of prescribing drugs to treat symptoms), they might be surprised to learn that many problems could be eliminated by adjusting hormone levels to fit the profile of a healthy 21-year-old.

One of the most misunderstood and mistakenly maligned hormones is testosterone. Body builders tarnished the reputation of testosterone by injecting large amounts of it into their youthful bodies. Testosterone abuse can produce detrimental effects, but this has nothing to do with the benefits a man over age 40 can enjoy by properly restoring his testosterone to a youthful level.

Doctors do not usually recommend testosterone replacement therapy because of studies showing it to be ineffective in treating the symptoms of aging. These studies often show a temporary benefit when testosterone is given, but within a few weeks the effects wear off. The problem is that these studies fail to identify that exogenously administered testosterone readily converts to estrogen in the body. The higher estrogen level negates the benefits of the exogenously administered testosterone. The solution to the estrogen-overload problem is to block the conversion of testosterone to estrogen in the body so that aging men can restore their strength, stamina, cognitive function, heart function, sexuality, and their outlook on life, i.e., alleviate symptoms of depression.

Testosterone is much more than a sex hormone. There are testosterone receptor sites in cells throughout the body, most notably in the brain and heart. Youthful protein synthesis for maintaining muscle mass and bone formation requires testosterone. Testosterone improves oxygen uptake throughout the body, helps control blood sugar, regulate cholesterol, and maintain immune surveillance. The body requires testosterone to maintain cardiac output and neurological function. Of critical concern to psychiatrists are studies showing that men suffering from depression have lower levels of testosterone than age-matched controls. For some men, elevating free testosterone levels could prove to be an effective antidepressant therapy.

(For any man suffering from depression, it is mandatory that they refer to the Male Hormone Modulation Therapy protocol. This describes safe ways of boosting free testosterone levels in a way that can alleviate or eliminate certain types of depression. Women should refer to the Female Hormone Replacement Therapy and the DHEA Replacement Therapy protocols for more information on what they can do to adjust their hormone status to improve their mood and alleviate depression.)

CAUTION: Although many depressed people benefit from natural treatments, none of the above therapies may be effective in patients suffering from serious clinical depression or manic depression. Such patients may require FDA-approved antidepressant drugs and/or lithium. Anyone suffering from clinical depression of any type should be under the care of a physician.

Summary

Although depression is a serious illness, it is possible to treat the underlying cause without taking synthetic drugs. Several natural remedies have brought relief to many people who suffer from depression.

1. SAMe works faster than most other antidepressants, but with no side effects. Dosages typically range from 400 to 1600 mg a day. However, as little as 35 mg a day has been used to treat depression.
2. Adrafinil can be imported from Europe for personal use. The dose is usually two tablets twice a day.
3. DHEA is a natural hormone that enhances brain functioning and promotes well-being. Dosages typically range from 50 mg (women) to 100 mg (men). Consult your physician if you are taking DHEA as an antidepressant.
4. Pregnenolone is another natural hormone that is often found in below-normal amounts in people with depression. Pregnenolone can be taken in doses of 50 to 200 mg daily. If more than 50 mg of pregnenolone is taken, it should be in divided doses. *(Refer to DHEA and Pregnenolone Precautions elsewhere in this volume.)*
5. DLPA (*dl*-phenylalanine) can boost endorphin levels in the brain to help lift a person out of a depressed state. The suggested dose is two 500-mg capsules of *dl*-phenylalanine in the morning on an empty stomach and one 500-mg capsule in midafternoon on an empty stomach (recommended to be taken in combination with Life Extension Mix).
6. DMAE (found in sardines and other foods) has been shown to elevate mood and is even more effective when taken with vitamin B_5 (pantothenate).
7. Tyrosine is used by the body to make the neurotransmitters dopamine, norepinephrine, and epinephrine, which play a role in elevating mood and keeping us alert; 500 to 1500 mg a day is recommended.
8. *L*-carnitine is an amino acid that can alleviate depression in some people in doses of 1000 mg twice a day.
9. NADH (nicotinamide-adenine dinucleotide) enhances brain cell energy and has alleviated depression in studies of people who took 5 to 10 mg a day.

10. Vitamin B_1 (thiamin) deficiency can lead to depression and fatigue; 50 mg a day is recommended.
11. Vitamin B_2 (riboflavin) deficiency can lead to depression; 50 mg twice daily is recommended.
12. Vitamin B_3 (niacin) converts tryptophan into serotonin, an important neurotransmitter that helps us stay happy. A single dose of 25 mg a day gradually increased incrementally to 100 mg 3 or 4 times a day is recommended. To avoid flush, use niacin in combination with the nutrient inositol. There are also "non-flush" combinations available.
13. Vitamin B_6 (pyridoxine) is also needed for conversion of tryptophan to serotonin. A deficiency of B_6 is often found in pregnant or lactating women and in alcoholics. Divided doses of 20 mg a day are recommended.
14. Vitamin B_{12} (cobalamin) helps fight depression by inhibiting monoamine oxidase (MAO), an enzyme that "attacks" and destroys certain neurotransmitters that help to elevate mood; 500 mcg sublingually, twice a day is recommended.
15. Choline plays an important role learning and memory; 2000 mg a day in divided doses is recommended.
16. Folic acid (a B vitamin) deficiency is common in many people with depression; 400 mcg a day is the RDA, however, people who are depressed may want to take 1000 mcg (1 mg) a day.
17. Vitamin C (ascorbic acid) deficiency has been found in many depressed people. Start with 1 gram (1000 mg) twice a day and gradually increase the dosage until you are taking at least 3000 mg twice a day.
18. Potassium is a mineral that has been linked to depression. Unless levels are dangerously low in the body, potassium should by replenished by natural foods such as bananas, nonfat milk, oranges, and fresh peas.
19. St. John's wort (hypericum) has recently gained prominence in the United States as a natural antidepressant; 300 mg 3 times daily (with a standardized concentration of 0.3% hypericin) in divided doses is recommended.

CAUTION: St. John's wort is contraindicated in people taking MAO inhibitors.

20. Ginseng is an overall tonic and rejuvenator, 400 mg daily in capsule form may be taken or brewed in a tea.

CAUTION: Women should consult a physician if vaginal bleeding occurs. People with high blood pressure or heart irregularities should not use ginseng.

21. Ginkgo biloba can improve cognition and increase vigor and lifespan; 50 to 100 mg a day in divided doses is recommended.
22. Omega-3 fatty acids (found in fish oil) may boost serotonin levels in the brain; 4 to 8 capsules of concentrated fish oil are recommended.
23. Testosterone levels may decrease in men over 40. Low levels of testosterone may lead to depression. (*Consult the Male Hormone Modulation Therapy protocol for indications and dosing recommendations.*)
24. *Women should consult the DHEA Replacement Therapy and Female Hormone Replacement Therapy protocols for more information on hormone levels and depression.*
25. Alcohol, caffeine, and sugar, which are known to cause abrupt changes in energy and mood, should be avoided.

For more information. Contact the National Depressive and Manic Depressive Association (800) 826-3632.

Product availability. SAMe, *dl*-phenylalanine, *L*-tyrosine, Life Extension Mix, St. John's wort extract, NADH, Rise & Shine, acetyl-*L*-carnitine, and other products are available by calling (800) 544- 4440 or order online at www.lef.org. Ask for a listing of offshore companies that sell adrafinil and KH3 to Americans by mail order.

DHEA REPLACEMENT THERAPY

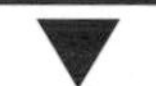

In 1981 the Life Extension Foundation introduced DHEA (dehydroepiandrosterone) through an article that described the multiple antiaging effects this hormone might produce. The general public learned about DHEA in 1996, as the benefits of DHEA were touted by the news media and in several popular books.

DHEA obtained credibility in the medical establishment when the New York Academy of Sciences published a book entitled *DHEA and Aging* and summarized in their journal, *Aging* (Dec. 29, 1995, 774:1–350). This highly technical book provided scientific validation for the many life extension effects of DHEA replacement therapy.

DHEA has been shown to improve neurological function (including memory, mood enhancement, and EEG readings), immune surveillance, and stress disorders. DHEA replacement therapy has become popular as an antiaging regimen and offers aging patients help in preventing diseases such as osteoporosis, fatigue, depression, atherosclerosis, and cancer.

DHEA replacement therapy involves the supplementation of the hormone to restore serum levels to those of a 21-year-old. DHEA is a precursor building block that allows our bodies to more easily create hormones that may be in decline because of age, disease, prescription medications, or other factors. Hormones such as testosterone and estrogen as well as serum DHEA levels begin to decline between 25 and 30 years of age and may be reduced by 95% of youthful peak levels by age 85.

The most remarkable finding about DHEA came from a human study by S. S. C. Yen and associates at the University of California, San Diego, in which 50 mg a day of DHEA over a 6-month period restored youthful serum levels of DHEA in both men and women. Dr. Yen showed that DHEA replacement was associated with an increase in perceived physical and psychological well-being for both men (67%) and women (84%). Increases in lean body mass and muscle strength were reported in men taking 100 mg a day, but this dose appeared to be excessive in women.

DHEA (50 or 100 mg a day) was also shown to significantly elevate insulin growth factor (IGF). Aging causes a decline in IGF levels that contributes to the loss of lean body mass, as well as to excess fat accumulation, neurological impairment, and age-associated immune dysfunction.

DHEA has been shown to protect against heart disease and atherosclerosis. A study using coronary artery angiography showed that low DHEA levels predispose people to more significant coronary artery blockage. Another study showed that DHEA inhibits abnormal blood platelet aggregation, a factor in the development of sudden heart attack and stroke. In contrast, some studies on DHEA do not show the cardiovascular disease protection.

In the journal *Drugs and Aging* (Oct. 1996), an analysis of previous studies on DHEA showed that

- In both humans and animals, the decline of DHEA production with aging is associated with immune depression, increased risk of several different cancers, loss of sleep, decreased feelings of well-being, and increased mortality.
- DHEA replacement in aged mice significantly improved immune function to a more youthful state.
- DHEA replacement has shown a favorable effect on osteoclasts and lymphoid cells, an effect that may delay osteoporosis. *(Editor's note: DHEA has been shown in other studies to promote the activity of bone-forming osteoblasts.)*
- Low levels of DHEA inhibit energy metabolism, thus increasing the risk of heart disease and diabetes mellitus.
- Studies in humans show essentially no toxicity at doses that restore DHEA to youthful levels.
- DHEA deficiency may expedite the development of some diseases that are common in the elderly.

Depression Responds to DHEA Treatment

Depression is a broad term for a host of unpleasant feelings, including emotional numbness, lack of energy, lack of motivation, feeling like a failure, and feeling undesirable. These feelings frequently show up for the first time in middle-aged people who feel like they're "over the hill." Elderly people, too, frequently get depressed, and they are particularly at risk of suicide. Depression is a growing problem among teenagers as well.

Doctors have long known that giving estrogen to women and testosterone to men during midlife can avert symptoms of depression, although the effects have never been phenomenal. Reports are stacking up that DHEA works better. DHEA turns into both estrogen and testosterone. And it just so happens that it goes south about the time people start thinking about being "over the hill."

DHEA is definitely a brain chemical. It's not only utilized by the brain, it's manufactured by it. Although researchers don't know what it's supposed to do yet, they *do* know that giving a person 500 mg of DHEA will cause them to have more REM (dream) sleep. This indicates a major role in brain chemistry.

DHEA is the only hormone besides cortisol that has consistently been linked with depression. It was studied as far back as the 1950s as an antidepressant. Back then, researchers reported that it gave people energy and confidence, and made them less depressed. While it seemed to work great, no one followed up on the studies.

DHEA emerged on the scene again in the 1980s when interest in antiaging hormones geared up. It was noted then that antidepressant activity was part of DHEA's overall antiaging benefits. Then, in 1996, a report suggested that DHEA's antidepressant effects might be direct, and not just a result of its antiaging benefits in older people. Researchers at Cambridge University discovered that young kids with major depression have abnormally low levels of DHEA (and abnormally high levels of cortisol).

In the late 1990s, this phenomenon was confirmed in a larger study. Researchers at the University of California at San Diego went back and analyzed old data from a large study that had been done on 699 older women living in Rancho Bernardo, California. That analysis is the largest study ever done on the association between levels of DHEA and depression. Nine different hormones had been measured during the study, which took place during the 1970s and 1980s. Included in the measurements were such things as bioavailable testosterone and sex-hormone-binding globulin. When the results were in, of all the hormones, only DHEA was associated with depression. (Low testosterone levels have been correlated with depression in men.)

Women at the lowest end of DHEA were far more likely to be depressed. This coincides with an earlier study where the percentage of women with depression was 21.7% if they had no detectable DHEA, versus 4.6% if DHEA could be detected in their blood. Interestingly, levels of DHEA in the Rancho study correlate with mood even within the normal range. In other words, the lower the DHEA, the worse the mood got. And DHEA correlated with mood irrespective of whether a person was taking antidepressants or not.

A group at the University of California, San Francisco went at the DHEA/depression question another way. They decided to give DHEA to people with depression and see if it would help. In the first double-blind, placebo-controlled study on DHEA's potential as an antidepressant, 11 patients with major depression were given up to 90 mg/day of DHEA for 6 weeks, and 11 were given a placebo. One week before the study actually began, all patients were given a placebo to weed out people who would respond to a sugar pill. People getting the real McCoy received 30 mg a day of DHEA for the first 2 weeks, 60 mg the second 2 weeks, and 90 mg the last 2 weeks. The idea of the graduated dose was to bring patients up to the DHEA levels they had when they were 20 to 30 years old (DHEA declines with age). Although the amount of DHEA wasn't adjusted individually, as it could have been, the graduated dose approximates what it takes to reach a "youthful" level in most people, according to Dr. Owen Wolkowitz, principle investigator on the study. Some of the participants were taking antidepressants. For these people, the antidepressants were either working partially, or not working at all. Only people who had been on the same antidepressant for at least 6 weeks without changing were allowed in the study, and no changes could be made in anyone's medication during the study.

After 6 weeks, psychological tests indicated that about half the participants responded to DHEA therapy, with an overall enhancement of mood scores by 30.5%. This is close to the response rate of antidepressant drugs.

An even better response was seen in another study conducted by researchers at the National Institute of Mental Health. In this study, participants were middle-aged people with dysthymia, a chronic, low-grade depression. They were given 90 mg of DHEA a day for 3 weeks, then 450 mg a day for 3 weeks more. Batteries of psychological tests were administered, including the Hamilton Depression Rating Scale, the Beck Depression Inventory, a visual analogue scale, and the Cornell Dysthymia Scale. (In addition, a day's worth of cognitive function tests was given, but DHEA didn't show a significant effect on cognition in this study. However, the researchers note a trend towards better cognition that could have played out if the study had lasted longer). None of the patients were taking any prescription drugs whatsoever except one man who was taking a hypertension drug. The study was set up in a very rigorous way; all participants got the drug or the placebo for 6 weeks, and then they were all secretly switched. All people involved in the study were blind to who was getting what. DHEA significantly alleviated the participants' depression. Seven symptoms in particular got much better: lack of pleasure, low energy, low motivation, emotional numbness, sadness, inability to cope, and excessive worry. DHEA worked for most people within 10 days. If the supplement was stopped, the symptoms came back. Overall, the response rate was 60%, which is better than what antidepressants usually do for dysthymia. Ninety milligrams a day was sufficient. No extra benefit was provided by the 450 mg dose.

Researchers have different theories about how DHEA alleviates depression. Both DHEA and DHEA-s can cross the blood–brain barrier and interact with the brain directly. DHEA can affect serotonin, GABA receptors, and other brain factors. A recent study indicates it might modulate the serotonin signaling pathway. In addition, DHEA is the precursor for estrogen and testosterone which have been reported to enhance mood.

DHEA also has antistress effects that may be part of its antidepressant action. Research shows that cortisol, the stress hormone, is elevated in major depression. DHEA counteracts cortisol. Calmness appears to be associated with higher levels of DHEA. People who practice transcendental meditation have higher levels of DHEA than those who don't. People who took part in a stress reduction program were able to increase their DHEA by 100%. At the same time, they reduced their stress hormone by 23%.

Exercise has been reported to enhance mood. This mood-enhancing effect may be due to DHEA. Exercise raises levels of DHEA, which also positively affects the heart. In a study published in the *American Journal of Cardiology,* depression and heart attack went together: women with depression are at greater risk of heart attack, and vice-versa. Exercise elevates DHEA, which, in turn, benefits the heart.

DHEA Inhibits Cancer Cell Proliferation

DHEA may be effective in preventing and treating cancer. In one study, DHEA inhibited tumor proliferation of rat liver cells by blocking the cancer cell promoting enzyme glucose 6-phosphate dehydrogenase (G6PDH). The human equivalent dose of 600 mg a day suppressed breast tumors in mice by 70%, yet these scientists showed that even human equivalent doses of 25 to 120 mg showed striking cancer prevention benefits, with no evidence of toxicity.

DHEA has been shown to inhibit chemically induced cancers in the colon, lung, breast, and skin. When DHEA is applied directly to the skin, DHEA prevented chemically induced skin cancer. DHEA had this effect by blocking the binding of carcinogens to skin cells and by inhibiting the enzyme *G6PDH*.

One study showed that patients with adult T-cell leukemia (ATL) had significantly decreased levels of DHEA compared to healthy controls. This has led some doctors to speculate that DHEA might be beneficial in treating this form of leukemia since DHEA has already been shown effective in treating hairy cell leukemia. Other cancer studies show DHEA inhibits cancer cell thymidine incorporation needed for cellular propagation and disrupts the oxidizing effects of chemical carcinogens. Scientists point out that DHEA functions not as an antioxidant, but as a modulator of the effects of chemical carcinogens on cells (*American Journal of Hematology*, 1996, 53[3]).

DHEA Protects against Brain Aging

Acetylcholine is a neurotransmitter that transmits nerve impulses from one brain cell to another. Acetylcholine is crucial for short-term memory and to protect brain cells against age-associated atrophy. Aging causes a decline in the release of acetylcholine into regions of the brain where it is needed for learning and memory.

In a study in *Brain Research* (Sept. 16, 1996), DHEA was administered to rats in order to measure the effect it produced on acetylcholine release into the hippocampus region of the brain. DHEA significantly increased acetylcholine release above pretreatment levels in all doses tested. At the highest dose, DHEA caused a fourfold increase in the release of acetylcholine compared to the control group. The scientists concluded that this was the first study to demonstrate a direct effect of DHEA in promoting the release of acetylcholine from brain cells in the hippocampus (a critical area for the storage of memory).

In a study published in *Behavioral Brain Research* (1997, 83[1–2]), DHEA interacted with certain neuronal receptors involved in short- and long-term memory storage. The results showed an improvement in memory in the Y-maze spatial leaning test that measures short-term memory and the step-down passive avoidance test that measures long-term memory in mice.

A study in *Life Sciences* (Oct. 4, 1996) showed that DHEA could protect against the precursor changes in brain cells that result in the pathological alterations associated with Alzheimer's disease.

DHEA Saves Skin

DHEA has powerful skin protective effects. A study published in the *Journal of Surgical Research* demonstrates that topically applied DHEA protects the skin's delicate blood vessels. Researchers found that if DHEA was applied after a serious burn, the blood vessels underlying the burned area were protected. Protecting the blood vessels saves the skin. Skin and blood vessels that would otherwise die and peel off can be saved by DHEA. No one knows for sure how DHEA saves skin this way, but its anti-inflammatory action no doubt has something to do with it. DHEA prevents destructive white blood cells and their biochemical cousins from gearing up. In particular, DHEA affects the blood vessel killer known as tumor necrosis factor (TNF). At the same time it's inhibiting the destructive process, it appears to be prolonging the healing process: DHEA causes edema (swelling) to last longer. This apparently helps save tissue.

Estrogen's skin-enhancing effects are well-known. It provokes collagen and a moisture factor known as hyaluronic acid. Aging decreases both estrogen and collagen. Enzymes that convert DHEA to estrogen also decline. Not surprisingly, women who take synthetic estrogen have scientifically proven thicker skin. Women who take both estrogen and testosterone have really thick skin—48% thicker than women who don't take either hormone. DHEA is converted to both estrogen and testosterone, providing the benefits of both hormones. DHEA is converted into estrogen and androgen-type metabolites found only in skin.

Studies show that DHEA is absorbed by skin when applied topically. A study from CHUL Research Center (in Canada) shows that the skin activity of DHEA applied topically is 85 to 90% greater than when taken orally (at least in rodents). No special carriers are needed to get DHEA into skin. A properly formulated topical preparation of DHEA will contain just enough hormone to benefit skin without providing enough to escape into circulation. It makes sense to apply the hormones directly to the skin if skin protection is the goal, since ingested hormones may end up everywhere *but* the skin.

DHEA has action against everyday insults as well. By maintaining skin immunity, DHEA preserves the ability of skin to react to cancer-causing, skin-destroying pollutants in air, food, and water. DHEA also has antioxidant action against peroxyl and superoxide free radicals.

Immune Function and DHEA

DHEA levels decline 80 to 90% by age 70 or later. DHEA has demonstrated a striking ability to maintain immune system synchronization. Oral supplementation with low doses of DHEA in aged animals restored immunocompetence to a reasonable level within days of administration. DHEA supplementation in aged rodents resulted in almost complete restoration of immune function.

DHEA has been shown in numerous animal studies to boost immune function via several different mechanisms. Only limited human studies have been done to measure DHEA's effect on the immune system.

In one study, scientists proposed that the oral administration of DHEA to elderly men would result in activation of their immune system. Nine healthy men averaging 63 years of age were treated with a placebo for 2 weeks followed by 20 weeks of DHEA (50 mg/day). After 2 weeks on oral DHEA, serum DHEA levels increased by three to four times. These levels were sustained throughout the study. Compared to the placebo, DHEA administration resulted in:

- ▼ An increase of 20% in IGF-1. Many people are taking expensive growth hormone injections for the purpose of boosting IGF levels. IGF stands for insulin-like growth factor and is thought to be responsible for some of the antiaging, anabolic effects that DHEA has produced in previous human studies.
- ▼ An increase of 35% in the number of monocyte immune cells.
- ▼ An increase of 29% in the number of B immune cells and a 62% increase in B-cell activity.
- ▼ A 40% increase in T-cell activity even though the total number of T-cells was not affected.
- ▼ An increase of 50% in interleukin-2.
- ▼ An increase of 22 to 37% in natural killer cells (NK) number and an increase of 45% in NK cell activity.
- ▼ No adverse effects noted with DHEA administration.

The scientists' conclusion: "While extended studies are required, our findings suggest potential therapeutic benefits of DHEA in immunodeficient states." (*Journals of Gerontology*, Series A, 1997, 52[1])

A study in the *Journal of Clinical Endocrine Metabolism* (June 1998) showed that when old female mice were treated with DHEA, melatonin, or DHEA + melatonin, splenocytes (macrophages) were significantly higher as compared to young mice. B-cell proliferation in young and in old mice significantly increased. DHEA, melatonin, and DHEA + melatonin helped to regulate immune function in aged female mice by significantly increasing cytokines, interleukin-2, and interferon-gamma and significantly decreasing cytokines, interleukin-6, and interleukin-10, thus regulating cytokine production.

Interleukin-6 (IL-6) is one of the pathogenic elements in inflammatory and age-related diseases such as rheumatoid arthritis, osteoporosis, atherosclerosis, and late-onset B-cell neoplasia. "Higher circulating levels of IL-6 predict disability onset in older persons," according to the report in the June 1999 issue of the *Journal of the American Geriatrics Society* (47:639–46, 755–56). The authors suggest that IL-6 may cause a reduction in muscle strength or contribute to specific diseases such as congestive heart failure, osteoporosis, arthritis, and dementia, which cause disability.

DHEA has consistently been shown to boost beneficial interleukin-2 and suppress damaging interleukin-6 levels. Interleukin-6 is overproduced in the aged, which contributes to autoimmune disease, immune dysfunction, osteoporosis, depressions in healing, breast cancer, B-cell lymphoma, and anemia. Chronic DHEA administration maintained immunocompetence in aged animals (by boosting interleukin-2 and other beneficial immune components and suppressing interleukin-6 and other detrimental immune components). Suppression of interleukin-6 with 200 mg a day of DHEA was shown to be effective against systemic lupus erythematosus (*J. Rheumatol.*, Feb. 1998, 25[2]:285–89).

Researchers compared levels of IL-6 in 283 subjects with a mobility or functional disability with IL-6 levels in 350 adults without a disability. The investigators found that adults in the highest third of values of IL-6 had a 76% higher rate for mobility disabilities and a 62% higher rate for inability to perform daily activities than subjects in the lowest third of values. "These data suggest that IL-6 is a global marker of impending deterioration in health status in older adults," wrote a team led by Dr. Luigi Ferrucci at the National Institute on Aging in Bethesda, Maryland.

In a study in the *Proceedings of the Society for Experimental Biology and Medicine* (May 1998; 218[1]:76–82), DHEA has been shown to restore normal cytokine production in immune system dysfunction induced by aging by suppressing the excessive production of cytokines (IL-6) by 75%, while increasing IL-2 secretion by nearly 50%, during a leukemia virus infection in old mice.

Another study in normal healthy individuals over the age of 40 found an opposite relationship between plasma DHEA levels and the presence of detectable levels of IL-6. Studies also revealed that low doses of DHEA and DHEA-s inhibited the production of IL-6 in unstimulated human spleen cell suspension cultures while enhancing its release by cultures transferred from organs of the same tissue (*Mech. Ageing Dev.*, Feb. 1997, 93:1–3, 15–24).

> The age-related increase in circulating IL-6 levels in humans which has been attributed to decline in DHEA production by the adrenal gland is currently attracting attention because of its possible relevance to the aetiology and management of a number of age-related clinical disorders. The potential importance of these observations and suggestions has prompted us to perform more detailed studies on the relationship between IL-6 and DHEA. Using immunoassay techniques we have found in normal healthy individuals over the age of 40 an inverse relationship between plasma DHEA levels and the presence of detectable levels of IL-6 (more than 1 pg/ml). In vitro, studies also revealed that low dose (10(-6)-10(-8) M) of DHEA and DHEA-s inhibited the production of IL-6 in unstimulated human spleen cell suspension cultures whilst enhancing its release by explant cultures of the same tissue. In contrast they had no effect on immunoglobulin production. These studies suggest that there is a real, but complex relationship between IL-6 production and DHEA levels which warrants further investigation.

DHEA Dosing and Safety Precautions

Properly managed DHEA therapy can be useful for most older men and women to increase energy, vitality, and to foster an overall youthful feeling. However, there are guidelines that should be followed for safe long-term use of DHEA.

When taking oral supplements of DHEA, it is important that antioxidants are available to the liver because DHEA can promote free radicals in liver cells. Animal studies have shown that extremely high doses (from 2000 to 10,000 mg DHEA daily in human terms) caused liver damage in mice and rats. When antioxidants were given along with the DHEA, liver damage did not occur despite the massive doses of DHEA being administered to these animals. It should be noted that the amount of DHEA shown to cause liver damage is 20 times more than is necessary to produce antiaging benefits. Green tea, vitamin E, and *N*-acetyl-cysteine (NAC) are antioxidants that have been shown to be especially effective in suppressing free radicals in the liver.

The Life Extension Foundation has evaluated thousands of DHEA blood tests to determine the ideal dose of DHEA for both men and women. The Foundation's findings indicate that the optimal dosage range for DHEA varies considerably between individuals. Prior recommendations to take DHEA 3 times a day are now being replaced with a general recommendation that men and women should consider taking a total of 15 to 75 mg a day in one to three divided doses. Most human studies use a daily dose of 50 mg, and this is the typical daily dose the majority of people use to restore serum DHEA to youthful levels. DHEA can be taken with or without food, though some believe that fat helps DHEA to assimilate better. Some people absorb DHEA better by taking it 20 to 30 minutes before meals.

A DHEA-s blood test should be taken 3 to 6 weeks after beginning DHEA therapy to help determine optimal dosing. Some people neglect to test their blood levels of DHEA and wind up chronically taking the wrong dose. When having your blood tested for DHEA, blood should be drawn 3 to 4 hours after the last dose. DHEA testing can save you money if it shows that you can take less DHEA to maintain youthful DHEA serum levels.

The standard blood test to evaluate DHEA status is one that measures DHEA-s (sulfate). The DHEA-s is calculated in micrograms per deciliter (mcg/dL) of blood. The youthful ranges of DHEA are as follows:

Men	Women
400 to 560	350 to 430

People over age 40 who do not supplement with DHEA usually have serum levels below 200, and many are way below 100. Chronic DHEA deficiency is a risk factor for developing the degenerative diseases of aging according to the preponderance of evidence existing in the scientific literature.

Some people obtain a baseline DHEA-s blood test before beginning DHEA replacement therapy. However, based upon numerous DHEA blood tests evaluated by the Life Extension Foundation, anyone over age 40 who does not supplement DHEA is already deficient in serum DHEA. Therefore, it may be more economical to have the first DHEA blood test 3 to 6 weeks after initiating DHEA replacement therapy. There are precautions that should be observed that are different for men and women.

Men

Before initiating DHEA therapy, men should know their serum PSA (prostate-specific antigen) level and have passed a digital rectal exam. Men with prostate cancer or severe benign prostate disease are advised to avoid DHEA since DHEA can be converted into testosterone (and estrogen). These sex hormones and their metabolites can promote benign and malignant prostate cell proliferation. It is important to understand, however, that well-controlled studies show that serum DHEA levels are usually lower in men with malignant prostate disease compared to healthy control subjects. Therefore, men are advised to have a PSA and digital rectal exam before initiating DHEA therapy to rule out existing prostate disease, not because DHEA causes the disease. To the contrary, there is evidence indicating that maintaining youthful levels of DHEA may protect against prostate cancer. To reduce the risk that hormone modulation with DHEA could contribute to a prostate problem, men taking DHEA are also advised to take

Vitamin E	400 to 800 IU a day
Selenium	200 to 600 mcg a day
Mega Soy Extract	135 mg 2 times a day (40% isoflavone extract)
Lycopene Extract	20 to 40 mg a day
Saw Palmetto Extract	160 mg, 2 times a day
Pygeum Extract	50 mg, 2 times a day
Nettle Extract	120 mg, 2 times a day

(An aromatase inhibitor should be considered if serum estrogen levels are high. Refer to the Male Hormone Modulation Protocol for complete information about suppressing excessive estrogen levels.)

Men over 40 should consider checking their PSA and DHEA-s serum levels every 6 to 12 months thereafter. Men should also periodically check their blood levels of free testosterone and estrogen to make sure that DHEA is following a youthful metabolic pathway. Men taking DHEA should refer to the Male Hormone Modulation Protocol to learn about additional hormone balance testing that can be done at the same time serum DHEA and PSA levels are being tested.

Women

DHEA can increase serum estrogen levels in women and eliminate the need for estrogen replacement therapy in some women. To help protect cells (especially breast cells) from excessive proliferation in response to estrogen, women taking DHEA should also take

Melatonin	500 mcg to 3 mg every night
Vitamin E Succinate	400 to 800 IU a day
Mega Soy Extract	135 mg, twice a day (40% isoflavone extract)
Indole-3-carbinol	200 mg, twice a day
Vitamin D_3	1000 to 1400 IU a day

Women should consider estrogen and testosterone testing when they take their DHEA blood test in order to evaluate DHEA's effect on their blood levels of estrogens.

Women who have been diagnosed with an estrogen-dependent cancer should consult their physicians before beginning DHEA therapy. Some studies indicate that higher serum DHEA protects against breast cancer, but no adequate studies have been done to evaluate the effects of DHEA in breast cancer patients. If DHEA were to elevate estrogen too much, this could theoretically increase the risk of breast cancer. (*Women taking DHEA should refer to the Female Hormone Replacement protocol for information about restoring youthful hormone balance.*)

Liver Disease

Men or women with existing liver disease (such as viral hepatitis or cirrhosis) should consider taking DHEA sublingually (under your tongue) or using a topical DHEA cream to reduce the amount of DHEA entering the liver. DHEA is converted by the liver into DHEA-s (dehydroepiandrosterone sulfate). Those with liver disease should carefully monitor liver enzyme levels to make sure that DHEA therapy is not making existing liver disease worse.

DHEA is best taken early in the day or possible insomnia could result. DHEA is normally produced by the adrenal glands early in the day and then converted by the liver to DHEA-s by midday when the DHEA/DHEA-s ratio is usually stabilized (10% DHEA/90% DHEA-s).

We again recommend that those taking DHEA have a DHEA blood test to make sure they are taking the precise dose to suit their individual biochemistry. Some people only need to take a small amount of DHEA in order to restore blood levels to that of a 21-year-old, while others need to take higher levels of DHEA. Those with existing prostate or breast cancers should not take DHEA unless closely supervised by a knowledgeable physician who understands DHEA's metabolic pathways.

Some people supplement with the hormone pregnenolone in lieu of, or in addition to DHEA. Since pregnenolone naturally converts into many of the same hormones as DHEA, some of the precautions we advise for DHEA may apply to pregnenolone.

DHEA tests often cost more than $100 at local laboratories, but the Life Extension Foundation offers low-cost DHEA-s and PSA (prostate-specific antigen) testing to members by mail order. *For complete information about the availability of discount blood testing in your area, refer to the Medical Testing protocols or call (800) 208-3444.*

If DHEA replacement sounds complicated, it is, compared to other preventive supplement programs. We suggest weighing the documented anti-aging benefits of maintaining youthful serum DHEA levels when deciding whether to embark on a DHEA replacement regimen. Or stated differently, review the degenerative effects of chronic DHEA deficiency to decide whether this program is worth your time and money.

Product availability. DHEA, melatonin, Saw Palmetto/Nettle Root Formula, selenium, Mega Soy Extract, and vitamins D_3 and E can be ordered by calling (800) 544-4440, or order online at www.lef.org.

DIABETES

Diabetes is a metabolic disorder that interferes with the body's ability to convert digested food into energy and growth. When we eat, the body converts food into glucose, a simple sugar that is our main source of energy. Once glucose becomes available in the bloodstream, it must enter the cells to provide this energy. The pancreatic hormone insulin is required to allow glucose to enter the cells. In a healthy person, the pancreas's beta cells produce exactly the amount of insulin needed to match the amount of food ingested. Blood sugar regulation is accomplished by the most finely controlled system in the body; blood sugar should remain in a very small range of approximately 70 to 120 mg/dl (milligrams per deciliter) even after a heavy meal.

When diabetes occurs, this metabolic process is altered. Depending on the type of diabetes, there is either insufficient insulin or an inability to utilize the insulin that is produced. In both cases, glucose builds up in the bloodstream and the cells starve. Once blood sugar levels pass a certain point, unused sugar spills into the urine as the body attempts to rid itself of the excess. This causes frequent urination and unquenchable thirst because of the continual dumping of fluids to transport the extra sugar into the bladder. The body is forced to turn to other sources of energy. Its solution is to break down stored fats for their small glucose contents. A by-product of this breakdown, ketone bodies, builds up in the blood and may be extremely dangerous. Ketoacidosis accounts for 10% of deaths due to diabetes. Besides thirst and frequent urination, some of the signs of diabetes are

- ▼ Extreme hunger (because food is not assimilated).
- ▼ Weakness (because the body lacks cellular energy).
- ▼ Weight loss (food eaten is just passed through the body)—this is not always seen in Type II diabetes.
- ▼ Tiredness (both because of the high blood sugar and because energy isn't absorbed).
- ▼ Frequent infection (partially due to high sugar levels acting as a growth medium for bacteria).
- ▼ Cuts and bruises slow to heal.
- ▼ Long-term complications that may become evident without other obvious causative agents (impotence, blurry vision, numbness, and pain in the extremities).
- ▼ Sweet-smelling breath (from ketoacidosis, a result of fat metabolism).

Diabetes has two primary forms, as well as some minor, transient ones.

TYPE I (ALSO KNOWN AS INSULIN-DEPENDENT DIABETES MELLITUS, IDDM)

This form of diabetes was once called juvenile diabetes because it commonly occurs in younger patients. It is considered an autoimmune disease and results when the immune system attacks the insulin-producing beta cells of the pancreas, destroying them. The result is a pancreas that produces little or no insulin. The exact cause of the attack on the beta cells is not known, but both genetic and viral factors are believed to be involved.

A person with Type I diabetes requires exogenous insulin (insulin from an outside source) to sustain life. This insulin must be injected daily, and often several times a day. Originally, insulin was obtained from pigs and cows, though today's purified forms are of recombinant DNA origin. Type I patients constitute only about 10% of all diabetics, but they often find the condition to be devastating in its impact, in both short- and long-term damage. There are currently several experiments in progress involving the prevention of Type I diabetes in those who have genetic predisposition to the disorder with beta cell antibodies present. The National Coordinating Center (800) 425-8361 has a list of screening sites around the country, in case you, or people you know, have an interest in participating.

TYPE II (ALSO KNOWN AS NON-INSULIN-DEPENDENT DIABETES MELLITUS, NIDDM)

This is the most common form of diabetes, affecting approximately 15 million people in this country alone. There may be an equal number of as-yet-undiagnosed Type II diabetics, because of the often subtle early signs of the disorder. It has been called adult onset diabetes because it commonly occurs after age 40, most often in the middle 50's and later. In the great majority of cases, the Type

II diabetic is overweight, putting additional demands on an aging organ system.

Type II patients usually produce insulin, but for some reason (either insufficient production or insulin resistance by the cells) their bodies are unable to process glucose efficiently. The resulting condition is similar to that of Type I: an excess of glucose in the blood and the lack of fuel for the cells. Type II may have varying effects in different people. The extreme levels of high blood sugar found in Type I are not as prevalent in Type II patients, and the short-term dangers are not as acute. However, unchecked or poorly controlled Type II will produce long-term damage similar to that found in Type I. Many Type II diabetics eventually take insulin because their disorder cannot be controlled without it.

Gestational Diabetes. Severe environmental and situational stressors, such as pregnancy, may produce high levels of blood sugar. This is similar to the effects of stress on other organ systems. (For example, temporary hypertension or tachycardia may be found among those in extreme situations.) Gestational diabetes is treated with insulin and usually disappears postpartum. However, women with gestational diabetes have a higher incidence of Type II in their later years.

Complications of Diabetes

Short-term complications. The short-term dangers of diabetes are most common among patients with Type I, though Type II patients taking the class of drugs known as sulfonylureas (Diabinese and Glucotrol, for example) may experience problems with hypoglycemia (low blood sugar). This is because the sulfonylureas act by directly stimulating the pancreas to produce additional insulin. Type II diabetics do not independently produce enough effective insulin, or insulin that successfully transports glucose into the cells.

One way of solving this problem is to increase the total amount of insulin available. These diabetics and those on injectable insulin are using treatments that directly increase the amount of glucose assimilation in the body. Taking too much insulin or oral medication, or eating fewer carbohydrates, will cause a precipitous drop in blood sugar. This may result in the body going into shock, a medical emergency. Shock may be treated through the ingestion of sugar, preferably in an easy to assimilate form. (This cannot be attempted if the person is unconscious.) These diabetics should carry glucose tablets or gels or similar products capable of quickly raising blood sugar.

The other short-term danger is of the opposite type: coma. This condition comes from extremely high levels of blood sugar and can result in death if left untreated. Note: if a diabetic is unconscious, never give insulin; wait for blood sugar tests given by a health care professional. To give insulin mistakenly to an unconscious diabetic in shock could be fatal.

Long-term complications. The cumulative effects of diabetes are systemwide. Because diabetes causes both vascular and neurological damage, the end results are enormously significant. This is true for diabetics of both major types. Be aware that diabetics may feel healthy and unaffected while these effects are developing. Type I diabetics, because of the greater number of years with the disease and because of the higher blood sugar levels often seen, may experience more damage at an earlier age. Poorly controlled Type II patients may see similar damage, however. Even well-controlled diabetics can suffer from some degree of these long-term complications:

- ▼ Kidney Failure

  Though most common in Type I cases, circulatory dysfunction may lead to difficulty or failure of this organ. Diabetes is the leading cause of end-stage renal disease.
- ▼ Stroke

  Diabetes is the major cause of strokes in the United States.
- ▼ Amputation

  Over 50% of amputations are diabetes related.
- ▼ Blindness

  Diabetes is the number one cause of blindness in the United States.
- ▼ Cardiovascular disease

  Diabetics are 2 to 4 times as likely to have heart disease as people without diabetes, according to the American Diabetes Association.

- ▼ Impotence
  Among diabetics, both vascular and neurological damage causes high rates of impotence.
- ▼ Neuropathy
  Peripheral neuropathy (pain and numbness in the extremities, usually in the feet and legs) is common in diabetes.

Medical Treatment of Diabetes

The diagnosis of diabetes is made with simple blood sugar (BS) tests. BS tests are often administered when a person sees a physician because of symptoms that suggest to the doctor that diabetes may be present. Other types of blood test are the fasting blood sugar (FBS) performed in the morning before any food is taken and the two-hour postprandial BS (performed 2 hours after a meal). Any BS reading over 140 mg/dl indicates a malfunction in the metabolic system. Besides these tests, factors that help determine the type and degree of diabetes, as well as the most appropriate treatment for each patient, include the level of hyperglycemia, age of onset, other existing medical conditions, and family history of diabetes.

Medicine also has an excellent measure of long-term diabetes control, superior to any blood sugar test that reflects only the patient's status at the moment. This is the hemoglobin A1c test, based on the level of glycosylated hemoglobin, a substance that accumulates over time in the blood. It is found in excessive amounts in poorly controlled diabetics. Because it is a test of an accumulated substance rather than an indicator of a momentary sugar level, the HbA1c indicates the level of control during the preceding two or three months.

The greater the level of blood glucose, the higher the production of glycosylated hemoglobin. An HbA1c score of 7 or less is the goal. (Nondiabetics usually score below 6.) Glycosylation is the chemical reaction that takes place when the body's proteins are exposed to elevated glucose levels. The products of glycosylation are called AGEs, or advanced glycosylation endproducts. Such "crosslinks" have been thought to be irreversible and create accelerated arterial aging. (For a further discussion of this process and its destructive results in diabetes, see Vlassara, 1994).

TYPE I (IDDM)

As its name clearly states, this form of diabetes requires regular and frequent subcutaneous injections of insulin to sustain life and prevent or delay long-term complications. Today's insulins are pure forms of the hormone without the minor problems of the older pork and beef varieties. Syringes are now extremely short and sharp (higher gauge), making injections relatively painless.

Insulin comes in short- and long-term release forms, which are combined in a typical regimen. The most common are R (regular) with an onset after 1/2 to 1 hour and a life of approximately 6 hours, and NPH/L (lente), slower release forms with an onset after approximately 3 hours, and a life of up to 24 hours. Insulins also come in very slow release forms (not commonly used) and several mixtures of R and L in one bottle. The most important advances in insulin therapy are the implantable pump (which releases insulin internally at the patient's remote-control direction) and Lispro (marketed as Humalog), a rapid release insulin that begins working within minutes and can be taken at the same time as a meal is served. Lispro's quick availability means that the critical problem of having to wait for several hours to reduce a high blood sugar level has now been partially solved. A high reading can be reduced to relatively normal levels in well under an hour. The active Type I diabetic can now limit the time his/her body suffers the damages of hyperglycemia by a significant amount.

It is important to realize that taking insulin does not remove the need to maintain proper dietary practices. Poor dietary control can overwhelm any insulin regime. Diet will be discussed below.

TYPE II (NIDDM)

The first treatment of Type II diabetes is always diet. In many cases, diet alone (with concomitant weight loss) may be the only thing needed to restore acceptable blood sugar levels. Even if medication is prescribed, and even if insulin is added, the patient must be aware of, and practice, dietary restraints.

Type II medications are of several classes, and may be combined in treatment:

- **Sulfonylureas.** These drugs were once the primary pharmaceutical treatment and still are used heavily (though Metformin/Glucophage now is the most widely prescribed pill).

  The sulfonylureas (Diabenese, for example) work by stimulating pancreatic production of insulin. They do contain the possibility of inducing hypoglycemic (low blood sugar) reactions, and the user must be prepared to counter such responses with sugar, juice, glucose tablets, etc. This also demands that meals be taken at the correct times. This class of drugs has a history of significant side effects, primarily cardiovascular.
- **Glucosidase Inhibitors.** Drugs such as Precose work by delaying the absorption of digested carbohydrates. This lowers the load placed on an inefficient metabolic system. The glucosidase inhibitors are taken with each meal and pose no risk of hypoglycemia since they do not artificially elevate insulin levels.
- **Biguanides (Metformin).** Marketed as Glucophage, this multi-action drug is the most widely prescribed Type II medication. It works by (1) reducing hepatic (liver) glucose production, thus stopping the body from adding to the blood's glucose levels, (2) reducing intestinal absorption of glucose, and (3) increasing insulin sensitivity, thus increasing glucose uptake. Because Glucophage does not increase the production of insulin, it also does not cause hypoglycemia. Side effects are usually minor gastric upsets such as nausea or diarrhea.

Rezulin. The newest Type II drug is Rezulin. This medication works directly on the core problem of this form of diabetes, the cells' resistance to insulin. Despite its effectiveness, Rezulin apparently has caused liver damage and death in enough people to have been nearly removed from the market. Though it remains available, physicians are closely monitoring the 1.2 million patients taking Rezulin.

Insulin. Some Type II patients find that diet and oral medications cannot control their blood sugar satisfactorily. In these cases, insulin may be added to the oral drugs, or may replace them entirely.

Medicines for common diabetes-related problems. There are numerous specialized pharmaceutical treatments for such diabetes complications as hypertension, high cholesterol, claudication (pain in the legs from vascular blockage) and impotence, as well as techniques for vision impairment, vascular blockage, and post-cardiac insult conditions.

Self-Treatment and Management of Diabetes

Of all the disorders common to human beings, diabetes is the one most affected by the patient's management. Not only does each person's fate directly rest on self-diagnosis and self-medication, but he/she controls the impact of the disorder on multiple bodily systems. A diabetic's diet, exercise, stress levels, personal habits, emotional states, and choice of vitamin, mineral, and other supplements taken will determine his/her immediate and eventual fate.

Self-testing and sugar management. Regular, home blood-glucose testing is at the core of diabetes control. Many years of research have proven, beyond a doubt, that the higher a person's average blood sugar, the more damage he/she will suffer. Reciprocally, the better the control, the fewer the complications (Morgensen, 1998; UK Prospectives Diabetes Study Group, 1998). Thus, it is not only how high blood sugar gets, but also how long it stays there. Testing your blood sugar frequently will help keep levels normalized and prevent high levels from remaining high. Physicians refer to this as "covering" a high sugar with additional insulin. If a diabetic "covers" a high reading with the new rapid-acting insulin (Lispro), the amount of time the body suffers damage may be significantly reduced.

In addition to glucose testing, diabetics should test for the presence of ketones in the urine if blood sugar exceeds 240 mg/dl. (Ketoacidosis is not a danger for Type II diabetics.) Diabetics should test even more frequently during periods of illness or injury, when blood sugar levels tend to rise dramatically, even in the absence of any food intake.

While glucose self-testing obviously is critical for those with IDDM, many Type II patients would benefit as well. They could respond to high sugars in a variety of ways, at the instructions of their physicians. These patients could be allowed to adjust their medications, reduce their next meal, or in some cases, add a small amount of insulin. When "covering" is not an option, having self-testing data allows the physician to adjust a patient's program properly. Even those Type II patients who are extremely well-controlled should test on a less frequent basis because of the numerous agents and events capable of elevating blood sugar.

Diet. As has been mentioned, even with well-designed medication regimes, diet is critical in many ways. On the most basic of levels, many diabetics must perform a delicate balancing effect with caloric/carbohydrate intake and medicine. This becomes even more important when the medications used have peaks of effectiveness (see below).

As also mentioned previously, diet and weight loss may be the only treatment required with Type II diabetes. Bringing intake down to the body's diminished digestive capacity is often the answer to this medical disorder.

More specifically, the following dietary recommendations may be made:

- Eat a cardiac patient's diet. Because degradation of the cardiovascular system is the root problem in diabetes, and so much of the resulting pathology is either in the heart and blood vessels or in organs with inadequate vascular supply, the basic rules of the cardiac diet should be followed. Diabetics typically have elevated cholesterol and high blood pressure. Therefore, fat intake should be kept low, and saturated fats should be avoided. Meals high in fiber and emphasizing complex carbohydrates are suggested. If blood pressure is not normal (120 over 80) or lower, salt intake should be reduced. Raw vegetables (as in salads) are absorbed slowly and are low in calories.
- Eat smaller meals. Even when properly medicated, it is difficult for the body of a diabetic to process large amounts of food at one time. Excessive food intake can cause blood sugar elevations. Smaller meals reduce the demand on an inadequate insulin supply system.
- Eat only small to moderate amounts of protein. Diabetes is a major cause of kidney disease. High-protein diets are difficult for the kidneys to process. The logical response is to restrict protein intake. Since proteins and fats are paired in red meats, it is recommended that sources of red meat be avoided as much as possible. Unfortunately, for many years diabetics were prescribed a diet in which carbohydrates were replaced with large amounts of proteins and fats. The long-term data concerning typical diabetes complications (with high incidences of vascular and renal disease) undoubtedly reflect that diet's errors.
- Meals should be timed to match the dosage curves of diabetes medications. All insulin and some oral drugs have periods of onset and peak activity. Diet plans should adjust to these pre-set times. If a patient cannot arrange to eat the appropriate amount of food at the correct times, then some accommodation must be made, for example, by altering medication times or adding a small meal to delay hypoglycemic reactions.
- Become familiar with the Glycemic Index (Thomas et al., 1994). This is an extremely useful tool to help regulate metabolic activity. The Glycemic Index lists the relative speed at which different foods are digested and raise blood sugar levels. Each food is compared to the effect of the same amount of pure glucose on the body's blood sugar curve. Glucose itself has a Glycemic Index rating of 100. Foods that are broken down and raise blood glucose levels quickly have high ratings. The closer to 100, the more that food resembles glucose. The lower the rating, the more gradually that food affects the blood sugar level. The Glycemic Research Institute ((202)-434-8270; e-mail

glycemic.com) publishes rating of hundreds of different foods, and issues a seal of approval on foods which elicit low responses. Here is a list of some common foods and their Glycemic Index ratings:

Baked potatoes, 95; White bread, 95; Mashed potatoes, 90; Carrots, 85; Chocolate candy bar, 70; Corn, 70; Boiled potatoes,70; Bananas, 60; White pasta, 55; Peas, 50; Unsweetened fruit juice, 40; Rye bread, 40; Dairy, 35; Lentils, 30; Fresh fruit, 30; Soy, 15; Green vegetables, tomatoes, <15.

- Know the facts about alcohol. The most important fact is that being out of control makes it difficult to manage diabetes, even masking the acute danger brought on by hypoglycemic reactions. If a person is capable of the moderate use of alcohol, other facts are important. Pure alcohol itself (scotch, vodka, rum, gin, etc.) contains no carbohydrates, despite what it is made from. Liqueurs, such as Amaretto and Kahlua, on the other hand, are high in carbohydrates. Another danger comes from the mixers used in cocktails, many of which have high sugar contents (colas, juices, tonic, margarita mix, etc.).

  One odd fact is that, under certain circumstances, alcohol can actually cause a low blood sugar reaction. If blood sugar is low and food is not eaten, plain alcohol alone may prevent the body's natural, protective response to hypoglycemia. In other words, when the body wants to release stored glycogen (sugar) to combat low blood sugar levels, alcohol prevents it from doing so.
- Diabetes' damage is increased tremendously by smoking. Tobacco usage causes severe damage to the vascular system, adding to a diabetic's already embattled health.

Stress. The problems of diabetes are compounded by stress. On a direct level, stress raises the blood sugar. This happens because of the primitive "fight or flight" response in which perceived dangers are met by the body's protective chemical reactions, including a release of adrenaline from the adrenal glands and dumping of glycogen (sugar) stores from the liver. In a healthy person, the reaction may be useful for the energy and alertness needed to deal with difficult situations. In a diabetic, the additional glycogen input cannot be utilized and results in elevation of the blood sugar. Such elevations can be extreme and may result from everything from bumping into an ex-spouse, to getting called by a doctor with the results of a blood test, to having to testify in court. Frequent and timely self-testing may help to mitigate this problem.

Stress also robs the body of necessary nutrient levels. All of the basic requirements of an individual are increased by stress.

When a diabetic's sugar levels become elevated, the body attempts to transport the excess sugar out through the kidneys by increasing urination. In the process of excreting fluids, water-soluble nutrients are lost, and must be replaced by regular supplementation.

Exercise. Exercise plays a direct role in the control of diabetes by increasing the efficiency of available insulin. Combined with diet, exercise may return some Type II diabetics to normal metabolic levels. An additional benefit accrues from the blood-pressure-lowering effect of exercise. As mentioned previously, diabetics typically suffer from hypertension, a major factor in some of the deadly and disabling complications discussed in this protocol.

Therapeutic Supplements for Diabetes

The use of supplements in the management of a complex disorder such as diabetes must be equally complex. Following the recommendations for diabetes presented below, the protocols for other, related medical problems will be suggested as well.

Note that the recommendations are directed primarily at the symptoms of diabetes, not at the disorder itself. Until a cure for the disorder is discovered, controlling its damage is paramount.

There are several major avenues of treatment for diabetes. All presume that the patient is taking a high-potency, easily assimilated, multivitamin-mineral complex as a basis for other specific, symptom-targeted supplements. The global objective of this approach is to limit, prevent, or in some cases reverse the vascular and neural damage seen in diabetes. This involves

- Improving the oxygen delivery capacity of the circulatory system by stopping, eliminating, or circumventing vascular blockage, thus improving cellular and neural health.
- Preventing diabetes-induced metabolic breakdowns.
- Reducing oxidative stress.
- Inducing angiogenesis (regenerating capillaries).
- Changing the lipid characteristics of blood corpuscles to make them less brittle and more capable of entering the small capillaries.
- Preventing endoneural hypoxia (oxygen deficiency in the tissues).

The following are the most important supplements for the aggressive treatment of diabetes:

Aminoguanidine. As described above, glycosylation is a major biological development that causes degenerative vascular disease. It is caused by the prolonged exposure of amino acids to elevated glucose levels. The ability of aminoguanidine to prevent this process makes it the single most important supplement for those with diabetes. Earlier reports of toxicity were investigated by the Life Extension Foundation, and safe levels of usage have now been determined. Still, regular liver tests should be performed.

Recommended dosage: 300 mg daily

The FDA currently prevents the purchase of aminoguanidine domestically. For a directory of offshore suppliers write to

International Society for Free Choice
9 Dubnoc Street
64368 Tel Aviv, Israel

Antioxidants. Oxidative damage plays critical roles in the complications of diabetes, including being part of the glycosylation process. Here are the most important antioxidants used to combat this oxidative stress:

Alpha-lipoic acid (aLA), also known as thioctic acid. Alpha-lipoic acid has also been shown to be useful in the maintenance of neural health (Garrett, 1997). It is suggested that vitamin B_{12} in the form of methyl-cobalamin be taken concurrently since aLA may cause B_{12} depletion. Recommended dosage: 250 mg 2 times daily.

Proanthocyanidins (grape seed/skin extract). These may be the most concentrated natural antioxidants available. They also inhibit a dangerous enzyme known as COX-2 that interferes with the body's levels of a beneficial substance called prostacyclin (discussed below). The newest and most effective form of proanthocyanidins is Biovin. Recommended dosage: 100 mg twice daily.

Vitamin E. This nutrient also protects prostacyclin, widens blood vessels, and thins the blood. Recommended dosage: 400 mg initially, gradually raised to 400 mg, 2 or 3 times daily.

Vitamin C. Recommended dosage: 2500 mg daily, in divided doses.

Coenzyme Q_{10}. CoQ_{10} is also an immune boosting agent. Recommended dosage: 30 to 100 mg daily.

Life Extension Mix. 3 tablets, 3 times a day provides broad-spectrum protection against free radicals.

Acetyl-L-Carnitine (ALC). This may be the single most important nutrient in the treatment of diabetic neuropathy, capable of demonstrating "a significant amelioration of symptoms" (Quatraro, 1995). Recommended dosage: 500–1000 mg twice daily.

Aspirin. This ubiquitous medication has numerous benefits for diabetics. Besides its blood-thinning (stroke preventing) properties, it is the painkiller that does not interfere with prostacyclin (Drvota, 1990). Even more significant was the finding of Malik and Meek (1986) that aspirin actually blocked glycosylation. Recommended dosage: One regular strength aspirin every other day.

Prostacyclin Enhancers. Prostacyclin is a major vasoprotective molecule that is central to the pathogenesis of diabetic neuropathy. Commonly used painkillers and anti-inflammatory agents interfere with the production of prostacyclin, adding to its inadequate supply in most diabetics. Several supplements previously mentioned help to potentiate its availability.

Because of the reduced amounts of prostacyclin among diabetics, their red blood corpuscles (the body's oxygen delivery mechanism) become brittle and rigid. This prevents oxygen from "squeezing" into them, causing particular damage to the smallest capillaries and the tissues they serve. Prostacyclin also inhibits the abnormal platelet aggregation that leads to clots and strokes.

The following supplements help to enhance the body's supply of prostacyclin:

Gamma-linolenic acid (GLA). This substance promotes the release of prostacyclin. GLA makes blood corpuscles more flexible, regenerates capillaries, and nourishes nerves. Combining GLA with vitamin C makes it more efficient.

Recommended dosage: 1500 mg daily, taken in divided doses. (Five borage oil capsules (MEGA GLA) provide 1500 mg of GLA.)

Eicosapentaenoic acid (EPA). This fish oil concentrate reduces abnormal blood clotting inside blood vessels and lowers triglyceride levels.

Recommended dosage: 1200 to 2400 mg daily.

Gingko Biloba. This is also a powerful antioxidant.

Recommended dosage: 120 mg daily.

Vanadium. Because this substance also mimics the action of insulin, Type II diabetics in particular should be aware of a possible reduction in medication requirements.

Recommended dosage: 7.5 mg 3 times daily.

Ginger. This prostacyclin inhibitor also directly inhibits abnormal platelet aggregation and reduces cholesterol (Bordia et al., 1997).

Recommended dosage: 500–2000 mg daily.

Other Nutrients to Consider

Niacin. Also known as vitamin B_3 and nicotinic acid, this substance has been found to preserve residual beta cell function (Pozzilli et al., 1996). It has multiple benefits for diabetics by dilating peripheral blood vessels and reducing cholesterol levels. It may be taken in a "no flush" formulation, while "timed release" niacin should be avoided.

Recommended dosage: 800 mg twice daily.

Chromium. Because of chromium's ability to enhance cellular absorption (increasing the efficiency of insulin), Type II diabetics should be aware of the possibility that their medications may need lowering.

Recommended dosage: 200 mcg twice daily.

Biotin. This vitamin may be helpful in the management of neuropathy and enhances glucose utilization (Koutsikos, et al., 1990).

Recommended dosage: 5 mg daily in divided doses.

Inositol and Taurine. These nutrients are depleted in diabetics, affecting a number of cardiovascular factors.

Recommended dosage: 1500 mg of each daily.

Magnesium. A deficiency in this mineral, common in diabetes, will cause severe vascular damage as well as neuropathy.

Recommended dosage: 500 mg daily.

L-lysine. This amino acid has some effectiveness in preventing glycosylation.

Recommended dosage: 500 mg daily.

Alternative Therapies

Chelation. The vascular complications of diabetes cause thickening, stiffening, and blockage of blood vessels. Obstruction is caused by free radical activity, lipid accumulation, and calcification. (The latter may easily be seen on X-rays of the feet, where diabetic circulation is at its worst, sometimes leading to infections and amputations.)

The technique of chelation involves introducing a substance called EDTA (ethylene-diamine-tetra-acetic acid) by intravenous drip over a period of several hours. This process is repeated several times (based on several factors including health and financial status; insurance will not reimburse for chelation). The purpose is to remove calcium deposits, normalize cholesterol levels, and decrease free radical activity, leading to less restriction of blood flow. This occurs when the EDTA bonds with the unwanted substances and carries them away to be discarded in the urine.

Though the technique is still controversial, more and more physicians are offering this treatment as reports of its success grow (Chappell and Stahl, 1993; Hancke and Flytlie, 1993). While i.v. chelation is most effective, some smaller preventive effects may be achieved though oral chelation. These products (such as the Life Extension Foundation's Pure-Gar) should contain EDTA to have any chance of success.

Relaxation Therapies/Meditation. Whether they are called relaxation, biofeedback, self-hypnosis, autogenic training, meditation, or any related name, these treatments all attempt to lower a person's stress levels (critically important in diabetes). Usually, this involves the focusing of attention on a stimulus, sound, or visualization. Once a subject is in this altered state, blood pressure and pulse rates are reduced and peripheral blood vessels are dilated, causing increased blood and oxygen delivery to deprived tissues.

These therapies may be done under the guidance of a professional such as a trained psychotherapist, in a group setting, or at home with books and tapes. However they occur, they *are* beneficial.

Acupuncture. Besides its sometimes effective assistance with smoking and weight loss cessation, acupuncture has been used to treat the pain and discomfort of peripheral neuropathy.

Related Disease Protocols

Because of its pervasive effects on health, diabetes must be regarded as a multitude of diseases. It is recommended that the following protocols be studied and incorporated into the regimen offered in this discussion as appropriate:

1. Anxiety and Stress
2. Cerebral Vascular Disease
3. Hypertension
4. Neuropathy
5. Stroke

Duration of Symptoms

At this time, diabetes is considered a lifelong condition. Most advances have occurred in the areas of home blood-glucose testing, insulin delivery, medications with fewer side effects, and the treatment of specific symptoms. Therefore, diabetics should take a long-term approach to health care, understanding that lifestyles and dietary cautions for the general public apply to them with greater urgency.

Summary

Self-treatment and management play a critical role in the control of diabetes. Regulation of diet, exercise, stress levels, and personal habits as well as vitamin, mineral, and other supplementation will strongly affect immediate and long-term wellness. Suggested supplements are

1. Aminoguanidine, to prevent degenerative vascular disease, 300 mg daily.
2. Alpha-lipoic acid (aLA) to reduce oxidative damage, 250 mg twice daily.
3. Proanthocyanidins such as grape seed-skin extract, 100 mg twice daily.
4. Vitamin E, to protect prostacyclin, 400 mg 2 or 3 times daily.
5. Vitamin C, another effective antioxidant, 2500 mg daily in divided doses.
6. Coenzyme Q_{10}, to boost the immune system and aid the cardiovascular system, 30 to 100 mg daily.
7. Acetyl-*L*-carnitine (ALC), an important nutrient in the treatment of diabetic neuropathy, 500–1000 mg twice daily.
8. Aspirin, for its blood thinning and painkilling properties and also its effectiveness in blocking glycosylation, one regular strength aspirin every other day.

9. Gamma-linolenic acid (GLA), to promote the release of prostacyclin, nourishing nerves, and regenerating capillaries, 1500 mg daily, taken in divided doses.
10. Eicosapentaenoic acid (EPA), a fish oil product to reduce abnormal blood clotting and lower triglycerides, 1200 to 2400 mg daily.
11. Gingko biloba, for its antioxidant effects, 120 mg twice daily.
12. Vanadium, because it mimics the effects of insulin (Type II diabetics should be aware of possible reduction in medication), 7.5 mg 3 times daily.
13. Ginger, to inhibit abnormal platelet aggregation and reduce cholesterol, found in the Life Extension Foundation's Herbal Cardiovascular Formula.
14. Niacin, to dilate peripheral blood vessels and reduce cholesterol levels, 800 mg twice daily.
15. Chromium, to enhance cellular absorption, 200 mg twice daily.
16. Inositol and taurine, which are depleted in diabetics, 1500 mg of each daily.
17. Magnesium, deficiencies of which cause severe vascular damage and neuropathy, 500 mg daily.
18. Life Extension Mix, 3 tablets, 3 times a day. Provides broad-spectrum protection against common diabetic pathologies.
19. *L*-lysine, to prevent glycosylation, 500 mg daily.
20. Chelation therapy, to remove calcium deposits, normalize cholesterol levels, and decrease free radical activity.
21. Relaxation therapies to lower stress levels.
22. Acupuncture, in the treatment of pain due to peripheral neuropathy.

For more information. Contact the American Diabetes Association, (800) 232-3472.

Product availability. Acetyl-*L*-carnitine, aLA, GLA, ginkgo biloba, vanadium, chromium, "no flush" niacin, *L*-lysine, proanthocyanidins, CoQ_{10}, and EPA are available by calling (800) 544-4448, or order online at www.lef.org.

DIGESTIVE DISORDERS

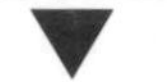

It is estimated that more than 100 million people in America are affected by some form of digestive disease. That's more than half of the U.S. population!

For some people, digestive disorders are a source of irritation and discomfort that may cause them to drastically limit their life styles and miss work frequently. For others, these disorders may be extremely crippling, and even fatal.

The Gastrointestinal Tract (GIT)

The gastrointestinal tract is a long muscular tube that functions as the food processor for the human body. The digestive system includes the following organs: the mouth and salivary glands, the stomach, the small and large intestines, the colon, the liver and pancreas, and the gall bladder.

Irritations or inflammation of the various sections of the gastrointestinal tract are identified as gastritis (stomach), colitis (colon), ileitis (ileum or small intestines), hepatitis (liver), and cholecystitis (gall bladder).

The gastrointestinal tract is not a passive system; rather it has the capability to sense and react to the materials that are passed through it. For a healthy digestive system, every person requires different food selections that match their gastrointestinal tract capacity.

The Digestive Process

The GIT breaks down foods by first using mechanical means such as chewing, and then by the application of a host of complex chemical processes. These chemical processes include everything from saliva to colon microbes. Since the GIT is the point of entry for the human body, everything eaten has an impact on the body. The food eaten and passed through the GIT contains nutrients as well as toxins. Toxins can be anything from food additives and pesticides to specific foods that induce a reactive response by the GIT.

The process of digestion is accomplished via the surface of the gastrointestinal tract using secretions from accessory glands. The two glands providing the majority of digestive chemicals utilized by the gastrointestinal tract are the liver and the pancreas. The function of the liver is to control the food supply for the rest of the body by further processing of the food molecules absorbed through the intestines. This is done by dispensing those food molecules in a controlled manner, and by filtering out toxins that may have passed through the gastrointestinal tract wall.

Another very important function of the gastrointestinal tract is as a sensory organ. By rejecting foods through objectionable taste, vomiting, and diarrhea or any combination of these symptoms, the sensing capacity of the GIT can protect the body. The surface of the GIT has a complex system of nerves and other cells of the immune system. The surface of the GIT, or mucosa, is part of a complex sensing system called the MALT (Mucosa Associated Lymphatic Tissue). The immune sensors in MALT trigger responses such as nausea, vomiting, pain, and swelling. Vomiting and diarrheas are abrupt defensive responses to MALT-sensing foods with a strong allergic or toxic component. This kind of food intolerance is responsible for many digestive problems. The gastrointestinal tract is "hard-wired" to the brain via hormonal, neurotransmitter-mediator chemical communication.

The gastrointestinal tract is a muscular tube that contracts in a controlled rhythm to move food through the different sections (peristalsis). Strength and timing variations in the contractions can cause cramping (very strong contractions) and diarrhea (contractions are very frequent).When the contractions are slow and irregular, constipation may occur. "Motility disorder" is the general term used to describe problems with peristalsis.

In all but a few cases, a food allergy is the primary cause of gastrointestinal tract problems. Chronic diseases have their origin in food allergies. The dysfunction, discomfort, and disease associated with GIT are the result of local immune responses to food selections or combinations of foods. Food selections are a result of personal tastes, social fads, ethnic culture, religion, and, to a larger degree, local and/or seasonal availability. The food selections made in modern affluent society are based on a developed taste for a rich diet centered on meats and dairy products that are loaded with fats, high concentrations of proteins, and fat-soluble toxins. Advertising and misinformation about "healthy" diets have overshadowed human nutritional needs in modern affluent diets.

Dietary Shifts and Digestive Disorders

Human evolutionary history clearly shows that we are primarily herbivores. Human saliva contains alpha-amylase, an enzyme specifically designed to break down complex carbohydrates into sugar compounds. Our teeth are designed to cut vegetable matter and to grind grains. The so-called canine teeth of humans bear no resemblance to the canines of even a domestic house cat. The human digestive system is long and the food is processed slowly to extract all the nutrients from plant material. Conversely, carnivores have short digestive tracts that digest flesh very quickly. The digestive systems of carnivores are able to eliminate the large amount of cholesterol consumed in their diets. Carnivores do not have alpha-amylase present in their saliva.

The effect of the shift in our diets during the last hundred years has resulted in 44% of Americans and Canadians being afflicted with heartburn; peptic ulcer disease appears in 5% of the population, and nonulcer dyspepsia plagues between 20 and 40% of Americans. Over-the-counter medications for these ailments are a multibillion-dollar industry. In nearly every hour of television advertising there is at least one spot selling an antacid or similar product.

If You Suffer from Ulcers

The medical community has discovered that most stomach ulcers are caused by the *Helicobacter pylori* (*H. pylori*) bacteria. A physician can have blood tested for the presence of the *H. pylori* antibody. Special antibiotic combinations can be used to eliminate this bacteria from the stomach within a matter of weeks. Those who fail to eradicate *H. pylori* are at a far greater risk for contracting stomach cancer.

Gastrointestinal Symptoms

There are five basic symptoms indicating a gastrointestinal tract problem. These symptoms are generally associated with dietary problems or specific food allergies. It is critical that anyone suffering from serious gastrointestinal tract problems work closely with a physician to test for the more developed and serious gastrointestinal tract diseases; that physician should also be experienced in working with dietary factors and food allergies.

Nausea and vomiting can vary between a squeamish feeling in the stomach to the violent action of immediate vomiting. Patients with nausea and vomiting symptoms should assume the ingestion of a reactive food (i.e., food containing toxins) or poisoning with a pathogen such as staphylococci. Vomiting immediately after eating is usually proceeded by excessive watery salivation. Some chronic low intensity nausea can occur for a protracted time due to sustained low-level food allergies or problems with food combinations. Patients with lower-level nausea usually have their symptoms disappear with diet revision. Nausea and vomiting are also linked with migraines caused by food allergies (*see the Migraine protocol*).

Bloating can result from excessive gas in the digestive system, failure of the digestive tract to sustain youthful peristaltic contractions, or a lack of sufficient quantities of digestive enzymes and bile acids required to rapidly break down food. Intestinal gas results from food fermentation and from swallowing air while eating. The bloating from intestinal gas is different from that which occurs in the colon.

Constipation is the decreased frequency or slowing of peristalsis resulting in harder stools. When the gastrointestinal tract is slowed down, feces can accumulate in the colon with attending pain and toxic reactions. A "spastic colon" results when the colon contracts out of frequency in painful spasms blocking movement of the stool. Some patients experience painful days of constipation followed by forceful diarrhea and watery stool, often accompanied with abdominal cramps.

Diarrhea is the increased frequency of bowel movement that is also loose or watery. If diarrhea increases, the possibility of celiac disease is considered. Celiac disease is a serious disease that allows certain macromolecules to pass through the intestinal wall. If blood appears in the stool, ulcerative colitis is likely. Protracted bouts with diarrhea can result in nutritional deficiencies due to the malabsorption of essential nutrients.

Abdominal pain appears in different patterns and with varying intensities. Cramping occurs because of muscle spasms of the abdominal organs. Severe cramping pain, often called colic, usually occurs from problems with food intakes that exhibit strong allergic response in the patient. Abdominal cramping near the navel is typically from the small intestine, and near the sides, top, and bottom of the lower abdomen, the pain is associated with the colon.

Diseases associated with central gastrointestinal tract disorders and diagnoses include depression, migraine, asthma, sinusitis, and fibromyalgia. These diseases have been identified with specific patterns of food allergic response. All of these diseases also have links to Irritable Bowel Syndrome (IBS). (IBS is more accurately referred to as RBS—reactive bowel syndrome.)

Steps to a Healthier Digestive System

Elimination diet plans are a good method of determining what foods are harmful to the GIT of a patient. Planning and following such diets are a safe starting point for anyone desiring to help themselves by tracking their gastrointestinal tract's response to food. Interview physicians to learn who may be most qualified to assist in planning an elimination diet. A very good indicator of a healthy gastrointestinal tract is a regular transit time for complete food digestion. Patients who are "regular" are usually in optimum health.

Aging causes many people to experience problems with complete digestion. This can be helped by the use of specific enzymes to improve the efficiency of digestion. Enzymes can be used to speed up the digestive process and to make more nutrients available for absorption.

Enzymes Are a Vital Component of the Digestive Process

Enzymes are essential to the body's absorption and full use of food. The capacity of the living organism to make enzymes diminishes with age, and some scientists believe that humans could live longer and be healthier by guarding against the loss of our precious enzymes.

Enzymes are responsible for every activity of life. Even thinking requires enzyme activity. There are two primary classes of enzymes responsible for maintaining life functions: digestive and metabolic. The primary digestive enzymes are proteases (to digest protein), amylases (to digest carbohydrate), and lipases (to digest fat). These enzymes function as a biological catalyst to help break down food. Raw foods also provide enzymes that naturally break down food for proper absorption. Metabolic enzymes are responsible for the structuring, repair, and remodeling of every cell, and the body is under a great daily burden to supply sufficient enzymes for optimal health. Metabolic enzymes operate in every cell, every organ, and every tissue, and they need constant replenishment.

Digestion of food takes a high priority and has a high demand for enzymes. When we eat, enzymatic activity begins in the mouth, where salivary amylase, lingual lipase, and ptyalin initiate starch and fat digestion. In the stomach, hydrochloric acid activates pepsinogen to pepsin, which breaks down protein, and gastric lipase begins the hydrolysis of fats. Without proper enzyme production, the body has a difficult time digesting food, often resulting in a variety of chronic disorders.

Poor eating habits, including inadequate chewing and eating on the run, can result in inadequate enzyme production and hence malabsorption of food. And this is exacerbated with aging, since that is a time of decreased hydrochloric acid production as well as of a general decline in digestive enzyme secretion.

Saliva is rich in amylase, while gastric juice contains protease. The pancreas secretes digestive juices containing high concentrations of amylase and protease as well as a smaller concentration of lipase. It also secretes a small concentration of maltase, which reduces to dextrose. Animals eating raw food often have no enzymes at all in saliva, unlike humans. However, dogs fed on a high carbohydrate, heat-treated diet have been found to develop enzymes in their saliva within a week in response to enzyme-depleting foods.

One of America's pioneering biochemists and nutrition researchers, Dr. Edward Howell, in his book *Enzyme Nutrition*, cites numerous animal studies showing that animals fed diets that are deficient in enzymes suffer from enlargement of the pancreas, as huge amounts of pancreatic enzymes are squandered in digesting foods that are devoid of natural enzymes. The result of this wasteful outpouring of pancreatic digestive enzymes is a decrease in the supply of crucial metabolic enzymes and impaired health.

How significant is an enzyme deficiency to overall health? For starters, organs that are overworked will enlarge in order to perform the increased workload. Those with congestive heart failure or aortic valvular disease often suffer from an enlarged heart, which is not a healthy condition. When the pancreas enlarges in order to produce more digestive enzymes, there results a deficiency in the production of life-sustaining metabolic enzymes, as available enzyme-producing capacity is used in digesting food instead of supporting cellular enzymatic functions. The tremendous impact that wastage of pancreatic enzymes can have on health and even life itself has been established in animal studies. The critical question is how this applies to human health.

For a good part of the 20th century, European oncologists have included enzyme therapy as a natural, nontoxic therapy against cancer. Almost all of the leading alternative cancer specialists treating Americans prescribe both food enzymes and concentrated enzyme supplements as primary or adjuvant cancer therapies. Nicholas Gonzalez, M.D., a New York City cancer specialist, uses very high doses of supplemental pancreas enzymes as a primary anti-tumor therapy. Dr. Gonzalez's clinical successes have led conventional drug companies to seek to duplicate these natural therapies and offer them as adjuvant drug therapies. One might assume that if pancreatic enzymes are efficacious in treating existing cancers, maintaining a large pool of these precious enzymes in the body would help to prevent cancer from developing in the first place. Epidemiological studies on human populations show that those who eat fresh fruits and vegetables that are loaded with natural enzymes have significantly reduced levels of cancer and other diseases. Whether the high enzyme content of these foods is partially responsible for their anticancer effect has not been proven, but the evidence is compelling.

Digestive organs such as the pancreas and liver produce most of the body's digestive enzymes, while the remainder should come from uncooked foods such as fresh fruit and vegetables, raw sprouted grains, seeds and nuts, unpasteurized dairy products, and enzyme supplements.

Eating food in its natural, unprocessed state is vital to the maintenance of good health, and a lack of it in the modern diet is directly responsible for much degenerative disease. Cooking of food, particularly if heat is prolonged and more than 118 degrees Fahrenheit, destroys enzymes in that food, leaving what is commonly consumed in the modern person's "enzyme-less" diet. This is one reason that by middle age, we become metabolically depleted of enzymes. The glands and major organs, including the brain, suffer most from this deficiency. The brain may actually shrink as a result of a cooked, overrefined diet devoid of enzymes the body so desperately needs. As stated earlier in this article, to try to meet the deficiency, the pancreas swells. Laboratory mice fed on heat-processed, enzyme-less foods have a pancreas 2 or 3 times heavier than that of wild mice eating their natural enzyme diet of raw food.

If foods are consumed uncooked, fewer of the body's digestive enzymes are required to perform the digestive function. The body thereby adapts to the plentiful, external supply by secreting fewer of its own enzymes, preserving these enzymes to assist in vital cellular metabolic functions. Frying is one of the worst cooking methods since it occurs at a much higher temperature than boiling, damaging protein as well as destroying enzymes. Many digestive disorders such as bloating may be related to an enzyme deficit that begins in middle age.

Enzymes can also be wasted by lifestyle factors. Enzymes do more work with increasing temperatures, and they are used up faster. For example, a fever induces faster enzyme action, and hence is unfavorable for bacterial activity. Enzymes have been found in the urine not only after fevers but also after strenuous athletic activity.

Animals harness the power of enzymes in food by burying or covering it, thereby allowing enzyme activity to begin predigesting food. In that manner, animals instinctively preserve their own enzyme supply. In fact, animals, and also the people of some native cultures, teach us not only about how to preserve our enzyme supply, but also about disease prevention through efficient use of enzymes. Although whales have up to 6 inches of fat keeping them warm, for instance, their arteries are unclogged. Similarly, Eskimos, who frequently eat large quantities of fat, are often not obese. Both these groups eat the fat-digesting enzyme, lipase, in the form of raw foods.

In vitro and controlled *in vivo* studies using internal and parenteral routes have examined the effectiveness of different types and sources of plant enzymes in a wide range of conditions, including mal-digestion, malabsorption, pancreatic insufficiency, steatorrhea, celiac disease, lactose intolerance, arterial obstruction, and thrombotic disease.

Enzymes derived from the *Aspergillus oryzae* fungus have been subjected to numerous studies evaluating their role in supporting healthy digestive function. Moreover, several human studies suggest the proteolytic enzymes derived from this fungus may play a role in anti-inflammatory and fibrinolytic therapy. These enzymes appear to be relatively heat stable, and they are also active throughout a wide pH range, important because most enzymes are deactivated in stomach acid. These enzymes, synthesized from fungus, contain no fungal residue even though that is their derivation. Modern filtration technology enables these fungal enzymes to be ideal for human consumption.

Oral supplementation of digestive enzymes taken just before or at mealtimes can assist digestion, according to Dr. Mark Percival. Writing in *Nutritional Pearls,* Dr. Percival says that although most supplemental enzymes are labile and will deactivate when exposed to stomach acid, some of the enzymes remain active if they are taken just before or with a meal. "The enzymes are physically protected" by the meal, allowing for some enzymatic activity to occur in the stomach. And those enzymes that make it through to the small intestine may help with digestion there as well. Because pH plays a major role in enzymatic activity, the enzymes derived from *Aspergillus* "may be highly useful as they appear to be remarkably stable, even when subjected to an acidic environment." Dr. Howell says he chews an enzyme capsule with his food in order to start the digestive process as soon as the food is consumed. Enzyme activity has been shown to begin even before the food is swallowed.

Dr. Arnold Renshaw, of Manchester, England, reported in *Annals of Rheumatic Disease* that he had obtained good results with enzyme treatment of more than 700 patients with rheumatoid arthritis, osteoarthritis, or fibrositis. "Some intractable cases of ankylosing spondylitis and Still's disease have also responded to this therapy." He went on to say that of 556 people with various types of arthritis, 283 were found to be much improved, and a further 219 were improved to a less marked extent. Of 292 cases of rheumatoid arthritis, 264 showed improvement of various degrees. The longer the duration of the disease, the longer time before improvement was observed, although most started to show improvement after just 2 or 3 months of enzyme therapy. Despite these favorable findings, digestive enzyme therapy in conventional medicine has been reserved for those diseases that directly result in a pathological deficiency of pancreas-derived digestive enzymes.

Common Digestive Disorders May Benefit from Enzyme Replacement

According to Schneider et al., in pathological digestive diseases the oral intake of exocrine pancreatic enzymes are of key importance in the treatment of mal-digestion in chronic pancreatitis with pancreatic insufficiency. They studied the therapeutic effectiveness of a conventional and an acid-protected enzyme preparation, and an acid-stable fungal enzyme preparation in the treatment of severe pancreatogenic steatorrhea. The results showed that a supplemental enzyme preparation is best for patients with chronic pancreatitis and those who underwent Whipple's procedure (a surgical procedure performed on pancreatic cancer patients), while patients with an intact upper gastrointestinal tract fare best with an acid-protected porcine pancreatic enzyme preparation.

Dr. Brad Rachman says that 58% of the population suffers from some type of digestive disorder, and a lack of optimal digestive function associated with enzyme inadequacy may lead to malabsorption and numerous related conditions. The problem is exacerbated in the elderly because their production of gastric hydrocholoric acid may be suboptimal. "This can be a significant factor that can impact nutrient absorption along with the creation of maldigestive-type symptoms. Bacterial production of hydrogen and methane are determined after a carbohydrate challenge. Excessive levels of these gases reflect overgrowth of bacteria in the upper gut." Help is at hand, he says, with enzyme replacement. Dr. Rachman says enzymes taken orally at meals may improve the digestion of dietary protein and thereby decrease the quantity of antigenic macromolecules leaking across the intestinal wall into the bloodstream. Such leaks may trigger the body's defenses against exposure to what it perceives as foreign protein or polypeptide invaders, producing the symptoms of allergies.

Dr. Howell agrees that allergies can also be helped by enzyme additions to the diet. So too can excessive cholesterol levels, he says. Discussing cholesterol and atherosclerosis, he quotes a 1962 study by three British doctors—C. W. Adams, O. B. Bayliss, and M. Z. Ibrahim, who set out to discover why cholesterol clogs arteries, ultimately manifesting in heart disease. They found that all enzymes studied became progressively weaker in the arteries as people aged, and the hardening became more severe. They suggested a shortage of enzymes is part of the mechanism that allows cholesterol deposits to accumulate in the inner part of arterial walls. Blood tests conducted by Stanford University researcher LO Pilgeram in 1958 demonstrated progressive decline in lipase in the blood of atherosclerotic patients with advancing middle and old age.

About the same time, Becker, Meyer, and Necheles at Michael Reese Hospital in Chicago found that enzymes in the saliva, pancreas, and blood became weaker with advancing age. They speculated that fat may be absorbed in the unhydrolyzed state in atherosclerosis. They also found definite improvement in the character of fat utilization following the use of enzymes.

Intravenous administration of brinase, a proteolytic enzyme preparation from *Aspergillus oryzae*, was found by an Irish research group, Fitzgerald et al., to be beneficial in the treatment of chronic arterial obstruction. Patients were observed for 3 months before receiving six intravenous infusions of either saline or brinase for more than 2 weeks. During the observation period, no changes were observed. After the infusion, 17 of the 27 obstructed arterial segments were found to have resumed blood flow, and the number of patent segments increased from 11 to 27. No improvements were observed in the placebo-treated patients.

Pancreatin is secreted from the pancreas and provides potent concentrations of the digestive enzymes protease, amylase, and lipase. Pancreatin is sold as a drug to treat those with pancreatic insufficiency. Pancreatin efficacy was demonstrated in a study conducted on patients who took pancreatin to maintain postoperative digestion. The effects of supplementation were determined by measuring the postoperative intestinal absorption and nutritional status in a randomized trial with patients receiving pancreatin or placebo. Before the trial, patients showed abnormal digestion of fats and protein, and total energy was low at baseline and 3 weeks after surgery. Pancreatin supplementation improved fat and protein absorption as well as improving nitrogen balance. However, those patients taking a placebo had worsened absorption after the surgery. The data suggest that long-term postoperative pancreatic enzyme supplementation is both efficacious and necessary in surgery patients who suffered from pancreatitis.

Considerable evidence exists to support the beneficial effects of enzymes, both natural and supplemental. And it is obvious that plant enzymes benefit specific conditions. Research dealing with intact absorption of food substrates shows that nondigested food substrates enter the blood and that plant enzymes break down different food substrates that would otherwise be passed into the blood without being fully digested.

The time when our normal ability to produce enzymes is greatest is in our youth, a time of rapid growth and in most cases a time of no serious illness. When we age and our food enzymes become depleted, we begin to suffer a broad range of health complaints.

How long we live and in what state of health is determined by our enzyme potential, according to Dr. Howell. Referring to a study by Dr. Meyer and his associates at Michael Reese Hospital in Chicago, Dr. Howell said the presence of enzyme of the saliva in young adults is 30 times greater than that in people aged over 69 years. Similarly, a German study by Eckardt of 1200 urine specimens found almost twice as much of the starch-digesting enzyme, amylase, in young people as in old.

So humans eating an enzyme-less diet use up vast quantities of their enzyme potential through secretions from the pancreas and other digestive organs, resulting in a possible shortened lifespan, illness, and lowered resistance to all types of stress.

G. A. Leveille, a University of Illinois researcher, discovered in the early 1970s that enzyme activities in the tissues become weaker with aging. Conducting experiments on rats, he found that at the age of 18 months—which is considered old age for rats—on enzyme-free fabricated diets, enzyme activity had shrunk to less than 20% of its level at one month of age. And Dr. Howell agrees: "the more lavishly a young body gives up its enzymes, the sooner the state of enzyme poverty, or old age, is reached."

The answer is substitution of raw food for cooked as much as possible. By eating foods with their enzymes intact and by supplementing cooked foods with enzyme capsules, Dr. Howell suggests we can stop abnormal and pathological aging processes. He singles out raw milk, bananas, avocados, seeds, nuts, grapes, and other natural foods as rich in food enzymes. He also suggests an enzyme supplement be taken with all cooked food and, under medical supervision, large doses in enzyme therapy to treat certain diseases.

We are what we eat. Few would disagree with this adage, but not everyone realizes it is not quite so simple. Enzymes make the digestion of food possible. This means we must make maximum use of enzyme activity, both internal enzymes and those we consume either in food or as supplements.

Benefits of Artichoke for Digestive Disorders

The artichoke plant is best known for its "heart," the bottom part of its spiky flower bud that many of us have learned to appreciate as both a delicacy and a nutritious vegetable. However, other parts of this tall thistle-like plant, which never reach the dinner table, have proven to be even more beneficial for our health. Clinical studies show its large basal leaves to be effective for improving digestion and liver function as well as cholesterol levels.

Since ancient times, humans have looked to nature for help to cure diseases. Up until modern times most remedies were derived from the plant kingdom, and even today a large percentage of our current pharmaceutical drugs are based on plant extracts from various parts of the world. Many old herbal remedies, however, have fallen into oblivion with the development of modern medicine.

Artichoke extract is one of the few phyto-pharmaceuticals whose experiential and clinical effects have been confirmed to a great extent by biomedical research. Its major active components have been identified, as have some of its mechanisms of action in the human body. In particular, antioxidant, liver-protective, bile-enhancing, and lipid-lowering effects have been demonstrated, which correspond well with the historical use of the plant. More research is needed to determine in detail the mechanisms of action for these effects. However, there appears to be evidence enough to suggest a potential role for artichoke extract in some areas where modern medicine does not have much to offer.

Artichoke has a long history. Used as a food and a medical remedy as early as the 4th century B.C., the artichoke plant has a long history. At the time, a pupil of Aristotle named Theophrastus was one of the first to describe the plant in detail. Enjoyed as a delicacy, an appetizer, and a digestive aid by the aristocracy of the Roman Empire, it later seems to have fallen into oblivion until the 16th century, when medicinal use of the artichoke for liver problems and jaundice was recorded. In 1850 a French physician successfully used extract of artichoke leaves in the treatment of a boy who had been sick with jaundice for a month and had made no improvement from the drugs used at that time. This accomplishment inspired researchers to find out more about the effects of this extract, and their research resulted in the knowledge we have today about the constituents of the extract and its mechanisms of action.

Artichoke leaf extract is made from the long, deeply serrated basal leaves of the artichoke plant. This part is chosen for medicinal use because the concentration of the biologically active compounds is higher here than in the rest of the plant. The most active of these compounds have been discovered to be the flavonoids and caffeoylquinic acids. These substances belong to the polyphenol group and include chlorogenic acid, caffeoylquinic acid derivatives (cynarin is one of them), luteolin, scolymoside, and cynaroside.

Cynarin was the first constituent of the extract to be isolated in 1934. Interestingly, it is found only in trace amounts in the fresh leaves, but is formed by natural chemical changes that take place during drying and extraction of the plant material. Cynarin was originally believed to be the one active component of the extract. Today the whole complex of compounds is considered important, since it has not yet been completely clarified which component is responsible for each effect. It is claimed that neither cynarin alone nor fresh plant material achieves the potency of the dried total extract (Kirchhoff et al., 1994).

Chlorogenic acid, another major component of the artichoke leaf extract, has recently become known as a powerful antioxidant with exciting potential in many applications. Laboratory investigations are ongoing all over the world with promising findings for future clinical application in areas such as HIV, cancer, and diabetes.

Most of the modern research on artichoke has been done with the German artichoke extract Hepar SL forte, standardized to contain 3% caffeoylquinic acids. A new, even more potent extract, standardized at 15% caffeoylquinic acids—calculated as chlorogenic acid—is now available on the American market.

Biological Effects

The original uses of artichoke since ancient times have been as an aid for indigestion and insufficient liver function. The mechanism of action, however, has been essentially unknown. Recent findings have provided a new foundation for our understanding and discovered additional benefits of the extract, such as antioxidant and lipid-lowering effects.

Effects on the Gastrointestinal System

The importance of effective liver function for overall health in general, and proper gastrointestinal function in particular, is rarely emphasized in health discussions in this country. One reason might be that there is neither laboratory evidence nor specific physical symptoms to reveal an overburdened liver in the beginning stages. The symptoms may be nonspecific, such as general malaise, fatigue, headache, epigastric pain, bloating, nausea, or constipation. Discomfort following meals and intolerance of fat are also notable indications of disturbances in the biliary system.

It is estimated that at least 50% of patients with dyspeptic complaints have no verifiable disease. Because of the liver's essential role in detoxification, even minor impairment of liver function can have profound effects. It is therefore important to take such chronic complaints seriously. In Germany and France, for example, physicians frequently prescribe herbal liver remedies such as artichoke extract with good results when presented with these chronic but nonspecific symptoms. We may have something to learn here.

The proven basis for the beneficial effects of artichoke leaf extract on the gastrointestinal system is the promotion of bile flow. Bile is an extremely important digestive substance that is produced by the liver and stored in the gall bladder. The liver manufactures about one quart a day of bile to meet digestive requirements. It is secreted into the small intestine, where it emulsifies fats and fat-soluble vitamins and improves their absorption. Any interference with healthy bile flow can create a myriad of immediate digestive disorders such as bloating.

Good bile flow is also essential for detoxification, which is one of the major tasks of the liver. The liver is constantly bombarded with toxic chemicals from the environment: the food we eat, the water we drink, and the air we breathe.

Bile serves as a carrier for these toxic substances, delivering them into the intestine for further elimination from the body. This is the major route for excretion of cholesterol. Yet another feature of the bile is helpful here: its promotion of intestinal peristalsis, which helps prevent constipation.

When the excretion of bile is inhibited for various reasons (gall stones or gall bladder disease), toxins and cholesterol stay in the liver longer with damaging effects. One of the causes of inhibited bile flow is obstruction of the bile ducts by the presence of gall stones. Other common reasons for impairment of the bile flow within the liver itself are, for example, alcohol ingestion, viral hepatitis, and certain chemicals and drugs. In the initial stages of liver dysfunctions, laboratory tests, such as serum bilirubin, alkaline phosphatase, SGOT, LDH, and GGTP, often remain normal, and it is not adequate to rely on such tests alone. Symptoms that may indicate reduced liver function are general malaise, fatigue, digestive disturbances, and sometimes increasing allergies and chemical sensitivities.

Excessive alcohol consumption is by far the most common cause of impaired liver function in the United States. It stimulates fat infiltration into the liver cells, causing the so-called fatty liver. Some livers are very sensitive to even minute amounts of alcohol; others are more tolerant. Recent research suggests that the fatty liver condition is more serious than previously believed, as it may develop to more advanced liver disease, such as inflammation, fibrosis, and cirrhosis.

Because of its long historical use for liver conditions, it seemed reasonable to investigate the artichoke plant scientifically, and the first clinical studies were conducted in the 1930s with encouraging results. In the 1990s the interest has been intensified, and several excellent clinical studies have been conducted during the last few years.

Realizing the importance of adequate bile flow for health, German researchers set out to confirm the earlier findings of bile-promoting effect of the artichoke plant in a controlled double-blind study on healthy volunteers (Kirchhoff et al., 1994). The participants were given a one-time dose of artichoke extract or placebo, and their bile secretion was measured with special techniques over the following hours. The bile secretion was found to be significantly higher in the group that received the artichoke extract.

Another clinical study showed an improvement of symptoms in 50% of patients with dyspeptic syndrome after 14 days of treatment with artichoke leaf extract. The study involved 60 patients with nonspecific symptoms such as upper abdominal pain, heartburn, bloating, constipation, diarrhea, nausea, and vomiting. In the placebo group, as a comparison, improvements of less distinct quality were noticed in 38% of the participants (Kupke et al., 1991).

Interesting results were also demonstrated in a large open label study of 417 participants with liver or bile duct disease. Most of these patients had long-standing symptoms, some of them for many years. They suffered from upper abdominal pain, bloating, constipation, lack of appetite, and nausea. These patients were treated with artichoke leaf extract for 4 weeks. After 1 week, around 70% of the patients experienced improvement of their symptoms, and after 4 weeks the percentage was even higher (approx. 85%) (Held 1991).

Even more remarkable improvement was shown in another recently completed open label study (Fintelmann, 1996), where 553 outpatients with nonspecific dyspeptic complaints were treated with a standardized artichoke leaf extract. The subjective complaints declined significantly within 6 weeks of treatment. Improvements were found for vomiting (88%), nausea (83%), abdominal pain (76%), loss of appetite (72%), severe constipation (71%), flatulence (68%), and fat intolerance (59%). Ninety-eight percent of the patients judged the effect of the extract to be considerably better, somewhat better, or equal to that achieved during previous treatment with other drugs. The dosage used in this study was 1 to 2 capsules 3 times daily of the preparation Hepar SL Forte. One capsule contains 320 mg of dry extract of artichoke leaves, standardized to provide 3% of caffeoylquinic acid.

The study by Fintelmann not only confirmed the efficacy of the artichoke extract for dyspepsia, but also demonstrated a significant effect of the extract on fat (lipid) metabolism. The researchers found a significant decline in both the cholesterol and triglyceride levels in the blood, which confirmed a discovery made as early as in the 1930s.

Artichoke leaf extract is well tolerated and has few side effects in recommended dosages. The use of the artichoke plant as food in many countries over hundreds of years supports its safety. More important, however, is that several rigorous studies report the absence of adverse effects when using a standardized extract compared to the placebo. In a large safety study, only one out of 100 subjects reported mild side effects such as transient increases in flatulence.

Local eczematous reactions have been reported after occupational exposure and skin contact with the fresh plant or its dried parts. Such an allergy should be considered a contraindication for external use of the extract, although no reactions to orally ingested extract have been observed so far. Because of its bile-stimulating effect, the extract should not be taken by individuals with gall stones or other bile duct occlusion.

A new artichoke extract is now available in the United States, giving Americans a chance to discover its merits. While the German artichoke products, cited in most European studies, typically contain 3% caffeoylquinic acids, this new artichoke extract is standardized to contain 15% caffeoylquinic acids, calculated as chlorogenic acid.

Artichoke leaf extract has proven to be a safe and natural way to maintain and improve general health, because of its many applications to essential physiological functions. As a nutritional supplement and antioxidant it can safely be used as an adjunct to conventional therapies.

How Eastern Europeans Cope with Digestive Disorders—Digest RC

The difference in life expectancy between the best and worst European countries is more than 10 years. In the early 1990s, overall Eastern European mortality was 20 to 100% higher than in the West. The reasons for these differences in mortality are attributed to poor diet, excess alcohol consumption, heavy smoking, and other dangerous health behaviors in Eastern Europe.

One dietary explanation for the decreased life span among Eastern Europeans is that their intake of antioxidants from fruits, vegetables, and nuts is much lower compared to the West. A severe deficiency of antioxidant vitamins, along with a low intake of folic acid and flavonoids, partially accounts for the high level of cardiovascular disease in Eastern Europe.

The traditional Eastern European diet consists of lots of animal fats and protein and very little in the way of fresh fruits and vegetables. This poor diet not only shortens life span, but also creates an epidemic of acute digestive disorders.

While digestive complications increase as people age, the bad health habits of the Eastern Europeans exacerbate common problems such as heartburn, bloating, gas, constipation, nausea, cramps, diarrhea, and irritable bowel syndrome.

In the United States, over-the-counter and prescription medications for digestive ailments are a multibillion-dollar industry. Most Eastern Europeans cannot afford the high-priced synthetic products sold by Western drug companies and instead rely on a natural herbal remedy. Rather than masking symptoms, this herbal preparation attacks the underlying cause of many forms of digestive disorder. Considering the magnitude of the digestive disorders caused by the poor health behaviors of the Eastern Europeans, the fact that this herbal remedy has such as strong track record makes it a fascinating potential solution for Americans.

A Popular Digestive Aid in Europe

Digest RC was introduced in Europe more than 45 years ago. Today, more than 100 million doses of the product are sold annually in Europe.

The mechanism of action of the formula is to stimulate peristalsis of the intestines, speed digestion of fats, and prevent stagnation of food in the digestive tract. The benefits the user finds are a reduction in esophageal acid reflux, alleviation of the feeling of fullness and bloating after eating, decreased digestive tract tension, alkalization of the gastric content, constipation relief, and normalized elimination.

Benefits of Black Radish Juice

Black radish juice extract is the primary active ingredient in Digest RC. Virtually unknown in the United States, the radish contains a variety of chemicals that increase the flow of digestive juices. The most important function of black radish extract is that it encourages the liver to produce fat- and protein-digesting bile and lowers the tension of the bile ducts. It also improves peristaltic movement. Constipation is another problem to benefit from radish consumption. Rich in fiber and digestive stimulants, regular consumption of radishes helps regulate the bowels. Since dehydration is a major cause of constipation, radishes help hydrate and lubricate the intestines and encourage relaxed bowel movements. The root juice extract of the black radish used in Digest RC is the most potent part of the plant.

A bonus is the radish's ability to assist the immune system, as it contains a variety of chemicals that possess natural antimicrobial actions. Regular consumption may lead to a significant improvement in the resistance against common microbial infections such as colds, sore throats, ear infections, and the flu.

A French study by Prahaveanu and Esanu in which liquid radish extract was administered to mice before they were inoculated with an influenza virus. There was a significant decrease in the mortality rate and a significant increase in the rate of survival as compared to the untreated controls. Another study, by Ivanocis and Horvath, found it to be protective against *E. coli*, more so than penicillin G.

A second ingredient of Digest RC is artichoke—which further increases production of bile and causes it to flow through bile ducts. Peppermint, another ingredient of Digest RC, increases secretion functions of the stomach and liver and production of enzymes.

Benefits of Charcoal

The charcoal in Digest RC is particularly useful in absorbing toxins. It is used in emergency departments to treat drug overdoses. It also calms a stressed digestive system, allowing digestive enzyme to be produced and released. Indigestion and nervous vomiting are also treated with this ingredient. The charcoal in Digest RC is actually a special herbal preparation of linden tree bark, traditionally used in Europe as a digestive aid. Unlike the specially prepared linden wood bark in Digest RC, ordinary activated charcoal is derived from materials such as peat or coconut shell. This special preparation has antibacterial properties, which when used as directed helps balance the digestive tract and supports the creation of the proper intestinal flora. At the same time it creates an inhospitable environment for parasitic infestation.

Benefits of Cholic Acid

Another key ingredient of Digest RC is cholic acid, or pure processed ox bile, a liver enzyme used for digestion. It is particularly helpful in digesting fats and meat protein. Also in Digest RC is calcium phosphate, which neutralizes stomach acid.

Digest RC uses a layered delivery system to ensure that the various herbal extracts perform their intended function in the right part of the digestive tract. The ingredients are cultivated in Europe in a pesticide-free environment and are standardized to ensure uniform potency. The safety profile and demonstrated efficacy of herbs such as artichoke, black radish, and peppermint, particularly in standardized pharmaceutical grade extract form, suggest that here is the answer to the digestive problems of millions of Americans.

Used extensively in Europe and hailed as a huge success, Digest RC uses a formulation that simultaneously relieves digestive disorders while strengthening the digestive system. While there are numerous products that work on individual symptoms of poor digestion and elimination, Digest RC stands out because it relieves more than one symptom at the same time. Digest RC also helps the liver function properly by enabling the organ to release toxins, and encouraging it to produce the correct amount of bile.

The Science behind Digest RC

Immunologist Dr. Mark Pasula, president and research director of Signet Diagnostic Corporation at Oxford Nutritional Center in Florida, believes the Digest RC formula works because of its two-pronged approach that relieves most digestive disorders while it helps to build a healthy digestive system.

In short, Digest RC has the capacity to rapidly relieve symptoms in the short term, while healing the source of the problems in the long run. Digest RC is the formula of choice for patients with digestive complaints who have not responded to food elimination therapy. Within a short time of regularly using the product, their digestive problems disappear and their digestive system actually strengthens.

Independent clinical research was conducted on Digest RC to analyze the therapeutic effectiveness of the product among patients with chronic digestive problems. Results showed statistically significant improvement in patients' symptoms during treatment. Digest RC was most successful in eliminating the most frequently occurring symptom, gas, in more than 95% of the cases. Symptoms such as constipation, intestinal pains and cramps, heartburn (reflux), and stomach pains and cramps were helped or completely eliminated in more than 90% of the cases. Bloating ceased in more than 80%, diarrhea in about 75%, and nausea and vomiting in approximately 65% of the cases. Digest RC was found to minimize the assimilation of undigested toxic products, which often stay in the gut for prolonged periods of time. Because of its cholepoietic and cholagogic abilities, Digest RC was particularly effective in preventing the stagnation of food and bloating in patients whose diet was rich in animal protein and fat. As there are no specific contraindications, Digest RC can be taken together with any medication and can be taken by patients suffering from different respiratory, cardiovascular, and musculoskeletal disorders. The only group of people who should avoid Digest RC are those with biliary tract obstruction or gall bladder disease because of the bile-stimulating effects of the black radish and artichoke extracts. It is not known how this product would affect those who have had their gall bladder removed.

Additional clinical studies relative to Digest RC are being initiated at a medical school in the United States to validate the results of the European studies.

What Conventional Medicine Offers

An FDA-approved prescription drug called Propulsid can be taken before a meal in order to initiate a quicker peristaltic movement of food out of the stomach. The dose of Propulsid is 10 mg, ideally taken 20 minutes before every meal and at bedtime. This drug can induce acute peristaltic contractions that can result in diarrhea and has been linked with several deaths when taken with certain cardiac medications. It is also difficult for some people to remember to take Propulsid 20 to 30 minutes before each meal.

Some of the most popular drugs prescribed to treat digestive complaints are Prilosec or Prevacid. These drugs are known as gastric acid-pump inhibitors because of the unique way in which they block the final metabolic step in the production of stomach acid. These drugs are quite expensive to purchase, but are more effective in suppressing disorders associated with excess stomach acid production than the older class of histamine 2 receptor antagonist drugs sold under the trade names Tagamet, Zantac, Pepcid, and Axid. Drugs such as Tagamet inhibit stomach acid secretion whereas Prilosec and Prevacid suppress virtually all stomach acid secretion.

Since most stomach ulcers are now thought to be caused by the *H. pylori* bacteria, special antibiotic regimens are now the therapy of choice in treating ulcers. The use of drugs that reduce stomach acid are therefore more frequently prescribed to treat esophageal reflux, where stomach acid regurgitates into the esophagus to cause heartburn. If left untreated, chronic esophageal exposure to stomach acid can cause esophagitis and esophageal cancer.

Some people with mild esophageal reflux may be able to use natural therapies to promote youthful peristaltic action and push food more rapidly out of the stomach, thereby alleviating reflux back into the esophagus.

Conclusion

Aging is a critical factor that negatively impacts the digestive system. As we age, we become acutely aware of the limitations now placed on our diets. Foods that were part of our carefree eating styles in younger years have become the culprits in our declining years. The variety of products marketed for digestive problems is astounding. Looking for relief, consumers purchase a myriad of remedies and yet continue to suffer.

The natural supplements mentioned within this protocol may prove to be a new potent and cost-effective treatment in helping halt the digestive disease epidemic. Here are some natural approaches to treating digestive disorders and improving overall health:

- Digestive Enzyme Supplements

  Choosing the right enzyme supplement can be difficult. Enzymes are very delicate and if not properly manufactured, they can easily lose their potency. Commercial enzyme supplements are often neutralized by varying pH levels of stomach acids. A digestive enzyme supplement should be broad-spectrum so that it can facilitate the digestion of protein, fat, carbohydrate, fiber, and milk lactose. The use of acid-protected enzyme formulas can enhance efficacy. One such formula that obtains its enzymes from fungus (but has no fungal residue) is called Super Digestive Enzyme Caps. This product is formulated to be effective in a broad spectrum of stomach acid pH conditions. Each capsule of Super Enzyme Caps contains a pancreatin and fungal enzyme concentrate that provides the following digestive activity

Amylase (carbohydrate enzyme)	40,000 USP units
Protease (protein enzyme)	40,000 USP units
Lipase (fat enzyme)	7,200 USP units
Protease II(6000 USP per milligram)	130 mg
Protease III (1000 FCC per gram)	130 mg
Amylase (25,000 FCC per gram)	140 mg
Lactase (5000 FCC per gram)	40 mg
Cellulase (4000 FCC per gram)	40 mg
Lipase (5000 FCC per gram)	20 mg
Whole fruit papaya powder	100 mg

Two to four dosages of an acid-protected enzyme supplement with the above potencies should be taken before or during meals. Digestive enzymes are quite reasonably priced compared to other supplements.

▼ Bile Acid–Stimulating Agents

While digestive enzymes facilitate the breakdown of food in the stomach, the impact of bile acids secreted from the liver into the small intestine may be even more important. A healthy liver makes about a quart of bile acid a day, and this bile should freely flow into the small intestine to digest fat and protein. European doctors believe that inadequate bile acid flow is a major cause of most digestive disorders.

Artichoke Extract facilitates the free flow of bile acid and also improves the overall health of the liver. The suggested dose is to take 300 to 600 mg of a standardized artichoke extract before, during, or after a heavy meal. The extract from artichoke used to measure pharmaceutical standardization is caffeoylquinic acid. Supplements can be found that contain as low as 3% and up to 15% caffeoylquinic acid. Higher concentration artichoke extracts are recommended. Artichoke extracts are quite affordable, and provide many ancillary health benefits in addition to improving bile acid flow and hence overall digestion. Those who want to optimize digestion should consider taking two to four digestive enzyme capsules before a meal along with 300 to 600 mg of a standardized artichoke extract.

A slightly more expensive way of stimulating bile acid flow is to use the European pharmaceutical preparation named Digest RC. Two to three tablets of Digest RC taken with meals provides standardized extracts from black radish and artichoke along with peppermint, cholic acid, and other digestive aids. Digest RC has a proven 45-year track record in Europe in treating a variety of common digestive disorders. After 3 weeks of using two to three tablets of Digest RC before every heavy meal, the dose can be reduced if symptoms of digestive discomfort dissipate.

WARNING: Those with gall stones or gall bladder disease should not take bile acid–stimulating agents such as artichoke or Digest RC.

Summary

1. Take two to four capsules of an acid-protected digestive enzyme supplement that provides standardized potencies of protease, amylase, and lipase. A supplement called Super Digestive Enzymes is suggested.
2. Take 300 to 600 mg of an artichoke extract standardized to contain a minimum 3% caffeoylquinic acid with each meal, or take two to three tablets of Digest RC with each meal.

For more information. Contact the Digestive Disease National Coalition, Chicago IL, (202) 544-7497; or the National Digestive Diseases Information Clearing House, Bethesda MD, (301) 654-3810, www.niddk.nih.gov/health/digest/nddic.htm.

Product information. Super Enzyme Caps, a 15% artichoke extract, and Digest RC tablets can be ordered by calling (800) 544-4440, or order online at www.lef.org.

DOWN SYNDROME

Down syndrome (DS) is one of the most frequent congenital multiple handicaps, occurring in 1 to 2 of every 1000 births. It is characterized as a chromosomal disorder, resulting in mental retardation and physical abnormalities. People born with DS have an extra chromosome, making three of a kind, known as trisomy. Ninety-five percent of all DS cases are caused by trisomy 21. People with this type of trisomy disorder generally live until their 30s or 40s. Down syndrome is characterized by delayed physical and mental development, with numerous physical abnormalities. Trisomy 18 (Edwards syndrome) occurs in 1 of every 3000 births. It is characterized by severe mental retardation and facial abnormalities. Other possible defects are cleft lip or palate, missing thumbs, webbed hands, club feet, heart defects, and genitourinary defects. Survival for more than a few months is rare. Trisomy 13 (Patau's syndrome) occurs in 1 of every 5000 births. It is characterized by severe mental retardation along with brain and eye defects. Other abnormalities may include cleft lip or palate, heart and genitourinary defects, and malformed ears. More than 80% of babies born with trisomy 13 do not survive past the age of 1 year. The remainder of this protocol will focus on a discussion of Down syndrome.

Characteristics and Diagnosis

Infants with Down syndrome are usually quiet, cry infrequently, and have poor muscle tone. Physical features include a small head, a broad flattened face, slanting eyes, and a short nose. Ears are small and set low on the head, and the tongue is large and often prominent. Hands and fingers are short with a single crease across the palm. The fifth finger in many instances has two rather than three sections and curves inward. About one-third of all children with DS have heart defects. Intelligence quotient (IQ) is about 50 compared with the normal IQ of 100, but some children with DS have a higher IQ.

Screening for DS is usually recommended for pregnant women over the age of 35. A diagnosis can often be made before birth by testing for low levels of alpha-fetoprotein in the mother's blood. If low levels are detected, a sample of the amniotic fluid will confirm the diagnosis. After the birth, the infant's blood will be sampled to confirm the presence of trisomy 21.

Physical and Developmental Problems

An increased risk of leukemia and heart disease is present in children with DS that will reduce the chance of survival until adulthood. Thyroid problems may also develop; they may not be detected unless appropriate blood testing is done. Hearing loss may occur due to chronic ear infections and the associated accumulation of inner ear fluid. Vision loss is also common due to deterioration of the cornea and lens. Adults with DS may begin to develop symptoms of dementia in their 30s such as memory loss, which further affects intelligence and personality. DS patients display motor and kinetic deficit. Their physical appearance is usually limp, with stooping shoulders, dropped lower jaw with mouth open, and a gawky and straddling gait. These conditions can be greatly improved when diligent physiotherapy is initiated in early infancy and continued through later years.

Treatment of DS

Historically, the treatment of Down syndrome has itself been the victim of profound prejudice and ignorance. It was considered hopelessly untreatable, a belief that dominated the scientific community and produced no new research on DS for more than 100 years. This prejudice manifested itself in the self-fulfilling prophecy of the label "incurable." The actual cause of Down syndrome was, and still is, unknown. Chromosomal aberrations are considered a symptom at the cellular level, and not a cause; therefore therapy should direct itself toward treating the clinical symptoms and the aberrations from different aspects of science. In addition, the immune system is usually weakened, requiring medical intervention. Inevitably, DS presents multiple handicaps in both the physical and mental development of the child. Many treatments for DS over the last hundred years have been considered failures because they were structured within very narrow parameters.

Modern DS treatment should be multidimensional, incorporating goals and requirements which would

1. Adjust the disturbance of the cellular metabolism.
2. Prevent brachymicrocephaly.
3. Adjust the disorders of vitamin, mineral, and enzyme metabolism.
4. Provide neurotransmitter precursor therapy.
5. Provide hormone replacement therapy when necessary.
6. Provide physical therapy and adequate education.
7. Provide immune augmentation.

Vitamins and Malabsorption

Schmidt has shown that malabsorption of B vitamins can occur in DS. Other studies show that multiple vitamin deficiencies can be present for long periods of time in patients with DS. Children with DS who were supplemented for the first three years of life with a combination of vitamin B_6 and 5-hydroxytryptophan improved in social maturity and accomplishment. DS patients would generally benefit by the daily consumption of a multinutrient formula such as Life Extension Mix. Recommended dosage would be just slightly below the adult dosage. Digestive enzymes can be included in this treatment since the supplementation will potentiate the absorption process.

It is believed the failure of the brain to develop, especially the hippocampal region (controlling memory), may be caused by vital nutrient deprivation. Proper nutrient assimilation combined with CT has increased brain growth in some DS patients. Addressing immune dysfunction is a crucial component of any DS protocol. Malnutrition/malabsorption is the number one cause of immune dysfunction in the world. Simply ensuring proper nutrient assimilation can be very effective at improving host defense mechanisms. Glutamine can be a potent healer of intestinal mucosa and thereby promote normal absorption of nutrients from the gastrointestinal tract. Glutamine utilization by the body is normally very high in all of us, but it can still have some psychotrophic effects in some individuals, so its usage is best monitored by a qualified physician. (Contact the Path Medical Center in Manhattan, (212) 213-6155, for more information detailing the use of amino acids as pharmaceutical agents in the treatment of brain dysfunctions.)

Thyroid Replacement Therapy

Conflicting conclusions have been reached concerning vitamin A levels in DS patients. Schmidt has reported one study showing DS patients had higher than normal levels of vitamin A and beta-carotene. These high levels of vitamin A may have been caused by a thyroid deficiency. This conflict may have been produced by not fully examining the role of thyroid hormone in the DS patient. Some scientists believe vitamin A should be supplemented, while other scientists would rather strive to increase thyroid hormone functioning as the means of potentiating vitamin A utilization at its site of action without raising vitamin A stores in the body.

Thyroid replacement therapy may be highly indicated as a means to reverse the impairment of the utilization of vitamin A at its site of action. Thyroid hormone is needed to produce transthyretin, which is required for the formation of retinol-binding protein. Retinol-binding protein stores about 99% of vitamin A in the blood until it is needed somewhere in the body. If thyroid deficiency is present while one is supplementing with vitamin A and Life Extension Mix, toxicity could occur because of the lack of retinol-binding protein necessary to store serum vitamin A. (Refer to an endocrinologist with DS competency when considering thyroid replacement therapy and vitamin A supplementation.)

Neurotransmitter Precursors

According to Schmidt in *Down Syndrome: Treatment and Care,* one of the manifestations of DS is a profound deficit in neurotransmitter functioning in the brain. Noradrenaline, serotonin, and choline acetyl transferase levels are severely lower in the brains of DS patients. Alzheimer's disease encompasses similar neuropathological abnormalities to DS. The same researcher states that phosphatidylcholine therapy has improved the neurophysiological and intellectual performance of DS patients. Choline bitartrate can have similar effects to phosphatidylcholine in most people.

Vitamin E seems to play a role in the progression of DS into Alzheimer's disease. Low levels of serum vitamin E correlated with progression, leading researchers in the *Journal of Mental Deficiency Research* to suggest that vitamin E supplementation may prevent premature Alzheimer's dementia in DS patients. The same study shows that vitamin B_6 alone, as well as 5-hydroxytryptophan, will raise the important neurotransmitter, serotonin, in the brains of DS patients.

The administration of 50 mg a day of 5-hydroxytryptophan and 250 mg of tyrosine can significantly raise serotonin and noradrenaline levels in the brain. Many DS patients have benefited from increased doses of vitamin B_6. This effect, as stated in *Down Syndrome: Treatment and Care*, may occur because of improved tryptophan metabolism. Schmidt has also shown that the incorporation of piracetam (a derivative of gamma-amino butyric acid) in the treatment of DS patients is most advantageous during the first 6 to 24 months of life. Even in older children, piracetam can have beneficial effects on motility, poor initiative, and weak attention spans. Piracetam is generally administered initially in doses of 800 mg a day over a 2-week period. The high end of the dose may reach 4800 mg a day for short periods of time.

A chemical synthesized from an amino alcohol called DMAE and *p*-chlorphenoxy-acetic acid is known as centrophenoxine. It has been credited with the ability to slow down brain aging and was used by Dr. H. Haubold as part of his basic treatment for DS. He incorporated centrophenoxine to increase neural metabolism and to delay the premature aging process in his patients. (Contact the Foundation for an overseas source of piracetam and centrophenoxine.)

Children's doses should be proportionately lower than those stated here. Compliance in small children may be difficult due to the bitter tastes of the vitamins and cholinergic enhancers. Simply combining the Life Extension Mix powder with a favorite fruit juice can improve the child's compliance.

Cell Replacement Therapy

The smallest common denominator of all aberrations found in DS is a disorder of the cell metabolism. Defective membrane transport was evident when B vitamin metabolism and mouth epithelium were studied by scientists F. Schmid, W. Rehm, and S. Christeller in 1975. These membranes were highly rigid, predisposing patients to infections of the respiratory tract and to enteral disorders of absorption in the intestinal tract. F. Schmid believes the exciting field of cell therapy (CT) offers positive benefits when applied in the treatment of DS. They believe the subcutaneous injection of fetal cell tissue provides the patient with high concentrations of biochemical substrates and enzymes that have corrected metabolic disorders. Controlled studies, using amounts of 200 to 300 mg of various lyophilisate combinations, to determine the optimal types of implantation tissue used for each specific DS symptom have been successful.

The term "cell therapy" means the use of cellular material for therapeutic purposes. In this context, CT encompasses some of medicine's oldest treatment methods. Within the last 20 years, the concept of CT has evolved to generally mean the use of fetal xenogenic tissue. In this more recent context, CT can be defined according to the same authors as: *an implantation by injection of xenogenic fetal or juvenile suspensions of cells or tissue in physiological solution. The implantation provides the organism of the recipient with a great number of biologically demonstrable substrates and enzymes, found in this concentration and composition only in juvenile tissue.* (For more information contact the International Association for Cytobiological Therapies, in Germany, 049-6227-63268. The association may also be able to provide you with information about other doctors and clinics that employ this valuable therapy.)

Sources of Additional Alternative Information

- **International Association for Cytobiological Therapies** (Dr. Fuchs): Robert-Bosch-Strausse 56a, D-69190 Walldorf, Germany; Tel: 049-6227-63268
- **Path Medical Center** (Dr. Eric Braverman): 274 Madison Ave, New York, NY; Tel: (212) 213-6155
- **Prof. Dr. med. F. Schmid**: Chefarzt der Stadtischen Kinderklinik (Chief, Municipal Pediatric Clinic); Am Hasenkopf 1, D-8750 Aschaffenburg, Germany
- **Dr. Sam Baxas**: 50 West Mashta Dr., Key Biscayne, FL 33149; Tel: (305) 361-3956; *and* Hauptstrasse 4, 4102 Binningen, Switzerland; Tel: 011-4161-422-1292; Fax: 011-4161-422-1289

Summary

Until recently, the birth defect that causes Down syndrome was thought to be untreatable. A search of the scientific literature, however, indicates that high-potency vitamin supplements, along with the European drug piracetam, can be effective in treating children with Down syndrome.

Another study found a causal relationship between cognitive decline in Down syndrome that could be related to undetected folate vitamin deficiency. Yet another study found value from thyroid replacement therapy, vitamin-mineral therapy, and 5-hydroxytryptophan in treating Down patients.

It has been suggested that malabsorption plays a role in a number of the vitamin and mineral deficiencies found in people with Down syndrome. A review of the published studies demonstrates that patients with Down syndrome are prone to suffer multiple deficiencies of vitamins and lifelong shortages of some trace metals. A significant reason for these deficiencies is malabsorption from the intestine. Treatment of vitamin deficiencies has shown success in some studies. In Down syndrome, the brain does not develop adequately. The hippocampal region of the brain, which is concerned with memory, is especially poorly developed. The deficiency of nutrients caused by DS may play a significant role in relation to the failure of the brain to develop.

Parents have been using high-potency vitamin supplements and piracetam to treat Down syndrome with astonishing results. Popular news reports have documented the before-and-after effects when Down syndrome children followed a protocol using high-dose nutritional supplements and the European medication piracetam.

Dosage Recommendations

One should keep in mind the mainstream treatment and prognosis of DS is bleak. The nutrients and drugs mentioned in this protocol can offer an alternative. Although these alternative treatments have produced remarkable results in many children in the last 10 to 20 years, these dosages, for the specific treatment of DS, have not been standardized during this time. Dosages were often experimentally determined by the physician/consultant or the primary care giver. When determining specific dosages for your child, keep in mind the child's individual constitution and his/her weight in relation to their peer age group (do they weigh less than other children in the age group, the same, or perhaps more?) and then moderate the recommended dosages offered below. Also consider the advice of a physician with experience in nutrient supplementation in DS children. Advisors at the Life Extension Foundation can also offer some guidelines concerning general children's dosages. None of the dosages listed below could be considered appropriate for all patient ages, or for all differing severities of DS. For this reason, it is crucial to review and formulate dosages with a qualified physician. The dosages listed below are offered as a guide, and should not be considered a replacement for competent medical consultation regarding nutrition for your child.

Life Extension Mix:

4 years old:	1/3 teaspoon powder 3x daily with meals
	or 1 tablet 3x daily with meals
	or 1 capsule 3x daily with meals
8 years old:	1/2 teaspoon powder 3x daily with meals
	or 2 tablets 3x daily with meals
	or 2 capsules 3x daily with meals
12 years old:	1 teaspoon powder 3x daily with meals
	or 3 tablets 3x daily with meals
	or 3 capsules 3x daily with meals

If headache occurs at any dosage, discontinue, then resume at a lower dosage.

Glutamine. 2 to 10 grams as a daily maintenance amount with water between meals. Most patients can safely take more, up to 40 grams. Consult the Path Medical Center in Manhattan for the pharmaceutical use of amino acids.

Enzymes. A high-quality digestive enzyme product can be employed at the normal dosages listed on its label, and can be lowered accordingly for children.

Thyroid replacement. Dosage should be determined by a competent endocrinologist experienced in treating DS.

Piracetam. Treatment of DS patients is most advantageous between the first 6 to 24 months of life. Even in older children, piracetam can have beneficial effects on motility, poor initiative, and weak attention spans. Piracetam is generally administered initially in doses of 800 mg a day over a 2-week period. The high end of the dose may reach 4800 mg a day for short periods of time. If headache is a side effect, discontinue, then resume with a lower dosage.

Centrophenoxine. One to three tablets daily, with water between meals. If headache occurs, discontinue, then resume at a lower dosage.

Phosphatidylcholine. 1 gram daily. If headache occurs, discontinue, then resume at a lower dosage.

Choline bitartrate. 500 mg to 2 grams daily with water or juice. If headache occurs, discontinue, then resume at a lower dosage.

5-Hydroxytryptophan. 50 mg daily with water, between meals.

Tyrosine. 250 mg daily with water in between meals. If headache occurs, discontinue, then resume at a lower dosage.

Vitamin E. 400 to 800 IU daily.

For more information. Contact the National Down Syndrome Congress, (800) 221-4602 or the Parent Assistance Committee on Down Syndrome, (914) 739-4085.

Product availability. Life Extension Mix powder and choline are available by phoning (800) 544-4440, or order online at www.lef.org. When calling the Foundation, ask for a listing of offshore suppliers of piracetam.

EMPHYSEMA AND CHRONIC OBSTRUCTIVE PULMONARY DISEASE

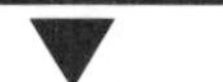

Several lung diseases are collectively known as Chronic Obstructive Pulmonary Disease (COPD), including asthmatic bronchitis, chronic bronchitis (with normal airflow), chronic obstructive bronchitis, bullous disease, and emphysema. About 11% of the population of the United States suffers from COPD, with the disease becoming increasingly common among older women. According to the Mayo Clinic, COPD kills 85,000 people a year in the United States.

The incidence of emphysema, the fourth leading cause of death in the United States, is up more than 40% since 1982. Emphysema ranks fifteenth among chronic diseases that contribute to limitation of physical activity. About 44% of those with emphysema report that their daily activities have been limited by the condition. According to the National Jewish Medical and Research Center in Denver, this chronic lung disease kills 13,000 people a year in the United States alone, but up to 2.4 million Americans are estimated to be suffering from this debilitating condition. Emphysema permanently enlarges and irreversibly damages the alveoli, damages the ends and walls of the smallest bronchioles (the tiny breathing tubes that branch off from the trachea and bronchi), and diminishes the elasticity of the lungs.

The alveoli (tiny air sacs whose walls are covered with minuscule blood vessels) remove carbon dioxide from the blood, releasing it into the lung to be breathed out, and also absorb oxygen, transferring it into the blood. This exchange is essential to survival and is the key function of the lungs. Alveoli have fragile, thin walls, which are easily damaged. Breakage of these walls makes the oxygen–carbon dioxide transfer much less efficient. The bronchioles distribute the air throughout the lung to the individual alveoli. Once damaged, the bronchioles tend to collapse, trapping stale air in the isolated sacs and no longer transmitting fresh air in.

As the alveoli and bronchial tubes are destroyed, more air is required to provide the same amount of oxygen to the blood via the parts of the lung that are still functioning. This need for more air eventually leads to lung overinflation. As the lung overexpands, it gradually enlarges, completely filling the chest cavity and causing a sense of shortness of breath. Because the lung can no longer expand or contract as completely as before, the "stale" air left in the lung is never completely replaced by fresh air. The combination of a larger, less elastic lung and damaged, nonfunctioning tissue means that the air flow out of the lung is much slower, resulting in the feeling of an obstructed airway.

Causes

Any lung disease that causes the narrowing of the respiratory airways (such as chronic bronchitis or asthma) may contribute to the onset of emphysema, but smoking is the primary cause. In addition to the irreversible damage smoking causes to lung tissue, it causes inflammation of the lungs, which resolves only when smoking is stopped. More than 80% of all emphysema is directly attributable to smoking. Tars, smoke, toxic chemicals added by tobacco companies for various reasons, and other gases combine to block the production of alpha-1-antitrypsin (AAT), leading to the destruction of the elastic fibers of the alveoli.

Smoking stresses the natural antioxidant defense system of the lung, allowing free radicals to damage tissue down to the cellular level. (Hand-rolled cigarettes have been implicated in a higher incidence of emphysema when compared to that of smokers of ready-made cigarettes.) Irritants contained in tobacco smoke tend to inhibit activity by the tiny cilia in the airways. The cilia are designed to expel foreign matter and mucus from the lung. Without their activity, it becomes difficult or impossible to cough up the mucus that accompanies pneumonia and other lung infections. It may be worth noting that one "drag" on a cigarette temporarily paralyzes the cilia. Smoking-induced emphysema usually becomes apparent after the age of 50.

About 2 out of every 1000 Americans have inherited an enzyme deficiency known as alpha-1-antitrypsin deficiency (A1AD or AAT deficiency). The deficiency leads to A1AD-related emphysema when the liver produces insufficient AAT to control a natural enzyme known as neutrophil elastase. Though neutrophil elastase plays an important role in fighting bacteria and cleaning up dead lung tissue, it eventually causes irreversible damage to the alveoli by damaging or destroying their elastic fibers, if there is not enough AAT to neutralize it. There are between 20,000 and 40,000 Americans with A1AD-related emphysema. For AAT-deficient individuals who smoke, the risk of developing emphysema is much greater than for the general population. A1AD-related emphysema usually strikes people in their thirties or forties and is very rarely seen in children. The earlier age of onset and the fact that A1AD-related emphysema often shows up first in the lower rather than upper lung are factors used to diagnose this variety of the disease.

Among other causes of emphysema are industrial pollutants, aerosol sprays, non-tobacco smoke, internal combustion engine exhaust, and physiological atrophy associated with old age (senile emphysema). Physical damage caused by an accident and followed by scarring can give rise to scar emphysema; severe respiratory efforts can rupture alveoli in cases of near suffocation, whooping cough, (child-bearing) labor, and acute bronchopneumonia. Tuberculosis and asthma can also give rise to lung overstretching, severely damaging the elastic fibers of the alveoli walls and bringing on emphysema. High altitude is associated with higher death rates among those suffering with COPD, but is not a proven causative factor at this time. Areas of high poverty also experience higher mortality rates among those suffering from COPD, possibly a reflection of inadequate medical care.

One study measured antioxidant levels in smokers and in a group of chronic obstructive pulmonary disease patients. Smoking, acute COPD attacks, and asthma were all associated with very low blood serum levels of antioxidants and evidence of increased oxidative stress. Another study measured free-radical injury from pulmonary oxygen and the protective role of antioxidant enzymes. Results suggest that increased free-radical toxicity and decreased glutathione peroxidase and catalase activities in red blood cells play a role in chronic obstructive pulmonary disease.

Symptoms

One tragedy of emphysema is that most patients lose 50 to 70% of their functional lung tissue before they become aware of the symptoms of the disease. Breathlessness (a feeling of being out of breath during routine physical activity) is usually the first symptom people notice. If walking up a flight of stairs takes your breath away, that could mean you have emphysema (but is also a symptom of heart disease and some types of cancer). Other common symptoms of emphysema are unexplained weight loss; increased chest size (barrel chest); wheezing or labored breathing (or reduced breath sounds); a productive cough yielding large amounts of dark, thick phlegm or mucus; and a lingering cough, often dismissed as "smoker's cough."

Other symptoms may be skipped breaths, insomnia or frequent nocturnal waking, memory loss, morning headaches, impotence, nasal flaring, blurred vision, increased breathing difficulty while lying down, chronic fatigue, impaired concentration, atypical irritability or loss of temper, excessive daytime sleepiness, and swelling of feet, ankles, or legs. If any of these symptoms persist, consult a doctor.

Diagnosis

There are many ways to diagnose emphysema, but the most accurate is the chest x-ray. Chest x-rays are also very useful in determining the amount of lung damage already sustained. Tapping on a patient's chest while listening with a stethoscope is a favorite technique of experienced doctors. Ruptured alveoli and overinflated lungs respond with a hollow sound. A registered respiratory therapist (RRT) can conduct a number of pulmonary function tests (PFTs). Spirometry measures the amount of air the patient can exhale in 1 second (forced expiratory volume, or FEV1) into a tube connected to the spirometer. The total amount of air the patient can exhale (forced vital capacity or FVC) is then compared to the FEV1 to determine the extent of airway obstruction.

A peak flow meter is a small, hand-held device that measures the severity of breathing impairment at a given moment. The patient takes a deep breath and blows into the machine as hard and long as possible. Arterial blood gas tests measure how well the lungs are oxygenating the blood stream and removing carbon dioxide from it, and pulse oximetry uses light waves to measure blood oxygen levels. Serum alpha-1-antitrypsin levels can be confirmed by blood workup, while urine pH test, pulmonary ventilation–perfusion scan, and chest MRI may all provide valuable indicators to a medical doctor or respiratory therapist.

Prevention

Don't smoke. If you smoke, quit. If you don't smoke, don't start. Avoid smoke-filled rooms and all sources of second-hand cigarette smoke. Your life depends on it. Avoid air pollutants such as fine particulate matter (lime dust, dry livestock waste dust, and the dust associated with the movement of stored grain), aerosol sprays, industrial pollutants, herbicides, pesticides, fumes from fuel and exhaust, smoke from bonfires or burning waste, and the dust stirred up while cleaning carpets and upholstery. An air purifier can help, and so can regular maintenance and cleaning of air conditioning and heating system ducts and filters.

Sound nutrition, including vitamin supplementation, may help to prevent emphysema. Special attention should be given to the intake of antioxidants to prevent the breakdown of functional lung tissue by free radicals. Regular aerobic exercise builds up lung capacity and helps cleanse the lungs of stale air. Walking is an excellent choice, if one avoids polluted areas. Unproven preventive measures often recommended by doctors include yearly pneumonia and influenza vaccinations.

Complications and Risks of Emphysema

Emphysema patients are at increased risk of contracting recurrent respiratory infections and lung cancer, and are at high risk for respiratory and coronary failure and for cor pulmonale, enlargement and strain on the right side of the heart. (Emphysema makes the heart work harder to keep the lungs supplied with blood because of damage to the lungs' circulatory system and other tissue damage.) This condition, which can also be caused by living at high altitudes for prolonged periods, often leads to failure of the right ventricle. Emphysema is a very serious disease that is greatly complicated and worsened by any type of lung infection. According to Dr. James Fisher, head of pulmonary and critical care at Wayne State University and the Detroit Medical Center, "Pneumonia is a very difficult thing to treat with emphysema, and it makes someone much sicker than if you just had pneumonia alone." Pneumovax is an easily obtainable pneumonia vaccine that protects against several types of bacterial pneumonia. It is given every 7 to 10 years.

E

Treatment

Emphysema is a pulmonary deficiency usually caused by years of free-radical damage that results in degenerative changes in the air sacs of the lung. Free radicals and changes of antioxidant enzymes are also thought to play a role in chronic obstructive pulmonary disease.

Pulmonary oxygen radical injury and the protective role of antioxidant enzymes in COPD were measured in one study. The results suggest that the increased free-radical toxicity and decreased glutathione peroxidase and catalase activities in red blood cells are involved in chronic obstructive pulmonary disease.

In another study, an imbalance between oxidants and antioxidants in smokers and in patients with airway diseases such as asthma was proposed. Antioxidants were measured in a group of chronic obstructive pulmonary disease patients. The results showed that smoking, acute COPD attacks, and asthma are associated with a marked oxidant/antioxidant imbalance in the blood, associated with evidence of increased oxidative stress.

The suggested daily dose of antioxidant nutrients for patients with these lung diseases is three tablets 3 times a day of Life Extension Mix and one capsule a day of Life Extension Booster. In order to help break up the thick mucus, 600 mg of *N*-acetylcysteine should be taken 3 times a day, along with 2 grams of vitamin C.

If the combination of these nutrients does not sufficiently break up the mucus, Pulmozyme, a drug used to treat cystic fibrosis, can be prescribed by your doctor. Pulmozyme is the most effective mucus-eradicating drug available. However, it is approved only for cystic fibrosis and, as a result, physicians often fail to prescribe it for acute mucus problems.

To restore energy production to damaged cells in the lungs, the following nutrients are suggested:

- Coenzyme Q_{10}, 100 mg, 3 times a day.
- Alpha-lipoic acid, 250 mg, twice a day.
- Acetyl-*L*-carnitine, 1000 mg, twice a day.
- NADH, 5 mg, twice a day.
- Taurine, 1000 mg, twice a day.
- Magnesium, 500 mg of elemental magnesium, once a day.
- Potassium, if needed.

Vitamin A Status Is Important

Epidemiologic studies have a shown the severity of COPD correlates with low vitamin A intake. Other reports indicate that serum levels of vitamin A (retinol) are below normal in patients with COPD.

The relationship between vitamin A status and COPD was further explored in a two-part study by researchers at the Faculty of Medicine of Botucatu UNESP in Sao Paulo, Brazil. In the first part of the study, 36 men, aged 43 to 74 years, were divided into five groups: healthy nonsmokers, healthy smokers, smokers with mild COPD, former smokers with moderate–severe COPD, and former smokers with severe, complicated COPD. All subjects underwent pulmonary function testing, and dietary intake of vitamin A was estimated from a food-frequency questionnaire. In addition, serum levels of retinol and other vitamin A–related compounds were determined from fasting blood samples. The results of this part of the study showed that serum levels of vitamin A were significantly lower in the two groups with moderate or severe COPD, although no group exhibited overt vitamin A deficiency.

In the second part of the study, 12 male smokers (45 to 61 years) with mild COPD were randomly assigned to receive either a placebo or a vitamin A supplement for 30 days. A comparison of pulmonary function tests performed at baseline and at the end of the study showed a significant improvement in forced expiratory volume in the vitamin A–supplemented group but only modest improvement in the group receiving the placebo. Interestingly, pulmonary function tests performed 30 days after the end of vitamin A supplementation were similar to baseline values.

These results support earlier findings of an association between low vitamin A status and COPD. In addition, the authors conclude that the improvement in pulmonary function observed following vitamin A supplementation suggests "the existence of a local vitamin A deficiency" in persons with COPD. Those with COPD may consider supplementation with 25,000 to 50,000 units of vitamin A a day.

Relieving Breathlessness

Most emphysema treatment is based on the concept that it can be treated but not cured. The administration to emphysema sufferers of theophylline and ipratropium bromide in combination has produced improvements in maximal oxygen consumption and maximal minute ventilation, and it has reduced several measures of breathlessness. British patients who had not responded to oral administration of corticosteroid (prednisone) were given budesonide (by inhalation). Researchers concluded that inhaled corticosteroids were of no benefit to patients with advanced COPD. Inhaled corticosteroids, while less dangerous than oral steroids, can still increase the risk of high blood pressure and diabetes. Other undesirable side effects reported by patients include edema, cataract development, bone brittleness, and premature skin aging sometimes known as "onion skin."

Researchers in New Zealand found that nebulized saline solution relieved breathlessness in patients at rest with COPD. Other conventional therapies include breathing techniques, aromatherapy, and oxygen therapy. Recent developments in lung reduction are very promising. Such surgery is called volume reduction surgery or lung shaving. Other experimental procedures showing some promise are the surgical removal of damaged alveoli, which reduces lung size, and laser removal of damaged lung tissue. Laser surgery has not been as effective as volume reduction therapy. Lung transplantation becomes more successful with each passing year, though there is a real shortage of donors. Research at the Mayo Clinic (1994) shows better survival with single lung transplants than when both lungs are replaced.

An old folk remedy that works well to loosen the phlegm in the lungs of those with damaged cilia is to inhale steam. Use of a steam or a hot mist vaporizer in a room can also be very helpful. (Avoid the use of cold water humidifiers as they often introduce mold, mildew, and harmful bacteria into the air, actually increasing the risk of lung infection.) Using a steam vaporizer in a small, enclosed space such as a bathroom can raise the level of humidity significantly and can be very useful. Adequate liquid intake enhances thinning and removal of lung secretions.

Postural drainage is a technique in which the lung segment to be drained is placed in the uppermost position relative to the rest of the body. There is also a very useful "clapping" technique in which someone "claps" the back or chest of the patient to loosen the built up phlegm. Also known as "percussion," the technique uses cupped hands clapping the chest wall in rapid succession, producing a series of hollow sounds. Both percussion and chest vibration (using a vibrator) can be used in combination with postural drainage as appropriate. Pillows are used to support the patient in the designated position. (Consult your medical caregiver for detailed instructions on the use of these techniques.)

Exercise and Nutrition

Though exercise before the onset of emphysema can increase lung capacity, it has not been demonstrated to have that effect in those suffering from the disease. Regular aerobic exercise does, however, help the patient to use available oxygen more efficiently, and also strengthens the heart. Protein therapy in those known to have AAT deficiency has significantly slowed the destruction of functional lung tissue. Use of protein therapy in smoking-induced emphysema has not been reported.

If sound nutrition is important in preventing emphysema, it is crucial once the disease has been diagnosed. Malnutrition may increase the risk of respiratory failure in patients with chronic obstructive pulmonary disease. French scientists found that the primary goal of a successful nutritional program for those with COPD should be to improve diaphragm strength by correcting mineral and electrolyte disturbances at the muscular level.

Pulmonary rehabilitation in emphysema patients has resulted in reduced hospitalization, improved well-being and exercise tolerance, and reduced shortness of breath. Such programs usually require physician referral, a cardiopulmonary stress test, and evaluation by an RRT (registered respiratory therapist). Substantial benefits are reported for those suffering from emphysema, asthma, bronchiectasis, chronic bronchitis, and sarcoidosis. It is also recommended for those planning to undergo lung reduction therapy as well as for those who have just completed that surgery. Residential programs last about 8 weeks and include smoking cessation, education on breathing exercises, nutrition, energy conservation, stress reduction, and the management of medication. Exercise includes such activities as walking on a treadmill, walking, stationary bicycling, stretching, and working out with light weights. Exercise programs are always tailored to individual needs. Regular exercise has been proven to improve the condition of the cardiopulmonary system.

Regenerating Alveoli

Scientists funded by the National Heart, Lung, and Blood Institute have demonstrated a remarkable regeneration of alveoli, which returned to their normal size and number. In research using rats at the Georgetown University School of Medicine, treatment with retinoic acid, a metabolite of vitamin A, resulted in a nonsurgical reversal of damage caused by emphysema for the first time. Not only was the number of alveoli increased in normal rats, but alveoli in rats with emphysema were repaired, and lung elasticity recoil was significantly improved. Though these studies have so far been conducted only in animals, results are very promising, leading a number of physicians to put their emphysema patients on retinoic acid therapy.

As human research studies are reported, many caregivers are confident that this remarkable therapy will be more widely adopted. In fact, the FDA has now approved the drug all-trans-retinoic acid for emphysema therapy. All-trans-retinoic acid must be prescribed by a physician. If the high cost of retinoic acid makes its cost prohibitive, consider taking four drops a day (100,000 IU) of emulsified liquid vitamin A. (*Refer to vitamin A precautions.*)

Summary

Emphysema is one of the diseases known collectively as COPD, Chronic Obstructive Pulmonary Disease. Though emphysema can be brought on by a number of situations and conditions that damage the lungs, the primary causative factor is smoking. Exposure to fine particulate matter, aerosol sprays, industrial chemicals, and air pollution can damage the lungs, leading to emphysema, or making the condition worse in those already suffering from the disease. Vitamin A and antioxidant supplementation, regular exercise, postural drainage and percussion, the use of steam and hot mist vaporizers, and lung reduction and transplant surgery are all useful therapies for emphysema.

1. Do not smoke, as smoking leads to emphysema and also makes emphysema worse.
2. Get regular exercise and eat a balanced, nutritious diet.
3. If you (or anyone in your family) are alpha-1-antitrypsin deficient, see your doctor about AAT supplementation.
4. Avoid industrial pollutants, second-hand tobacco smoke, grain dust, and other air pollutants. This applies to everyone, but is especially important for emphysema patients.
5. The suggested dose of high-potency vitamins for COPD patients is three tablets, 3 times a day of Life Extension Mix and one capsule a day of Life Extension Booster.
6. To help break up thick mucus in the lungs, drink plenty of fluids and take 600 mg a day of *N*-acetyl cysteine and 2 grams of vitamin C 3 times a day.
7. In patients for whom the *N*-acetyl cysteine and vitamin C do not provide sufficient relief from the thick mucus, Pulmozyme, a drug used to treat cystic fibrosis, can be prescribed by your doctor. As it is only approved for cystic fibrosis, it is unlikely to be prescribed for emphysema unless requested by the patient.
8. In order to restore energy to damaged lung cells, the following nutrients are suggested:
   - Coenzyme Q_{10}, 100 mg, 3 times a day.
   - Alpha-lipoic acid, 250 mg, twice a day.
   - Acetyl-*L*-carnitine, 1000 mg, twice a day.
   - NADH, 5 mg, twice a day.
   - Taurine, 1000 mg, twice a day.
   - Elemental magnesium, 500 mg, twice a day.
   - Potassium, if needed.
9. *N*-Dimethylglycine (DMG) can be taken at the rate of one or two tablets (125 to 250 mg) under the tongue immediately before exercise. It has been demonstrated to help in oxygenation.

For more information. Contact the American Lung Association, (800) 586-4872.

Product availability. Life Extension Mix, Life Extension Booster, *N*-acetyl cysteine, vitamin C, Coenzyme Q_{10}, acetyl-*L*-carnitine, NADH, taurine, magnesium, potassium, and DMG can be obtained by phoning (800) 544-4440, or order online at www.lef.org.

ESOPHAGEAL REFLUX

Description

What the English have called dyspepsia or heartburn is actually esophageal reflux. The problem is caused by the backflow of stomach acid upward into the lower esophagus. In normal digestion, the valve that separates the esophagus and stomach, the lower esophageal sphincter (LES), opens to allow food to pass into the stomach and then closes to prevent the food and acidic stomach juices from flowing back up. Esophageal reflux occurs when the LES relaxes more often than it should and/or at inappropriate times causing the stomach contents to back up. Sometimes, particularly in obese people, the opening through the diaphragm that allows the esophagus to pass from the chest to the abdomen becomes large. This is called a hiatal hernia and may result in esophageal reflux.

The stomach has a lining that protects it from the effects of the acid and because the esophagus lacks this lining, the stomach acid that refluxes will cause pain, inflammation (esophagitis), and damage. Excessive backflow of the stomach contents into the esophagus causes gastroesophageal reflux disease (GERD). Untreated GERD can result in precancerous changes called Barrett's esophagus.

Causes

Esophageal reflux can occur in persons who are overweight, pregnant, or smokers. A person who eats fried, fatty, or spicy food, eats chocolate, peppermint, and citrus fruits, or drinks coffee, tea, alcohol, and carbonated drinks can also suffer reflux because these substances may increase the tendency of the LES to relax. Gastritis, the inflammation of the stomach itself, ulcer disease, and taking nonsteroidal antiinflammatory drugs such as aspirin and ibuprofen may result in reflux.

Symptoms

The most obvious symptom of esophageal reflux is heartburn. Heartburn occurs after eating and can last from a few minutes to a few hours. The person who experiences heartburn feels a burning sensation that can begin in the pit of the stomach or lower breastbone region and which can then move upward into the chest and throat, causing a bitter acid taste. Heartburn can also be called acid regurgitation, indigestion, or sour belching. A person can experience heartburn from bending over or lying down. Belching can also sometimes be a symptom of heartburn.

Persons suffering from GERD have the same symptoms as those with esophageal reflux, but there can be long-term complications. GERD may cause esophageal scarring, esophageal cancer, or Barrett's syndrome, a chronic irritation from acid reflux that causes the normal esophageal lining cells to be replaced by the intestinal lining cells. When these cells are present in the esophagus, there is an increased risk of developing cancer.

Pain during swallowing and slight bleeding can be caused by the inflammation of the esophagus. Peptic esophageal ulcers are open sores on the esophageal lining with the pain occurring behind or just below the breastbone. The pain can be relieved by antacids, taken 40 minutes to 1 hour after eating. Peptic ulcers can be healed by using drugs to reduce the stomach acid over a 4- to 12-week period. These ulcers heal slowly and tend to recur. The esophagus can become more narrow, making swallowing solid food painful.

A number of tests can be given to a person suffering from esophageal reflux, including x-rays, endoscopy, manometry of the lower esophageal sphincter (LES), or the Bernstein test. Before an x-ray is taken, the person drinks a barium solution, then lies on an incline with the head lower than the feet. This will cause the reflux of the barium from the stomach to the esophagus. The x-rays will also reveal any esophageal ulcers or a narrowed esophagus. Esophagoscopy involves examining the esophagus through a flexible viewing tube which can also take a biopsy to correctly identify acid reflux. Manometry is a pressure measurement taken of the LES that will indicate its strength and will distinquish a normal sphincter from one that is poorly functional. The Bernstein test involves placing an acid solution into the lower esophagus. If the symptoms appear quickly then disappear when a salt solution is placed in the lower esophagus, the problem is acid reflux. If diagnosis of esophageal reflux is difficult, the doctor may measure the acid levels inside the esophagus using a pH test.

CAUTION: X-rays to evaluate upper–digestive tract disease expose the patient to tremendous amounts of radiation. Ask your doctor for nonradiation diagnostics such as endoscopy rather than CAT scans, which use x-rays.

Treatment

The reason for treating esophageal reflux is to prevent gastric contents in the stomach from entering the esophagus, allowing this area to heal. There are a number of things people can do on their own. Maintain a reasonable weight; avoid eating tomatoes, garlic, onions, chocolate, peppermint, citrus fruits, and fatty and oily foods; and avoid coffee, tea, alcohol, and any drinks that are carbonated. Instead of eating three large meals a day, eat smaller meals more frequently, maybe four or five a day, and don't lie down after these meals. Don't eat for at least 2 to 3 hours before bedtime, and when going to bed, elevate the head of the bed 4 to 6 inches to facilitate gravity in keeping the gastric contents in the stomach. Also, sleep on the left side because this will cause less pressure on the LES, and therefore the stomach contents will not back up. Get a lot of rest and exercise. Don't smoke because nicotine relaxes the esophageal sphincter. Don't take aspirin, ibuprofen, and other nonsteroidal antiinflammatory drugs.

Conventional management of symptoms in patients with mild to moderate esophageal reflux without erosive esophagitis, in which the lining of the esophagus breaks down, requires a systematic approach beginning with lifestyle modification plus over-the-counter H2 antagonists (Tagamet, Pepcid, Zantac, Axid) and/or antacids (Tums, Maalox, etc). If these measures do not suppress heartburn, then prescription pharmacologic management with more potent prescription H2 antagonists drugs is warranted.

For persons suffering from GERD, long-term therapy might be required and should be individualized according to the severity of symptoms, the degree of esophagitis, and the presence of other acid reflux complications. In most patients, maintenance therapy is vital. In the last decade, two proton pump–inhibiting drugs, omeprazole (Prilosec) and lansoprazole (Prevacid) have become potent acid-suppressing drugs taken by people who were previously unresponsive to other medications. They completely suppress hydrochloric acid production, and normally provide relief after 1 week. The benefits, safety, and costs of the available therapeutic alternatives must be considered in choosing acute and long-term therapy. Appropriate use of endoscopy and other diagnostic tests is important in ruling out erosive esophagitis, Barrett's syndrome, esophageal cancer, stomach ulcers, or stomach cancer. Cisapride (Propulsid) is a promotility drug that improves some of the motility defects present in GERD and increases the peristaltic movement of the esophagus, which moves food down into the stomach. For those who are at high risk for developing esophageal cancer (those with Barrett's syndrome), the long-term use of drugs such as Prilosec or Prevacid may reduce the risk of esophageal cancer.

Persons who don't respond very well to, or don't want to take, medication, might opt for a surgical procedure known as Nissen fundoplication. This procedure wraps the stomach around the esophagus, creating a new valve to prevent acid from refluxing into the stomach. A laparoscope is used in this minimally invasive surgery, which will dramatically reduce the discomfort and recuperative time, with the patient staying hospitalized for 2 nights and returning to full activity in 1 to 2 weeks.

Alternative Treatment

One of the difficulties with the chronic administration of H2 blockers is that the stomach is not meant to have a weak acid environment. One of the functions of the hydrochloric acid in the stomach is to break down proteins for digestion. The failure of the stomach to perform this task may result in improper digestion and the absorption of so-called digestive remnants into the blood through the wall of the intestine. Normally, proteins are broken down into individual amino acids. If the proteins are not entirely broken down, and proteins get into the blood, this can set up allergies mediated by certain white cells called T-cells resulting in a host of problems such as autoimmune disease.

The constant irritation of stomach acids on the lining of the esophagus can result in an increased risk of esophageal cancer and esophagitis. Antioxidant nutrients can protect against esophageal inflammation and, according to published studies, they may lower the risk of esophageal cancer. If you suffer from heartburn, you should consider taking 3 tablets of Life Extension Mix with each meal to help reduce your risk of esophageal cancer and esophagitis. Life Extension Mix, is a high-potency multi-nutrient formula containing nutrients that have been shown to reduce the risk of gastric and esophageal cancers.

Summary

Esophageal reflux occurs when the lower esophageal sphincter malfunctions, allowing the backward flow of acid from the stomach into the esophagus. Being overweight or pregnant, overeating, smoking, and eating fatty and spicy foods and specific foods like citrus fruits, peppermint, and chocolate will cause reflux as will drinking alcohol, coffee, and carbonated drinks. The main symptom of esophageal reflux is heartburn, which feels like a burning sensation beginning in the stomach and sometimes moving upward into the chest and throat.

Taking an antacid after a meal will usually reduce the risk of heartburn. Maintaining a reasonable weight, avoiding the foods mentioned above, eating smaller meals more often (four or five meals a day instead of three large ones), and sleeping on the left side with your head elevated 4 to 6 inches above the rest of your body are a few measures you can take to avoid heartburn.

If heartburn persists, esophagoscopy, manometry of the LES, x-rays, or the Bernstein test might have to be performed on the patient to find out what is causing the problem. Alternative medications or a surgical procedure known as Nissen fundoplication might be helpful.

For more information. Contact the Consumer Nutrition Hotline of the National Center for Nutrition and Dietetics, (800) 366-1655, Monday to Friday, 9 to 4 o'clock CST. A dietitian will answer questions about heartburn and refer you to a registered dietitian in your area. The National Digestive Diseases Information Clearinghouse, 2 Information Way, Bethesda, MD 20892-3570, will send out their publications list as well as a packet on gastroesophageal reflux disease.

Product availability. Life Extension Mix can be ordered by phoning (800) 544-4440, or order online at www.lef.org. Zantac, Tagamet, Pepcid, and Axid are now sold over the counter.

FEMALE HORMONE MODULATION THERAPY

Concern about the life-threatening side effects of synthetic hormone drugs has caused many women to be deprived of the benefits of safe natural hormone replacement therapy.

Proper hormone modulation can prevent degenerative disease and improve functioning in both the physical and emotional spheres of life, both at menopause and throughout life. For example, many sexual "dysfunctions," including lack of desire, can be mitigated when hormone levels are naturally restored to a youthful profile. Menopause might also be delayed and be less traumatic if hormone adjustments are made in time. Numerous female health problems are tied to inadequate hormone balances, as we will show.

Forty-five million women are menopausal in the United States today; another 3.5 million women will become menopausal this year. Based on life expectancy trends, women face the prospect of spending the last one-third to one-half of their lives in a state of hormonal imbalance. The quality and quantity of life for these women will be determined by how well they (and their doctors) manage their hormone replacement.

Hormone Deficiencies: Estrogen

Starting around age 45 to 50, women face a perplexing dilemma regarding estrogen, one of the primary sex hormones. The amount of estrogen naturally produced by their bodies dwindles. This estrogen deficiency causes a wide variety of menopausal miseries, including hot flashes, depression, vaginal dryness, anxiety, and forgetfulness. The menopausal decline in estrogen production is a direct cause of premature aging.

Estrogen replacement therapy (ERT) remains controversial. FDA-approved estrogen drugs have been documented to cause cancer. The most conclusive report showed that women taking estrogen and a synthetic progestin drug had a 32 to 46% increase in their risk of breast cancer (*New England Journal of Medicine,* June 15, 1995). These estrogen and progestin drugs carry warning labels listing a shocking array of dangerous side effects.

Although estrogen increases the risk of some types of cancer, it also has critical antiaging benefits, including the prevention of osteoporosis and heart disease and the reversal of some aspects of neurological decline. Many doctors don't believe that estrogen causes cancer, while others think that combining estrogen with a synthetic progestin neutralizes the risk. Some studies show that estrogen does not cause cancer in the short-term, but in women taking estrogen and/or a synthetic progestin for more than 10 years, there appears to be a significantly elevated risk of breast, ovarian, and uterine cancers.

The report that women had a 32 to 46% increase in their risk of breast cancer while using estrogen alone, or estrogen and a synthetic progestin, was based upon data from the famous Nurses' Health Study conducted at Harvard Medical School. This study showed that the carcinogenic risk of estrogen–progestin replacement therapy became most pronounced when it was used for 10 or more years.

Increased breast cancer risk is not the only danger of using estrogen drugs. A report published in the *American Journal of Epidemiology* (May 1995) showed that long-term estrogen replacement therapy increased the risk of fatal ovarian cancer. This 7-year study included 240,073 pre- and post-menopausal women. After adjusting for other risk factors, women who used estrogen for 6 to 8 years had a 40% higher risk of deadly ovarian tumors, while women who used estrogen drugs for 11 or more years had a startling 70% higher risk of dying from cancer of the ovaries. The increased carcinogenic risk from estrogen is a serious concern. Cancers of the breast, uterus, and ovaries account for 41% of cancer incidence in U.S. women. Breast cancer is running at epidemic levels, striking 1 in 9 women, up from 1 in 30 women in 1960. Conventional estrogen replacement therapy and estrogen-based oral contraceptives have been used extensively since 1960. Clearly, an alternative is needed to provide the antiaging and health-enhancing benefits of estrogen, while protecting against its cancer-causing effects.

Dangerous Estrogen Drugs

The most popular estrogen drug in the United States is Premarin, which contains estrogens derived from the urine of pregnant mares. Besides the fact that the process of collecting mares' urine is an inhumane and cruel procedure, the form of estrogen it produces is the most dangerous kind. In humans, estrogen has three different forms, one of which, estriol, is safe and effective. Premarin contains no estriol. Instead it is a "conjugated" estrogen, never intended for human bodies. Other popular estrogen drugs are sold under the names Estrace and Estraderm. Provera is the name of a popular synthetic progestin often given with Premarin to help prevent estrogen-induced uterine cancer. Unfortunately it does not prevent estrogen-induced breast or ovarian cancer.

Estrogen and progestin drugs have well-documented side effects that cause many women to avoid using them. In addition to increased cancer risks, some of the other risks of estrogen/progestin drugs include

- ▼ Weight gain.
- ▼ Abnormal blood clot formation (thrombosis).
- ▼ Increased risk of gallstones, fibroid tumors, and headaches.
- ▼ Premenstrual-type symptoms (irritability, fluid retention).

Despite these unpleasant and sometimes lethal side effects, many women use estrogen drugs because of their ability to reduce the unwanted effects of menopause and for their antiaging properties. Estrogens are steroid hormones that promote youthful cell division in target organs of the body. The antiaging benefits of estrogen replacement therapy include

- Enhanced skin smoothness, firmness, and elasticity.
- Enhanced moistness of skin and mucous membranes.
- Enhanced muscle tone.
- Reduced genital atrophy and enhanced sex drive in women.
- Reduced menopausal miseries such as hot flashes and anxiety.
- Reduced risk of heart disease and osteoporosis.
- Reduced risk of colon cancer.
- Improved memory and neurological function.
- Protection against Alzheimer's disease.
- Enhanced immune function.
- A greater feeling of well-being.

Estrogen's benefits make it desirable for most menopausal women to maintain youthful levels of this hormone. The question is, can the antiaging benefits of estrogen be obtained without increasing the risk of cancer and arterial blood clots? There are preferable alternatives to these synthetic hormones. Estrogen supplements may be produced from plant sources. These safe and effective estrogens are known as "phytoestrogens," and they have been studied in great detail. A review of the published literature reveals some interesting findings about plant-derived estrogens. Phytoestrogens from soy have been documented to reduce hot flashes and protect against age-related diseases such as osteoporosis, heart disease, and cancer. There are additional plant-derived extracts that have been shown effective in alleviating menopausal symptoms such as depression, anxiety, insomnia, and vaginal atrophy, and we need to look at them as well.

Soy Estrogens Versus Dangerous Estrogen Drugs

A soy extract that provides at least 50 mg of soy phytoestrogens is a key ingredient for effective natural estrogen replacement therapy. Compelling research findings show that soy phytoestrogens may be safer and as effective as FDA-approved estrogen drugs.

Based upon records of dietary soy consumption in Japan, where breast cancer incidence is very low, daily soy isoflavone intake has been estimated at 50 mg a day. The typical Western diet, on the other hand, only provides 1 to 5 mg a day of the soy isoflavones that may protect against several forms of cancer.

At a conference in Brussels, Belgium (Sept. 15–17, 1996), entitled "The Role of Soy in Medicine," numerous clinical studies were presented, showing that soy phytoestrogens in doses ranging from 40 to 160 mg a day produced rapid and significant reductions in menopausal symptoms. Other studies presented at this conference showed that, in countries where soy is a major constituent of the diet, women do not suffer discomforting menopausal symptoms the way Western women do.

According to peer-reviewed scientific studies, soy isoflavones protect against menopausal disorders that are normally treated by FDA-approved estrogen drugs. Unlike these dangerous drugs, phytoestrogens from soy have been shown to

- Prevent cancer at multiple sites.
- Prevent gallstones.
- Protect kidney function.
- Stimulate bone formation.
- Lower cholesterol levels.
- Inhibit the oxidation of LDL cholesterol.
- Inhibit the development or progression of atherosclerosis.

Unlike estrogen drugs, phytoestrogens have a balancing effect on the body. When estrogen levels are too low, their very mild estrogenic effect raises total estrogenic activity. When estrogen levels are too high, they compete with estrogen at cell membrane receptor sites, thus lowering total estrogenic activity.

In a study in the *American Journal of Clinical Nutrition* (1994, 60: 333–40), 27 women with a mean age of 56 years were studied in a double-blind cross-over trial to assess whether supplementation with soy phytoestrogens could reduce the frequency of hot flashes. These women were given 80 mg of soy phytoestrogens or placebo for 2 months. The authors concluded that soy phytoestrogens demonstrated greater estrogenic hormonal activity and reduced hot flashes compared to placebo.

Phytoestrogens Prevent Osteoporosis

At the University of Kentucky in Lexington, Dr. Paolo Fanti studied the effects of genistein (from soy) on bone loss in ovariectomized rats. Dr. Fanti found the mechanism of action of genistein (the most abundant soy phytoestrogen) appears to differ from that of estrogens. The protective action of genistein seems to depend on stimulation of bone formation rather than estrogen's effect of suppressing bone resorption.

A 6-month study on 66 postmenopausal women was conducted at the University of Illinois at Urbana-Champaign to investigate bone density and bone mineral content in response to soy therapy. In this study, postmenopausal women received, on a daily basis, either phytoestrogens derived from soy protein or milk-derived protein (that contained no phytoestrogens).

The results showed significant increases in bone density and bone mineral content for the lumbar spine in the women receiving the phytoestrogens derived from soy protein diets compared to the control diet. Increases in other skeletal areas also were noted in the women on the soy diets. Dr. Erdman, the lead scientist, concluded that soy isoflavones show real potential for maintaining bone health.

More Benefits of Soy Estrogens

A major cause of the breast cancer epidemic may be widespread use of insecticides, fungicides, manufacturing chemicals, and chlorine-based substances that mimic and mutate estrogen. These fat-soluble substances called "hormone modulating pollutants" accumulate in the body over time, and are being recognized as a contributing factor in the development of hormone-related cancers. Women with breast cancer have high levels of estrogen-altering pesticide residue in their breast fat cells compared to women who do not have breast cancer. Soy contains "friendly estrogens" that block estrogen-receptor sites on cells that are vulnerable to attack by carcinogenic "mutated" estrogens.

Kenneth D. Setchell, Ph.D., of Children's Hospital and Medical Center in Cincinnati, Ohio confirmed the estrogenic activity of the principal soy isoflavones daidzein, genistein, and glycitein. Dr. Setchell conducted research on the chemical structure and metabolism of soy phytoestrogens, and concluded that consuming modest amounts of soy protein results in relatively high blood concentrations of phytoestrogens and that this could have a significant hormonal effect in many individuals.

Dr. Sulistiyani of the Primate Research Center at Bogor Agricultural University in Indonesia stated that, in his opinion, one of the reasons estrogen replacement therapy is so effective in helping to reduce the risk of coronary heart disease in postmenopausal women may be in part because of its antioxidant properties. Considering the increased risk of breast cancer and uterine cancer in women using estrogen drugs, the researcher suggested that one alternative is to take phytoestrogens, such as genistein, which have been shown to protect the heart against cardiovascular disease. In studies using Cynomolgus female monkeys who had their ovaries removed to simulate postmenopausal women, it was shown that genistein inhibited LDL (the harmful form of cholesterol) oxidation by 48%. When used in combination with vitamin E this effect was even more pronounced!

Soy Estrogens Are Readily Available

While the health benefits of soy are well documented in the scientific literature, it has been difficult and expensive, up until now, to obtain the amount of genistein and other soy isoflavones that scientists say may treat menopausal symptoms and prevent age-related diseases.

The Life Extension Foundation introduced a soy extract (Mega Soy) in October, 1997 that contains enough phytoestrogens from soy to provide double the amount of genistein, daidzein, and glycitein found in the typical Japanese diet. This soy extract is so concentrated that only a small amount is needed to obtain enough phytoestrogens to potentially provide effective estrogen replacement for many women. This concentrated soy extract is now available in several commercial formulations.

Black Cohosh—Another Safe Phytoestrogen

An important and widely studied plant component used to treat menopause is a standardized extract from the black cohosh plant, also known as *Cimicufuga racemosa*. This black cohosh extract is approved by the German Ministry of Health for the treatment of menopausal symptoms related to estrogen deficiency. Standardized black cohosh has been trademarked under the name Remifemin for sale as a drug in countries throughout the world. More than 1.7 million women in Europe and Australia have used this natural herbal extract to treat menopausal symptoms. Clinical studies show that Remifemin alleviates not only hot flashes, but also depression, anxiety, vaginal atrophy, and a host of other menopausal-related disorders.

A fascinating study involved 60 women who were given either standardized black cohosh extract, Valium, or Premarin (synthetic estrogen) for menopausal symptoms. The women in the black cohosh group were relieved of depression and anxiety more effectively than the women in the Valium or Premarin group. This study was published in a German language medical journal (*Med. Welt*, 1984, 36: 871–74).

Premarin and Valium have been among the best selling drugs on the U.S. market for decades, yet produce terrible side effects. European women, on the other hand, have been using a safe natural herbal extract that's been shown to work better in alleviating depression and anxiety than these two widely prescribed FDA-approved drugs.

Another study on black cohosh extract involved women under age 40 who produced very little natural estrogen or progesterone because their ovaries had been removed (by hysterectomy). One group received estriol (a weak, but safe form of estrogen); the second group received Premarin; the third took Premarin and a progestin drug; the fourth was given black cohosh extract; and the fifth group received a placebo. This 24-week study rated women according to symptoms that included hot flashes, irritability, heart palpitations, etc. The results of the study showed that women experienced a 30% improvement in all groups receiving different forms of estrogen–progestin and black cohosh extract. There was no improvement in the placebo group. At the conclusion of the study, the majority of women receiving the estrogen drugs or black cohosh extract were symptom-free. But, most importantly, the women receiving the black cohosh extract reported fewer side effects. This study showed that phytotherapy with standardized black cohosh worked as well as estrogen drugs, but produced fewer uncomfortable and dangerous side effects. This research was published in a German journal (*Zent bl. Gynakol.*, 1988, 110:611–18).

The most impressive study on the benefits of this phytoestrogen was carried out by 131 physicians on 629 menopausal women. This study showed that black cohosh extract produced clear improvement in over 80% of patients within 6 to 8 weeks. Both physical and psychological symptoms improved. Here were the results of the changes in specific menopausal symptoms:

Symptom	Percent of women who became symptom-free	Percent who showed improvement
Hot flashes	43.3%	86.6%
Profuse perspiration	49.9%	88.5%
Headache	45.7%	81.9%
Vertigo	51.6%	86.8%
Heart palpitation	54.6%	90.4%
Tinnitus	54.8%	92.9%
Nervousness/irritability	42.4%	85.6%
Sleep disturbances	46.1%	76.8%
Depressive moods	46%	82.5%

Most patients in the above clinical study reported noticeable benefits within 4 weeks. After 6 to 8 weeks, complete resolution of symptoms was reported in a high number of patients (*Gynecology,* 1982, 1: 14–16).

A placebo-controlled study published in a German journal (*Planta Med.*, 1991, 57) investigated the hormonal mechanisms by which black cohosh alleviates menopausal symptoms. The doctors conducting the study pointed out that hot flashes correspond closely with a surge of luteinizing hormone released from the pituitary gland in response to estrogen deficiency. Black cohosh was shown to suppress increased luteinizing hormone secretion in menopausal women and this effect was specifically linked with a reduction in the incidence of hot flashes.

Black cohosh extract has shown estrogenic effects within the body in several studies, but it does not elevate estrogen levels in the blood. Black cohosh extract appears to bind to estrogen receptors in order to mimic the hormonal effects of the weak estrogen, estriol. Estriol has been shown to protect against the types of cancers that more potent forms of estrogen (estradiol and estrone) appear to cause. Black cohosh extract has been referred to as being "estriol-like" because of the rejuvenating effect it exerts on the vaginal, rather than the uterine, lining.

Because of the impressive safety record of standardized black cohosh extract, it is has become a popular natural alternative to FDA-approved estrogen drugs.

More Estrogenic Plants

There are other, important plant-derived hormone modulators that are used by alternative physicians to treat menopausal symptoms. It is important to understand that estrogens are continually being modified as they circulate in the body. They are converted from one form to another and are outfitted with numerous other compounds that cause their biological activity to vary considerably. While it may appear that the combination of soy phytoestrogens and standardized black cohosh may provide complete estrogen replacement, there are other hormonal factors to adjust for if the metabolism of youth is to be maintained (or restored).

An extract from the licorice root called glycyrrhetic acid (GA) stimulates the natural conversion of testosterone to estrogen in the body. Glycyrrhetic acid is an antioxidant that is often used to protect the liver and suppress viral activity in hepatitis patients. Offshore cancer clinics prescribe high doses of GA in injectable form to patients because of studies showing that it modulates immune function and suppresses cancer cell replication. It is interesting to note that while FDA-approved estrogen drugs can cause abnormal blood clotting, the GA contained in licorice root inhibits the clotting factor thrombin, thus reducing the risk of a heart attack or stroke. Licorice root extracts have many disease-fighting applications, but for menopausal women, the most important factor is that glycyrrhetic acid extracted from licorice is a safe source of natural estrogen. Numerous studies indicate that GA is an effective estrogen replacement therapy in humans. The Chinese have successfully used licorice extracts for more than 3000 years to treat menopausal disorders.

Dong Quai extract is the supreme female tonic in traditional Chinese medicine. It has been used successfully to alleviate PMS (premenstrual syndrome) and menopausal symptoms by helping to normalize estrogen levels. Dong Quai extract has shown to have a muscle relaxant effect, and has been used as an analgesic and antiinflammatory agent. Scientists believe that one unique mechanism of action of Don Quai is to promote natural progesterone synthesis. Progesterone, which will be discussed in more detail below, is another hormone whose production declines at menopause. Progesterone is more important than estrogen for preventing and treating osteoporosis because progesterone is directly involved in the production of bone-forming cells called osteoblasts. Many menopausal women use a topical natural progesterone cream to provide for direct absorption of progesterone into the bloodstream.

Another hormone imbalance that women encounter as they grow older is excessive prolactin secretion from the pituitary gland. Prolactin interferes with the beneficial effect of estrogen and may promote the development of estrogen-induced cancers. Prolactin secretion may be suppressed by a natural extract called vitex agnus castus. In a study in a German medical journal (*Arzneim. Forsch./Drug Res.,* (1993, 43 [II]: 7), vitex agnus castus extract was shown to suppress excessive prolactin secretion and promote natural progesterone synthesis over a 3-month period. As with the other plant hormone-modulating extracts, no side effects were observed.

WARNING: Prolactin is so dangerous in patients with hormone-dependent cancers that the Life Extension Foundation advocates prolactin suppression drug therapy for breast and prostate cancer patients.

A Natural Estrogen Replacement Approach

When choosing a natural estrogen replacement program, make sure the ingredients are standardized to meet pharmaceutical potency. An investigation conducted in 1998 of natural estrogen products sold in health food stores showed that many companies were not using the standardized plant extracts that had been used in the published studies to treat menopausal symptoms. Phone calls to these companies confirmed that many extracts were "one-to-one" ratios, which means that relatively little of the active ingredient was present. It should be pointed out that this investigation also found that respected brand-name supplement companies were using pharmaceutical-grade standardized extracts in their products to treat menopausal symptoms.

An ideal multi-ingredient phytoestrogen supplement should contain concentrated pharmaceutical extracts. If the active ingredients are not standardized, one cannot expect to obtain consistent biological activity.

Several natural hormone replacement formulas are available to Americans. A product called Natural Estrogen was formulated by the Life Extension Foundation to provide the complete hormone-modulating effects that can be obtained from plant sources. The Natural Estrogen formula provides phytoestrogens from soy, estrogenic plants such as licorice extract, and hormone-modulating plant extracts such as black cohosh (*Cimicifuga racemosa*), Dong Quai (*Angelica sinensis*), and vitex extract. More about how to safely use natural estrogen supplements will appear later in the protocol.

When Natural Estrogen is Not Enough

Some women experience such severe menopausal symptoms that natural, safe forms of estrogen supplements do not provide sufficient relief. If this occurs, and a woman is afraid of the cancer risks and side effects of long-term therapy with estrogen drugs approved by the FDA, there is a third option. Estriol is used extensively in Europe for estrogen replacement therapy in menopausal and postmenopausal women, but to date has rarely been used for that purpose in the United States. It can, however, be obtained in the U.S. from compounding pharmacies with a doctor's prescription.

Evidence suggests that estriol offers many of the benefits of more traditional estrogen-replacement therapies, but without the harsh side effects or longer term dangers often encountered by other substances and trademarked products. First, some background. The primary forms of estrogen include three substances: estrone, estradiol and estriol. Estrone sulphate is the form of estrogen found in Premarin, while 17-α estradiol is the form of estrogen found in the products Estrace and Estraderm. Estrone and estradiol, known as "conjugated estrogens," significantly increase the risk of breast and ovarian cancer when taken for more than 10 years. According to the Merck Manual, conjugated estrogens are substances that even have been listed as known carcinogens, yet they are the unquestioned choices of too many physicians.

Estriol, on the other hand, is a weak estrogen that provides the antiaging benefits of estrogen replacement therapy, apparently without the risk of cancer. Consider this evidence of its benignity: during pregnancy, huge amounts of estriol are secreted by the placenta to protect the fetus. Urinary assay of estriol is used to assess the fetus' viability.

Since estriol is a weak estrogen, larger amounts must be used for estrogen replacement therapy. Estriol is used in doses of 2 to 8 mg a day. A dose of 2 to 4 mg of estriol is equivalent to, and as effective as, 0.6 to 1.25 mg of conjugated estrogens such as Premarin. One of the most common side effects of standard estrogen therapy is endometrial hyperplasia, or hyperproliferation of the cells of the uterine lining, a condition that often turns into uterine cancer. This condition, which sometimes occurs at younger ages, will be described in more detail later. However, most investigators have found that the use of the alternative estriol therapy, even at the high dose of 8 mg a day, does not cause endometrial hyperplasia.

In one study by scientists at the Medical College of Georgia in Augusta, 52 women with severe menopausal symptoms were given estriol succinate continuously for 6 months in doses of 2 to 8 mg a day. Significant improvements in symptoms were noted within 1 month of the start of the study, and they persisted as long as estriol therapy was continued. The degree of symptom improvement was directly related to the dose. Symptom relief was moderate at 2 mg a day, but marked at 8 mg a day.

Estriol therapy also reversed vaginal atrophy and improved the quality of cervical mucus. No breakthrough bleeding occurred in any of the subjects and biopsies of the inner mucous membrane of the uterus failed to show endometrial hyperplasia in any case, regardless of the dose of estriol used. The scientists concluded, "Estriol therapy may be employed in dosages up to 8 mg/day continuously, especially in those patients in whom other estrogens induce undesired side effects such as nausea, breakthrough bleeding, or endometrial hyperplasia, and the recurrence of hot flashes during cyclic therapy of more potent estrogens. . . . Being a weak estrogen, it does not induce endometrial proliferation or breakthrough bleeding of any consequence, while modifying menopausal symptoms."

A large, long-term study of estriol therapy for the symptoms of menopause was conducted by C. Lauritzen at the University of Ulm in Germany. The investigators concluded, "Estriol therapy was successful in 92% of all cases. In 71%, hot flashes and sweating were completely eliminated, in 21% they were ameliorated, becoming weaker and occurring more seldom. . . . Depressive moods were abolished in 24% of the cases, and in 33% they were ameliorated, so that an overall improvement occurred in 57%." The study also found that forgetfulness, loss of concentration, irritability, and heart palpitations were remarkably improved towards normal. Also, the number of patients suffering from migraine headaches decreased from 33 to 12, and atrophying of the vulva was completely eliminated in 44 of 61 cases, and showed improvement in 12 cases.

"Remarkably," the scientists added, "the quality of the skin improved according to the subjective impression of patients and physicians in a high percentage of cases. . . . In no case, did a deterioration of symptoms occur."

As described above, one of the major benefits of estrogen therapy is prevention of the bone loss associated with menopause. Postmenopausal women taking estrogen experience 50% fewer bone fractures than women of comparable age who have not taken estrogen.

Although no studies have yet been conducted in the U.S. to determine whether estriol therapy can prevent osteoporosis, a prospective double-blind study was conducted in 136 postmenopausal women at the Chinese Great Wall Hospital in Beijing, China using nylestriol (CEE), a long-acting estriol derivative. The doctors found that the placebo group had significantly greater loss of bone mass and higher low-density lipoprotein levels when compared with the treated group. They concluded, "CEE is an effective estrogen for preventing bone loss and lipid disorders in postmenopausal women, just as is the more popular conjugated estrogen (Premarin), but is more convenient. Long-term CEE medication, its effects on the endometrium and the regimen of progestin combination await further study."

There also is direct evidence from animal studies, and indirect evidence from human studies, that estriol can prevent breast cancer. Much of this work has been done by Dr. H. M. Lemon and associates of the Department of Internal Medicine at the University of Nebraska Medical Center in Omaha. In one study, they induced mammary tumors by radiation in female rats. In the control group, 75% developed tumors.

However, among those animals receiving estriol, just 48% developed tumors. In another study by the Lemon team, estriol was shown to have "the most significant anti-mammary carcinogenic activity of 22 tested compounds [because]. . . estriol is less likely to induce proliferative changes in the target organs of cancer-prone women than estrone or estradiol."

Because of these anticancer effects of estriol in animals, Lemon looked at the question of whether estriol is related in any way to breast cancer in humans. He found that women with breast cancer have low levels of estriol relative to other forms of estrogen. The evidence about estriol as a safe alternative estrogen therapy can be summed up well by the Medical College of Georgia scientists, who concluded, "Estriol deserves a place in our therapeutic resources."

The Epidemic Deficiency of Progesterone

Throughout mature life, women will experience a gradual loss of another critical hormone, progesterone. This decline becomes significant as women get closer to menopause. Symptoms of a progesterone deficit include premenstrual discomfort, night sweats, and hot flashes, along with a loss of the sense of well-being (depressed feelings). During and after menopause, natural progesterone synthesis often grinds to a halt, setting the stage for a host of menopausal miseries and degenerative diseases.

Scientific studies indicate that progesterone may have potential in the hormonal prevention of breast cancer. At a recent scientific conference, persuasive evidence was presented showing that the correct use of natural progesterone could result in a significant reduction in the risk of breast cancer. Progesterone has many beneficial properties, such as the activation of natural killer cells, but one factor of special relevance is that progesterone diminishes the production of a cancer-causing form of estrogen called 4-hydroxyestrone, while increasing the production of cancer-preventing estriol. In other words, estrogen may be made safe through the concomitant use of progesterone, particularly when taken in natural forms.

In addition to making people feel better, progesterone may help to prevent the mental decline that occurs with aging. Progesterone has been shown to increase neuronal energy production and to protect brain cells.

Progesterone and Estrogen Prevent Osteoporosis

Interestingly, the combined effects of these two critical hormones lead to the prevention of bone loss at all ages, though progesterone deficiencies appear to be a more significant factor as women age.

There are two types of bone regulating cells. The osteoclasts function to dissolve older bone and leave tiny unfilled spaces behind. The osteoblasts then move into these spaces and produce new bone. This process of dissolving older bone mass by osteoclasts and new bone formation by osteoblasts is the mechanism for the repair and continuing strength of bone.

Like all living cells, osteoblasts and osteoclasts require hormonal guidance to properly function. Osteoblasts depend primarily on progesterone and testosterone, while osteoclasts need estrogen-like hormones. In the absence of these hormones, osteoblasts and osteoclasts cease to function properly and rapid deterioration of the bone occurs. Osteoporosis can occur when osteoclasts dissolve more bone than what the osteoblasts are able to replace.

Estrogen regulates the activity of osteoclasts, which results in a slowing of dissolving older bone. Progesterone, on the other hand, promotes the production of osteoblasts, which are required to effect new bone formation. Natural progesterone has been shown to stimulate the new bone formation required to prevent and reverse osteoporosis.

Osteoporosis can be caused by mineral and vitamin deficiencies, corticosteroid drugs, poor eating habits, lack of exercise, too much cortisol, and too little testosterone (two other important hormones). The major influence on age-associated bone deterioration, however, would appear to be a severe deficiency of ovarian-secreted progesterone.

An Antiaging Hormone

In 1994, the Life Extension Foundation introduced a natural progesterone cream to help prevent osteoporosis, menopausal symptoms, depressed feelings, and breast cancer. Over the last year, a number of studies have appeared indicating that topically applied progesterone cream works better than what was originally published.

Three years ago, the FDA approved a clinical study entitled, "Use of Natural Progesterone Cream in the Prevention of Osteoporosis: A Randomized Double-Blind Placebo Controlled Trial." A double-blind study is one in which the researchers are unaware of which group is given the substance being studied or placebo. This ongoing study is being conducted by Dr. Helene Leonetti, M.D., of the Bethlehem Obstetrics Clinic in Bethlehem, PA. The women being studied are in the immediate postmenopausal phase (1 to 5 years after menopause), which is when bone loss is most rapid. After the first year, the positive effects of progesterone became so apparent, that the doctors overseeing the study were "unblinded." In other words, it became apparent to the doctors which women were receiving progesterone compared to the placebo. The women in the progesterone group experienced the disappearance of lumps and bumps in their breasts, were less depressed, and had fewer hot flashes and better bone densities (though the time interval was too short for this to be significant). An important point brought out was that no women using progesterone cream experienced loss of bone density, while the placebo group showed slight bone loss. The study is about to complete its second year and it will continue for 1 more year. The expectation is that the women on the progesterone will have significantly greater bone density tests compared to the placebo.

New research indicates that progesterone may help prevent mental decline in the elderly. Dr. John Lee, one of the world's foremost experts on progesterone therapy, has found studies showing that the brain cells concentrate progesterone 20 times higher than blood serum levels. Recovery after brain trauma is better if progesterone levels are higher. Dr. Lee also has pointed out that progesterone has been shown to increase brain cell energy production while suppressing hyper-excitotoxicity. "Excitotoxicity" occurs when too much (or too little) of neurotransmitters such as glutamate are released from brain cells. This type of toxicity is now considered a cause of brain aging and degenerative neurological disease. Life Extension members are taking supplements such as methyl cobalamin and vinpocetine to help prevent nerve cell damage caused by excitotoxicity. It now appears that progesterone also protects against this type of brain cell damage.

Progesterone May Prevent Breast Cancer

A large base of evidence suggests that progesterone is protective against, as well as a potential treatment for, breast cancer (Cowan, 1981; Hagen, 1998.) A study by Chang (1995) showed transdermal estradiol increased cell proliferation rate by 230%, while transdermal progesterone decreased the cell proliferation rate by over 400%. A combination estradiol/progesterone cream maintained the normal proliferation rate. This is direct evidence that estradiol (a potent estrogen) stimulates hyperproliferation of breast tissue cells and progesterone prevents hyperproliferation.

A second study by noted researcher Bent Formby, Ph.D. (1998) was published with insightful results. To determine the biologic mechanism of why progesterone inhibits the proliferation of breast cancer cells, a variety of cancer cell lines with different receptors and different expression of genes were exposed to progesterone. Exposure to progesterone induced a maximal 90% inhibition of cell proliferation in T47-D breast cancer cells and no measurable response in MDA-231 progesterone-receptor negative breast cancer cells. Further research along the same lines should be able to specify exactly when progesterone therapy would be most effective.

Previous retrospective studies have shown that women undergoing breast cancer operations during the luteal phase of the menstrual cycle (the span between ovulation and the start of menstruation), when progesterone is higher, have much longer survival times. Angiogenesis (new blood supply) is essential for tumor growth and vascular endothelial growth factor (VEGF) is one of the most potent angiogenic factors. Heer and colleagues (1998) suggest that since progesterone seems to lower VEGF expression, its lowering could possibly decrease the potential for tumor spread. Dr. P. E. Mohr in the *British Journal of*

Cancer (1996) reported that women with a progesterone level of 4 mg/mL or more at the time of their breast cancer surgery had a significantly better survival rate at 18 years than those with a lower serum level of progesterone. In those women with good progesterone levels at the time of their surgery, it was revealed that approximately 65% were surviving 18 years later, whereas only 35% of the women with low progesterone levels survived.

A study done by Cowan et al. in 1981, published in the *American Journal of Epidemiology,* showed that the incidence of breast cancer was 5.4 times greater in women with low progesterone than in women who had good progesterone levels. Some final evidence confirming progesterone-protective effects on breast tissue comes from a study by J. M. Foidart in *Fertility and Sterility* (April, 1998.) Either a placebo gel, an estrogen gel, a progesterone gel, or a combination estrogen/progesterone gel was applied to women's breasts for 14 days prior to breast surgery. After surgery, the breast tissue was analyzed and it was found that estradiol increased breast cell proliferation and that progesterone greatly decreased proliferation.

As Dr. Lee explains, "The goal of progesterone supplementation is to restore normal physiologic levels of bioavailable progesterone." That is why testing saliva or blood progesterone levels is important, especially for premenopausal women who are using progesterone cream to alleviate premenstrual syndrome (PMS) symptoms. In women whose doctors are prescribing excess amounts of supplemental estrogen, the administration of progesterone may enable the dose of estrogen to be reduced, since progesterone restores sensitivity to estrogen receptors on cell membranes. Saliva tests are available to ascertain progesterone and other hormone levels in the body. The Life Extension Foundation may be offering these tests in the future, subject to further validation studies.

Potential Dangers of FDA-Approved Synthetic Progesterone Drugs

The issue of synthetic versus natural hormones is as important with progesterone as it is with estrogen. Just as the pharmaceutical industry created their dangerous estrogen drug Premarin, they produced a pseudo-progesterone named Provera. As with Premarin, the warning label on Provera is full of dangers including the possibility of birth defects, breast cancer, blood clots, fluid retention, acne, rashes, weight gain, and depression. Such drugs as Provera are classified as "progestins," not as progesterones. The side effects of Premarin and Provera may be the main reason women stop taking their replacement hormones, and are definitely the reason that HRT has such a questionable and spotty reputation.

An alternative to artificial progestins is the option of using natural progesterone products. Products like the Life Extension Foundation's Pro-Fem use progesterone derived from soybeans. Not only are such soy-based or wild yam–based natural progesterones far safer than synthetic drugs, they are as easily utilized as the real progesterone manufactured within the human body. The preferable forms of natural progesterone are creams that are rubbed in to appropriate areas. This route of administration bypasses the liver and allows hormone delivery to the place where it is needed the most. For example, progesterone cream applied to the breasts slows cell proliferation and eases breast pain. As to safety, according to Northrup (1994), "There is virtually no danger of overdose." (Note that a woman cannot simply eat wild yams or wild yam products. The human body does not have the means of converting plants into progesterone molecules. Processing is a requirement, though processed phytohormones are still "natural.")

In addition to the established and dangerous progestins such as Provera, the FDA has just approved a drug called Prometrium, which is an oral pill containing 200 mg of natural progesterone to be taken daily. This is overkill because your liver will go into overdrive trying to excrete this acute, overabundant supply of progesterone. Most of this oral progesterone drug that is not detoxified by the liver will be unavailable for cellular use. Progesterone cream is better utilized and much more economical. Dr. Foidart, in another study in May 1998 on transdermal replacement hormone therapy, states that avoidance of the "first passage effect" (through liver) is ensured by the transdermal application of hormones and probably explains the superiority of this route of hormone administration. Natural progesterone should not be confused with the synthetic FDA-approved progestins that cause many side effects. Synthetic progestins do not provide the broad spectrum of benefits that have been documented for natural progesterone.

Hormone Deficiencies: DHEA

DHEA (dehydroepiandrosterone) is a precursor of estrogen and testosterone, so taking DHEA might raise the levels of these hormones. DHEA is a good starting place for hormone modulation in the aging female.

While there have been contradictions in the research on DHEA, it appears to be a true rejuvenative hormone to at least a moderate degree, improving mood, neurological functions, immune system functioning, bone growth, energy, and feelings of well-being. In a review of research, the journal *Endocrine News* (1996) reported that DHEA, given until the patient's blood levels matched those found in their teenage years, resulted in "remarkable improvement of physical and psychological well-being in both genders. This finding in addition to the absence of side effects provides great promise for the replacement strategy." It should be noted that because DHEA may raise estrogen levels, the Life Extension Foundation recommends that it be taken with melatonin to provide a safeguard against breast cell proliferation. (Melatonin is a pineal hormone with multiple benefits and no significant side effects. Most importantly, it appears to protect against breast cancer.)

Though women usually have less DHEA than do men, both sexes lose it at about the same rate, suggesting that it is an age-related decline, not just a result of menopause. Peak levels are typically reached when women are in their third decade of life, following which they begin to lose approximately 2% per year (Wright and Morganthaler, 1997). As with all hormones, blood levels are only one criterion to establish in supplementation. The ultimate goal is individual functioning.

Hormone Imbalances Affect All Ages

While the need to supplement hormones becomes critical at menopause, many health problems are caused by hormonal imbalances. There is no need to wait until menopause to improve your physical and emotional state by spending some time modulating the levels of these substances with safe and natural supplements.

Hormonal dysfunctions are found to be the cause of many menstrual complaints, the most prominent being premenstrual syndrome, commonly called PMS. For many years, women had their PMS complaints diminished, ignored, or attributed to psychosomatic causes. In truth, the complex hormonal interactions required to produce a "normal" menstrual cycle are easily disturbed by a variety of biochemical, environmental, and psychological sources. There are dozens of uncomfortable and painful symptoms of PMS, and their appearance may occur from a few days before menstruation begins, to several weeks before bleeding starts. Women with PMS tend to have relatively high levels of estrogen coupled with relatively low levels of progesterone. This estrogen–progesterone balance is critical to most of the health problems discussed in this protocol. Other factors associated with PMS are diet, obesity, vitamin and mineral deficiencies, and an imbalance in hormone-like compounds called eicosanoids (which may be corrected with dietary and supplement alterations, to be discussed later).

Menstrual cramps are not the same as PMS. It is common to have PMS and painless periods, while women without PMS may have severe cramping during their periods. Cramps are caused by uterine contractions, and have been treated with birth control pills (hormones) to eliminate the ovulation-related hormonal changes that lead to cramping. Since excess prostaglandin production causes contractions of the smooth muscles, another treatment is to use medications such as ibuprofen that inhibit prostaglandins. Prostaglandins are chemicals that regulate involuntary muscles: blood vessels, uterus, and intestines. They are one form of eicosanoids, mentioned as causative agents in PMS.

Irregular Menstruation

When a woman regularly misses her period or commonly bleeds (spots) between periods, she has a condition called "dysfunctional uterine bleeding," which frequently is associated with an estrogen–progesterone imbalance, though thyroid or pituitary problems are other possible causes. Conventional medical treatment utilizes standard birth control pills to regulate periods. It should be noted that modern contraceptive pills are far safer than they once were, plus they offer a quick and easy solution to the problem. Unfortunately, they don't act precisely or individually in the manner of true hormone modulation.

Excessive menstrual bleeding, named "menorrhagia," always is uncomfortable and often is an incredibly inconvenient problem, interfering with the natural patterns of life. In its most severe forms, menorrhagia can lead to anemia, requiring nutritional supplements just for that deficit alone. Treatment may include raising progesterone levels and taking prostaglandin inhibitors to decrease the flow of blood forced out by uterine contractions. The most common form of benign breast pain comes from the hormonal changes of the menstrual cycle. Breast tissue is affected by cyclic change, just like the uterus. Fluid buildup occurs premenstrually, but has no way of being discharged in the way the uterus releases its menstrual flow. Breast fluid must be reabsorbed, and sensitivity and pain may result. In other cases, breast pain seems unrelated to menstrual patterns and the causes aren't always clear, but alterations in hormones such as estrogen, progesterone, and prolactin (a hormone whose function is to stimulate lactation) have been implicated. Of the most concern is that breast tissue is extremely sensitive to estrogen. High estrogen levels lead to tissue growth, cyst formation, and pain (as well as cancer, to be discussed later). Because progesterone balances estrogen by "down-regulating" the estrogen receptor cells in the breast, it blocks estrogen's "grow" signals. The result is to decrease the proliferation of cell tissues, protecting them from the dangerous, negative effects of even modest amounts of estrogen.

Too Many Sex Hormones Cause Excessive Tissue Growth

Benign fibroid uterine tumors are the number one reason for hysterectomies in the United States (Hutchins, 1990). Their cause is unknown and they often prove asymptomatic, depending on their size and location. However, some may lead to excessive bleeding, pelvic pressure, and frequent urination. Fibroids causing health problems such as anemia must be treated, often with different levels of surgery. In some cases, fibroids may be managed with the help of progesterone. Typically, fibroids shrink after menopause because of the reduction in endogenous (self-produced) estrogen that occurs. As we have mentioned, estrogen is a growth-stimulating hormone.

Polycystic ovaries is a condition directly caused by a hormone imbalance. Because of an excess of androgens (the "male" hormone), normal egg development is prevented. When eggs are underdeveloped, numerous small cysts are formed. Standard medical treatment includes prescription birth control pills, antiandrogenic medications, or synthetic progestin to prevent the uterine lining from suffering from excessive hormonal stimulation. Alternatively, natural progesterone may reduce symptoms without the side effects of progestins.

Another tissue-growth health concern is endometrial hyperplasia, an excess of glandular tissue in the uterine lining. This condition is most common in women with irregular periods, irregular egg production, and irregular sloughing of the lining of the uterus. Usually it is not dangerous and often simply goes away. Physicians monitor hyperplasia to make sure that abnormal cells are not present and that the condition does not become chronic. Traditional treatment involves giving a synthetic progesterone such as Provera to cause the uterine lining to slough off, removing the excess tissues. If this fails, a D and C (dilation and curettage) may be performed. Again, the safe alternative of natural progesterone will decrease estrogen receptor cells, often clearing up the problem.

Endometriosis is a condition involving the migration of endometrial tissue to other areas of the body, typically within the pelvis (but occasionally even further away from its point of origin). It may lead to pelvic pain, menstrual dysfunction, bowel pain, or infertility. Endometriosis is hormone-dependent, involving high levels of estrogen. Its actual causes are only theoretical at this time, though its pain is extremely factual. Again, conventional treatment is hormonal, using birth control pills, synthetic progesterone, or drugs such as Lupron, which make a woman temporarily menopausal. The goal is to reduce the level of estrogen in the system, leading to a drop in "grow" signals to the endometrial tissues. The Life Extension Foundation prefers the use of natural progesterone, either in creams such as ProFem, or, in some cases, a more concentrated cream from a compounding pharmacist (one who individually makes compounds by prescription) or natural progesterone capsules.

Possibly the most controversial area involving the use of exogenous (produced outside the body) hormones is the effect such treatment has on breast tissue. The concerns regard birth control pills as well as standard menopausal hormone replacement therapy and range from enlarged, tender breasts to deadly breast cancer. Breast tissue may be the most estrogen-sensitive area of the body. Combine this with eicosanoid imbalances and possible links to the growth hormones used in the dairy industry, and there are multiple reasons why breast cancer rates rise with age and are the leading cause of death in women in the menopausal years (National Center for Health Statistics, 1987).

Again, primary focus is on the relative balance of estrogen and progesterone. While the breasts are saturated with estrogen receptor cells, the presence of sufficient progesterone "down-regulates" such receptors, protecting against the powerful "grow" signals of estrogen. In addition, a compound called I3C (indole-3-carbinol) affects estrogen metabolism in ways that reduce the risk of breast cancer (Telang et al., 1997). The Life Extension Foundation offers a safe IC3 product in pill form.

The shortsighted and sometimes antifemale model of traditional medicine is best represented by the "therapeutic" technique of prophylactic breast and ovary removal. Women born with a gene labeled "BRCA 1" have a significantly increased risk of breast cancer because the gene causes an excessive ovarian production of estrogen (Stratton et al., 1997). As we have learned, estrogen is a stimulator of breast cancer cells. The response of many physicians is to surgically remove the potentially dangerous organs. While that may be a last-ditch necessity in some cases, it seems both appropriate and less damaging to attempt first to lower estrogen's dangerous effects through other means, including IC3 and progesterone supplements.

The cause of ovarian cancer is far less evident than the causes of breast cancer, but hormonal levels do appear to have a role. For example, Helizisouer et al. (1995) discovered a strong connection between ovarian cancer and the "male" hormone androgen. Another hormonal connection involves birth control pills. Women taking these medications have a lower risk of getting ovarian cancer, possibly because of the decrease in ovarian stimulation. Conversely, fertility drugs increase ovarian activity and are linked to higher rates of ovarian cancer.

The most important fact about uterine cancer is straightforward and the same as in other malignancies of the reproductive system: estrogen encourages the growth of uterine tissue.

Lack of Libido Is Not Just in Your Head

Most of the discussion of loss of sexual desire has centered on the problems of menopause. Yet this problem is far more common in women of all ages than is recognized, largely because of the societal pressure on women to be sexual and from their individual needs to please their partners. Many of the situations thus have psychological roots and are beyond the intent of this protocol. However, hormones play a significant and often undiscovered role.

Research with menopausal women has been the origin of much of our knowledge in this area. Davis (1998) points out that while using androgens with postmenopausal women successfully increases their sexual desire, the bigger picture is that androgen levels fall significantly throughout the reproductive years and probably affect desire from an early age. In addition, research by Braunstein, reported as a Reuters Health news release, indicated that testosterone delivered through a transdermal patch increased women's perception of orgasmic pleasure. Some androgens in particular (DHEA and DHEA-sulfate) decline steadily from early adulthood (Longcope, 1998). Other androgens show more decline closer to menopause. Treatment with androgens is safe and effective for these dysfunctions when given at low levels and paired with progesterone (Slayden, 1998). Many women lose their sexual desires after giving birth. Many of these sexual problems are directly tied to general postpartum depression. The goal is to modulate the estrogen–progesterone balance to reach earlier, healthier levels, reducing as many negative postpartum outcomes as possible, including loss of libido. Also available as treatments are antidepressant medications, the most successful of which are the SSRIs (specific serotonin reuptake inhibitors) such as Prozac, Zoloft, and Paxil.

Alzheimer's and Hormone Deficits

Alzheimer's, like osteoporosis, is looked at as a condition of old age. However, some forms of dementia do occur at younger ages (for instance, by definition, presenile dementia). The dementing process of Alzheimer's is associated with a variety of socioeconomic factors as well. There is some evidence that estrogen may protect against Alzheimer's because those women with the highest estrogen levels have the lowest rate of occurrence of the disease. (Northrup, 1998). In addition, the biochemical actions of estrogen, as well as those of two other hormones, DHEA and pregnenolone, increase connections among brain cells, and enhance memory (Flood et al., 1992). Wright and Morganthaler (1997), in their book *Natural Hormone Replacement*, specifically call for hormone replacement as a means of preventing senility and Alzheimer's disease. These researchers also emphasize the significant differences between synthetic and natural hormones, both in safety and effectiveness.

Hormone Modulation

The process of achieving proper female hormonal balance is not a one-step procedure. This protocol will describe a series of events that will optimize the benefits available to all women who empower themselves in their personal health care. It is possible to take shortcuts in regulating hormones, and many positive outcomes may be achieved even without careful modulation. However, it is recommended that these concerns be addressed as much as possible.

Both natural and synthetic hormones come with synthetic instructions: the dosages specified on the labels are for the "average" woman, one who doesn't exist. While these dosages may achieve much of the symptom relief these products advertise, it would be unusual to realize optimal hormone modulation for all the hormones discussed using only the amounts listed. While this protocol will offer dosages to be taken, these should be considered as starting points, not as final goals. The individualization that offers the greatest amount of long-term health improvement is based on testing and feedback.

People do not regulate the temperature in their homes by simply setting the air conditioning thermostat on a "recommended" number and leaving it there indefinitely. They check the actual temperature, assess their own comfort levels, and make adjustments for time of day and season of the year. If we are this careful with air conditioning, why would we be reluctant to adjust such a critical matter as hormone level? Adjustment only can be achieved by self-evaluation and testing before and after hormone-affecting supplements are taken. Despite labels recommending "one capsule a day," only personal symptom change and blood level differences can determine what actually works well. Most of this testing takes place at the initiation of supplements, though periodic reevaluation is a necessity. Testing before any supplements are taken is called "baseline" measurement, and may be invaluable in the future. When new medical problems arise, knowing these earlier baseline standards allows for more accurate diagnosis and treatment. Testing may be performed in several ways.

Blood Testing

This measurement technique has the advantage of widespread established technology and standards, plus the capability of being done by mail. (The Life Extension Foundation offers such a service.) It is critical to remember that different labs have different standards. For example, Laboratory A has methods of testing that lead it to declare that a given hormone for a 30-year-old, nonpregnant woman has a "normal range" of 4 to 7. Laboratory B may use different specimen collection methods or measurement techniques, and declares the "normal range" of scores to be between 3.2 and 6.4. One lab's standards should not be used to evaluate testing by another source. In addition, it is impossible to give a representative sample of all the possible optimal or even average scores because these figures change based on age, pregnancy status, menopausal status, the particular day within each woman's menstrual cycle, and time of day. For example, cortisol norms may have substantial differences based on whether the sample was taken in the morning or the afternoon. In the end, each woman must compare her current scores with the average scores for a desired age from the same lab's norms.

Saliva Testing

This measurement technique does not have the standards that blood testing enjoys, but it is available by mail order and offers a degree of convenience. Standards are important when attempting to emulate the results of published studies. Some argue that saliva testing is more accurate than blood testing; others disagree.

Urine

The use of the 24-hour urine test may be the most accurate form of measurement because hormones are secreted in "bursts" rather than steadily throughout the day (Wright and Morganthaler, 1997). By collecting a full day's worth of urine, a woman gets a more complete picture of her actual levels. The shortcoming of this test is the difficulty involved in its collection: every drop of urine must be gathered during the 24-hour period.

When evaluating the effectiveness of either a new supplement or a change in dosage of an ongoing supplement, it is recommended that testing intervals of 45 days be used. Because some hormones gradually convert into other hormones (known as a "cascade"), waiting 45 days ensures accuracy.

Making Choices That Are Right for You

While a positive doctor–patient interaction always is beneficial, such cooperation is even more important for women dealing with hormonal issues. Some women insist on having female health care providers, fearing that their PMS or menopausal complaints may be dismissed too easily or treated too routinely. Their fears are sometimes warranted. But the key to choosing and keeping a physician is finding someone (male or female) who listens and includes you in the health feedback loop. Symptom improvement may be accomplished with minimal effort, but achieving true hormone modulation requires time and patience.

The selection of hormone modulation goals is a complex decision based on personal philosophy, resources, time, and fortitude. Philosophically, a woman must strike a personal balance between acceptable methods and acceptable outcomes. Choices involve types of hormones used, their sources, the costs, side effects, desired results and both short- and long-term benefits and risks. In addition, there is a choice to be made in terms of outcome priorities: is symptom reduction sufficient by itself or are optimal blood levels also required? Is it more important to use only plant hormone sources or to change blood hormone levels back to those of a younger age? These are the types of decisions to be made by each woman.

This protocol now offers generalized recommendation concerning the modulation of hormones. The choices presented will include, whenever possible, the most natural forms of supplements available.

Priming the Hormonal Pump

Before individual sex hormones are supplemented it is suggested that a "priming" procedure be used.

This priming is based on the "cascade" effects of DHEA as it gradually converts into all of the other hormones. To protect against the possible over-conversion of estrogen, women should add melatonin and soy extracts as a cancer safeguard. The priming dosages are as follows:

- DHEA, 15 mg once or twice daily.
- Melatonin, 3 mg at bedtime.
- Mega Soy extract, one capsule twice a day (110 mg of soy isoflavones).

This simple hormone priming may bring hormones back to the desired levels and eliminate any symptoms. If this does not occur, specific recommendations are now made for individual hormone adjustment. Remember, wait 45 days before testing to determine the effect of each new supplement or new supplement dose.

Estrogen Supplementation

A product called Natural Estrogen contains plant-derived phytoestrogens and nutrients that have been shown to favorably alter estrogen metabolism in the body. The recommended initial dose is one capsule of Natural Estrogen, twice a day. While postmenopausal women may start at any time, premenopausal women should begin on the fifth day of their menstrual cycle. It is recommended that women already taking estrogen drugs such as Premarin should wean themselves off the synthetic hormones gradually over several months as follows, using equivalent amounts of Natural Estrogen:

- 1st month—Natural Estrogen every other day, previous medication every other day.
- 2nd month—Natural Estrogen 2 days in a row, previous medication for 1 day.
- 3rd month—Natural Estrogen 3 days in a row, previous medication for 1 day.

Thereafter, take Natural Estrogen in the cyclic pattern described above. Please note that Natural Estrogen provides the same amount of phytoestrogens as MegaSoy, so most women will not need to take MegaSoy Extract if they are taking Natural Estrogen. If Natural Estrogen plus the previous doses of pregnenolone, DHEA, and melatonin do not achieve adequate symptom relief and blood levels, the use of estriol is recommended. The dosage for estriol, the safest form of estrogen, is between 2 and 8 mg a day, based on the ratio of 2 mg of estriol to 0.6 mg of Premarin. Again, trying and evaluating different dosages is the way to achieve the important goal of taking the least amount of estrogen that attains the desired blood or symptom level. Estriol creams in varying potencies may be tried for localized problems like vaginal dryness and thinning.

Should estriol alone not achieve a woman's goal, the next step is the utilization of a compound estrogen drug such as Tri Est, the medication described earlier as having three forms of estrogen in the same proportion found in human females. Typically, women are prescribed 1.25 mg of estriol twice daily for mild menopausal symptoms. Stronger symptoms may require double the dosage. If Tri Est is not adequate, it is possible to have a cooperative physician order individualized estrogen mixtures from formulary pharmacies. In this way, if the Tri Est with only 20% of the more dangerous estradiol and estrone fails to alleviate symptoms, a drug may be made with 40 or 60% estradiol. This is still a better choice than the standard medications with 80% estradiol. This graduated protocol is appropriate for any situation requiring supplemental estrogen. A natural product such as Natural Estrogen is recommended for PMS, menopause, and hormonally related health concerns related to estrogen deficit.

Progesterone Supplementation

The steps for progesterone supplementation are the same for both situations in which progesterone is needed to balance estrogen and those specifically calling for progesterone because it is the treatment of choice.

Natural progesterone is more beneficial than synthetic "progestin" drugs that are often prescribed to balance the negative effects of synthetic estrogen drugs. Natural progesterone in the form of transdermal creams is extremely safe. Overdoses have not been reported.

The Life Extension Foundation's ProFem and similar products offering natural forms of progesterone should be the starting (and hopefully final) type of treatment.

The recommended starting dosages are as follows:

- For severe osteoporosis
  - 1st jar: ½ teaspoon morning and night
  - 2nd jar: ¼ teaspoon morning and night
- For premenopausal women
  - Days 1 to 14 of cycle: no application
  - Days 15 to end of cycle: ⅛ to ¼ teaspoon daily
- For postmenopausal women
  - Apply ⅛ to ¼ teaspoon daily

An alternative to artificial progestins is the option of using natural progesterone products. Not only are such soy-based natural progesterones far safer than synthetic drugs, they are as easily utilized as the real progesterone manufactured within the human body. The preferable forms of natural progesterone are creams that are rubbed into different areas of the skin. This route of administration bypasses the liver and allows hormone delivery to the place where it is needed the most.

Dosages should be adjusted/increased as required when attempting to balance estrogen levels. The cream should be massaged into soft tissue areas such as breasts, underarms, and inner thighs on a rotating basis to avoid the oversaturation of cells.

DHEA Supplementation

DHEA is a precursor of estrogen and testosterone, so taking DHEA might raise the levels of these other hormones. It has been recommended previously in this protocol that DHEA is a good starting place for hormone modulation because of this ability. (See Priming the Hormonal Pump above.)

At the start of the section, it was recommended that women utilize a starting dose of 15 mg once or twice a day. Since DHEA is a precursor of testosterone as well as estrogen, many woman find both hormones will rise to more youthful levels by supplementing DHEA alone. As needed, women may adjust DHEA dosages to 25 mg twice daily. On a cautionary note, women with reproductive cancers should not take DHEA. In fact any woman with a family history of ovarian cancer, or a high score on an ovarian cancer blood screening test known as CA 125, should avoid all androgen supplements. As always, the best judge of dosage level is a test of blood level. The objective of DHEA supplementation is to achieve the blood levels that are considered normal for a 20- to 30-year-old woman (Yen, 1990). A DHEA blood test will greatly assist in proper dosing.

Hormone Modulation: Supportive Lifestyle and Nutrients

Every hormone discussed in this protocol is influenced by both environmental and nutritional factors. Here are some of the most important of these factors:

- Stress. There are strong correlations between excessive stress and such problems as adrenal insufficiency, lack of menstrual cycle, PMS, vaginitis, urinary incontinence, bone loss, and infertility.
- Smoking. Obviously, the link between cancer and smoking is well documented. Less well known is smoking's connection to bone loss, cervical dysplasia, miscarriage, and Alzheimer's disease.
- Exercise. The obvious connection here is to osteoporosis. But lack of regular exercise plays a role in adrenal disease, cardiopulmonary disorders, loss of libido, and menstrual problems.
- Obesity. Some menstrual disorders are found more often in overweight women. In fact, a diet that lowers body fat may lower estrogen levels as well.
- Nutrition. Here are some areas in which dietary supplements play an important role in the development and treatment of hormonally related diseases:
  - Vitamin E. Research at Johns Hopkins Medical School demonstrated 600 IUs a

day of vitamin E raised both estriol and progesterone levels in a group of women with fibroid breast disease. Both estriol and progesterone help to protect against estrogen's possible tumor-creating effects.

- Calcium, magnesium, and vitamin D_3. Any women with bone loss should supplement her diet with at least 1000 mg of elemental calcium, 600 mg of elemental magnesium, and 400 IUs of vitamin D_3 a day. A product such as Mineral Formula for Women contains the necessary amounts of these nutrients. *For more information on this topic, please refer to the Osteoporosis protocol in this book.*
- Antioxidants. The addition of such antioxidants as vitamin C, vitamin E, CoQ_{10}, grape seed-skin extract (proanthocyanidins) and alpha-lipoic acid may be of great assistance when treating a number of the disorders in this protocol, including cardiac problems and cancers.
- Fats. Diets high in saturated fats lead to heart disease, cancers, and an imbalance in the eicosanoid hormones (an important factor in fibroid cysts.) In contrast, diets high in essential fatty acids help to balance eicosanoids. Other eicosanoid imbalance links include uterine cramps, pelvic pain, and breast pain.
- High-potency B-complex vitamins. Various B vitamins have been examined by researchers. Abraham (1983) found vitamin B_6 to be helpful in reducing menstrual cramps. More recently, Mills (1996) showed that supplementing the B-complex group in women with endometriosis produced a significant decrease in symptoms.
- Bioflavonoids. Supplements of this member of the vitamin C complex appear to actually inhibit excessive estrogen synthesis (Kellis and Vickery, 1984).

Summary

The need to modulate the relative levels of the primary female hormones is of critical importance throughout life. Beyond the well-publicized hormone replacement therapy for menopausal symptoms, such disorders as PMS, endometriosis, several types of cancer, sexual dysfunctions, fibroid tumors, osteoporosis, cardiac disease, and Alzheimer's disease are closely related to hormonal imbalances. Many disorders are linked to either excessive or deficient estrogen levels, particularly as they compare to the amount of progesterone available. Not only should hormones be modulated regularly, but natural sources for hormone supplementation should be used. Synthetic and nonhuman analogue hormones carry with them unwanted, even deadly side effects. Hormone modulation requires individualization, and works best when carefully monitored through laboratory testing. Both lifestyle and nutritional variables play an important role in hormone modulation.

Estrogen is an antiaging hormone that provides many beneficial effects throughout the body. The major drawback to conventional estrogen replacement therapy is the increased risk of certain cancers. FDA-approved estrogen drugs have other adverse side effects that preclude many women from effectively using them. Natural plant extracts provide the body with safe and possibly more effective estrogen replacement.

Menopause is not just an estrogen deficiency. Numerous hormone imbalances threaten the health of menopausal women. The published literature has identified several plant extracts that favorably modulate hormone balance in aging women.

The decline in progesterone production is correlated with increased bone loss and increased risk of cancer. Many of the effects associated with normal aging can be attributed to a progesterone deficiency, so progesterone replacement therapy may be another missing link to solving the human aging process. The beneficial effects of natural progesterone have now been shown in women and men. Progesterone protects against many of the detrimental changes of aging, and the only downside is that too much can make a person feel sleepy or even euphoric. Please note that it usually takes 2 to 4 weeks for topically applied progesterone to build up to sufficient levels in the body to cause noticeable effects.

Individual symptomatic improvement and blood analysis of estrogen, progesterone, testosterone, prolactin, luteinizing hormone, and follicular stimulating hormone (FSH) by a physician can help determine how well natural hormone modulation therapy is working.

The proper intake of hormone-modulating plant extracts, phytoestrogens, DHEA, natural progesterone, and other natural hormones may provide significant health benefits to the aging female.

The following nutrients and drugs are suggested to restore hormone balance in aging women or women with symtoms of an imbalance:

1. Natural progesterone cream (ProFem): Apply topically to the skin (follow directions as outlined in this protocol).
2. Natural Estrogen: Take one capsule, 2 times a day.
3. DHEA: Take one 15-mg capsule, 1 to 2 times a day.
4. Life Extension Mix (multivitamin supplement): Take 3 tablets, 3 times a day.
5. Melatonin: Take 2 to 3 mg only at bedtime.
6. Consider supplementation with fish, flax, or Perilla oil to restore fatty balance.
7. Consider estriol or TriEst if menopausal symptoms are not alleviated by nonprescription therapies. Blood or saliva testing may also indicate the need for additional estrogen or progesterone.

Blood or saliva testing after 45 days is mandatory to verify you are taking the proper dosages.

For more information. Contact the National Institute on Aging, (800) 222-2225.

Product availability. Individual blood testing by mail, Natural Estrogen, ProFem, black cohosh, DHEA, Mega Soy Extract, melatonin, perilla oil, fish oil, flaxseed oil, and Life Extension Mix (multiple vitamin-mineral capsules and tablets) may be ordered by phoning (800) 544-4440, or order online at www.lef.org.

FIBRINOGEN AND CARDIOVASCULAR DISEASE

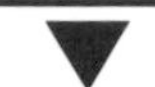

Most heart attacks and strokes are caused by a blood clot that obstructs the flow of blood to a portion of the heart or the brain. Blood clots that form inside arteries are the leading causes of death in the Western world. Blood clots kill almost 700,000 Americans every year.

High levels of the blood-clotting agent fibrinogen predispose a person to coronary and cerebral artery disease, even when other known risk factors such as cholesterol are low. The role of fibrinogen in the development of cardiovascular disease has been confirmed in several well controlled studies.

In 1996, Life Extension was the first research group to recognize the importance of fibrinogen as an independent risk indicator for cardiovascular disease. A new study in the *Journal of the American College of Cardiology* (1999, 33:1347–52) validates the LEF position on fibrinogen as an independent indicator and cause of heart attack, stroke, and cardiovascular disease risk. This published report examined data on nearly 400 male physicians participating in the Physicians' Health Study. Blood fibrinogen levels of 199 subjects who experienced heart attacks during the study period were compared with those of 199 control subjects who did not suffer heart attacks. The investigators report that patients with heart attacks had significantly higher fibrinogen levels compared with healthy controls. In fact, subjects with especially high fibrinogen levels had a risk of heart attack twice that of men with lower levels of fibrinogen. These findings remained unchanged regardless of the presence or absence of other coronary risk factors, including high cholesterol. The authors stated that these findings "support the conclusion from other prospective studies that fibrinogen is a strong and independent predictor for ischemic heart disease."

Further support of this proposition was reported in another 1999 study regarding the reduction of fibrinogen levels using a European drug called Bezafibrate. The study reported that a patient's baseline fibrinogen was associated with age, gender, behavioral lifestyle variables, lipid profile, and presence or severity of coronary heart disease. Furthermore, baseline fibrinogen emerged as an "independent predictor of cardiovascular events in patients with coronary artery disease." Additionally, in patients with high baseline fibrinogen levels, the reduction of fibrinogen was associated with a decrease in the incidence of primary endpoints, cardiac death, and ischemic strokes (*Blood Coagul. Fibrinolysis*, 1999 [Feb] 10 Suppl. 1: S41–3). (*Refer below for more information regarding the benefits of Bezafibrate in the reduction of fibrinogen and cardiovascular disease*).

Fibrinogen and Its Impact on Your Health

Fibrinogen is a blood protein that has a critical role in the normal and abnormal clot-formation process (coagulation) in the body. During coagulation, fibrinogen reacts with thrombin, releasing four small fibrinopeptides to produce fibrin, which in turn produces an insoluble fibrin network generally referred to as a scab.

Fibrinogen also participates in the cellular phase of coagulation, acting to promote platelet aggregation, which may lead to diminished blood flow and delivery of oxygen to the body. Fibrinogen can also cause blood platelets to bind together, initiating abnormal arterial blood clots.

Fibrinogen contributes to atherosclerotic disease in two ways. First, fibrinogen may initiate the development of plaque by combining with LDL cholesterol; second, it may then convert to fibrin and serve as a base for further LDL cholesterol buildup, contributing to or causing an atherosclerotic plaque buildup, which slowly occludes arteries.

Most heart attacks occur because a blood clot forms inside a coronary artery and strangles the blood supply to the heart. Most strokes, or brain attacks, occur because a blood clot forms inside a cerebral artery and reduces or blocks the blood supply to the brain. Since high levels of fibrinogen can cause abnormal arterial blood clotting and contribute to atherosclerosis, it is crucial to keep serum fibrinogen levels in a safe range (under 300 mg/dL).

Fibrinogen elevation in cigarette smokers, for example, has been identified as a primary mechanism causing heart disease and stroke. Cigarette smoking increases cardiovascular disease risk, and it also raises fibrinogen levels in the blood. Published studies documenting the dangers of cigarette smoking show those cigarette smokers who suffer from cardiovascular disease also have high fibrinogen levels. In fact, high fibrinogen levels may be a more powerful predictor of cardiovascular mortality than cigarette smoking itself.

Traditional Therapy

Anticoagulant Drug Therapy

Anticoagulant drugs work either to reduce fibrin formation or to inhibit abnormal platelet aggregation.

Warfarin (Coumadin) and heparin are commonly prescribed to reduce the risk of abnormal blood clotting. However, these drugs only address some of the factors that may precipitate coagulation. Too many people still suffer heart attack or stroke even though they properly took their medication. Prescription anticoagulation drugs fail to modulate all the mechanisms involved in causing blood clots to form inside blood vessels.

The goal of anticoagulant therapy is to administer the lowest possible dose of the anticoagulant to prevent clot formation or expansion, while minimizing the risk of bleeding. Warfarin is the most frequently prescribed oral anticoagulant, the fourth most prescribed cardiovascular agent, and the overall eleventh most prescribed drug in the United States.

Unfortunately, the antithrombotic effect of warfarin is not present until about the fifth day of drug therapy. While warfarin therapy is being initially administered, patients who require a rapid anticoagulation should also be given heparin. Heparin and warfarin therapies should overlap for approximately 4 to 5 days.

All these drugs are to be carefully monitored as they may easily be overdosed or cause adverse reactions.

CAUTION: Some of these reactions or secondary bleeding episodes may be worse than the blood clotting that the therapy is trying to prevent.

Depending upon FDA-approved prescription drugs to lower disease risk associated with high fibrinogen levels may cause problems. For example, the popular cholesterol-lowering drug Lopid (gemfibrozil) actually increases fibrinogen levels by 9 to 21%. Other FDA-approved heart medications have shown little effect on fibrinogen levels.

Integrated and Alternative Therapy

Some nonpharmacologic approaches of lowering fibrinogen include stopping smoking, avoiding obesity, lowering LDL cholesterol and homocysteine levels, and avoiding exposure to cold.

Low-dose aspirin and certain nutrients can provide partial protection against abnormal blood clots, but if you have high fibrinogen levels, additional measures should be taken to prevent heart attack and stroke.

Platelet-aggregation inhibitors reduce the risk of fibrinogen causing an abnormal blood clot. Some effective nonprescription platelet-aggregation inhibitors include low-dose aspirin, green tea, ginkgo biloba, garlic, and vitamin E.

High vitamin A and beta-carotene serum levels have been reported to reduce fibrinogen levels in humans. For example, animals fed a vitamin A–deficient diet have an impaired ability to break down fibrinogen, but when they are injected with vitamin A, they produce tissue plasminogen activators that break down fibrinogen. A study in the October 1997 *Diabetes Care Journal* indicates that no one antioxidant may be effective, and that total antioxidant capacity is important in reducing the risk associated with fibrinogen and cardiovascular disease.

Additionally, both fish and olive oil have been shown to lower fibrinogen in women with elevated fibrinogen levels. The minimum daily amount of fish oil required to produce a fibrinogen-lowering effect is 6 grams, which equals about five capsules of Mega EPA fish oil concentrate capsules. In more recent study results reported in the July 1997 issue of the *American Journal of Nutrition*, researchers at Louisiana State University in Baton Rouge indicated, based on two randomized, double-blind, placebo-controlled, parallel studies conducted in human subjects, that increasing the amount of fish oil consumed to 9 grams a day "decreased fibrinogen concentrations."

Therapeutic Effects of Vitamins

Elevated homocysteine levels have been shown to block the natural breakdown of fibrinogen by inhibiting the production of tissue plasminogen activators. Folic acid, trimethylglycine (TMG), and vitamins B_{12} and B_6 significantly reduce elevated homocysteine levels.

The therapeutic benefits of vitamins B_6 and B_{12} were discussed in a 1998 *Cardiovascular Reviews and Reports* (United States), reinforcing the use of these vitamins as part of an integrated therapy or disease prevention approach. Another study in 1998 based on data from 80 clinical and epidemiological studies that included more than 10,000 patients suggested that supplementation with B vitamins, in particular with folic acid, is an efficient, safe, and inexpensive means to reduce the elevated homocysteine levels implicated in cardiovascular risk and disease (*Annu. Rev. Med.* [United States], 1998).

Vitamin C has been studied and reported beneficial relative to the reduction of fibrinogen levels since the 1980s. In a report published in the journal *Atherosclerosis*, heart-disease patients were given either 1000 or 2000 mg a day of vitamin C to assess its effect on the breakdown of fibrinogen. At 1000 mg a day, there was no detectable change in fibrinolytic activity (fibrinogen breakdown) or cholesterol. At 2000 mg a day of vitamin C, however, there was a 27% decrease in the platelet-aggregation index, a 12% reduction in total cholesterol, and a 45% decrease in fibrinolytic activity.

Interestingly, researchers have found that exposure to cold increases fibrinogen levels by 23%, and mortality from heart attack and stroke is higher in winter than in summer. A study in 1997 reported in *Fibrinolysis and Proteolysis* (United Kingdom) indicated that increased winter cardiovascular mortality is related to a winter rise in concentrations of fibrinogen. Also, winter increases in infection markers and hemostatic blood factors appeared to be due to a winter decline in dietary vitamin C intake.

For additional fibrinogen-lowering effect, the proteolytic enzyme bromelain derived from the pineapple plant may also be effective for coagulation inhibition (*Planta Med.*, 1990 [June] 56 [3]: 249–53). For those seeking to lower elevated fibrinogen levels and inhibit coagulation, two to six capsules a day of Herbal Cardiovascular Formula containing a standardized bromelain concentrate should be considered.

Niacin

Low-dose niacin was reported effective in reducing plasma fibrinogen in a 1998 *American Journal of Cardiology* study that "demonstrated that niacin supplementation decreases plasma fibrinogen and low-density lipoprotein cholesterol in subjects with peripheral vascular disease." And they reported further, those changes in fibrinogen levels are highly correlated with changes in low-density lipoprotein cholesterol in subjects taking niacin (*Am. J. Cardiol.*, 1998 [Sept] 1; 8 [5]: 697–99, A9).

Another earlier study of niacin's effect in hypertriglyceridemic men has shown that long-term treatment with nicotinic acid not only corrects serum lipoprotein abnormalities, but also reduces the fibrinogen concentration in plasma and stimulates fibrinolysis (*Journal Cardiovascular Risk* [United States], 1997 [June] 4 [3]: 165–71).

Niacin (vitamin B_3) also improves cholesterol profiles when given in doses well above the vitamin requirement. Nicotinic acid lowers total cholesterol, LDL cholesterol, and triglyceride levels, while raising HDL cholesterol levels. Most people cannot use the high doses (1000 to 3000 mg a day) of niacin required to suppress cholesterol levels. However, if tolerated, niacin can be very effective. Niacin causes a flushing effect, resembling an acute allergic reaction, that many people find intolerable. While niacin is considered relatively safe, like cholesterol-lowering prescription drugs, it can cause liver toxicity when taken in high doses. Monitoring liver enzymes every 6 months is important when taking more than 1000 mg of niacin day. Those with hepatitis should avoid niacin to avoid complications.

Bezafibrate—A Choice in Europe

A European drug called Bezafibrate has been shown to lower fibrinogen levels by 25% in patients with fibrinogen levels between 300 and 415 mg/dL. In patients whose fibrinogen levels were more than 600, Bezafibrate lowered fibrinogen levels by 45%. Bezafibrate has been used extensively in Europe since 1978 to lower LDL cholesterol by 20 to 30%, and to increase beneficial HDL cholesterol. It has more than 9 million patient-years of safety documentation. In 1998, two studies reported that in 3122 patients with high cardiovascular risk, Bezafibrate and a placebo added to a hypolipemic (low fat) diet decreased plasma fibrinogen. "Bezafibrate lowered significantly the levels of triglycerides in these patients." (*Rev. Invest. Clin.*, 1998 [Nov–Dec] 50 [6]: 491–96) and (*Eur. Heart J.*, 1998 [July] 19 Suppl. H: H42–47).

The fact that Bezafibrate still is not approved by the FDA reflects a serious lack of concern on the part of our government about the health care of its citizens.

For those with cardiovascular vascular disease, please refer to the Atherosclerosis, Cholesterol Reduction, Hypertension, and Stroke protocols for additional suggestions and treatment information.

Summary

The following supplements offer synergistic benefits to assist in the reduction of fibrinogen levels (over 300 mg/dL) and the risk of cardiovascular disease:

1. Aspirin, 81 mg every day, with the heaviest meal of the day.
2. Vitamin B_6, 250 to 500 mg daily.
3. Vitamin C, 3000 to 5000 mg daily.

4. Vitamin E, 400 to 800 IU daily.
5. Folic acid, 800 mg with every meal. Use a folic acid supplement that also contains at least 1000 mg of vitamin B_{12}. Folic acid works synergistically with vitamin B_{12} to lower homocysteine levels.
6. Ginkgo biloba, 120 mg daily.
7. Green tea, 350 mg a day of green tea, 95% polyphenol extract.
8. Herbal Cardiovascular Formula (contains bromelain), two capsules, 2 times a day.
9. Mega EPA, 6 to 9 grams a day (six to eight Mega EPA capsules).
10. Niacin, 1500 to 3000 mg a day (if tolerable). Consider flush-free niacin (inositol hexanicotinate) to avoid a "red face."

For more information. Contact the National Heart, Lung, and Blood Institute (301) 251-1222.

Product availability. Healthprin (low-dose aspirin), green tea, ginkgo biloba, vitamin E, Mega EPA, folic acid, vitamin C, vitamin B_6, flush-free niacin, and Herbal Cardiovascular Formula are available by phoning (800) 544-4440, or order online at www.lef.org. Call for a list of offshore pharmacies if you are interested in obtaining the drug Bezafibrate.

FIBROMYALGIA

Fibromyalgia is an illness characterized by severe muscle pain, that is associated with poor sleep and often depression. It shares some of the features of chronic fatigue syndrome (CFS). Indeed, 70% of patients diagnosed with fibromyalgia meet all of the diagnostic criteria for CFS. The major difference between the two is the presence of musculoskeletal pain in fibromylagia. In medicine, a disease exists when an illness has very specific symptoms and physical exam and laboratory findings. An illness that cannot be as definitively defined and may mimic other conditions is called a syndrome. Fibromylagia (FMS) is such an illness.

Fibromyalgia is one of the more common problems seen in a general family medical practice. It is characterized by muscle pain, which may be generalized, and tender points, which are localized to known specific locations. Unlike arthritis, no inflammation is present and joints are not directly affected. The associated pain may cause aching or burning and is unpredictable in nature. In some people, the pain can be severe and disabling; in others there is only mild discomfort.

Although there is no known cause of fibromylagia, its onset may be related to physical or mental stress, inadequate sleep, injury, exposure to cold and dampness, infections, and occasionally rheumatoid arthritis. The condition seems to run in some families although no genetic component has yet been identified. Current thinking suggests that patients with the disease may have lower levels of serotonin, which explains the problem with sleep and an exacerbation of the response to pain. It may affect 4% of the general population.

The stiffness and pain associated with FMS usually appear gradually with worsening due to fatigue, physical straining, and overuse. The soft tissue and muscle of the neck, shoulders, chest and rib cage, lower back, and thighs are especially vulnerable. The diagnosis requires that all three major and four or more of the following minor criteria be present:

Major Criteria

1. Generalized aches or stiffness of at least three anatomical sites for at least 3 months
2. Six or more typical, reproducible tender points
3. Exclusion of other disorders that can cause similar symptoms

Minor Criteria

1. Generalized fatigue
2. Chronic headache
3. Sleep disturbance
4. Neurological and psychological complaints
5. Numbing or tingling sensations
6. Irritable bowel syndrome

7. Variation of symptoms in relation to activity, stress, and weather changes
8. Depression

The following is a more detailed list of potential symptoms that patients may experience:

Sleep disturbances. Sufferers may not feel refreshed, despite getting adequate amounts of sleep. They may also have difficulty falling asleep or staying asleep.

Stiffness. Body stiffness is present in most patients. Weather changes and remaining in one position for a long period of time contribute to the problem. Stiffness may also be present upon awakening.

Headaches and facial pain. Headaches may be caused by associated tenderness in the neck and shoulder area or soft tissue around the temporomandibular joint (TMJ).

Abdominal discomfort. Irritable bowel syndrome including such symptoms as digestive disturbances, abdominal pain and bloating, constipation, and diarrhea may be present.

Irritable bladder. An increase in urinary frequency and a greater urgency to urinate may be present.

Numbness or tingling. Known as parasthesia, symptoms include a prickling or burning sensation in the extremities.

Chest pain. Muscular pain at the point where the ribs meet the chest bone may occur.

Cognitive disorders. The symptoms of cognitive disorders may vary from day to day. They can include "spaciness," memory lapses, difficulty concentrating, word mix-ups when speaking or writing, and clumsiness.

Environmental Sensitivity. Sensitivities to light, noise, odors, and weather are often present, as are allergic reactions to a variety of substances (see below).

Disequilibrium. Difficulties in orientation may occur when standing, driving, or reading. Dizziness and balance problems may also be present.

Substantial overlap between chemical sensitivity, fibromyalgia, and chronic fatigue syndrome exists. The latter two conditions often involve chemical sensitivity and may even be the same disorder. Those agents associated with symptoms and suspected of causing onset of chemical sensitivity with chronic illness include gasoline, kerosene, natural gas, pesticides (especially chlordane and chlorpyrifos), solvents, new carpet and other renovation materials, adhesives/glues, fiberglass, carbonless copy paper, fabric softener, formaldehyde and glutaraldehyde, carpet shampoos and other cleaning agents, isocyanates, combustion products (poorly vented gas heaters, overheated batteries, etc.), and medications (dinitrochlorobenzene for warts, intranasally packed neosynephrine, prolonged antibiotics, and general anesthesia with petrochemicals, for example).

Multiple mechanisms of chemical injury that magnify response to exposures in chemically sensitive patients can include neurogenic inflammation, kindling and time-dependent neurologic sensitization, and autoimmune activation. The scientific literature suggests that there may be a marked correlation between the body's ability to effectively detoxify xenobiotic (foreign) substances and the presence of chronic disease processes such as fibromyalgia.

Epidemiological studies have shown that the tendency toward depression in patients with fibromyalgia may be a manifestation of a familial depressive spectrum disorder (alcoholism and/or depression in the family members) and not simply a "reactive" depression secondary to pain and other symptoms.

Diagnosis

There is currently no diagnostic or laboratory test to identify fibromylagia. A diagnosis is made by first ruling out other conditions that may mimic its symptoms such as thyroid disease, lupus, Lyme disease, and rheumatoid arthritis. A study of thyroid function showed that 63% of a group of FMS patients suffered from some degree of hypothyroidism. This percentage is much higher than for the general population. Fibromyalgia patients were shown either to suffer from a thyroid hormone

F

deficiency or from cellular resistance to thyroid hormone. (*Refer to the Thyroid Deficiency protocol for suggestions that could correct a thyroid hormone defect as a possible underlying cause of fibromyalgia.*)

The diagnosis is made based upon the patient's historical and physical findings. A history of generalized muscle pain and malaise coupled with the finding of the specific tender points is suggestive. The patient will often state that the symptoms developed after a viral infection. A history of poor sleep is also suggestive. It is important to consider other conditions including depression and chronic viral infection. It is the latter that overlaps with chronic fatigue. Sometimes treating the poor sleep resolves the condition, which would not be true for depression. On physical exam, in addition to tender points, the patient may have a particular type of skin and soft tissue consistency that may be best described as "doughy."

Both fibromylagia and CFS not only overlap, but describe a vague constellation of symptoms. That is why one of the major criteria is exclusion of other disorders that can cause similar symptoms. A truly thorough workup would include things that most conventional physicians do not look at, such as the yeast syndrome (*see the Candida protocol*), for example. A complementary physician, Dr. Ed McDonagh, has a very extensive protocol for the diagnosis and treatment of both fibromyalgia and CFS, which he groups together.

His workup includes dark-field (specialized) microscopy of the blood; routine blood chemistries; sedimentation rate for inflammation; antinuclear antibody test for lupus; antioxidant assay; intracellular mineral diagnostics for mineral status; comprehensive digestive stool analysis for digestion; DHEA level; ELISA-ACT for T-cell mediated allergy; hair analysis for minerals looking for heavy metals; amino acid analysis of urine; basal temperature for thyroid function (*see the Thyroid Deficiency protocol*), antibodies for candida; antibodies for Epstein Barr, CMV, Herpes, Chlamydia, and Heliobacter to look for chronic infection; and other testing as needed.

Drug Treatment

Treatment consists of managing the symptoms to the greatest possible extent. It may be necessary to try several approaches before a satisfactory regimen is found. Various medications and nutritional supplements that have been studied in clinical trials have provided pain relief and improved sleep quality in FMS patients.

One study found that 55% of FMS patients suffered from sleep disturbances, and that these sleep disturbances were not caused by pain. Alleviating insomnia with antidepressant medication, melatonin, and/or prescription sleep-inducing drugs could alleviate pain.

Antidepressant drugs have been used with varying degrees of success in treating fibromyalgia. Begin with a tricyclic antidepressant. If this does not work, a SSRI antidepressant such as Celexa (20 to 40 mg) replaces the tricyclic. Celexa has a much better side-effect profile than Prozac. Tryptophan is now available from some compounding pharmacies and may be taken by itself up to 3000 mg a day. If it is combined with either a tricyclic or SSRI antidepressant, the dosage must be reduced.

One European study showed that the combination of monoamine oxidase (MAO) inhibiting drugs such as Nardil or Parnate along with the nutrient 5-hydroxytryptophan significantly improved fibromyalgia syndrome, whereas other antidepressant treatments yielded poorer benefits. The doctors who conducted this study stated that a natural analgesic effect occurred when serotonin levels and norepinephrine receptors were enhanced in the brain. The monoamine oxidase inhibiting drugs did produce some side effects. European doctors combine 5-hydroxytryptophan with a decarboxylase inhibitor in order to make it available to produce serotonin in the brain. It is difficult for Americans to get 5-hydroxytryptophan with a pharmaceutical decarboxylase inhibitor. The vitamin B_6 Americans use also inhibits the ability of 5-hydroxytryptophan to enhance brain levels of serotonin. One of the reasons these agents work is by improving the quality of sleep, which is also mediated by serotonin.

CAUTION: Anyone who has been taking a tricyclic or SSRI antidepressant such as

Prozac or Celexa must wait at least 14 days (this is called wash out) prior to beginning an MAO inhibitor. Fatal reactions have occurred when MAO inhibitors have been mixed with these antidepressants. Additionally, patients taking MAO inhibitors must avoid certain foods and medications. Your doctor or pharmacist will give you a list of these items. It is also very important to boost magnesium levels by supplementation.

Natural Treatment

The European antidepressant drug *S*-adenosylmethionine (SAMe) has been shown in several published studies to be specifically effective as a therapy to reduce the chronic pain and depression associated with fibromyalgia. The suggested dose is 400 to 800 mg twice a day.

SAMe is currently sold as a dietary supplement in the United States.

Recently, in a study conducted on 12 fibromyalgia and chronic fatigue syndrome (CFS) patients, researchers found a vitamin B_{12} deficiency in all test subjects, which correlated positively with an increase in homocysteine levels found in their cerebrospinal fluid. They concluded that the elevated homocysteine levels are directly related to symptoms of fatigue found in both FMS and CFS patients.

In addition to drug and nutritional supplementation, certain approaches may help patients feel better and improve the quality of life: (1) physical therapy including massage, myofascial release, cranio-sacral therapy, mild electrical stimulation, the application of heat or cold, ultrasound, posture and movement training, and chiropractic treatment; (2) gentle exercise to ease sore muscles by increasing blood circulation and range of motion; (3) alternative approaches such as biofeedback, yoga, Tai chi, stress management, nutritional counseling, and acupuncture. (4) Swimming in a heated pool allows for greater mobility with greater ease than most other activities. (5) Massage properly done is also helpful. (6) Hot soaks with one half pound of Epsom salt added to the hot bath water are great for pain.

Acupuncture may be of variable benefit with its greatest impact upon treating painful muscle. In the experience of many complementary physicians, orthomolecular therapy with the intravenous administration of up to 50 mg of vitamin C 2 to 3 times a week for 4 to 24 weeks may be helpful. Some patients benefit from chelation therapy. Oral or intravenous NADH has also been found to be clinically useful. The ultraviolet irradiation of blood (UBI) has been found to be useful for some patients.

Dr. Ed McDonagh also considers natural hormone replacement, DHEA, immune enhancers such as thymus and rejuvenators such as cell therapy, medications to control yeast or other bacteria if present, allergy desensitization if indicated, thyroid replacement if necessary, and Heidelburg testing if gastric dysfunction is suspected.

A Pain-Suppressing Drug

For patients with persistent symptoms or those with severe symptoms at the outset, the author may prescribe the drug buprinorphine, a mild narcotic with agonist and antagonist properties that has a very low addiction liability, if any. Patients can use it for a long time without developing serious withdrawal symptoms when the drug is discontinued. The drug is virtually unknown among most physicians.

Of special interest, particularly since depression compounds and confounds FMS, buprinorphine is a very rapidly acting antidepressant that works when other antidepressants fail. In addition, it helps patients sleep, probably as a result of pain reduction. This makes buprinorphine particularly useful in FMS where pain, sleep abnormalities, and depression predominate the constellation of symptoms. The dosage is variable. The drug is commercially available only as an injectable .3 mg ampule, which is a small dose even for injection.

Since the drug is poorly absorbed orally, larger dosages must be used. When used orally, the liquid is withdrawn or shaken from the ampule and held under the tongue as long as possible. Compounding pharmacies can make up buprinorphine for sublingual use as a troche. Both forms, the ampules and the troches, are not inexpensive. For pain that prevents sleep, start with two to six ampules sublingually or .5 to 2 mg of a sublingual troche. For treating pain associated with depression throughout the day, begin with two to six ampules or .5 to 2 mg every 4 to 6 hours. As with most medications, begin with a low dose and increase until the smallest dose that proves effective is reached. *Do not worry about addiction.* (*See the Pain protocol for more information.*)

Duration of Symptoms

A study to ascertain the long-term natural history of fibromyalgia syndrome was conducted on a group of patients seen in an academic rheumatology referral practice. These patients were originally surveyed soon after onset of symptoms, and were again interviewed 10 years later. Of the original 39 patients, there were four deaths, and of the remaining 35 patients, 29 (83%) were re-interviewed. Mean age at the follow-up interview was 55 years, and mean duration of symptoms was 15.8 years. All patients had persistence of the same fibromyalgia symptoms, although almost half (48%) had not seen a doctor for them in the last year. Moderate to severe pain or stiffness was reported in 55% of patients; moderate to a great deal of sleep difficulty was noted in 48%; and moderate to extreme fatigue was noted in 59%.

These symptoms showed little change from earlier surveys. In 79% of the patients, medications still were being taken to control symptoms. Despite continuing symptoms, 66% of patients reported that symptoms were a little or a lot better than when first diagnosed. Fifty-five percent of patients said they felt well or very well in terms of symptoms, and only 7% felt they were doing poorly. With the exception of sleep trouble, which was persistent, baseline survey symptoms correlated poorly with symptoms at the 10-year follow-up. The conclusion was that fibromyalgia symptoms last, on average, at least 15 years after illness onset. However, most patients experience some improvement in symptoms after FMS onset.

Summary

1. Try addressing the sleep problem first.
2. *S*-adenosylemethionone (SAMe) 400 to 800 mg, twice a day (the most important single nutrient or drug therapy according to the published studies).
3. If 2 fails, add one of the tricyclic antidepressants (*see the Insomnia protocol*).
4. If 3 fails, consider combining 5-hydroxytryptophan with an SSRI antidepressant such as Celexa 20 to 40 mg.
5. Tryptophan up to 3000 mg a day may be substituted for the 5-hydroxytryptophan.
6. *Consult the Insomnia protocol.*
7. If the above suggestions fail, consider combining an MAO inhibitor such as Nardil, 15 to 75 mg a day, with 5-hydroxytryptophan, 20 to 100 mg a day. The MAO is taken in divided doses throughout the day and the 5-hydroxytryptophan is taken at night.

CAUTION: The dosing must be carefully supervised by a physician. Discontinue any tricyclic or SSRI antidepressant at least 14 days prior to beginning an MAO inhibitor. Fatal reactions have occurred when MAO inhibitors have been combined with certain antidepressants and drugs. Your physician or pharmacist will advise you of potential MAO food and drug interactions.

8. Magnesium supplementation with a good chelated product.
9. Gentle daily exercise, in particular, swimming.
10. Consider acupuncture.
11. Consider massage.
12. If homocysteine levels are increased, *refer to Homocysteine protocol.*
13. Nightly hot soaks in bathtub with one half pound of Epsom salt.
14. Consider orthomolecular therapy with intravenous vitamin C, 50 mg 2 to 3 times a week.
15. Consider ultraviolet blood irradiation.
16. Consider oral or intravenous NADH.

17. Consider DHEA. (*See the DHEA Replacement Therapy Protocol.*) Dosage is best titrated by blood or saliva testing in concert with a physician knowledgeable about DHEA.
18. Consider higher dose pregnenolone, 100 to 400 mg a day.
19. Consider buprinorphine, two to six ampules sublingually or sublingual troches .5 to 2 mg before bed for night pain and poor sleep.
20. Consider buprinorphine two to six ampules sublingually or sublingual troches .5 to 2 mg every 4 to 6 hours for daytime pain and depression.

Product availability. DHEA, magnesium, SAMe, and pregnenolone are available by calling (800) 544-4440, or order online at www.lef.org.

GINGIVITIS

Description

Gingivitis is an inflammation of the gums usually caused by plaque buildup that is the result of inadequate brushing and flossing, causing the gums to become inflamed, swollen, and to bleed easily. If it isn't treated, tooth loss can occur. Plaque, a soft, sticky film primarily made up of bacteria, will harden after 72 hours into tartar, which can't be removed by brushing or flossing. This is why the best defense against gingivitis is brushing and flossing after meals, as well as professional cleaning by a dental hygienist every 3 to 4 months depending upon the individual tendency to build up plaque. Plaque buildup occurs between the teeth and gums, in faulty fillings, and around the teeth near poorly cleaned partial dentures, bridges, and braces. Even though the main cause of gingivitis is plaque buildup, there are other causes for the disease. Birth control pills, cyclosporine (taken by people who have had organ transplants), and nifedipine (taken to control blood pressure and disturbances in the heart rhythms) are just a few of the medications that can cause gingivitis. Vitamin C and niacin deficiency can also result in gingivitis.

Treatment

If gingivitis is left untreated it can lead to periodontal disease, which affects the gum tissue, bone, and the supporting tissues of the teeth. The warning signs of the disease are a bad taste in the mouth, bad breath, red or swollen gums, tender gums, bleeding gums, loose teeth, sensitive teeth, pain when chewing, pus around teeth and gums, and brown, hard deposits, called calculus, on the surface of the teeth. The best treatment for gingivitis is prevention with good dental hygiene as described above.

It's best to start instilling good oral hygiene in a child as early as infancy. Before the teeth start to come in, the infant's gums should be thoroughly cleaned after each feeding with a water-soaked washcloth to stimulate the gum tissue and remove food. When the baby's teeth begin to come in, the teeth should be brushed gently with a small, soft-bristled toothbrush using a small amount of fluoridated toothpaste. At the age of 2 or 3, the child can be taught the proper brushing techniques. Because the child doesn't have the dexterity to do it alone, the parent should follow it up with brushing and gentle flossing until the age of 8. The child should start seeing a dentist about the age of 1 so the primary teeth can be checked for cavities and any other problems.

Studies show that adolescents should exercise proper oral hygiene care at home because three quarters of all 13- to 17-year-olds have gums that bleed. Teens should brush thoroughly after all meals and floss daily. Choosing a proper diet should help maintain and preserve their teeth. For those teens who wear braces, special attention should be paid to keeping the spaces between the teeth and archwires clean by using floss threaders.

Adults should practice good oral hygiene and see the dentist every 6 months because periodontal disease is the most common cause of tooth loss. These regular visits are usually painless and the dentist will be able to detect any periodontal disease an adult may have that's in the early stages.

Seniors can suffer from a wide range of problems, including root decay. Older people who suffer from arthritis should adapt their toothbrush for easy use, for instance, by enlarging the handle. This can be done by inserting the handle into a rubber ball, inserting it into a sponge hair curler, or gluing it into a bicycle grip. Studies confirm that electric toothbrushes are excellent at removing plaque and effective in stimulating the gums.

An Oral Spray for Gingivitis

Specific nutrients have been shown to prevent and alleviate gingivitis. Up until now, no one has put all of these nutrients into one topical form that could be effectively applied directly to the gums.

A pioneering physician, Dr. Jonathan Wright, and his associate, Dr. Donald Carter, have formulated a topical mouth spray that has produced significant results in those suffering from periodontal disease. Dr. Jonathan Wright gained national fame after his offices were ransacked by the FDA in 1993. Dr. Wright's political retaliation against the agency helped motivate Congress to pass the bill in 1994 that kept the FDA from turning dietary supplements into drugs. Drs. Wright and Carter have codeveloped a topical nutritional therapy for the prevention and treatment of periodontal diseases. The active ingredients in this oral spray are substantiated in peer-reviewed scientific studies. Many of the "inactive" ingredients have been successfully used by nutritionally oriented dentists to treat various gum diseases.

The Japanese have long used Coenzyme Q_{10} as a therapy to treat gingivitis, and some people apply the oil from CoQ_{10} soft gel capsules directly to the lining of their gums. CoQ_{10} reduces swelling, bleeding, pain, and helps promote the attachment of gum tissue to the bone. A special oil-based suspension has been developed for this oral spray that enables the CoQ_{10} to adhere to the gums.

If CoQ_{10} were the only ingredient in this oral spray, it would be a uniquely effective product. Drs. Wright and Carter have taken the extraordinary step of designing a formula that contains eight active ingredients that are documented to prevent and treat gum disease, plaque formation, and tooth decay. There are 21 additional ingredients that have been used in nutritional dentistry to prevent and treat a wide range of oral diseases. These ingredients are emulsified into a patented delivery system that guarantees stability and resultant action. A number of studies published in several well known journals and documented in *Life Extension Magazine* attest to the effectiveness of these active ingredients.

Folic acid has been clinically tested in mouthwash solutions to assess its benefit in treating gingivitis. One study showed that after 4 weeks of using a folic acid mouthwash, significant improvement occurred compared to placebo. In this controlled study involving 60 patients, dietary folic acid intake did not correlate with treatment results, suggesting the importance of applying folic acid topically to the gums (*Journal of Clinical Periodontology,* 1984 11:619–28).

In a double-blind study on 30 pregnant women, the effects of folic acid mouthwash, folic acid tablets, or placebo were evaluated. After 28 days, folate serum levels increased significantly in both groups receiving folic acid, but only the group receiving the folic acid mouthwash showed a highly significant improvement in a Gingival Index. There were no significant changes in the Plaque Index (*Journal of Clinical Periodontology,* 1982, 9[3]:275–80).

Thirty patients with normal blood folate levels were studied in a clinical setting. One group rinsed their mouths daily with a folate solution and the other used a placebo mouth rinse. After 60 days, the group receiving the folic acid rinse showed significant improvement in gingival health compared to the placebo group (*Journal of Oral Medicine,* 1978, 33[1]:20–22).

An experimental study on contraceptive users with normal plasma folate levels demonstrated improved gingival health after receiving supplementation with topical folic acid for 60 days (*Journal of Preventive Dentistry,* 1980, 6:221). A double-blind study was conducted on 30 patients comparing supplementation with 4000 mcg of ingested folic acid to placebo. After 1 month, based on plaque and gingival indices, folic acid supplementation appeared to increase the resistance of the gingiva to local irritants leading to a reduction in inflammation (*Journal of Periodontology,* 1976, 47[11]:667–68).

Green tea extract was shown to topically inhibit concentrations of *Streptococcus mutans* bacteria, which have been implicated in the development of dental caries (the decay and breaking down of teeth and their bone support). The scientists suggested that certain extracts from green tea might be especially helpful in preventing tooth decay by preventing the development of bacterial plaque (*Chem Pharm Bull-Japan*, Mar 1990, 38[3]). In a Chinese study, green tea extract was used to rinse and brush the teeth. The study demonstrated that *S. mutans* could be inhibited completely after contact with green tea extract for 5 minutes. There was no drug resistance after repeat cultures. The clinical effects showed that the Plaque Index and Gingival Index decreased significantly after green tea extract was used to rinse and brush the teeth. The scientists concluded that green tea extract is an effective agent to prevent dental caries (*Chiang Hsueh Tsa Chih* [*China*], Jul 1993, 28 [4]).

The name of this new oral spray is MistORAL. It contains a broad spectrum of nutrients that function by a variety of mechanisms to help prevent diseases of the mouth, including gingivitis and tooth decay. We have heard from consumers that gum bleeding stops just 4 days after using this new oral spray. Some people carry these 2-ounce bottles with them when dining out so that they can spray their mouths clean after each meal.

MistORAL contains the following impressive list of ingredients to support the health of the mouth:

Coenzyme Q_{10}. To promote the attachment of the tissue to the tooth and reduce gum bleeding. Considered the #1 therapy to treat periodontal disease.

Vitamin K_1. A specific bleeding gum therapy. Dr. Jonathan Wright uses vitamin K_1 as a major tooth preservative and gum support facilitator.

Propolis extract. A natural antibiotic to reduce gum inflammation.

Eucalyptol oil. An antiseptic gum stimulant.

Menthol. A cleanser and stimulant.

Folic acid. A specific antigingivitis therapy when applied topically according to five published studies.

Aloe vera extract. To sooth and heal sore inflamed gums.

Green tea. Neutralizes free radicals in the mouth and protects against infections.

Stevia/rebaudiana. The new herbal natural noncaloric sweetener.

Calcium ascorbate. Improves blood circulation and strengthens the walls of the blood vessels.

Citrus seed extract. A natural broad-spectrum antiinfective with important bioflavonoids.

Myrrh oil. Used as a mouthwash for 1000 years, antiinflammatory, antibacterial, relieves painful flare-ups. Tightens gums and prevents pyorrhea.

Gotu-Kola extract. Another natural antibiotic.

Echinacea extract. Antiinflammatory, anti-infective, and antiseptic.

Calendula extract. Heals inflammation and is a botanical antioxidant.

Chamomile extract. Eases sore teeth and gums, and is a mild antimicrobial.

Chaparral extract. Contains NGDA, which is a natural antibiotic.

Lemon grass extract. A detoxifying, natural astringent.

Vitamin E. Prevents free-radical damage to gums and mucus membranes caused by infection and abrasion.

Parsley extract. Freshens mouth.

Pau D'Arco extract. An antiinfective.

Spearmint oil. Cleanses and stimulates.

Peppermint oil. Cleanses and refreshes mouth.

Citric acid. Reforms detrimental periodontal exudation.

Goldenseal extract. Antiinfective agent.

Red thyme oil. Antimicrobial action, fights infection.

Tea tree oil. Powerful antiseptic.

Cool cayenne extract. Enhances circulation to gums and functions as an herbal catalyst (makes them work better).

Vitamin B_6. Works with vitamin K_1 to stop bleeding.

Zinc. Helps inhibit dental plaque formation and protects gums against numerous insults.

Many dentists recommend Coenzyme Q_{10} for periodontal and gum disease. MistORAL provides CoQ_{10} plus B vitamins such as folic acid to keep the gums healthy and vital; a broad-spectrum antibacterial combination to kill the bacteria that are the root cause of gum disease; specific nutrients to overcome inflammation; and vitamin K_1 to tame excessive bleeding, protect against decay, and facilitate healthy gum metabolism.

The best documented area of preventative medicine is modern dentistry. MistORAL adds a potent new weapon to the arsenal of oral hygiene therapies available to maintain healthy gum tissue. The suggested use is twice a day after brushing and carried on person when away from home.

Other Alternative Treatments

Proper oral hygiene is still required for the relief of gingivitis. Vitamin supplements, Coenzyme Q_{10}, and green tea can also alleviate the symptoms.

Grapefruit seed extract (GSE) can be used as an oral rinse (3 drops into a small glass of water and swishing vigorously in the mouth for 30 seconds or more) or on the toothbrush, with or without toothpaste. GSE can kill the bacteria that cause plaque and gingivitis.

The standard dose of Life Extension Mix (3 tablets, 3 times a day) can improve the health of your gums. Life Extension Mix provides more than 2500 mg of vitamin C. Also, Coenzyme Q_{10} in oil-filled capsules should be taken in 100- to 200-mg daily doses. Green tea beverages provide direct bacteria-killing, plaque-inhibiting effects for the gums. Standardized green tea capsules providing 200 mg a day of polyphenols can be used to help deliver gingiva-protecting nutrients.

For people suffering from chronic gingivitis, the regular use of Life Extension Mouthwash provides every nutrient shown to be of benefit topically for the health of your gums. One study showed that zinc and folic acid can inhibit gingivitis, and Life Extension Mouthwash contains the identical amount of zinc and folic acid used in this study. Life Extension Mouthwash also contains a chlorophyll extract, sanguinaria extract, vitamin E, aloe vera, and caprylic acid. All contribute to the health and healing of the gums via different mechanisms.

Of interest, the antiseizure medication dilantin, also called phenytoin, over long use can cause thickening of the gums. It was discovered that the reason for this is that phenytoin speeds up healing and cell proliferation. As a consequence people taking phenytoin who have even a mild amount of chronic gingivitis sometimes develop gum thickening. Therefore, phenytoin can be used short-term along with the other modalities to speed up healing.

Summary

Gingivitis is an inflammation of the gums in which the gums get red and swollen and bleed easily. Plaque buildup along the gum line of the teeth is the usual cause of gingivitis. Simple gingivitis can be prevented with the daily use of a toothbrush and dental floss, and with visits to the dentist every 3 to 6 months. If left untreated, gingivitis can cause periodontal disease and tooth loss.

1. MistORAL, twice a day after brushing and carried on person when away from home.
2. Grapefruit seed extract, 3 drops in water as an oral rinse.
3. Life Extension Mix, 3 tablets, 3 times a day.
4. Coenzyme Q_{10}, 100- to 200-mg daily doses.
5. Green tea to kill bacteria and inhibit plaque.
6. Life Extension Mouthwash for health and healing of the gums.
7. Consider phenytoin 100 mg 3 times a day.

For more information. Contact the American Dental Association, Dept. of Public Education and Information, 211 E. Chicago Ave., Chicago, IL 60611.

Product availability. Life Extension Mouthwash, MistORAL, Coenzyme Q_{10}, Life Extension Mix, and green tea capsules can be ordered by calling (800) 544-4440, or order online at www.lef.org.

GLAUCOMA

Glaucoma is a leading cause of blindness throughout the world, affecting over 60 million people. Glaucoma is an optic neuropathy in which the pressure within the eye becomes elevated due to blockage of the normal flow of fluid between the cornea and lens. In the course of the disease, axons of the optic nerve die and the plates of lamina cribosa collapse leading to deterioration of the optic-nerve tissue. When axonal deterioration progresses to a certain point, peripheral vision begins to decline, with central vision becoming affected much later.

Glaucoma may be classified as two main types: (1) primary, open-angle glaucoma (POAG) is the most common form in whites and blacks with incidence increasing with age; (2) angle-closure glaucoma is more widespread in the Far East, primarily China.

Primary Open-Angle Glaucoma

In POAG, intraocular pressure (IOP) rises slowly and painlessly, often going undetected until the later stages. Watery fluid known as aqueous humor constantly circulates through the anterior chamber of the eye, flowing between the iris and the lens. The trabecular meshwork, serving as a drain, is located in the angle where the iris and cornea meet. When the trabecular meshwork becomes clogged, the aqueous humor cannot drain, causing fluid to back up, which in turn causes pressure to build up within the eye. The fluid is forced out of the weakest part of the eye, the sclera, where the optic nerve leaves the eye. The extremely thin optic nerve cells become compressed, damaged, and eventually die. This results in permanent vision loss.

Symptoms of POAG are a progressive loss of peripheral vision, blurred vision, tearing watery eyes, and occasional headache. POAG is primarily a diagnosis of exclusion, indicating that upon examination, it cannot be identified as another specific disorder. Specialists often believe it is idiopathic in nature and there are various theories concerning the cause of elevated IOP. These include abnormal cell function in the trabecular meshwork, fewer cells in the trabecular meshwork due to aging, a structural defect in the eye's drainage system, or an enzymatic abnormality. Juvenile POAG presents by the age of 35 and is most often a familial disorder. Researchers have localized the gene in a number of families on the short arm of chromosome 1. This gene has been identified as producing a protein that affects the "stickiness" of the fluid pathways in the trabecular meshwork.

Angle-Closure Glaucoma

Angle-closure glaucoma has a familial tendency and is also more common in farsighted individuals. Individuals with angle-closure glaucoma have a narrower than normal angle in which the trabecular meshwork and iris are located. Upon aging, the lens grows larger and the ability of aqueous humor to pass between the iris and lens while flowing into the anterior chamber becomes decreased. This causes a fluid buildup and narrows the angle even more. When the space between the iris and the trabecular meshwork becomes completely blocked, an acute angle-closure glaucoma attack ensues. An acute attack will be characterized by severe, sudden eye pain, blurred vision, nausea, headaches, and rainbow-like halos around lights.

Treatment

Glaucoma must be diagnosed and treated early to prevent further degeneration of eyesight. Using a simple procedure called tonometry, an ophthalmologist or optometrist will measure fluid pressure in the anterior chamber of the eye. To reduce IOP, the amount of aqueous humor must be decreased or the outflow through the trabecular meshwork must be increased. Treatment usually begins conservatively with a long-term topical drug (eye drops) such as a beta-adrenergic antagonist. If needed, other treatments may be given either topically or systemically. These include prostaglandin analogs, adrenergic agonists, carbonic anhydrous inhibitors, and cholinergic agonists. Patients must be monitored closely for pulmonary and cardiac side effects. When drugs are no longer effective in keeping IOP under control or when new or worsening optic nerve damage occurs, treatment will be intensified. Laser surgery may be used if appropriate, to unblock clogged drainage channels or to surgically create a new pathway for the outflow of aqueous humor.

New Approaches to Understanding Glaucoma

New research in the field is leading specialists to consider nonpressure-related factors in the treatment of glaucoma. While IOP is the most important risk factor, other related conditions are being discovered as well. Researchers are studying a pigment dispersion syndrome in which the iris rubs against the zonules, which hold the lens in place, causing disruption of the pigmented cells in the back of the iris and releasing pigment, which clogs the trabecular meshwork. Uveitis, in which inflammation gradually kills off the trabecular cells, may also play a role. Further research on inflammation and the immune system is needed to treat the effects of uveitis.

Abnormal or insufficient blood flow to the optic nerve head and retina is also under investigation as a risk factor for glaucomatous damage. Other hemorheologic factors may include increased erythrocyte agglutinability, increased serum viscosity, and decreased erythrocyte deformability. Other possible risk factors include low blood pressure, abnormal (inherited or acquired) connective tissue of the lamina cribosa, low intracranial pressure, primary ganglion cell degeneration, and the effect of excitotoxins such as aspartate and glutamate.

A recent study reported in the *Proceedings of the National Academy of Sciences* that the drug aminoguanidine may help save the vision of patients with hard-to-treat glaucoma by inhibiting buildup of NOS-2. Researchers studied the effects of nitric oxide synthase 2 (NOS-2), an enzyme that appears to collect on the optic nerves of glaucoma patients. NOS-2 stimulates the emission of nitric oxide, a compound implicated in the retinal nerve damage associated with glaucoma. Researchers testing the effectiveness of aminoguanidine on rats with raised IOP over a 6-month period reported that no cupping of the optic disk occurred in those rats treated with aminoguanidine compared with rats left untreated. Intraocular pressure remained elevated throughout the study—whether animals received aminoguanidine or not. According to researchers: "That is important, because it means that lowering the pressure is not what protected the [retina]." Researchers concluded that this is an important finding for "those 'hard-to-treat' patients who do not respond to traditional therapies."

The Benefits of Nutritional Supplementation

Maintaining collagen integrity can play an important role in both treatment and prevention of glaucoma. Vitamin C is known to improve the condition of collagen structure throughout the body. In clinical studies, it has also reduced IOP levels in some patients who were unresponsive to standard glaucoma drugs. Dosage may be administered orally or intravenously and patients must be monitored to achieve optimal dosing benefits. Intravenous administration is the most effective means of reducing IOP, but must be done on a continued basis.

Bioflavonoids also aid collagen metabolism. These compounds have been shown to improve capillary integrity, prevent free-radical damage, and inhibit cross-linking with collagen fibers to form a more stable collagen matrix. European bilberry (*Vaccinium myrtillus*), an anthocyanoside, has been used in Europe for a variety of eye problems, with very good results. Rutin, a citrus bioflavonoid, has been used successfully as an adjunct to lower IOP. Subclinical hypothyroidism (*see Thyroid Deficiency protocol*) should be evaluated and treated if found to further lower intraocular pressure.

Ginkgo biloba extracts, standardized to 24% ginkgo flavonglysides, demonstrated some improvement in reducing IOP and improving visual field in glaucoma patients at dosages of 160 mg a day for 4 weeks and then 120 mg a day thereafter. Although only mild improvements were seen, the severity of the condition deemed the results relevant.

The effects of magnesium are similar to those of drugs used as "channel blockers" in the treatment of glaucoma. Channel blockers block the entry of calcium to produce relaxation of the arteries. Glaucoma patients given magnesium at a dose of 121.5 mg twice a day for 4 weeks showed improvement in blood supply and visual field due to the effects of relaxing constricted blood vessels.

Other dietary supplements shown to contribute to a reduction in IOP are chromium and omega-3 oils. Chromium aids in the ability of eye muscles to focus. In a study of 400 eye patients, deficiencies in either vitamin C or chromium were associated with elevated IOP. In animal studies, cod liver oil was shown to significantly reduce IOP when administered orally or intramuscularly. When removed from dosing, IOP levels returned to baseline.

The herbal extract forskolin lowers intraocular pressure by enhancing the energy cycles that are necessary to move aqueous humor into and out of the eye. It is suggested that you try the herbal extract forskolin at a dose of 10 to 60 mg a day. Check your blood pressure to make sure that forskolin is not causing low blood pressure.

CAUTION: If you have prostate cancer, do not use forskolin.

Hydergine also improves energy factors via the same mechanism as forskolin. A dose of 5 to 20 mg a day of Hydergine could be effective in lowering intraocular pressure. It is mandatory that you have regular intraocular pressure tests administered by an ophthalmologist if you are trying to use forskolin or Hydergine as a treatment for glaucoma.

Supplemental thiamine should be considered by the glaucoma patient as well. In two separate studies conducted in the U.S. and Russia, glaucomatous patients were found to have significantly lower thiamine levels than controls. Thiamine, in daily dosages of up to 20 mg, was administered both parenterally and orally with improvement of visual functions observed between days 2 and 6.

As stated earlier, aminoguanidine may help save the vision of patients with hard-to-treat glaucoma, according to the August 17, 1999 issue of the *Proceedings of the National Academy of Sciences* (1999; 96:9944–48). This study showed that only 10% of crucial vision cells in the retina were lost in a group of aminoguanidine-supplemented rats compared to a 36% loss of retinal cells in the group not receiving aminoguanidine. The study was funded by the National Eye Institute and the Glaucoma Foundation. Dr. Robert Ritch, chair of the Foundation's scientific advisory board, said, "Although the current investigations do not yet translate into clinical use, this [study] is the sort of breakthrough research that could eventually lead to a stemming of vision loss from glaucoma."

The recommended safe dose of aminoguanidine is 300 mg a day. Aminoguanidine is especially important for diabetics, who suffer from greatly accelerated glycosylation throughout their body. It appears that the glycosylation mechanism of damage is responsible for vision problems caused by cataracts and glaucoma.

Summary

1. Glaucoma requires prompt diagnosis and treatment because of the potential to lead to blindness.
2. Patients require continued follow-up.
3. Take aminoguanidine, 300 mg a day.
4. Consider Hydergine, 5 to 20 mg a day.
5. Take Life Extension Mix, a high-potency nutrient formula containing magnesium, thiamine, and other nutrients that may be of benefit.
6. Ginkgo biloba, 160 mg a day for 4 weeks and then 120 mg a day thereafter.
7. Chromium, 200 mcg/day, and omega-3 oils, 3000 to 7000 mg a day.

For more information. Contact the Glaucoma Research Foundation, (800) 826-6693.

Product availability. You can order thiamine, vitamin C, rutin, bilberry and ginkgo biloba extracts, magnesium, chromium, omega-3 oils, and forskolin by calling (800) 544-4440, or order online at www.lef.org. Call for a list of offshore suppliers who sell high-potency Hydergine tablets and aminoguanidine by mail order for personal use, or ask your physician to prescribe Hydergine for you.

HAIR LOSS

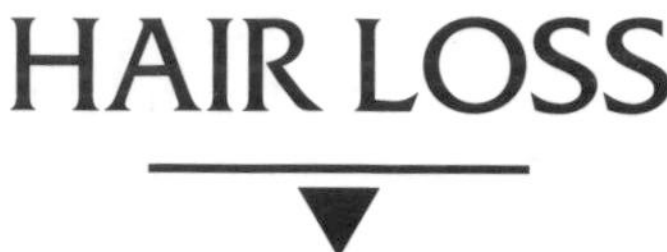

(See Baldness)

HEARING LOSS

Hearing loss affects about one third of all adults between the ages of 65 and 74. The percentage increases to 50% for adults ages 75 to 79. Hearing loss may result from dysfunction of any part of the auditory system. Causes of hearing loss include diseases, noise exposure, ototoxicity, tumors, and injury to the cochlear nerve and brain. The most common type of hearing loss in elderly persons is presbycusis, a term that describes hearing loss that is attributed to aging, with the specific cause being unknown.

Detecting Hearing Loss

Screening for hearing loss is the first step in determining the type and degree of hearing loss. Today's technology makes a hearing screening in a physician's office a quick procedure. In a matter of just seconds, a screening audiometer can identify patients who need to be referred to an otolaryngologist or audiologist for further examination.

Many elderly patients are reluctant to admit a loss of hearing due to embarrassment or fear. It is extremely important that adults over the age of 65 be screened regularly, however. A recent study of elderly patients has shown that untreated hearing loss increases psychosocial difficulties and reduces functional health. These physical and psychological problems might be easily avoided by treating the problem of hearing loss properly.

Treatment

Hearing aids. Amplification provided by a hearing aid is the best rehabilitative strategy for hearing loss that cannot be treated medically or surgically. Approximately 95% of hearing-impaired patients can be significantly helped through hearing aids, assistive listening devices, and/or rehabilitation. Hearing aids have evolved from cumbersome, highly visible devises to amazingly sophisticated and discreet minicomputers. There are more than 1000 models of hearing aids available. An audiologist or hearing-instrument specialist will help you select the hearing aid that is right for you based on your preferences and degree of hearing loss.

Cochlear implants. Surgery is the appropriate treatment for a minority of patients suffering from profound hearing loss. The cochlear implant is an option for those patients who derive no benefit from the most powerful hearing aid. Implantation of this device involves mastoid surgery and brief hospitalization. Cochlear implants are only recommended to a limited population of patients who would be totally deaf otherwise. For these patients, the implant can make a tremendous difference in hearing capacity.

Alternative Treatments

Alpha-lipoic acid. There is evidence that agents such as alpha-lipoic acid which reduce free-radical formation play an important role in reducing auditory toxicity caused by aminoglycosides, cisplatin, and noise. New studies show that the "universal" antioxidant alpha-lipoic acid lessens nerve damage induced by ototoxic aminoglycoside antibiotics. It has also been shown to protect against cisplatin auditory toxicity. Patients undergoing treatment with drugs that have aminoglycoside antibiotics. It has also been shown to protect against cisplatin auditory toxicity. Patients undergoing treatment with drugs that have ototoxic side effects may benefit from a dose of 250 mg twice a day of alpha-lipoic acid.

Hydergine. The drug Hydergine is considered to be an all-purpose "brain booster" and may help improve hearing. While the FDA has approved doses of only 3 mg a day of Hydergine, doses of 12 to 20 mg a day may be required to help improve hearing. Hydergine is nontoxic and relatively safe. Its potential side effects include mild nausea and some gastric disturbance. It is not recommended for people with psychosis, low blood pressure, or abnormally low heartbeat.

Hydergine was originally produced and distributed by Sandoz Pharmaceuticals. The original patent has since expired, and generic versions are now available in various strengths by prescription. Hydergine is available by prescription only in the United States; however, many people choose to obtain low-cost 5-mg Hydergine from overseas pharmacies.

Ginkgo biloba. Ginkgo biloba has helped some people with the hearing disorder tinnitus. Ginkgo provides a wide range of health benefits, including improving neurological function. Ginkgo biloba has also been shown to have a protective effect against cisplatin auditory toxicity. People with hearing loss should consider taking 120 mg per day of ginkgo extract.

Summary

Hearing loss is most common in adults over 65 years of age. In order to determine the degree of hearing loss and appropriate treatment, your physician will administer a hearing test and make the necessary referrals to an otolaryngologist or audiologist for further examination. Most patients experiencing hearing loss can be treated extremely effectively through use of a hearing aid. For others suffering more profound hearing loss, surgery involving cochlear implants may be an option. Alternative treatments may help in preventing age-related hearing loss and ototoxicity.

1. Hearing aids provide effective treatment for approximately 95% of patients.
2. Cochlear implants may be recommended for patients with profound deafness.
3. Alpha-lipoic acid, 250 mg 2 times a day, can reduce hearing loss from ototoxic drugs.
4. Hydergine, 12 to 20 mg a day, may help restore hearing.
5. People with hearing loss should consider taking 120 mg a day of ginkgo extract.

For more information. Contact the League for the Hard of Hearing, 71 West 23rd Street, New York, NY 10010-4162; (917) 305-7700; Fax: (917) 305-7888.

Product availability. Hydergine is a prescription drug in the United States. For a list of suppliers who sell low-cost, high-potency Hydergine from offshore pharmacies, phone (800) 544-4440. Alpha-lipoic acid and Ginkgo biloba extract are available from that number, or order online at www.lef.org.

HEART VALVE DEFECTS

(See Valvular Insufficiency/Heart Valve Defects)

HEMOCHROMATOSIS

Hemochromatosis is a genetic disease of abnormal iron metabolism. The person suffering from hemochromatosis absorbs too much iron from an ordinary diet. Consequently, this condition is sometimes called "iron overload" or "iron storage overload." If untreated, hemochromatosis can damage major organs in the body. Iron is a catalyst for the generation of free-radical activity that has been identified as an underlying cause of cancer, atherosclerosis, liver cirrhosis, neurologic disease, and other aging-related disorders. Approximately 32 million Americans are carriers for hemochromatosis, but approximately 1 out of every 200 people actually manifests the disease.

Symptoms and Diagnosis

Though hemochromatosis can, rarely, be acquired through massive doses of iron pills or supplements or through blood transfusions, the genetic form of the disease is far more common. Genetic hemochromatosis (GH), also known as hereditary hemochromatosis (HH), can be found through screening.

The following are symptoms of HH:

- Chronic fatigue
- Cirrhosis of the liver (with or without history of alcohol use)
- Liver cancer (with or without history of alcohol use)
- Arthritis or joint pain
- Impotence/low libido
- Sterility
- Early menopause/irregular menses
- Hair loss
- Diabetes, in particular "bronze diabetes," which is characterized by blue or gray skin tone
- Weight loss
- Cancer
- Abdominal pain/swelling
- Frequent colds and flu and other signs of weakened immune system
- Headaches
- Hypothyroidism
- Always feeling "cold"
- Heart irregularities/heart failure/heart attack (particularly in younger men)

Screening for HH involves multiple tests. It is also important to know that a person can be anemic and still have this iron overload condition. Hemochromatosis can be a "silent carrier" as well as a silent killer. "Low iron" cannot be relied upon to determine if someone is suffering from HH. The following tests, however, can help screen for HH:

- Total Iron Binding Capacity (TIBC)
- Serum Iron Test

In addition, the gene for hemochromatosis was discovered in the mid-1990s. A relatively new DNA test called HLA-H, or more commonly HFE or Hfe, is available. The patient's physician may also want to test liver enzymes, run an EKG, order a CT of the abdomen, and investigate the family history in order to confirm a diagnosis of the genetic disorder. A liver biopsy can also show exactly how much excessive iron the liver is storing. However, with the advent of the DNA test for HH, liver biopsies are not taken as frequently. A study published in the October issue of *Gastroenterology* examined 197 French HH patients with the C282Y homozygous gene. The aim of the study was to define noninvasive predictors of severe fibrosis (a complication involving bridging fibrosis or cirrhosis). Ultimately, simple biochemical and clinical variables such as serum aspartate aminotransferase, serum ferritin, and hepatomegaly were just as predictive as liver biopsies except for the diagnosis of severe fibrosis.

Conventional Treatments

Traditionally, the fastest and most efficient way to rid the body of excessive iron is through phlebotomy. Identical to donating blood at a blood bank, the person "gives" blood once or twice a week. If anemia is also present, however, drugs in the form of iron chelators may be prescribed. The number of phlebotomies necessary to "de-iron" the body varies, depending on the disease's severity at diagnosis. Phlebotomies are usually needed periodically throughout life as well.

In addition to phlebotomies, in conventional treatment the patient may be told to avoid alcohol, vitamin C with meals, cast-iron cookware, breakfast cereals containing 100% of the recommended daily allowance of iron, and raw shellfish. The person may also be told to drink coffee or tea with meals in order to help block iron in the foods eaten.

An Alternative Approach

Using Calcium to Block Iron Absorption

A practical way of lowering iron is to interfere with its absorption from food. *The American Journal of Clinical Nutrition* (1998; 68:3–4) stated that if 300 mg of calcium were taken with a meal, the amount of iron absorbed would be reduced by 40%. That's a simple and inexpensive way to reduce iron in the blood. In order to obtain 300 mg of calcium, it is necessary to take a calcium supplement that supplies 300 mg of *elemental* calcium. The best way of doing this is to take one to two 1000-mg capsules of calcium citrate with every meal that contains iron. Each 1000-mg calcium citrate capsule provides 220 mg of elemental calcium. Another calcium supplement called Bone Assure would provide 333 mg of elemental calcium (and other important minerals) per 2-capsule dose. According to the published studies, the maximum amount of calcium that will inhibit iron absorption is 300 mg with each meal. Amounts of calcium greater than 300 mg do not cause any additional interference with iron absorption. It is important to note that some people become tolerant to calcium-induced iron-absorption blockage after several months, so if calcium provides a sudden reduction in serum iron levels, make sure it continues to work by having regular blood tests. Soluble fibers such as psyllium seed husks (Metamucil), guar gum, and the pectins also help to block iron (and other mineral) absorption.

Tea Drinking

A recent study in the U.K. journal *Gut,* indicates that drinking black tea rich in tannin with meals can reduce iron absorption. The control group drank water with meals; the study group drank tea with meals. Intestinal iron absorption was measured by studying serum iron binding capacity and serum ferritin. Results showed a significant reduction in the study group as opposed to the control group. The goal then is to use the drinking of black tea to reduce phlebotomy frequency in the management of patients with hemochromatosis.

A potent iron-chelating agent is green tea extract. Green tea is an antioxidant that helps to remove excess iron from the liver. Hemochromatosis patients should take 4 to 10 green tea extract capsules with at least 250 mg of active polyphenols per capsule.

Diet

A Norwegian study examined the effects of diet on primary hemochromatosis. Health professionals as well as patients have indicated a strong desire to try to reduce the number of phlebotomies necessary per year through following a specialized diet. This study indicated the following items should be avoided:

- Ascorbic acid–rich fruit juice (particularly when taken with meals)
- Ascorbic acid–rich fruit (particularly when taken with meals)
- Alcohol
- Meat (quantities should be limited)
- Norwegian brown whey cheese (an iron-supplemented cheese common in the Norwegian diet)

Recommendations included following a diet rich in the following:

- Bread and cereals (non–iron fortified)
- Fruits (non–ascorbic acid varieties)
- Fresh vegetables

A recent Swedish study printed in the *European Journal of Clinical Nutrition* also recommended following a diet in which foods were not fortified with iron. Sweden formerly had the highest iron fortification of its food in the world. In January of 1995, the iron fortification program was withdrawn because of the uncertain effects and benefits of such fortification. Sixteen men with hemochromatosis were then studied as to the effects of the fortification withdrawal. The study indicated iron absorption was significantly reduced; these effects were measured through quantitative phlebotomy. The study further concluded that those persons suffering with hemochromatosis will have a slower rate of clinical disease progression when their food is not iron-fortified.

Vitamin Supplementation

Iron is a catalyst for many enzymatic reactions as well as for massive free-radical damage to cells. Because hemochromatosis patients suffer from chronic high iron levels, they are at risk for a host of free-radical-generated diseases, including cancer and heart disease. Therefore, it is crucial to inhibit these free radicals by consuming large amounts of antioxidants on a regular basis.

One problem that hemochromatosis patients must face is that the potent antioxidant vitamin C, when taken in the presence of iron-containing foods, can increase the absorption of iron from the digestive tract into the bloodstream. Therefore, hemochromatosis patients should take one 500-mg *buffered* vitamin C capsule 3 times per day between meals. Published findings demonstrate that in iron-overloaded plasma, vitamin C acts as a potent antioxidant against lipid peroxidation. Some doctors, on the other hand, suggest that hemochromatosis patients should avoid vitamin C altogether.

To combat liver damage, vitamin E is an important weapon. Vitamin E is a vital lipid-soluble antioxidant that has been shown to be decreased in patients with hereditary hemochromatosis and in experimental iron overload. Iron loading has been shown to significantly decrease hepatic and plasma vitamin E, which can be overcome by vitamin E supplementation. Free-radical index markers increase three- to fivefold in the iron-loaded livers, but supplementation with vitamin E has been shown to reduce these levels of free-radical activity by at least 50%.

It should be noted that copper overload induces similar free-radical-induced damage as does iron overload. Iron-overload disease causes severe depletion of liver glutathione. Glutathione is an important antioxidant, and its depletion in iron overload causes additional free-radical damage.

We therefore recommend that hemochromatosis patients take, in divided doses 2 or 3 times and day and with meals, the following:

- 400 IU of vitamin E
- 200 mcg of selenium
- A complete vitamin B complex
- 800 mcg of folic acid
- 30 mg of zinc
- 100 mg of grape seed skin extract
- 120 mg of ginkgo extract
- 800 to 1000 mg of garlic
- 250 mg of alpha-lipoic acid
- 300 IU of gamma-tocopherol
- 600 mg of *N*-acetyl-cysteine (NAC)
- 300 mg of elemental calcium
- 200 mg of elemental magnesium

In addition, patients should take 500 mcg to 3 mg of melatonin (this supplement should be taken at *bedtime only*).

Other Alternative Treatments

Hemochromatosis patients may also consider intravenous chelation therapy administered by a knowledgeable physician. In addition, the prescription drug deferoxamine has been shown to reverse both the biochemical indicators and the clinical manifestations of iron overload over a 2-year time period.

One interesting anti-aging and immune-boosting therapy involves administering one's own youthful blood during a state of disease or severe aging. If affordable, the Life Extension Foundation recommends that hemochromatosis patients have their blood frozen for future use.

Nutritionist Carmen Fusco has successfully helped patients with the most severe form of hemochromatosis. Her regimen includes tea with every meal for the tannins that bind iron, and extra calcium because calcium competes with iron and prevents some of its absorption.

If a glass of wine is desired once the liver improves, red wine with the tannins and chromium found in the grape skins is preferable to white wine.

Summary

1. Phlebotomy treatment is the fastest and most efficient conventional route to rid the body of excess iron. The goal of most patients is to

reduce the number of phlebotomies necessary per year or month.

2. Tannin-rich tea should be taken with every meal for its iron-reducing capabilities.
3. Patients should avoid alcohol, iron-fortified food, and ascorbic-rich food and drink.
4. Buffered vitamin C should be taken 3 times a day between meals.
5. Take in divided doses, 2 or 3 times a day and with meals, the following:
   - 400 IU of vitamin E
   - 200 mcg of selenium
   - A complete vitamin B complex
   - 800 mcg of folic acid
   - 30 mg of zinc
   - 100 mg of grape seed–skin extract
   - 120 mg of ginkgo extract
   - 800 to 1000 mg of garlic
   - 250 mg of alpha-lipoic acid
   - 300 IU of gamma-tocopherol
   - 600 mg of *N*-acetyl-cysteine (NAC)
6. Take the following to reduce iron absorption with each meal that contains iron:
   - 300 mg of elemental calcium.
   - 6 to 10 grams of soluble fiber (psyllium, guar gum, and/or a pectin fiber).
7. Melatonin, 500 mcg to 3 mg, taken nightly at bedtime.
8. Green tea extract capsules, 4 to 10 per day. These should provide at least 300 mg of active polyphenols per capsule.

For more information. Contact the Hemochromatosis Foundation, P.O. Box 8569, Albany, NY 12208, (518) 489-0972.

Product availability. Vitamin C, vitamin E, selenium, folic acid, zinc, grape seed–skin extract, *N*-acetyl-cysteine, garlic, ginkgo biloba, alpha-lipoic acid, vitamin B-complex, green tea, gamma-tocopherol, and melatonin can be ordered by calling (800) 544-4440, or order online at www.lef.org. Ask for a list of physicians in your area who are knowledgeable in the administration of chelation therapy.

HEPATITIS B

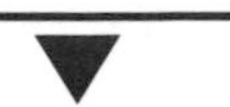

Hepatitis B is a potentially fatal liver disease and is 100 times more infectious than HIV. It can live on a dry surface for at least 7 days, making it one of the most communicable diseases and the ninth most common cause of death worldwide.

Hepatitis B (HBV) causes inflammation of the liver. This inflammation can cause liver cell damage, which can lead to liver cirrhosis and a significant increased risk of liver cancer.

According to the Centers for Disease Control and Prevention (CDC), there are approximately 1.25 million carriers of hepatitis B in the United States. There are up to 320,000 new hepatitis B infections reported in the United States every year. Seventy percent of new cases occur among people between the ages of 15 and 39. Hepatitis B is also a major cause of liver cirrhosis deaths in the United States. Additionally, 22,000 pregnant women in the United States are infected with HBV and can transmit it to their newborns.

Hepatitis B can be prevented. Hepatitis B vaccine provides immunity in more than 95% of young healthy adults. About 93% of adults who contract the disease will recover within 6 months and not contract HBV again. However, the blood tests of those individuals will always show that they have been infected with Hepatitis B virus, and blood banks will not accept their blood.

Approximately 5 to 10% of adults and 75 to 90% of children under the age of 5 who are infected with HBV are unable to clear the virus within 6 months and are considered to be chronically infected. These individuals are commonly called hepatitis B carriers.

Signs and Symptoms

Hepatitis B is most commonly spread by physical contact with contaminated blood as in the sharing of nonsterilized needles or by sexual relations. Symptoms of hepatitis B range from loss of appetite, weakness, body aches, nausea, vomiting, diarrhea, fever, hives, joint pains, yellowing of the skin and eyes (jaundice), and dark urine, to a "unique" distaste for tobacco. The latter symptom often characterizes a "full-blown" hepatitis infection.

Hepatitis can be a cause of liver cirrhosis. Cirrhosis slows the blood flow through the liver and causes greatly increased pressure in the portal vein that carries nutrients from the stomach and intestines to the liver. As a result, varicose veins may develop in the stomach and esophagus and, without warning, these large veins can break, causing a person to vomit blood or have black, tarry stools (bowel movements).

Drug Therapies

The FDA-approved treatment for HBV is the drug alpha-interferon. Less than 50% of patients with chronic hepatitis B are candidates for interferon therapy. Initially, 40% of HBV patients treated will respond; however, a number will relapse when the treatment is stopped. In the long term, approximately 30 to 35% of eligible patients will benefit. The treatment, given by injection for several months, may have a number of side effects including flu-like symptoms, headache, nausea, loss of appetite, diarrhea, fatigue, and thinning of hair. Some patients experience depression. The type and severity of side effects differ for each individual. Interferon may interfere with the production of white blood cells and platelets by depressing the bone marrow. Blood tests are needed to monitor blood cells, platelets, and liver enzymes. Some HBV patients with advanced cirrhosis might be considered for a liver transplant. Many new treatments are under investigation.

The malaise and aching associated with the treatments vary in severity among recipients and may be lessened by the *Immune Enhancement protocol,* antioxidant support, and favorable lifestyle. The drug ribavirin (800 to 1200 mg per day) may be considered in combination with alpha-interferon in view of its effectiveness against hepatitis C.

Isoprinosine has been used effectively in Europe against hepatitis B. The dose used is 2000 to 3000 mg per day for a period of 2 months followed by a rest period of 2 months followed by another 2 months of isoprinosine. Isoprinosine is not approved by the FDA, but can be ordered from offshore pharmacies.

Treatment by an infectious-disease specialist is essential. One third of all people infected by this virus can expect total remission after 2 to 4 months of treatment with alpha-interferon.

Benefits of Selenium

The protective role of selenium against hepatitis B viruses was reported in early January of 1997 in the *Journal Biological Trace Element Research.* The study reported that in areas of China with high rates of hepatitis B and primary liver cancer, high levels of dietary selenium reduce liver-cancer incidence and hepatitis B infection. In a 4-year trial on 130,471 Chinese, those who were given a selenium-spiked table salt showed a 35.1% reduction in primary liver cancer, compared with the group given salt without selenium. In the same journal report, another clinical study of 226 hepatitis B–positive people showed that a 200-mcg tablet a day of selenium reduced primary liver cancer incidence down to zero. Upon cessation of selenium supplementation, primary liver cancer incidences began to rise, indicating that viral hepatitis patients should take selenium on a continuous basis.

These human trials have been duplicated in animal studies showing that selenium supplementation reduced hepatitis B infection by 77.2% and precancerous liver lesions by 75.8%.

Another report in the *Journal of Trace Elements and Medical Biology* discussed the role of trace minerals for diseases such as liver disease and hepatitis. The report indicates that while there is still some debate regarding the specific role of trace minerals, minerals such as selenium and zinc are of benefit to those with diseases such as hepatitis *(J. Trace Elem. Med. Biol.,* 1997 [Nov.] 11 (3):158–61).

A 3-year study investigated whether supplementation of sodium selenite could prevent hepatitis B in a population of 20,847 persons in Jiangsu Province, China. The researchers concluded that *The incidence of virus hepatitis infection in the test population was significantly lower than that of controls provided with no selenium"*

(*Biol. Trace Elem. Res.*, 1989 [Apr–May] 20 (1–2): 15–22).

Based on these studies, those infected with hepatitis B should take at least 200 mcg of selenium every day. Optimal doses of selenium would range as high as 600 to 800 mcg a day. Selenium is a low-cost dietary supplement sold everywhere.

Nutritional Support

Antioxidants in amounts that do not place stress on the liver may be of benefit for hepatitis B patients. According to a report in the June 1998 issue of the *Gastroenterol. Clin. Journal,* investigators showed that nutritional antioxidants (which help neutralize the damage of oxidative stress) are potential therapeutic and preventive agents for diseases such as hepatitis. Other investigators reported at the same time that oxidative stress (free-radical damage) is often seen in hepatitis B and may contribute to the emergence of a hepatocellular carcinoma, a tumor seen in patients after years of chronic inflammation of the liver. They stated that antioxidants that down-regulate oxidative damage may be a useful complement to specific antiviral drugs in the therapy of viral diseases (*Biol. Trace Elem. Res.,* 1997 [Jan] 56 (1): 107–16).

In a related study, vitamin E was reported in a randomized, double-blind, placebo-controlled study to be a successful adjunct approach when combined with alpha-interferon therapy in the treatment of hepatitis due to its strong antioxidant activity (*Free Radic. Res.,* 1997 [Dec] 27 (6):599–605).

In Europe, the herb *Silybum marianum* (milk thistle) has been given German Commission E status as a supportive agent in the treatment of inflammatory liver diseases (hepatitis and cirrhosis). In Japan, *Glycyrrhiza glabra* (licorice root) has found widespread use in the treatment of hepatitis B. This herb has the ability to decrease serum liver enzymes, aspartate aminotransferase (AST), and alanine aminotransferase (ALT).

Precautionary Steps to Avoid Infecting Others

If you are diagnosed as a hepatitis B carrier, the following precautions will reduce the risk of transmitting the disease to others:

- Remind your doctor, dentist, or healthcare providers that you are an HBV carrier.
- All cuts and open sores should be covered with a bandage. Wipe up your blood spills. Then reclean the area with a solution of one part household bleach to ten parts water.
- Do not share toothbrushes, razors, needles, syringes, nail files, clippers, scissors, or any object which may come into contact with your blood or body fluids. Do not share food which has been in your mouth, and do not prechew food for babies.
- Do not donate blood, plasma, body organs, tissue, or sperm.
- If pregnant, tell your physician you are an HBV carrier. A child born to a carrier mother needs to receive the hepatitis B immunoglobulin and the first hepatitis vaccine injection within 12 hours of birth.
- Avoid or severely restrict alcohol intake. Your liver may be further damaged by alcohol, particularly if taken with acetaminophen, found in Tylenol or other cold and headache remedies.
- Be careful not to spread the HBV virus to others. Hepatitis B is transmitted by contact with infected blood, serum, semen, and vaginal fluids. Wash your hands with soap after touching your own blood or body fluids. Throw personal items such as tissues, menstrual pads, tampons, or bandages away in a plastic bag. HBV is not spread by sneezing, coughing, or casual contact.
- Tell sexual partners you have hepatitis B. Partners should be tested for HBV, and if they are not immune to the virus, they should receive the vaccination series of three shots. Until protection from HBV has been guaranteed, use a condom.

- People living in the same household as a carrier should see their doctor for hepatitis B testing and vaccination. If anyone is exposed to your blood or body fluids, hepatitis B immunoglobulin given within 2 days to 2 weeks can prevent the infection.

Blood Testing

Sometimes the signs of illness for hepatitis may be so minor that one may be unaware that an infection is in process. In some cases the only way to detect the presence of hepatitis B is via blood testing. These blood tests can be used to determine if you have hepatitis B or have been infected at one time. Blood testing can also reveal if the hepatitis B infection is progressing toward chronic hepatitis, or if you have developed an immunity to the disease.

Here is a summary of the various blood tests for hepatitis B and a brief description of what they indicate:

- Anti-HBs +: Shows that the individual has been vaccinated, has received immunoglobulin, is immune, or is an infant who has received antibodies from its mother.
- Anti-HBc +: Means past or present infection and lasts indefinitely; also may be detected in someone who has received immunoglobulin, or an infant who has received antibodies from its mother.
- IgM anti-HBc +: Indicates recent infection with HBV, usually within 4 to 6 months.
- HBeAg +: Indicates active viral replication and high infectivity.
- Anti-HBe +: Indicates decreasing infectivity.
- HBsAg +: Acute or chronic HBV; persistence for 6 months after acute infection indicates progression to chronic hepatitis B.

Source: Hepatitis Foundation 1999.

If the HBsAg (hepatitis B surface antigen) test is positive or reactive, this means you are infected with HBV and are infectious. If the anti-HBc or HBc-Ab (antibody to hepatitis B core antigen) test is positive, it means you are currently infected with HBV or have been infected some time in the past. If the anti-HBs (antibody to HBsAg) test is positive, it means that you are immune to hepatitis B either as a result of having had the disease or from having had hepatitis B vaccine.

Summary

In addition to conventional drug therapy, broad-spectrum antioxidant supplementation is recommended. A popular supplement used by Foundation members is the 67-ingredient Life Extension Mix formula in the dose of 3 tablespoons 3 times a day. Some hepatitis B patients cannot tolerate the beta-carotene, vitamin A, or niacin in Life Extension Mix, and this can be determined by blood tests that measure liver enzymes (ALT, AST, GGTP). Patients who cannot take Life Extension Mix may have to take individual supplements to provide optimal nutritional support. Additional herbal support with licorice and silymarin extracts can be obtained by taking 1 tablespoon early in the day of Life Extension Herbal Mix powder.

The best possible diet for the individual with hepatitis is a diet that features chemical-free (organic) foods. Strict attention to optimal bowel evacuation must also be carried out in order to avoid any unnecessary toxic bowel load upon the immune system and the liver. All alcohol should be avoided. As in the case with all liver disease, one must be certain that the body load of iron is not excessive because excessive iron, itself, is a liver toxin. Measurements of serum iron, total iron-binding capacity, percent saturation, complete blood count, blood ferritin, and sometimes bone marrow analysis for iron stores may be needed and should be discussed with your physician.

The following are important in the integrated treatment of hepatitis:

1. Selenium, 200 mcg, 2 to 3 times a day.
2. Milk thistle extract, 100 to 200 mg, 3 times a day.
3. Licorice root extract, 500 mg, 3 times a day (monitor blood pressure for any untoward increase).
4. Garlic, 4000 mg a day in divided doses.
5. Vitamin C, 5000 to 10,000 mg a day in divided doses.

6. Vitamin E, 400 to 800 IU should be taken daily.
7. Glutathione (reduced), 500 mg, and/or *N*-acetylcysteine (NAC), 600 mg, 3 times a day.
8. Whey protein, 30 grams, once a day.
9. Alpha-lipoic acid, 250 mg, 2 times a day.
10. Grape seed–skin extract, 100 mg, 2 or 3 times a day.
11. Green tea polyphenols, 600 to 800 mg early in the day, either from green tea extract capsules or from drinking 5 to 10 cups of green tea (some people cannot tolerate the caffeine in tea beverages and have to use decaffeinated green tea extract capsules).

(See the *Immune Enhancement protocol* from Life Extension for more information regarding the possible benefits of supplements and/or an integrated therapy treatment approach. Also see the *Hepatitis C protocol* for additional suggestions.)

For more information. Contact the American Liver Foundation, (800) 223-0179.

Product availability. Selenium, milk thistle extract, licorice root extract, kyolic garlic, vitamin C, vitamin E, glutathione, whey protein, alphalipoic acid, grape seed–skin extract, green tea, and Life Extension Mix and Herbal Mix can be ordered by phoning (800) 544-4440, or order online at www.lef.org. Call for a list of offshore companies that supply isoprinosine or ribavirin to Americans by mail for personal use. Interferon is a drug that must be prescribed, administered, and supervised by a physician experienced and knowledgeable in its use.

HEPATITIS C

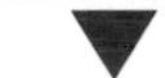

Ray C. Wunderlich, Jr., M.D.

According to the Centers for Disease Control (CDC), approximately 4 million Americans are infected with the hepatitis C virus. The CDC has estimated that 20 to 50% of infected hepatitis C patients will develop liver cirrhosis, and 20 to 30% of those will go on to develop liver cancer or liver failure requiring a liver transplant. Hepatitis C infection contributes to the deaths of 8000 to 10,000 Americans every year. This toll is expected to triple by the year 2010 and exceed the number of annual deaths due to AIDS, according to the CDC. There are also other nonliver diseases associated with hepatitis C viral infection.

Infection with the hepatitis C virus occurs from blood transfusions, needle sharing, working in a medical environment, and sexual contact. Often, the infected individual does not know how he or she acquired this potentially lethal virus that has a high affinity for liver cells.

Hepatitis C used to be called non-A/non-B hepatitis and was not considered a significant health risk. The growing awareness of this new viral epidemic has resulted in more research being conducted on hepatitis C than on any other cause of liver disease.

Diagnosis

People are diagnosed with hepatitis C when a blood test reveals a positive reading for the hepatitis C antibody. While the hepatitis C antibody test can diagnose whether one may have the disease, the blood test that identifies and measures the overall viral load is the *polymerase chain reaction test* (PCR). Standard tests to measure hepatitis C activity include the liver function tests SGOT, SGPT, GGTP, and alkaline phosphatase. Hepatitis C antibody tests can accurately diagnose hepatitis C infection, but they are not always precise in evaluating the success of treatments.

How Hepatitis C Damages the Liver

The hepatitis C virus does most of its damage by latching onto molecules of iron and delivering massive free-radical damage to liver cells. These free radicals can mutate cellular DNA to cause hepatocellular carcinoma, and they can kill large numbers of liver cells. Liver dysfunction wreaks havoc throughout the body. Successful eradication of the hepatitis C virus from the body requires that iron levels in the liver and blood be at very low levels, and thus it can be said that high stores of iron in the liver preclude successful therapy against the hepatitis C virus. It is mandatory to reduce iron levels in the body before initiating treatment with interferon-ribavirin combination therapy.

Hepatitis viruses have been shown to induce liver inflammation, cirrhosis, and primary liver cancer via free-radical attacks on liver cells. The ensuing liver dysfunction causes havoc throughout the body. Antioxidant supplements, in addition to antiviral therapies, are used by innovative physicians to protect against the liver-destroying free radicals generated by the hepatitis C virus.

In areas of China with high rates of hepatitis B and primary liver cancer, epidemiological surveys demonstrated that high levels of dietary selenium reduce liver-cancer incidence and hepatitis B infection. Animal studies showed that selenium supplementation reduced hepatitis B infection by 77.2% and precancerous liver lesions by 75.8%. In a 4-year trial on 130,471 Chinese, those who were given a selenium-spiked table salt showed a 35.1% reduction in primary liver cancer, compared with the group given salt without selenium added. A clinical study of 226 hepatitis B–positive people showed that one 200-mcg tablet a day of selenium reduced primary liver-cancer incidences down to zero. Upon cessation of selenium supplementation, primary liver cancer incidences began to rise, indicating that viral hepatitis patients should take selenium on a continuous basis. Selenium also appears to be effective in suppressing the hepatitis C virus.

In patients with hepatitis C, particularly those who are HIV-positive, a systemic depletion of glutathione is present, especially in the liver. This depletion may be a factor underlying the resistance to interferon therapy. This finding represents a biological basis for *N*-acetylcysteine (NAC) and glutathione supplements as adjuvant (assisting) therapies. Hepatitis C patients should also consider taking 30 to 60 grams a day of whey-protein isolate concentrate to boost liver glutathione levels to help protect liver cells against hepatitis C–induced free-radical liver damage. High-quality whey-protein supplements can also help to boost immune function. The fact that hepatitis C often becomes active in the body after age 40 indicates that age-associated immune decline plays an important role in the progression of the disease.

Conventional Therapy

The FDA-approved therapy to treat hepatitis is a 6-month regimen of injectable alpha-interferon. The standard treatment consists of 3 million IU injected subcutaneously 3 times a week for 6 months, always prescribed and supervised by an infectious-disease specialist. Even in patients who do not respond to interferon therapy by itself, inasmuch as there still is viral activity in the liver, there is a significant reduction in primary liver cancer. Many hepatitis C patients have refused interferon therapy because of its toxic side effects and low rate of response (20%), but the fact that a recent study showed that interferon therapy confers a 75% reduction in the risk of lethal primary liver cancer in hepatitis C patients warrants consideration of a 6-month therapy with interferon (combined with ribavirin).

About half of patients with chronic hepatitis C treated with interferon will not have a biochemical or virological response. In an attempt to improve that statistic, one study showed that the removal of a pint of blood every 2 weeks until iron deficiency was produced led to an improvement of 15% in the interferon treatment. Furthermore, elevation of storage iron in chronic hepatitis C has been associated with a poor response to interferon. Currently, however, the overall evidence shows that iron removal (via phlebotomy) lowers the transaminase blood tests but may not substantially improve responsiveness to alpha-interferon treatment. Nevertheless, iron reduction could delay the progression of liver injury to fibrosis and cirrhosis. Therefore, phlebotomy is usually recommended for even mildly iron-loaded patients with hepatitis C virus infection. (The production of anemia, whether by ribavirin or by phlebotomies, always must be considered a potential risk to patients struggling to obtain health.) Forty to fifty percent have an initial response to alpha-interferon treatment, but most relapse. Only 15 to 20% of patients with chronic hepatitis C have a sustained response to interferon therapy.

The Rationale for Using Ribavirin with Interferon

Hepatitis C patients exhibit, at best, only a 20% response to treatment with alpha-interferon. (Initially, 40 to 50% may have a response, but most relapse). When the antiviral drug ribavirin is combined with interferon, the response rate improves two- to tenfold. The standard regimen consists of 800 to 1200 mg a day of orally administered ribavirin taken in 3 divided doses for 6 months (200 to 400 mg, 3 times a day). At this time, however, the FDA says that ribavirin can be used only after a patient has already failed a 6-month regimen of alpha-interferon therapy. The FDA's concern about ribavirin stems from the appearance of anemia seen in 10% of treated patients. (The anemia disappears after cessation of ribavirin therapy but could have a deleterious effect upon already sick individuals.)

Ribavirin can be bought over-the-counter in many countries and has been safely used by millions of people for more than 10 years. The FDA insists, however, that ribavirin is a dangerous drug. The experience of the Life Extension Foundation indicates otherwise. Ribavirin is a broad-spectrum, antiviral drug that Foundation members have used safely since 1983 to suppress acute and chronic viral infections. There has been no report of the toxicity that the FDA warns about. Perhaps it is the simultaneous use of folic acid, vitamin B_{12}, and melatonin (along with the other nutrients) that have protected these individuals against anemia. Published studies show that folic acid and vitamin B_{12} are especially effective in treating anemia and that the hormone melatonin can protect against chemotherapy-induced anemia. It might be a good idea for those taking ribavirin to also take at least 500 mcg of melatonin at night in addition to the daily intake of folic acid (800–1600 mcg a day) and vitamin B_{12} (1000–3000 mcg a day).

There are numerous studies showing ribavirin to be a relatively safe agent. Both the FDA and Life Extension Foundation agree that all who take ribavirin should have blood testing done first and repeatedly thereafter at 2-week intervals while on the drug in order to detect anemia at an early stage (and to either treat it successfully or to withdraw the medication). Those who use ribavirin for less than 14 days to treat acute influenza (or just plain flu) have little reason to be concerned about anemia.

The published research shows that 10% of hepatitis patients taking ribavirin for 6 months will develop anemia. Anemia can pose a serious risk for those with coronary artery disease, pulmonary disease, or pre-existing blood disease. The FDA, however, mandates that hepatitis C patients first fail the brutal 6-month regimen of alpha-interferon therapy *before* being allowed to try ribavirin, even though interferon appears to be the more toxic agent. The brutal side effects of interferon treatment include aches, pains, malaise, gastrointestinal symptoms, and depression, which has led to suicidal behavior and actual suicides. These and other adverse reactions are contained in the standard warnings for the use of the drug.

Based upon the review of published studies about ribavirin toxicity, it is the Life Extension Foundation's position that the FDA exaggerates the potential adverse effects of ribavirin and denies this drug to hepatitis C patients for reasons that are not scientifically based. One example of ribavirin's lack of toxicity can be read in the conclusions of a study by French investigators who stated, "long-term administration of ribavirin is well tolerated and may be beneficial in controlling the progression of chronic hepatitis C." (Zoulin et al. in the *J. Viral Hepat.* [England], May 1998, 5 [3]:193–98).

If anemia is already present, ribavirin should not be used. Ribavirin use must also be avoided in a pregnant or lactating woman, as well as in a woman seeking to become pregnant and in a man seeking to impregnate a woman. Individuals with coronary artery disease, severe pulmonary disease, and kidney disorders should be closely monitored for ribavirin-induced anemia and kidney toxicity.

Using Interferon and Ribavirin Together

At the University of Florida, Gainesville, the effectiveness of interferon alone versus interferon and oral ribavirin was studied in patients with relapses of chronic hepatitis C (after standard interferon treatment). There were 172 patients who received interferon and placebo, while 173 patients received interferon and oral ribavirin, 1000 to 1200 mg a day (depending on body weight) for 6 months. At the end of the study, 82% of those treated with interferon *and* ribavirin had no detectable hepatitis C virus in their serum, compared to only 47% in the interferon-placebo group. The investigators concluded that in patients with chronic hepatitis C who relapse after treatment with interferon, therapy with interferon and oral ribavirin results in higher rates of sustained virological, biochemical, and histological response than treatment with interferon alone. The researchers' comments on the "toxicity" of ribavirin further support the view of the Life Extension Foundation: "Combined therapy caused a predictable fall in hemoglobin concentrations but otherwise had a safety profile similar to that of interferon alone." In other words, no toxicity except the known anemia effect of ribavirin was encountered. One strongly suspects that these medically managed patients, too, failed to receive the folic acid, vitamin B_{12}, and melatonin that, for the most part, has characterized those Foundation members who have used oral ribavirin to treat a variety of viral disorders since 1983 without a single report of the toxicity about which the FDA warns.

When interferon and ribavirin were used together for *initial* treatment of chronic hepatitis C, investigators, using similar criteria of response and similar doses to the previous study, found a 38% response rate with interferon and ribavirin versus a 13% response with interferon alone. The best response rate was obtained with 48 weeks (rather than 24 weeks) treatment duration.

The hepatitis C virus inflicts massive damage to liver cells, which often leads to cirrhosis and primary liver cancer. It is crucial for those infected with the hepatitis C virus to eliminate the virus from their bodies before it causes irreversible liver damage. Since interferon therapy *by itself* is only effective in 20% of cases, the FDA's ban on using combination interferon-ribavirin therapy sentences 80% of hepatitis C patients to treatment failure and severe liver damage.

The scientific literature supports the use of ribavirin *and* interferon as the primary treatment for most hepatitis C infections, yet the FDA chooses to ignore the science, thus condemning tens of thousands of hepatitis C patients to liver degeneration and death.

The Life Extension Foundation believes that the FDA's suppression of ribavirin provides a commonsense example of just how incompetent this agency is at evaluating scientific data. The Foundation has spent hundreds of thousands of dollars exposing the FDA's failure to approve of ribavirin because this issue provides blatant evidence of FDA fraud and incompetence.

Additional Ribavirin Studies

In a double-blind study published in the *Lancet* (1998, 351 [9096]:83–87), 100 patients were randomly assigned to treatment with interferon in combination with ribavirin or placebo for 24 weeks. The primary endpoint to the study was eradication of the hepatitis C virus. The findings of this study showed that 36% of patients in the interferon-and-ribavirin group experienced elimination of the virus from the blood compared with 18% of patients in the interferon-and-placebo group. The scientists concluded that the patients with high levels of the hepatitis C virus in their blood should be treated with interferon *and* ribavirin.

The *Lancet* study showed that the addition of ribavirin to interferon therapy doubled the number of hepatitis C patients who experienced eradication of the virus from their blood. This new *Lancet* report confirms previous studies showing a consistent 50% improvement in hepatitis C therapy when ribavirin is added to standard interferon therapy.

While the FDA has not approved ribavirin as the primary therapy to treat hepatitis C, your doctor can legally prescribe it to you. You probably won't get insurance reimbursement, however, since the FDA doesn't approve of ribavirin until after interferon therapy fails. The brand name for the FDA-approved ribavirin drug is Rebetol.

Most people use ribavirin by itself for short periods (2 to 10 days, 600 to 1200 mg a day) to knock out common flu viruses, or to treat lethal infections such as viral cardiomyopathy, Hanta virus, viral encephalitis, or influenza. There are over 2000 published studies that discuss ribavirin, and only 261 of these studies mention toxicity problems. Here are summaries of some of the published literature concerning ribavirin and toxicity:

> Long-term therapy in humans using combination ribavirin and interferon to treat hepatitis C enhances the therapeutic efficacy two- to threefold *without increasing the toxicity* (*Scandinavian Journal of Gastroenterology,* Supplement [Norway], 1997, 32 [223]:46–49).

> Treatment of measles patients with ribavirin resulted in shorter and less severe disease, as well as fewer complications, compared with patients in the placebo group. *Ribavirin was well tolerated. There were no side effects or changes in laboratory values that could be associated with drug-related toxicity* (*Clinical Therapeutics* [USA], 1981, 3 [5]:389–96).

> Ribavirin enhances the efficacy, but not the adverse effects, of interferon in chronic hepatitis C. A meta-analysis of individual patient data from European centers shows that the sustained response rate was significantly higher for the interferon-ribavirin combination therapy than for interferon or ribavirin mono-therapy. *No serious adverse events were observed.* The efficacy of interferon-ribavirin therapy appears to be enhanced two- to threefold over interferon mono-therapy in all major subgroups of chronic hepatitis C patients tested. *In view of its acceptable toxicity profile,* interferon-ribavirin combination therapy is a candidate for the new standard therapy for chronic hepatitis C (*Journal of Hepatology* [Denmark], 1997, 26 [5]:961–66).

The FDA wants hepatitis C patients to first fail interferon therapy before being allowed to use ribavirin and interferon, despite the above three studies showing little or no toxicity.

> The efficacy and toxicity of ribavirin (and of another antiviral drug called *ddl*) given for 6 weeks were investigated in the murine acquired immunodeficiency syndrome model. The results showed a *significant protection* against splenomegaly, lymphadenopathy, and hypergammaglobulinemia in mice treated with ribavirin by itself at the human equivalent dose of *1800 mg a day.* Ribavirin (and the other antiviral drug) *protected* against the loss of T cells in spleen and *restored the capacity* of splenocytes to proliferate after activation with a mitogenic agent. Moreover, the drug combination resulted in a *protection* of the spleen and cervical lymph node architectures and a regression of germinal centers. Toxicity to the blood appeared at a human equivalent dose of *9000 mg a day* of ribavirin (*Journal of Pharmacology and Experimental Therapeutics* [USA], 1996, 279 [2]:1009–17).

This study shows that *7 to 14 times more ribavirin* than what is administered to humans produces blood cell toxicity. Humans usually take 600 to 1200 mg a day of ribavirin.

> Ribavirin protects mice against the effects of retrovirus infection at doses of less than or equal to the human equivalent dose of 3,600 mg a day, but induces severe blood cell toxicity at doses less than or equal to the human equivalent dose of 7,200 mg a day (*Journal of Acquired Immune Deficiency Syndromes and Human Retrovirology* [USA], 1996, 12 [5]:451–61).

> The effects of testicular toxicity of ribavirin and its reversibility in mice were evaluated. At the human equivalent dose of 2,520 mg a day, there was mild testicular damage after six months. At the human equivalent dose of 5,400 to 10,800 mg a day there was significant testicular damage after six months. Upon cessation of treatment, *essentially total recovery* from ribavirin-induced testicular toxicity was apparent within one to two spermatogenesis cycles, which was consistent with *negligible effects* (*Toxic Substances Journal* [USA], 1994, 13 [3]:171–86).

The FDA uses this study to support its position that most hepatitis C patients should not receive 1200 mg a day of ribavirin.

> To evaluate the efficacy of oral ribavirin, 24 patients with chronic active hepatitis B were put on a course of treatment with 800 to 1000 mg a day ribavirin and/or interferon. Ribavirin, alone and in combination with interferon-beta, decreased hepatitis B virus levels in most patients to approximately half of baseline levels. Interferon alone exerted the most inhibitory effect on hepatitis B virus activity. Ribavirin was well tolerated, but the dose was transiently reduced in *two cases* because of mild anemia, although all patients completed the treatment schedule. *The combination of interferon and ribavirin did not appear to result in greater toxicity.* These results indicate that ribavirin suppresses hepatitis

B virus replication, although its effect is less than that of interferon, and that it may be useful as adjunctive therapy for chronic hepatitis B (*Hepatology* [USA], 1993, 18 [2]:258–63).

When developmental toxicity of ribavirin was examined, few if any developmental malformations were present that could be related with confidence to the drug. Several malformed fetuses were present in the highest dose level tested in rats (only 720 mg a day human equivalent) from days 6 through 15 of pregnancy. When evaluated for effects on reproduction and postnatal survival in rats, ribavirin at human equivalent doses of 4,320 to 6,480 mg a day produced statistically significant and/or clearly dose-related increased incidences of fetal resorptions, abnormalities, and reduced postnatal survival. Most significantly, pregnant baboons (most similar to humans) given ribavirin orally at human equivalency levels of 4,320 mg to 8,640 mg a day during critical periods of differentiation and organogenesis were reported to have produced *no adverse effects on in utero development* (*Journal of the American College of Toxicology* [USA], 1990, 9 [5]: 551–61).

CAUTION: Nevertheless, based on contradicting studies, pregnant women should avoid antiviral drugs.

The FDA says that ribavirin has produced embryonic damage in *all* "adequate" studies, but clearly there are studies showing that ribavirin does not always produce teratogenic effects.

Ribavirin was tested to determine its effects on the offspring of male rats. Human equivalent doses of 3,600 to 14,400 mg a day were administered for five days. Ribavirin was regarded as being *devoid of any mutagenic potential* demonstrable by a rat-dominant lethal assay (*Mutation Research* [Netherlands], 1987, 188 [1]:29–34).

CAUTION: Despite this positive study, humans involved in reproduction should avoid antiviral drugs such as ribavirin.

To assess safety, tolerance, and the clinical and laboratory effects of oral ribavirin in patients with AIDS, the AIDS and the AIDS-related complex (tests) were performed. Nine of ten patients with AIDS had a CD4 count of less than 100, and all patients with the AIDS-related complex had a CD4 count of less than 200. Oral ribavirin was administered in the high dose of 1200 mg twice daily for 3 days followed by 600 mg a day for up to one year. *Ribavirin treatment was well tolerated,* with anemia requiring transfusion in one of the ten patients with AIDS [who was] receiving the drug for 8 weeks; no other significant toxicity occurred. Six of nine patients initially positive for HIV-1 in blood became negative during ribavirin treatment. Six of nine patients with AIDS had a twofold improvement in lympho-proliferative response with ribavirin treatment. The conclusions were that 600 mg a day of *ribavirin was well tolerated and safe* in the patients with severe AIDS and the AIDS-related complex (*Annals Internal Medicine* [USA], 1987, 107 [5]:664–74).

HIV infection can itself induce anemia, so it is not surprising that 10% of patients required a transfusion. To reiterate, there are now more effective drugs than ribavirin approved by the FDA to treat HIV.

Based on a review of the published studies about ribavirin toxicity, it is clear that the FDA is grossly exaggerating the potential side effects of ribavirin and is denying this drug to hepatitis C victims for reasons that are not scientifically based.

Summary

Complementary Therapies

The Life Extension Foundation's protocol for hepatitis C includes

1. The standard dose of alpha-interferon (3 million IU injected subcutaneously 3 times a week for 6 months) prescribed by an infectious-disease physician. Interferon is the FDA-approved therapy for treatment of hepatitis C. However, it works only in a minority of patients when used without ribavirin.
2. 1000 to 1200 mg a day of ribavirin (taken in 3 doses) for 6 months. Ribavirin increases the effectiveness of interferon therapy by up to tenfold.
3. The standard doses of Life Extension Mix and Life Extension Herbal Mix. Please note that some hepatitis C patients encounter liver

enzyme elevations in response to the moderate doses of vitamin A, niacin, and beta-carotene in Life Extension Mix. If your liver-enzyme levels elevate after starting Life Extension Mix, discontinue it and take separately the other nutrients contained in Life Extension Mix. Beta-carotene possesses unique immune-enhancing benefits that could help suppress the hepatitis C virus, but some hepatitis C patients cannot tolerate it.

4. High doses of green tea polyphenols (300 to 900 mg/day and garlic (2000 to 4000 mg/day of a high-allicin garlic supplement) to reduce serum and liver iron levels to a minimum. Iron promotes hepatitis virus–induced liver injury and precludes successful treatment with interferon. Verify that liver iron levels have been reduced before starting interferon therapy. Some people must donate blood before going on interferon-ribavirin therapy in order to sufficiently reduce iron levels.
5. Liver-protecting nutrients and immune-boosting therapies such as 200 mg of milk thistle extract, twice a day; 500 mg of licorice extract, 3 times a day (monitor blood pressure to make sure licorice does not elevate it); 800 mcg a day of selenium; 1200 mg a day of *N*-acetylcysteine; and vitamin C ranging from 4000 to 10,000 mg a day.
6. *S*-adenosylmethionine (SAMe) for the purpose of protecting and restoring liver cell function destroyed by the hepatitis C virus. SAMe is in clinical trials in the United States for treating liver cirrhosis, and published research shows a significant benefit. The high cost of SAMe may preclude some hepatitis C patients from being able to afford it. The suggested dose of SAMe is 200 mg, 3 times a day to be taken with the methylation-enhancing agents trimethylglycine (TMG), in a dose of 1000 mg, twice a day; folic acid in the dose of 800 mcg, 3 times a day; and methyl cobalamine (a form of vitamin B_{12}) in the dose of 5 mg, twice a day (taken by sublingual administration).
7. Alpha-lipoic acid, 250 mg 2 times a day to boost glutathione levels in liver cells.
8. *L*-glutathione, 500 mg, 3 times a day.
9. Whey protein concentrate/isolate powder, 30 to 60 grams a day (to boost immune function and liver cell glutathione levels).
10. Grape-seed extract (85 to 95% proanthocyanidin) 100 mg, 2 to 3 times a day (to protect against free radicals in the liver).
11. Make sure serum iron levels are at the lowest possible tolerable levels (ideally below 60 mcg/dL of blood). As long as anemic symptoms do not appear, lower iron as much as possible, under physician's supervision (refer to *Hemochromatosis protocol* for iron-lowering suggestions).
12. Melatonin, 500 mcg to 6 mg at bedtime.

Folic acid and vitamin B_{12} may also protect against ribavirin-induced anemia, which occurs in 10% of hepatitis C patients being treated with ribavirin. If anemia does develop using ribavirin, discontinue ribavirin until blood cell counts return to normal, then resume ribavirin therapy. Refrain from alcohol consumption. The liver of a hepatitis C patient is especially vulnerable to the damaging effects of alcohol.

(*See the Life Extension Immune Enhancement protocol for additional suggestions.*)

For more information. Contact the American Liver Foundation, (800) 223-0179.

Product availability. Milk thistle, licorice, garlic capsules, selenium, alpha-lipoic acid, glutathione, whey powder, *N*-acetylcysteine, vitamin C, Life Extension Mix, Green Tea capsules (regular and decaffeinated) are available by calling (800) 544-4440, or order online at www.lef.org. Ask about availability of Ribavirin, which can be obtained from Mexican pharmacies and imported for personal use. A directory of offshore companies that ship ribavirin to Americans for personal use may also be obtained by writing the International Society for Free Choice, 9 Dubnoc Street, 64368, Tel Aviv, Israel.

HIV AND AIDS (ACQUIRED IMMUNE DEFICIENCY SYNDROME)

A controversy continues to exist in the scientific community as to whether the Human Immunodeficiency virus (HIV) is the sole agent responsible for the decline in immune function that is clinically defined as Acquired Immunodeficiency Syndrome (AIDS). In 1985, the Life Extension Foundation proposed that the decline in the immune function might be prevented or slowed down via the daily use of high-potency dietary supplements. Since 1985, several thousand medical papers have provided evidence that HIV-related immune-system destruction directly correlates with deficiencies of specific hormones, vitamins, minerals, and amino acids (*AIDS, 1997; Proc. Natl. Acad. Sci. USA*, 1997; *J. Nutr.*, 1994). In fact, it appears that the proper combination of hormones and nutrients may be a safe and highly effective method of restoring immune competence to those who are HIV positive, or who are in the early stages of displaying symptoms indicating that they are at risk for developing clinically defined AIDS (VIIIth Int. Conf. AIDS, 1992). When reviewing medical studies relating to AIDS and nutrition, it appears that HIV infection is a controllable disease if the appropriate steps are taken to protect against deficiencies of critical nutrients and hormones that the delicate immune system requires for optimal function (*Lancet,* 1989).

The Critical Importance of Glutathione

The HIV virus severely depletes the cells of an amino acid called glutathione. Numerous studies reveal that the lack of glutathione causes lymphocytes to become weak in their immunological "efficiency," thereby contributing to the immune cell impairment characteristic of AIDS (*FASEB J.,* 1997). The depletion of cellular glutathione also helps explain the decrease in protein synthesis that results in the catabolic (wasting) state that affects so many AIDS patients. Glutathione plays an important role in maintaining cellular integrity throughout the body, including the epithelial lining of the intestines. The intestinal impairment caused by glutathione deficiency often manifests as inflammatory bowel disease, a common problem in AIDS patients that prevents effective absorption of vital nutrients into the body (*Gut,* 1998).

Free radicals have been linked to much of the immune system destruction caused by HIV. The HIV-induced cellular depletion of glutathione is associated with free-radical injury to numerous immune-system components. A wide range of antioxidants have been shown to protect immune function, and nutrients that maintain cellular levels of glutathione are especially important in preventing or slowing the progression of HIV infection. T-helper lymphocytes require adequate levels of glutathione to function normally, and HIV induces oxidative stress that depletes T-helper cells of glutathione (*Res. Immunol.,* 1992).

Macrophages are another component of the immune system which relies on glutathione. The macrophages are very large immune cells that protect the body by swallowing and destroying foreign particles and cancer cells. The production of a substance called leukotriene C by macrophages is essential for them to reach invading organisms. When glutathione levels are low, the macrophages' production of leukotriene C is inhibited, resulting in diminished macrophage function.

It is now widely understood that AIDS is associated with a deficiency of glutathione that leads to the generation of enormous levels of oxidative stress that damage and kill otherwise-healthy cells throughout the body.

Substances That Boost Glutathione Levels

HIV-induced free-radical oxidation occurs in the presence of low levels of glutathione (*H. S. Biol. Chem.,* 1989). Free radicals impair and destroy immune cells, and scientific studies consistently show glutathione deficiency to be a critical factor in the pathogenesis of immune suppression (AIDS). This suggests that supplementation with nutrients to boost cellular glutathione is crucial to protect against a primary mechanism by which HIV destroys immune function.

The following glutathione-enhancing nutrients are recommended in their order of importance:

Nutrient	Dose
N-Acetylcysteine (NAC)[1]	600 mg, 3 times a day
Vitamin C	2000 mg, 3 times a day (take with NAC)
Selenium	200 mcg, 3 times a day
Alpha-lipoic acid	250 mg, 2 times a day
Whey protein isolate	30 to 60 grams of powder once a day
S-Adenosylmethionine (SAMe)[2]	400 to 800 mg a day
Glutathione[3]	500 mg, 2 times a day

[1] *N*-acetylcysteine is well-tolerated by most people, however some may be sensitive to it as it is a sulfur containing compound. It is recommended to consume vitamin C in a dose of 3 times the amount of cysteine to mitigate cysteine's oxidation to cystine. Vitamin C is included in the appropriate dose in the list suggested above. Please remember if your liver is in a weakened state, it may not be able to convert NAC to glutathione. Taking NAC under these conditions may further suppress lymphocyte functions. A solution may be to consume glutathione supplements directly even though they are poorly absorbed, and also to detoxify the liver under the guidance of a qualified health care practitioner. NAC can be resumed after liver toxicity has been resolved.

[2] Anyone taking SAMe should also take on a daily basis 800 mcg of folic acid, 500 mcg of vitamin B_{12}, and at least 100 mg of vitamin B_6 to protect against excess homocysteine accumulation in the blood.

[3] Controversy surrounds oral glutathione supplementation as some research has shown that this form of ingestion has not been efficacious, while other research contradicts this. Glutathione is strongly recommended for HIV patients who can afford this relatively expensive supplement.

Blood Tests

Regular blood tests are an essential part of an HIV treatment program. The chemistry profile includes iron, glucose, liver and kidney function, WBC, RBC, platelet count, and other important tests. These tests can detect blood changes that may indicate the presence of, or predisposition to, a wide range of abnormalities. They are a crucial source of information to assess the effects of drugs or nutrients which may be causing liver toxicity and kidney or heart muscle damage. These tests should be performed at least semi-annually. Specific tests could be repeated more often to monitor the efficacy of the current therapies you are using. Test information is a valuable component of the therapy decision-making process and should be utilized by all people with HIV undergoing prescription antiviral medication. The Foundation would like to remind you that correct test result interpretations depend on the knowledge and experience of trained clinical scientists. Therefore, it is recommended that you work closely with your primary care physician or qualified laboratory scientist when evaluating test results.

Immune Cell Subset Testing

In order to assess the effectiveness of immune-boosting therapies, a complete immune cell subset test should be performed monthly or bimonthly. This test will measure CD4 (T-helper) total count, CD4/CD8 (T-helper to T-suppressor) ratio, and NK (natural killer cell) activity. The CD4 test and the CD8 tests are important, but one should remember they are just counts—they are not measuring function, which is more important. High counts in these cells are desirable, but if they are not functional cells they are useless and would offer no immune system activity.

Cell-Mediated Immunity Tests

Helper T-cells, also known as CD4 or T4 cells, sound the emergency alarms and assist the cytotoxic T-cells in their action. T-cells determine cell-mediated responses to disease. Another test known as Multitest CMI measures CMI (Cell-Mediated Immunity). Sometimes this test is also called DTH, or Delayed Type Hypersensitivity-Type IV, and it is a direct indicator of antigen presentation. Antigen presentation is absolutely the first event that must take place before the immune system can mount an immune response. Cell-mediated immunity is then activated and is crucial to fighting viruses, fungi, yeast, bacteria, and parasites, especially those that reside within cells. CMI enables immune cells to patrol the body on a seek-and-destroy mission. The Multitest CMI is an excellent way to determine how a person's immune system is functioning. Multitest CMI is a skin patch with seven inactivated antigens which include tetanus, candida, diphtheria, proteus, and others along with glycerin, which is used as a control or neutral value. The patch pricks the skin surface, and a small amount of antigen enters. If a person was exposed to an antigen, there should be a strong reaction in the form of a welt, which can become red and itchy.

The formation of a welt is direct proof antigen presentation is taking place. Without antigen presentation, the CD4 helper cells can never become aware of the presence of an antigen and then inform other immune cells. The Multitest CMI is a direct measure of an immune response to an antigen. The degree of skin reaction to the test antigens is known as Delayed Cutaneous Hypersensitivity, or DCH. After 48 to 72 hours, the test is read by evaluating the presence and size of a welt if the person was previously exposed to an antigen. If no response (anergy) occurs on the Multitest CMI immune function test, in the case of a known re-exposure, this would indicate a high degree of immune dysfunction and/or suppression. Very minor responses (less than 2-mm size welts) are not desirable and would also indicate a very weak immune system. The larger the welt, the greater the strength of the immune system. As the size of the welts become larger, this correlates with stronger immune systems. Multitest CMI should be used every time blood tests are done to determine if immune function is improving or declining. It could inform you when and if changes to your protocol are necessary.

Natural Killer Function

Unlike other immune cells which must first obtain information from CD4 Helper cells, the Natural Killer (NK) cell can target and kill antigens both inside and outside of cells without conferencing with other immune cells. Acting on their own volition, NK cells can target and kill viruses, cancer cells, bacteria, and many other antigens. However, NK cell function can be impaired by the failure of some infected cells to present antigens on their cell surfaces which signal the NK cell. This disables the NK cell from "seeing" the infected cell directly, thereby diminishing its ability to destroy it. Multitest CMI is especially valuable in this situation when used with an NK Function test. A high NK Function score of 100 or more lytic units indicates the NK cells can see the infected cells and have the energy to destroy them. A high lytic unit value implies correct NK function, but coupled with a low Multitest CMI score, or anergy, would still indicate immune dysfunction since diminished antigen presentation will blind the NK cells from seeing all the infected cells which need to be destroyed.

In this way, both tests are used synergistically for a broader evaluation of immune function. Multitest CMI and NK Function tests may be considered the polygraph test for the efficacy of all AIDS treatment protocols. High CD4 counts and low PCR viral loads are used as immune markers, but they are not always indicators of actual immune function. High CD4 counts and low PCR viral loads without correct immune functioning will not protect you from PCP, CMV, TB, or other opportunistic infections (OI). Actual, measurable improvements of immune function may, even with low CD4 cells and high PCR viral loads, offer protection from OI.

DHEA Test and Treatment

Several significant studies have shown that HIV infection progresses when serum levels of the hormone DHEA begin to decline (*J. Infect. Dis.*, 1991, 1992; *AIDS Res. Hum. Retrovir.*, 1994). Many people with HIV have incorporated DHEA into their treatment program because maintaining healthy blood levels of DHEA might prevent immune degradation from progressing to general immune system collapse. Its beneficial mechanism of action may not be due to any direct antiviral effect, but rather to DHEA's ability to protect immune functions against a wide variety of insults.

The Foundation recommends that all people with HIV and most people over 40 have their DHEA blood level tested to determine their baseline level. DHEA supplementation should then be initiated and monitored to bring their serum level up to that of a healthy 21-year-old. An appropriate dosage for men is 25 mg, 2 to 3 times a day.

DHEA can possibly increase liver damage in people who already have hepatitis and cirrhosis. Before starting DHEA replacement therapy, please consult with your physician and refer to the DHEA-Pregnenolone Precautions in the *DHEA Replacement Therapy protocol.* After prudent medical counsel, if DHEA replacement therapy is still indicated in those with liver dysfunction, it can be taken in the following way: the DHEA powder capsule should be opened, and the powder poured under the tongue, remaining there for 10 to 20 minutes before being swallowed. In this fashion, much of the hormone enters directly into the blood-stream before reaching the liver.

TSH Test and Treatment

Proper levels of thyroid hormones are crucial for optimal immune function. Blood tests do not always accurately detect a thyroid hormone deficiency. One method of determining if thyroid deficiency is present would be to take your body temperature about 30 minutes before lunch. If your temperature is consistently below normal, you may want to take a thyroid hormone supplement. The TSH (thyroid stimulating hormone) test is extremely sensitive to both hypo- and hyperthyroid conditions, often showing even subclinical disorders. Popular prescription thyroid replacement drugs are Synthroid (synthetic thyroid hormone); Armour, Forest Pharmaceuticals (natural thyroid hormone); and Cytomel (T3 thyroid fraction). One must be careful not to overdose on thyroid hormone, as it has a fairly long half-life in the body. Thyroid hormone replacement therapy requires the supervision of a knowledgeable endocrinologist.

Cortisol Test and Treatment

There are many studies which show the correlation of elevated cortisol levels present in people with HIV (*J. Acq. Immune Defic. Syndr.,* 1992). Excessive cortisol production from the adrenal glands is immunosuppressive and usually closely correlates with autoimmune dysfunction. When cortisol levels remain high, the immune system persists in a Th-2 type response of the $CD4^+$ helper cells. Therefore, it is important to suppress excessive cortisol production. Testing cortisol levels in the blood is difficult because adrenal surges of cortisol can occur erratically throughout the day. Possibly for this reason, mainstream doctors have ignored this valuable tool in the treatment of HIV. However, a resting morning level of cortisol, taken before 9 a.m., may be quite significant in determining overall cortisol status in the body. The European procaine drug KH3 is believed to be the best way to block the effects of elevated cortisol levels in people with HIV and also in cancer patients. One or two tablets of KH3 can be taken first thing in the morning on an empty stomach, repeating the same dose an hour before dinner. Also, melatonin replacement therapy, vitamin C, and aspirin can lower elevated cortisol.

Antioxidant Therapy

Thousands of research studies have proven the positive effect antioxidants have in managing immune suppression. The Life Extension Foundation (in 1985) was the first organization to propose that decline in the immune function of people with HIV might be prevented or slowed down by taking high-potency antioxidant supplements. According to Marianna Baum, Ph.D., from the University of Miami Medical School, "multiple nutritional abnormalities occur relatively early in the course of HIV infection and appear to facilitate disease progression" (VIIIth Int. Conf. AIDS, 1992).

Most people with HIV use a high-potency multinutrient supplement such as Life Extension Mix that contains the nutrients most often deficient in those who are immune compromised. Upon a diagnosis of immune suppression, the Foundation recommends this aggressive comprehensive antioxidant "cocktail" that comprises high levels of nutrients to prevent the progression of immune suppression due to oxidative cell damage. People with HIV should consume 3 tablets of Life Extension Mix, 3 times a day with meals.

H

S-Adenosylmethionine

Apart from raising glutathione levels, a particular form of methionine known as *S*-adenosylmethionine (SAMe) serves as a methyl donor for a host of methylation reactions in the body. In this capacity, it may prevent and reverse liver disease as studies have shown it may be the most effective substance known to regenerate damaged liver tissue. This should be an important consideration, as it may offer great protection against hepatotoxic antiretroviral medications, even possibly reversing their damage (*Drugs [N.Z.],* 1989, 1990).

CoQ_{10}

A popular supplement used by HIV-positive patients is Coenzyme Q_{10}. Studies indicate that Coenzyme Q_{10} boosts immune function. In a pilot study in AIDS patients, Coenzyme Q_{10} provided significant benefits. Coenzyme Q_{10} has been shown to be deficient in HIV-infected people. It is suggested that HIV patients take at least 200 mg a day of Coenzyme Q_{10} (*Biochem. Biophys. Res. Commun.,* 1988, 1991, 1993; *Anal. Biochem.,* 1997).

Vitamin C

Vitamin C (ascorbic acid) is required for normal host defense and functions. An analysis of vitamin C uptake and its effects on virus production and cellular proliferation was performed. Exposure to high concentrations of vitamin C preferentially decreased the proliferation and survival of HIV-infected cells, and caused decreased viral production. This study showed high concentrations of vitamin C were preferentially toxic to HIV-infected host cell lines *in vitro* (*Am. J. Clin. Nutr.,* 1991). When plasma levels were measured for all antioxidant micronutrients in PWHIV (PW = People With) and in controls, it was observed that PWHIV showed a significant depletion of all carotenoids (lutein, lycopene, alpha-carotene, etc.) and vitamin C. The Life Extension Mix contains water-soluble ascorbic acid, an ascorbate complex, fat-soluble ascorbyl palmitate, and a natural vitamin C juice powder complete with synergistic bioflavonoids. It is considered the most comprehensive vitamin C complex ever developed in a nutrient product.

Beta-Carotene

Besides being very important to vitamin A production, the main function of the lipophilic antioxidant beta-carotene is to prevent damage to membrane and plasma polyunsaturated lipids (*AIDS,* 1993).

The rapidly proliferating cells of the immune system are very rich in polyunsaturated lipids. In a study in the January–April 1995 issue of the *Yale Journal of Biology and Medicine,* PWA (People With AIDS) were given 100,000 IU a day of beta-carotene. After 4 weeks of beta-carotene treatment, total lymphocyte counts rose by 66% and T-helper cells rose slightly. Six weeks after beta-carotene treatment, the immune-cell measurements returned to pretreatment levels.

While this study demonstrated no toxicity associated with high-dose beta-carotene supplementation, the Life Extension Foundation recommends against high-dose beta-carotene in PWA who also have hepatitis. For some people with hepatitis, long-term use of beta-carotene may cause liver enzyme elevation, indicating potential liver damage. Many PWA have also been infected with hepatitis B or C. PWA (People With AIDS) who do not have hepatitis or other liver damage should consider consuming 25,000 to 100,000 IU of beta-carotene daily. Healthy people seeking to boost overall immune function should consider consuming 25,000 IU of beta-carotene daily, along with other lipophilic antioxidants. The Life Extension Mix contains alpha- and beta-carotene along with an expensive natural carotenoid complex that appears to be more potent than synthetic beta-carotene in preventing disease.

Vitamin B_{12}

Vitamin B_{12} is essential to everyone for good health. Vitamin B_{12} is crucial to many enzymatic processes in the body and functions synergistically with folic acid and TMG to enhance DNA methylation and reduce toxic homocysteine in the blood. Vitamin B_{12}, together with folic acid, is very effective at increasing the oxygen-carrying capacity of red blood cells. This is of crucial importance to those taking most antiretroviral medications, as these drugs are notorious for destroying the rapidly-dividing red blood cells causing severe anemia. Vitamin B_{12} has been used by many PWHIV as a treatment for peripheral neuropathy caused by prescription medications. Severe neurological impairment can result, in the elderly as well, if vitamin B_{12} is deficient. Vitamin B_{12} exerts a regulatory influence on T-cells, may increase appetite, and contributes to an overall sense of well-being. Studies have shown PWA suffer from vitamin B_{12} deficiency as a result of severe malabsorption syndrome (*Eur. J. Hematol.* [Denmark], 1991; *AIDS Patient Care,* 1991). Using a sublingual form or nasal gel can circumvent this problem. Incorporating glutamine into your program can help to heal the intestinal tract and treat a malabsorption syndrome. The Foundation's latest, most advanced form of this essential nutrient is methylcobalamin, which research has shown may function better than conventional forms of vitamin B_{12} and is readily available by calling the Foundation. Three 500-mcg sublingual vitamin B_{12} tablets taken daily are recommended. If a blood test reveals a continuing vitamin B_{12} deficiency, weekly vitamin B_{12} injections may be indicated.

Pharmaceuticals

Naltrexone

In 1984, the FDA approved naltrexone (Revia) as a "narcotic antagonist," a treatment to keep heroin and other opiate addicts off addictive substances, and in 1995, the FDA approved it for the treatment of alcoholism. It has also been used in trials for treating obesity. Naltrexone works by temporarily blocking the opiate receptors, part of the endorphin system. As a treatment for addictions, it blocks the pleasurable effects of alcohol, eliminates the "high," and reduces the craving for more.

Naltrexone, however, has another very interesting effect: it increases the amount of endorphins in the brain. Endorphins are hormonal neurotransmitters and are immune modulators, which function as a major link in the communication between the brain and the immune system. Naltrexone increases the natural brain endorphin metenkephalin, which in turn enhances NK cell function and stimulates cytotoxic lymphocytes. Endorphins also serve as a natural "up-regulator" for the immune system, thus working as an immune enhancer. The up-regulation of endorphins is believed to reduce the abnormally high level of alpha-interferon found in persons with AIDS, which seems to interfere with the normal functioning of the immune system.

Dr. Bernard Bihari in New York City uses naltrexone in his practice for HIV treatment. He also employs antiviral medications as he believes they are of benefit in the management of HIV. We have already illustrated that HIV has never been proven to exist or to cause AIDS; notwithstanding, we strongly believe naltrexone has been proven to greatly improve the functioning of the immune system, and we wish to inform you of Dr. Bihari's great success with it. He has also used naltrexone to treat lymphoma, pancreatic cancer, and hepatitis C, leading to remission of these illnesses. Dr. Bihari has conducted clinical trials of naltrexone and other HIV/AIDS therapies, and articles about his work have been published in several gay magazines and newsletters (see the reference list for details on specific publications).

Naltrexone for HIV infection is taken in a very low dose (about 3 mg an evening), enough to sustain the up-regulation of the endorphin system, and it appears to have no negative side effects when taken at these low doses. In higher dosages, such as the dosages used in the treatment of alcoholism and the obesity trials, there were side effects. Some patients experienced nausea, difficulty sleeping, anxiety, nervousness, abdominal pain and cramps, vomiting, low energy, joint and muscle pain, and headaches. Incredibly, no negative side effects have been documented or reported for naltrexone when used as a treatment for HIV/AIDS. Dr. Bihari has led two studies in which 3-mg doses of naltrexone completely stopped the progression of AIDS and the decline of the immune system in 85% of patients who took it consistently. His patients had stable T4 counts for as long as 7 to 8 years. All of his patients using naltrexone had no opportunistic infections, and their levels of acid labile alpha-interferon declined. Naltrexone has no side effects, never causes resistance, and is currently available in the United States with a prescription. Dr. Bihari strongly suggests naltrexone at the top of the list of any protocol being considered by persons living with HIV. Naltrexone is an FDA-approved medication which must be dispensed from a pharmacy with a doctor's prescription. Call the Foundation for information about doctors who offer this therapy.

Isoprinosine and Diethyldithiocarboliate

Isoprinosine is a drug shown to be capable of slowing down the progression of AIDS, and since 1986, the Foundation recommended that PWHIV add this antiviral to their treatment program. Isoprinosine therapy can beneficially boost thymus gland activity. Isoprinosine is approved by every regulatory agency in the world except the Food and Drug Administration in the United States. A study published in the *New England Journal of Medicine* in 1990, is one of hundreds showing that isoprinosine can boost immune function in PWHIV, cancer patients, and even healthy people.

In 1985, the Foundation recommended PWHIV take isoprinosine to slow down the progression of immune suppression which can lead to full immune-system collapse. Isoprinosine and some other immune-boosting drugs work best when taken on an alternating dosing schedule, 2 months on and 2 months off.

Researchers in 1985 and in later years have shown how a reducing agent, diethyldithiocarboliate (Imuthiol), which has been used as an immunomodulator—and has also inhibited tumor production—could be useful to improve the immune response in PWHIV by preventing and treating AIDS (*Cancer Res.,* 1985; *Lancet,* 1985, 1988, 1990; *Life Sci.,* 1989; *JAMA*, 1991).

Biostim

A French drug, Biostim, was studied with regard to its effect on modulating varying immune responses. In response to staph infection, Biostim therapy significantly increased the critical phagocytic component of immune attack. Biostim also modulated synthesis of human polymorphonuclear granulocytes.

The immunological effect in aged humans was studied to understand which specific immune components were affected by oral administration of Biostim. The results showed significant restoration of cell-mediated immunity, an increased percentage of $CD3^+$, $CD2^+$, $CD4^+$, and $HNKI^+$ immune cells, and increased phagocytic activity.

Pre-incubation of immune cells with Biostim resulted in augmentation of natural microbicidal activity. Nonspecific activation of host defenses may have a significant impact on the outcome of infections in the immunocompromised patient. Biostim was shown to be effective in increasing resistance to experimental infections in animals. It also exhibited anticandida effects.

Alveolar macrophages are issued from circulating monocytes and stand at the front line defenses of the lung. The effectiveness of Biostim in respiratory infections is due to its action in deep lung cells and, in particular, alveolar macrophages. This drug has been shown to stimulate phagocytosis, increase enzymatic activities, and promote interleukin-1 secretion. These activities have been demonstrated *in vitro* as well as in animal and human subjects.

Biostim is an immunomodulator of organic origin acting on cells on the immune system (B-cells, T-cells, phagocytic cells) and on mediators (IL1-CSG). Its mode of action has been explored by means of experimental infections. The types of defenses involved differed according to whether the experimental infection was caused by an extracellular or intracellular microorganism. *Candida albicans* and *Saccharomyces cerevisiae* were used to produce fungal infections, while bacteria infections were produced with *Staph, E. coli, Strep,* pneumonia, and other organisms. The influenza virus was used to produce a viral infection. In these experimental models, Biostim increased the survival time of the infected animals and reduced bacterial, fungal, and viral proliferation. These effects were observed even in immunocompromised mice. These studies have demonstrated Biostim as an effective immune adjunct *in vitro* and *in vivo.*

People with HIV should consider using Biostim in 3-month dosing schedules as follows: 2 tablets daily for 8 days, then discontinue for 3 weeks; 1 tablet daily for 8 days, then discontinue for 3 weeks; 1 tablet daily for 8 days, then discontinue for 9 months.

Hormones

Melatonin

Melatonin is a hormone secreted by the pineal gland during sleep. It is considered a master hormone, as it is a neuroendocrine modulator and can exert a regulatory effect over many different areas in the body. Evidence suggests HIV immune suppression may be slowed by nightly intake of melatonin. Melatonin enhances the production of T-helper cells. It also stimulates the production of other immune system components, including NK cells; interleukin-2, -4, and -10; gamma-interferon; eosinophils; and red blood cells. In addition to enhancing different modalities of the immune system, melatonin is a formidable antioxidant in its own right and can prevent immune system cell loss directly through this mechanism.

Dr. George Maestroni, a pioneer in melatonin immunotherapy, conducted a pilot AIDS study in Italy wherein 11 PWHIV were given 20 mg of melatonin every night. After a month of treatment, the patients had a 35% increase in T-helper cells, a 57% increase in natural killer cells, and a 76% increase in lymphocyte production.

In spite of these remarkable findings, this line of research has not been pursued because melatonin cannot be patented and will consequently never generate enormous profits for the pharmaceutical giants. However, melatonin appears to benefit PWA in many other ways, including providing protection against AZT toxicity and wasting syndrome. The Foundation suggests that PWHIV read *Melatonin,* by Dr. Russell Reiter and Jo Robinson. It is a timely and valuable work of great benefit to all and especially to PWHIV. The Life Extension Foundation suggests using 3 to 30 mg nightly.

Growth Hormone

When HIV patients lose a significant amount of body weight, usually more than 10%, they may have AIDS wasting. Muscle mass in these individuals may constantly be broken down as an effect of dysfunctional metabolism. Instead of using nutrients from food and or body fat reserves for energy, the body uses the energy stored in lean muscle mass. Without medical intervention, this can progress to a life threatening condition. Recombinant DNA human growth hormone (somatotropin) can shift the body's metabolism from catabolic to anabolic and reverse weight loss.

Many insurance companies can underwrite the cost of this treatment. A stipulation of eligibility for this treatment is the concurrent use of antiretroviral medication. Information about using antiretroviral medications has been discussed in a previous section and may be useful when forming your decision. Remember, although you may be written a prescription for antiretroviral medications and verified as to taking possession of them, it is not tantamount to actually consuming them, as that is still, of course, your own personal decision. If you do not have insurance or the finances to pay for human growth hormone (HGH) therapy and you and your physician still feel you are a candidate for this treatment, please call NORD (National Organization of Rare Disorders), which can inform you of several drug manufacturers' Compassionate Care Programs.

NORD also has its own program in place. Call NORD at (888) 628-6673 for more information, eligibility requirements, and application materials. The Life Extension Foundation can also provide a list of doctors and clinics around the world who offer this promising therapy to those medically eligible, regardless of HIV status.

(*Refer to the Male Hormone Modulation Therapy protocol and the DHEA Replacement protocol for more information on the use of testosterone and DHEA.*)

Amino Acids

L-Glutamine

We have already discussed the medical causes of immune suppression that have been proven to create a malabsorption syndrome in the intestinal tract. Malabsorption syndrome is a component of the vicious cycle of immune suppression because it can be viewed as both a cause and an effect of immune suppression. Not being able to utilize ingested foods and nutrients can be one specific cause of malnutrition. At this point it is necessary to break the cycle of malabsorption, antioxidant

H

depletion, oxidative stress, immunosuppression, and more malabsorption. It can be helpful to remember that the majority of the immune system components and activity in the body is located in the intestinal tract. It has a predominant presence in the mucosal lining since that is the area of the body that must assimilate matter entering from the environment.

The amino acid glutamine plays a major role in the health and well-being of the gastrointestinal tract and its supportive organs (stomach, small and large intestine, liver, pancreas, and gall bladder). Glutamine is vital to the functioning of intestinal cells called enterocytes located in the finger-like projections of the mucosal villi. These cells which make up the mucosal lining of the small intestines are some of the most rapidly-dividing cells in the body and have higher energy requirements. Glutamine is the primary nutrient for enterocytes. The enterocyte cells break down glutamine to form glutamate, which is then converted to ATP and used as the cells' energy supply. Studies have confirmed that glucose sugar is simply not utilized as a fuel source for the intestine (*Metabolism,* 1998; *JPEN,* 1985, 1990; *Q. J. Eper. Physiol.,* 1985).

WARNING:

a. Glutamine supplementation in individuals with severe cirrhosis of the liver, Reye's syndrome, or any other metabolic disorder that can lead to an accumulation of ammonia in the blood is clearly not indicated and can present an increased risk for encephalopathy or coma. Under these conditions, the body is unable to metabolize excess nitrogen, which converts to ammonia and can cause brain swelling and brain death. When the liver is severely damaged or when hepatic coma is imminent, glutamine is not effective and can cause further brain damage.

b. Wasting is a life-threatening condition which should not be self-treated. If you involuntarily have lost more than 10% of your body weight, you should suspect wasting is taking place and seek the care of a knowledgeable physician. Bio Impedance Analysis can determine lean body mass and establish a baseline for you, against which future treatments' efficacy can be judged. In addition to glutamine, please review the information about Life Extension's Whey Isolate, which is extremely bioavailable and tissue-sparing. In addition to these treatments, your physician may wish to employ anabolic steroids such as testosterone and nandrolone and/or growth hormone. These treatments are very well grounded and medically prudent in cases of wasting and should be highly considered when necessary.

L-Carnitine

Another nutrient often overlooked by people with HIV is *L*-carnitine, which has been shown to boost immune function, via several different mechanisms, to protect the heart against AZT toxicity and to enhance essential fatty-acid and glucose uptake. Protease inhibitors can raise triglycerides. *L*-carnitine can be an appropriate treatment for this side effect. High doses of *L*-carnitine have also enhanced immunological and metabolic functions in people with HIV who were deficient in *L*-carnitine. The recommended dose is 3 to 4 grams daily in 2 divided doses on an empty stomach.

Additional Suggestions

Olive Leaf Extract

Olive leaf extract is a nonprescription, over-the-counter food supplement that has been used as a natural means to treat viral, bacterial, fungal, and parasitic infections, skin diseases, arthritis, heart disease, and many other illnesses. The ethnopharmacology of the olive tree enjoys a colorful historical past as it has been thought to be the tree referred to as the "Tree of Life" in the Book of Genesis. The ancient Egyptians may have been the first to employ the olive leaf as a tool in the mummification of their royalty. Hippocrates, the father of medicine, used olive oil to treat ulcers, cholera, and muscle pains over 2500 years ago. In later cultures, it was used as a popular folk remedy for the treatment of fevers. In the 1850s, the first formal medical documentation was done using olive leaves to treat severe cases of fever and malaria. In 1854, a healing remedy of olive leaves was published in the *Pharmaceutical Journal,* England's leading medical journal of the day. Italian researchers discovered olive leaf extract could lower blood pressure in animals. It was also confirmed that olive leaf extract increased blood flow to the coronary arteries, relieved arrhythmias, and treated intestinal muscle spasms. In addition, olive leaf extract is thought to have powerful antioxidant properties. Countless studies illustrate that antioxidant activity is crucial to the management of HIV disease.

Olive leaf extract contains a phenolic glucoside known as oleuropein, which has been shown to be the source of its extremely powerful disease-resistant properties (unpubl. study, 1994; *GMHC Treat. Issues,* 97 [98]; www.oliveleafextract.com; *Antimicrob. Agents Chemother.,* 1970; www.Biosyna.com/resch-1.html; *Nature [New Biol.],* 1972; *Olive Leaf Extract,* 1997). Olive leaf extract was tested by Upjohn Pharmaceuticals in the late 1960s and found to kill a large number of viruses. According to Jim Van Sweden of Upjohn, Dr. H. E. Renis was a prolific researcher of olive leaf extract, working in Upjohn's Department of Virology. His study "In Vitro Antiviral Activity of Calcium Elenolate," published in the peer review journal *Antimicrobial Agents and Chemotherapy,* revealed calcium elenolate's formidable antiviral activity, as it inactivated almost all the viruses tested against it.

Calcium elenolate is a chemical compound of oleuropein found in olive leaves. William Fredrickson, Ph.D., a researcher and CEO of F+S BioGenesis Group Inc., has also studied olive leaf extract extensively and believes the compound (+)-2-epienolic acid found in olive leaf extract is a natural reverse transcriptase inhibitor. He cites S. Z. Hirschman's study "Inactivation of DNA Polymerases of Murine Leukemia Viruses by Calcium Elenolate," published in *Nature (New Biology),* as documentation of olive leaf extract's reverse transcriptase mechanism of action. He also believes it is a natural protease inhibitor, and he has seen 100% protease inhibition activity *in vitro* while conducting a laboratory screen of oleuropein. There is no documentation, however, to support his observation. At this time, Fredrickson is conducting preliminary efforts for a clinical study to confirm (+)-2-epienolic acid's protease inhibition activity. As an alternative to the ingesting of toxic pharmaceutical protease inhibitors, in 1996 the PWA community discovered this believed natural source of protease inhibitors known as olive leaf extract. It has been shown to be nontoxic in all animal studies even when given in doses of 3 grams per kilogram of body weight. By functioning as a reverse transcriptase inhibitor and a believed protease inhibitor, it is selectively cytotoxic to virus-infected cells but has never shown any toxicity to human DNA alpha-, beta-, or gamma-polymerases.

Olive leaf extract has been taken by PWA in doses ranging from 1 capsule or tablet 4 times a day, to ½ cup of extract twice a day. If you wish to take more or less, please consult a Life Extension adviser or your health care professional. Make sure of the correct potency of the product. Olive leaf extract products sold by Life Extension will have the recommended 23% oleuropein content and be guaranteed fresh.

Olive leaf extract does not have any side effects per se, though some people may experience a "die-off" effect, also called the Herxheimer Reaction. A die-off effect is caused by a rapid increase in volume of waste material and pathogens being brought into the lymph system. Reactions to the die-off effect include extreme fatigue, diarrhea, headaches, muscle and joint achiness, and flu-like symptoms. These reactions are temporary and will pass once the body has expelled the circulating toxins. If these detoxifying symptoms are too uncomfortable, reduce the amount of olive leaf extract taken or discontinue use temporarily. Upon feeling better, resume the supplement at a lower amount and increase it to your desired dose slowly. A source of testimonials about olive leaf extract can be obtained from Mark Konlee, director of Keep Hope Alive, P.O. Box 27041, West Allis, Wisconsin 53227, (414) 548-4344.

SPV-30

SPV-30 is an herbal extract derived from the European boxwood tree (*Buxus sempervirens*), a species of evergreen. The proprietary extract is manufactured by Arkopharma, of Nice, France, the largest phytopharmaceutical company in Europe dedicated to natural herbal products. Research scientists have identified 20 active alkaloids in SPV-30 out of a total of nearly 100 using HPLC and gas chromatography. The five most active alkaloids are buxtaurine, cyclobuxine D, boxamine, cyclovirobuxine D, and cyclovirobuxine C.

SPV-30's potential as a natural antiretroviral was first identified by Jacques Durant, M.D., head of the Infectious Diseases Department of the Hospital de l'Archet in Nice. He learned of it from a PWA who took SPV-30 and was able to maintain high CD4 levels over a sustained period of time despite her episodic intravenous drug abuse and bouts of opportunistic infections.

In a double-blind, placebo-controlled Phase I trial in France, patients taking SPV-30 had an average increase of 94 CD4 cells after 30 weeks. The placebo group saw an average loss of 43 CD4 cells after 30 weeks. No toxicities were noted and no serious side effects were reported. These results encouraged Professor Luc Montagnier, co-discoverer of the HIV virus and one of the world's leading AIDS researchers, to act as scientific advisor and chief virologist for an 18-month multicenter, Phase II/Phase III study in France. The French Ministry of Health had classified the study as an antiretroviral trial. Of the 22 trials listed in the Ministry of Health's 1995 Clinical Trials Directory, SPV-30 is the only natural herbal product listed in an antiretroviral trial. An American study was also performed using SPV-30 in 1996. The current evidence suggests SPV-30 is working primarily as an antiretroviral, as well as an antioxidant, which favorably alters overexpressed cellular transcription factors (*Int. J. Phytother. Phytopharmacol.*, 1998). SPV-30 inhibits HIV by targeting the reverse transcriptase enzyme, the same enzyme that AZT and other nucleoside agents target. There is evidence SPV-30 reduces a cellular messenger, tumor necrosis factor alpha, which becomes elevated in PWHIV. Many studies have shown that this elevation, associated with an inflammatory response, correlates with increased viral replication and cell loss.

One of the more remarkable results of the SPV-30 was the noticeable quality-of-life improvement in many of the participants. They were asked to comment on many factors affecting them, such as energy levels, ability to fall asleep, appetite, digestion, and overall sense of well-being. Nearly half of the participants reported "much improved" energy, and 98.2% of the participants believed their energy levels were either much improved or about the same. About 45% reported their overall sense of well-being had greatly improved also. We think these findings are significant enough to warrant investigation by PWHIV, as so much of the taken-for-granted components of a person's quality of life begin to slowly erode after an HIV diagnosis.

AIDS Buyers Clubs around the country have anecdotally reported on a specific SPV-30 treatment regime that has produced the most beneficial results and is included here:

Upon rising, on an empty stomach, take 5 to 500 mg bitter melon capsules with 2 large glasses of water. Wait 30 minutes before eating.

Consume the following 3 times daily, with or without meals, and with 1 large glass of water:

- ▼ Glycyrrhizinate Forte (licorice)—300 mg, Jarrow Formulas (Note: This product can elevate blood pressure.)
- ▼ 1-SPV-30 (boxwood extract)—330 mg, Arkopharma

Consume the following at the end of the evening, 2 hours after eating:

- ▼ Bitter melon capsules—5 to 500 mg, with 1 large glass of water

Thymic Immune Factors

Thymic Immune Factors is a synergistic formula that contains herbal activators and a full complement of homeopathic nutrients in addition to fresh, healthy thymus, lymph, and spleen tissues, which produce white blood cells to fight invading organisms and cancer cells. The immunological tissue extracts in this product are raw, concentrated, toxin-free, and freeze-dried to preserve their biological activity. People with HIV may consider using a unique product such as Thymic Immune

Factors to potentiate white blood-cell production and activity.

Silymarin

Milk thistle extract, or silymarin, is a unique type of bioflavonoid that exerts a protective effect on the liver. This is of importance to PWHIV because they may be ingesting hepatotoxic antiviral medications, and also because silymarin supports the liver's activities, one being the production of glutathione, which is extremely crucial in correcting immune system functioning. Silymarin is only one of several products the Foundation offers that promote healthy liver function. Please refer to the glutathione information in the antioxidants section of this protocol for more information concerning products which promote healthy liver function.

Enzymes

Proper digestion of nutrients is necessary for maintaining good health in all of us. PWHIV and PWA have an elevated necessity for life-sustaining nutrients. In many cases, even the consumption of all the correct nutrients for these individuals simply does not produce nourishment because of malabsorption. A comprehensive digestive-enzymes formula should be used to offer the greatest possible digestive activity. Some digestive-enzymes are also used by the body to dissolve tumors, which can also be of consideration to those who are immunocompromised. The Foundation carries several excellent digestive enzymes products that can maximize nutrient absorption.

Conventional Drug Therapies Approved by the FDA

The FDA has approved several cytotoxic antiviral drugs to slow the progression of HIV infection. The most popular of these drugs are AZT, ddI, ddC, and 3TC. There is enthusiasm in some parts of the AIDS community that various combinations of these antiviral drugs could enable those with HIV infection and clinically diagnosed AIDS to maintain long-term remissions.

The published research shows that the proper combination of these antiviral drugs and a protease inhibitor works far better than AZT alone. A combination of AZT and 3TC, along with one of the new, relatively nontoxic protease inhibitors, may be the ideal combination to try first in AIDS patients who do not respond to natural therapies.

In several studies published in 1994, AZT was compared to a placebo with no difference in overall survival rates. In some cases, AZT caused an *increase* in mortality. Recognizing that AZT monotherapy is clearly not the solution to AIDS, some of the AIDS support groups are suggesting that aggressive combinations of almost every antiviral drug available be tried in AIDS patients. These combination therapies can, in the short-term, produce a significant reduction in the PCR (viral load testing) and even an increase in CD4 (T-helper cells). Regular blood tests would be needed to monitor the toxicity of these antiviral drugs to determine when to switch from one toxic combination to another.

Our concern is that if combination antiviral therapy produces irreversible damage to the immune system, there could very well be no increase in survival time, even though the therapy might kill a large number of HIV viruses and infected immune cells. It is interesting to note that, in two studies documenting the benefits of combination antiviral drug and protease-inhibitor therapy, those who had never taken an antiviral drug had higher survival rates than those who had previously taken AZT. One reason for the better effect on these "antiviral virgins" was that not as much resistance to antiviral drugs had developed in them. The use of AZT results in the development of drug-resistant strains of HIV within 1 to 2 years.

Another reason the "antiviral virgins" did better is that their immune systems may not have been previously damaged by toxic drugs such as AZT and ddI. Since HIV is a slow-progressing disease, and since blood tests enable you to monitor the benefits of the Foundation's protocol, HIV patients may consider following a nontoxic protocol first before resorting to combination antiviral-drug and protease-inhibitor therapy. Other scientists believe that the toxic drug combination should be used as soon as HIV infection is diagnosed in order to try to eradicate the HIV from the body before too many viruses are produced.

The bottom line is that expensive FDA-approved drugs produce toxicities that may limit their long-term use. If HIV infection can be controlled with natural therapies while a person is healthy, the toxic drugs could theoretically be reserved for future use in the event HIV begins to proliferate out of control.

A Critique of the Protease Inhibitors

Protease inhibitors are the newest class of AIDS drugs which burst onto the scene at the 1996 Conference of Retroviruses and Opportunistic Infections and have been making front page news ever since. Protease inhibitors were approved following the fastest and most lenient approval process in FDA history. They were described as the "great hope" in the war on AIDS. *The New England Journal of Medicine,* September 11, 1997, edition contained the first published report showing clinical data on protease inhibitors. The one cited trial included no patient data, used no control group, allowed no reporting of any AIDS-defining event other than recurrent pneumonia, and was prematurely terminated when emerging mortality statistics favored the protease inhibitor group. AIDS doctors have overlooked a remarkable lack of documented information concerning what protease inhibitors can do (and can't do) for a patient's health. This has not stopped them from embracing the new treatment options offered by protease inhibitors. While bold-type headlines praise protease inhibitors, the tiny type in pharmaceutical ads and product inserts tell a far different story about drug-induced diabetes, disfiguring fat migration, and sudden death.

Protease inhibitors function by breaking an enzymatic link necessary for the reproduction of HIV. Reverse transcriptase and protease are two of HIV's enzymes. Protease inhibitors block the actions of the protease enzyme. The enzyme becomes dysfunctional and cannot cut apart proteins, which is a crucial requirement for the reproduction of HIV. AZT, which is a nucleoside analog, is similar in function to protease inhibitors because it too can cause an enzyme to become dysfunctional; in AZT's case, that enzyme is reverse transcriptase. Nucleoside analogs are extremely effective at blocking the formation of HIV DNA, by blocking the functioning of all reverse transcriptase in the body. Unfortunately, the proper functioning of reverse transcriptase and protease within normal healthy cells is a vital prerequisite for the construction of human DNA, and therein lies these drugs' devastating toxicity. When protease inhibitors are used in conjunction with older nucleoside analog drugs such as AZT and ddI, the treatment is called a "combo cocktail." The AIDS establishment claims this cocktail of drugs achieves unprecedented and incredible results.

Lifelong therapy with protease inhibitors is furiously promoted even though Crixivan's manufacturer, Merck, openly states in its product insert, . . . *"The long-term effects of protease inhibitors are unknown."*

Merck further states, *"Since Crixivan has been marketed, other side effects have been reported including rapid breakdown of red blood cells, kidney stones and kidney failure. In some patients with hemophilia, increased bleeding has been associated with protease inhibitor use."*

"It is not yet known whether taking Crixivan will extend your life or reduce your chances of getting illnesses associated with HIV [since information about Crixivan is based on] *clinical studies up to 24 weeks."*

Even one of the governments top AIDS scientists, Dr. Anthony Fauci, was moved to express serious concern over the use of protease inhibitors "by otherwise healthy people," in the July 10, 1996, edition of the *Journal of the American Medical Association, JAMA.* Fauci said, "We do not know whether early intervention in asymptomatic individuals will result in a long-term clinical benefit or whether the cumulative toxicity over years of drug administration will outweigh the potential benefits." Dr. Robert Gallo has also warned, "these drugs are toxic; the longer you take the drugs, the greater the toxicity." Articles have appeared in *Newsday* magazine listing protease inhibitors' toxic side effects, such as diarrhea, nausea, fungal infections, bloody urine, kidney stones, weakness, headaches, and liver inflammation requiring "doctor visits and additional medicines." Other side effects reported include CMV retinitis, diabetes, liver failure, "buffalo humps" (large fat deposits at the base of the neck), acute renal failure, acute pancreatitis, grade-four diarrhea, and sudden death.

Patients using protease inhibitors are admonished to adhere to a strict dosing schedule under the threat that their HIV virus will mutate into a new drug-resistant strain. Dr. David Rasnick, an organic chemist who holds a Ph.D. in chemistry and was a pioneer in the development of protease inhibitors and holds eight patents on them, states that "no one has ever found a resistant HIV protease in any patient. The only inhibitor-resistant HIV proteases ever examined have been produced in the lab using genetic engineering" (*HIV Protease and Its Inhibitors,* 1997).

The media's reporting of miraculous recoveries are based on unpublished manufacturers' studies so brief that they are measured in weeks instead of months and tote the end result of reduced viral load, which has never been proven to correlate with actual health benefits. Dr. Michael Lederman was the protocol chairman and author of the AIDS Clinical Trials Group 315 at the National Institutes of Health. He said the study was never designed to consider the patients' overall health; instead it measured the surrogate marker known as viral load, a lab test which he believes does not diagnose health or measure or isolate active virus (*The Big Tease,* 1997; *What's Up with the Viral Load Theory,* 1996).

The AIDS mainstream celebrates the ability of protease inhibitors to decrease viral load, sometimes to undetectable levels, as an unprecedented occurrence. AZT has been doing this for many years without curing AIDS. The February 1997 edition of *POZ Magazine* states, "in the European Delta study, fully 40% of participants became 'undetectable' on AZT/ddI; another 5% did so on AZT alone. We have been reducing viral load to undetectable levels for a decade. But if becoming 'undetectable' on nucleoside combos hasn't prevented progression to disease and death, why is 'undetectable' on protease combinations impervious to failure—except for the fact that we haven't followed patients long enough to see it?" The AIDS mainstream also pretends protease inhibitors are responsible for decreasing AIDS deaths, but the Centers for Disease Control and Prevention (CDC) illustrates year after year in its own surveillance publications that AIDS mortalities have steadily decreased every year since 1983. According to the CDC's own statistics, mortality rates have consistently declined from 92% in 1986 to 23% in 1995, a long time before protease inhibitors came into use (HIV/AIDS Surveillance Rep.).

The release of protease inhibitors as the latest "great hope" in the war on AIDS is strikingly familiar to the release of AZT in 1986. Protease expert Dr. David Rasnick has said, "Once again, all we have are researchers talking to reporters about incomplete studies that haven't been scrutinized by the scientific review process. And the researchers involved are funded by the companies that make the drugs in question. There is no justification for the claims coming from these sources, particularly when we've seen it all before." AZT's declarations of success were based on abbreviated trials of less than 6 months. These trials were sponsored by the drug's manufacturer, which only published those trials that had favorable outcomes, and were measured by the end result of increased T-cells, which have been proven to be of questionable human value (*The Truth Behind T-Cell Counts,* 1996; *How Your Immune System Works,* 1994; *A Critical Analysis of the HIV-T4-Cell AIDS Hypothesis,* 1995).

Similarly, early elation over protease inhibitors was the result of, again, unpublished manufacturer's studies, measured in weeks not months, and which used reduced viral load as the end result, which has not been correlated with actual health benefits (*Reappraising AIDS,* 1996).

An alternative to the ingesting of toxic pharmaceutical protease inhibitors, discovered by the People with AIDS Community in 1996, is a believed natural source of protease inhibitors known as olive leaf extract, which is nontoxic and only targets the protease enzyme of viruses and is available over the counter without a prescription. Olive leaf extract was discussed in the preceding section.

H

Other Causes of Immune Suppression

The number one cause of immune deficiency in the world has been known to be malnutrition. Those with intestinal diseases often fail to absorb critical nutrients, while letting other immune-suppressing agents into their bodies. That is why maintaining intestinal health is such an important aspect of long-term HIV therapy. A second known cause of immune suppression can be pharmaceutical and recreational drug use. The immunosuppressive effects of many drugs have been well documented for many decades. Pneumonias, mouth sores, fevers, swollen lymph glands, night sweats, and bacterial infections are all conditions which can be indicative of immunosuppression and have been recorded in the medical literature for over 50 years. Antibiotics, steroids, and antiviral drugs such as AZT, ddI, ddC, 3Tc, and D4T, are well-known to cause damaging effects to the immune and digestive systems. Many HIV/AIDS treatment drugs are immunosuppressive when used on a daily basis. Bactrim and Septra (also known as TMP/SMX) antibiotics are a double chemotherapeutic folic-acid inhibitor and are very effective at destroying digestive flora. The American Medical Association's *Encyclopedia of Medicine* states they "may cause a folic-acid deficiency resulting in anemia." It also states that adverse effects may be nausea, vomiting, diarrhea, loss of appetite, headache, dizziness, muscle and joint pain, and rash.

Folic acid is a common B vitamin present in most normal diets and required by several kinds of bacteria present in a healthy intestinal colony. A perfectly well-looking person may actually have a drug-induced, subclinical state of malnutrition as a result of the ingestion of antibiotics, thus promoting the end result of immune suppression. SMX is a powerful sulfonamide derivative. Together with nitrite, which is found in amyl nitrite and isobutyl nitrite (a recreational drug known as "poppers"), sulfon amide is a very strong electrophilic oxidizing agent. The immunosuppressive effects of recreational drug use have been recorded in the medical literature going back to the turn of the century. Many male homosexuals in large urban areas in Western countries share patterns of behavior that encompass the recreational use of nitrites along with the long-term prophylactic use of antibiotics. Both chemicals—pharmaceutical SMX and recreational nitrites—reduce the oxygen-carrying capacity of red blood cells by oxidizing ferrous iron in hemoglobin to ferric. This causes a condition known as methemoglobulinemia, a progressively life-threatening deficiency of the oxygen supply of the respiration chain of the mitochondria (*Am. J. Int. Med.*, 1979; *J. Foren. Sci.*, 1981; *The Mitochondrion in Health and Disease,* 1992).

Treatment Options

Whatever conventional antiviral therapy you have chosen to use, remember that FDA-approved antiviral drugs such as nucleoside analogs (AZT, ddI) and the protease inhibitors are extremely toxic. If you are healthy, we recommend that natural therapies be tried first.

Blood tests. Blood Chemistry Profile & Complete Blood Count, Immune Cell Subset, Multitest CMI, Natural Killer Function, DHEA Test & Treatment, TSH Test & Treatment, Cortisol Test & Treatment.

Antioxidants. Life Extension Mix, *N*-acetylcysteine, whey protein, *S*-adenosylmethionine, selenium, alpha-lipoic acid, CoQ_{10}, vitamin C, beta-carotene, B_{12}, glutathione.

Hormones. Melatonin, growth hormone, DHEA, testosterone.

Amino acids. *L*-glutamine, *L*-carnitine.

Additional supplements. Olive leaf extract, SPV-30, Thymex, silymarin, enzymes.

Sources of Additional Alternative Information

Organizations

The Life Extension Foundation

This nonprofit, medical research foundation is politically activated to promoting freedom of choice in American health care. The Foundation, as the world's strongest critic of the FDA, is the only nonprofit, member-driven organization to successfully sue this government agency, whose main purpose is to protect the financial interests of the pharmaceutical industry. The fastest and easiest source for comprehensive health and nutritional information, longevity, research, and pharmaceutical-grade nutritional products and herbals.

Group for the Scientific Reappraisal of the HIV/AIDS Hypothesis

Members of this organization are scientists, researchers, and leaders of the debate about etiology of AIDS from all over the world. They publish a monthly newsletter, *Reappraising AIDS,* which offers readable and highly informative insights into the polemic.

The Group
7414 Girard Ave. #1-331
La Jolla, CA 92037
Tel: (810) 772-9926
Fax: (619) 272-1621

HEAL (Health Education AIDS Liaison)

A nonprofit, community-based education network with independent chapters located throughout the United States. Originally founded in 1982 as an AIDS support group, under the direction of Dr. Michael Ellner, President, and Dr. Frank Buincouckas, Science Advisor, HEAL New York became in 1985 the inspiration for an international movement challenging the validity of the HIV/AIDS hypothesis and the efficacy of HIV-based treatments. For more than a decade, HEAL New York has been a leading source of comprehensive information on effective, nontoxic, and holistic approaches to recovery from AIDS and has served as a consistent voice calling for honesty in AIDS issues. There are presently chapters in twenty North American cities and seven countries worldwide.

New York, NY Tel: (212) 873-0780
Los Angeles, CA Tel: (213) 896-8260
Ft. Lauderdale, FL Tel: (954) 473-1704

Continuum

A bimonthly magazine published in London. It features extensive articles on alternatives to pharmaceutical therapies and standard AIDS-think while covering AIDS news and events around the world.

Continuum
172 Founding Court
Brunswick Centre
London, WC1N 1QE, England
Tel: (44)(0) 171-713-7071
Fax: (44)(0) 171-713-7072

Internet Sites

www.lef.org

The Life Extension Foundation hosts the fastest and easiest source for comprehensive health and nutritional information, longevity research, and pharmaceutical-grade nutritional products and herbals. Join immediately and add your voice to the 50,000 members of the Life Extension Foundation who have changed the course of medicine in the world by demanding freedom of choice in health care.

www.virusmyth.com

The Group for the Scientific Reappraisal of the HIV/AIDS Hypothesis came into existence as a group of signatories of an open letter to the scientific community. This Web site contains more than 250 web pages with over 200 articles.

www.epcnet.com/heal and www.aliveandwell.org

HEAL Los Angeles' free educational forums inspire a will to live, participate in life, and cultivate a healthy future. The scientific data HEAL makes available help people separate fear from facts and provide a solid foundation upon which to base important health decisions. HEAL's forums emphasize personal independent understanding of medicine and science, and individual responsibility in health management.

www.healsf.org

This is the HEAL San Francisco chapter Web site. What if everything you thought you knew about AIDS was wrong? This site examines the mounting body of evidence that much of what the general public has been told about AIDS is wrong. If you or a loved one are HIV positive, this site offers an alternative.

The Foundation can provide the most advanced life-extension information available in the world. We invite you to participate in this process. We have become aware of many great therapies due to our members' input, and we are grateful for having been able to, as a direct result, impact many more lives. If you are aware of an alternative treatment or information that you feel may warrant further investigation, we encourage you to bring it to our attention by faxing our office at (954) 761-9199. Because the study of immune suppression has proved to be very profitable in the last two decades, this field of research has become extremely prolific. We appreciate the studies you have already made us aware of and thank you in advance for your future contributions, which may be incorporated into next year's HIV protocol.

HOMOCYSTEINE

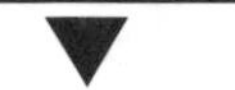

Cardiovascular disease causes 44% of all deaths in the United States. Alzheimer's dementia affects 4 million Americans now, and is expected to increase sharply as the population ages. Both cardiovascular and Alzheimer's disease have now been linked to the accumulation of a toxic amino acid called *homocysteine*. Vitamin supplement users have assumed they are being protected against homocysteine overload, but this article will expose that fallacy and recommend a scientific course of action to follow.

The medical establishment woke up to the dangers of homocysteine when the *New England Journal of Medicine* (April 9, 1998) and the *Journal of the American Medical Association* (*JAMA,* Dec. 18, 1996) published articles suggesting that vitamin supplements be used to lower homocysteine levels. This same message was published by the *Life Extension Foundation* 18 years earlier (*Anti-Aging News,* Nov. 1981, 85–86).

Some cardiologists suggest that coronary artery disease patients take a multivitamin supplement to lower their homocysteine levels. Patients who follow this advice, but fail to have their blood tested for homocysteine, could be making a fatal mistake.

The Life Extension Foundation has uncovered a flaw in the theory that a person can blindly take vitamin supplements to adequately reduce homocysteine levels. While folic acid, vitamin B_{12}, B_6, and trimethylglycine (TMG) all lower homocysteine levels, it is *impossible* for any individual to know if he or she is taking the proper amount of nutrients without a homocysteine blood test.

The clear message from new scientific findings is that there is no safe "normal range" for homocysteine. While commercial laboratories state that normal homocysteine can range from 5 to 15 micromoles per liter of blood, epidemiological data reveal that homocysteine levels above 6.3 cause a steep, progressive risk of heart attack (the American Heart Association's journal *Circulation,* Nov. 15, 1995, 2825–30). One study found each 3-unit increase in homocysteine equals a 35% increase in myocardial-infarction (heart-attack) risk (*American Journal of Epidemiology,* 1996, 143[9]:845–59).

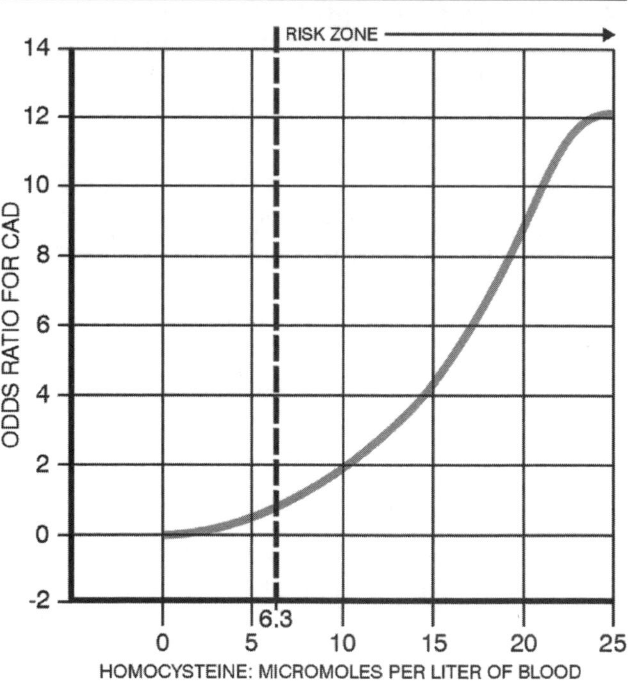

A Lethal Misconception

People taking vitamin supplements think they are being protected against the lethal effects of homocysteine when, in reality, even supplement users can have homocysteine levels far above the *safe* level of 6.3 to 7.0.

The Foundation has identified several cases in which people who were suffering from coronary artery disease had lethal levels of homocysteine despite taking the recommended dose (and higher) of vitamin supplements.

One case involved a 60-year-old man who previously had bypass surgery, but who was again suffering angina pain with significant restenosis (reclogging of the coronary arteries) verified by angiography. This man knew about the dangers of homocysteine and had been taking more than 15,000 mcg a day of folic acid, along with other homocysteine-lowering vitamins. Because of the angina pain and restenosis, the Foundation recommended a homocysteine blood test. The results came back showing that this man had a shockingly high homocysteine reading of 18 in his blood. (Homocysteine levels over 15 have been shown to be extremely dangerous.) The Foundation immediately suggested this man take 6 grams a day of TMG (trimethylglycine), and within one month, his homocysteine level dropped to 4. This case was a wake-up call that one or more homocysteine-lowering factors are not always the solution to keeping homocysteine levels in the safest range (below 7). It was also a confirmation of our position that people who want to lower homocysteine must take in account all of the factors involved.

Another case involved a healthy person who took everyday a 500-mg TMG supplement, 4000 mcg of folic acid, and high doses of many other vitamins. A homocysteine blood test revealed a reading of 11.3, which is far above the safe range of under 7. Six grams of TMG and 500 mg of vitamin B_6 were added to his daily program, and the homocysteine level dropped to under 6 within 60 days.

In response to these individual cases, the Foundation analyzed all the homocysteine tests it had conducted on Foundation members and discovered that 62% of members tested have too much homocysteine in their blood. The following chart shows the breakdown of members and their coronary risk factors based on serum homocysteine readings:

Risk for Coronary Heart Disease*

	Serum Homocysteine (micromoles per liter of blood)	Percentage of members in this range
Lowest risk	0–6.3	38%
Moderate risk	6.3–10	52%
Highest risk	Over 10	10%

**Circulation,* 1995, 92:2835–930.

The most recent survey (*Cardiologia,* 1999, Apr, 44[4]:341–45) shows that the average American's homocysteine level is 10, so the fact that 90% of Foundation members are below 10 is a testament to the effectiveness of dietary supplements in suppressing dangerously high homocysteine levels *(Annals of Epidemiology,* May 1997, 7[4]:285–93).

The problem is that certain members are not being protected against the damaging effects of homocysteine, and the only way of finding out is to have a blood test. When homocysteine is too high, the addition of extra amounts of vitamin B_6 and/or TMG (trimethylglycine) has reduced levels to the safest range in every case we have worked with. The Foundation has found that the addition of extra folic acid produces only a moderate reduction in elevated homocysteine levels. Folic acid is a critical component of a homocysteine-lowering program, but there is a limit to how much homocysteine can be reduced by folate and vitamin B_{12}. Cardiologists are increasingly recommending folic-acid supplements to their coronary artery disease patients, but the results from the Foundation's laboratory indicate that it takes more than folic acid to reduce serum homocysteine to a level where it ceases to be a risk factor for causing a heart attack.

Mechanisms of Homocysteine Detoxification

Elevated homocysteine can be reduced (or detoxified) in two ways. The most common pathway is via the *remethylation* process, where *methyl groups* are donated to homocysteine to transform it into methionine and *S*-adenosylmethionine (SAMe).

A potent remethylation agent is TMG, which stands for *trimethylglycine*. The *tri* means there are three *methyl* groups on each *glycine* molecule that can be transferred to homocysteine to transform (remethylate) it into methionine and SAMe. The remethylation (or detoxification) of homocysteine requires the following minimum factors: (1) folic acid, (2) vitamin B_{12}, (3) zinc, and (4) TMG.

Choline is another "methyl donor" that helps to lower elevated homocysteine levels, and this conversion doesn't require cofactors. However, choline only enhances remethylation in the liver and kidney, which is why it is so important to take adequate amounts of remethylating factors such as folic acid and vitamin B_{12} to protect the brain and the heart. The published literature emphasizes that folic acid and vitamin B_{12} are critical nutrients in the remethylation (detoxification) pathway of homocysteine.

The other pathway in which elevated homocysteine is reduced is via its conversion into cysteine and eventually glutathione via the *trans-sulfuration* pathway. This pathway is dependent on vitamin B_6. The amount of vitamin B_6 required to lower homocysteine has considerable individual variability. Methionine is the only amino acid that creates homocysteine. People who eat foods that are high in methionine (such as red meat and chicken) may need more vitamin B_6. Elevated homocysteine can occur when there are insufficient vitamin cofactors (such as folate and vitamin B_6) to detoxify the amount of methionine being ingested in the diet.

Elevated homocysteine can also be caused by a genetic defect that blocks the trans-sulfuration pathway by inducing a deficiency of the vitamin B_6–dependent enzyme cystathionine-*B*-synthase. In this case, high doses of vitamin B_6 are required to suppress excessive homocysteine accumulation. Since one would not want to take excessive doses of vitamin B_6 (greater than 300 to 500 mg a day for a long time period), a homocysteine blood test can help determine whether you are taking enough vitamin B_6 to keep homocysteine levels in a safe range. There are some people who lack an enzyme to convert vitamin B_6 into its biologically active form, pyridoxal-5-phosphate. In this case, if low-cost vitamin B_6 supplements do not sufficiently lower homocysteine levels, then a high-cost pyridoxal-5-phosphate supplement may be required.

For many people, the daily intake of 500 mg of TMG, 800 mcg of folic acid, 1000 mcg of vitamin B_{12}, 250 mg of choline, 250 mg of inositol, 30 mg of zinc, and 100 mg of vitamin B_6 will keep homocysteine levels in a safe range. But the only way to really know is to have your blood tested to make sure your homocysteine levels are under 7. If homocysteine levels are too high, then up to 6 grams of TMG may be needed along with higher amounts of other remethylation cofactors. Some people with cystathione-B synthase deficiencies will require 500 mg a day or more of vitamin B_6 to reduce homocysteine to a safe level. For the prevention of cardiovascular disease, you would want your homocysteine blood level to be under 7. For the prevention of aging, some people have suggested that an even lower level is desirable, but more research needs to be done before any scientific conclusions can be reached.

Elevated Homocysteine Is a Sign of Other Degenerative Diseases

Elevated homocysteine can be a sign of a methylation deficiency throughout the body. Methylation is fundamental to DNA repair. If DNA is not adequately repaired, mutations and strand breaks will result. This will lead to accelerated aging, as greater amounts of faulty proteins are synthesized from the damaged DNA. The liver depends on methylation to perform the numerous enzymatic reactions required to detoxify every drug and foreign substance that the body is exposed to. Methylation is also required for the growth of new cells. Without it, new cells cannot be made.

A study published in the journal *Medical Hypothesis* (1998, 51[3]:179–221) provides evidence that aging may be exclusively a result of cellular "demethylation," or, said differently, the aging process is caused by the depletion of enzymatic "remethylation" activity that is required to maintain and repair cellular DNA. This study suggests that aging may be reversible if aged cells could be programmed to remethylate rather than demethylate.

Homocysteine induces cellular damage by interfering with the methylation process. Methylation will be compromised if homocysteine is elevated, and elevated homocysteine is a warning sign that the methylation cycle is not functioning properly. Homocysteine may also damage cells directly by promoting oxidative stress.

There is a growing consensus that deficient methylation is the major cause of the degenerative diseases of aging. The consumption of methylation-enhancing nutrients like TMG, choline, folic acid, and vitamin B_{12} may be one of the most readily available and effective anti-aging therapies presently known. However, it is important to tailor the intake of methylation-enhancing nutrients to one's individual biochemistry. The best way of assessing your body's rate of methylation is to measure blood levels of homocysteine. Elevated serum homocysteine is the classic sign of a methylation deficiency (or demethylation) that is correctable with the proper intake of methylation enhancing nutrients such as TMG, folic acid, and vitamin B_{12}.

Homocysteine and Alzheimer's Disease

Recent studies show that people with dementia of the Alzheimer's type have elevated levels of homocysteine in their blood. At an international scientific conference held in The Netherlands the week of April 27, 1998, a team of scientists unveiled findings showing a definitive link between elevated homocysteine and Alzheimer's disease. The scientists advocated that people have their blood tested for homocysteine in order to determine how much folic acid should be taken to drop homocysteine levels to the safe range.

While the scientists speculated that Alzheimer's disease could be avoided if people reduced their homocysteine levels, it has not yet been determined whether homocysteine itself contributes to Alzheimer's disease. A more likely explanation is that elevated homocysteine is an indication of the severe disruption in the methylation pathway that occurs in the brains of Alzheimer's patients. It has been reported that people with Alzheimer's disease have virtually no *S*-adenosylmethionine (SAMe) in their brains. SAMe is required for DNA methylation (maintenance and repair) of brain cells. Thus, while homocysteine itself may not cause Alzheimer's disease, it appears to represent an important measurable biomarker of a methylation deficit that could cause Alzheimer's and a host of other degenerative diseases.

Research reported at Tufts University in 1995 documented the same finding linking elevated homocysteine and Alzheimer's disease and recommended supplementation with folic acid and vitamin B_{12}. It should be noted that dementia can be caused by a deficiency of vitamin B_{12}, folic acid, and other nutrients, so another reason for people with dementia of the Alzheimer's type have to elevated homocysteine levels could be that they are suffering from a common vitamin deficiency. Numerous studies conducted on the elderly show that deficiencies of folic acid, vitamin B_{12}, and other nutrients are epidemic in elderly people who do not take vitamin supplements. Since both elevated homocysteine and vitamin deficiencies have been linked to dementia, the best approach to preventing and treating dementia (including Alzheimer's dementia) would appear to be testing the blood for elevated homocysteine *and* taking methylation enhancing nutrients such as folic acid, TMG, and vitamin B_{12}.

A review of the published literature provides compelling evidence that elevated homocysteine is common in people suffering from dementia of the Alzheimer's type. Since Alzheimer's disease cannot be positively diagnosed until after death, it is impossible to state whether all the people in a scientific study are really suffering from Alzheimer's disease. Dementia can be caused by multi-infarct cerebrovascular disease or even by simple vitamin deficiencies.

In a study published in the *International Journal of Geriatric Psychiatry* (April 1998, 235–239), Dr. McCaddon and his group were able to confirm that patients diagnosed with senile dementia of the Alzheimer's type have significantly elevated levels of homocysteine compared to age-matched controls. An earlier study published in the *Journal of Gerontology and Biological Sciences* (March 1997, 76–9) also showed that homocysteine levels were significantly elevated in Alzheimer's disease patients compared to controls. This study found that folic acid and vitamin B_{12} deficiencies were present in both the Alzheimer's disease patients and the age-matched case controls.

The reason that homocysteine levels are so high in people suffering from dementia of the Alzheimer's type is not fully understood. Scientists speculate that severe aberrations in the methylation cycle might be involved in the disease process and that elevated homocysteine is a sign of the breakdown of the methylation cycle (*European Neuropsychopharmacol.* (June 1995, 107–14). Other researchers report that abnormal amino acid metabolism early in Alzheimer's causes elevated homocysteine levels. This may lead to neuronal damage that occurs as the disease progresses (*Journal of Neural Transmission* (1998, 105:[2–3]:287–94). Remember, the repair and maintenance of cellular DNA is dependent on healthy methylation processes. Methylation deficiencies result in severe damage to brain cells. Under-methylation can cause severe damage to brain cells. Methylation is required for the maintenance of the myelin sheath and the repair of DNA in the brain. Elevated levels of homocysteine in the blood indicate some degree of methylation deficiency that is correctable with an individualized supplement program.

The studies showing that homocysteine is a biomarker for the development of dementia of the Alzheimer's type mandates that those seeking to avoid senility should have their blood tested in order to ascertain their homocysteine levels. While it was apparent in the year 1969 that homocysteine was a major cause of vascular disease, the evidence that homocysteine represents a marker of brain cell degeneration is of very recent origin, and has been overlooked by many conventional neurologists.

Despite the evidence linking elevated homocysteine to methylation deficiencies that are involved in the Alzheimer's disease process, the Alzheimer's Disease Society has criticized the recommendation that people take folic acid supplements to lower their homocysteine levels. What follows is a direct quote from that organization, *"No one knows whether taking (folic acid) supplements will help prevent the disease or whether it will affect the rate at which the disease progresses. The only way this will be discovered is by doing further studies on many, many more patients over a long period of time."* The Life Extension Foundation finds perplexing the concept that anybody would warn against taking folic acid supplements at a time when the conventional medical establishment has acknowledged that taking folic acid lowers homocysteine and protects against heart attack, stroke, and colon cancer.

The Critical Need for Homocysteine Blood Testing

Measuring blood levels of homocysteine is a new and potentially life-saving test that provides information about vitamin and methylation status, in addition to determining levels of toxic homocysteine. Those with a family history of heart disease, stroke, or Alzheimer's disease are at a particular risk for elevated homocysteine. Elevated homocysteine has also been linked to complications in diabetes, lupus, and other chronic diseases. While many people have assumed that because they are taking vitamin supplements, their homocysteine levels will be in a *safe* range, The Life Extension Foundation has discovered that this might not always be the case.

The only way of knowing for sure is to get tested. Homocysteine testing used to be expensive, but prices have come down as consumer interest has increased.

Summary

The newest scientific evidence indicates that there is no safe "normal range" for homocysteine. However, epidemiological data reveal that homocysteine levels above 6.3 cause a steep progressive risk of heart attack. Homocysteine levels should be medically tested to ensure that the proper combination and dosages of supplements are taken. Dosages should be adjusted based on individual needs. The following supplements have demonstrated effectiveness in lowering homocysteine levels either alone or in combination:

1. Folic acid, 800 to 5000 mcg a day.
2. Vitamin B_{12}, 1000 to 3000 mcg a day.
3. Vitamin B_6, 100 to 600 mg a day.
4. Zinc, 30 to 90 mg a day.
5. Choline, 500 to 5000 mcg a day.
6. Trimethylglycine, 500 to 9000 mg a day.
7. SAMe, 200 to 800 mg a day.
8. Inositol, 250 to 1000 mg a day.

Product availability. The nutritional supplements discussed in this protocol are available by phoning (800) 544-4440, or order online at www.lef.org.

HYPERTENSION

A startling statistic in the May 4, 1999, edition of *The New York Times* revealed that only 18% of people with high blood pressure (hypertension) are successfully treated to achieve normotensive ranges. Untreated hypertension carries enormous health risks, such as increased risk of heart disease, stroke, kidney disease, and eye disease, yet fear of medication side effects and improper prescribing by physicians are contributing to an epidemic of hypertension-induced disease.

"Blood pressure" can be defined as the pressure or force that is applied against the artery walls as blood is carried through the circulatory system. It is recorded as a measurement of this force in relation to the heart's pumping activity, and is measured in millimeters of mercury (mmHg). The top number, or systolic pressure, is the measurement of the pressure that occurs when the heart contracts or beats. The bottom number, or diastolic pressure, is the measurement recorded between beats, while the heart is at rest. The systolic number is placed over the diastolic number. For example, 110/70 (read as "110 over 70") means a systolic pressure of 110 mmHg and a diastolic pressure of 70 mmHg. The systolic number is always the higher of the two numbers.

"Hypertension" is an indicator that the force required for blood flow is greater than normal. A blood pressure measurement of less than 130/85 is considered "normal," while 130–140/85–90 is defined as "high normal." A large study reported in the March 1997 issue of the journal *Circulation* indicates that "even borderline blood pressure readings represent a risk factor for atherosclerosis and stroke." Blood pressure is considered to be elevated when repeated measurement shows a systolic pressure greater than 140, a diastolic pressure greater than 90, or both.

Because the heart is working harder than normal, high blood pressure increases the risk of coronary heart disease, heart attack, stroke, aneurysm, kidney failure, and atherosclerosis. When the heart works harder than normal over an extended period of time, it tends to enlarge. High blood pressure also causes the arteries and arterioles to become scarred, hardened, and less elastic. This, in turn, can limit the amount of blood flowing to the organs; can cause blood clots in the arteries; and can ultimately damage the heart, brain, and kidneys.

Disease Cause

The cause of hypertension is unknown in 90 to 95% of all cases. People who have a family history of high blood pressure may be more likely to suffer from it. People who suffer from stress, worries, fear, pressure from events from daily life, and nervous stress can also suffer from hypertension.

Because persons with hypertension may not exhibit any symptoms, they often go undiagnosed until complications occur. Regular (yearly) blood-pressure screening can facilitate early diagnosis and treatment and reduce the risk of further complications associated with hypertension.

Hypertension is generally classified as primary or secondary. Primary or essential hypertension has no known cause; however, certain lifestyle factors such as body weight and salt intake are involved. Ninety-five percent of persons diagnosed with hypertension fall into this category. The diagnosis is made when no other cause is found. Secondary hypertension is caused by some other medical diagnosis or problem, such as kidney disease, Cushing's syndrome, pregnancy, oral contraceptive use, chronic alcohol abuse, or the use of certain medications.

There are several factors that put people at risk for hypertension. Gender, age, heredity, and race are factors that cannot be controlled. As people age, their chances of developing hypertension increase. Men are generally at greater risk than women. However, as women age, their risk increases with the onset of menopause, and later in life it exceeds that of men. Heredity can be a risk factor if one or more parents have been diagnosed with hypertension. African Americans are at higher risk for contracting hypertension than Caucasians are.

According to the journal *Ethn. Dis.,* (winter 1998), other risk factors that can be controlled are lifestyle related: obesity, lack of exercise, diet, stress, the use of certain medications, smoking, and excessive alcohol consumption.

Disease Symptoms

Hypertension usually has no evident symptoms. Many people can have high blood pressure for years without knowing it, and that is why it can be so dangerous. The only way a person can find out if he or she has hypertension is to have his or her blood pressure checked at least once every 2 years by a doctor or other health professional. Some of the warning signs of hypertension can include nosebleeds, an irregular heartbeat, headaches, and dizziness; however, if a person does not have these warning signs, it does not necessarily mean he or she does not suffer from it.

Hypertension can occur in children or adults. It occurs predominantly in middle-aged and elderly people, obese people, heavy drinkers, blacks, and women who are taking oral contraceptives. Called the silent killer, there may not be any symptoms for many years until a vital organ is damaged. A person can be calm and relaxed and still have high blood pressure, even though tension or nervousness also causes hypertension.

Blood pressure may rise as people get older. Males suffer from hypertension earlier than females and are more likely to develop high blood pressure than females in early adulthood into early middle age. By the time women reach the age of 55, their chances of getting hypertension even out with men. Three fourths of all women past the age of 75 suffer from hypertension.

Conventional Treatment

There is no cure for hypertension, but conventional doctors treat it in one or both of two ways: (1) by changing the patient's lifestyle and eating habits and (2) by prescription medications. The change of lifestyle is preferable to taking medication. Alternative doctors seek to address the underlying cause of hypertension and correct it.

Change in Lifestyle and Eating Habits

A January 1998 Harvard Medical School study sums up the impact of excess weight or small weight gains relative to the risk of hypertension: "Excess weight and even modest adult weight gain substantially increase risk for hypertension. Weight loss reduces the risk for hypertension."

An earlier Harvard 1996 study that included 41,541 female nurses, published in *Hypertension Journal,* stated that "these results support hypotheses that age, body weight, and alcohol consumption are strong determinants of risk of hypertension in middle-aged women. They are compatible with the possibilities that magnesium and fiber as well as a diet richer in fruits and vegetables may reduce blood pressure levels."

If a person is overweight, or only a little overweight, it is suggested he or she lose weight. Losing 2 pounds can cause a 1 to 2 point drop in blood pressure. Brisk walking or bike riding for 30 to 40 minutes, 3 times a week, can lower blood pressure a few points. Strenuous exercise can lower blood pressure even more. (Also refer to the section "The DASH Diet" in this protocol, for a diet that many people say "requires them to eat too much.")

Integrated and Alternative Treatments

A New, Rational Approach for Hypertension Therapy

Several basic concepts are often ignored despite being relevant to the treatment of hypertensive patients and associated cardiovascular disease.

Although people often consider hypertension as a disease, it is not itself a disease but, rather, one warning manifestation of a disease. Approximately 90% of the time, the underlying cause(s) of hypertension are unknown; thus, the condition itself is named according to its sign, as essential hypertension.

Commonly, physicians are told that by eliminating the hypertension—i.e., by merely reducing blood pressure—the increased risk and mortality associated with underlying cardiovascular disease will be reversed. Unfortunately, the cumulative experience of over two decades of worldwide clinical trials indicates that getting rid of only one aspect of hypertensive disease, the elevated blood pressure, reduces only part of the cardiovascular risk associated with hypertension.

We must appreciate that what we call "hypertension" is a powerful indicator of disease in other body systems, such as left ventricular hypertrophy, that may exist prior to and progress independently of the hypertension itself and insulin resistance, reflecting the same underlying pathophysiology in skeletal muscle, fat, and other tissues. Thus, the disease we call hypertension is not just a blood pressure reduction or numbers game. We must consider the treatment of associated disease to treat hypertension successfully.

Ultimately the goal would be to identify underlying disease—not only the elevation of blood pressure, but also the other multisystemic aspects of hypertensive cardiovascular disease—and implement an integrated medical approach as well. Focusing on such underlying factors would allow treatment of the disease process itself, rather than just the elevated blood pressure.

A second concept is also often overlooked but quite obvious: people are different. By analogy with an elevated temperature, the same elevation of blood pressure that leads to the diagnosis of "essential" hypertension may result from many different "primary" causes, which just happen to have hypertension as one shared clinical manifestation. This immediately implies that when we ask, "Is this drug or integrated therapy good, or preferred for hypertension?" the answer should be, "It depends." As an obvious example, the salt-sensitive hypertensive patient responds to dietary salt recommendations and to different drug classes differently from an individual who is not salt sensitive.

Therefore, it is worthwhile to consider associated underlying cardiovascular disease and treatment protocols present in the cardiovascular section of this book when treating hypertension as well as an individual's unique response to various conventional and integrated therapies. Working closely with your physician to monitor your individual response to integrated therapies is recommended.

There are nutrients that may reduce or eliminate the need for antihypertensive medications. However, nutrients may not work immediately to lower blood pressure the way drugs do, so it is important to carry nutritional blood pressure–lowering therapy through over a period of 4 to 12 weeks. Also, physician cooperation is crucial if you are to reduce your intake of blood pressure–lowering drugs safely. Routine, ongoing blood pressure monitoring is mandatory to determine whether the nutritional or integrated medical regimen you are following is controlling or reducing your blood pressure or not.

Benefits of Coenzyme Q_{10}

Coenzyme Q10 (CoQ10) and garlic provide aid in the reduction of blood pressure. These supplements may also mitigate the underlying disease that may be the cause of hypertension.

In March 1999, the results of a randomized, double-blind trial among patients receiving antihypertensive medication was published. Patients known to have essential hypertension and presenting with coronary artery disease were given 60 mg of CoQ_{10} twice a day. The doctors conducting the study stated,

> Findings indicate that treatment with Coenzyme Q_{10} decreases blood pressure, possibly by decreasing

> oxidative stress and insulin response in patients with known hypertension receiving conventional antihypertensive drugs (*Journal of Human Hypertension,* 1999 [March], 13 [3]:203–8).

Another study using higher doses of CoQ_{10} concluded,

> Patients treated with an average of 200 mg/day of CoQ_{10} showed improvement in symptoms of fatigue and dyspnea with no side effects noted. Previous observations on the improvement in diastolic function and left ventricular wall thickness through the therapeutic administration of coenzyme Q_{10} in patients with hypertensive heart disease prompted the investigation (*Molecular Aspects of Medicine,* 1997, 18 Suppl:S145–51).

CoQ_{10} was tested in 109 cardiology patients presenting with hypertension for at least 1 year. An average dose of 225 mg/day orally of CoQ_{10} was administered along with antihypertensive medication. The aim was to attain blood levels greater than 2.0 mcg/mL (average 3.02 mcg/mL on CoQ_{10}). Rather than being fixed, dosage was adjusted according to clinical response and blood CoQ_{10} levels. Researchers reported, "A definite and gradual improvement in functional status was observed with the concomitant need to gradually decrease antihypertensive drug therapy within the first one to six months." A remarkable 51% of patients were completely removed from between one and three antihypertensive medications an average of 4.4 months after starting CoQ_{10} administration. A highly significant improvement was seen in left ventricular wall thickness and diastolic function in those patients (9.4% of total) who were monitored by echocardiogram before and during treatment.

In a study conducted to clarify the mechanism of the antihypertensive effect of CoQ_{10}, 26 patients with essential arterial hypertension were treated with oral CoQ_{10}, 50 mg twice daily for 10 weeks. Plasma CoQ_{10}, serum total and high-density lipoprotein (HDL) cholesterol, and blood pressure were determined in all patients before and at the end of the 10-week period. At the end of the treatment, systolic pressure decreased from 164.5 ± 3.1 to 146.7 ± 4.1 mmHg, and diastolic pressure decreased from 98.1 to 86.1 mmHg. Plasma CoQ_{10} values increased from 0.64 mcg/mL to 1.61 mcg/mL. Serum total cholesterol decreased from 222.9 mg/dL to 213.3 mg/dL, and serum HDL cholesterol increased from 41.1 mg/dL to 43.1 mg/dL ± 1.5 mg/dL.

Fish Oil

High doses of fish-oil concentrates have lowered blood pressure in some people. There are cardiovascular as well as other health benefits associated with taking fish oil.

A study published in the October 1997 *American Journal of Clinical Nutrition* stated that "fish oils have been shown to lower blood pressure in hypertensive subjects." According to a January 1999 *Journal of Nutrition* study, the fatty acid DHA (docosahexaenoic acid, obtained directly from fish oil) was shown to alter the membrane fatty acid composition as well as the amount of ATP released from vascular endothelial cells, and also decrease plasma noradrenaline. The doctors who conducted this study stated that these factors may ameliorate the rise in blood pressure normally associated with advancing age. The *Journal of Vascular Research* (January 1998) corroborated these findings by showing that the EPA (eicosapentaenoic acid) fatty acid fraction of fish oil, when administered to aged rats, increases the release of ATP from the vascular endothelial cells, leading to repression of the blood pressure rise seen with advancing age. The October 1997 *American Journal of Clinical Nutrition* stated that "fish oil has a mild blood pressure–lowering effect in both normal and mildly hypertensive individuals."

Fish oil has been shown to reduce high levels of triglycerides by an average of 35%; however, fish oil does not reduce cholesterol as originally thought. Fish oil supplements do lower triglycerides dramatically, however.

If your gastrointestinal tract can tolerate high daily doses of fish oil, then you may lower your blood pressure and gain other benefits. One consideration is to start with a half dosage and then slowly increase to the dosage that will be recommended.

The Effects of Garlic on Hypertension

Several studies suggest that garlic may have protective effects against cardiovascular diseases. One cross-sectional observational study reported in *Circulation,* October 1997, tested the hypothesis that regular garlic intake would delay the stiffening of the aorta related to aging. Chronic garlic powder intake was shown to attenuate age-related increases in aortic stiffness. Arterial stiffening with age is one cause of hypertension. The doctors conducting this study stated,

> These data strongly support the hypothesis that garlic intake had a protective effect on the elastic properties of the aorta related to aging in humans.

As reported in the June 1998 *Journal of Cardiovascular Pharmacology,* garlic preparations have also been shown to have a beneficial effect on lipids, blood pressure, and platelet function.

An April 1998 study (*Prostaglandins Leukotrienes, and Essential Fatty Acids,* Scotland) reported the effect of garlic on blood lipids, blood sugar, fibrinogen, and fibrinogenic activity of 30 patients who received 4 grams of garlic daily for 3 months. The patients were monitored at 1.5 and 3 months when it was determined that garlic had significantly reduced total serum cholesterol and triglycerides and increased the beneficial HDL cholesterol fraction. With regard to fibrinogenic activity, it was determined that the garlic inhibited platelet aggregation.

To analyze the effect of garlic on blood pressure, researchers in Australia reviewed published literature on randomized controlled trials of garlic preparations that were at least 8 weeks in duration. The researchers identified eight trials using Kwai, a dried garlic powder preparation involving 415 subjects. In seven trials that compared garlic to placebo, three showed a significant reduction in systolic blood pressure (SBP) and four showed a reduction in diastolic blood pressure (DBP). The overall pooled mean difference in the absolute change (from baseline to final measurement) of SBP was greater in subjects treated with garlic than in those treated with placebo. In DBP subjects, the corresponding reduction was slightly smaller. The researchers concluded that there may be some clinical use in patients with mild hypertension and recommended that more thorough and rigorously designed trials be conducted.

Another randomized, placebo-controlled, double-blind trial was conducted on 47 nonhospitalized patients using Kwai garlic preparation. The patients who were admitted had diastolic blood pressures between 95 and 104 mmHg after a 2-week acclimatization phase. Blood pressure and plasma lipids were monitored during treatment after 4, 8, and 12 weeks. Researchers found significant differences between the placebo and Kwai groups. Systolic blood pressure fell from 102 to 91 mmHg after 8 weeks and again to 89 mmHg after 12 weeks in the drug group. Researchers also reported a significant reduction in serum cholesterol and triglycerides in the same group. No significant changes were noted in the placebo group.

Other researchers evaluated a garlic preparation containing 1.3% allicin (2400 mg) in nine patients with relatively severe hypertension (DBP $\geq$ 115 mmHg). At peak effect, about 5 hours after dosing, sitting blood pressure fell 7/16 ($\pm$ 3/2 standard deviations) mmHg, with a significant decrease in diastolic blood pressure from 5 to 14 hours after dosing. Researchers concluded that the garlic preparation reduced blood pressure with no evident side effects.

Dosage Recommendations

Studies continue in this area, with investigations pointing strongly toward the benefits of garlic, fish oil, and CoQ_{10} aiding in the treatment of hypertensive disease. The amount of standardized garlic extract needed to lower blood pressure is 1500 to 6000 mg per day. The amount of coenzyme Q_{10} needed to lower blood pressure is 200 to 300 mg per day.

A popular combination of supplements to take three times a day is

- 2 to 3 MEGA EPA fish oil capsules (each capsule contains 400 mg EPA/300 mg DHA)
- 1 CoQ_{10} (100 mg) supplement
- 2 garlic powder (900 mg) capsules
- 2 vitamin C (1000 mg) capsules (more about vitamin C later in this protocol)

H

Coenzyme Q_{10} should be taken in a liquid oil capsule for optimal assimilation. The garlic powder should contain a high allicin content (greater than 8000 parts per million). Consideration should also be given to diet changes during this same period to maximize results. After 4 weeks, consult your physician about your blood pressure, and depending on its drop, your physician may be able to reduce the dosage of your antihypertensive medication. The rationale and objective is to be able to reduce your intake of drugs slowly as the natural antihypertensive properties of garlic/coenzyme Q_{10} begin to take effect.

IMPORTANT NOTE: It is crucial to monitor your blood pressure closely, since the garlic/coenzyme Q_{10} combination does not work for everyone. Consult your physician on how you might integrate this therapy as part of your hypertensive treatment. (We recommend that you refer to the *Atherosclerosis, Congestive Heart Failure, and Cholesterol Reduction protocols* for more information relative to taking an integrated medical approach to hypertension.)

Benefits of Dietary Mineral Intake

A report in the *American Journal of Clinical Nutrition* stated that there is growing evidence that maintaining an adequate dietary mineral intake protects against high blood pressure. The report specifically noted the beneficial effects of meeting or exceeding dietary allowances of calcium, magnesium, and potassium in controlling elevated arterial pressure due to high intake of dietary sodium chloride. The report further noted that educating individuals to maintain adequate levels of these minerals may be a more valid health recommendation than simply reducing sodium intake. Another report in the *Annals of Medicine* stated that "in certain patients potassium, calcium, and magnesium may be protective electrolytes against hypertension." The report went on to suggest that "with appropriate dietary modifications, it is possible to prevent the development of high blood pressure and to treat hypertensive patients with fewer drugs and with lower doses. In some patients antihypertensive medication may not be at all necessary."

Anyone with elevated blood pressure should be taking 500 to 1500 mg of elemental magnesium per day. About 80% of Americans are magnesium-deficient, and low levels of magnesium are associated with hypertension and arterial disease. Even if magnesium fails to lower your blood pressure, it can reduce the risk of complications, such as stroke.

Benefits of Vitamin C

In the early 1990s, several large population studies showed a reduction in cardiovascular disease in those who consumed vitamin C. The most significant report emanated from UCLA in 1992, where it was announced that men who took 800 mg a day of vitamin C lived 6 years longer than those who consumed the FDA's recommended daily allowance of 60 mg a day. The study, which evaluated 11,348 participants over a 10-year period of time, showed that high vitamin C intake extended average life span and reduced mortality from cardiovascular disease by 42%. This study was published in the journal *Epidemiology* (1992 3 [3]:194–202).

In 1998, several well-controlled studies showed that vitamin C enables the arterial system to expand and contract with youthful elasticity. Enhancing the elasticity of the arterial system is one method of reducing blood pressure. Cardiologists often prescribe nitroglycerin and longer-acting nitrate drugs to dilate the coronary arteries and relieve angina pain. Nitrate drugs not only improve coronary blood flow but also lower the oxygen demand of the heart by reducing peripheral vascular resistance. Unfortunately, nitrate drugs also produce negative effects. The main limiting factor to the nitrate drugs is tolerance: the vascular system stops responding to the dilating effects of the drugs, and angina is no longer controlled. Nitrate drugs may also cause a progressive weakening of the heart muscle cells' ability to produce energy. When vitamin C is administered to coronary artery disease patients, the vasodilating effects of the nitrate drugs may be significantly prolonged and the energy-producing capacity of the cells maintained.

A double-blind study published in the *Journal of the American College of Cardiology* (1998, 31 [6]:1323–29) compared the effects of nitrate drugs in people receiving vitamin C to a placebo group not receiving vitamin C. The doctors administered nitrate drugs to healthy people and patients with coronary artery disease and then measured vasodilation response and cellular levels of cGMP (cyclic guanosine monophosphate), an energy substrate that is depleted by nitrate drugs. At day zero, all participants were measured to establish a baseline. After 3 days of vitamin C administration (2 grams, 3 times daily), there was no change in either group. After 6 days of vitamin C therapy an impressive 42% improvement in vasodilation response was observed and a 60% improvement in cellular cGMP levels was measured in coronary artery disease patients receiving vitamin C compared to placebo. A similar improvement occurred in the healthy subjects taking vitamin C compared to the placebo group. The doctors concluded the study by stating, "These results indicate that combination therapy with vitamin C is potentially useful for preventing the development of nitrate tolerance."

Another study published in the *Journal of Clinical Investigation* (1998, [July 1]) looked at the effects of nitrate drug therapy on human patients. Tolerance development was monitored by changes in arterial pressure, pulse pressure, heart rate, and activity of isolated patients. All patients experienced the deleterious effects of nitrate tolerance. However, when vitamin C was coadministered with the nitrate drugs, the effects of nitrate tolerance were virtually eliminated. The most significant improvement was a 310% improvement in the arterial conductivity test. The nitrate drugs induced a dangerous up-regulated activity of platelets, but this too was reversed with vitamin C supplementation. The doctors who conducted this study indicated that vitamin C may be of benefit during long-term, nonintermittent administration of nitrate drugs in humans.

An especially damaging effect of nitrate drugs is that they cause a decrease in the intracellular (inside the cells) production of cGMP, an energy substrate that is required to maintain cellular energy levels. Vitamin C has been shown to protect against nitrate-induced depletion of cGMP. In a study published in the May 22, 1998, issue of *FEBS Letters* (Netherlands), kidney cells exposed to 5 hours of pretreatment with a nitrate drug showed a substantial depletion of intracellular cGMP. When vitamin C was present during pretreatment with nitrate drugs, cGMP levels were 3.1-fold higher.

Chronic heart failure is associated with reduced dilating capacity of the endothelial lining of the arterial system. Scientists tested heart failure patients by high-resolution ultrasound and Doppler to measure radial artery diameter and blood flow. Vitamin C restored arterial dilation response and blood flow velocity in patients with heart failure. The scientists determined that the mechanism of action was that vitamin C increased the availability of nitric oxide, an important precursor to cGMP. This study was published in the February 1998 issue of the journal *Circulation*.

Also in 1998, another aspect of vitamin C's effect on coronary artery disease was discovered. A study published in the *Journal of the American College of Cardiology* (1998, 41 [5]:980–86) showed that low plasma ascorbic acid (vitamin C) levels independently predict the presence of an unstable coronary syndrome in heart disease patients. According to the doctors, the study's results showed that the beneficial effects of vitamin C in treating coronary artery disease may result, in part, by an influence on arterial wall lesion activity rather than a reduction in the overall extent of fixed disease.

The Institute of Public Health, Cambridge, UK, conducted one of the first systematic reviews of epidemiological studies of vitamin C and blood pressure in 1997. The scientists reviewed published cross-sectional studies, prospective studies, and trials in humans that examined the association between vitamin C intake or plasma vitamin C levels and blood pressure. Relevant references were located by MedLine search (1966–1996) and EMBASE search (1980–1996), by searching personal bibliographies, books and reviews, and from citations in located articles. The conclusion from this analysis of the published literature was as follows:

> We found a consistent cross-sectional association between higher vitamin C intake or status and lower BP, though no study controlled adequately for confounding by other dietary factors. Further cross-sectional studies are required to establish whether an independent association exists. If this is shown to be the case, larger and longer-term trials will be needed to confirm the association is causal. Potentially, the impact on cardiovascular disease of a modest change in mean population vitamin C intake is large (*Journal of Human Hypertension,* 1997 [June], 11 [6]:343–50).

A British Medical Research Council in Cambridge, UK, reported the benefits of vitamin C in 1998 from a large national survey as follows:

> Plasma ascorbate concentration was inversely correlated to systolic and diastolic blood pressures and pulse rate. Other covariates of blood pressure included age, sex, domicile, plasma retinol, fibrinogen and gamma-tocopherol concentrations, erythrocyte count, prothrombin time, and urine sodium:creatinine ratio. Covariates of pulse rate included sex, domicile, plasma fibrinogen and platelet count. Blood pressure was also correlated to intake of vitamin C. CONCLUSIONS: Plasma ascorbate concentration and intake of vitamin C are covariates of blood pressure in older people living in Britain (*Journal of Hypertension,* 1998 [July]).

Vitamin C clearly has a role to play in the integrative approach to controlling hypertension. The suggested dose for vitamin C is 2000 mg, 3 times a day.

Benefits of Arginine

Arginine can work synergistically with such ACE-inhibiting antihypertensive drugs as Vasotec, Capoten, and Zestril (see more on ACE inhibitors under the "Currently Prescribed Drugs" section of this protocol). This is important for those with chronic hypertension who fail to respond to conventional or alternative therapies.

Since the Life Extension Foundation's original recommendations about using arginine to treat hypertension were made in 1991, numerous new studies have been published indicating that arginine may be even more effective as an antihypertensive agent than was previously reported. Here is a summary of these new studies:

> The *l*-arginine-nitric oxide pathway appears to play an important role in systemic hypertension, progressive renal disease, nephrotoxicity (lead poisoning), inflammation and atherosclerosis (*Current Opinions in Nephrology and Hypertension,* 1998 [Sept], 7 [5]:547–50). These results support the roles of both increased endothelin synthesis and decreased nitric oxide activity in the pathogenesis of cyclosporin A–induced hypertension (*Journal Human Hypertension,* 1998 [Dec], 12 [12]:839–44).
>
> *l*-arginine supplementation improved the urinary NOx excretion and prevented hypertension. We conclude that hypoxia-induced sustained arterial hypertension is associated with depressed NO production and can be mitigated by *l*-arginine supplementation (*Kidney Int.*, 1998 [Jul], 54 [1]:188–92).
>
> Supplementation of *l*-arginine normalized the abnormality of renal hemodynamics accompanying salt-induced hypertension (*American Journal of Hypertension,* 1997 [May], 10 [5 Pt 2]:89S–93S).
>
> These findings demonstrated that *l*-arginine ameliorated adverse cardiovascular effects of hypertension in aged spontaneously hypertensive rats (SHRs) as demonstrated by reduced arterial pressure and total peripheral resistance, diminished left ventricular mass and collagen content, and improved coronary hemodynamics (*Hypertension,* 1999 [Jan], 33 [1 Pt 2]:451–55).
>
> University of Southern California researchers in Los Angeles reported a fall in blood pressure using *l*-arginine for hypertension in African Americans. The researchers pointed out that a defect in nitric oxide production may be a possible mechanism of hypertensive disease. Arginine enhances the body's natural synthesis of nitric oxide (*Journal of Human Hypertension,* 1997 [Aug], 11 [8]:527–32).

The suggested dose of arginine to lower blood pressure is 4500 mg, 3 times a day.

WARNING: If you'd like to see whether any of the nutritional antihypertensive agents can help you reduce the dosage or replace your antihypertensive drugs, extreme caution is mandatory and physician cooperation is essential. You should reduce the dosage of your antihypertensive drug very slowly while increasing your intake of the nutrient supplement(s). Monitor your blood pressure on a daily basis. If you do not exercise caution, an acute hypertensive event could occur, resulting in a stroke.

The DASH Diet

The DASH Diet enables many people to experience a blood pressure drop in 2 weeks, and many complain about having to eat too much food! What a diet! What a way to lower blood pressure without drugs.

High blood pressure affects one in four Americans, yet very few dietary guidelines have been promoted to control its effects on the body. However, a recent study known as the DASH trials, published in the *New England Journal of Medicine,* has provided evidence of a diet that seems to lower blood pressure quickly. The low-fat diet is high in fruits and vegetables and includes low-fat dairy products. The trials were funded by the National Heart, Lung, and Blood Institute (NHLBI) and supported by the other two branches of the National Institutes of Health (NIH).

The DASH trials began with 459 adults with systolic blood pressure of less than 160 mmHg and diastolic blood pressure between 80 and 95 mmHg. Of the participants, 133 had Stage I hypertension (140–159 mmHg systolic and 90–99 mmHg diastolic) for which no medication was taken. One half of the subjects were women; 60% were African Americans, who seem to develop hypertension earlier and more frequently than other racial groups. High blood pressure is defined as a systolic measure equal to or greater than 140 mmHg, a diastolic pressure greater than 90 mmHg, or both.

At the start of the study, all participants were given a control diet for 3 weeks that was low in fruits and vegetables, included low-fat dairy products, and approximated the daily fat intake of the average American. After this initial period, the subjects were divided into three groups. One continued with the control diet, one was given a "fruit and vegetable" diet, and one was given the "combination" diet: high in fruits and vegetables together with low-fat dairy products, and low in saturated and total fat.

Both noncontrol diets had about 8 to 10 times the average American's intake of fruits and vegetables, and the "combination" diet had about 2 to 3 times the normal intake of low-fat dairy products. The diets did not focus on a reduction in salt intake. In fact, the three diets had a sodium intake of about 3 grams per day, which is just slightly lower than that consumed by the average American. None of the diets was vegetarian or used any kind of fat substitutes, and all included a variety of foods that were fresh, dried, frozen, or canned. All three of the diets controlled for sodium levels, a possible confounding factor of the study because of its traditional role in blood pressure elevation.

Throughout the trials, blood pressures were monitored, and after 8 weeks the final levels were recorded. The "fruit and vegetable" diet produced a 2.8/1.1 mmHg reduction in blood pressure overall as compared to the control: among the 133 subjects with hypertension, it produced a reduction of 7.2/2.8 mmHg. The combination diet caused the most dramatic reduction in blood pressure, with an overall reduction of 5.5/3.0 mmHg and, in hypertensive participants, an overall reduction of 11.4/5.5 mmHg. An interesting phenomenon that was observed during the trials was that blood pressure reductions for the most part occurred within the first 2 weeks of the diet program, and subjects maintained these levels for the rest of the trials.

The principal complaint that subjects had about the diet was that they were required to eat too much food. A sample dinner might consist of 3 ounces of baked cod, 1 cup of rice, 2 cups of broccoli, 2 cups of stewed tomatoes, a small spinach salad, one whole-wheat dinner roll with a teaspoon of margarine, and 2 cups of melon balls. Participants said that they were not used to eating this much food. In a real-world situation, where a person is not required to maintain a constant body weight as the participants were in the DASH trials, the person would lose some weight.

The DASH trials produced some promising results. Blood pressure reductions were seen not only in those with hypertension, but also in those with normal-high blood pressure—in other words, those at risk of developing hypertension. These results suggest that the diet may be helpful not only in treating hypertension but in preventing it.

Furthermore, the diet's results in hypertensive subjects were similar to what one might expect from single-drug therapy, suggesting that the DASH diet may be a suitable substitute for drug treatment in some patients.

Although DASH researchers believe the diet to be a possible alternative to drug treatment, they warn that personal physicians should always be consulted before any kind of treatment modification is made. They also estimate that if all Americans adopted this diet, heart disease would decrease by 15% and strokes would decrease by 27%. The most sound advice that DASH supporters can give is to start to eat the DASH way gradually. Try to structure meals around vegetables and carbohydrates instead of around foods high in protein. Also remember that 8 to 10 servings of fruits and vegetables are not as much as one would think, because the recommended serving sizes are half of what the average American would consider to be a "serving."

More information on the DASH Diet can be found at [http://www.nih.gov/news/pr/apr97/Dash.htm].

DASH Diet sources: National Institutes of Health, press release, April 16, 1997; (*The New York Times,* June 4, 1997; *New England Journal of Medicine,* [April 17], 336:1117–18; National Institutes of Health, "The DASH Diet," April 3, 1997.

Currently Prescribed Drugs

People can control hypertension by using a wide variety of prescription drugs, with the medication being tailored to the individual. Some doctors will start with one type of drug and add others if necessary. Other doctors will start with one drug and, if it is ineffective, stop using it and prescribe another. In prescribing a drug, the doctor will consider factors such as age, sex, and race and will also consider the severity of the hypertension and other conditions such as high cholesterol and diabetes. Persons should notify their doctor about any side effects they are experiencing caused by the drugs so that the doctor can adjust the dosage or switch to another drug. It is important that people follow the directions of their doctor to the letter, and it is also important to have regular blood pressure monitoring to make sure that it is under control.

The first drug commonly given to a person with high blood pressure is a diuretic. This helps the kidneys eliminate salt and water, thereby decreasing the fluid volume throughout the body. Diuretics also dilate the blood vessels. Potassium and magnesium supplements or potassium-retaining drugs should sometimes be taken along with the diuretics. Blacks, the elderly, obese people, and people with heart or kidney failure should take diuretics.

Adrenergic blockers (including alpha- and beta-blockers, and alpha-beta-blockers) block the effects of the sympathetic nervous system, which causes stress and raises blood pressure. White people, young people, and people who have had heart attacks, chest pain, or migraine headaches should take adrenergic blockers.

Angiotensin-converting enzyme inhibitors (ACE inhibitors) block an enzyme that constricts the arteries. White people, young people, people suffering from heart failure, and people suffering from chronic or diabetic kidney disease should take these drugs.

Other drugs that can be taken by people suffering from hypertension are vasodilators and calcium antagonists. The vasodilators cause the muscle in the walls of the blood vessels to relax, allowing the blood vessels to dilate. This drug is added as a second drug when the first drug does not sufficiently lower the blood pressure. Calcium antagonists reduce the heart rate and relax the blood vessels by reducing the amount of calcium that is able to enter the cells.

The latest class of antihypertensive drugs consists of the angiotensin II receptor antagonists, sold under brand names such as Atacand, Cozaar, or Hyzaar. Ask your doctor about this new class of antihypertensive medication if you are not satisfied with the drugs you currently are using.

For those patients currently taking hypertensive drugs (or now being recommended to take drugs), several new recommendations from the *Journal of the American Medical Association (JAMA),* June 1998, may be of value, especially to those who have been taking drugs long-term, those not receiving adequate declines in blood pressure, or those encountering adverse side effects.

Diuretics have again been recommended by the Sixth Joint National Committee on

Prevention, Detection, Evaluation, and Treatment of High Blood Pressure (JNC VI) as one of the *first-choice medications in the management of hypertension*. This recommendation is based on the results of numerous randomized, diuretic-based, long-term controlled clinical trials, involving a total of 16,164 elderly patients, that have demonstrated a reduction in both cerebrovascular and cardiovascular morbidity.

Despite this and other national recommendations, the use of diuretics has steadily decreased over the past 15 years. Reasons include heavy promotion of other medications, as well as many physicians' perception that diuretics produce adverse metabolic effects and do not reduce coronary heart disease events. Data, however, now indicate that (1) changes in glucose and cholesterol metabolism are minor, especially with the smaller doses now being used; (2) cardiovascular morbidity and mortality have been reduced in hypertensive patients, even in those with hyperlipidemia or diabetes, when diuretics are used; and (3) concerns about hypokalemia-induced arrhythmias have been overstated.

> While special indications exist for other medications in the treatment of hypertension, diuretics should be used more, not less frequently; use of diuretics would reduce the number of resistant hypertensive patients (*JAMA* 1998 [Jun 10]; 279 [22]:1813–16).

The antihypertensive drug Hyzaar is both an angiotensin II receptor–antagonist and a diuretic. Many new antihypertensive drugs are advertising once-a-day dosing. What patients don't know is that some people need to take these drugs more often for 24-hour a day control of hypertension. Learn how to take your own blood pressure so that you can determine whether your "one-a-day" drug is really providing 24 hours of benefit. (Some hypertensives may need to take their medications twice a day.)

Aspirin Reduces Cardiovascular Complications Associated with Hypertension

Despite treatment, there is often a higher incidence of cardiovascular complications in patients with hypertension than in normotensive individuals. Inadequate reduction of their blood pressure is a likely cause, but the optimum target blood pressure has not been known. A 1998 study to determine the impact of aspirin as an integrated therapy for hypertension was investigated. A total of 18,790 patients from 26 countries, aged 50 to 80 years (mean 61.5 years) with hypertension and diastolic blood pressure between 100 mmHg and 115 mmHg (mean 105 mmHg) were randomly assigned a target diastolic blood pressure. The study was designed to assess the optimum target diastolic blood pressure for hypertensive patients and the potential benefit of a low dose of aspirin in the treatment of hypertension. The doctors discovered:

> Intensive lowering of blood pressure in patients with hypertension was associated with a low rate of cardiovascular events. The [study] shows the benefits of lowering the diastolic blood pressure down to 82.6 mmHg. Acetylsalicylic acid (aspirin) significantly reduced major cardiovascular events with the greatest benefit seen in all myocardial infarction. There was no effect on the incidence of stroke or fatal bleeds, but non-fatal major bleeds were twice as common (*Lancet,* 1998 [June 13], 351 [9118]:1755–62).

Please refer to newly added recommendation for aspirin, as part of an integrated hypertension therapy listed below in the protocol.

Conclusions and Precautions

Our general precaution is that is if you're going to attempt to use any of the nutrients the Foundation recommends to replace antihypertensive drugs, you must do so with the cooperation of your physician. You cannot assume that any nutrients will be able to replace a drug that already is effectively controlling your blood pressure. Daily blood-pressure monitoring is mandatory to ensure that the nutrient regimen you are following is really keeping your blood pressure under control.

If nutrients fail to keep your blood pressure under control, our favorite class of antihypertensive drugs continues to be the angiotensin II receptor antagonists, such as Cozaar or Hyzaar. Ask your doctor about this new class of antihypertensive medication if you are not satisfied with the drugs you currently are using. Many new antihypertensive drugs are advertising once-a-day dosing. What patients don't know is that some people need to take these drugs more often for 24-hour a day control of hypertension. Learn how to take your own blood pressure so that you can determine whether your "one-a-day" drug is really providing 24 hours of benefit.

NOTE: Those with hypertension often have artery disease (*see the Atherosclerosis protocol for additional suggestions*).

Summary

1. Have your blood pressure checked regularly.
2. Stop smoking.
3. Avoid sodium (salt) intake. About a third of the people who have hypertension can be helped by lowering salt intake. Try to reduce your salt intake to about 1 to 12 teaspoonsful a day.
4. Eat more fresh fruits, vegetables, and foods high in fiber and food that has less fat.
5. Reduce stress on and off the job.
6. Moderate alcohol intake. It is now known that a moderate amount of alcohol can help decrease your risk for heart problems, but it should not exceed 3 ounces a day.
7. Exercise regularly and keep weight within normal limits.
8. Take garlic, 1500 to 6000 mg a day, and Coenzyme Q10, 200 to 300 mg a day, in combination to lower blood pressure.
9. Take magnesium, 500 to 1500 elemental milligrams a day.
10. Take calcium, 1000 elemental milligrams a day.
11. Take potassium, to be prescribed by your doctor: often 400 to 500 mg a day.
12. Take fish oil concentrate, 8 to 10 capsules of Mega EPA fish oil capsules a day.
13. Take vitamin C, 2000 mg, 3 times a day.
14. Take arginine in doses of 4500 mg, 3 times a day.
15. Take low-dose aspirin: 1/4 aspirin tablet every day with the heaviest meal of the day, to reduce possible cardiovascular complications associated with hypertension.
16. Precisely follow your doctor's prescribed drug regimen.

Diuretics, beta-blockers, central-acting sympatholytics, alpha-blockers, vasodilators, angiotensin-converting enzyme inhibitors, and calcium-channel blockers, among others, are drugs that can be prescribed to lower blood pressure. It cannot be stressed enough that you should be sure to follow the doctor's directions exactly if the doctor prescribes medicine to lower your blood pressure and also make sure the doctor knows all the prescribed and over-the-counter medicines you are taking.

For more information. Contact the American Heart Association, 7272 Greenville Ave., Dallas, TX 75231; (800) 242-8721, Monday to Friday, 8:30 A.M. to 5:00 P.M. CST; the National Heart, Lung, and Blood Institute Information Center, P.O. Box 30105, Bethesda, MD 20824-0105; (800) 575-WELL, 24-hr recorded information, (301) 251-1222, Monday to Friday, 8:30 A.M. to 5:00 P.M. EST.

Product availability. CoQ_{10}, Mega EPA, garlic, vitamin C, Life Extension Mix, garlic, potassium, calcium, magnesium, and arginine are available by calling (800) 544-4440, or order online at www.lef.org. Prescription drugs cited should be prescribed by a doctor who treats hypertension.

HYPOGLYCEMIA

Definition

Hypoglycemia literally means "low blood sugar" and is often mistaken for a disease when it is actually a symptom. Ingested sugars and carbohydrates trigger a release of the hormone insulin from the pancreas. Insulin helps the body turn sugars into energy and stored fats. In some people, the amount of insulin released is too high for the amount of carbohydrates ingested, resulting in too much sugar being burned up too quickly. A net loss of blood sugar results. In hypoglycemia attacks, there is too much insulin and not enough blood sugar, causing fatigue, weakness, loss of consciousness, and even death. There are three general types of hypoglycemia. Two of them are rare organic forms involving the pancreas. The third and most common form is called functional hypoglycemia (FH) and is usually caused by an inadequate diet too high in sugar and refined carbohydrates. Hypoglycemia may be better described as carbohydrate intolerance: the body is unable to absorb certain carbohydrate loads effectively without adverse consequences. Different people react differently to ingested sugars and carbohydrates, with some having a higher tolerance level than others.

Although predisposition to FH may be an inherited condition and is most often due to dietary factors, it can also be found in people with such disorders as schizophrenia, alcoholism, drug addiction, juvenile delinquency, hyperactivity, diabetes, and obesity. In some people, severe FH can contribute to other illnesses such as epilepsy, allergies, asthma, ulcers, arthritis, impotence, and mental disorders.

Symptoms of Hypoglycemia

Symptoms include

- Fatigue, dizziness, shakiness, and faintness
- Irritability and depression
- Weakness or cramps in feet or legs
- Numbness or tingling in the hands, feet, or face
- Ringing in the ears
- Swollen feet or legs
- Tightness in chest
- Frequent heart pounding or palpitations
- Anxiety, nightmares, and panic attacks
- Night sweats
- Constant hunger
- Headaches and migraines
- Impaired memory and concentration
- Blurring of vision
- Nasal congestion
- Abdominal cramps, loose stool, or diarrhea

FH may be considered subclinical, meaning that symptoms are subtle, episodic, and difficult to diagnose. Patients may have a low but acceptable blood sugar level that does not drop until the last hours of a prolonged test. Glucose tolerance tests often miss the lowest blood sugar levels that had triggered acute symptoms. Severe regular attacks of hypoglycemia may have diabetes as the underlying cause. If symptoms persist, see your doctor.

Hypoglycemia and Diet

A perfectly regulated diet can help to control hypoglycemia. Usually a regime high in protein, unrefined carbohydrates (slow to be absorbed such as whole-grain products and vegetables), and moderate fats is recommended. Heavily sugared foods should be avoided, and foods high in natural sugars should be restricted. Alcohol, caffeine, tobacco, and other stimulants should be avoided, because they are capable of precipitating an attack. Small meals taken often during the day are recommended to control the amount of carbohydrates entering the system.

Short-term treatment focuses on raising the blood sugar level without delay. Any substance containing simple sugars, such as fruit juice, soft drinks, or candy—if taken at the onset of a hypoglycemic episode—will help to raise blood sugar quickly and ease the severity of the attack. Sugar combined with a protein source, such as a glass of milk or a piece of cheese, will help slow the absorption of glucose into the system, avoiding the "seesaw" effect caused by rapidly changing blood sugar levels.

The Role of Nutritional Supplementation

Hypoglycemia may damage brain cells. When hippocampal brain-cell cultures are deprived of glucose, a massive release of lactate dehydrogenase (LDH) occurs, which is an indicator of neuronal death. The addition of the vitamin B_6 metabolite pyridoxal 5-phosphate has been shown to inhibit the LDH release. When pyridoxal 5-phosphate is given before glucose deprivation, a more potent inhibitory effect on LDH release has been observed. Scientists have suggested that pyridoxal 5-phosphate protects neurons from glucose deprivation-induced damage. These scientists recommend that pyridoxal 5-phosphate be used prophylactically to protect against brain-cell death induced by metabolic disorders such as hypoglycemia.

Another possible cause of low blood sugar is the inability to release glycogen (stored sugar in the liver), secondary to vitamin B_6 and chromium deficiency. Some hypoglycemics are helped by the daily administration of 100 to 250 mg of pyridoxal 5-phosphate and 200 mg of chromium. Chromium is a mineral found in brewer's yeast, whole-grain breads and cereals, molasses, cheese, and lean meats and as a dietary supplement.

Too much insulin in the blood can be partially neutralized by taking the amino acid cysteine along with vitamin B_1 and vitamin C. Hypoglycemics should start with once-a-day doses of 500 mg of cysteine along with 250 mg of vitamin B_1 and 1500 mg of vitamin C. This dose should be administered twice daily during the second week and 3 times a day by the third week. The objective is to prevent hypoglycemic attacks by neutralizing excess insulin. Every hypoglycemic is slightly different, so the dosage ranges will vary from person to person.

Hypoglycemia and Diabetes

Hypoglycemia can also be a common complication of diabetes. Diabetes occurs when the body cannot use glucose for fuel because either the pancreas is not able to make enough insulin or the insulin that is available is not effective. As a result, glucose builds up in the blood instead of getting into body cells. The aim of treatment in diabetes is to lower high blood sugar levels. To do this, people with diabetes may use insulin or oral drugs, depending on the type of diabetes they have or the severity of their condition.

Summary

1. A perfectly regulated diet can help to control hypoglycemia.
2. Fruit juice, soft drinks, or sweets, if taken at the onset of a hypoglycemic episode, help to ease the severity of the attack quickly.
3. Some hypoglycemics are helped by the daily administration of 100 to 250 mg of the vitamin B_6 metabolite pyridoxal 5-phosphate and 200 mcg of chromium.
4. Hypoglycemics should start with once-a-day doses of 500 mg of cysteine along with 250 mg of vitamin B_1 and 1500 mg of vitamin C. Increase this regimen to 2 to 3 times a day.

For more information. Contact the Hypoglycemia Association, Inc. (HAI), (202) 544-4044, Box 165, Ashton, MD 20861-0165.

Product availability. The amino acid cysteine, vitamin B_1, vitamin B_6, pyridoxal 5-phosphate, vitamin C capsules, and chromium picolinate are available by calling (800) 544-4440, or order online at www.lef.org.

IMMUNE ENHANCEMENT

The Life Extension Foundation's Immune Enhancement protocol is designed to enhance immune function in aging patients, in patients receiving cancer chemotherapy, and in those suffering from chronic viral or bacterial infections.

The Harmful Role of Free Radicals

Free radicals have been linked to immune system damage that accompanies normal aging. A strong immune system is critical to the prevention of infection by viruses, fungi, and bacteria. It is thought that cancer cells form regularly, and that a vigilant immune response is therefore required to kill or deactivate these deformed cells before they become malignant tumors. Members of the Life Extension Foundation have long been encouraged to follow a daily antioxidant regimen that protects against immune-suppressing free radicals.

The incidence of cancer and new infectious diseases increases every year in the United States. In addition, many dangerous bacteria have become resistant to the antibiotics that once kept them in check. These virulent, antibiotic-resistant strains of bacteria are increasingly becoming a threat to our lives. There is strong scientific evidence showing that antioxidants and other natural therapies can play an important role in maintaining and enhancing immune function.

Nutritional Immunology

The concept that appropriate nutrients can enhance the human immune response is known as nutritional immunology. The foundation of this field of study was laid in the early 1800s when physicians discovered that severe malnutrition led to thymic atrophy. For most of that century, the evidence of a relationship between malnutrition and the immune system was based on anatomical findings. With the discovery of vitamins, it became evident that essential nutrients played a critical role in maintaining immune function.

Studies published in the 1980s and 1990s clearly show specific immune-enhancing effects of the proper use of nutritional supplements, proteins, hormones, and certain drugs. Micronutrients are now known to play a key role in many of the metabolic processes that promote survival from critical illnesses. The paragraphs that follow discuss nutrient supplements, proteins, and hormones, and examine their role in enhancing the human immune system.

The Role of Vitamins

Vitamins are essential for oxidative phosphorylation and protection against oxidants. Dietary supplementation with ascorbic acid, tocopherols, and vitamin B_6 enhances several aspects of lymphocyte function. Benefits are most evident in the elderly.

Vitamin A

During the 1920s and 1930s, vitamin A became known as the *anti-infective* vitamin, and the first attempts were made to use vitamin A therapeutically during the course of infectious illnesses. The first systematic studies of immunonutritional interrelationships in laboratory animals were initiated in 1947 by Abraham E. Axelrod and his students. Human studies soon followed—and, by the late 1970s, the field of nutritional immunology was well established. Newer research into vitamin A shows its importance to overall good health and its protective effects against tumor growth.

I

Beta-Carotene

Beta-carotene has been shown to have a powerful effect in boosting natural killer (NK) cell activity in elderly men. In a controlled, double-blind study, the effects of 10 to 12 years of beta-carotene supplementation on NK cell activity were evaluated. While no significant difference was seen in NK cell activity in the middle-aged groups, elderly men supplemented with beta-carotene had significantly greater NK cell activity than the corresponding control group (of elderly men) who were receiving placebo.

Results show that long-term beta-carotene supplementation may be beneficial for immune viral and tumoral surveillance. A French study using mice concluded that, though beta-carotene supplementation resulted in a nonsignificant increase in NK cells in the spleen, their killing capacity was significantly enhanced after beta-carotene supplementation. The treatment had no adverse effects.

Vitamin E

The best-publicized study of the use of vitamin E to boost immune function appeared in the *Journal of the American Medical Association (JAMA),* 1997, 277 17 [1380–86]: The double-blind, placebo-controlled study looked at healthy humans at least 65 years of age. Supplementation with vitamin E for 4 months improved certain clinically relevant indices of cell-mediated immunity. These results clearly show that a level of vitamin greater than that currently recommended by the FDA enhances certain clinically relevant *in vivo* indices of T-cell-mediated immune function in healthy elderly persons.

Oral alpha-tocopherol supplementation at the rate of 100 mg per day significantly increased natural killer (NK) cell activity in a 16-month-old Japanese boy with Shwachman syndrome (associated with severe vitamin E deficiency). The study—published in the *European Journal of Pediatrics,* 1997, 156 6 [444–8]: shows that severe vitamin E deficiency causes impaired NK cell activity, but that the condition is reversible with alpha-tocopherol supplementation.

Vitamin E's antioxidant activity is also crucial to cardiovascular health. Large amounts of vitamin E have been shown to lower cholesterol levels and protect arteries from free-radical damage. The natural platelet adhesion-inhibitory properties of vitamin E make it a potential antithrombotic agent as well.

Vitamin C and Ascorbic Acid

High levels of vitamin C can protect levels of vitamin E in tissue and may contribute to the immunoenhancement of vitamin E.

A steady supply of vitamin C is vital to good health. Because the human body can neither manufacture nor store vitamin C, our requirements must be met from dietary sources such as fruit, vegetables, and supplements. Vitamin C's antioxidant protection is especially important to healthy lungs. Numerous studies have shown that vitamin C protects the airways against inhaled (environmental) and internal oxidants. Individuals suffering from asthma, allergies, and sensitive respiratory systems will receive significant protection from adequate doses of vitamin C.

Trace Elements

It is now understood that trace elements are essential not only for their direct antioxidant activity, but also for their role as cofactors for a number of antioxidant enzymes. Wound healing and immune function are highly dependent on adequate levels of trace elements, as well as vitamin levels. Dietary supplements of trace elements are crucial to compensate for mineral-depleted soils providing much of the food we eat.

Zinc

The trace element zinc has many roles in basic cellular function. These include DNA replication, RNA transcription, cell division, and cell activation. Zinc also functions as an antioxidant and stabilizes membranes. Zinc-deficient patients display reduced resistance to infection. Zinc's importance in many aspects of the immune system—from skin barrier to lymphocyte gene regulation—may be based on its importance in cellular function. Zinc is also needed for the normal development and function of the cells which mediate nonspecific immunity (such as neutrophils and natural killer cells). Zinc deficiency is known to enhance the development of acquired immunity by preventing the outgrowth of and certain functions of T-lymphocytes such as activation, cytokine production, and B-lymphocyte help.

Immune dysfunction and susceptibility to infection have been observed in zinc-deficient human subjects. A study investigated the production of cytokines and characterized the T-cell subpopulations in three groups of mildly zinc-deficient subjects. These included head and neck cancer patients, healthy volunteers found to have a dietary deficiency of zinc, and healthy volunteers in whom a zinc deficiency was induced by dietary means.

The study demonstrated that zinc status affects cytokine levels. Production of interleukin-2 and gamma-interferon was decreased even when the zinc deficiency was mild. Natural killer cell activity was also decreased in zinc-deficient subjects. T-cell formation was decreased even in mildly zinc-deficient subjects. The study demonstrates the crucial role of zinc in promoting specific immune responses.

Copper, Manganese, Selenium

In addition to zinc, copper, manganese, and selenium act as cofactors of antioxidant enzymes to protect against oxygen free radicals produced during oxidative stress. Though all are essential, selenium is found to be most deficient in traumatized patients. In recent years the benefits of selenium have been recognized by researchers as an effective protector against certain cancers—such as breast, lung, liver, urogenital, colorectal, prostate, and ovarian—by removing harmful lipids and hydroperoxides from the body.

A convenient way of obtaining most of the nutrients needed for healthy immune function is to take 3 tablets, 3 times a day, of the 63-ingredient Life Extension Mix. One capsule a day of Life Extension Booster provides additional amounts of the nutrients that protect immune system cells against damaging free radicals.

Echinacea and Ginseng

Echinacea is also known as purple cornflower and is a member of the daisy family. Echinacea's ability to fight cold viruses and respiratory infections has long been known. Studies have shown that echinacea increases antibody production, reduces inflammation, and enables white blood cells to migrate to the infection site.

There are many varieties of the herb ginseng which is found primarily in Asia and the United States studies by Chinese researchers have demonstrated that red panax ginseng (*Panax ginseng*) cuts the risk of many types of cancer, including lung, liver, ovarian, pancreatic, colorectal, and stomach cancers. Some users of ginseng claim that it boosts energy and it may improve mental functioning, especially under stress.

CAUTION: Ginseng should not be taken with monoamine oxidase inhibitors, certain antipsychotic medications, or in addition to hormone replacement therapy.

In a controlled study at the Irvine Medical Center of the University of California, *Echinacea purpurea* and *Panax ginseng* were evaluated for their capacity to stimulate cellular immune function in normal individuals, as well as in patients with either chronic fatigue syndrome or acquired immunodeficiency syndrome (AIDS). Both extracts significantly enhanced the NK function of all test groups, both in combination and separately. Supplementation with either herb increased other measurements of immune competence. The study shows that extracts of echinacea and ginseng enhance cellular immune function in normal individuals, as well as in patients with depressed cellular immunity.

Grape Seed–Skin Extract

The effects of the proanthocyanidins found in grape seed–skin extract on immune dysfunction were studied in mice. The proanthocyanidin enhanced *in vitro* interleukin-2 production and natural killer cell cytotoxicity.

In addition, grape seed–skin extract strengthens weak and diseased blood vessels, making it effective in the treatment of cardiovascular disease. In patients with diabetes, grape seed–skin extract has lessened capillary hemorrhaging, which leads to diabetic retinopathy.

The powdered Life Extension Herbal Mix incorporates 27 different herbs into one daily drink. Many of these herbs have shown immune-enhancing effects. The suggested daily dose is 1 tablespoon taken first thing in the morning.

Rice Bran Extract—Arabinoxylane (MGN-3)

In research at the Department of Otolaryngology of Drew University of Medicine and Science, MGN-3 was examined for its effect on human NK cell activity. During 2 months of supplementation, NK activity was shown to have increased significantly, leading to the conclusion that MGN-3 could be used as a new biological response modifier with possible therapeutic effects against cancer. More research is needed into the benefits of this supplement.

Whey Protein Concentrate

Whey protein concentrate dramatically raises glutathione levels. Glutathione protects immune cells and detoxifies harmful compounds in the body. Glutathione is intimately tied to immunity. Reduced glutathione levels have been associated with AIDS and other viral diseases, and raising glutathione levels appears to be one way of modulating immunity.

In one study, glutathione in animals was raised to higher-than-normal levels by whey protein better than by other proteins, including soy. A study involving HIV-positive men fed whey protein concentrate found dramatic increases in glutathione levels, with most men reaching their ideal body weight. Whey protein improves immune function and fights infections. Immune response also was dramatically enhanced in animals fed whey protein concentrate when exposed to such immune challenges as salmonella, streptococcus pneumonia, and cancer-causing chemicals. Again, this effect on immunity was not seen with other proteins.

Studies have examined the impact of whey protein concentrate on preventing or treating cancer. When different groups of rats were given a powerful carcinogen, those fed whey protein concentrate showed fewer tumors and a reduced pooled area of tumors (tumor mass index). The researchers found that whey protein offered "considerable protection to the host" over that of other proteins. It should be noted that not all whey protein concentrates are created equal. Processing whey protein to remove the lactose and fats without eliminating its biological activity requires special care by the manufacturer. The process must use low temperature and low acid conditions so as not to "denature" the protein. Maintaining the natural state of the protein is essential to its biological activity. Immune-suppressed patients should consider taking 30 grams a day of specially designed whey protein concentrate.

L-Carnitine

L-carnitine is an amino acid compound produced within the body that has been shown to be effective in lessening memory loss and mental alertness due to aging and Alzheimer's disease. *L*-carnitine initiates a cascade effect of chemical activity within the brain, acting as an antioxidant to prevent free-radical damage and assisting in energy supply. It also assists in the production of acetylcholine, an important chemical messenger within the brain.

Several studies in the published literature have shown that *L*-carnitine can help memory and alertness in those suffering from age-related cognitive functioning and also in those suffering from memory loss due to alcoholism. In Alzheimer's patients, *L*-carnitine has been shown to slow the disease progression, especially at early onset (*see the Alzheimer's Disease protocol*).

In addition to its memory-enhancing effects, *L*-carnitine may also provide cardiac protection to cancer patients. Researchers have studied the effect of *L*-carnitine on doxorubicin-induced damage in the perfused rat heart. Doxorubicin is a cytotoxic antibiotic derived from *Streptomyces* and used in the treatment of sarcoma, acute leukemia, malignant lymphoma, and other cancers. In the study presented in *Pharmacology Research,* doxorubicin-induced metabolic damage was carried out in isolated cardiac myocytes and in isolated heart mitochondria, causing a significant 70% inhibition of palmitate oxidation in cardiac myocytes. Researchers found, however, that perfusion of the heart with *L*-carnitine after 10 minutes perfusion with doxorubicin caused an 88% reversal of induced inhibition of palmitate oxidation in cardiac cells. In addition, *L*-carnitine treatment did not interfere with the cytotoxic effect of doxorubicin against the growth of solid Ehrlich carcinoma. Researchers concluded that "inhibition of fatty acid oxidation in the heart is at least a part of doxorubicin cardiotoxicity and that *L*-carnitine can be used to prevent the doxorubicin-induced cardiac metabolic damage without interfering with its antitumor activities."

Coenzyme Q_{10}

Coenzyme Q_{10} is an important antioxidant produced in the body and found in small amounts in some foods. Researchers are not yet in agreement on whether CoQ_{10} should be classified as a vitamin. CoQ_{10} is found in high concentrations in the healthy heart, where it plays an important role in initiating cell-produced energy. Studies have documented its effectiveness in improving the quality of life in people with advanced heart disease, congestive heart failure, angina, and arrhythmia.

Researchers concluded in the January 1999 *International Journal of Cardiology* that serum concentration of lipoprotein-*a* decreases on treatment with hydrosoluble Coenzyme Q_{10} in patients with coronary artery disease. In a randomized double-blind, placebo-controlled trial, subjects with clinical diagnosis of acute myocardial infarction, unstable angina, angina pectoris with moderately raised lipoprotein-*a* received either Coenzyme Q_{10}, 60 mg twice daily, or placebo for a period of 28 days. Serum lipoprotein-*a* showed significant reduction in the Coenzyme Q_{10} group compared with the placebo group (31.0% vs. 8.2% $p < 0.001$), with a net reduction of 22.6% attributed to Coenzyme Q_{10}. HDL cholesterol (the good type) showed a significant increase in the CoQ_{10} group without affecting total cholesterol, while LDL cholesterol (the bad type) and blood glucose showed a significant reduction. As an added benefit, Coenzyme Q_{10} was also associated with significant reductions in thiobarbituric acid reactive substances, and malon/dialdehyde and diene conjugates, indicating an overall decrease in oxidative stress.

Coenzyme Q_{10} administration increases brain mitochondrial concentrations and exerts neuroprotective effects. Coenzyme Q_{10} is an essential cofactor of the electron transport chain as well as a potent free-radical scavenger in lipid and mitochondrial membranes. This was demonstrated by studies published in the *Proc. Natl. Acad. Sci. (USA)*. Feeding rodents with Coenzyme Q_{10} resulted in increased mitochondrial concentrations in the cerebral cortex. Oral administration of Coenzyme Q_{10} also markedly weakened striatal lesions produced by systemic administration of 3-nitropropionic acid in a mouse model with familial amyotrophic lateral sclerosis (ALS), significantly increasing life span. These results show that oral administration of Coenzyme Q_{10} increases both brain and brain mitochondrial concentrations and provides further evidence that Coenzyme Q_{10} can exert neuroprotective effects that might be useful in the treatment of neurodegenerative diseases.

CoQ_{10} has also shown promise in clinical trials on breast cancer patients in which tumor spread and mortality rate were significantly lowered with trial dosages. Additional research is needed to determine long-term toxicity in cancer treatment.

DHEA

DHEA levels decline 80 to 90% by age 70 or later. DHEA has demonstrated a striking ability to maintain immune system synchronization. Oral supplementation with low doses of DHEA in aged animals restored immunocompetence to a reasonable level within days of administration. DHEA supplementation in aged rodents resulted in almost complete restoration of immune function.

DHEA has been shown in numerous animals studies to boost immune function via several different mechanisms. Only limited human studies have been done to measure DHEA's effect on the immune system.

In a 1997 study, scientists proposed that the oral administration of DHEA to elderly men would result in activation of their immune systems. Nine healthy men averaging 63 years of age were treated with a placebo for 2 weeks followed by 20 weeks of DHEA (50 mg/day). After 2 weeks on oral DHEA, serum DHEA levels increased by three to fourfold. These levels were sustained throughout the study. Compared to the placebo, DHEA administration resulted in

- An increase of 20% in IGF-1. Many people are taking expensive growth hormone injections for the purpose of boosting IGF levels. IGF stands for insulin-like growth factor and is thought to be responsible for some of the anti-aging, anabolic effects that DHEA has produced in previous human studies.
- An increase of 35% in the number of monocyte immune cells.
- An increase of 29% in the number of B immune cells and a 62% increase in B-cell activity.
- A 40% increase in T-cell activity even though the total number of T-cells were not affected.
- An increase of 50% in interleukin-2.
- An increase of 22 to 37% in number of natural killer (NK) cells and an increase of 45% in NK cell activity.
- No adverse effects were noted with DHEA administration.

The scientists concluded, "While extended studies are required, our findings suggest potential therapeutic benefits of DHEA in immunodeficient states" (*Journal of Gerontology,* Series A, 1997, 52 [1]).

A study in the *Journal of Clinical Endocrine Metabolism* (June 1998) showed that when old female mice were treated with DHEA, melatonin, or DHEA plus melatonin, splenocytes (macrophages) were significantly higher as compared to young mice. B-cell proliferation in young and in old mice significantly increased. DHEA, melatonin, and DHEA plus melatonin helped to regulate immune function in aged female mice by significantly increasing cytokines, interleukin-2, and interferon-gamma and significantly decreasing cytokines, interleukin-6, and interleukin-10, thus regulating cytokine production.

Interleukin-6 (IL-6) is one of the pathogenic elements in inflammatory and age-related diseases such as rheumatoid arthritis, osteoporosis, atherosclerosis, and late-onset B-cell neoplasia. "Higher circulating levels of IL-6 predict disability onset in older persons," according to their report in the June 1999 issue of the *Journal of the American Geriatrics Society* (47:639–46, 755–56). The authors suggest that IL-6 may cause a reduction in muscle strength or contribute to specific diseases such as congestive heart failure, osteoporosis, arthritis, and dementia, which cause disability.

DHEA has consistently been shown to boost beneficial interleukin-2 and suppress damaging interleukin-6 levels. Interleukin-6 is overproduced in the aged, which contributes to autoimmune disease, immune dysfunction, osteoporosis, depressions in healing, breast cancer, and B-cell lymphoma and anemia. Chronic DHEA administration maintained immunocompetence in aged animals by boosting interleukin-2 and other beneficial immune components, and by suppressing interleukin-6 and other detrimental immune components. Suppression of IL-6 with 200 mg a day of DHEA was shown to be effective against systemic lupus erythematosus (*J. Rheumatol.,* 1998 Feb., 25:2, 285–89).

Researchers compared levels of IL-6 in 283 subjects with a mobility or functional disability, with IL-6 levels in 350 adults without a disability. The investigators found that adults in the highest third of values of IL-6 had a 76% higher rate for mobility disabilities and 62% higher rate for inability to perform daily activities than subjects in the lowest third of values. "These data suggest that IL-6 is a global marker of impending deterioration in health status in older adults," writes a team led by Dr. Luigi Ferrucci at the National Institute on Aging in Bethesda, Maryland.

In a study in the *Proceedings of the Society for Experimental Biology and Medicine* (1998 [May]; 218 [1]:76–82), DHEA was shown to restore normal cytokine production in immune system dysfunction induced by aging by suppressing the excessive production of cytokines (IL-6) by 75%, while increasing IL-2 secretion by nearly 50%, during a leukemia virus infection in old mice.

For DHEA dosing information and safety precautions, refer to the *DHEA Replacement Therapy protocol.*

Melatonin and KH3

Aging, cancer, AIDS, chemotherapy, and infectious agents can all stimulate excessive cortisol production from the adrenal glands, decimating immune function, and leading to immune system destruction and desynchronization. It is crucial to inhibit excessive cortisol production. (*As has been noted in the HIV Infection (AIDS) protocol, there are 17 European studies showing that HIV causes the destruction of the immune system by stimulating excessive cortisol production.*)

DHEA and melatonin work together to suppress cortisol levels. High doses of the European procaine drug KH3, taken at least twice per day, is suggested as the best way of protecting against the effects of elevated cortisol levels so often seen in cancer, AIDS, and stressed-out patients. One to two tablets of KH3 can be taken first thing in the morning on an empty stomach, with the same dose taken again 1 hour before dinner on an empty stomach. It is difficult to test cortisol levels in the blood because adrenal surges of cortisol can occur erratically throughout the day, which is one reason why this important cause of immune system destruction has been largely ignored by American doctors.

The most effective hormone therapy to protect and improve immune function is melatonin, which enhances the production of T-helper cells, which are necessary to identify cancer cells, viruses, fungi, and bacteria. Melatonin enhances the production of other immune components, including natural killer cells, interleukin-2, interleukin-4, interleukin-10, gamma-interferon, and eosinophils. The latest evidence suggests that melatonin is even more effective than nutrient antioxidants in suppressing immune cell-killing free radicals.

Biostim

Influenza and other infectious diseases tend to be more severe in older patients. Despite immunization, elderly people often lack the immune capacity to generate an antibody response to prevent infection from the influenza virus. As many as 69,000 Americans have died from influenza in a bad epidemic year. Biostim is a French drug that has been shown to prevent infectious diseases in the elderly. It is used in Europe to boost immune function and treat certain infectious diseases.

An examination of the published literature reveals that if Biostim were available in the United States, thousands of American lives could be saved every year. These studies also indicate that Biostim would dramatically reduce the need for antibiotic therapy, thereby saving untold millions of dollars in prescription drug costs.

A double-blind trial was conducted to evaluate the capacity of Biostim to diminish the frequency of infectious episodes in chronic bronchitis. The study duration was 9 months. Of the 73 subjects selected, 38 received Biostim and 35 a placebo. By the ninth month, the duration in days of infectious episodes was 60% lower in the Biostim group compared with the placebo group. The use of antibiotic therapy was reduced by 81% in the Biostim group compared with the placebo group. Prewinter administration of Biostim to subjects significantly diminished the frequency of infectious episodes, and thus the consumption of antibiotics.

In another study, 314 elderly subjects admitted to hospitals were given either Biostim or a placebo. The subjects were regularly examined every 3 months for 1 year. The incidence of acute infectious episodes was evaluated in both groups. The number of subjects with infection in the group receiving the Biostim was significantly lower than in the placebo group. In the group receiving the Biostim, the number of infectious episodes was reduced throughout the 12 months of the trial. Finally, there was a significant decrease in the duration of antibiotic therapy. Biostim was well tolerated. This study shows that Biostim is effective in protecting elderly, and therefore fragile, subjects against respiratory infections.

An evaluation of the safety of Biostim given with an antibiotic to treat acute infections was performed in three double-blind, placebo-controlled studies on fragile institutionalized or hospitalized patients. Two of the studies showed that in acute respiratory infections, Biostim was well tolerated and resulted in a more rapid improvement. The third study showed that Biostim produced a more rapid improvement in the most severely ill patients. It was concluded that Biostim can be initiated safely during acute episodes occurring in subjects with recurrent respiratory infections, and that it results in a faster improvement of clinical symptoms.

Biostim therapy (3-month dosing schedule): 2 tablets daily for 8 days, then stop for 3 weeks; 1 tablet daily for 8 days, then stop for 3 weeks; 1 tablet daily for 8 days, then stop for 9 months. Repeat Biostim therapy once a year.

Thyroid-Stimulating Hormone

Aging, cancer, and AIDS often generate suboptimal levels of thyroid hormone production. Proper levels of thyroid hormones are crucial for optimal immune function. Blood tests do not always detect a thyroid hormone deficiency. However, a TSH (thyroid-stimulating hormone) test is recommended. If your temperature 30 minutes before eating is consistently below normal, you may want to start taking a thyroid hormone supplement, as directed by your physician. Popular prescription thyroid replacement drugs are Synthroid (synthetic thyroid hormone, T4) and Cytomel (T3 thyroid hormone). You must be careful not to overdose on thyroid hormones, so the advice of a knowledgeable physician is important when you are considering thyroid hormone therapy.

Thymic Immune Factors

Thymic Immune Factors is a glandular compound prescribed by many alternative doctors that provides extracts of fresh, healthy tissue from the thymus, lymph nodes, and spleen. These glands produce the disease-fighting cells of our immune system and the white blood cells that engage in life-or-death combat with invading organisms in our bloodstream under the "instruction" of the thymus gland. The primary ingredient is immunologic tissue from the thymus gland.

Thymic Immune Factors contains herbal activators (echinacea, goldenseal root, and clove). It has been used extensively to amplify the immune-potentiating effect of DHEA replacement therapy. According to a physician familiar with DHEA, thymus extract is required to produce the immune-system-boosting benefit of DHEA.

T-cells mature in response to hormones secreted by the thymus gland. Aging causes a shrinkage of the thymus, and the resulting reduction in the production of thymic hormones is a major cause of the progressive decline in immune function that occurs with aging. By taking 2 to 4 capsules a day of Thymic Immune Factors, you can replace some of the thymic hormones lost to aging.

Exercise

Japanese studies reviewed in the *Exercise and Immunology Review,* 1997, 3 (68–95) show that regular physical activity may enhance NK cell activity. Given the many other health benefits, regular exercise should be on everyone's health agenda. There is research evidence that vitamin supplementation becomes increasingly important with exercise, as physical activity raises oxygen demand, causing an increase in the formation of oxygen radical species. Vitamins are involved in energy metabolism or free-radical scavenging.

Danger from Chronic Alcohol Ingestion

Research suggests that those who routinely consume significant quantities of alcohol may damage their immune systems and are thus at greater risk for the stimulation of carcinogenesis, the onset of cancer.

Summary

The immune system is the body's protection against damage from invading bacteria, viruses, and cancers. In order for it to function properly, it must have the support of proper nutrition. Nutritional immunology is the field of study dealing with this support. Free radicals have been linked to the immune system damage that accompanies normal aging. Vitamins play a critical role along with trace elements in maintaining the human immune system. Several herbs have demonstrated the ability to enhance and strengthen the immune system. These include echinacea, ginseng, and grape seed–skin extract. Other nutrients that have shown a positive effect on immune function are soy protein extract, whey extract, *L*-carnitine, and Coenzyme Q_{10}. Useful hormones and extracts are melatonin, DHEA, KH3, and thyroid-stimulating hormone. Biostim, a European medication, enhances the immune system as shown by carefully conducted trials.

Here is a review of the most important supplements that have been shown to protect and enhance immune function:

1. Life Extension Herbal Mix incorporates 27 different herbs into a powder designed to make one daily drink. Two of the extracts are from echinacea and ginseng, which significantly enhance NK function, both separately and together. Another beneficial ingredient of this formula is grape seed-skin extract. The suggested daily dose of Life Extension Herbal Mix is 1 tablespoon taken first thing every morning.
2. Life Extension Mix provides the vitamins, trace minerals, amino acids, and herb extracts that have documented benefits to the immune system. The recommended dose of Life Extension Mix is 9 tablets per day (3 with each meal).
3. Whey protein concentrate dramatically raises glutathione levels. (Glutathione protects immune cells and detoxifies harmful com-

pounds in the body.) Immune-suppressed patients should consider taking 30 grams per day of specially designed whey protein concentrate.

4. Life Extension Booster contains grape seed–skin extract, three forms of selenium, vitamin E (gamma- and alpha-tocopherol), and other important nutrients. Suggested dose is 1 capsule per day with any meal.
5. Biostim is a European medication widely prescribed on the continent and proven effective in protecting elderly people against respiratory infections. The Life Extension Foundation can provide information on offshore suppliers of Biostim.

Product availability. The Life Extension Foundation has several products especially formulated for maximum immune function. These are Enhanced Life Extension Protein, Thymic Immune Factors, and Ultimate Whey Designer Protein (which contains riboflavin). Goldenseal, echinacea, thymus, lymph, and spleen extract are all ingredients of Thymic Immune Factors. Life Extension Mix, Life Extension Booster, Coenzyme Q_{10}, *L*-carnitine, melatonin, DHEA, and vitamin B_6, as well as the other products listed here are available by calling (800) 544-4440, or order online at www.lef.org. Ask for a listing of offshore companies that sell Biostim and KH3.

INFLUENZA VIRUS (FLU)

Definition

Influenza or flu is an acute respiratory infection capable of sweeping through entire communities. Flu season begins in November or December and may last until April or May. Primarily affecting children 5 to 14 years of age, schools are infamous for transmission of flu viruses, and families with school-aged children have the highest rate of infection. Although the word "flu" is often applied to almost anything that makes us feel unwell, influenza should not be mistaken for the common cold or other airborne viruses. The flu differs significantly from the common cold (*refer to Common Cold protocol*) in both the rapid onset of the illness and in the potentially life-threatening complications that can develop, especially in the elderly. Although most people recover within a week, serious complications can occur in newborn babies, people with certain chronic illnesses, and the elderly. A "flu shot" or vaccination is made available each year to help combat or prevent flu in the most vulnerable of the population; however, elderly people often lack the immune capacity to generate an antibody response to prevent infection from the influenza virus. As many as 69,000 Americans have died from influenza in a bad epidemic year. Colds generally do not exhibit the severe symptoms that accompany influenza.

Symptoms and Diagnosis

Influenza is a respiratory disease spread via airborne droplets of infected respiratory fluid (from the coughing and sneezing of an infected person). Influenza almost never causes gastrointestinal symptoms and should not be mistaken with "stomach flu" characterized by vomiting, nausea, and diarrhea. Doctors diagnose influenza by the presence of flu symptoms in the community and whether the patient's complaints fit the current pattern. Rarely is laboratory testing used to identify the virus. Flu viruses can be classified into three groups: types A, B, and C. Type A is the most prevalent and associated with the most serious epidemics. Type B is milder and has rarely been associated with epidemics, and type C has never been associated with epidemic outbreaks. Usual flu symptoms include:

- Fever and chills
- Weakness and aching in legs, arms, back
- Headache
- Nasal congestion
- Loss of appetite

- ▼ Sore throat
- ▼ Dry cough
- ▼ Burning eyes

Complications

Newborns recently out of intensive care are particularly vulnerable to complications from the flu such as fever-related convulsions, croup, and ear infections. In a small number of children and adolescents, a complication known as Reye's syndrome (associated with the use of aspirin to treat flu symptoms) sometimes develops. Reye's syndrome is a neurological disease characterized by the onset of nausea, vomiting, confusion, and delirium. Although fewer than 3 children per 100,000 with flu develop Reye's syndrome, you should consult your physician before administering aspirin to children.

Complications from bacterial infections of the lower respiratory tract producing pneumonia or bronchitis are most common among people with chronic respiratory illnesses and the elderly. Symptoms of complications usually occur after the patient has begun to feel better. A brief period of improvement is quickly followed by high fever, shaking chills, chest pain with each breath, and coughing, which produces thick, yellowish-green sputum. Although pneumonia usually reacts well to antibiotics, some pneumonia-causing bacteria are resistant to these drugs.

Recent research findings on 55 adult volunteers indicate that cold and flu symptoms are intensified by stress. Interleukin-6, a protein which provides a biologic pathway for immune responses, was shown to be present in higher concentrations in nasal secretions of test subjects reporting greater psychological stress before inoculation with influenza type A virus. (As will be discussed later in this protocol, the supplemental hormone DHEA can suppress elevated levels of interleukin-6.) The subjects also presented with more intense flu symptoms and increased mucous production. The researchers from Carnegie-Mellon University in Pittsburgh concluded that "this is the first study to provide evidence . . . that psychological stress influences upper respiratory infectious illness through a biological pathway."

Flu Vaccine

Influenza viruses are difficult to treat because they are constantly changing. A global network of laboratories coordinated by the World Health Organization identifies and monitors new virus strains around the world. Based on the strains in circulation at the time, a new vaccine is formulated. Sometimes an unpredicted virus may emerge after the vaccine has been manufactured and distributed resulting in infection even among those vaccinated. Viruses for vaccine production are incubated in chicken eggs. People with allergies to eggs should not take the vaccine since some egg protein may be present. The following high-risk groups should consult their physicians about receiving the vaccine:

- ▼ All people 65 years of age and older
- ▼ People with chronic medical conditions including respiratory illnesses, diabetes, or cancer
- ▼ Residents and employees of any age living in nursing homes or chronic care facilities
- ▼ Children receiving long-term aspirin therapy
- ▼ Children 6 months or older with respiratory disorders
- ▼ Physicians, nurses, and other caregivers who have contact with high-risk patients

Treatments

The most common treatment for influenza is bed rest, plenty of fluids, and aspirin or acetaminophen to relieve fever and discomfort. Antibiotics are not effective against viruses but can be used to treat bacterial infection that results from influenza virus (see "Complications"). There are also alternative therapies that can shorten the duration and severity of the illness and help avoid complications.

Rimantadine (a derivative of Amantadine) can be used to treat influenza type A but has no effect on influenza type B. Given within the first 48 hours of the disease, it can be used to reduce the severity of the illness, and to protect those who have been in contact with an infected person or who respond poorly to influenza vaccination.

Ribavirin is a broad-spectrum, antiviral drug that is especially effective against influenza-like viruses. Ribavirin is approved in almost every country to treat influenza except the United States (though it can be purchased at U.S. compounding pharmacies with a doctor's prescription or from offshore pharmacies). When you first develop the symptoms of the flu, take 200 mg of ribavirin every 3 to 4 hours. In many cases, this can prevent the full development of the flu because of ribavirin's ability to interfere with influenza virus replication. Do not take ribavirin for more than 2 weeks without having a blood test to make sure the ribavirin is not causing a reduction in red blood cell production (anemia). Those with preexisting anemia may want to avoid ribavirin as about 10% of those taking ribavirin for 6 continuous months develop anemia within that 6-month period. Those with coronary artery disease or pulmonary insufficiency have to be especially concerned about anemia and should not take ribavirin for more than 1 to 2 weeks. Those with pre-existing kidney disease have been advised to use caution when taking ribavirin even though the published research does not indicate that ribavirin is especially toxic to the kidneys.

Biostim

Biostim is a French drug that has been shown to prevent infectious diseases in the elderly. Biostim is used in Europe to boost immune function and treat certain infectious diseases. An examination of the published literature reveals that if Biostim were available in the United States, thousands of American lives could be saved every year. These studies also indicate that Biostim would dramatically reduce the need for antibiotic therapy, thereby saving untold millions of dollars in prescription drug costs. A double-blind trial was conducted to evaluate the capacity of Biostim to diminish the frequency of infectious episodes in chronic bronchitis. The study duration was 9 months. Of the 73 subjects selected, 38 received Biostim and 35 a placebo. By the ninth month, the duration in days of infectious episodes was 60% lower in the Biostim group, compared with the placebo group. The use of antibiotic therapy was reduced by 81% in the Biostim group, compared with the placebo group.

Prewinter administration of Biostim to subjects significantly diminished the frequency of infectious episodes, and thus the consumption of antibiotics. In another study, 314 elderly subjects admitted to hospitals were given either Biostim or a placebo. The subjects were regularly examined every 3 months for 1 year. The incidence of acute infectious episodes was evaluated in both groups. The number of infected subjects in the group receiving the Biostim was significantly lower than in the placebo group. In the group receiving the Biostim, the number of infectious episodes was reduced throughout the 12 months of the trial. Finally, there was a significant decrease in the duration of antibiotic therapy. Biostim was well tolerated. This study showed that Biostim is effective in protecting elderly, and therefore fragile, subjects against respiratory infections.

An evaluation of the safety of Biostim given with an antibiotic to treat acute infections was performed in three double-blind, placebo-controlled studies on fragile institutionalized or hospitalized patients. Two of the studies showed that, in acute respiratory infections, Biostim is well tolerated and resulted in a more rapid improvement. The third study showed that Biostim produced a more rapid improvement in the most severely ill patients. It was concluded that Biostim can be initiated safely during acute episodes occurring in subjects with recurrent respiratory infections, and that it results in a faster improvement of clinical symptoms.

Other Herbal Extracts

There also are herbal extracts that have antiviral effects. When flu symptoms occur, it is suggested that you take echinacea liquid herbal extract at a dose of 6 full droppers in a small amount of water, followed by 2 full droppers every 2 waking hours until the 2-ounce bottle is empty. You also may want to consider taking 300 mg of astragalus extract, as well as 4 capsules a day of Sports ginseng, a standardized extract containing both Korean and Siberian ginseng.

A new extract from the elderberry called sambucol has been shown to keep the influenza virus from entering the cells. Sambucol should be taken in doses of 1 tablespoon 4 times a day.

DHEA is an adrenal hormone that has shown antiviral and immune-boosting benefits. When flu symptoms occur, 100 mg of DHEA should be taken 3 times a day until flu symptoms subside. Refer to DHEA-Pregnenolone Precautions in the *DHEA Replacement Therapy protocol* before taking DHEA. Melatonin has immune-enhancing benefits and possible antiviral effects, and it helps you get the sleep you need to fight the flu virus. Melatonin should be taken in doses of 10 mg before going to sleep for the duration of the flu attack.

High-potency vitamin formulas such as Life Extension Mix and other nutrients cited in the *Immune Enhancement protocol* should be considered. Also refer to the *Common Cold protocol* for additional suggestions.

Summary

1. Influenza almost never causes gastrointestinal symptoms and should not be mistaken with "stomach flu."
2. The flu differs significantly from the common cold in both the rapid onset of the illness and in the potentially life-threatening complications that can develop.
3. The most common treatment for influenza is bed rest, plenty of fluids, and aspirin (see "Complications" for information about Reye's syndrome in children) or acetaminophen to relieve fevers and discomfort.
4. Rimantadine (a derivative of Amantadine) can be used to treat influenza type A but has no effect on influenza type B.
5. Ribavirin, 200 mg taken every 3 to 4 hours, can prevent full development of the flu because of ribavirin's ability to interfere with influenza virus replication.
6. Echinacea liquid herbal extract at a dose of 6 full droppers in a small amount of water, followed by 2 full droppers every 2 waking hours until the 2-ounce bottle is empty, should be considered.
7. Consider 300 mg of astragalus extract, as well as 4 capsules a day of Sports ginseng.
8. Sambucol should be taken in doses of 1 tablespoon 4 times a day.
9. DHEA (100 mg taken 3 times a day until flu symptoms subside) and melatonin (taken in doses of 10 mg before going to sleep for the duration of the flu attack) have both shown antiviral and immune-boosting benefits.
10. Biostim has been shown to prevent infectious diseases in the elderly.
11. High-potency vitamin formulas such as Life Extension Mix and other nutrients should be considered as prophylaxis.

For more information. Contact the NIAID, Office of Communications and Public Liaison, Building 31, Room 7A-50, 31 Center Drive MSC 2520, Bethesda, MD 20892-2520.

Product availability. Rimantadine and amantadine are available by prescription. Ribavirin can be obtained in Mexico, or you can call (800) 747-0149 for a list of offshore suppliers who will mail it to you. If you already have the flu, it will take too long to obtain ribavirin by mail to be of any help; echinacea liquid herbal extract, elderberry (sambucol), and astragalus extract can be ordered by calling (800) 544-4440, or order online at www.lef.org.

INSOMNIA AND DAYTIME SLEEPINESS

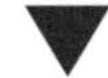

Sleep is absolutely essential for repair and rejuvenation, and those with chronic insomnia must find a solution in order to maintain quality of life. Most people don't know that chronic insomnia predisposes people to early death. Therefore, from a life extension perspective, it is absolutely essential that good sleep patterns be restored.

Insomnia is a frequent symptom indicative of overt or underlying depression. In this case, it is essential to treat the depression in order to produce healthier sleep patterns. Improving sleep often alleviates depression, and vice versa.

Insomnia can be described as either difficulty initiating or maintaining sleep or both. It affects millions of people and is often difficult to treat. Those who suffer from insomnia feel as though they have not had sufficient sleep when they awaken. Over the long term it may cause fatigue, irritability, and decreased concentration just to name a few symptoms. Elderly people require less sleep than younger adults, on average 6 to 8 hours per day or even less. This is a normal age-related change and should not be considered a sleep disorder in a healthy individual.

Sleep is not a static condition but actually a fluid condition with changes occurring through the sleep period. These stages demonstrate different brain wave patterns. In particular, the period of so-called rapid eye movement (REM) sleep is when we dream. There are about five periods of REM during the night. The deepest periods of sleep, stages 3 and 4, occur earlier in the night. It is the deeper phases of sleep which decrease in duration as we age.

Diagnosis and Treatment

The diagnosis of insomnia is based on a person's individual needs for sleep. It may be classified as primary insomnia, a condition with no apparent relationship to stress or other upset, or secondary insomnia, a condition related to another cause. Treatment will depend on the underlying cause, if any, and the severity of the sleeplessness. The more common reasons for difficulty initiating sleep are anxiety, stress, and depression.

A difficulty maintaining sleep may be caused by the same factors just mentioned as well as a sleep disorder caused by obstructive or central apnea where a disturbance in breathing wakes the individual up. Another common condition is nocturnal myoclonus, which causes the individual to "twitch" large muscle groups periodically resulting in awakening.

Often people will complain of being tired and having poor sleep yet they do not recall awakening. This is because not all awakenings are full awakenings. In the language of those who study sleep, this refers to full versus partial arousals. A person's sleep may be grossly disturbed with multiple partial arousals even in the absence of full arousals.

To find the cause of insomnia, one first attempts to find out whether it is initiation maintenance of sleep which is the problem. One looks for the more common reasons such as new things leading to stress. An increase in caffeine consumption includes not only tea and coffee, but carbonated beverages as well. Shift workers often have a problem resetting their biological clock to deal with a topsy-turvy schedule. The use of alcohol as a sedative before bed can have the opposite effect, resulting in further impaired sleep.

It is good to ask one's bed partner about heavy snoring or periods where there is gasping for air or kicking of arms and legs. Your physician may refer you for a sleep study which monitors your brain waves and limb movements as well as looking for sleep apnea.

How to Properly Use Melatonin

A common cause for insomnia in people over the age of 35 or 40 is deficiency of the hormone melatonin. Melatonin is the hormone released by the pineal gland that induces drowsiness, and enables the body to enter the deep-sleep patterns characteristic of youth.

After darkness, young pineal glands secrete melatonin slowly for about 5 hours to enable the body to enter the various stages of deep sleep, so people can feel revitalized and rejuvenated the next morning. Further, melatonin supplementation has been shown in many scientific studies to be a safe and effective sleep-enhancing therapy.

The optimal dose of melatonin has considerable individual variability. Many people find as little as 500 mcg is ideal, while others take 3 to 6 mg of melatonin before bedtime to solve their sleep problems. Too much melatonin can interfere with some people's sleep, so the lowest effective dose of melatonin to get to sleep and stay asleep is often the best course of action to follow.

Natural Sleep

Some people still wake up too frequently during the night or too early in the morning, even after taking melatonin. In order to duplicate the mechanisms by which the young pineal gland induces youthful sleep patterns, a formula called Natural Sleep was developed in 1995, and it has produced a good track record in helping alleviate chronic insomnia problems. This formula contains two different melatonin delivery systems that work together to generate the same kind of secretion of melatonin that occurs naturally in young people.

First, the Natural Sleep capsule bursts open in the stomach within 5 minutes after swallowing to provide immediate-release melatonin. That induces the drowsiness needed to get to sleep. Then, Natural Sleep gradually introduces tiny beadlets of sustained-release melatonin into the digestive tract, to enable the person to stay asleep and avoid the nocturnal tossing and turning characteristic of age-related sleep disturbances.

Each capsule of Natural Sleep contains 2.5 mg of immediate-release melatonin plus 2.5 mg of sustained-release melatonin. Many people find this dose effectively enables them to enjoy a complete night's rest every night. Natural Sleep also contains vitamin B_{12} because of studies showing that it can normalize circadian rhythms, thereby enabling people to enter sleep without stress or tension. Also, chromium picolinate and chromium polynicotinate are included in the new formula to help lower blood sugar levels that can inhibit the ability to fall asleep. Niacinamide ascorbate, magnesium, calcium, and inositol are included as well in Natural Sleep to help induce a state of relaxation.

Natural Sleep does not contain any potentially toxic herbal extracts. Insomnia often is a lifelong affliction, requiring the continuous need for nightly self-medication. The ingredients in Natural Sleep have been thoroughly investigated for long-term safety, and can be taken for an indefinite period of time without any risk of toxicity or tolerance.

Some people who occasionally wake up in the middle of the night will take another dose of melatonin to get back to sleep.

Other Natural Sleep-Inducing Therapies

Some people find that commercially available GABA taken before bedtime is helpful. Tryptophan is now available at compounding pharmacies and can be taken before bed. 5-Hydroxytryptophan is now available at most health food stores and can be taken before bed as well. Avoid taking vitamin B_6 supplements within 6 hours of taking 5-hydroxytryptophan (5-HTP) because B_6 can cause the conversion of 5-HTP to serotonin in the blood before it has a chance to cross the blood-brain barrier to increase serotonin in the brain. Excessive serotonin in the blood can be dangerous, which is why it may be safer to use tryptophan rather than 5-hydroxytryptophan (5-HTP). Both of these compounds can be converted to serotonin in the brain which plays a role in sleep. Patients taking SSRI antidepressants such as Prozac should consult with their physicians prior to taking these agents because the dose of antidepressant may need to be reduced. This is true for St. John's Wort as well.

While the long-term administration of valerian is not recommended, passion flower taken in moderation for short- to medium-term treatment of insomnia in conjunction with the other therapies mentioned may be helpful. It is available as a tea, in capsules, and as a tincture.

Some people use the herb valerian to fall asleep. Valerian produces a drug-like hypnotic effect within the central nervous system similar to benzodiazepine drugs such as Valium and Halcion. Since valerian-containing products often are promoted as natural herbal remedies, the public mistakenly believes they are safe to take on a regular basis. Studies indicate, however, that there is a possible toxicity risk when taking valerian over an extended period of time. Since a tolerance effect occurs with valerian due to its Valium-like properties, people often need to take greater and greater amounts of it as time goes by in order to continue to obtain the desired hypnotic (sleep-inducing) effect.

Use of Prescription Drugs

The use of tranquilizing drugs to solve chronic insomnia is not recommended by conventional or alternative medicine. The first problem cited by critics is addiction. It's not that the patient necessarily gets addicted to the drugs themselves; the problem arises when the insomniac becomes accustomed to the good night's sleep the drugs induce, and doesn't want to stop taking the medication. The other problem is tolerance, which means the drug slowly stops working, even when higher doses are taken. The dual problems of addiction and tolerance cause physicians to be extremely cautious when prescribing sleep medications. Other reasons for avoiding these drugs include increasing the risk of sudden death for the following individuals: (1) sleep apnea patients, (2) those who consume alcohol, and (3) some elderly people. Elderly people slowly metabolize sedative drugs, meaning that clearance from their body can take too long, and they experience fatigue the next day. It should also be noted that benzodiazepine drugs frequently used to induce a sedative effect can impair mental function.

Having said all of the above, we want to make the argument that for the chronic insomniac who cannot find relief by safer natural therapies, long-term, prescription drug therapy should be considered.

Insomnia induces a state of depression, lost productivity, and a shortened life span. One study showed that elderly people who suffered from chronic insomnia where more likely to die sooner than if they were cigarette smokers. Depression can cause insomnia and insomnia can exacerbate the miseries of chronic depression, chronic pain, and aging.

The Life Extension Foundation believes that a chronic insomniac should do almost anything to alleviate his/her problem, even to the point of taking sleeping pills under the guidance of a cooperating physician. One reason the Foundation suggests this is that within the next 10 years, there is a chance that a drug could be developed that safely helps people to sleep without any side effects or tolerance problems. If this were to happen, then those chronic insomniacs who avoided prescription sleeping pills would have suffered needlessly, since once the "cure" was discovered, they would no longer need their sleep medication. There is also the quality of life issue. If the judicious use of prescription sleeping pills buys the chronic insomniac 5 to 10 years of good sleep, it is worthwhile.

One way of avoiding the tolerance problem is to alternate the type of sleeping pill used. Here is a suggested prescription drug schedule to treat chronic insomnia for the person who has never taken prescription sleeping pills:

1. Valium, 2.5 mg taken *only* at bedtime for 30 days.
2. During the next 30-day cycle, switch to 5 to 10 mg of Ambien, taken *only* at bedtime.
3. During the next 30-day cycle, switch to Klonopin,1 to 2 mg taken *only* at bedtime.

This cycle may be repeated, using a wide variety of tranquilizing drugs for many years without the tolerance factor occurring.

At some point, a person may find that they do better by taking the Valium one night, Ambien the next night, and Klonopin the third night. If heavy alcohol is ever consumed, these types of drugs should be avoided on that night. It should be noted that chronic alcohol intake in and of itself is a major cause of poor sleep patterns.

An "old" drug frequently prescribed to induce a state of deep sleep is a tricyclic antidepressant drug called Elavil (amitriptyline hydrochloride). This drug normally puts people to sleep fast, but induces many side effects such as severe dry mouth, weight gain, constipation, and host of other problems. Newer tricyclic antidepressant drugs produce fewer side effects, but do not work as well in inducing deep sleep patterns. A typical dose of Elavil taken a few hours before bedtime is 10 to 25 mg. Some people use Elavil until the side effects become too pronounced, and then discontinue it for months or years.

There are a number of prescription drugs that will induce a state of sleep. Halcion seems to produce the most severe side effects and is not recommended. A person with chronic insomnia must develop a close relationship with a physician who understands that some people need sleep medications on a routine basis or their lives will be miserable, and that they are also at a higher risk of contracting a serious degenerative disease.

Other Sleep Disorders

Nocturnal myoclonus (abrupt spasm of a group of muscles) and restless leg syndrome are both related. The latter is exactly what it sounds like. It is a familial disorder characterized by the irresistible urge to kick the legs around. Many patients have both conditions. Patients with a family history are likely to benefit from higher dose therapy with folic acid, around 50 mg per day. Dosages this high require a prescription from your physician. Another consideration is low blood iron even in the presence of anemia. This can be determined by testing the ferritin level which, if low, reflects low iron. Treatment with simple ferrous sulfate, 200 mg 3 times per day; should do the trick. However, one must watch for excessively high iron levels because of the free-radical-promoting nature of iron, which contributes to aging. Another supplement to try is magnesium citrate at doses of about 250 mg taken at night.

If no abnormality is found to be causing sleeplessness, another test known as a sleep latency study is conducted the day after a sleep study. The person is asked to take little naps during the day, and the period of time it takes prior to falling asleep is measured. This is how narcolepsy may be diagnosed. Narcolepsy is a disorder in which people fall asleep during the day very suddenly despite normal night-time sleep.

Another, less commonly diagnosed disorder is pathological daytime sleepiness. Again, the person sleeps normally during the night but feels sleepy during the day. People who have this disorder may feel sleepy, but they don't fall asleep on the spot as patients with narcolepsy do.

Once a diagnosis is made, treatment options can be sought. Sleep apnea may be corrected with CPAP, which is assisted breathing preventing collapse of the airway during sleep. There are a number of other treatments, including surgery. Central apnea—where breathing is not obstructed but results from a failure of the brain to tell the person to breathe—is more difficult to treat. We know of no alternative therapies for treating central apnea at this time.

It is very important to recognize that one of the early signs of depression is a change in sleep pattern. A person may not have all of the classic symptoms of a major depressive illness and yet have disturbed sleep. When the depression is treated, the sleep normalizes. (Please see the *Depression protocol*.)

Summary

1. Avoid caffeine at least 6 hours before bedtime.
2. Avoid alcohol or smoking 2 hours before bedtime.
3. Get regular exercise, but at least 3 hours before bedtime.
4. Establish regular bedtime hours, waking up each morning at the same time.
5. Ensure that your bedtime routine is calming; read or listen to soft music.
6. Don't use the bedroom to do work.
7. Learn to meditate.
8. Consider using a light sound machine to relax.
9. Consider using cranioelectroneural stimulation.
10. Consider specialized sleep tapes and CDs.
11. Try differing doses of melatonin.
12. When all else fails, consider the judicious use of prescription drugs.

For more information. Contact the National Sleep Foundation, 1367 Connecticut Ave. NW, Dept. SCM, Washington, DC 20036. *GHB The Natural Mood Enhancer,* Ward Dean, MD, John Morgenthaler, Steven Wm. Fowkes is recommended reading.

Product availability. To order Natural Sleep or other melatonin products, call (800) 544-4440, or order online at www.lef.org. For tryptophan compounding, contact the Tryptophan Medical Center Pharmacy (800) 723-PILL. Call (800) 456-9887 for Sleep Tapes—Tools for Exploration.

JET LAG

Jet lag occurs when there is a disruption of the body's internal 24-hour clock, known as the circadian rhythm cycle. The cycle is controlled by the release of the hormone melatonin from the pineal gland located in the brain. This disturbance can produce physical and psychological stress. The rapid change in time zones causes jet lag, but it can also occur when a person starts working the night shift after keeping a daytime work schedule; this is known as *industrial jet lag*.

Jet lag mainly occurs in people who rapidly traverse multiple time zones. Children under 3 years of age don't seem to suffer jet lag badly because they are more adaptive and less set in their ways. Adults who can easily adjust to changes in routine are less susceptible to jet lag, while those who stick to a fixed daily routine often suffer more.

Causes

A person who is overtired, excited, stressed, nervous, or hung over before the flight is usually the person who suffers the most from jet lag. This person should get a good night's sleep prior to departure. Jet lag is also more likely to occur in a person who doesn't exercise.

Because the air aboard an airplane is dry, people who normally live in more humid conditions suffer headaches, dry skin, and dry nasal and throat membranes. This can create a condition for catching colds, coughs, sore throats, or the flu. To combat this, it's suggested that passengers drink plenty of water. Coffee, tea, alcoholic drinks, and fruit juices are not recommended. Coffee and tea have a high caffeine content and are abrasive on the stomach, while orange juice is just as abrasive. The impact of alcohol on the body is 2 to 3 times more potent when flying.

Aircraft are pressurized to near 8000 feet, and unless the passenger is acclimated to this pressure, they may suffer from swelling, tiredness, and lethargy. Stale air in the aircraft is another cause for headaches, irritability, and fatigue; many airlines don't supply constant fresh air.

Symptoms

Fatigue will occur in a person who travels across multiple time zones. It usually takes 1 day to recover from each time zone that is crossed. The person will be worn out and tired for days after arriving at his or her destination. Fatigue is usually accompanied by a lack of concentration and motivation. It's hard to deal with an activity that requires effort or skill, such as driving, reading, or discussing a business deal. Poor concentration, insomnia, daytime sleepiness, slowed reflexes, indigestion, hunger at odd hours, irritability, depression, lack of resistance to infections, headaches and muscle aches, mood disturbance, and loss of mental efficiency are other symptoms of jet lag.

Treatments to Minimize Jet Lag

There are a number of techniques that can be used to reduce jet lag with the most important taking place before the person gets on the airplane. Before leaving, make sure that all business and personal affairs are taken care of. The person should make sure he or she isn't stressed out by being excited or worried, and shouldn't be hung over from the night before. He or she should get plenty of exercise in the days prior to departure and a good night's sleep the night before.

Taking a daytime flight is better than flying at night, while a nonstop flight is also better for reducing jet lag. Traveling east to west also reduces the effects of jet lag.

Sleeping aids such as blindfolds, ear plugs, neck rests, and blow-up pillows are helpful in getting quality sleep during the flight. Being barefoot also eases the pressure on the feet. Walking around the airplane, along with standing for a while and doing stretching exercises in the seat, reduces swelling of the legs and the feet as well as the possibilities of blood clots and other trauma.

If there is an extended layover, taking a shower, if available, is good for reducing jet lag. A shower will loosen up the muscles and get the circulation going again.

Alternative Treatments to Minimize Jet Lag

Melatonin, an over-the-counter product, is a substance that is naturally produced in humans at night. It tricks the body into resetting its own biological clock. If taken in the morning, melatonin delays the body clock and allows the person to stay up later. If melatonin is taken at night, it encourages sleep.

One study looked at the effects of melatonin during the rapid deployment of Army aviation personnel across time zones. The soldiers suffered the combined insult to their systems of going on missions beginning immediately upon arrival, which resulted in desynchronization of physiological and cognitive performance rhythms. The benefits of melatonin (10 mg) in maintaining stable sleep/wake cycles of Army air crews was tested during a training mission involving rapid deployment to the Middle East and night operations. Cognitive performance was tested before and after travel. Activity rhythms were recorded continuously for 13 days. Melatonin treatment advanced both bed times and rise times, and maintained sleep durations between 7 and 8 hours. Placebo treatment mostly was associated with longer advances in rise times than bed times, resulting in shorter sleep durations (5 to 7 hours).

Upon awakening, the melatonin group exhibited significantly fewer errors (mean 7.5) than the placebo group (mean 14.5) in a dual task-vigilance test. This study demonstrated the value of melatonin for the prevention not only of sleep disruptions but also of cognitive degradation, even in uncontrolled sleeping environments characteristic of military deployments.

The best way of using melatonin to alleviate jet lag is to take one 3-mg capsule of melatonin the night before you leave, and another 3-mg capsule on the first night you go to sleep in your new destination. The melatonin will adjust your circadian rhythm to the new time zone, and you should wake up feeling as if you were home. If you are able to sleep on the plane, taking melatonin at that time could enable you to arrive at your new destination fully refreshed.

Additionally, there are specialized music tapes and CDs which can alter brain wave patterns, aiding in sleep disturbed by jet lag.

Summary

1. Consider melatonin, as directed above.
2. Consider CES.
3. Consider light/sound technology.
4. Consider Specialized music tapes and CDs.

For more information. See *GHB—The Natural Mood Enhancer,* by Ward Dean, M.D., John Morgenthaler, and Steven William Fowkes.

Product availability. Pharmaceutical-grade melatonin supplements in a wide range of potencies are available by calling (800) 544-4440, or order online at www.lef.org. Tryptophan Medical Center Pharmacy (800) 723-PILL CES; light/sound technology [drbaer.com]. Specialized music tapes and CDS: Tools For Exploration, (800) 456-9887.

KIDNEY DISEASE

For many years, kidney disease has been included in the top ten causes of death by a disease, according to the Centers for Disease Control (CDC). Kidney disease also plays a significant role in hypertension and diabetes, two other diseases that are included in the top ten causes of death in America each year (*see the Hypertension and Diabetes protocols*). End-stage renal (kidney) disease (ESRD) is growing at a rate of 4 to 8% each year in the United States. ESRD patients with advanced disease may require either therapeutic or regular dialysis (or both), or eventually may require a kidney transplant to save their lives. ESRD patients are put on dialysis or placed on kidney transplant waiting lists when kidney function has been reduced to 10 to 15% or less.

Kidneys are bean-shaped organs that act as sophisticated trash filters to scavenge organic waste products from the blood. Kidneys also help to control blood pressure. These organs are located on either side of the lower back just below the rib cage. Each day the kidneys filter approximately

200 quarts of blood, ridding the body of waste products and extra water. The extra water is passed through the ureters and then briefly stored in the bladder before being eliminated as liquid waste.

Filtered waste products include normal organic material from the breakdown of cells, proteins, excess food by-products, and various minerals, as well as the individual waste excretions from cells of the body. Alcohol, drugs, excess protein, minerals, and other ingested toxins are also passed through the kidneys and can have a dramatic effect on kidney health.

Kidney function is normally measured using simple tests to determine gross problems. These include blood and urine tests to measure creatine levels, possible blood in the urine, blood urea nitrogen (BUN), protein leakage, and mineral content— including calcium, magnesium, phosphorus, sodium, potassium, oxalic acid, and other elements.

Urinary tract infections (UTIs) are common health problems that are caused by kidney damage, various urinary systemic infections, sexual contact, kidney stone blockages, and bacteria carried to the kidneys via the bloodstream or the urethra. Infection can be one of the major causes of impaired kidney function and should be treated immediately to prevent more serious disease.

Kidney Dialysis

Dialysis is a treatment method that uses a kidney dialysis machine (dialyzer) to filter out waste products contained in the blood. Dialysis is a proven technique used to remove wastes and extra fluid from the body. There are currently 200,000 patients receiving dialysis treatment in the United States. The treatment allows patients to live relatively normal lives within the limitations of their disease.

There are two types of dialysis methods used. The most common dialysis technique is hemodialysis. It accounts for 85% of all dialysis patients, whereas the remaining 15% use a method known as peritoneal dialysis. Neither method is painful, and both are equally effective in removing wastes and extra fluids from the body. The choice is usually one of preference or convenience desired by the patient with consultation of the appropriate medical professionals.

Dialysis is usually performed at special dialysis clinics or hospitals, but some machines are installed for home use. Once the dialysis patient has had either a pair of needles inserted semi-permanently into the forearm (for hemodialysis) or has had an abdominal catheter placed into the abdominal wall (for peritoneal dialysis), she or he can receive treatment with minimal help.

Even for patients using dialysis, ESRD can cause other problems over time. These problems can include high blood pressure (including a latent nocturnal factor), bone disease, anemia, and nerve damage. As kidney function declines past the minimum threshold, kidney transplant becomes the only hope for patients with advanced ESRD.

Studies on human dialysis patients indicate that a high number of free radicals are formed in response to dialysis and that antioxidant dietary supplements can protect against this damage.

Renal Transplantation

Kidney transplantation accounts for more than 10,000 organ transplant operations each year. Today there are 60,000 patients with functioning kidney transplants living in the United States. Approximately 2000 patients (1900 in 1998) die each year while awaiting a matching donor kidney. Potential candidates for kidney transplantation must have kidney function estimated to be below 15%, and these patients must not be positive for certain diseases such as unstable coronary artery disease, infection, or glomerulonephritis.

Transplanted kidneys come from three general classifications: living related donors, living unrelated donors, and cadavers. The total number of transplanted kidneys in 1997 was 10,800. Living related donors are blood relatives. They may offer the only option for some patients. Living unrelated donors are persons who make one of their kidneys available to a needy patient who has the same blood type and who is in good health. Living unrelated donors accounted for 4% of kidney transplants in the United States in 1994. From 1987 through 1994, kidneys harvested from cadavers accounted for 73% of all transplanted kidneys, with 93.4% of patients surviving for at least 1 year and 87.7% surviving for 3 years or more. Over this time period, recipients of kidneys from living donors had a survival rate of 97.3% after 1 year and 94.3% after 3 years. "Rejections today are often milder, occur later, and are more reversible," says Dr. Thomas R. Schwab, M.D., a nephrologist at the Mayo Clinic Dialysis Center in Rochester, MN.

Can Renal Replacement Be Deferred?

A study was conducted to determine whether a very-low-protein diet could defer renal replacement therapy (RRT) to patients with chronic renal failure. High protein intake is known to stress the kidneys and, over time, can be a contributing factor to a slow pervasive decline in kidney function. Two groups of patients (23 patients and 53 patients, respectively) were put on a very-low-protein diet (0.3 g/kg) combined with supplemental amino acids. The patients in these groups were well-motivated renal replacement therapy (RRT) candidates who were closely monitored for nearly 1 year. During the course of the study, indications of malnutrition did not occur, and patients were able to maintain acceptable kidney function, GFR < 10 ml/ml/min (or < 15/ml/min for diabetic patients).

L-Carnitine Adjuvant Therapy

For patients who are predialysis, undergoing dialysis, or post-transplant, nutritional supplementation of *L*-carnitine lost during dialysis may reduce the effects of common renal problems—such as cardiomyopathy, and blood platelet aggregation—and may also help improve the patients' perception of general quality of life.

General muscle weakness indicated by low serum *L*-carnitine is a common complaint among patients undergoing hemodialysis. One study measuring the serum amount of *L*-carnitine found that hemodialysis lowered *L*-carnitine levels and posed new problems for patients. This study measured muscle atrophy via nerve conduction and velocity testing, and found indications of "neurogenic atrophy of the muscles." This well-known muscle weakness was further studied by doctors in Japan who reported that low dosages of *L*-carnitine (500 mg/day) showed improvement in two thirds of 30 patients studied for 12 weeks. The patients reported less incidences of muscle weakness, general fatigue, and cramps/aches. This study concluded that low dosages of *L*-carnitine could improve muscle weakness and should be considered for prolonged adjuvant therapy for dialysis patients.

The improvement of the patient's quality of life is very important to dialysis patients. In one study, patients were tested before taking *L*-carnitine. After 3 months' supplementation, patients reported an "improved vitality and general health." This double-blind study was conducted on 101 patients who received *L*-carnitine just before and immediately after dialysis. It was noted that serum albumin levels correlated with the patients' feelings of well being.

A recent study of *L*-carnitine therapy on erythropoiesis and blood platelet aggregation was conducted on patients with chronic renal failure, and it was found that *L*-carnitine caused a "significant rise in collagen-induced platelet aggregation." The 22-month study divided the patients into three groups. Group I received erythropoietin, Group II received erythropoietin and *L*-carnitine, and Group III received *L*-carnitine. Iron concentration and platelet count measured in urea concentration were relatively unchanged. The rise of collagen was observed after only 2 months of *L*-carnitine therapy.

Hereditary and Acquired Renal Tubular Disorders

Autosomal dominant polycystic kidney disease (ADPKD) is one of the most common human genetic diseases. It is also one of the most serious genetic diseases, and it is ultimately responsible for many kidney transplants each year, as kidney function wanes over the years. (Because ADPKD is of genetic origin, patients who receive kidney transplants do not re-acquire the genetic mutation with the transplanted kidneys.) Worldwide, the disease is responsible for 8 to 10% of end-stage kidney disease, and results show chronic kidney failure in 45% of patients under the age of 60. Patients with the disease develop cysts in both kidneys. These cysts grow over the lifetime of the patient and ultimately lead to renal failure and hypertension. Patients suffering from ADPKD can benefit from a kidney transplant operation. There are approximately 60,000 kidney transplants in the United States each year.

Polycystic Kidney Disease (PKD) is characterized by autonomous cellular proliferation, pockets of fluid accumulation within the cysts, and intraparenchymal fibrosis of the kidney. Clinical observations include renal failure, liver cysts, and cardiac valve abnormalities.

The traditional method of detecting ADPKD was by ultrasound, computed tomography (CT), or magnetic resonance imaging (MRI) of kidneys for the presence of renal cysts. The problem with detecting ADPKD is that patients who are carrying the defective gene may not have developed symptoms, may not show any developed cysts, and may therefore not be diagnosed with ADPKD. Recent methods of DNA testing can now identify individuals who carry the defective gene but are not symptomatic. For example, every member of four Chinese families with a known history of ADPKD showed unique DNA patterns. This new diagnostic method has value for patients with developed ADPKD as well as for presymptomatic patients.

ADPKD progresses to end-stage renal insufficiency before age 73 in about half of affected patients. The mechanism by which some patients are affected by numerous cysts that form inside the proximal and distal tubules, although other patients are spared, is a mystery. The formation of cysts begins in early childhood, affecting less than 1% of tubules as a consequence of mutated DNA. The risk factors associated with PKD (polycystic kidney disease) include gender (males progress more quickly than females), race (black patients progress more rapidly than whites), and other contributing factors such as hypertension and proteinuria. These factors aggravate and can accelerate PKD through to end term.

Hypertension can create a significant risk factor for kidney failure, and for those with ADPKD the risk factor is amplified. In a study conducted in the UK, ambulatory patients were tested over a 24-hour period to measure the nocturnal fall of blood pressure. For ADPKD patients, the reduction in nocturnal blood pressure was attenuated, showing increased risk. Further studies are needed to evaluate the contribution nocturnal hypertension makes on the overall progression of renal failure. In another related study of untreated children however, it was found that the nocturnal hypertension was a major risk factor for renal deterioration.

Doppler ultrasonography is used to assess renal vascular resistance (RVR) by measuring resistive and pulsatility indices. In a study of 42 patients with ADPKD and 65 control subjects, it was found that Doppler indices do reflect increased RVR in those patients with ADPKD and that renal function disturbance did manifest systemic arterial hypertension. Hypertension is a common and serious factor of ADPKD that usually occurs early in the disease before renal function begins to decrease. The abnormality of the kidneys in these patients was easily observed using ultrasound; however this method did not show ADPKD potential for patients if renal cysts were not present. DNA testing is required to determine whether a patient carries the PDK1 and PDK2 chromosomes. The occurrences of cardiovascular complications are a very common cause of death for patients with ADPKD.

Acquired kidney disorders are caused by factors that include several groups of toxic materials such as heavy metals, protein metabolism disorders, light chain proteinuria, prescription drugs such as ifosfamide, out-dated tetracyclines, aminoglycosides, and toluene inhalation (industrial toxins exposure and glue sniffing). The possibility is now being explored that ADPKD may have an emerging infectious disease component as well. Recent research has shown fungal DNA in kidney tissue and cyst fluid of PKD patients, but not in healthy kidneys without ADPKD.

At the University of Illinois College of Medicine, a differential activation protocol assay showed bacterial endotoxin and fungal beta-*D*-glucans in cyst fluids from human kidneys with PKD. Tissue and cyst fluids were examined for fungal components, and the serological tests showed *Fusarium, Aspergillus,* and *Candida* antigens. It was concluded that "endotoxin and fungal components, sphingolipid biology in PKD, the structure of PKD gene products, infection, and integrity of gut function [will establish a mechanism] for microbial provocation of human cystic disease."

Tubular disorders such as glomerular impairment may be alleviated by taking taurine, an amino acid shown to protect against experimentally induced lipid peroxidation of the renal glomerular and tubular cells. Taurine (1000 mg) should be taken 2 to 3 times a day.

The kidneys can be protected from free-radical damage, a major factor in renal health, by supplementing with vitamin E. Vitamin E has been shown to restore tubular flow to rats with severe kidney disease by suppressing the free radicals that cause tubulointerstitial damage.

Homocysteine can be very damaging to kidneys. Dialysis patients often require high levels of homocysteine-lowering nutrients such as folic acid, vitamin B_{12}, TMG (also known as betaine or trimethylglycine), and vitamin B_6. Folic acid was used in an important study conducted on 82 patients undergoing dialysis (70 used hemodialysis and 12 used peritoneal dialysis) 3 times a week for 4 weeks. The results showed that both groups had homocysteine concentration reduced by 35% after taking 2.5 to 5 mg folic acid after each dialysis treatment. Although dialysis had the effect of lowering homocysteine levels, folic acid further reduced homocysteine levels and, more importantly, had long-term effects even after folic acid supplementation was withdrawn. "Homocysteine concentrations remained decreased in 20 patients four weeks after withdrawal of folic acid supplementation."

The established dosages for these critical nutrients are as follows:

- Folic acid (800 mcg)
- TMG or betaine (500 mg) taken twice each day
- Vitamin B_{12} (300 mcg)
- Vitamin B_6 (150 mg minimum) taken throughout the day

Kidney Stones (Calculi)

The occurrence of kidney stones is one of the most common of all kidney problems. Kidney stones are also one of the most painful of all health problems. It is estimated that of all people in the United States, 10% will pass a kidney stone at some time during their lives, with men being more affected than women and white people being more prone to stone formation than black people.

Kidney stones are solid, rock-like materials that form from the mineral substances contained in the urine. Most kidney stones consist of calcium combined with either oxalate or phosphate. Less common types of kidney stones include a struvite, or infection, stone and the uric acid stone. Even more rare are kidney stones that are made up of cystine. Evidence shows that cystine-based stones tend to run in families.

Kidney stones can grow to a size that can be life threatening or require surgery to remove. Some large kidney stones cannot be surgically removed due to the age of the patient and the danger of the associated trauma to a vital organ. The size of kidney stones can vary widely from the size of a grain of sand to a golf ball, however most kidney stones are quite small.

The symptoms of a kidney stone "attack" include the following: sudden extreme pain in the lower back, side, or groin; blood in the urine; fever and chills; vomiting; a bad odor or cloudy appearance to the urine; and a burning sensation during urination. These types of symptoms require a doctor's help. Such pain can be an indication of movement of the stone or a serious urinary tract blockage requiring immediate medical intervention. Frequently, kidney stone episodes include urinary tract infections. Recurrent untreated UTIs can eventually cause permanent kidney damage and reduced kidney function.

Kidney stones are usually yellow or brown in color and the structure and texture of the stones can be smooth or jagged. Several other visual characteristics are common, such as a crystalline appearance with different mineral striations appearing throughout the structure of the stone. Examination and testing of a kidney stone by a urologist can determine much about the possible cause of and remedy for patients with the potential to form more kidney stones.

Most kidney stones are formed as a result of limited water intake, dietary choices, mineral imbalances, and metabolic factors that create high concentrations of calcium and oxalate or cystine within the kidney itself. Sufficient water intake is both a preventive as well as a therapeutic measure.

Kidney stones tend to run in families and can be associated with geographic factors as well. Those people living in tropical climes may be more susceptible to kidney stone formation due to a shift in the body's water management in a tropical setting. Perspiration becomes prevalent as a percentage of the body's water management and urination declines slightly as the urine is in storage longer throughout the urinary tract. Perspiration can also be an even more significant factor for those performing hard physical labor under hot conditions. Water loss through perspiration can approach a gallon, as is the case for most NFL lineman during a football game—some lose 10 pounds of water weight during a 4-hour game. Although it may seem obvious, the fact is that most people do not drink enough water every day, and in tropical areas this is even more critical.

Passing or removing lodged or problem kidney stones can be as simple as drinking large amounts of liquid and running up and down stairs vigorously, or as complex as focusing shock waves passed through the lower abdomen in a process called extracorporeal shock wave lithotripsy (ESWL). Whatever method used to tackle the problems of a kidney stone that is lodged, increased water intake is the first step. As silly as it may sound, running up and down stairs or jumping up and down vigorously can be effective in passing a recalcitrant kidney stone. This practice is simply using the basic physics of gravity to get the stone moving so that it can be passed normally.

When a kidney stone is firmly lodged in the ureters, bladder, or urethra, other measures must be taken to pass or remove the stone. In the past, problem stones represented a significant problem because the only way to remove the stone was invasive surgery with a high risk of postsurgical infection. Now it is possible for most urologists to avoid surgery unless there is no alternative. The newer methods used to remove kidney stones include the extracorporeal method known as shock wave lithotripsy, ureterscope calculus removal, and tunnel surgery.

Lithotripsy is a noninvasive procedure that uses shock waves to break up the stone into smaller pieces enabling the urine to carry the kidney stone debris out of the body. Two types of machines are used to create shock waves of the right frequency and amplitude necessary to fracture the stones without causing injury to the patient. The original machines use a water tank in which the patient sits while the machine pulses the adjacent water. Since water cannot be compressed, the shock waves exert great force on very hard objects such as a kidney stone. Newer machines operate without a tank, and the patient simply lies on a table during the procedure. After lithotripsy, copious amounts of water must be taken to pass the broken pieces of the stone. Some patients experience localized bruising after litho-tripsy.

Tunnel surgery or percutaneous ephrolithotomy is a surgical technique characterized by the doctor cutting a narrow "tunnel" through the skin to reach the stone inside the kidney. Using this "tunnel" the doctor passes a special instrument through the tunnel to find and remove the kidney stone.

Kidney Stone Prevention

Research into the prevention of recurrent kidney stones has produced many helpful dietary guidelines, nutritional protocols, and lifestyle changes that can reduce or eliminate the potential for future kidney stones. Using several effective protocols can significantly reduce the chance of kidney stones occurring again after a first episode and may help pass a recurrent stone quicker with less difficulty.

In 1997 a research division of a health care provider conducted a double-blind study with a group of 64 patients who had a history of renal calculi to determine if potassium-magnesium citrate would prevent the recurrent formation of calcium oxalate kidney stones. The patients were given 42 mEq (milliequivalent) potassium, 21 mEq magnesium, and 63 mEq citrate or a placebo daily for 3 years. New renal calculi formed in 63.6% of patients receiving the placebo; however, patients receiving the potassium-magnesium citrate protocol presented with 12.9% recurrent renal calculi. The study concluded that "potassium-magnesium citrate effectively prevents recurrent calcium oxalate stones, and this treatment given for up to 3 years reduces risk of recurrence by 85%."

Two major studies have shown that, contrary to the "common sense" thinking of the past, calcium should not be reduced for patients with a history of kidney stones. It was originally postulated that patients with a history of renal calculi should limit their intake of calcium. In fact, current recommendations from the National Institutes of Health published on the Internet continue to call for calcium-restricted diets. Such dietary changes also affect the alkali and pH of the body by calling for the restriction of such foods as apples, beets, parsley, broccoli, pineapples, and spinach. The new findings contradict these dietary restrictions and offer new scientific evidence that uncombined intestinal oxalic acid is the real culprit for calcium oxalate kidney stones.

Harvard researchers studied nearly 92,000 nurses over a period of 12 years to determine the relationship between calcium intake and the occurrence of renal calculi (Nurses' Health Study). The conclusion of this massive study showed that those nurses who ate diets that were higher in calcium were at lower risk for kidney stones! The reason this type of dietary modification reduced the chance of kidney stones was relatively simple.

The highest percentage of kidney stones is comprised of calcium and oxalic acid forming calcium oxalate inside the kidneys. Oxalic acid is able to pass through the intestinal wall into the blood and travel to the kidneys, where it has the chance to combine with calcium. Calcium oxalate (calcium and oxalic acid), when normally combined inside the digestive tract, does not pass through the intestinal wall into the blood but is eliminated with other waste products. Therefore, when oxalic acid combines with dietary calcium or supplemental calcium inside the intestinal tract, oxalic acid will never reach the kidneys, and calcium oxalate kidney stones cannot be formed.

The Nurses' Health Study presented the following important new findings:

- ▼ Dietary calcium intake from food or supplements reduced the risk for renal calculi.
- ▼ Calcium supplementation must be taken with food and in small dosages (< 400 mg).
- ▼ Plant foods high in calcium, fiber, vitamins, minerals, antioxidants, and some protein were an excellent source for dietary phytochemicals.

Another study conducted in South Africa found that "mineral water containing calcium and magnesium deserves to be considered as a possible therapeutic or prophylactic agent in calcium oxalate kidney stone disease." A French mineral water containing calcium (202 ppm) and magnesium (36 ppm) was selected as the delivery method. Twenty men and twenty women who had previously formed calcium oxalate renal calculi participated in the study. The mineral water was ingested over a 3-day period and then switched to tap water. The male participants received the most benefit, showing nine risk factors that were favorably affected by the mineral water protocol.

Drugs

Over-the-counter (OTC) and prescription drugs can cause kidney damage. Regular blood tests to assess kidney function are recommended for anyone taking medications known to damage the kidneys.

Summary

Kidney disease includes ADPKD, a genetic disease that slowly reduces kidney function over the years. ADPKD requires dialysis when renal function is reduced to less than 10 to 15%. When dialysis is unable to support kidney function, kidney transplantation is the only recourse. New research into gene therapy is being planned now that the PKD1 gene has been characterized. The PKD1 gene is responsible for 85% or more of all ADPKD disease.

1. Kidney stone prevention should be centered on increased water intake, increased calcium intake using dietary factors, and appropriate

calcium-magnesium supplementation to be taken only with food.

2. Glomerulonephritis may be improved by supplementing with taurine.
3. Homocysteine levels may be lowered by supplementing with the nutrients folic acid, vitamin B_{12}, vitamin B_6, vitamin E, and TMG betaine.
4. Dialysis patients should be taking antioxidant supplements like *N*-acetylcysteine, lycopene, and vitamins C and E to protect against dialysis-induced free radicals.

For more information. Contact the National Kidney Foundation, (800) 622-9010, and the National Kidney and Urologic Diseases Information Clearinghouse, (301) 654-4415.

Product availability. Taurine, vitamin E, B-complex vitamins, folic acid, TMG betaine, and magnesium are available by phoning (800) 544-4440 or by ordering online at www.lef.org.

KIDNEY STONES

(See Kidney Disease)

LEARNING DISORDERS

(See Age-Associated Mental Impairment and Attention Deficit Disorder protocols.)

LEUKEMIA AND LYMPHOMAS (HODGKIN'S AND NON-HODGKIN'S)

Leukemias are cancers of the blood-forming organs, and lymphomas are cancers of the lymphatic tissues. In general, leukemias and lymphomas respond well to the conventional treatment methods of chemotherapy and radiation therapy. Because there are many different types of these cancers, treatment is based on the specific diagnosis of the disease.

Leukemia

In the United States, more than 30,000 new cases of leukemia will be diagnosed in the coming year, and adult onset of the disease will account for 90% of these cases. Leukemia is not a single disease but a group of related diseases. There are no specific symptoms for leukemias; instead, symptoms are more generalized and include fatigue, weakness, unexplained weight loss, and pain. Most cases of leukemia are found during routine laboratory tests such as complete blood counts (CBC), white blood counts (WBC), and platelet counts. Once the initial diagnosis of leukemia is made, further testing includes bone marrow aspiration, lumbar puncture, and excisional biopsies to determine the specific type of leukemia. When leukemias are detected, they are not classified by stages because they are systemic diseases, and other organs such as the spleen, lymph nodes, liver, and central nervous system are already involved.

Leukemias are classified into acute and chronic forms. Cancerous cells rapidly reproduce and accumulate in both types of the disease, crowding out normal white blood cells. The difference between the two types of leukemia is that in the acute form, bone marrow cells do not reach maturity and immature cells accumulate. In the chronic form, the cells appear mature but are abnormal and live longer than normal white cells. If left untreated, the majority of patients with an acute form of the disease have a life expectancy of 1 year.

Leukemias are further classified according to the type of affected bone marrow cells. The cancer is *myelogenous* if the involved blood cells are granulocytes or monocytes. The cancer is *lymphocytic* if the affected cells are lymphocytes. Leukemias are divided into four main types: acute myelogenous (AML), chronic myelogenous (CML), acute lymphocytic (ALL), and chronic lymphocytic (CLL). There are also several subtypes of these diseases based upon the French-American-British (FAB) classification system for acute leukemias. Prognosis and treatment are based on the diagnosis of the type and subtype of the disease.

Leukemias respond well to chemotherapy and radiation therapy, and these treatment methods are often used in combination. The treatment of leukemia involves the use of a combination of cancer medications given over a period of time. As a general rule, AML will be treated with high doses of chemotherapy agents over a short period of time, whereas ALL is treated with lower doses of chemotherapy over a longer period of time. Chemotherapy agents attack rapidly dividing cells; however, they also interfere with the production of white blood cells, thereby exposing the patient to the risk of infection. Medications known as growth factors increase white blood counts and are often given in combination with chemotherapy. Interferons (IFN) are a group of naturally occurring biologic response modifiers that are sometimes used in the treatment of chronic leukemias. The most commonly used of these substances is Interferon-alpha.

Interferon reduces the growth of cancerous cells, inhibits their replication, and enhances the immune system's response to the cancer. Interferon appears to be particularly useful when it is used as a maintenance therapy in patients with minimal residual disease (postremission) or complete remission. In addition, all-transretinoic acid (a vitamin analogue), when used in combination with Interferon, may be useful in prolonging the lives of patients with promyelocytic leukemia and other forms of the disease. A cautionary note to the use of this therapy is that the patient may be at risk for thrombosis (blood clots). However, heparin therapy or the use of certain nutrients may reduce this risk (*consult the Thrombosis Prevention protocol*).

Other therapies for the treatment of leukemias include stem-cell therapy. Stem-cell therapy involves removing stem-cells from the patient either by bone marrow aspiration or by a procedure called *apheresis* (also called peripheral blood stem-cell [PBSC] transplant), where the cells are removed from the peripheral blood system. Stem-cells may be obtained from the patient or from a donor who is a close tissue match to the patient. In this therapy, high doses of chemotherapy and radiation therapy destroy the patient's bone marrow, and the collected stem-cells are then transplanted into the patient to restore normal blood cell production. This type of therapy is still in the experimental stage. As a result it is very expensive and may not be covered by insurance.

Hodgkin's Lymphoma

Hodgkin's lymphoma is a cancer of the lymph nodes. The American Cancer Society estimated that over 7000 new cases of the disease would be diagnosed in 1998. However, Hodgkin's disease has an overall cure rate of 75% in newly diagnosed cases. Slightly more than half of all newly diagnosed cases will occur in men.

Although it may affect any lymph tissue, Hodgkin's disease most commonly affects the supra-clavicular, high cervical, or mediastinal nodes. Some patients exhibit no symptoms of the disease, while others may have fever, night sweats, or weight loss, among other symptoms. Most patients have one or more slow-growing enlarged lymph nodes, but because swollen lymph nodes are more often associated with infections, patients often ignore this symptom. It is important to have any lymph node over one inch in size checked by a physician, particularly if the node enlargement is not associated with infection. If Hodgkin's disease is suspected, the patient may undergo magnetic resonance imaging (MRI) or computed tomography (CT) to determine the location(s) of enlarged nodes inside the body and detect any abnormalities of the spleen or other organs that may be associated with the disease. Diagnosis is confirmed by any one of a number of biopsy techniques, including fine needle aspiration, excisional biopsy, or incisional biopsy. A bone marrow aspiration may also be used to stage the disease.

Once the diagnosis is made, it is important to stage the disease. Staging determines the disease's extent of involvement. This information is used to plan a treatment program, and will affect the survival rate. Clinical staging consists of a thorough patient history and physical examination, X-rays, and laboratory tests. Other diagnostic tools for staging include gallium scans and lymphangiograms (a type of X-ray). Some patients require pathological examination, which involves a surgical procedure called a laparotomy (sometimes referred to as a staging laparotomy). The current staging system for Hodgkin's disease is the Ann Arbor Staging Classification system. Four stages (I, II, III, IV) of the disease are recognized, based upon the degree of involvement. Stage I disease is the least serious and stage IV the most serious.

Hodgkin's lymphoma is treated using a combination of chemotherapy agents. There are two common chemotherapy combinations: mechlorethamine (Mustargen), vincristine (Oncovin), prednisone (Deltasone, Meticorten), and procarbazine (Matulane), or Adriamycin, bleomycin (Blenoxane), and dacarbazine (DTIC). The type of chemotherapy used will depend upon a number of factors, including the stage of the disease and the patient's age.

Radiation therapy is often used in combination with chemotherapy. Depending on the severity of the disease, radiation may involve the use of a focused beam of radiation or total nodal irradiation. As with all types of lymphomas, bone marrow transplantation or peripheral blood stem-cell transplantation may be considered in patients who do not respond to chemotherapy or radiation therapy.

Non-Hodgkin's Lymphoma (NHL)

The American Cancer Society estimated that nearly 57,000 new cases of non-Hodgkin's lymphoma (NHL) would be diagnosed in 1998. NHL is the fifth most common type of cancer in the United States. The disease is difficult to treat, with an average 1-year survival rate of 70% and a 5-year rate of 51%. Approximately 90% of all non-Hodgkin's lymphomas are diagnosed in adults. The average age at diagnosis is in the early 40s, and the disease is slightly more common in men than in women. The risk for the disease increases throughout life. Other potential risk factors for the disease may include adult onset diabetes of long duration and a history of previous cancers, according to a British study. Survival rates for non-Hodgkin's lymphoma are variable, depending on the type of cell involved and the stage of the disease.

Non-Hodgkin's lymphomas are cancers that also affect the lymphatic system, particularly the lymphocytes—the cells responsible for maintaining the body's immune system. There are two major types of lymphocytes: B-cells and T-cells. B-cells are more common and are involved in approximately 85% of all non-Hodgkin's lymphomas.

Generalized symptoms of the disease include unexplained weight loss, fever, profuse sweating, and severe itchiness. The disease may affect the lymph nodes close to the body's surface (e.g., in the neck, groin, or underarm). These nodes become swollen and are usually noticeable to the patient. If lymph nodes in the abdomen are affected, the patient may experience abdominal swelling resulting from accumulating fluid or tumor growth. If lymph nodes near the intestines are affected, the patient may have difficulty with the passage of stools. When the lymphoma originates in the thymus, the growth of the tumor may block the trachea or the superior vena cava may become compressed, resulting in a life-threatening condition known as superior vena cava (SVC) syndrome.

The disease is diagnosed by either fine needle aspiration, incisional biopsy, or excisional biopsy. Other techniques used to assist in the diagnosis include X-rays, CT scans, and bone marrow aspiration. Because there are a number of different types of malignancies in non-Hodgkin's lymphomas, the types are classified according to two systems. The Working Formulation classifies these lymphomas based on prognosis: the categories are low-, intermediate-, and high-grade. The Revised European American Lymphoma (REAL) system divides NHL into types according to clinical behavior. The categories are indolent, aggressive, and highly aggressive. High-grade and highly aggressive tumors are the most difficult to treat.

Treatment for non-Hodgkin's lymphoma depends on the type of lymphoma (e.g., indolent or aggressive), the stage of the disease, the age of the patient, and the patient's overall health. As in Hodgkin's lymphomas, chemotherapy and radiation therapy are used to treat the disease. Bone marrow transplantation may be considered for patients who do not benefit from other forms of therapy. In one recent study, Interferon was found to be an effective treatment for low-grade lymphomas; however, intermediate- and high-grade tumors did not respond as well. A recent French study of B-cell non-Hodgkin's lymphomas also indicated that Interferon-gamma and -alpha may be useful in the treatment of certain types of the disease.

Other Beneficial Treatments for Leukemia and Lymphoma

Although leukemia and lymphomas respond well to the conventional treatment methods of chemotherapy and radiation therapy, other potentially beneficial treatments are available. Vesanoid, a vitamin A analogue, has been approved for the treatment of promyelocytic leukemia. The medication inhibits cell division and allows cells to reach maturity and function normally. Although Vesanoid is approved in the treatment of only a specific type of leukemia, it may be beneficial in the treatment of other types of leukemia (but probably not CLL) and some types of lymphoma. Although vitamin A therapy can help to induce remission in patients with promyelocytic leukemia, the duration of the response to the medication is short-lived. Additional therapy with Vesanoid is often less effective, suggesting that patients may develop some resistance to the medication.

Research has demonstrated that drug resistance may be overcome by using retinoic acid in combination with other medications, such as vitamin D_3 and its analogs. Patients with other forms of leukemia or lymphoma should consult with their physician regarding the potential benefits of this treatment. If the patient's physician does not recommend Vesanoid for treatment of the disease because the FDA has not approved the medication for their type of cancer, patients can consider water-soluble vitamin A as an alternative. The recommended dose of vitamin A supplement is 100,000 to 300,000 International Units (IU) daily. Monthly blood testing is necessary to monitor vitamin A liver toxicity.

CAUTION: Prior to considering vitamin A therapy, refer to the symptoms of vitamin A toxicity in Appendix A.

Vitamin D_3 and its analogs may induce certain leukemia and lymphoma cancer cells to differentiate into normal cells. For patients with multiple myeloma, data demonstrate that vitamin D_3 may function to

- Induce arrested growth of cancerous cells.
- Induce programmed cell destruction (apoptosis) when used with conventional therapy and cytokines (e.g., Interferon).
- Suppress the expression receptor on malignant plasma cells.
- Inhibit the side effects of conventional therapies that enhance cancer cell gene expression.

This evidence suggests that vitamin D_3 and its analogs may be beneficial to patients with multiple myeloma when used in conjunction with conventional chemotherapy. Monthly blood tests to monitor serum calcium, kidney function, and liver function are necessary to prevent vitamin D_3 toxicity. Although not specifically recommended for patients with chronic lymphocytic leukemia, vitamins A and D_3 may be beneficial because of their effects against a wide range of cancer cells.

Curcumin, a spice and food color additive, may have antioxidant, anti-inflammatory, and antitumor properties. In patients with promyelocytic leukemia, curcumin may promote apoptosis or induce cell death. The recommended daily dose of curcumin is 2000 mg taken with a heavy meal. Because the other antioxidants mentioned in this protocol can interfere with the apoptic properties of curcumin, they should not be taken in conjunction with it.

CAUTION: Patients with biliary tract obstruction should avoid using curcumin.

Another beneficial treatment for certain types of leukemia and lymphoma uses soy extracts with a high *genistein* content. Genistein is an inhibitor of protein tyrosine kinase, the enzyme that cancer cells require in order to replicate. A study conducted to assess the effects of genistein in several types of cancer showed that protein kinase C activity was inhibited, subsequently retarding the growth of cancer cells. Patients undergoing radiation therapy must avoid taking soy extracts for one week prior to, during, and following radiation therapy because radiation therapy uses protein kinase C to generate free radicals for cancer cell destruction.

Because genistein appears to inhibit cancer cell growth, it may be useful for purging the bone marrow in several types of leukemia. Some studies suggest that genistein may enhance the effects of some chemotherapy agents. Other studies have shown that genistein induces a significant suppression of cancer cell colony formation and apoptosis in patients with chronic myelogenous leukemia. In patients whose tumor cells have mutant p53 oncogenes, the benefits of soy extracts may be significant. The presence of mutant p53 genes is determined by pathologic examination of the cancer cells. An immunohistochemistry test for the presence of p53 can be performed by the following:

IMPATH Laboratories
1010 Third Avenue, Suite 203
New York, N.Y. 10021
Phone: 1-800-447-5816

If the test for mutant p53 is positive, then mutant p53 is present and soy extract therapy may be very beneficial. If the test is negative, functional p53 is present and it is less likely that soy extracts will provide any benefit. The Foundation realizes that many cancer patients desiring to use soy extracts may not be able to have immunochemistry testing for mutant p53. Patients may wish to consult their physicians to determine if mutant p53 was discovered during diagnosis of their disease.

The most concentrated form of soy extract available is Mega Soy Extract. The recommended dose for cancer patients is five 700-mg capsules taken four times a day in evenly spaced doses.

An interesting study (*Proc. Soc. Exp. Biol. Med.*, 1998 [May] 218[1]:76–82) showed that the hormone DHEA (dehydroepianstrosterone) favorably modulated the immune dysfunction that occurred during murine leukemia retrovirus infection in old mice. Leukemia is associated with dysregulated cytokine production. When leukemic mice were given DHEA supplements, loss of the cytokines Interleukin-2 and Interferon-gamma was prevented. DHEA also suppressed the excessive production of the dangerous cytokines interleukin-6 and interleukin-10. This preliminary study indicates DHEA might be effective in treating the immune dysfunction in those leukemia patients with a DHEA deficiency (especially older people). Please refer to the *DHEA Replacement Therapy protocol* for complete information on the proper use of DHEA supplements.

At this juncture, the hormone melatonin is not recommended in the treatment of lymphoma and leukemia. Patients should avoid the use of this product until more information is available.

CAUTION: If patients do choose to use melatonin, monthly blood testing for tumor markers should be closely monitored to determine if melatonin is promoting leukemic or lymphatic cell proliferation.

Because all cancer therapies produce individual responses based on factors such as the type of disease, patient's age, and the presence of other diseases, the Foundation recommends monthly blood markers to monitor the benefits of any supplemental therapies. The results of these blood tests provide critical information to evaluate the effectiveness of nonconventional therapies. If tumor markers do not decrease after the initiation of any nonconventional therapy, patients should discontinue their use and seek other alternatives immediately.

Conclusion

Leukemia, Hodgkin's lymphoma, and non-Hodgkin's lymphoma generally respond well to conventional therapies. There are many different types of these diseases; therefore chemotherapy and radiation therapy are individualized. Patients who do not respond well to chemotherapy and radiation therapy may benefit from other treatments such as bone marrow transplantation or a peripheral blood stem-cell transplant. In addition to conventional treatment there are a number of alternative therapies available. Patients with certain types of leukemia or lymphoma may derive beneficial effects from Vesanoid, vitamin A, vitamin D_3, curcumin, and soy extracts. It is imperative that patients have monthly monitoring of blood tumor markers to assess the usefulness of any treatment. Consult your hematologist or oncologist prior to initiating alternative treatments.

Summary

1. Early diagnosis and treatment of leukemias and lymphomas are essential. Symptoms of leukemia and lymphoma are generalized and include fatigue, weight loss, fever, and night sweats. In Hodgkin's and non-Hodgkin's lymphomas, swollen lymph nodes may be present.
2. Diagnosis of the specific disease may include X-rays, CT scans, and biopsy.
3. Chemotherapy and radiation therapy are usually used in combination to treat these diseases. The actual course of therapy depends on the specific type of disease.
4. Interferon, a biologic response modifier, has been proven effective in the treatment of some leukemias and low-grade lymphomas.
5. Patients who do not respond to chemotherapy and radiation therapy may be considered for peripheral blood stem-cell transplants or bone marrow transplants.
6. Vesanoid, a vitamin A analog, has proven effective in patients with chronic promyelocytic leukemia and may be beneficial for other types of cancers.
7. Water-soluble vitamin A may provide a useful alternative to Vesanoid for some cancer patients. The recommended dosage of this vitamin is 100,000 to 300,000 IU daily.

   CAUTION: Monthly blood tests are necessary to avoid vitamin A toxicity.

8. Vitamin D_3 and its analogs may induce differentiation of cancer cells into normal cells in certain types of lymphomas and leukemias.

   CAUTION: Serum calcium, kidney function, and liver function should be monitored monthly to avoid vitamin D toxicity.

9. Curcumin may induce cancer cell death in promyelocytic leukemia. The recommended daily dosage is 1800 to 2700 mg taken with a heavy meal.

   CAUTION: Patients with biliary tract obstruction should not take Curcumin.

10. Soy extract high in genistein, such as Mega Soy Extract, may inhibit cancer cell growth for a number of types of cancer. Recommended daily dosage of Mega Soy Extract is four 700-mg 40% isoflavone extract capsules spaced evenly throughout the day.

    CAUTION: Patients must avoid the use of soy extracts one week prior to, during, and following radiation therapy because soy extracts may inhibit the generation of free radicals that are essential to this type of therapy.

11. Patients who are positive for mutant p53 oncogenes may receive substantial benefits from the use of soy extracts.
12. At this time, melatonin is not recommended for the treatment of leukemia and lymphoma because it may promote cancer cell growth. DHEA replacement therapy may be considered.

For more information. Contact the American Cancer Society, (800) ACS-2345.

Product availability. Water-soluble vitamin A liquid, vitamin D_3 capsules, and Mega Soy Extract are available by phoning (800) 544-4440, or order on-line at www.lef.org. Vesanoid is a prescription drug and should be prescribed by your oncologist or hematologist.

LEUKOPENIA

(See Anemia/Thrombocytopenia/ Leukopenia)

LIVER CIRRHOSIS

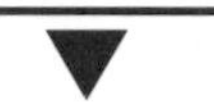

The Liver

The liver is the largest organ (about the size of a football and averaging about 3.5 pounds) and has more functions than any other human organ. A person's entire blood supply passes through the liver several times a day, and at any given time there is about a pint of blood there. The liver produces and secretes bile (to be stored in the gallbladder until needed) that is used to break down and digest fatty acids. It also produces prothrombin and fibrinogen, both blood-clotting factors, and heparin, a mucopolysaccharide sulfuric acid ester that helps keep blood from clotting within the circulatory system.

The liver converts sugar into glycogen, which it stores until the muscles need energy and it is secreted into the blood stream as glucose. The liver synthesizes proteins and cholesterol and converts carbohydrates and proteins into fats, which are stored for later use. It also produces blood protein and hundreds of enzymes needed for digestion and other bodily functions. As it breaks down proteins, the liver also produces urea, which it synthesizes from carbon dioxide and ammonia. (Urea, the primary solid component of urine, is eventually excreted by the kidneys.) The liver also stores critical trace elements such as iron and copper, as well as vitamins A, D, and B_{12}.

Cirrhosis

Cirrhosis of the liver is a chronic, diffuse (widely spread throughout the organ), degenerative liver disease in which the parenchyma (the functional organ tissue) degenerates, the lobules are infiltrated with fat and structurally altered, dense perilobular connective tissue forms, and areas of regeneration often develop. The first scientist known to have diagnosed the disease was Gianbattista Morgagni, who published 500 autopsies in 1761. Laennec named the disease in 1826, using the Greek word for orange color because cirrhotic livers turn a yellowish to tan color.

Cirrhosis is the seventh leading cause of death by disease in the United States, with about 25,000 dying from it each year (down from 50,000 in 1979). About a third of the cases are *compensated,* meaning there are no clinical symptoms. Such cases are usually discovered during routine tests for other problems, or during surgery or autopsy. In most cases, though, there is a loss of liver cell function, and an increased resistance to blood flow through the damaged liver tissue (a condition known as portal hypertension) leading to esophageal varices (enlarged, swollen veins at the lower end of the esophagus). Severe cirrhosis leads to ammonia toxicity, hepatic coma, gastrointestinal hemorrhage, and kidney failure. As liver cells are destroyed, they are systematically replaced by scar tissue.

Symptoms

Symptoms of cirrhosis include nausea or indigestion and vomiting, constipation or diarrhea, flatulence, anorexia, weight loss, ascites (the accumulation of serous fluids in the peritoneal cavity), light-colored stools, weakness or chronic dyspepsia, dull abdominal aching, varicosities, nosebleeds, bleeding gums, other internal and external bleeding, easy bruising, extreme dryness of skin, and spider angiomas. Psychotic mental changes such as extreme paranoia can occur in cases of advanced cirrhosis. Other symptoms are testicular atrophy, gynecomastia (enlargement of the male breast), and loss of chest and armpit hair.

Complications

When blood flow in the cirrhotic liver is restricted, blood can "back up" in the spleen, causing enlarged spleen and sequestered blood cells. In this condition the platelet count typically falls, and abnormal bleeding can result. In extreme cases blood can actually flow backward from portal circulation to systemic circulation, leading to varicose veins in the stomach (gastric varices), esophagus (esophageal varices), and rectum (hemorrhoids). Ruptured varices bleed massively and are often fatal. Bilirubin levels may build up in the blood, causing jaundice and bright yellow to dark brown urine. Cirrhosis can also cause insulin resistance and diabetes mellitus. Brain injury can result from inadequate filtering of blood toxins. Such brain damage can have symptoms that range from poor concentration to coma, swelling of the brain, stupor, and even death. Cirrhosis is often associated with osteomalacia (the adult form of rickets, a softening of the bones that often leaves them brittle) and osteoporosis (a reduction in bone mass).

The Alcohol Factor

The most common cause of cirrhosis is believed to be alcohol (ethanol) abuse (about 10% of American men and about 3% of American women chronically abuse alcohol). Though it affects many organs, alcohol is especially harmful to the central nervous system and the liver, and is a factor in about three-fourths of the cases of cirrhosis in the United States. Alcohol must be metabolized, and the liver performs most of that job, suffering serious damage in the process. Not only does alcohol destroy liver cells, it also robs them of their ability to regenerate.

Such cofactors as hepatitis C virus can increase the risk of cirrhosis in those whose intake of alcohol is excessive. Alcohol-induced cirrhosis is among the ten leading causes of death in the United States. Women are at much higher risk for drinking-related cirrhosis than are men. This may be true because less of the alcohol consumed is metabolized in the stomach in women before being absorbed into the blood stream. Autopsies indicate that from 10 to 15% of American alcoholics suffer from cirrhosis at the time of death. About a third of those consuming one cup to one pint (8 to 16 ounces) of hard liquor a day (or the equivalent in other drinks) over a 15-year period will develop cirrhosis.

In addition to cirrhosis, alcohol abuse can lead to fatty liver, which can lead to stearohepatitis (or steatohepatitis, the older term), scarring of the liver, and eventually to cirrhosis. Overuse of alcohol can also lead to acute, chronic hepatitis. Complications can include liver dysfunction, abnormal blood clotting, jaundice, and hepatic encephalopathy (neurological dysfunction brought on by failure of the liver). Chronic abusers of alcohol often need significant vitamin supplementation to correct vitamin deficiencies caused as much by neglect and poor eating habits as by damage from the alcohol. An acute thiamin (vitamin B_1) deficiency is typical.

Other Risk Factors and Causes

Cirrhosis patients are at high risk for obesity, fatal bacterial infections, stomach ulcers, kidney problems, gallstones, and diabetes mellitus. They are also at increased risk for liver cancer. Risk factors for cirrhosis include nutritional deficiencies (lack of proteins, vitamins, choline, trace elements, or methionine), hepatitis (B, C, or D) and other bacterial and viral infections, and severe reactions to prescription or "recreational" drugs. Vitamin B_1 (thiamin) deficiency may directly cause alcoholic cirrhosis. One study concluded that vitamin B_1 deficiency is a greater risk factor for liver cell death than heavy alcohol consumption.

Congestive heart failure and poisons (including alcohol, phosphorus, and carbon tetrachloride) pose a serious threat to the liver and can lead to cirrhosis. Genetic disorders, inherited metabolic diseases such as hemochromatosis (marked by excessive iron absorption and accumulation) and Wilson's disease (in which the liver stores too much copper), advanced syphilis, exposure to blood flukes, other parasitic infections (such as schistosomiasis), and blocking of the common bile duct are all factors that can lead to cirrhosis. Liver injury from an accident or from cystic fibrosis can also bring on cirrhosis.

Diagnosis

Positive diagnosis of cirrhosis must be made by liver biopsy, but X-ray, blood tests, and physical examination are all used in diagnosis, as is observation of the symptoms mentioned earlier. CAT (computerized axial tomography) scans, radioisotope liver scans, and ultrasound can all be used to diagnose cirrhosis. Early diagnosis is critical in order to establish the cause of the disease and determine the amount of damage to the liver.

Two symptoms of cirrhosis are the loss of healthy, functioning liver cells and the scarring and distortion of the liver that eventually take place. As fewer cells function, less albumin (a protein) is manufactured. Lowered albumin levels permit water retention (edema) in the legs and abdomen (ascites). Easy bruising and bleeding result, and, in some cases, vomiting of blood. Intense skin itching can also result from excessive bile product deposits in the skin, often accompanied by jaundice or yellow skin.

Gallstones are more likely to form in cirrhosis patients because there is not enough bile reaching the gallbladder. Toxins that the liver would normally remove build up in the blood, dulling mental functions and bringing on personality changes. Drugs the patient is taking, normally filtered out and disposed of in urine, may remain in the bloodstream for a much longer period and act longer than expected or even build up in body tissue. A liver with cirrhosis is usually much larger than a healthy liver.

Precautions and Prevention

Once cirrhosis has been diagnosed, sodium and fluids should be restricted, and all alcohol consumption must cease. Antiemetics, diuretics, and supplemental vitamins are prescribed. Cirrhosis patients should avoid straining at the bowel, violent sneezing and coughing, and nose blowing, and should use stool softeners as prescribed by a qualified medical caregiver. Untreated cirrhosis can be fatal; patients should avoid exposure to infections and eat small but frequent meals of nutritious foods, carefully following caregiver instructions. The liver is the only organ that can generate healthy, new tissue in response to injury or disease. It is therefore possible to regenerate a cirrhosis-damaged liver if extraordinary therapies are followed and the underlying cause of the cirrhosis is eliminated.

More than half of all liver disease could be prevented if we acted on the knowledge we already have. Avoiding or limiting the use of alcoholic beverages is a good place to start, because it is well documented that alcohol destroys liver cells. Man-made chemicals also pose an extreme threat to the liver, so take recommended precautions. Remember that all ingested, inhaled, and absorbed toxins must be processed by the liver. When working with hazardous chemicals use adequate ventilation; follow product instructions; do not mix chemicals; wear protective clothing and breathing equipment; avoid inhalation and ingestion of hazardous materials; avoid skin contact and flush (wash) affected areas immediately; if necessary, call your poison control center or your emergency number (such as 911). A complete listing of toll-free poison control center numbers can be obtained online [http://www.medicinenet.com/Script/Main/hp.asp].

Treatments

When varices result, they can be treated with a reduction of salt intake and with diuretics, which help eliminate excess salts and fluids from the body. Coma and encephalopathy are treated by a reduction of protein intake, and hemorrhage from varices can be stopped by sclerotherapy (injection of a scarring chemical into the bleeding vein). Varices can also be compressed by the use of a special balloon that is inflated around the enlarged vein, squeezing it as the balloon is inflated. There is a new procedure (using radiology)—transjugular intrahepatic protosystemic shunt (TIPS)—that shows some promise.

Interferon-alpha, a powerful antiviral, may reduce the risk of cancer in some cirrhosis patients. In cases of total liver failure, transplantation has been successful. Over 80% of liver transplant patients are still alive 5 years after the surgery. Japanese researchers found evidence that malotilate prevented both damage to liver cells and cirrhosis they attempted to induce in rats.

Natural Therapies

The liver can often perform its essential functions in spite of serious damage. It also has more ability to self-repair than do most other organs. It is important to give the liver the nutrients it needs to function and to regenerate and detoxify itself. Research done at the Center for Biomedical Research at the Hospital of St. Joan in Reus, Spain, in 1992 shows that supplementation of zinc lessens the effects of fibrogenesis in rats with induced cirrhosis. German research shows that zinc deficiencies are implicated in liver cirrhosis and concludes that zinc substitution should be provided to all cirrhosis patients when deficiency and corresponding symptoms are found. (Long-term supplementation of zinc should not exceed 90 mg a day.) Selenium deficiencies have also been found in the blood of cirrhosis patients, leading to recommendations for selenium supplementation. Ursodeoxycholic acid, a widely tested bile acid, has been found effective in slowing the progress of cirrhosis, preventing gallstone formation, and preventing the formation of varices.

Research has shown decreased blood serum levels of vitamins E and K_1, and increased levels of vitamin A and iron in some cirrhosis patients. These patients should not directly supplement vitamin A or beta carotene, and should also avoid niacin (vitamin B_3) and supplements containing extracts from the chaparral shrub. (Some research found absolutely no correlation between cirrhosis and vitamin A levels in the liver and concluded that cirrhosis patients were not at increased risk from vitamin A supplementation, while other studies showed decreased vitamin A levels in cirrhosis patients. More research is needed, but cirrhosis patients should consider vitamin A supplementation only under direct medical supervision.) Japanese studies showed that moderate intake of caffeine (in coffee) helped to counteract some of the negative effects of alcohol on the liver. Consumption of caffeine in green tea showed no such effect.

In Russian studies, supplementation with ascorbic acid (vitamin C) and alpha-tocopherol (vitamin E) improved the liver function of chronic liver disease patients. In a 1998 American study it was found that a high level of supplementation of vitamins B_2 (riboflavin) and B_{12} (cyanocobalamin and hydroxycobalamin, associated with folate metabolism) reduced the risk of cirrhosis associated with alcohol consumption above 50 grams (1.75 ounces) a day.

Recommended supplements for a seriously damaged liver are the amino acids acetyl-*L*-carnitine (2000 mg a day), *N*-acetylcysteine (600 mg twice a day), *L*-arginine (5 to 10 grams a day), leucine (1200 mg a day), isoleucine (600 mg a day), and valine (600 mg a day). Silymarin (at about 600 mg a day) is effective in cirrhosis patients, even in alcoholic liver cirrhosis. It is especially helpful for diabetics with cirrhosis because it reduces the lipoperoxidation of cell membranes and insulin resistance, decreasing the need for insulin supplementation. *L*-Arginine (up to 5 to 10 grams a day) and glutamine (2000 mg a day) are only effective when there is still at least 20% liver function remaining. (*L*-arginine should be taken under a doctor's supervision.)

Because ethanol damages the liver at least in part by the generation of free radicals, and because it depresses an enzyme needed to convert methionine into SAMe (*S*-adenosylmethionine), SAMe supplementation can help regenerate normal liver function. Periodic blood testing is required to monitor the effectiveness of patient therapy. Doses of 400 to 800 mg twice a day have shown promise in reversing alcoholic cirrhosis. A less expensive alternative is twice-a-day supplementation with 500 mg of TMG (trimethylglycine, or betaine), folic acid (800 mcg), and vitamin B_{12} (500 mcg per day). Supplementation with phosphatidylcholine (2000 mg per day) may provide protection against alcohol-induced septal fibrosis, cirrhosis, and lipid peroxidation.

Because anemia is a common complication in cirrhosis patients, iron deficiency is a possibility. Iron supplementation should only be used under direct medical supervision with close monitoring because excessive iron can cause severe liver damage, especially when combined with alcohol, porphyrogenic drugs, or chronic viral hepatitis. Iron can also enhance the disease-producing abilities of viruses, adversely affect immune function, and enhance fibrogenic pathways, all of which may increase liver injury. Iron may also be implicated as a cocarcinogen or promoter of hepatocellular carcinoma, even in patients without hepatitis C or cirrhosis.

Ongoing Research

There is a large amount of research and study into causes and cures of cirrhosis of the liver. Patients and healthcare providers should stay abreast of research findings for the latest developments in cirrhosis treatment and therapy.

Summary

Cirrhosis of the liver can be caused by excessive alcohol consumption, accidental, bacterial, or viral liver damage, exposure to toxic chemicals, and severe reaction to prescription or "recreational" drugs. Supplementation of antioxidants, branched-chain amino acids, and all except B_3 (niacin) of the B complex of vitamins has been shown to be beneficial. For specific antiviral therapies to help eradicate hepatitis B or C, refer to our *Hepatitis B* and *Hepatitis C* protocols.

1. Drink alcohol in moderation if at all. If diagnosed with cirrhosis, do not drink.
2. Studies on alcoholic cirrhosis patients have shown benefits from supplementing valine, leucine, and isoleucine. These branched-chain amino acids can enhance protein synthesis in liver and muscle cells and are used by body builders to produce an anabolic effect. Four capsules of Branch Chain Amino Acids (free form) provide 200 mg of *L*-leucine, 600 mg of *L*-isoleucine, 600 mg of *L*-valine, and 10 mg of vitamin B_6 (pyridoxine). The suggested dose is 2 to 4 capsules per day between meals with fruit juice or before eating.

WARNING: These capsules are only to be used by adults who are fully grown, and not by anyone afflicted with pellagra.

3. Patients with depleted SAMe levels should take from two to four 200-mg tablets a day of SAMe, spread throughout the day. Patients must adhere to physician-prescribed blood testing schedules to assess the effectiveness of this therapy. A cost-effective alternative to SAMe supplementation is TMG (trimethylglycine). The suggested dose is two 500-mg tablets after meals, twice a day, or as directed by a physician.
4. The vitamin B complex is extremely important for liver health. Therefore, daily supplementation of vitamins B_1 (500 mg), B_2 (75 mg), B_5 (1500 mg), and B_6 (200 mg) is strongly recommended (though vitamin B_3 [niacin] should be avoided by cirrhosis patients).
5. Other recommended daily supplements are 1500 mg of choline, 1600 mg of folic acid, 500 mg of vitamin C, 800 IU of vitamin E, 300 micrograms of selenium, and 100 mg of Coenzyme Q_{10} (for its antioxidant and blood flow-enhancing properties).
6. Acetyl-*L*-carnitine should be taken in two daily doses of 1000 mg each. Take two 600-mg doses per day of *N*-acetylcysteine. Drink green tea, or take 4 to 10 standardized 100-mg capsules of green tea extract a day to lower toxic levels of iron (which may exacerbate free radical damage to the liver).
7. 5 to 10 grams of *L*-arginine and 2000 mg a day of glutamine may help lower blood levels of toxic ammonia permitted to build up by a damaged liver. *L*-arginine can help facilitate liver regeneration if the liver still has at least 20% functional reserve capacity.
8. Silymarin treatment (about 600 mg a day) is appropriate for all alcoholic liver disease patients, and has reduced insulin resistance in diabetic patients with cirrhosis.
9. Zinc should be supplemented in cirrhosis patients at a rate of at least 30 mg per day (not to exceed 90 mg a day), while selenium should be supplemented according to your doctor's instructions.

For more information. Contact the American Liver Foundation, (800) 223-0179.

Product availability. SAMe; vitamins B_1, B_2, B_5, and B_6; folic acid; choline; vitamins C and E; Coenzyme Q_{10}; acetyl-*L*-carnitine, *N*-acetyl-cysteine, green tea, *L*-arginine, curcumin, silymarin, and the branched-chain amino acid complex

L

(valine, leucine, and isoleucine) can be ordered by calling (800) 544-4440, or order on-line at www.lef.org.

LIVER DEGENERATIVE DISEASE (GENERAL)

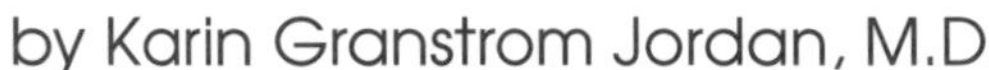

by Karin Granstrom Jordan, M.D.

In spite of increasing health consciousness in our society, it is striking how comparatively little attention is given to the liver and its vitality in our discussions about health and disease.

This article presents the intriguing facts about the central role of the liver, and explains why a well functioning liver is crucial for our overall health. It points to the environmental hazards that constantly challenge the liver's detoxification capacity and presents recent research on the effects of alcohol on the liver. It tells you what you can do to support and optimize the function of your liver—and thus your future health.

Hepatoprotection—protection of the liver—is a subject that should be close to heart for all of us. The reason is the liver's critical role in all aspects of metabolism and its central role in overall health.

In Europe and Asia herbal liver tonics have been in common use for decades or even centuries. The effectiveness of the herbs used in these remedies has been validated during the last decades through modern research and clinical studies. These herbs generally contain antioxidants, membrane stabilizing and bile enhancing compounds or compounds that prevent depletion of sulfhydryl compounds such as glutathione, as we will see in the review below.

First let us take a look at the liver.

What Does the Liver Do?

The liver is a remarkable organ with multiple functions. Weighing about four pounds, it is the largest organ of the body, located on the right side in the upper abdomen. The liver quietly does an extraordinary job in keeping us alive and healthy by metabolizing the food we eat, i.e. breaking it down to useful parts, and protecting us from the damaging effects of the numerous toxic compounds that we are exposed to on a daily basis. It has impressive restorative capabilities, and is the only organ that will regenerate itself, when part of it is damaged.

This regeneration capacity is one of the intriguing survival mechanisms of the body and very fortunate for us, as our health to a large extent depends on a well-functioning liver. While being exposed to a tremendous amount of potential damage, the liver is responsible for a multitude of essential functions related to metabolism, filtration, bile production, detoxification, and immune function.

The metabolic functions of the liver are countless, as the liver is intricately involved in carbohydrate, fat and protein metabolism, in storage of vitamins and minerals and in many essential physiological processes. So, for example, the liver is involved in several regulatory mechanisms that control blood sugar levels and hormone levels. It synthesizes proteins (such as plasma albumin, fibrinogen and most globulins), lipids and lipoproteins (phospholipids, cholesterol) as well as bile acids that are excreted in the detoxification process.

Detoxification is an essential part of the human body's metabolism, and the liver plays a key role in this process. Toxic chemicals, both of internal and external origin, are constantly bombarding the liver. Our normal everyday metabolic processes actually produce a wide range of toxins that need to be taken care of by neutralizing mechanisms in the liver. Nutritional deficiencies and imbalances add to the production of toxins, as do alcohol and many prescription drugs, which increases the stress on the liver by requiring a strong detoxification capacity. Even unprocessed organic foods, however, have naturally occurring toxic components and require an effective detoxification system.

It is our external environment, however, that contributes the most to the load of toxins that the liver has to detoxify. The burden on the liver today is heavier than ever before in history. Toxic chemicals are found in the food we eat, in the water we drink and the air we breathe both outdoors and indoors. Chemicals such as p-xylene, tetrachloroethylene, ethylbenzene and benzene were documented as "everywhere present" in the air, in a study by the Environmental Protection Agency (EPA) (Wallace LA et al., 1989). Others listed as "often present" were chloroform, carbon tetrachloride, styrene, and p-dichlorobenzene. A visit to the gas station or the dry cleaner as well as smoking resulted in elevated breath levels of toxins.

The FDA has found the level of chlorinated pesticides in food to be alarming (Total Diet Survey). DDE was found in 63% or more of the 42 food samples, although DDT and DDE have been banned for use in this country since 1972. Unfortunately, toxic chemicals used all over the world move easily around the globe with the winds.

There is enough evidence today of a connection between chemical exposure and chronic health problems to understand that our herbicides, pesticides, household chemicals, food additives etc. create a serious health problem.

Now, what happens when the liver's detoxification system is overloaded? The reason is simple. When the liver cannot do its work, the toxins that we are exposed to accumulate in the body and make us sick in various ways. They have damaging effects on many body functions, particularly the immune system, and cause many chronic health problems. An overburdened and undernourished liver is known to be a root cause of many chronic diseases.

A majority of cancers are thought to be due to the effects of environmental carcinogens (cigarette smoke is one of them), particularly if combined with deficiencies of nutrients that are needed for optimal functioning of the detoxification and immune systems. It was recently demonstrated in a study of chemical plant workers in Turin, Italy, that people with the poorest detoxification systems were the ones who developed bladder cancer (Talska G et al. 1994).

Detoxification Pathways

The liver has three main detoxification pathways: 1/Filtering of the blood to remove large toxins. 2/ breaking down enzymatically unwanted chemicals. This usually occurs in two steps, with Phase I modifying the chemicals to make them an easier target for the Phase II enzyme systems. 3/ synthesizing and secreting bile for excretion of fat-soluble toxins and cholesterol.

Filtering of the blood is one of the liver's primary functions. Approximately 2 quarts of blood pass through the liver every minute to be detoxified. This is critical as the blood is loaded with bacteria, endotoxins and antigen-antibody complexes and various other toxic substances from the intestines. A healthy liver clears almost 100% of the bacteria and toxins from the blood before it joins the general circulation.

The liver's second main role in detoxification involves an ***enzymatic process in two steps*** for the neutralization of unwanted chemical compounds, such as drugs, pesticides and enterotoxins from the intestines. Even normal body compounds such as hormones get eliminated this way. Phase I enzymes directly neutralize some of these chemicals, but many others are converted to intermediate forms that are then processed by phase II enzymes. These intermediate forms are often much more chemically active and therefore more toxic than the original substance, so if the Phase II detoxification systems aren't working adequately, these intermediates linger and cause damage.

Phase I detoxification involves a group of fifty to one hundred enzymes that has been named the cytochrome P450 system. These enzymes play a central role in the detoxification of both exogenous (such as drugs and pesticides) and endogenous (such as hormones) compounds and in the synthesis of steroid hormones and bile acids.

A side effect of this metabolic activity is the production of free radicals, which are highly reactive molecules that will bind to cellular components and cause damage. The most important antioxidant for neutralizing these free radicals is glutathione, which is needed both for Phase I and Phase II. When exposure to high levels of toxin produce so many free radicals from Phase I detoxification that all the glutathione is used up, Phase II processes dependent on glutathione stop. This causes an imbalance between Phase I and Phase II activity, which results in severe toxic reactions, due to build-up of toxic intermediate forms.

Phase II detoxification involves conjugation, which means that a protective compound becomes bound to the toxin. Besides glutathione conjugation there are essentially five other pathways: amino acid conjugation, methylation, sulfation, sulfoxidation, acetylation and glucoronidation. These enzyme systems need nutrients and metabolic energy in order to work. If the liver cells are not functioning properly, phase II detoxification slows down and increases the toxic load by allowing the build-up of toxic intermediates.

The third major role of the liver is synthesis and secretion of bile. The liver manufactures approximately one quart of bile every day, which serves as a carrier for toxic substances to be effectively eliminated from the body. In addition, the bile emulsifies fats and fat-soluble vitamins in the intestine, improving their absorption. When the excretion of bile is inhibited (cholestasis), toxins stay in the liver longer with damaging effects.

Cholestasis has several causes, one of which is obstruction of the bile ducts by the presence of gallstones. Bile flow can also be impaired within the liver itself. By far the most important cause of cholestasis and impaired liver function in the United States is the consumption of alcohol. Other common causes are viral hepatitis and side effects from various drugs, particularly steroidal hormones including estrogen and oral contraceptives.

These conditions often cause alterations of liver function tests indicating cellular damage. In the initial stages of liver dysfunction, however, standard tests (serum bilirubin, alkaline phosphatase, SGOT, LDH, GGTP, etc.) are usually not sensitive enough to be of value. The measurement of serum bile acids, on the other hand, has proven to be a safe and sensitive test to determine the functional capacity of the liver.

Symptoms that may indicate reduced liver function are general malaise, fatigue, and digestive disturbances including constipation, allergies and chemical sensitivities. Generalized pruritus and nausea and vomiting during pregnancy can also be a result of impaired hepatofunction.

Fatty Liver (Steatosis)/ Steatohepatitis/Cirrhosis

Fatty liver or steatosis is a common finding in human liver biopsies. It is a condition where fat has accumulated within liver cells (hepatocytes) without causing any specific symptoms. (It has been defined either as more than 5% of cells containing fat droplets or total lipid exceeding 5% of liver weight.).

Fatty liver as a longstanding chronic condition can occur in association with a wide range of diseases, toxins and drugs, although in clinical practice, the majority of cases are due to alcohol excess, diabetes and obesity. Much less common are occurrences of acute fatty liver of pregnancy and as a response to administration of tetracyclines, acetaminophen and other drugs and toxins.

The understanding of steatosis has advanced considerably in recent years. Fatty liver was believed to be a benign reversible condition. Careful clinical studies, however, demonstrate that fatty liver of either alcoholic or non-alcoholic origin can lead to inflammation, cell death and fibrosis (steatohepatitis), and eventually even cirrhosis. Cirrhosis is the irreversible end result of fibrous scarring, a response of the liver to a variety of kinds of long-standing inflammatory, toxic, metabolic, and congestive damage.

Alcohol is by far the commonest cause both of steatosis and cirrhosis in the Western world. As we know it, however, there is a considerable interindividual difference in the degree of liver damage produced by excessive alcohol intake. There seem to be no correlation between the incidence and severity of fatty liver and either the amount, type or duration of alcohol abuse. It has been unclear why in some individuals steatosis, whatever its etiology, never progresses to steatohepatitis and cirrhosis.

A growing body of evidence supports a role for lipid peroxidation in the further development of liver damage. In other words it requires additional exposure to toxins that produce free radical damage (Pessayre et al.).

Free radicals have been demonstrated to have an important role in the hepatotoxic effect of many substances as well in the pathological processes of inflammation, atherosclerosis, cancerogenesis and aging.

Lipid oxidation is a chain reaction which is started by the attack of unstable free radicals on membrane lipids (unsaturated fatty acids) with the formation of lipidic free radicals and, in presence of oxygen, of lipoperoxides. The end products of the chain reaction are of various types depending on the fatty acids involved. The peroxidation damage impairs the anatomical and functional integrity of membranes and creates new toxic substances that further extend the damage.

Cytochrome P450 (CYP) 2E1, an enzyme in the P450 system which is known to be induced in both alcoholic and non-alcoholic steatohepatitis (Weltman MD et al., 1997), seems to play a role here through its generation of free radicals. In light of this recent research it seems likely that the individual susceptibility to advanced alcoholic liver disease can be explained by differences in the amount of exposure to environmental toxins and to the dietary intake of anti- or pro-oxidants (Berson A, 1998, Vol 114, No 4).

Obesity and Liver Disease

Among the causes for non-alcoholic steatohepatitis (NASH), obesity is considered to be the most common. There is evidence to suggest that liver disease actually can be considered a complication of obesity. No major prospective longitudinal studies of NASH have been carried out. It seems, however, that the risk of progression to cirrhosis generally is low for non-obese individuals but significant among obese individuals. There is no predictable correlation between symptoms (or lack of them), abnormality of liver function tests and severity of liver tissue damage.

In a study of 50 unselected, obese (21-130% above ideal body weight) subjects admitted to hospital for weight reduction, Braillon et al (1985) found that 10% had normal livers, 48% fatty livers, 26% steatohepatitis, 8% fibrosis and 8% cirrhosis.

Interestingly, it has been observed among patients with fatty liver related to obesity, that rapid weight loss caused by dieting and intestinal bypass surgery increase the risk for developing steatotohepatitis. The resulting increase in the concentration of fatty acids and/or ketones within the liver severely augments the generation of free radicals (Day CP et al.: 1994).

A study by Yang et al (1997) indicates that obesity also increases susceptibility to endotoxin-mediated liver injury. Endotoxins are cell wall components produced by intestinal gram-negative bacteria, thought to play a role in liver injury induced by alcohol and other hepatotoxins. Under normal conditions they are absorbed into the portal venous circulation and detoxified in the liver. Hepatic dysfunction will interfere with this clearing mechanism and amplify the negative activities of endotoxin, such as lipid peroxidation, reduced P-450 function and impairment of the immune system.

Berson et al. 1998 summarizes the insights from the new research on the mechanisms of steatohepatitis well:

> "Its development requires a double hit, the first producing steatosis, the second a source of oxidative stress capable of initiating significant lipid peroxidation. This concept provides a rationale for both the treatment and prevention of disease progression in steatosis of alcoholic and non-alcoholic causes. Management strategies should ideally be directed at reducing the severity of steatosis and at avoiding and removing the triggers of inflammation and fibrosis. ***Specific treatment modalities for at-risk individuals might include sensible weight reduction, cessation of exposure to toxins and treatment with antioxidants and inhibitors of peroxisomal b-oxidation."***

As conventional medicine does not have much to offer in the treatment of chronic liver conditions, we may benefit from looking at alternative possibilities. Several natural remedies have long been used in Europe for liver support and are validated by recent scientific research. Some of the most valued are extracts from ancient plants such as milk thistle and artichoke. Also green tea and phospholipids extracted from the soybean have proven to be extremely valuable.

Phosphatidylcholine

Phosphatidylcholine (PC), the main component of lecithin) is a phospholipid, a kind of fat that is found throughout the body as an integral part of cell membranes, essential for their structural and functional integrity.

Cell membranes act like gatekeepers, allowing nutrients into the cells but blocking damaging toxins from gaining entrance. Supplemental phosphatidylcholine in the form of polyunsaturated phospholipid extract from soybeans (PPC) has been shown to enhance this function. It has been shown to protect against various types of experimental liver damage in animal models (see below) and to accelerate liver regeneration after partial hepatectomy (Holecek M et al., 1992). Clinical studies have proven it to be a promising agent for the treatment and prevention of liver cirrhosis, and PPC is approved for the treatment of chronic liver diseases in many European countries and is actually listed in the PDR of the United States. PPC is well absorbed in humans and animals when taken orally (by mouth). There are no known contraindications, side effects or interactions with other drugs, even with consumption of large quantities of phosphatidylcholine or commercially available (less pure) lecithin.

Although it has not been clearly established how PPC exerts its protective effect, it is believed that it is based on its ability to be incorporated into normal and damaged liver cell membranes. Animal studies have indicated that poly*unsaturated* phosphatidylcholine becomes incorporated into the membranes of hepatocytes as a substitute for endogenous *saturated* phosphatidylcholine molecules (Stoffel W et al., 1978). This substitution is shown to result in an increase in membrane fluidity and active transport activity. Another mechanism seems to be increased collagen breakdown by stimulating collagenase activity in hepatic stellate cells preventing the development of fibrosis and cirrhosis (Li et al., 1992). Surprisingly, recent evidence gathered in rodents and non-human primates revealed striking antioxidant effects as well. Despite its rich content in polyunsaturated linoleic acid, PPC was shown to prevent lipid peroxidation and associated liver damage from alcohol or carbon tetrachloride (CCl_4). (Aleynik SI et al., 1995). Similarly it was shown that PPC can prevent or minimize the liver damage induced by adriamycin treatment (Biagi PL, 1993).

Membrane alterations have been described in a variety of liver diseases and are particularly prominent in alcoholic liver disease. (Yamada S et al., 1985). A characteristic feature of liver disease, regardless of its cause, is the increased deposition of collagen, the connective tissue protein. This increased collagen accumulation could result from enhanced collagen biosynthesis and/or decreased collagen breakdown. Several studies have focused on PPC and its effect on collagen and fibrosis.

A baboon study (Lieber C, 1994) confirmed earlier results (Lieber C 1990) showing that in the baboon, feeding of ethanol results in hepatic fibrosis and cirrhosis even when associated with an adequate diet. This effect could be prevented by supplementing the diet with a 94-96% pure PPC preparation. None of the 8 animals fed alcohol with PPC for up to 6.5 years had progression to fibrosis or cirrhosis as had 10 of 12 unsupplemented baboons, a highly significant difference.

Another study (Ma X, Lieber C et al., 1996) revealed that PPC reduces hepatic fibrosis induced by either CCl4 or human albumin in rats, and that PPC not only prevents the development of fibrosis but accelerates the regression of pre-existing fibrosis. The study further suggested that the protective effect exerted by PPC against fibrosis is due, at least in part to increased collagen breakdown.

Lieber's team further showed (Aleynik S, 1997) that PPC extracted from soybeans opposes hepatic oxidative stress induced by CCl4 in rats and chronic alcohol consumption in baboons. In 1998 the same team showed that the oxidative stress caused by alcohol in the pancreas can be fully prevented by the administration of PPC. It was further observed that alcohol feeding caused depletion of pancreatic glutathione, which was fully restored by PPC.

The above mentioned animal studies have led to ongoing double-blind clinical studies, where alcohol-consuming patients are given PPC with the aim of finding out to what extent PPC may affect lipoprotein changes and the development of arteriosclerosis. While waiting for these results in humans, a study was undertaken on ethanol-fed rats to examine whether PPC, with or without alcohol consumption, affects serum lipoprotein. (Khursheed P et al., 1997). PPC supplementation of the diet markedly decreased postprandial triglyceride and LDL-cholesterol levels, whereas it maintained high levels of HDL-cholesterol (the good cholesterol). There was also a marked reduction of alcoholic fatty liver.

If these changes in serum proteins produced by PPC in ethanol-fed rats can be extrapolated to men, they may add a great additional benefit to alcohol consumers in preventing atherosclerosis and coronary heart disease.

High serum lipids are common also in diabetic patients (approx. in 50%), and the incidence of coronary heart disease is high. In a double-blind study on the lipoprotein profile in diabetic patients (Kirsten R., 1994), 30 non-insulin-dependent diabetics with secondary hyperlipidemia received 2.7 g PPC or placebo daily over a 2-month period. LDL-cholesterol and triglyceride levels decreased significantly when compared with the placebo group, and HDL cholesterol levels increased. In the control group the values did not change throughout the trial.

Another clinical trial of interest was designed to evaluate the effects of PPC in combination with interferon alpha (IFN) in chronic hepatitis B and C. IFN is the standard treatment for these diseases, however only 50% of patients with Hepatitis B and 20-30% of patients with hepatitis C respond to this anti-viral drug with long term normalization of serum enzymes. Of patients with hepatitis C who do respond to IFN while under treatment, there is at least a 50% relapse rate. Thus more effective treatment is needed. 176 patients completed the study protocol. All patients were given the same amount of interferon during the 24-week test period. In addition patients were randomly assigned to receive either PPC or placebo for the same 24 weeks. The results show that PPC increased the response rate to IFN in chronic viral hepatitis C (71% versus 51% in the placebo group). Prolonged PPC therapy given to responders 24 weeks beyond the cessation of interferon therapy tended to increase the rate of sustained responders in patients with hepatitis C (41% versus 15%). In contrast, PPC did not alter the biochemical response to interferon in patients with hepatitis B. The reason why PPC showed a beneficial effect in hepatitis C and not in hepatitis B is not clear and will be further investigated.

In addition to hepatoprotective qualities of phospholipids, a study by Lichtenberger et al. (1995) pointed to their possible use in prevention and reversal of NSAID-induced gastrointestinal injury. The consumption of non-steroidal anti-inflammatory drugs (NSAIDs) in our society is greater than any other drug class because of their relative effectiveness in the treatment of pain and inflammation. A major concern, however, with these drugs relates to their well-established ability to induce gastrointestinal injury in the forms of bleeding and ulcers. Efforts to reduce their injurious effects by means of enteric coating have had limited success because of the resulting delay of therapeutic action.

It has become clear over the last few years, according to Lichtenberger, that the gastrointestinal tract has hydrophobic "non-wettable" properties that protect the underlying epithelium from gastric acid and other toxic substances. This characteristic seems to be attributable to an extracellular lining of phospholipids, which are synthesized in surface mucus cells of the stomach. It has been observed that aspirin and other NSAIDs have the ability to rapidly transform the gastric mucosa from a non-wettable to a wettable state and thereby increasing the tissue's susceptibility to the corrosive actions of gastric acid.

A study using phosphatidylcholine on experimentally induced gastric ulcers in rats (Dunjic BS 1993) showed that mucosal lesions were significantly reduced by a single dose of PPC given before or after the injury factor, which in this study was ethanol or NSAID.

Another experimental study (Lichtenberger LM et al. (1995) showed evidence that aspirin and other NSAIDs chemically bind with the major surfactant phospholipid, dipalmitoylphosphatidylcholine (DPPC) in the gastric mucosa. When the NSAID is bound to the phospholipid before administration, the injurious potential of NSAIDs is significantly reduced. These observations clearly demonstrated that the tendency of NSAIDs to induce acute and/or chronic GI lesions and bleeding was remarkably decreased if the drugs were administered as a complex with DPPC or related phospholipids. It was also shown that the antipyretic and anti-inflammatory activities of aspirin were consistently enhanced when associated with phospholipids. This unexpected finding was attributed to the increase in lipid permeability and solubility of the aspirin complex, which would promote its movement across the membranes into the target cells. These are intriguing research findings, and its clinical use has yet to be assessed in completion of human studies.

Green Tea

Catechins are another group of plant polyphenols of potential therapeutic significance. These flavonoids are for example found in high concentrations in green tea, which is made from the unfermented leaves of the tea plant. Green tea has been in common use among Chinese people for thousands of years. During he last decades it has become widely used in Europe in the treatment of hepatic disease and other conditions.

As with many other flavonoids, catechin has been shown to possess antiviral activity and to have several immune stimulating properties. (Kaul T et al., 1985, Sipos J et al., 1981, Valloton J 1981). It has furthermore been shown to prevent hepatotoxicity from carbon tetrachloride, ethanol and bromotrichloromethane intoxication (Ritter J et al., 1985) in experimental studies. Its hepatoprotective effect has been related to its properties as a powerful free radical scavenger and antioxidant as well as its anti-endotoxin effect and its ability to stabilize membranes.

An international workshop in 1981 on the use of catechin in diseases of the liver concluded that the flavonoid has much promise for the treatment of many types of hepatic disease, particularly acute and chronic viral hepatitis. Catechin has been shown, in numerous double-blind clinical studies, to decrease serum bilirubin levels in patients with all types of acute viral hepatitis (A, B and C) and to give significantly more rapid relief of clinical symptoms (i.e., nausea, anorexia, fatigue, abdominal discomfort, and pruritus) and a greater improvement in liver function tests than in control groups.

An interesting study from 1998 (Sai K et al.) was performed on rats that were given green tea in the drinking water one week before and throughout a 2 week exposure to 2-nitropropane. 2-nitropropane has been detected in tobacco smoke, is widely used as an industrial solvent (Hoffman and Rathkamp 1968), and has been demonstrated to induce hepatotoxicity (Lewis et al., 1979), cell proliferation (Cunningham and Matthews 1991) and carcinogenesis (Fiala et al., 1987) in the liver of rats. In humans, hepatotoxicity and liver cancer are considered to be the major risks from this toxin. The findings of the study showed that treatment with green tea effectively inhibited hepatotoxic changes induced by 2-nitropropane treatment such as lipid peroxidation, oxidative DNA damage and cell proliferation, suggesting that green tea intake may be effective for prevention of hepatic injuries after chronic exposure to 2-nitropropane.

The role of endotoxins in the development of liver disease (particularly all types of hepatitis and alcohol-induced cirrhosis) has been mentioned before. Catechin has a direct degradation effect on endotoxins and indirectly stabilizes cell membranes by preventing free radical–induced damage by (the lipid portion of) the endotoxin molecule.

Catechin affects collagen metabolism in various ways and offers anti-ulcer activity both in animal and human studies (Wendt P et al., 1980). This effect is due to catechin's ability to inhibit histidine decarboxylase, an enzyme responsible for the conversion of histidine to histamine, which may have wide clinical applications also for allergic conditions and inflammations.

Another interesting application is its potential use after abdominal surgery, where the formation of adhesions is a common and severe problem. (Catechin is an inhibitor of procollagen and collagen biosynthesis (Pontz B, 1982).) When catechin was given within the first five days of surgery in an animal (rat) study it substantially inhibited adhesion formation following experimental adhesion induction (Rivkind A et al., 1983). Catechin has also been shown in a double blind, human study to significantly reduce postoperative edema (Baruch J, 1984).

For most people drinking green tea daily seems to be one of the most practical and readily available means for preventing chronic toxicity or cancer, induced by oxidative stress from environmental chemicals. It is estimated that about one cup of green tea corresponds to the preventive dose used in the above-mentioned animal study. The dosages used for hepatic diseases in clinical studies have typically been one gram three times a day.

Milk Thistle

Silybum Marianum or milk thistle is a medicinal plant known since ancient times, and widely used in traditional European medicine. Since 1975, silymarin, and its main constituent silybin in particular, have been the subject of numerous experimental, pharmacological and clinical studies, which have provided support for its current clinical use in Europe in the treatment of liver disease.

Silybum marianum is a member of the aster family, to which the artichoke plant also belongs (see below). The plant is native to the Mediterranean area, where it has been in common use for more than 2000 years. Currently it is grown commercially throughout the Unites States as well as in Africa and South America. The name "milk thistle" is surrounded with several myths, but could simply be due to its characteristic spiked leaves with white veins.

The active extract of milk thistle is silymarin, a mixture of flavolignins, including silydianin, silychristine, and silybin, with the latter being the most biologically active. Silymarin has proven to be one of the most potent liver-protecting substances known, although the mechanisms are not yet fully understood. Its main routes of protection appear to be prevention of free–radical damage, stabilization of plasma membranes and stimulation of new liver cell production.

Silymarin acts as an antioxidant and free radical scavenger, many times more potent than vitamin E. (Hikino H et al., 1984). It has been shown to inhibit lipid peroxidation and to prevent glutathione depletion induced by alcohol and other liver toxins and even increase the total glutathione level in the liver by 35% over controls (Valenzuela et al., 1989). Silymarin has also been shown to inhibit the formation of liver-damaging leukotrienes by being a potent inhibitor of the enzyme lipoxygenase. This enzyme is a needed catalyst for the transfer of oxygen to polyunsaturated fatty acids (Fiebrich F et al., 1979, Dehmlow C, 1996). Silymarin has furthermore been reported to decrease the activity of tumor promoters (Agrawal R et al., 1994, Zi X et al., 1997) and protect against radiation-induced suppression of hepatic and splenic DNA and RNA synthesis (Hakova H et al., 1993). Perhaps the most interesting effect of silymarin on the liver is its ability to stimulate protein synthesis (Sonnenbichler J et al., 1986), which results in production of new liver cells to replace damaged old ones. Interestingly, silybin does not have a stimulatory effect on malignant hepatic tissue.

Experimental liver damage in animals can be produced by numerous toxic chemicals, such as carbon tetrachloride and ethanol. Silymarin has been shown to be very effective in protecting the liver from these toxins. Most interesting is its effect against the poisoning of Amanita phalloides (the toadstool mushroom). The toxins in this mushroom are the most powerful liver-damaging substances known, and ingestion causes severe poisoning and leads to death in approximately 30% of the cases. In experimental models silymarin was 100% effective in preventing toxicity, when it was administered *before* amanita poisoning, Even if given 10 minutes after the amanita toxin, it completely counteracted the toxic effects. If given within 24 hours, silymarin would still prevent death and greatly reduce the amount of liver damage. (Vogel G et al., 1984; Desplaces A et al., 1975). Observation of human cases with Amanita poisoning has demonstrated similar results. In 60 patients who were treated with silybin 20 mg/kg/day starting 24-36 hours after ingestion of the mushroom, the survival rate was 100% (Vogel G 1977). Another European trial involving 220 patients resulted in a mortality rate of 12.8%, versus a 22.4% in patients who had not received silymarin therapy.

The effectiveness of silymarin to protect the liver against chemical-induced damage is true also for alcohol. In a double blind trial of patients who chronically abused alcohol and had histologic documentation of chronic alcoholic hepatitis, the patients were given silymarin 140 mg twice a day for 6 months. Several liver function tests normalized and others decreased significantly, as compared to the levels in the control group (Feher J, 1989). Positive effects on histology, lymphocyte proliferation and lipid peroxidation were also described.

Another study involving ninety-seven patients with persistent liver function test abnormalities after one month of alcohol abstinence, showed impressive results. The patients were given either silymarin or placebo for a period of 4 months. At the end of therapy mean serum levels of AST and ALT had fallen by 30% and 41% respectively in the silymarin group, compared to an increase of 5% and 3% respectively in the placebo group. Significantly more patients returned to a normal bromsulphalein retention with treatment, and there was significantly more reversal of tissue damage (histological injury) (Salmi HA, 1982).

Ferenci P et al., (1989) asked 170 patients (92 alcoholic and 78 non-alcoholic) with biopsy-confirmed cirrhosis (the most severe form of liver scarring) to abstain from alcohol. He then treated 87 with silymarin 140 mg three times a day and 83 with placebo for a period of 2-6 years. The study showed a reduction of mortality in the treated group, particularly in the patients with cirrhosis of alcoholic origin. Silymarin has also been shown to improve immune function in patients with cirrhosis, the mechanism of which has yet to be determined (Deak G, 1990).

Silymarin is also reported to be effective in both acute and chronic viral hepatitis. A study of 29 patients with acute viral hepatitis (Magliulo E et al., 1978) showed a significantly higher rate of normalized laboratory parameters in the silymarin group after 3 weeks of treatment compared to the placebo group. In a study on chronic viral hepatitis, silymarin treatment resulted in a remarkable improvement (Berenguer J et al., 1977). Used in a dose of 420 mg/day for 3-12 months the effects achieved were: reversal of liver cell damage (as noted by biopsy), increase in plasma protein levels, a lowering of liver enzymes and improvement of common hepatitis symptoms.

Interestingly some studies on phosphatidylcholine-bound silymarin indicate an even greater effectiveness, which most likely is due to enhanced absorption across the gastrointestinal mucosa (Barzaghi N et al., 1990). In a small short-term study of 20 patients with chronic hepatitis due to either virus or alcohol, phosphatidyl-bound silymarin was given for two weeks with significant decrease in bilirubin and liver enzyme levels (Vailati A et al., 1993).

In animal studies it has recently been demonstrated that silymarin from milk thistle can inhibit the development of diet-induced hypercholesterolemia (Krecman V et al., 1997) as well as inhibit cholesterol biosynthesis (Skottowa et al., 1998). This potential characteristic is not surprising, as the same is known to be true for artichoke, which is a close relative to the milk thistle.

Artichoke

Artichoke extract has demonstrated a strong antioxidant potential and hepatoprotective effect in recent research on animals. It protects the liver and the animal from the damaging effects of toxins, such as carbon tetrachloride and other environmental chemicals in a manner similar to that of silymarin from the milk thistle. Like milk thistle artichoke extract is also able to stimulate regeneration of damaged liver tissue. The usefulness of artichoke for preventing or reducing buildup of fat in the liver from chronic alcohol consumption is noteworthy.

The regenerative effect of artichoke leaf extract was studied in rats after removal of part of the liver. (Maros et al., 1966, 1968). Clear signs of regeneration were observed, such as increase in liver tissue and liver cell content of RNA, stimulation of cell division, and increase of blood circulation in the liver.

Studies of hepatoprotective action have been done only in animals, as the common procedure involves exposure to toxins. The basic research method for this type of investigation is to give the test substance, in this case artichoke leaf extract, to the animal prior to or simultaneously with administration of a toxic substance and observe the results.

Such studies were undertaken by Adzet et al. (1987) using artichoke leaf extract against carbon tetrachloride-induced poisoning in rats and indicated a clear reduction of liver injury. Another investigation by Adzet (1987) on isolated rat liver cells (hepatocytes) exposed to the same chemical tested the activity of the different polyphenolic compounds in artichoke extract. Cynarin, which is a caffeoylquinic acid and a major constituent of the extract, was found to be responsible for the main cell-protective action.

In another study on ethanol treated rats by Samochowiec (1971) a significant reduction (28%)

of fatty acid esters was found with cynarin treatment. Cynarin also reduced levels of serum and liver cholesterol in ethanol-intoxicated rats according to a study by Wojiciki (1978).

More recently Gebhardt (1995) demonstrated hepatoprotective effects against carbon tetrachloride-induced toxicity on liver cells from rats, and again cynarin was found to be the compound responsible for the cell protective effect. When studying rat liver cells exposed to t-BHP (tertiary butylhydroperoxide), Gebhardt (1997) found that artichoke leaf extract significantly prevented oxidative damage to hepatocyte membranes and that chlorogenic acid and cynarin were the main contributors to this strong antioxidant effect. The findings also suggested that the cell protection should not be limited to the hepatocytes, opening the possibility that inhibition of low-density lipoprotein oxidation and other atherosclerosis-preventing actions may occur.

Who Can Benefit From Liver Protection?

Modern living unfortunately involves daily exposure to substances that are toxic to our bodies, which imposes a heavy load to carry for the liver. Therefore it is logical to think that all of us can benefit from some kind of liver support in prevention of free radical damage and development of disease. Individuals with a substantial alcohol consumption, with obesity, diabetes or with high exposure to environmental toxins have an even greater reason to protect the liver because of the documented risk of developing a serious liver condition.

Knowing that in its earliest stages, malfunction of the liver rarely causes any symptoms and that conventional medicine has very little to offer in treatment of liver disorders, it seems wise to remember that prevention is the best cure. We are fortunate today to have access to natural liver-protecting remedies that are safe, effective and without significant side effects.

And it is good to know that hepatoprotection is beneficial not only for the liver, but for the overall health and vitality of our body.

Summary

The following steps are important in preventing liver disease.

1. Poly*unsaturated* phosphatidylcholine has been shown to increase liver cell membrane fluidity, enhance transport activity, stimulate collagenase activity to prevent the development of fibrosis and cirrhosis, and protect against free radicals. Despite its rich content in polyunsaturated linoleic acid, polyunsaturated phosphatidylcholine has been shown to prevent lipid peroxidation and associated liver damage from alcohol, carbon tetrachloride or adriamycin chemotherapy treatment. Take 1800 to 2700 mg of polyunsaturated phosphatidylcholine.
2. Studies on liver and alcoholic cirrhosis patients have shown benefits from supplementing valine, leucine, and isoleucine. These branched-chain amino acids can enhance protein synthesis in liver and muscle cells and are used by body builders to produce an anabolic effect. Four capsules of Branch Chain Amino Acids (free form) provide 200 mg of *L*-leucine, 600 mg of *L*-isoleucine, 600 mg of *L*-valine, and 10 mg of vitamin B_6 (pyridoxine). The suggested dose is 2 to 4 capsules per day between meals with fruit juice or before eating. Warning: These capsules are only to be used by adults who are fully grown, and not by anyone afflicted with pellagra.
3. Patients with depleted SAMe levels should take from 2 to 4 200-mg tablets a day, spread throughout the day. Patients must adhere to physician-prescribed blood testing schedules to assess the effectiveness of this therapy. A cost-effective alternative to SAMe supplementation is TMG (trimethylglycine). The suggested dose is two 500-mg tablets, twice a day after meals, or as directed by a physician. Do not take this supplement on an empty stomach.
4. The vitamin B complex is extremely important for liver health; therefore daily supplementation of vitamins B_1 (500 mg), B_2 (75 mg), B_5 (1500 mg), and B_6 (200 mg) is strongly recom-

mended (though vitamin B_3 [niacin] should be avoided by cirrhosis patients).

5. Other recommended daily supplements are 1500 mg of choline, 1600 mg of folic acid, 500 mg of vitamin C, 800 IU of vitamin E, 300 micrograms of selenium, and 100 mg of coenzyme Q10 (for its antioxidant and blood-flow-enhancing properties) and
6. Acetyl-*L*-carnitine should be taken in two daily doses of 1000 mg each. Take two 600-mg doses per day of *N*-acetylcysteine and three 300 mg doses of a standardized artichoke extract that contains a minimum of 3% caffeoylquinic acid concentration.
7. Drink green tea, or take 2-4 green tea extract capsules per day that provide at least 300 mg each of a 95% standardized extract per day.
8. Five to ten grams of *L*-arginine and 2000 mg per day of glutamine may help lower blood levels of toxic ammonia permitted to build up by a damaged liver. *L*-Arginine can help facilitate liver regeneration if the liver is still at least 20% effective.
9. Silymarin (300-900 mg per day) is appropriate for alcoholic liver disease patients, and has reduced insulin resistance in diabetic patients with cirrhosis. The most active flavonoid in silymarin is *silybin*. Some silymarin products are standardized to provide a high concentration of silybin, which provides greater efficacy than the typical milk thistle extract sold as silymarin
10. Zinc should be supplemented in cirrhosis patients at a rate of at least 12 mg per day (not to exceed 45 milligrams a day).

For specific anti-viral therapies to help eradicate hepatitis B or C, refer to our Hepatitis B or Hepatitis C protocols within this book or at www.lef.org.

For specific information on treating liver cirrhosis, refer to *Liver Cirrhosis protocol*.

For more information on conventional therapies: Contact the American Liver Foundation, (800) 223-0179.

Product availability. Polyunsaturated phosphatidylcholine (PPC), *S*-adenosyl methionine (SAMe); vitamins B_1, B_2, B_5, and B_6; folic acid; choline; vitamin C and vitamin E; Coenzyme Q_{10}; acetyl-*L*-carnitine, *N*-acetyl-cysteine, green tea, *L*-arginine, curcumin, silymarin, and the branched-chain amino acid complex (valine, leucine, and isoleucine) can be ordered by calling (800) 544-4440, or by ordering on-line at www.lef.org.

LUPUS

Lupus is an autoimmune, inflammatory disease with multiple acute and chronic manifestations. In its most common and serious form, Systemic Lupus Erythematosus (SLE), it is a potentially fatal dysfunction of the autoimmune system. Instead of defending against invading viruses and bacteria, the body's multitude of immune agents mistakenly identify our own tissues as the enemy and attack the organs, blood, skin, joints, and gastrointestinal tract. In its most life-threatening form, SLE produces kidney, brain, heart, and lung inflammation. Even in milder forms, this inflammatory process leads to arthralgia (joint pain), fever, fatigue, mood changes, and other symptoms that may become disabling.

It should be noted that there are two other common forms of this disease, Discoid Lupus Erythematosis (DLE), a less serious form primarily causing disc-shaped skin lesions, and Drug Induced Lupus Erythematosis (DILE), which is transient and subsides when the causal agent is withdrawn. A further discussion of DILE will be provided later in this protocol.

The epidemiology of lupus reveals it to be primarily a disease of younger women, although men and children are represented as well. The Lupus Foundation of America estimates that as many as 2,000,000 U.S. residents have SLE. Lupus is a many-faceted disease, with a range of impact from minor to life-threatening, and with a multitude of symptom areas throughout the entire body. It is an unpredictable disorder, capable of long remissions and sudden unexplained "flareups" (sudden activation of apparently quiescent disease states). Fortunately, the recognition and treatment of SLE has improved dramatically in recent years. Once under reasonable control, many lupus patients have normal life expectancies. The key is to prevent, or quickly deal with any inflammatory organ involvement.

The causes of SLE are not entirely clear, but most experts believe there is a genetic predisposition involved, although on a polygenetic level "there doesn't appear to be a single causative gene" (DeHoratius, 1999). Because of this, lupus does not often occur in multiple generations of a family. Researchers previously have identified chromosome 6 (the human leukocyte area—HLA) as an important genetic marker, and in 1997, Tsao, et al., identified a significant area on chromosome 1 as well. In either case, the low correlation between genetic factors and active lupus indicates that environmental triggers must play a critical role in the development of SLE. These environmental factors may be infections, nutritional deficits, stress, or some unsuspected agent. It is accepted that these same factors (infections, nutrition, and stress) can exacerbate lupus and even induce flareups.

The biochemistry of lupus is important in the understanding of how traditional medical and alternative/supportive treatments work. Basically, the body has a vast array of cells at its disposal to deal with infections, depending on the type of invader it detects. Some cells focus on this detection process, telling other cells what to do and what to attack, by labeling foreign substances (antigens) as enemies, and choosing the appropriate disease-fighting agent from the dozens available. Cells called antibodies attack and inflame those cells labeled antigens. Other groups of cells, including the complement system, are charged with regulating and cleaning up excess antibodies. If antibodies are present in excess while mediating substances are at low levels, inflammation may be excessive and unchecked. (A complete description of the body's defense system is beyond the scope of this protocol, but may be found in Wallace, 1995). Depending on which antigens are identified, specific antibodies will be activated to destroy them. In lupus, the question is which tissues were misidentified? The body's systems are so disrupted that they begin manufacturing "autoantibodies" (antibodies that attack the person's own tissues). The autoantibodies produced lead to the multitude of symptoms in SLE, and help explain why the disease is so varied. As will be seen, medical tests for lupus search for excessive amounts of different key antibodies and are used to chart the course of the disease.

Symptom Areas and Dangers

The following are brief descriptions of the most common areas of lupus activity:

Joints. Approximately 90% of patients have some form of musculoskeletal symptoms, typically pain in the hands, wrists, knees, and shoulders (arthralgia).

Kidneys. Nearly 50% of lupus patients have significant renal disease, and can suffer kidney failure.

Lungs. The most common involvement is pleuritis, an inflammation of the membrane surrounding the lungs, with or without pleural effusion (buildup of fluids).

Cardiac. As with the lungs, inflammation of the lining of the heart (pericarditis) is the most common symptom.

Blood. Lupus inflammation may produce anemia and leukopenia (a dangerous reduction in white blood cells which leaves the body easily susceptible to infection).

Central nervous system. SLE frequently produces brain dysfunctions, including strokes, seizures, headaches, and dementia.

Mouth and nose. Mucosal ulcers are seen in approximately 30% of patients (Belmont, 1996), but rarely are serious threats to overall health.

Skin. Various dermatological disruptions are extremely common, varying from facial rash (the famous "butterfly" pattern of lupus that is similar to the facial markings of a wolf, giving rise to the name "lupus"), to photosensitivity (which may initiate a system flareup), to discoid skin lesions, to hair thinning.

Gastrointestinal tract. Outbreaks here may be as a direct result of the disease itself, or as a consequence of the use of anti-inflammatory medications, especially steroids.

The vascular system. Besides the effects on the blood supply of the brain, kidneys, and other organs, SLE causes a specific and dangerous complication for the blood vessels themselves, called vasculitis.

The immune system. Despite its over-reactivity to its own tissues, the immune system in SLE patients is inefficient against external disease-causing organisms. As a result, people with lupus are particularly susceptible to infection.

Bones. Osteoporosis is seen in lupus both as a direct result of the disease itself (when chronic inflammation and inactivity lead to demineralization), and as a side effect of corticosteroid therapy.

Medical Diagnosis of SLE

Despite its many facets, lupus has been misdiagnosed for many years. Many lupus patients look healthy, and even after being obviously ill, have brief remissions that make it appear as if they have recovered from whatever they had. Of course, the historic prevalence of SLE in females has produced a lack of research, interest, and funding. Even today, patients may wait for years before an accurate diagnosis is made (Wallace, 1995).

In 1971 (revised in 1982), the American College of Rheumatology devised 11 criteria for the presence of SLE. A person with four of the eleven may be diagnosed with lupus. The first four are symptoms of the skin: photosensitivity, mouth sores, butterfly rashes, and discoid (disc- shaped) lesions. The next four criteria describe inflammatory reactions in the joints, the central nervous system, the kidneys, and the linings of the lungs or heart.

The final three criteria are blood test abnormalities:

1. Positive ANA testing. A positive antinuclear antibody result is found in nearly all lupus patients, although some people with positive ANA's do not have lupus. They may have a related disorder, such as arthritis, or they may have no signs of any active disease state. This test measures the presence of immune system agents (antibodies) which falsely identify the nucleus of our own cells as enemies and proceed to attack and inflame them. Physicians can use ANA results as a measure of current lupus activity.
2. Altered blood count. Low red or white blood cell levels are common.
3. Other abnormal antibody counts. These include a positive LE (Lupus Erythematosis antibodies), Anti-DNA (antibodies that attack genetic material), false-positive syphilis tests, and tests with such names as anti-Sm, complement, anti-Ro, and rheumatoid factor. Each of these antibodies, when elevated in the blood, produces a specific, different symptom in the body.

It is possible for lupus patients to manifest such symptoms as fatigue and depression without concomitant blood abnormalities. This may be caused by stress, medication, or another group of blood proteins called cytokines.

Medical Management of SLE

Fortunately for present day lupus patients, the survival and quality of life statistics continue to improve dramatically as newer, more sophisticated techniques become available. This section of the protocol will describe the primary pharmacological treatments in current usage.

Steroids. Despite their negative consequences, steroids are a critical intervention for lupus, particularly when the disease threatens an organ. Steroids (cortisone, prednisone, dexamethazone, and their cousins) are hormones that have a number of functions in the body, including the stabilization of inflammatory cells and the decrease of the white blood cells responsible for immunologic memory. Steroids may be administered orally, intravenously, intra-articularly (into the joint), intramuscularly, or locally (for skin involvement).

If there is heart, lung, kidney, liver, or blood involvement, high dose steroids are necessary. Other severe flareups often require a lower dosage.

In all cases, whenever it is possible to discontinue steroid treatment, it is preferable to do so. Side effects include palpitations, agitation, tachycardia (rapid heart rate), insomnia, impaired wound healing, impaired response to infection, loss of bone calcium, avascular necrosis (bone death), glucose intolerance (leading to or exacerbating a diabetic state), water retention, hypertension, heartburn, and a number of other unpleasant results.

It should be noted that topical steroid creams do not cause these side effects. Additionally, with oral and injectable administration, some people have only a few side effects, and the impact is dose dependent. For those with inflammation of the gastrointestinal tract, there is a new steroid named Budesonide, which offers far fewer side effects.

Immunosuppressive therapies. These treatments typically are used in organ-threatening cases when steroids have failed, or are not tolerated by the patient. In truth, these regimens are forms of chemotherapy, also referred to as cytotoxic therapy, and may involve some of the same drugs used in treating cancer. As such, they offer the same powerful positive and negative consequences of most chemotherapy. As with steroids, immunosuppressants, because of their toxicity, should be utilized only when other treatments are ineffective. The most common drugs used are cytoxan and methotrexate.

NSAIDS. The nonsteroidal anti-inflammatory drugs are an excellent substitute for steroidal medications whenever they provide sufficient suppression of SLE activity. These drugs (from simple aspirin and ibuprofen to Naprosyn, Indocin, Lodine, and Daypro) are less expensive, safer, and are often as effective as the previously mentioned therapies. They relieve fever, arthralgias, headaches, fatigue, pain, and various inflammations. NSAIDS have some particular benefits and side effects that make careful selection very important. One concern is the kidney-liver "profile" of each drug. Because they often are taken for long periods of time, kidney and liver complications are cumulative. Fortunately, new NSAIDS without the same side effects became available in 1999. Consult a physician for the appropriateness of the new medicines regarding your case.

Antimalarials. This class of drugs is remarkable for its effectiveness, safety, and multiple benefits. However, antimalarials are not useful in organ-threatening SLE, and they take months to reach their full effectiveness. These medications, most often Plaquenil, may be used in combination with other treatments, or in some mild cases, may be the only drug required. The antimalarials decrease inflammation, protect the skin from ultraviolet light damage, inhibit blood clotting, provide energy, block cytokines (which promote inflammation), and, as a bonus, lower cholesterol. Aside from a rare buildup in the eyes which can be monitored easily, Plaquenil has no major drawbacks other than possible gastrointestinal intolerance. Choice of medication is important because some other antimalarials (chloroquine) may cause permanent eye damage.

Related medical treatments. Some of the less-used therapies for SLE include dialysis (for advanced kidney damage), gold (for its antirheumatic properties), cyclosporin A (for inflammatory arthralgia), antileprosy drugs for skin and joint problems), retinoids (vitamin A derivatives), gamma-globulin (for recurrent infections), DMSO (for lupus related urinary tract cystitis [Sotolongo, et al., 1984]), and antidepressants for the frequent emotional disturbances commonly found with SLE patients.

Drug-Induced Lupus

Mentioned previously, DILE (drug induced lupus) requires medical treatment to identify and discontinue the provocative agent. These are some of the drugs capable of causing lupus, according to Wallace (1995):

- Hydralazine
- Methyldopa (Aldomet)
- Tegretol
- Phenothiazines (Thorazine and other antipsychotics)
- Quinidine
- Sulfasalazine

Further, the following drugs may exacerbate lupus:

- Antibiotics (particularly sulfa drugs and tetracycline)
- Oral contraceptives
- Oral diabetes drugs
- Cimetidine (Tagamet)
- Sulfa-based medications

These lists are far from complete. Any patient with lupus-like symptoms should be removed from potentially causative substances for an adequate period of time to assess their possible role in the disease state.

New medical treatment thalidomide. This previously shunned drug has been found to be useful in lupus, and specifically for the treatment of ankylosing spondylitis, a related rheumatic syndrome. Research (Breban, et al., 1999) has shown that thalidomide suppresses an important inflammatory agent named TNF-alpha.

GL 701. The FDA recently gave "Fast Track" status to this new SLE medication. As reported on the Internet in the Doctor's Guide, GL 701 was found to be effective in maintaining or improving lupus patients' conditions while steroid dosage was reduced. "Fast Track" designation means that the drug may be approved for public use in less time than would be expected.

Kiel Synchronization protocol. This procedure, developed by a German clinic, is a variation on the NIH (National Institutes of Health) protocol for the treatment of severe SLE. The NIH protocol uses Cytoxan (an immunosuppressant/chemotherapy drug), and cortisone on a frequent and long-term basis (Gourley, et al., 1996). In contrast, the Kiel protocol uses smaller and less frequent doses of the same powerful drugs, but combines them with a blood filtration technique called plasmaphoresis which removes undesirable proteins and antibodies. This is reported to have achieved a long-term, treatment-free remission in 64% of their 28 patients (Schroder et al., 1997). The Kiel protocol reports are promising and warrant further scrutiny. For the most recent developments, use the Internet address: www.Kielaid.org.

Collagen. Research in rheumatoid arthritis (Trentham, 1993) pointed to the potential of using oral collagen (a protein that is a major component of joints and skin) to signal the body to reduce inflammation.

Leumedins. This is a new class of drugs capable of blocking inflammation.

Monoclonal antibodies. Findings regarding these substance also come from arthritis research. One such substance blocks the protein TNF-alpha, an important part of the inflammatory chain reaction mentioned above in thalidomide treatment research.

Lifestyle Management of SLE

The individual lupus patient can play an important role in minimizing the impact of the disease on both longevity and quality of life. The recommendations in this section relate to either reducing the "triggers" of lupus flareups or making the body more capable of withstanding the assaults of this complex disease.

1. Environmental Triggers. Some of the substances encountered in everyday life that may exacerbate SLE:
   - Aromatic amines. Commonly used in hair dyes.
   - Silicone and silica dust.
   - Alfalfa sprouts.
   - Hydrazines. These are found naturally in some mushrooms and tobacco smoke.
   - Tartrazines. These are used as preservatives in food dyes such as FD&C yellow #5.
2. Ultraviolet Light. Although people believe they look healthier with a tan, SLE patients may find that flareups are induced by exposure to the sun. Specifically, ultraviolet A and B (UVA and UVB) are strongly related to lupus through several biochemical reactions. Even on cloudy days, ultraviolet light is present in sufficient amounts to provoke a reaction. Not all lupus patients are photosensitive, although some are hyperreactive. Sunscreens help (with at least an SPF of 15), but they only reduce the

negative responses, rather than eliminating them. An individual's own history is the best predictor of the effects of the sun.

3. Rest. Lupus is typified by reduced energy levels. Some ways of coping with this problem is to get sufficient sleep, pace yourself as much as possible, and rest when necessary. Failure to rest when tired is a formula for longer periods of exhaustion. It is just as bad to remain in bed too long, which leads to the next recommendation.
4. Exercise. As important as exercise is for the average person, it is even more critical for those with SLE. Aerobic exercises such as walking or swimming build desperately needed endurance, and help to deter the muscle atrophy which so easily occurs if a patient doesn't take advantage of those times when energy is available. Most people with lupus have such good periods, particularly if they utilize the peak of medication activity. In addition to aerobic exercise a muscle-building regimen is recommended strongly. If lupus robs you of a percentage of strength and endurance, it makes sense to have a greater capacity on which to draw.
5. Stress. Although medical personnel debate whether or not stress can cause the onset of lupus, it generally is accepted that both physical and emotional stress are capable of producing flareups. There is a firm physiological basis for this statement. Stress increases the secretion of the hormones corticotrophin and cortisol, and research in psychoneuroimmunology has identified pathways connecting the brain to the immune system (Berk and Tan, 1994). This same research also describes the positive effects of relaxation and laughter on interferon-gamma, an important immunoregulator, suggesting that patients' mood states play a role in the autoimmune process. Cohen et al. (1994) demonstrate that the immune system is responsive to basic Pavlovian conditioning, and provide a summary of successful behavioral interventions.

Additional reports of the interaction of psychological factors on immune functioning may be found in O'Leary and Miller (1991) and Ader et. al. (1995).

Such a wealth of evidence for the role of stress leads to the obvious recommendation that SLE patients alter their lives to reduce stress. Unfortunately, reality intrudes far too often, seemingly preventing positive changes. Despite this, patients must assert this as a priority, because their long term health and survival are at stake.

Besides radical change, people can begin to learn simple relaxation techniques, try biofeedback training, or seek psychological help in coping with their stress.

Nutritional Management of SLE

General Nutrition

People living with chronic illnesses have nutritional requirements well beyond those of the general public. The disease process places excessive demands on the entire system while interfering with the ability of the body to assimilate basic nutrients. It is hardly possible to nourish a chronically ill person with the best of diets. Add the fact that SLE patients frequently have gastric distress and variable appetites, and the nutritional task becomes even more daunting. An early study by Cook and Reading (1985) demonstrated the beneficial effects of nutritional supplementation of SLE patients. It is essential for those with lupus to take a regimen of a high- potency, easily assimilated, vitamin-mineral product such as Life Extension Mix. Avoid the commercial one-a-day formulations. Despite the public's fascination with finding a single magic pill, it takes a number of nutrients to produce improved health, and that cannot be combined into one tablet.

SLE patients must also plan to avoid the most common serious complications of their disease. Certainly, the possible vascular involvement would weigh heavily in favor of a low saturated fat diet, the benefit of which is shown in early research in animals with lupus-like disease (Corman, 1985). Likewise, the potential kidney problems suggest a diet relatively low in protein as well as low in salt (because kidney malfunctions lead to high blood pressure).

Steroid Therapy Side Effects

Many lupus patients have no choice in the use of steroid therapy: They must take these drugs or suffer catastrophic organ involvement. Some side effects of steroids may be mitigated with the proper supplements. The most significant example is the loss of calcium leading to osteoporosis. Proper nutritional treatment of osteoporosis involves a delicate balance of minerals, far beyond simply taking calcium. *For a thorough discussion of such treatment please refer to the Osteoporosis protocol.*

Additionally, steroids may cause potassium levels to decrease. When this occurs, oral replacement is required. Because steroids can release clots of fat into the blood stream, nutritional supplements which break down fats are recommended. *For a complete description of how to deal with this problem, see the Thrombosis Prevention protocol.* Another possible result of steroid therapy is cognitive confusion and loss of concentration. If this occurs, there are many supplements available. *Again, the reader is referred to another section, the Age-Associated Mental Impairment protocol, for a listing of the treatments available.* Finally, steroids may deplete vitamin B_6, vitamin D, and zinc. These substances require supplementation. Note that B-complex vitamins also are depleted by aspirin and indomethacin (Lupus Alert, 1988), common anti-inflammatory medications.

Specific Symptom Treatment

The complexity of SLE causes symptoms in many sites, in many ways. It is possible to treat some of these with supplements:

Osteoporosis. Besides being a side effect of steroid use, osteoporosis can occur as a direct result of lupus. (*As mentioned above, see the Osteoporosis protocol for details.*)

Pain. There are several supplements recommended for the chronic achiness common in lupus. Two amino acids, dl-phenylalanine and tyrosine (500 mg taken 2 or 3 times a day) are capable of elevating brain endorphin levels. Endorphins are the body's natural pain killers, and raising their availability can reduce pain. Another substance used to limit pain is melatonin. Not only does melatonin have analgesic effects, but it also appears to potentiate the effects of other analgesics. The best usage of melatonin is at bedtime, when 500 mcg to 10 mg help to lower pain and improve sleep.

Arthritis. Because most lupus patients have some form of arthritic symptoms, from mild to disabling, SLE may be treated with many of the same supplements used in the Arthritis protocol. These substances include antioxidants, glucosamine, chondroitin, and essential fatty acids (particularly, gamma-linolenic acid or GLA). In addition to the recommendations for pain listed above, there are specific natural arthritic pain products such as ArthroPro and Natural Pain Relief for Arthritis, that utilizes agents used in European clinics as the primary treatment for joint inflammation.

Systemic Inflammation. Earlier studies have also shown the efficacy of essential fatty acids such as those contained in perilla, flax, or fish oil supplements. Alexander, et al. (1987) demonstrated a reduction in glomerulonephritis (kidney disease), and a significant rise in longevity in a fish oil supplemented group of lupus-prone animals, as compared to groups given either saturated fat or corn oil supplements. Robinson et al. (1985) stated that fish oil "had the most striking protective effect seen thus far in any animal model of inflammatory disease." These results were supported by Kelly, et al. (1985), who showed that fish oil suppressed lupus in mice, delaying renal disease and prolonging survival.

DHEA. Dehydroepiandrosterone (DHEA) is a hormone that the body may convert into both androgens and estrogens for various uses. DHEA has multiple interactions with the body's immune system and the excess or lack of this substance produces significant effects on an autoimmune disease such as SLE. In one study (Araghi-Niknam, et al., 1998), supplemental dietary DHEA restored normal functioning to the dysregulated cytokine (immune-modulating proteins) production in mice. Other research (Yang et. al., 1998) demonstrated that DHEA delayed the activity of a key inflammatory agent, interleukin-6 (IL-6) and prolonged the survival of mice with lupus-like disease. Similarly, Suzuki et al. (1995) showed that DHEA significantly increased production of IL-2 (an interleukin that moderates the system's inflammatory responsiveness), while reversing autoimmune disease in laboratory animals. An even broader statement of the importance of DHEA came from Jiang et al. (1998). These researchers concluded that DHEA restored IL-2 secretion, decreased the inflammatory agent interferon-gamma, and normalized IL-6 activity. In addition, they discovered that DHEA and antioxidant nutrients (vitamins E and C, curcumin, alpha-lipoic acid, and others mentioned previously) have a synergistic effect upon one another, emphasizing the need for a complex nutritional approach.

An impressive study on the effects of DHEA on SLE was conducted by researchers at Stanford University Medical Center. The study group consisted of 50 females, 37 premenopausal and 13 postmenopausal, with mild to moderate SLE. Test subjects were treated with long term (up to 1 year) therapy of 50 to 200 mg daily of oral DHEA. The results showed that DHEA therapy was associated with a decrease in SLE disease activity as measured by the SLE Disease Activity Index Score, patient global assessment, and physician global assessment compared to baseline. Prednisone doses were concurrently reduced. These improvements were sustained over the entire treatment period. Thirty-four patients (68%) completed 6 months of therapy, and 21 patients (42%) completed 12 months of therapy. Mild acne was the most common side effect, affecting 54% of the study group. Researchers reported that efficacy was similar in both pre- and postmenopausal women, and that DHEA was well tolerated and clinically beneficial in patients who maintained therapy.

Testosterone. This hormone appears to play a significant role in the body's autoimmune system. Kanda et al. (1996) studied the effects of testosterone on several inflammation-causing agents. They found that it reduced IL-6 and two immunoglobulins, IgG and IgM. In mice with lupus, Kiesler, et al.(1995) discovered low levels of testosterone and high levels of estradiol (estrogen), suggesting a causal relationship. When testosterone was given to these animals, longevity increased. This evidence indicates that hormone balances in SLE patients may be disrupted, and that proper regulation may be therapeutic. *This treatment is discussed in great detail in the Male Hormone Modulation Therapy protocol.* Females must be more careful about using testosterone as there may be a more narrow therapeutic dosage range.(*See Female Hormone Modulation Therapy protocol.*)

Summary

Systemic Lupus Erythematosis is a complex disorder of the immune system that may affect multiple systems of the body, and symptoms range from mild to fatal. Its causes are not fully understood, but probably involve genetic and environmental factors. Medical treatment for lupus utilizes a variety of pharmaceutical approaches from aspirin to steroids to chemotherapy, some of which produce side effects nearly as bad as the illness itself. To support and enhance treatment, this protocol suggests lifestyle adjustments and nutritional supplements to mitigate specific symptoms and systemic inflammation.

The prognosis for SLE patients has improved dramatically in the last several decades, and newer, safer drugs are becoming available. An overall cure awaits some major breakthrough, probably in the field of genetic engineering.

1. Aromatic amines, silicone and silica dust, alfalfa sprouts, hydrazines, tartrazines, and UV light are environmental triggers that exacerbate the condition and should be avoided.
2. Regular aerobic exercise to build up endurance, and rest as needed.
3. Avoidance of both physical and emotional stress which may cause flareups.
4. Life Extension Mix, 3 tablets 3 times a day, for high potency, easily assimilated, multi-nutrient benefits.
5. A low salt, low saturated-fat diet.
6. Calcium and magnesium supplementation to offset bone loss (especially important when taking steroids).
7. Potassium, vitamins B_6, D, and E, and zinc to offset nutritional depletion due to the use of steroids. These nutrients are contained in Life Extension Mix, but additional potassium may be needed.

8. Melatonin, 500 mcg to 10 mg, to lower pain and induce sleep.
9. For arthritic symptoms, antioxidants, glucosamine, chondroitin, and essential fatty acids such as gamma-linoleic acid.
10. DHEA, to boost autoimmune function and decrease disease activity. (*Refer to DHEA Replacement protocol* for dosage information.)

For more information. Contact the Lupus Foundation of America, (800) 558-0121.

Product availability. DHEA, Natural Pain Relief for Arthritis, *dl*-phenylalanine, tyrosine, essential fatty acids (Mega GLA and Mega EPA), melatonin, alpha-lipoic acid, vitamins B_6, D, and E, calcium, Life Extension Mix, and Mineral Formula for Women and for Men are available by calling (800) 544-4440, or order on-line at www.lef.org.

MACULAR DEGENERATION

The macula is the central and most vital area of the retina. It records images and sends them via the optic nerve from the eye to the brain. The macula is responsible for focusing central vision that is needed for seeing fine detail, reading, driving, and recognizing facial features.

Age-related macular degeneration (AMD) is the leading cause of blindness in people over the age of 55, affecting more than 10 million Americans. It is a condition in which the central portion of the retina (the macula) deteriorates. It is equally common in men and women and more common in whites than blacks. The cause is unknown, but the condition tends to run in some families. Macular degeneration affects more Americans than cataracts and glaucoma combined.

There are two forms of macular degeneration: atrophic (dry) and exudative (wet). Approximately 85 to 90% of the cases are the dry type. Both forms of the disease may affect both eyes simultaneously. Vision can become severely impaired, with central vision rather than peripheral vision affected. The ability to see color is generally not affected, and total blindness from the condition is rare.

There is little that can be done within conventional medical treatment protocols to restore lost eyesight with either form of the disease. Leading researchers, however, are documenting the benefits of a more holistic approach in the treatment of AMD. Patients are being encouraged to increase physical fitness, improve nutrition (including a reduction in saturated fats), abstain from smoking, and protect their eyes from excessive light. Dietary supplementation of trace elements, antioxidants, and vitamins is recommended for improving overall metabolic and vascular functioning. Early screening and patient education offer the most hope for reducing the debilitating effects of the disease.

DRY MACULAR DEGENERATION

In the dry type of macular degeneration, the retina deteriorates in association with the formation of small yellow pigment-like deposits, called drusen, that form under the macula. The formation of these deposits leads to a thinning and drying out of the macula. Vision loss is related to the location and amount of retinal thinning caused by the drusen.

The dry type of macular degeneration tends to progress more slowly than the wet type, with vision being lost painlessly. The first symptom is usually a distortion in one eye, causing straight lines to look wavy. Blank spots will occur as the macula continues to degenerate. A vision test will sometimes reveal physical deterioration before symptoms occur.

The Benefits of Nutritional Supplementation

Nutrients that may improve micro capillary circulation in the eye and thus slow down deterioration of the macula include ginkgo biloba at 120 mg a day, grape seed-skin extract at 200–300 mg a day, and bilberry extract at 150 mg a day.

A double-blind case-controlled study showed that those with macular degeneration had decreased intake of vitamin E, magnesium, zinc, vitamin B_6, and folic acid. This study identified 14 specific antioxidant components that could stabilize, but not improve, dry macular degeneration when consumed for a period of 1.5 years. Supplementation with the Life Extension Mix and Life Extension Booster formulas provides these specific antioxidant components. Also, Life Extension Mix and Booster contain other nutrients, such as lutein, which have been shown to prevent wet macular degeneration.

Hydergine in doses of 4 to 5 mg a day and higher has shown benefit in treating dry macular degeneration. The following antioxidant nutrients should also be considered: alpha-lipoic acid, 500 mg a day, and glutathione, 500 mg a day.

The standard daily dose of Life Extension Mix—3 tablets, 3 times a day—provides adequate levels of vitamin B-complex, zinc, and other nutrients that are crucial for ocular function.

Anyone with dry macular degeneration also should refer to the Wet Macular Degeneration section, since those with dry macular degeneration are at a high risk of developing the more debilitating wet macular degeneration.

The Effects of UV Sunlight and Smoking

The daily application of the vitamin A–based Viva Drops can provide antioxidant protection to the lens of the eye. Also, wrap-around UV-blocking sunglasses provide significant protection against UV sun rays. Exposure to sunlight without wearing UV blocking sunglasses is a risk factor in developing macular degeneration.

Cigarette smoking among women has been shown to increase the risk of macular degeneration by 2.4-fold, compared with women who never smoked. Those who quit smoking still had a two-fold increased risk relative to those who had never smoked. Even among those who had quit smoking for 15 or more years, little reduction in risk was shown, compared with current smokers. Cigarette smoking has been determined to be an independent and avoidable risk factor for age-related macular degeneration among women.

WET MACULAR DEGENERATION

In the wet type of macular degeneration, abnormal subretinal blood vessels grow under the retina and macula: this is known as angiogenesis. These newly formed blood vessels will bleed or leak, causing the macula to bulge or form a mound, often surrounded by small hemorrhages. Central vision will thus become distorted. Vision loss may be rapid and severe under these circumstances. Individuals suffering from wet macular degeneration may see a dark spot or spots within their central vision due to the blood leakage under the retina. Because the macula is no longer smooth, straight lines will appear wavy.

Laser surgery may be recommended in the early stages of deterioration to save further vision loss. It is not always successful and may even cause scarring and additional vision loss. Successful laser surgery may slow the rate of vision loss and preserve some sight, but will not stop a recurrence. Low-dose radiation therapy has shown promising results in decreasing neovascularization associated with the disease.

In a new study, researchers at Johns Hopkins University, led by Dr. Neil M. Bressler, have reported that verteporfin (Visudyne), a new drug that is expected to be available in early 2000, has prevented vision loss in 61% of wet AMD patients receiving it in experimental trials. The drug will help millions of sufferers who have been offered little hope with conventional therapies.

The Benefits of Nutritional Supplementation

The phytochemicals that protect against wet macular degeneration are lutein and zeaxanthin. Life Extension Mix and Chloroplex both contain lutein. Those with early-stage wet macular degeneration should also use a product called Lutein Plus, which provides potent concentrations of both zeaxanthin and lutein. One tablespoon a day of Lutein Plus powder is suggested to prevent or slow the progress of wet macular degeneration.

Soy contains the phytochemical genistein, which has anti-angiogenesis properties. Those with wet macular degeneration may want to take two 700-mg capsules, 2 times a day, of Mega Soy Extract in order to obtain enough genistein to possibly inhibit blood-vessel growth in the eye.

Also, there are several new anti-angiogenesis drugs being developed, primarily to treat cancer. An FDA advisory panel has approved thalidomide to treat leprosy. Thalidomide is an extremely potent anti-angiogenesis drug that could slow or possibly stop the progression of wet macular degeneration. It would be legal for doctors to prescribe thalidomide to treat wet macular degeneration, even though it will only be officially approved to treat leprosy.

CAUTION: Thalidomide causes severe birth defects and must not be used by pregnant women or women who may become pregnant.

Protection against Free Radical Damage

Free radical damage has been implicated in the development of wet macular degeneration. Zinc, vitamin C, and vitamin E deficiencies have been found in many people who develop wet macular degeneration. It should be noted that these vitamins have not yet been shown to slow the progression of the disease once it has been clinically manifested. The daily dose of Life Extension Mix—3 tablets, 3 times a day—will provide broad-spectrum antioxidant protection against free radical damage to the eye. An additional 30 mg of zinc should also be considered.

Summary

Age-related macular degeneration is the leading cause of irreversible vision loss in the United States, occurring as a result of deterioration of the central portion of the retina known as the macula. Approximately 85 to 90% of the cases are of the dry type. Although the cause of AMD remains unknown, researchers continue to find a positive correlation between the onset of the disease with genetic susceptibility, the effect of normal aging, and low levels of serum and dietary antioxidants.

1. Ginkgo biloba, 120 mg a day (dry type).
2. Grape seed-skin extract, 200–300 mg a day (dry type).
3. Bilberry extract, 150 mg a day (dry type).
4. Hydergine, 4 to 5 mg a day (dry type).
5. Life Extension Mix and Life Extension Booster for antioxidant properties and lutein (wet and dry type).
6. Lutein Plus, 1 tbsp., for lutein and zeaxanthin (wet and dry types).
7. Mega Soy Extract for genistein to help inhibit blood-vessel growth in the eye (wet type).
8. Viva Drops for antioxidant protection to the lens of the eye (wet and dry type).
9. Zinc, 30 mg (wet type).

For more information. Contact the Association for Macular Diseases, (212) 605-3719.

Product availability. Ginkgo biloba extract, proanthocyanidins (grape seed-skin extract), bilberry extract, selenium, alpha-lipoic acid, glutathione, lutein powder, Mega Soy Extract, Life Extension Mix, zinc, Lutein Plus, and wraparound UV blocking sunglasses are available by phoning (800) 544-4440, or order on-line at www.lef.org.

MALE HORMONE MODULATION THERAPY

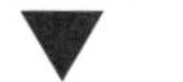

A Hormonal Attack on Aging

Controversy and the Life Extension Foundation have long been considered synonymous by both supporters and critics. In terms of complexity and instant effect, the protocol you are about to read surpasses any Life Extension program ever discussed in these pages.

The age-reversal premise we are espousing is the subject of three books written by highly respected medical doctors. These books provide a persuasive compilation of research findings and clinical experience to document the safety and efficacy of using this approach to treat aging. The books fail, however, to lay out an aggressive therapeutic plan of action. In this protocol, the Foundation provides a novel step-by-step program to enable members to immediately take advantage of this new information.

In writing this protocol, the Life Extension Foundation reviewed several thousand published scientific studies to validate safety and anti-aging efficacy. We also received input from experts who have personally followed this system for several years.

Foundation members are getting impatient. They don't want to see their bodies ravaged by age if a documented therapy is available that can control or reverse this devastating process. In this case, proven therapies exist and many are FDA-approved.

Implementing this protocol requires diligent medical testing, but the potential for significant age reversal is compelling.

Male Hormones and Aging

As men age past year 40, hormonal changes occur that perceptibly inhibit physical, sexual, and cognitive function. The outward appearance of a typical middle-aged male shows increased abdominal fat and shrinkage of muscle mass, a hallmark effect of hormone imbalance. A loss of feeling of well-being, sometimes manifesting as depression, is a common psychological complication of hormone imbalance (94–97, 271).*

Until recently, these changes were attributed to "growing old," and men were expected to accept the fact that their bodies were entering into a long degenerative process that would someday result in death.

A remarkable amount of data has been compiled indicating that many of the diseases that middle-aged men begin experiencing, including depression, abdominal weight gain, and prostate and heart disease, are directly related to hormone imbalances that are correctable with currently available drug and nutrient therapies. To the patient's detriment, conventional doctors are increasingly prescribing drugs to treat depression, elevated cholesterol, angina, and a host of other diseases that may be caused by an underlying hormone imbalance.

If doctors checked their male patients' blood levels of estrogen, testosterone, thyroid, and DHEA (instead of prescribing drugs to treat symptoms), they might be surprised to learn that many problems could be eliminated by adjusting hormone levels to fit the profile of a healthy 21-year-old.

Few physicians know what hormone blood tests to order for men, nor do they have the experience to properly adjust hormones to reverse the degenerative changes that begin in mid-life.

This protocol will provide the patient and physician with the information necessary to safely modulate hormone levels for the purpose of preventing and treating many of the common diseases associated with growing older.

Too Much Estrogen

The most significant hormone imbalance in aging men is a decrease in free testosterone, while estrogen levels remain the same or increase precipitously. As men grow older, they suffer through a variety of mechanisms from the dual effects of having too little testosterone and excess estrogen. The result is a testosterone-estrogen imbalance that directly causes many of the debilitating health problems associated with normal aging (1–12, 28).

One cause of hormone imbalance in men is that their testosterone is increasingly converted to estrogen. One report showed that estrogen levels of the average 54-year-old man are higher than those of the average 59-year-old woman (1, 5, 13–18, 48).

The reason that testosterone replacement therapy does not work by itself for many men is that exogenously administered testosterone may convert (aromatize) into even more estrogen, thus

*Numbers in parentheses are references. Please refer to the reference section.

M

Testosterone Metabolic Pathways

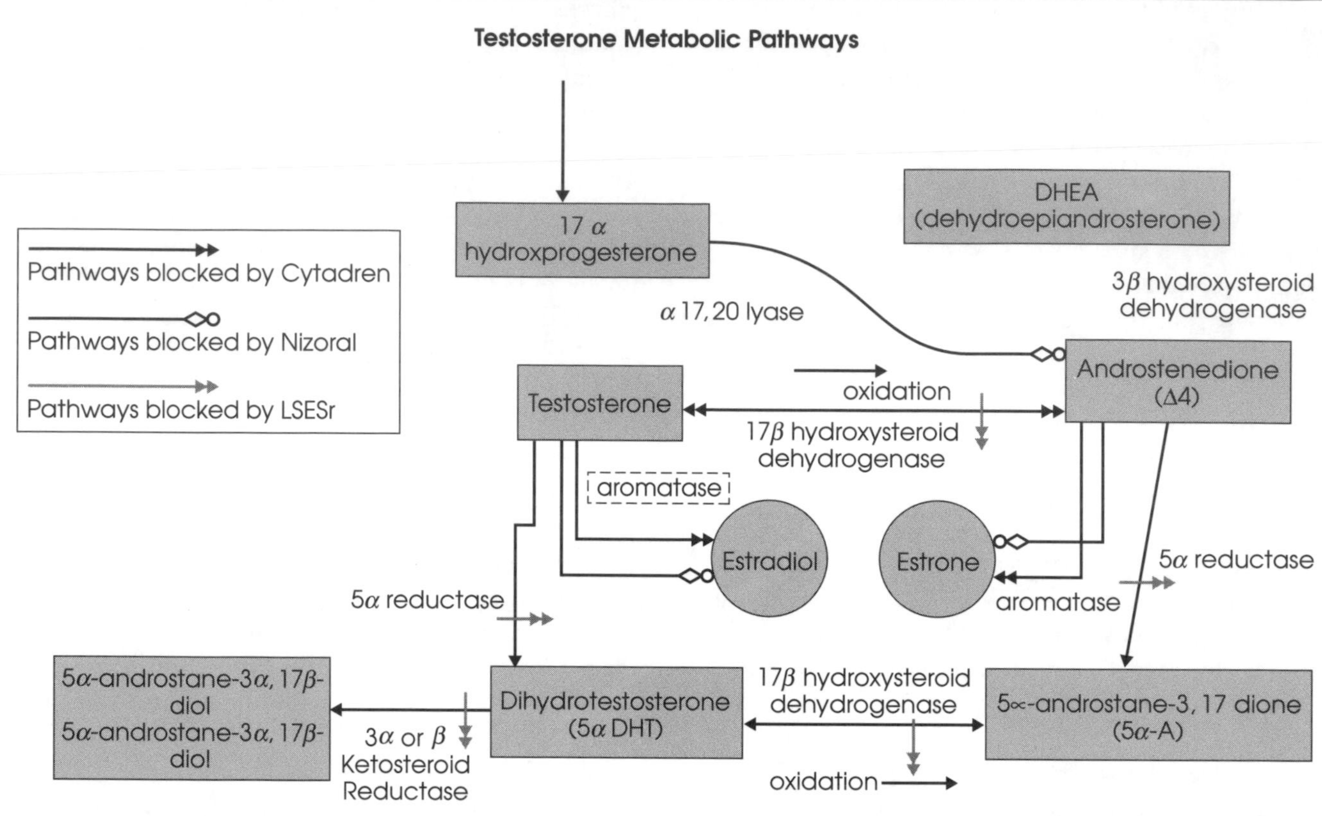

Graph provided courtesy of Stephen Strum, M.D.

potentially worsening the hormone imbalance problem in aging males (i.e., too much estrogen and not enough free testosterone) (21, 26). While there are studies showing that testosterone replacement therapy does not increase estrogen beyond normal reference ranges, we are going to show later how the standard laboratory reference ranges do not adequately address the issue of estrogen overload (4, 8, 9, 17, 22–25, 27, 29–32).

Estrogen is an essential hormone for men, but too much of it causes a wide range of health problems. The most dangerous acute effect of excess estrogen and too little testosterone is an increased risk of heart attack or stroke (39–43, 261–270). High levels of estrogen have been implicated as a cause of benign prostatic hypertrophy (BPH) (35–44, 46, 47). One mechanism by which nettle extract works is to block the binding of growth-stimulating estrogen to prostate cells (42–44, 48, 49, 50).

When there is too little testosterone present, estrogen attaches to testosterone cell receptor sites throughout the body and creates many problems in aging men. In youth, low amounts of estrogen are used to turn off the powerful cell-stimulating effects of testosterone. As estrogen levels increase with age, testosterone cell stimulation may be locked in the "off" position, thus reducing sexual arousal and sensation and causing the loss of libido so common in aging men (94, 99, 259).

High serum levels of estrogen also trick the brain into thinking that enough testosterone is being produced, further slowing the natural production of testosterone. This happens when estrogen saturates testosterone receptors in the hypothalamus region of the brain. The saturated hypothalamus then stops sending out a hormone to the pituitary gland to stimulate secretion of luteinizing hormone, which the gonads require to produce testosterone. High estrogen can thus shut down the normal testicular production of testosterone (1, 53, 54, 271–276, 277).

One further complication of excess estrogen is that it increases the body's production of sex hormone–binding globulin (SHBG) (280). SHBG binds free testosterone in the blood and makes it unavailable to cell receptor sites (51–52, 55, 56).

Based on the multiple deleterious effects of excess estrogen in men, aggressive action should be taken to reduce estrogen to a safe range if a blood test reveals elevated levels. We will discuss the appropriate blood tests and steps that can be taken to lower estrogen levels later in this protocol.

The Critical Importance of Free Testosterone

Testosterone is much more than a sex hormone. There are testosterone receptor sites in cells throughout the body, most notably in the brain and heart (60, 180). Youthful protein synthesis for maintaining muscle mass and bone formation requires testosterone (57, 59, 61–74, 87–90, 261–264, 287). Testosterone improves oxygen uptake throughout the body, helps control blood sugar (68, 75–80), regulate cholesterol (67, 69, 81), and maintain immune surveillance (82, 83). The body requires testosterone to maintain youthful cardiac output and neurological function (58, 65). Testosterone is also a critical hormone in the maintenance of healthy bone density (59, 66, 67, 84–86), muscle mass (65–67, 87–90, 287), and red blood cell production (67, 69, 91–93, 98).

Of critical concern to psychiatrists are studies showing that men suffering from depression have lower levels of testosterone than do control subjects (94–98). For some men, elevating free testosterone levels could prove to be an effective antidepressant therapy. There is a basis for free testosterone levels being measured in men suffering from depression and for replacement therapy being initiated if free testosterone levels are low normal or below normal.

Testosterone is one of the most misunderstood hormones. Body builders tarnished the reputation of testosterone by putting large amounts of synthetic testosterone drugs into their young bodies. Synthetic testosterone abuse can produce detrimental effects, but this has nothing to do with the benefits a man over age 40 can enjoy by properly restoring his natural testosterone to a youthful level.

Conventional doctors have not recommended testosterone replacement therapy because of an erroneous concern that testosterone causes prostate cancer. As we will later show, fear of prostate cancer is not a scientifically valid reason to avoid testosterone modulation therapy.

Another concern skeptical doctors have about prescribing testosterone replacement therapy is that some poorly conducted studies showed it to be ineffective in the long-term treatment of aging. These studies indicate anti-aging benefits when testosterone is given, but the effects often wear off. What doctors fail to appreciate is that exogenously administered testosterone can convert to estrogen in the body. The higher estrogen levels may negate the benefits of the exogenously administered testosterone. The solution to the estrogen-overload problem is to block the conversion of testosterone to estrogen in the body. Numerous studies show that maintaining youthful levels of free testosterone can enable the aging man to restore strength, stamina, cognition, heart function, sexuality, and outlook on life, i.e., to alleviate depression (261–70).

Why Testosterone Levels Decline

Testosterone production begins in the brain. When the hypothalamus detects a deficiency of testosterone in the blood, it secretes a hormone called gonadotrophin-releasing hormone to the pituitary gland. This prompts the pituitary to secrete luteinizing hormone (LH), which then prompts the Leydig cells in the testes to produce testosterone.

In some men, the testes lose their ability to produce testosterone, no matter how much LH is being produced. This type of testosterone deficiency is diagnosed when blood tests show high levels of LH and low levels of testosterone. In other words, the pituitary gland is telling the testes (by secreting LH) to produce testosterone, but the testes have lost their functional ability, so the pituitary gland vainly continues to secrete LH because there is not enough testosterone in the blood to provide a feedback mechanism that would tell the

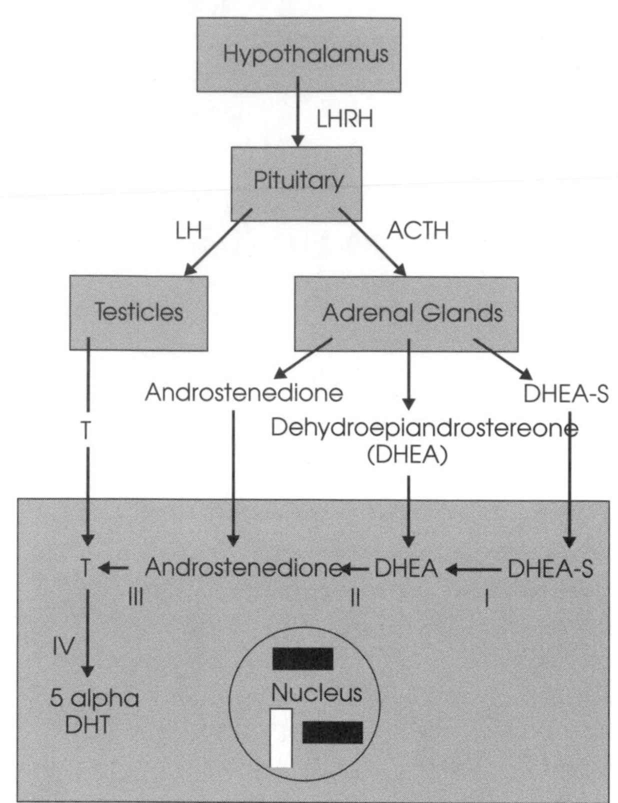

The Prostate Cell & Intra-Prostatic Synthesis of Androgens

Legend I = Sulfatase
II = 3 beta hydroxysteroid dehydrogenase
III = 17 beta hydroxysteroid dehydrogenase
IV = 5 alpha reductase
Androgen receptor
Androgen receptor blocked

Courtesy of Stephen Strum, M.D.

pituitary to shut down. In other cases, the hypothalamus, or pituitary gland, fails to produce sufficient amounts of LH, thus preventing healthy testes from secreting testosterone. Blood testing can determine whether sufficient amounts of LH are being secreted by the pituitary gland and help determine the appropriate therapeutic approach.

If serum (blood) testosterone levels are very low, it is important to diagnose the cause, but no matter what the underlying problem, therapies exist today to safely restore testosterone to youthful levels in any man (who does not already have prostate cancer).

As indicated earlier in this article, a major problem aging men face is not low production of testosterone, but excessive conversion of testosterone to estrogen. Specific therapies to suppress excess estrogen and boost free testosterone back to youthful physiological levels will be discussed later.

The Effects of Testosterone on Libido

Sexual stimulation and erection begin in the brain when neuronal testosterone-receptor sites are prompted to ignite a cascade of biochemical events that involve testosterone-receptor sites in the nerves, blood vessels, and muscles. Free testosterone promotes sexual desire and then facilitates performance, sensation, and the ultimate degree of fulfillment.

Without adequate levels of free testosterone, the quality of a man's sex life is adversely affected and the genitals atrophy. When free testosterone is restored, positive changes can be expected in the structure and function of the sex organs. (It should be noted that sexual dysfunction can be caused by other factors unrelated to hormone imbalance. An example of such a factor is arteriosclerotic blockage of the penile arteries.)

The genital-pelvic region is packed with testosterone receptors that are ultra-sensitive to free testosterone-induced sexual stimulation. Clinical studies using testosterone injections, creams, or patches have often failed to provide a long-lasting, libido-enhancing effect in aging men (98). We now know why. The testosterone can be converted to estrogen. The estrogen is then taken up by testosterone receptor sites in cells throughout the body. When an estrogen molecule occupies a testosterone receptor site on a cell membrane, it blocks the ability of serum testosterone to induce a healthy hormonal signal. It does not matter how much serum free testosterone is available if excess estrogen is competing for the same cellular receptor sites.

Estrogen can also increase the production of sex hormone–binding globulin (SHBG), which binds the active free testosterone into a nonactive "bound testosterone." Bound testosterone cannot be picked up by testosterone receptors on cell membranes. For testosterone to produce long-lasting, libido-enhancing effects, it must be kept in the "free" form (not bound to SHBG) in the bloodstream. It is also necessary to suppress excess estrogen, as this hormone can compete for testosterone receptor sites in the sex centers of the brain and the genitals.

Restoring youthful hormone balance can have a significant impact on male sexuality (99–102).

Testosterone and the Heart

Normal aging results in the gradual weakening of the heart, even in the absence of significant coronary artery disease. If nothing else kills the elderly male, at some point his heart just stops beating.

Testosterone is a muscle-building hormone, and there are many testosterone-receptor sites in the heart (57). The weakening of the heart muscle can sometimes be attributed to testosterone deficiency (103–108). Testosterone is not only responsible for maintaining heart muscle protein synthesis, it is also a promoter of coronary artery dilation (109–113) and helps to maintain healthy cholesterol levels (81, 114).

There are an ever-increasing number of studies indicating an association between high testosterone and low cardiovascular disease rates in men (81). In the majority of patients, symptoms and EKG measurements improve when low testosterone levels are corrected. One study showed that blood flow to the heart improved 68.8% in those receiving testosterone therapy (9). In China, doctors are successfully treating angina with testosterone therapy (9, 115, 116).

The following list represents the effects of *low* testosterone on cardiovascular disease:

- ▼ Cholesterol, fibrinogen, triglycerides, and insulin levels increase (30–33).
- ▼ Coronary artery elasticity diminishes.
- ▼ Blood pressure rises.
- ▼ Human growth hormone (HGH) declines (weakening heart muscle).
- ▼ Abdominal fat increases (increasing the risk of heart attack).

Those with cardiovascular disease should have their blood tested for free testosterone and estrogen. Some men (with full cooperation from their physicians) may be able to stop taking expensive drugs to stimulate cardiac output, lower cholesterol, and keep blood pressure under control, if they correct a testosterone deficit or a testosterone-estrogen imbalance.

Despite numerous studies substantiating the beneficial effects of testosterone therapy in treating heart disease, conventional cardiologists continue to overlook the important role this hormone plays in keeping their cardiac patients alive (9, 30, 31, 77, 93, 111–113, 115, 116, 261–270).

Testosterone and the Prostate Gland

Many doctors will tell you that testosterone causes prostate disease. The published scientific literature indicates otherwise.

As readers of *Life Extension Magazine* learned in late 1997, estrogen has been identified as a primary culprit in the development of BPH (117–119). Estrogen has been shown to bind to SHBG in the prostate gland and cause the proliferation of epithelial cells in the prostate (124, 182–184). This is corroborated by the fact that as men develop benign prostate enlargement, their levels of free testosterone are plummeting, while their estrogen levels remain the same or are rising. As previously discussed, aging men tend to convert their testosterone into estrogen. The published evidence shows that serum levels of testosterone are not a risk factor for developing benign prostate disease (8, 36, 41, 117–137).

The major concern that has kept men from restoring their testosterone to youthful levels is fear of prostate cancer. The theory is that since most prostate cancer cell lines need testosterone to proliferate, it is better not to replace the testosterone that is lost with aging. The problem with this theory is that most men who contract prostate cancer have low levels of testosterone, and the majority of published studies show that serum testosterone levels do not affect one's risk for contracting prostate cancer.

Since there is such a strong perception that any augmentation of testosterone can increase the risk of prostate cancer, we did a MEDLINE search on all the published studies relating to serum testosterone and prostate cancer. The appendix at the end of this article provides quotations from the published literature as it relates to the issue of whether testosterone causes prostate disease. Out of 27 MEDLINE studies we found, five indicated that men with higher testosterone levels had a greater incidence of prostate cancer, whereas 21 studies showed that testosterone was not a risk factor. One study was considered neutral.

Before anyone starts a testosterone replacement program, he should have a serum PSA test and a digital rectal exam to rule out prostate cancer. Nothing is risk free. A small minority of men with low testosterone and prostate cancer will not have an elevated PSA or palpable lesion detectable by digital rectal exam. If these men use supplemental testosterone, they risk an acute flare-up in their disease state. That is why PSA monitoring is so important every 30 to 45 days during the first 6 months of any type of testosterone augmentation therapy. If an underlying prostate cancer is detected because of testosterone therapy, it is usually treatable by nonsurgical means.

Please remember that testosterone does not cause acute prostate cancer, but if you have existing prostate cancer and don't know it, testosterone administration is likely to boost PSA sharply and provide your doctor with a quick diagnosis of prostate cancer (and an opportunity for very early treatment). We acknowledge that some aging men will not want to take this risk.

As stated above, the MEDLINE score was 21 to 5 against the theory that testosterone plays a role in the development of prostate cancer. None of these studies took into account the prostate cancer prevention effects for men who take lycopene, selenium, and vitamins A and E (135–144), nor did they factor in possible prostate disease preventives such as saw palmetto, nettle, soy, and pygeum (42–44, 145–170, 172).

In Dr. Jonathan Wright's book, *Maximize Your Vitality and Potency*, a persuasive case is made that testosterone and DHEA actually protect against the development of both benign and malignant prostate disease. Dr. Wright also points out that natural therapies such as saw palmetto, nettle, and pygeum provide a considerable degree of protection against the alleged negative effects that higher levels of testosterone might have on the prostate gland.

We eagerly await the results of more studies, but the fear of developing prostate cancer in the future should not be a reason to deprive your body today of the life-saving and life-enhancing benefits of restoring a youthful hormone balance.

Once a man has prostate cancer, testosterone therapy cannot be recommended because most prostate cancer cells use testosterone as a growth promoter. This, regrettably, denies prostate cancer patients the wonderful benefits of testosterone therapy. Men with severe BPH should approach testosterone replacement cautiously. It would be prudent for those with BPH who are taking testosterone replacement therapy to also use the drug Proscar (finasteride) to inhibit 5-alpha-reductase levels, thereby suppressing the formation of dihydrotestosterone (DHT) (171–182). DHT is 10 times more potent than testosterone in promoting prostate growth, and suppressing DHT is a proven therapy in treating benign prostate enlargement. Saw palmetto extract suppresses some DHT in the prostate gland, but its effectiveness in alleviating symptoms of BPH probably has more to do with

- ▼ Its blocking of alpha-adrenergic receptor sites on the sphincter muscle surrounding the urethra. (This is how the drug Hytrin works.)
- ▼ Its inhibition of estrogen binding to prostate cells (like nettle).
- ▼ Its inhibition of the enzyme *3-ketosteroid* (which causes the binding of DHT to prostate cells).
- ▼ Its anti-inflammatory effect on the prostate.

It is unfortunate that many people still think that restoring testosterone to youthful levels will increase the risk of prostate disease. This misconception has kept many men from availing themselves of this life-enhancing and life-saving hormone.

While it is clear that excess estrogen causes benign prostate enlargement, the evidence for excess estrogen's role in the development of prostate cancer is uncertain (8, 41, 117–134, 182–217, 236). Some studies show that elevated estrogen is associated with increased prostate cancer risk, while other studies contradict this finding. For more information on testosterone, estrogen, and the prostate gland, refer to the February 1999 issue of *Life Extension Magazine* (182–217).

Testosterone and Depression

A consistent finding in the scientific literature is that testosterone replacement therapy produces an increased feeling of well-being. As stated earlier, newly published studies show that low testosterone correlates with symptoms of depression and other psychological disorders (94–97, 272).

A common side effect of prescription antidepressant drugs is the suppression of libido. Those suffering with depression either accept this drug-induced reduction in quality of life, or get off the antidepressant drugs so they can at least have a somewhat normal sex life. If more psychiatrists tested their patients' blood for free testosterone and prescribed natural testosterone therapies to those with low free testosterone, the need for libido-suppressing antidepressant drugs could be reduced or eliminated. As previously described, testosterone replacement often enhances libido, which is the opposite effect of most prescription antidepressants.

One study showed that patients with major depression experienced improvement that was equal to that achieved with standard antidepressant drugs (97).

Androderm is one of several natural testosterone-replacement therapies that can be prescribed by doctors. A 12-month clinical trial using this FDA-approved drug resulted in a statistically significant reduction in the depression score (6.9 before versus 3.9 after). Also noted were highly significant decreases in fatigue from 79% before the patch to only 10% after 12 months (218).

According to Jonathan Wright, M.D., author of the book *Maximize Your Vitality & Potency,* the following effects have been reported in response to *low* testosterone levels:

- Loss of ability to concentrate
- Moodiness and emotionality
- Touchiness and irritability
- Great timidity
- Feeling weak
- Inner unrest
- Memory failure
- Reduced intellectual agility
- Passive attitudes
- General tiredness
- Reduced interest in surroundings
- Hypochondria

The above feelings can all be clinical symptoms of depression, and testosterone replacement therapy has been shown to alleviate these conditions. Testosterone thus has exciting therapeutic potential in the treatment of depression in men.

Testosterone and Aging

We know that many of the degenerative diseases of aging in men such as Type II diabetes, osteoporosis, and cardiovascular disease are related to a testosterone deficiency. We also know that common characteristics of middle age and older age such as depression, abdominal fat deposition, muscle atrophy, low energy, and cognitive decline are also associated with less than optimal levels of free testosterone (58, 219).

A consistent pattern that deals with fundamental aging shows that low testosterone causes excess production of a dangerous hormone called cortisol. Some anti-aging experts call cortisol a "death hormone" because of the multiple degenerative effects it produces. Some of these effects are immune dysfunction, brain cell injury, and arterial wall damage.

A group of scientists conducted two double-blind studies in which they administered supplemental testosterone to groups of aging men and observed the typical responses of lower levels of cholesterol, glucose, and triglycerides, reductions in blood pressure, and decreased abdominal fat mass. The scientists showed that excess cortisol suppressed testosterone and growth hormone production and that the administration of testosterone acted as a "shield" against the over-production of cortisol in the adrenal gland (289).

It is important to point out that testosterone is an anabolic (or protein building) hormone while cortisol is a catabolic hormone that breaks down proteins in the body. Normal aging consists of a progressive decrease in free testosterone with a marked increase in cortisol. As men age past 40, cortisol begins to dominate, and the catabolic effects associated with growing older begin to dominate.

These findings have significant implications in the battle to maintain youthful hormone balance for the purpose of staving off normal aging and its associated degenerative diseases.

The Testosterone Doctor

Eugene Shippen, M.D., authored a book in 1998 called *The Testosterone Syndrome*. He was a speaker at the American Academy of Anti-Aging Medicine Conference held in December 1998, where he provided extensive evidence documenting the pathology of the testosterone deficiency syndrome in men. Here are some excerpts from Dr. Shippen's presentation that appeared in the March 1999 issue of *Life Extension Magazine*:

> "First, Testosterone is not just a "sex hormone." It should be seen as a "total body hormone," affecting every cell in the body. The changes seen in aging, such as the loss of lean body mass, the decline in energy, strength, and stamina, unexplained depression, and decrease in sexual sensation and performance, are all directly related to testosterone deficiency. Degenerative diseases such as heart disease, stroke, diabetes, arthritis, osteoporosis, and hypertension are all directly or indirectly linked to testosterone decline (220–223). Secondly, testosterone also functions as a prohormone (99). Local tissue conversion to estrogens, dihydrotestosterone (DHT), or other active metabolites plays an important part in cellular physiology.
>
> Excess estrogen seems to be the culprit in prostate enlargement. Low testosterone levels are in fact associated with more aggressive prostate cancer (201, 205, 224–229). While fear of prostate cancer keeps many men from testosterone replacement, it is in fact testosterone deficiency that leads to the pathology that favors the development of prostate cancer.
>
> Testosterone improves cellular bioenergetics. It acts as a cellular energizer. Since testosterone increases the metabolic rate and aerobic metabolism, it also dramatically improves glucose metabolism and lowers insulin resistance (76, 80, 230).
>
> Another myth is that testosterone is bad for the heart. Actually, low testosterone correlates with heart disease more reliably than does high cholesterol (19, 231). Testosterone is the most powerful cardiovascular protector for men. Testosterone strengthens the heart muscle; there are more testosterone receptors in the heart than in any other muscle (232). Testosterone lowers LDL cholesterol and total cholesterol (69, 81, 111), and improves every cardiac risk factor. It has been shown to improve or eliminate arrhythmia and angina (9, 106, 113–115, 233–234, 266). "Testosterone replacement is the most underutilized important treatment for heart disease."
>
> Testosterone shines as a blood thinner, preventing blood clots (32). Testosterone also helps prevent colon cancer (235–236).
>
> Previous research on testosterone used the wrong form of replacement. Injections result in initial excess of testosterone, with conversion of excess to estrogens. Likewise, total testosterone is often measured instead of free testosterone, the bioavailable form. Some studies do not last long enough to show improvement. For instance, it may take six months to a year before the genital tissue fully recovers from atrophy caused by testosterone deficiency, and potency is restored.
>
> Physicians urgently need to be educated about the benefits of testosterone and the delicate balance between androgens (testosterone) and estrogens. Each individual has his or her own pattern of hormone balance; this indicates that hormone replacement should be individualized and carefully monitored."

Dr. Shippen's book, *The Testosterone Syndrome,* retails for $21.95. Foundation members can purchase it for $15.00 by calling (800) 544-4440. The book provides a persuasive argument in favor of hormone modulation in the aged male, and contains many interesting case histories. Dr. Wright's and Dr. Ullis's books on this subject are also available.

Obesity and Hormone Imbalance

A consistent finding in the scientific literature is that obese men have low testosterone and very high estrogen levels. Central or visceral obesity (pot belly) is recognized as a risk factor for cardiovascular disease and type II diabetes. New findings have shed light on subtle hormone imbalances of borderline character in obese men and often fall within the normal laboratory reference range. Boosting testosterone levels seems to decrease the abdominal fat mass, reverse glucose intolerance, and reduce lipoprotein abnormalities in the serum. Further analysis has also disclosed a regulatory role for testosterone in counteracting visceral fat accumulation. Longitudinal epidemiological data demonstrate that relatively low testosterone levels are a risk factor for development of visceral obesity (7,237).

One study showed that serum estrone and estradiol were elevated twofold in one group of morbidly obese men. Fat cells synthesize the aromatase enzyme, causing male hormones to convert to estrogens (278). Fat tissues, especially in the abdomen, have been shown to literally "aromatize" testosterone and its precursor hormones into potent estrogens (80, 237–242).

Eating high-fat foods may reduce free testosterone levels according to one study that measured serum levels of sex steroid hormones after ingestion of different types of food. High-protein and high-carbohydrate meals had no effect on serum hormone levels, but a fat-containing meal reduced free testosterone levels for 4 hours (243).

Obese men suffer from testosterone deficiency caused by the production of excess aromatase enzyme in fat cells and also from the fat they consume in their diet (240). The resulting hormone imbalance (too much estrogen and not enough free testosterone) in obese men partially explains why so many are impotent, and suffer from a wide range of premature degenerative diseases (45).

Factors Causing the Estrogen-Testosterone Imbalance in Men

If your blood tests reveal *high* estrogen and *low* testosterone, here are the common factors involved:

Excess "aromatase" enzyme. As men age, they produce larger quantities of an enzyme called aromatase. The aromatase enzyme converts testosterone into estrogen in the body (17, 240, 241, 244, 245). Inhibiting the aromatase enzyme results in a significant decline in estrogen levels while often boosting free testosterone to youthful levels (279). Therefore, an agent designated as an "aromatase inhibitor" may be of special value to aging men who have excess estrogen.

Liver enzymatic activity. A healthy liver eliminates surplus estrogen and sex hormone-binding globulin. Aging, alcohol, and certain drugs impair liver function and can be a major cause of hormone imbalance in aging men. Heavy alcohol intake increases estrogen in men and women (54, 246, 285).

Obesity. Fat cells create aromatase enzyme and especially contribute to the buildup of abdominal fat (241, 242). Low testosterone allows the formation of abdominal fat (47, 239, 248), which then causes more aromatase enzyme formation and thus even lower levels of testosterone and higher estrogen (by aromatizing testosterone into estrogen). It is especially important for overweight men to consider hormone modulation therapy.

Zinc deficiency. Zinc is a natural aromatase enzyme inhibitor (247). Since most Life Extension Foundation members consume adequate amounts of zinc (30 to 90 mg a day), elevated estrogen in Foundation members is often caused by factors other than zinc deficiency.

Lifestyle changes (such as reducing alcohol intake) can produce a dramatic improvement in the estrogen-testosterone balance, but many people need to use aromatase-inhibiting agents to lower estrogen and to improve their liver function to remove excess SHBG. Aromtase converts testosterone into estrogen and can indirectly increase SHBG. SHBG binds to free testosterone and prevents it from exerting its biochemical effects in the body.

Correcting a Hormone Imbalance

A male hormone imbalance can be detected through use of the proper blood tests and can be corrected using available drugs and nutrients. The following represents a step-by-step program to safely restore youthful hormone balance in aging men:

Step 1: Blood testing

The following initial blood tests are recommended for any man over age 40:

- Complete blood count and chemistry profile to include liver-kidney function, glucose, minerals, lipids, and thyroid (TSH)
- Free and Total Testosterone
- Estradiol (estrogen)
- Progesterone
- DHEA
- PSA
- Luteinizing hormone (LH)
- Homocysteine

Step 2: Interpretation of estrogen-testosterone ratio and free testosterone test results

One of the difficulties in offering standardized interpretations at this time is that blood testing laboratories are using varying test methodologies and reference ranges for testosterone and other hormones.

The following guidelines should be followed when interpreting serum testosterone-estrogen (estradiol) levels:

Free testosterone should be at the high-normal reference range. We define high-normal range as the upper one-third of the highest number on the reference range. Under no circumstances should free or total testosterone be above the high-normal range.

Estrogen (estradiol) should be in the mid- to lower-normal range. If estradiol levels are in the upper one-third of the normal reference range, or above the normal reference range, this excessive level of estrogen should be reduced.

What is most surprising is how "standard laboratory reference ranges" can fool a man (and his physician) into believing he has proper hormone balance simply because he falls within the "normal" range. The following charts compare the conventional normal ranges for a man aged 20 to 49 with the optimal ranges for most men over age 40:

Reference Ranges used by LabCorp and Life Extension's Laboratory

Hormone	Conventional Normal Range	Optimal Range
Free Testosterone	12.4–40 pg/mL	26–40 pg/mL
Estradiol	0–44 pg/mL	15–30 pg/mL
Total Testosterone	300–1000 ng/dL	600–000 ng/dL

Reference Ranges used by SmithKline

Hormone	Conventional Normal	Optimal Range
Free Testosterone	34–194 pg/mL	128–194 pg/mL
Estradiol	0–50 pg/mL	15–30 pg/mL
Total Testosterone	194–833 ng/dL	500–833 ng/dL

Reference Ranges used by Quest Laboratories

Hormone	Conventional Normal	Optimal Range
Free Testosterone	50–210 pg/mL	138–210 pg/mL
Estradiol	0–60 pg/mL	15–30 pg/mL
Total Testosterone	260–1000 ng/dL	500-1000 ng/dL

Please remember that the conventional "normal" ranges stated above are for men aged 20 to 49. Conventional medicine does not expect a man over age 50 to have much testosterone, so the laboratories use a much lower reference range for men over 50. For instance, the reference range used by LabCorp for men over 50 for free testosterone is only 10.8 to 24.6, yet we have strong reason to believe the optimal range for a man over 50 should be 26 to 40. This low reference range shows how conventional medicine expects and accepts that a man over 50 will have suboptimal free testosterone levels (and suffer all of the negative consequences of a testosterone deficiency that we have discussed thus far). We presume that no one reading this article wants to be in that "normal" range of free testosterone for men over age 50.

Also note that these reference ranges indicate that it can be normal for a man to have no estrogen. The fact that most aging men have too much estrogen does not mean it is acceptable for a man to have *no* (or virtually no) estrogen. Estrogen is used by men to maintain bone density, and abnormally low estrogen levels may increase the risk for prostate cancer and osteoporosis (37, 117, 132, 184, 249). The objective is to achieve hormone balance, not to create sky-high testosterone levels without enough estrogen. The problem is that, if we do nothing, most men will have too much estrogen and far too little testosterone.

There are five possible reasons why *free testosterone* levels may be *low*-normal (below the upper third of the highest number of the reference range):

- Too much *testosterone* is being converted to *estradiol* by *excess aromatase enzyme* and/or the *liver* is failing to adequately detoxify surplus estrogen. Excess aromatase enzyme and/or liver dysfunction is likely the cause if estradiol levels are over 30. Remember, aromatase converts testosterone into estradiol, which can cause estrogen overload and testosterone deficiency.
- Too much *free testosterone* is being bound by *SHBG* (sex hormone-binding globulin) (281–284). This would be especially apparent if *total* testosterone levels were in the high normal range, while *free* testosterone was below the upper one-third range. (On LabCorp's scale, this would mean a number below *26*.)
- The *pituitary* gland fails to secrete adequate amounts of *luteinizing hormone* (LH) to stimulate *testicular* production of testosterone. *Total testosterone* in this case would be in the bottom one-third to one-half range. (On LabCorp's scale, this would be a number below *333* to *500*.)
- The *testes* have lost their ability to produce testosterone, despite adequate amounts of the testicular-stimulating *luteinizing hormone*. In this case, LH would be above normal, and total testosterone would in very low normal or below normal ranges.
- Inadequate amounts of *DHEA* are being produced in the body. (DHEA is a precursor hormone to testosterone and estrogen) (250).

Step 3: What to do when results are less than optimal

If *estradiol* levels are *high* (above 30), *total testosterone* is *mid- to high-normal* and *free testosterone* levels are *low or low-normal* (at the bottom one-third of the highest number on the reference range), you should

- Make sure you are getting 80 to 90 mg a day of *zinc*. (Zinc functions as an aromatase inhibitor for some men.)
- Consume 110 mg of *soy isoflavones* (phytoestrogens) each day. (High levels of phytoestrogens compete with estradiol on cell receptor sites and stimulate the liver to remove estrogens from the blood.) Cruciferous vegetables such as broccoli and cauliflower can also stimulate the liver to metabolize and excrete excess estrogen.
- Reduce or eliminate alcohol consumption to enable your liver to better remove excess estrogens. (*Refer to the Foundation's Liver Degeneration protocol to learn about ways to restore healthy liver function.*)
- Review all drugs you are regularly taking to see if they may be interfering with healthy liver function. Common drugs that affect liver function are the NSAIDs: ibuprofen, acetaminophen, aspirin, the "statin" class of cholesterol-lowering drugs, some heart and blood pressure medications, and some antidepressants. It is interesting to note that drugs being prescribed to treat the symptoms of testosterone deficiency such as the statins and certain antidepressants may actually aggravate a testosterone deficit, thus making the cholesterol problem or depression worse.
- Lose weight. Fat cells, especially in the abdominal region, produce aromatase enzyme, which converts testosterone into estrogen (242).
- If all of the above fail to increase free testosterone and lower excess estradiol, ask your doctor to prescribe the potent aromatase inhibiting drug *Arimidex* (anastrozole) in the very low

dose of one-half mg (0.5 mg), twice a week. Arimidex is prescribed to breast cancer patients at the dose of 1 to 10 mg a day. Even at the higher dose prescribed to cancer patients, side effects are rare. In the minute dose of 0.5 mg twice a week, a man will see an immediate drop in estradiol levels and should experience a rise in free testosterone to the optimal range.

If *free testosterone* levels are in the *lower two-thirds* of the highest number in the reference range, but *total testosterone* is *high-normal*, and *estradiol* levels are not over *30,* you should

- Consider following some of the recommendations in the previous section to inhibit aromatase, since many of the same factors are involved in excess SHBG activity.
- Take 320 mg a day of the super-critical extract of saw palmetto and 240 mg a day of the methanolic extract of nettle (*Urtica dioica*). Nettle may specifically inhibit SHGB (42–44,251–252), while saw palmetto may reduce the effects of excess estrogen by blocking the nuclear estrogen receptor sites in prostate cells, which in turn activate the cell-stimulating effects of testosterone and dihydrotestosterone. Saw palmetto also has the effect of blocking the oxidation of testosterone to androstenedione, a potent androgen that has been implicated in the development of prostate disease (253).

If *total testosterone* is in the lower one-third of the reference range or below normal, and *free testosterone* is low, you should

- See if your luteinizing hormone (LH) is below normal. If LH is low, your doctor can prescribe an individual dose of *chorionic gonadotropin (HCG)* hormone for injection. Chorionic gonadotropic hormone functions similarly to LH and can re-start testicular production of testosterone. Your doctor can instruct you on how to use tiny 30-gauge needles to inject yourself 2 to 3 times a week. (Editor's note: Some scientists think HCG may cause cancer. If this concerns you, consider using a testosterone patch, cream, or pellet.)
- After one month on chorionic gonadotropic hormone, a blood test can determine whether total testosterone levels are significantly increasing. You may also see your testicles growing larger. If total testosterone levels are restored, monitor blood levels of estradiol and free testosterone every 30 to 45 days for the first 5 months to make sure the exogenous testosterone you are putting into your body is following a healthy metabolic pathway, i.e., is raising your levels of *free testosterone*, but *not* increasing *estradiol* levels beyond *30*.

If *total testosterone* remains low in spite of several months of chorionic gonadotropic hormone therapy, this indicates that your testicles are not capable of producing testosterone. In that case, initiate therapy with the testosterone patch, pellet, or cream. Do not use testosterone injections or tablets.

Before initiating testosterone replacement therapy, have a PSA blood test and a digital rectal exam to rule out detectable prostate cancer. Once total testosterone levels are restored to a high-normal range, monitor blood levels of estradiol, free testosterone, and PSA every 30 to 45 days for the first 6 months to make sure the exogenous testosterone you are putting into your body is following a healthy metabolic pathway and not causing a flare up of an underlying prostate cancer. The objective is to raise your levels of *free testosterone* to the upper third of the reference range, but to not increase estradiol levels beyond *30*.

Excess estrogen (estradiol) blocks the production and effect of testosterone throughout the body, dampens sexuality, and increases the risk of prostate and cardiovascular disease. Once you have established the proper ratio of free testosterone (upper one-third of the highest number in the reference range) and estradiol (not more than *30*), make sure your blood is tested every 30 to 45 days for the first 5 months. Test every 6 months thereafter for free testosterone, estradiol, and PSA. For men in their 40s to 50s, correcting the excess level of estradiol is often all that has to be done. Men over 60 sometimes need the chorionic gonadotropin injection, and may need to use a testosterone patch, cream, or pellet later in life.

Therapies

The Testosterone Patch and PSA

An oncologist affiliated with the Life Extension Foundation reports that some men on the testosterone patch will show an elevated PSA that then drops upon cessation of the exogenously administered testosterone. There are published studies that contradict this finding (185, 254–257). Elevation of PSA could be caused by the conversion of exogenous testosterone to estrogen or DHT.

Therapies have been discussed that can prevent testosterone from cascading into estrogen and DHT. This oncologist noted that prostate cancer patients with low testosterone levels have a more aggressive disease, most likely related to the development of tumor cells that are androgen independent, and thus more resistant to therapy. This observation is substantiated by the published literature (185, 186, 201, 205, 224–229, 254–256, 286, 288).

"Andro" Supplements

Androstenedione is a precursor to both testosterone and estrogen. Early studies showed that "andro" supplements could markedly increase testosterone levels, but more recent studies cast doubt on this concept. A study in the Journal of the American Medical Association (*JAMA*) reported on an 8-week study showing that androstenedione supplements increased estrogen levels in 30 men. No increase in strength, muscle mass, or testosterone levels was observed. Meanwhile, home run hitter Mark McGwire, who made androstenedione a media sensation, says he stopped taking the supplement in April 1999. Perhaps combining androstenedione with an aromatase inhibitor that would prevent it from converting to estrogen would make this precursor hormone work better in men. In the meantime, we suggest avoiding androstenedione until more definitive research is published (258).

Testosterone Drugs

Synthetic testosterone "steroid" drugs are chemically different from the testosterone your body makes and do not provide the same effect as natural testosterone. Here is a listing of some of the synthetic testosterone drugs to avoid using on a long-term basis: Methyltestosterone, Danazol, Oxandrolone, Testosterone propionate, cypionate, or enanthate.

The fact that testosterone is marketed as a "drug" does not mean it is not the same natural hormone your body produced. Scientists learned decades ago how to make the identical testosterone that your body produces, but, since natural testosterone could not be patented, drug companies developed all kinds of synthetic testosterone analogs that could be patented and approved by the FDA as new drugs. Here is a listing of currently available recommended natural testosterone drugs:

- Androderm Transdermal System (Smith Kline Beecham's testosterone patch)
- Testoderm Transdermal System (Alza's testosterone patch)
- Testosterone creams, pellets, and sublingual tablets (available from compounding pharmacies)

Both synthetic and natural testosterone drugs require a prescription, and a prescription should only be written after blood or saliva tests reveal a testosterone deficiency.

Alternative physicians usually prescribe testosterone creams and other types made at compounding pharmacies, whereas conventional doctors are more likely to prescribe a box of ready-made, FDA-approved testosterone patches. All forms of natural testosterone are the same and all will markedly increase free testosterone in the blood or saliva.

If you interact with children, you may want to avoid testosterone creams. There is a report of a young male child going through pre-mature puberty after he made contact with the testosterone cream on his father's body and on weightlifting equipment in the home. This unique case is a testament to the powerful effects that testosterone exerts in the body.

CAUTION: Do not use testosterone replacement if you have prostate cancer.

Men with existing prostate cancer should follow an opposite approach as it relates to testosterone. Prostate cancer patients are normally prescribed testosterone *ablation* therapy (using a drug that blocks the pituitary release of LH and another drug that blocks testosterone-receptor sites on the cells). Early state prostate cancer cells can often be controlled by totally suppressing testosterone in the body. Late-stage prostate cancer patients are sometimes put on drugs that produce estrogenic effects to suppress prostate cancer cells that no longer depend on testosterone for growth. Regrettably, prostate cancer patients put on testosterone ablation therapy often temporarily suffer many of the unpleasant effects of low testosterone that have been described in this article. Before initiating a therapy that boosts your free testosterone level, a blood PSA (prostate specific antigen) test and digital rectal exam are recommended for men over age 40. While restoring free testosterone to healthy physiological levels (25 to 40 pg/mL) does not cause prostate cancer, it can induce existing prostate cancer cells to proliferate faster.

Mandatory Testing

When embarking on a hormone modulation program, medical testing is critical. First, a baseline blood PSA must be taken to rule out existing prostate cancer. Then free testosterone and estradiol tests are needed to make sure that too much testosterone is not being converted into estradiol (estrogen). If estrogen levels are too high, the use of aromatase inhibitors can keep testosterone from converting (aromatizing) into estrogen in the body. Follow-up testing for testosterone, estrogen, and PSA are needed to rule out occult prostate cancer and to fine tune your program. It's possible that testosterone patches and creams can increase testosterone levels too much. In that case, blood or saliva testing could save you money by allowing you to use less of the testosterone drug.

There are now natural dietary supplements in development that boost free testosterone levels and suppress excess estrogen. Even when these supplements become available, PSA testing is still mandatory, since any substance that increases testosterone should be avoided by most prostate cancer patients.

More Information

Over the last year, three new books have been written about testosterone replacement therapy. The best place to read about actual case histories of men who successfully used hormone modulation is Dr. Eugene Shippen's book *The Testosterone Syndrome* (260). Dr. Shippen's book provides many interesting details that could not be covered in this concise protocol. Dr. Jonathan Wright's book, *Maximize Your Vitality and Potency,* contains historical and more technical data about the benefits of testosterone that again, could not be fit into this concise protocol. Dr. Karlis Ullis's book, *Super T,* deals primarily with dietary and supplement modifications related to testosterone deficiency.

The Testosterone Syndrome, Eugene Shippen, M.D., cover price: $21.95, member price: $15.00. *Maximize Your Vitality and Potency,* Jonathan Wright, M.D., cover price: $14.95, member price: $11.00. *Super T,* Karlis Ullis, M.D., cover price: $12.00, member price: $8.50.

You can expect updates to this protocol in future issues of *Life Extension Magazine* as more information becomes available. The Foundation will be monitoring the effects of this program intensely, based on reports from clinical physicians and Foundation members. As always, worldwide data base searches will be conducted routinely to uncover new studies relating to the effects of hormone modulation and aging.

Studies

Due to the highly controversial nature of this article, we have taken the unprecedented step of publishing over 180 pages of scientific abstracts on our Web site [www.lef.org] that are numerically matched to the statements made in this article. This may be the first time for such a massive undertaking, and it reflects the urgent need to convey this information to skeptical physicians so that they will prescribe testosterone and aromatase-inhibiting drugs to Foundation members whose blood tests indicate a need for these therapies.

Updates to this protocol can be found on the Foundation's website at www.lef.org.

What the Published Literature Says about Testosterone and Prostate Cancer

Studies indicating that testosterone does not cause prostate cancer

Study 1. "This nested case-control study was based on the cohort of men who donated blood to the Janus serum bank at Oslo University Hospital between 1973 and 1994. Cancer incidence was ascertained through linkage with the Norwegian Cancer Registry. The study included sera from 59 men who developed prostate cancer subsequent to blood donation and 180 men who were free of any diagnosed cancer in 1994 and were of similar age and had similar blood storage time. Neither testosterone, DHT, nor the ratio of testosterone to DHT was associated with risk of developing prostate cancer. These results showed no association, positive or negative, between androgens measured in serum and the subsequent risk of developing prostate cancer." (*Cancer Epidemiology Biomarkers Prev.,* 1997 [Nov]; 6[11]:967–69). Study conducted at Department of Community Medicine and General Practice, University Medical Center, Trondheim, Norway [lars.vatten@medisin.ntnu.no].

Study 2. "We conducted a nested case-control study in a cohort of 6860 Japanese-American men examined from 1971 to 1975. At the time of examination, a single blood specimen was obtained, and the serum was frozen. After a surveillance period of more than 20 years, 141 tissue-confirmed incident cases of prostate cancer were identified, and their stored sera and those of 141 matched controls were assayed for total testosterone, free testosterone, dihydrotestosterone, 3-alpha-androstanediol glucuronide, androsterone glucuronide, and androstenedione. The findings of this study indicate that none of these androgens is strongly associated with prostate cancer risk" (*Cancer Epidemiol. Biomarkers Prev.,* 1996 [Aug]; 5[8]:621–25). Study conducted at Japan-Hawaii Cancer Study, Kuakini Medical Center, Honolulu 96817, USA.

Study 3. "Prostate cancer was identified in 14% (11/77) of the entire group and in 10 men (29%) aged 60 years or older. The median age for men with cancer was 64 years. No significant differences were noted between the cancer and benign groups with regard to PSA level, PSA density, prostate volume, total testosterone level, or free testosterone level. A high prevalence of biopsy-detectable prostate cancer was identified in men with low total or free testosterone levels despite normal PSA levels and results of digital rectal examination. These data suggest that (1) digital rectal examination and PSA levels are insensitive indicators of prostate cancer in men with low total or free testosterone levels, and (2) PSA levels may be altered by naturally occurring reductions in serum androgen levels" (*Journal of the American Medical Association* [*JAMA*], 1996 [Dec. 18]; 276[23]:1904–6). Study conducted at Division of Urology, Beth Israel Hospital, Harvard Medical School, Boston, Massachusetts 02215.

Study 4. "We conducted a prospective nested case-control study to evaluate the relationships of serum androgens and estrogens to prostate cancer using serum collected at baseline for the Alpha-Tocopherol, Beta-Carotene Cancer Prevention Study. None of the individual androgens or estrogens was significantly related to prostate cancer. These results do not support a strong relationship of serum androgens and estrogens with prostate cancer in smokers" (*Cancer Epidemiology and Biomarkers Prev.,* 1998 [Dec]; 7[12]:1069–74). Study conducted at Division of Cancer Epidemiology and Genetics, National Cancer Institute, Bethesda, Maryland 20892-7374 [jd7g@nih.gov].

Study 5. "We report a nested case-control study of serum biomarkers of 5-alpha-reductase activity and the incidence of prostate cancer. From a cohort of more than 125,000 members of the Kaiser Permanente Medical Care Program who underwent multiphasic health examinations during 1964–1971, we selected 106 incident prostate cancer cases. A control was pair matched to each case on age, date of serum sampling, and clinic location. The adjusted odds ratios and 95% confidence intervals for a one quartile score increase were 1.00 for total testosterone (1.00 = no increased risk), 1.14

M

for free testosterone, 1.13 for androsterone glucuronide, and 1.16 for 3-alpha-diol G" (*Cancer Epidemiology Biomarkers Prev.,* 1997 [Jan]; 6 [1]:21–24). Study conducted at Department of Epidemiology, School of Public Health, University of North Carolina, Chapel Hill 27599-7400.

Study 6. "Serum samples were obtained from 6860 men during their study examination from 1971 to 1975. After a surveillance period of about 14 years, 98 incident cases of prostate cancer were identified. Their stored sera and that of 98 matched controls from the study population were tested for the following: testosterone, dihydrotestosterone, estrone, estradiol, and sex hormone globulin. There was a suggestion that serum dihydrotestosterone levels were lower and the testosterone/dihydrotestosterone ratios were higher in the prostate cancer cases compared with their controls. However, none of these associations or that of the other hormones was strongly significant" (*Cancer Research,* 1988 [June 15]; 48[12]:3515–17). Study conducted at Japan-Hawaii Cancer Study, Kuakini Medical Center, Honolulu 96817.

Study 7. "A case-control study of prostatic cancer was carried out to examine the association between selected physical characteristics and factors related to sexual development and behavior and the risk for this disease. The levels of testosterone (T), dihydrotestosterone, salivary testosterone and T/SHBG (sex hormone–binding globulin) did not vary with age. Older men had higher oestradiol (estrogen) levels. Further, little association between hormone levels and risk factors was found, except for married subjects having increased serum androgens and heavy subjects having decreased serum androgens (not significant)" (*European Journal of Cancer Prev.,* 1992 [April]; 1[3]:239–45). Study conducted at Department of Urology, Erasmus University, Rotterdam, The Netherlands.

Study 8. "A population-based nested case-control study was conducted to determine the relation of prediagnostic serum levels of testosterone, dihydrotestosterone, prolactin, follicle-stimulating hormone, luteinizing hormone, estrone, and estradiol to the risk of subsequent prostate cancer. Serum specimens of study subjects were available from a blood collection campaign in Washington County, Maryland, in 1974. There were no significant differences in levels of these hormones between cases and controls, although elevated levels of luteinizing hormone and of testosterone/dihydrotestosterone ratios were associated with mild increased risks of prostate cancer" (*Cancer Epidemiology Biomarkers Prev.,* 1993 [Jan–Feb]; 2[1]:27–32). Study conducted at National Cancer Institute, Division of Cancer Etiology, Bethesda, Maryland 20892.

Study 9. "The possible relationship between changes in peripheral hormone levels and the occurrence of prostatic pathology was studied in a case-control study involving estimation of various plasma hormones in 368 Dutch and 258 Japanese men, who were grouped as controls and patients with benign prostatic hyperplasia, focal prostatic carcinoma, or clinically evident prostatic carcinoma. There were no significant differences in plasma androgen levels between Japanese or Dutch prostate cancer cases and their respective control subgroups.

These findings do not support a correlation between the lower plasma testosterone levels and a lower incidence of prostate cancer in the Japanese men. Furthermore, no significant differences were found between salivary levels of testosterone or the ratio between testosterone and SHBG in the various Dutch subgroups. In Japanese benign prostatic hyperplasia patients, the testosterone to SHBG ratio was significantly increased. In conclusion, the results of this retrospective, cross-sectional study do not indicate that hormonal levels play a primary role in the origin or promotion of prostatic abnormalities" (*Cancer Research,* 1991 [July 1]; 51[13]:3445–50). Study conducted at Department of Endocrinology and Reproduction, Erasmus University, Rotterdam, The Netherlands.

Study 10. "Frozen serum samples were analysed for PSA, DHT, testosterone and SHBG, and compared to the diagnosis and tumor stage, grade and ploidy. DHT levels were slightly lower in patients with prostate cancer but the difference was not statistically significant. There was a trend towards lower DHT values in more advanced tumors. Testosterone levels were lower in patients with cancer than in the control group, but the differences were not significant. There was no correlation between testosterone levels, tumor stage, and ploidy. The testosterone/DHT ratio tended to be higher in patients with more advanced tumors. SHBG levels were lower in patients with cancer than in controls, but the differences were not statistically significant. There were no systematic variations of tumor stage, grade, and ploidy. Within a group, DHT levels tended to be lower among cases and in those with more advanced tumors. No systematic variation was found in the levels of testosterone or SHBG" (*British Journal of Urology,* 1996 [March]; 77[3]:433–40). Study conducted at Department of Urology, Karolinska Institute at Stockholm Soder Hospital, Sweden.

Study 11. "Index cases and their brothers and sons had a significantly lower mean plasma testosterone content than controls of comparable age. Preliminary data suggest that the metabolic clearance rate of testosterone and the conversion ratio of testosterone to estradiol are relatively high in probands. The observations indicate that familial factors are potent risk factors for the development of prostatic cancer. They also suggest that plasma androgen values in families with prostatic cancer cluster in the lower range of normal and that plasma sex-steroid content is more similar in each brother with or without prostatic cancer than among nonbrothers" (*Prostate,* 1985; 6[2]:121–28).

Study 12. "Baseline sex hormone levels were measured in 1008 men ages 40 to 79 years who had been followed for 14 years. There were 31 incident cases of prostatic cancer and 26 identified from death certificates with unknown dates of diagnosis. In this study, total testosterone, estrone, estradiol, and sex hormone-binding globulin were not related to prostate cancer, but plasma androstenedione showed a positive dose-response gradient" (*Cancer Research,* 1990 [Jan 1]; 50[1]:169–73). Study conducted at Department of Community and Family Medicine, University of California, San Diego, La Jolla 92093.

Study 13. "The hypothesis that serum concentrations of pituitary hormones, sex steroid hormones, or sex hormone–binding globulin (SHBG) affect the occurrence of prostatic cancer was tested in a consecutive sample of 93 patients with nowly diagnosed, untreated cancer and in 98 population controls of similar ages without the disease. Remarkably close agreement was found for mean values of total testosterone (15.8 in cases and 16.0 in controls), and free testosterone (0.295 and 0.293 respectively), with corresponding odds ratios for the highest vs. lowest tertile of 1.0 (1.00 = no increased risk) for testosterone and 1.2 for free testosterone. Similar close agreement between cases and controls was found for serum concentrations of estradiol, androstenedione, and SHBG, although the mean estradiol level was nonsignificantly lower among cases" (*British Journal of Cancer,* 1993 [July]; 68[1]:97–102). Study conducted at Department of Urology, Orebro Medical Center Hospital, Sweden.

Study 14. "Modest depression of serum testosterone and estradiol was noted for prostate cancer patients compared to clinic controls, although the differences were not statistically significant. This depression was interpreted to be a likely result of the malignant process rather than a cause of it" (*Prostate,* 1987; 11[2]:171–82). Study conducted at Department of Epidemiology, School of Public Health, University of North Carolina at Chapel Hill, 27514.

Study 15. "The prostate cancer patients had a slightly lower mean free testosterone and mean estradiol/free T ratio than the BPH patients. The mean estradiol/free testosterone ratio was significantly higher in the BPH patients and in the PC patients than in the young controls. It seems possible that the observed age-dependent significant increase in plasma estrogen concentration in the BPH patients may act as a protective factor against prostatic cancer" (*Prostate,* 1983; 4[3]:223–29).

Study 16. "A fourfold higher relative risk for the development of prostatic cancer was observed for brothers of prostatic cancer cases compared to their brothers-in-law and males in the general population of the state of Utah. Probands and their brothers, and sons of the patients with the disease, had significantly lower plasma testosterone levels than controls of comparable age. This is the first documentation indicating that familial (possibly genetic) factors are potent risk factors for predisposing men to the development of prostatic cancer and in regulating the plasma content of androgens. Our results indicate that plasma androgen levels in families with prostatic cancer are clustered in the lower range of the normal population. They also suggest that plasma androgen content is more similar within each family with the cancer than among the families without cancer" (*Journal of Clinical Endocrinology and Metabolism,* 1982 [Jun]; 54[6]:1104–8)

Study 17. "Pretreatment hormone levels were determined in 222 patients with prostatic cancer and their prognostic value assessed. The patients were grouped into yearly survival categories and only those whose cause of death was due to the disease were included in the study. Low concentrations of testosterone in plasma at the time of diagnosis related to a poor prognosis. Patients who died within 1 year of diagnosis had the lowest mean plasma levels of this steroid. The pretreatment mean plasma testosterone concentrations were found to be higher as the survival period of the various groups lengthened. The indications from this study are that poor testicular function is associated with early death from prostatic carcinoma and that the measurement of blood levels of testosterone at diagnosis could provide a prognosis of subsequent life span" (*European Journal of Cancer Clinical Oncology,* 1984 [April]; 20[4]:477–82).

Study 18. "Pretreatment plasma concentrations of total testosterone, prolactin, and total estradiol were measured in 123 prostatic cancer patients who were categorized into groups according to the UICC classification. The mean follow-up time was 48 months. Higher pretreatment estradiol and testosterone levels were associated with better survival" (*Scandinavian Journal of Urology and Nephrology Supplmental,* 1988; 110:137–43). Study conducted at Second Department of Surgery, Helsinki University Central Hospital, Finland.

Study 19. "This cross-sectional study was undertaken to determine whether serum hormones (free testosterone, androstenedione, luteinizing hormone, or prolactin) have any influence on serum prostate specific antigen (PSA) levels in patients with stage A–C prostate cancer. None of the hormones in any of the analyses showed any association to serum PSA values. Serum free testosterone, androstenedione, and luteinizing hormone appeared to have no influence on serum PSA values in nonmetastatic cancer patients" (*JAMA,* 1995 [Nov]; 87[11]:813–19). Study conducted at Department of Radiation Oncology, Michael Reese Hospital, Center for Radiation Therapy, University of Chicago, Illinois.

Study 20. "Serum levels of testosterone, DHT, androsterone, 5 alpha-androstane-3 alpha, 17-beta-diol (5 alpha-diol), and estradiol were measured by radioimmunoassay in the sera of 9 patients with untreated prostatic cancer and in 11 with benign prostatic hypertrophy (BPH). Although no specific changes in steroid hormone levels in either disease group were found, response patterns of serum T, DHT, and E2 were shown to be those characteristic of male senescence, suggesting a relative predominance of estrogens over androgens" (*Prostate Supplemental,* 1981; 1:19–26).

Study 21. "We studied the effect of exogenous testosterone administration on the serum levels of PSA (prostate-specific antigen) and PSMA (prostate-specific membrane antigen) in hypogonadal men. Serial serum PSA, serum PSMA, and serum total testosterone levels were obtained at intervals of every 2 to 4 weeks in 10 hypogonadal men undergoing treatment with exogenous testosterone, delivered as testosterone enanthate injection or by testosterone patch. A two-tailed, paired t-test failed to demonstrate a significant correlation between serum PSA or PSMA and serum testosterone levels. This study suggests that in hypogonadal men, neither PSMA nor PSA expression is testosterone-dependent" (*Journal of Surgical Oncology,* 1995 [Aug]; 59[4]:246–50). Study conducted at Department of Surgery, Walter Reed Army Medical Center, Washington, D.C. 20307-5001.

Neutral study

Study 22. "Blood samples were collected from 52 incident cases of histologically confirmed prostate cancer and 52 age- and town of residence- matched healthy controls in Athens, Greece. DHT was associated inversely, significantly, and strongly with the risk of prostate cancer, whereas testosterone was associated marginally positively, and E2 was associated nonsignificantly inversely with the disease" (*Cancer Causes Control,* 1997 [July]; 8[4]:632–36). Study conducted at Department of Epidemiology and Harvard Center for Cancer Prevention, Harvard School of Public Health, Boston, Massachusetts 02115.

Studies indicating that testosterone causes prostate cancer

Study 1. "We conducted a prospective, nested case-control study to investigate whether plasma hormone and sex hormone–binding globulin (SHBG) levels in healthy men were related to the subsequent development of prostate cancer. No clear associations were found between the unadjusted levels of individual hormones or SHBG and the risk of prostate cancer. However, a strong correlation was observed between the levels of testosterone and SHBG (r = .55), and weaker correlations were detected between the levels of testosterone and the levels of both estradiol (r = .28) and DHT (r = .32) (all P < .001). When hormone and SHBG levels were adjusted simultaneously, a strong trend of increasing prostate cancer risk was observed with increasing levels of plasma testosterone (ORs by quartile = 1.00, 1.41, 1.98, and 2.60 [95% CI = 1.34–5.02]; P for trend = .004), an inverse trend in risk was seen with increasing levels of SHBG (ORs by quartile = 1.00, 0.93, 0.61, and 0.46 [95% CI = 0.24–0.89]; P for trend = .01), and a non-linear inverse association was found with increasing levels of estradiol (ORs by quartile = 1.00, 0.53, 0.40, and 0.56 [95% CI = 0.32–0.98]; P for trend = .03). No associations were detected between the levels of DHT or prolactin and prostate cancer risk. High levels of circulating testosterone and low levels of SHBG—both within normal endogenous ranges—are associated with increased risks of prostate cancer. Low levels of circulating estradiol may represent an additional risk factor" (*Journal of the National Cancer Institute,* 1996 [Aug]. 21; 88[6]:1118–26). Study conducted at Department of Medicine, Brigham and Women's Hospital, Harvard Medical School, Boston, MA.

Study 2. "Basal serum concentrations of sex steroids, sex hormone–binding globulin (SHBG), and gonadotrophins, and the basal levels and response to adrenocorticotropic hormone (ACTH) of adrenocortical steroids, were measured before treatment in 72 patients with prostate cancer and in 42 age-matched healthy controls. Patients aged < 60 years with prostate cancer had significantly elevated levels of total testosterone and unconjugated (E1) and total (tE1) oestrone, while patients aged > or = 60 years had significantly elevated levels of total and non-SHBG-bound testosterone (NST), 17-alpha-hydroxyprogesterone and tE1. Gonadotrophins, SHBG levels and relationships between total testosterone and SHBG were normal in both age groups of patients, as were basal levels and ACTH-induced increments of adrenocortical steroids. The patients had normal age-related variations in SHBG and NST and in basal levels and ACTH-induced increments of adrenocortical steroids. There was a significant age-related increase in serum E1 in the control subjects but not in the patients. Patients with metastatic disease had significantly lower E1 levels than had patients without metastases. The results suggest an increased sensitivity of the testis to gonadotrophic stimulation, as well as an increased peripheral oestrogen synthesis in patients with prostate cancer, the latter being most pronounced in younger subjects. Men developing prostate cancer may have been exposed to a combination of elevated endogenous oestrogen and androgen levels for a long time. These findings support the theory of a synergism between oestrogens and androgens as an important factor in the aetiology of prostate cancer" (*British Journal of Urology,* 1997 [March]; 79[3]:427–31). Study conducted at Department of Obstetrics and Gynaecology, Karolinska Institute, Huddinge University Hospital, Sweden.

Study 3. "A blinded, case-control study was undertaken to determine if hair patterning is associated with risk of prostate cancer, as well as specific hormonal profiles. The study accrued 315 male subjects who were stratified with regard to age, race, and case-control status (159 prostate

M

cancer cases/156 controls). Free testosterone was greater among cases than in controls (16.4 +/–6.1 vs. 14.9 +/–4.8 pg/ml, P = 0.02). Conversely, DHT-related ratios were greater among controls. Data suggest that increased levels of free testosterone may be a risk factor for prostatic carcinoma" (*Journal of Andrology,* 1997 [Sep–Oct]; 18[5]:495–500). Study conducted at Division of Urology, Duke University Medical Center, Durham, North Carolina 27710.

Study 4. "We present the case of a hypogonadal patient in whom a 20-fold increase in prostate-specific antigen and a palpable prostatic nodule developed 6 months into the administration of intramuscular testosterone" (*Urology,* 1999 [Feb]; 53[2]:423–24). Study conducted at Department of Urology, Lahey Clinic Medical Center, Burlington, Massachusetts 01805.

Study 5. "The metabolic clearance and production rates of testosterone were significantly higher in (prostate cancer) patients than in controls. These results indicate that men with prostatic cancer have elevated clearance and production rates of testosterone without an alteration of estradiol production or clearance" (*Journal of Steroid Biochemistry,* 1989 [July]; 33[1]:19–24 r). Study conducted at Department of Internal Medicine, University of Utah School of Medicine, Salt Lake City 84132.

More studies can be found on the Foundation's website at www.lef.org.

MEDICAL TESTING PROTOCOLS

The Life Extension Foundation has advocated regular medical testing since 1983 for the purpose of optimizing your personal life extension program. Regular blood testing enables you to detect

- Abnormalities that may predispose you to diseases that are treatable if caught at an early stage, such as cancer, diabetes, and cardiovascular disease.
- Toxicities that could be counteracted to prevent organ damage—for example, liver damage caused by hepatotoxic drugs, vitamin A, iron overload, etc.—by adjusting your nutrient or drug intake.
- Hormone imbalances—e.g., DHEA deficiency or cortisol overload—that can accelerate your rate of aging if not corrected.
- A positive cancer profile, indicating the development of cancer.
- Other imbalances that could be adjusted to enable you to become healthier, more energetic, sexier, and stronger.

Here are some of the important tests that can be used to assess your health and longevity, and the results you should strive to attain:

Glucose: optimal level should be under 100. A consistent effect of calorie restriction is a reduction in serum glucose levels to a low normal range. Calorie restriction is the only documented method of extending maximum life span. Calorie-restricted people often have serum glucose levels between 70 and 80. When glucose levels are greater than 100, accelerated aging can occur via several mechanisms.

Glucose-lowering nutrients include 200 mcg of chromium with every meal, and/or 7.5 mg of vanadyl sulfate 3 times a day, and/or 4 decaffeinated green tea capsules with every meal, and/or fiber supplements. Thyroid hormone level should be checked yearly. If it is too low, you should consider thyroid hormone supplementation under a doctor's supervision. Another method of improving thyroid function is to take 6 to 30 grams of a highly concentrated soy extract, iodine, and tyrosine. These can help to normalize your thyroid hormone levels.

Iron: Optimal level should be under 100. Iron is a catalyst for free-radical activity that increases the risk of heart disease, Alzheimer's disease, cancer, and a host of degenerative diseases. Low iron levels have been shown to protect against cancer and heart disease in large human populations.

Iron-lowering nutrients include 4 decaffeinated green tea capsules and/or 4 garlic/EDTA capsules, and/or 300 clemental milligrams of calcium with meals that contain iron. Donating a pint of blood to yourself for future use is another way of lowering serum iron levels.

Cholesterol: Optimal LDL cholesterol level below 100–120. Optimal HDL cholesterol level above 50. Oxidized LDL cholesterol adheres to the inner linings of arteries, a condition which contributes to atherosclerosis. It also promotes abnormal arterial clotting. HDL cholesterol removes excess fat and other types of cholesterol from the arterial system.

Nutrients that favorably alter cholesterol levels—i.e., lower dangerous LDL cholesterol and elevate HDL cholesterol—include 200 mcg of chromium twice a day, 30 grams a day of soluble fiber, 1000 to 3000 mg a day of niacin with meals, and 2000 mg a day and higher of vitamin C. Herbal extracts such as curcumin and gugulipid have dose-related cholesterol-lowering effects.

At the American Heart Association's annual stroke conference (February 1999), a report was presented showing that people with cholesterol levels under 180 doubled their risk of hemorrhagic stroke compared to those with cholesterol levels of 230. Hemorrhagic stroke occurs when a blood vessel in the brain breaks open and is different than the more common thrombotic stroke caused by an abnormal blood clot. This study showed that the risk of thrombotic stoke was twice as likely in those with cholesterol levels over 280 compared to those at 230. The report concluded that optimal cholesterol level for overall stroke prevention was around 200.

Some overzealous Foundation members have been pushing their cholesterol levels way below 180. In the few reports of hemorrhagic stroke suffered by Foundation members, their cholesterol levels have all been far below 180 mg/dL. Based on a review of the published data, no one wants chronic high levels of cholesterol in their blood, but optimal ranges for overall disease prevention may be between 180 to 210 and not "as low as you can get!"

Triglycerides: optimal triglyceride level is below 100. Triglycerides combine a fatty acid and glycerol. Elevated triglyceride levels predispose a person to atherosclerosis and abnormal platelet aggregation. Nutrients that may lower elevated triglyceride levels include high doses of fish oil, garlic, and niacin.

Why Blood Tests Are Not Used Regularly

The high cost and inconvenience of regular blood testing prevents many people from being tested as often as they should be. Another problem with blood testing is that different labs often produce varying readings from the same blood specimen, making the results of regular testing difficult to interpret.

The Life Extension Foundation receives blood-test results for evaluation from members who sometimes use different laboratories every time they are tested. In many cases, the member is not even aware that different laboratories had been used in testing.

Another problem is that commercial testing laboratories seldom perform the unique tests that Foundation members request, which means, for example, that a lab technician may be doing his first-ever DHEA serum test on your blood.

In order to standardize the methods used for all blood tests, the Life Extension Foundation has made an arrangement with a nationwide testing laboratory to perform all basic blood testing. For specialized tests to measure DHEA, growth hormone, and cortisol, the Foundation has contracted with a reputable specialty laboratory which has been performing these unique tests for 15 years. Here are descriptions for the most popular blood tests:

Blood Chemistry/Complete Blood Count

This testing panel includes LDL; HDL; total cholesterol; triglycerides; iron; glucose; liver and kidney function; and many more important tests. These tests detect blood changes that may predispose you to a wide range of degenerative diseases. They also provide information to assess whether or not the drugs and nutrients you may be taking are causing liver, kidney, or heart damage.

We suggest that this battery of tests be performed annually. If a serious abnormality is detected—such as elevated glucose, cholesterol, or iron—testing should be repeated more often to determine the benefits of whatever therapy you are using to correct the potentially life-shortening abnormality.

Homocysteine

Measuring blood levels of homocysteine is a new and potentially life-saving test that provides information about vitamin and methylation status in addition to determining levels of toxic homocysteine. Those with a family history of heart disease, stroke, or Alzheimer's disease are at a particular risk from elevated homocysteine. Elevated homocysteine has also been linked to complications in diabetes, lupus, and other chronic diseases. While many people have assumed that because they are taking vitamin supplements their homocysteine levels will be in a "safe" range, the Life Extension Foundation has discovered that this might not always be the case. Refer to the Foundation's *Homocysteine protocol* to learn about the lethal effects of elevated serum homocysteine and what you can do to lower it.

Fibrinogen

Elevated levels of fibrinogen predispose you to arterial clotting that can cause a heart attack or a stroke. Elevated fibrinogen may be at least as great a risk factor for coronary artery disease as elevated LDL cholesterol. Optimal fibrinogen levels should be under 300.

Fibrinogen-lowering nutrients include bromelain in doses of 250 to 1000 mg twice a day, and/or 8 fish oil capsules a day, and/or beta-carotene in doses of 25,000 to 100,000 IU a day, and/or vitamin C in doses exceeding 2000 mg a day, and/or taking a European drug called Bezafibrate.

Prostate-Specific Antigen (PSA)

The PSA and free PSA tests are more than 80% accurate in detecting prostate cancer and measuring the effectiveness of prostate cancer therapies. The Life Extension Foundation believes that men over 40 should have a PSA test annually, and men over 60 should have this test every 6 months. Individuals with prostate cancer should have a PSA test every 30 days in order to measure the efficacy of the prostate cancer therapy they are using.

Immune Cell Subset Test

For people with cancer, HIV infection, chronic herpes outbreaks, hepatitis, autoimmune disorders, and other diseases that suppress immune function, or who have declining immune function due to normal aging, the immune cell subset test shows your T-helper to T-suppressor cell ratio, your total T-helper cell count, and natural killer cells. This information can be used to help develop an immune system–boosting program that could put these diseases into long-term remission.

The immune cell subset test should be repeated several months after the initiation of such immune-boosting therapies as isoprinosine, melatonin, gamma-linolenic acid (GLA), and DHEA with the objective of restoring your immune system to normal, healthy function.

Hormone Profiles

If you are considering hormone replacement therapy, we suggest that you take one or more of the tests below. Low DHEA levels can be raised to youthful levels by taking DHEA. We suggest that, after you take your initial DHEA sulfate test to determine the dosage you need, further DHEA testing be done 3 weeks and 6 months after commencing DHEA-replacement therapy and every 6 months thereafter.

Men who take DHEA or pregnenolone should have a PSA test done because DHEA may elevate testosterone levels, which can cause existing prostate cancer cells to hyperproliferate. DHEA and pregnenolone usually are contraindicated in men with prostate cancer. However, some scientists favor their limited use in prostate cancer patients.

Men (and women, to a lesser extent) should consider testing to determine if DHEA is elevating their testosterone levels, which in turn could produce an anti-aging effect. Women (and men, to a lesser extent) should consider testing for total estradiol to see if DHEA is elevating their estrogen levels, which might reduce or eliminate their need for estrogen replacement therapy, and which may become undesirably elevated in men, possibly evoking prostate problems.

Ovarian and breast cancer patients should consider that DHEA supplementation may increase estrogen levels in some individuals, and that estrogen may be a contributing factor to these disorders. In this respect, the estrogen receptor-blocking properties of melatonin may prevent estrogen from causing such a problem.

New findings indicate that growth hormone plays an important role in maintaining many functions of youth, including the formation of new bone matrix and the maintenance of normal protein synthesis in brain cells. Hence, there is the test for IGF-1 (somatomedin C). Aging is associated with the excess secretion of cortisol from the adrenal glands. Cortisol is a glucocorticoid hormone that suppresses immune function, inhibits healthy brain-cell metabolism, promotes atherosclerosis, and accelerates aging. The drawback of cortisol testing is that it needs to be done twice in the same day, around 9 a.m. and 4 p.m., to obtain reliable results.

Cortisol-reducing therapies include the following:

- ▼ Vitamin C (at least 4 grams a day)
- ▼ Aspirin
- ▼ DHEA or pregnenolone replacement therapy
- ▼ Double doses of the procaine formulas KH3 or GH3

If you have elevated cortisol, we suggest trying several of the therapies above and then repeating the cortisol test monthly until you find the right combination of therapies to reduce your cortisol levels adequately.

- ▼ Refer to *Male Hormone Modulation Therapy protocol* or *Female Hormone Modulation Therapy protocol* for information about testosterone, estrogen, and progesterone testing.

Cancer Profile

Emil Schandl, Ph.D., a clinical biochemist and oncobiologist with the Center for Metabolic Disorders and American Metabolic Testing Laboratories, has developed a battery of blood tests designed to predict your risk of developing cancer (CA) long before symptoms occur. This CA Profile© includes the HCG and HCG b hormones, PHI (phosphohexose isomerase) and GGTP (*g*-glutamyl transpeptidase) enzymes, CEA (carcinoembryonic antigen), TSH (thyroid stimulating hormone), and DHEA-S (dehydroepiandrosterone, the "anti-stress, immunity, and longevity hormone"). Dr. Schandl also suggests a PTH (parathyroid hormone) test to evaluate calcium status in the bones.

The CA Profile© yields 90 positives out of 100 pathologically established malignancies. Because of its capacity to foretell the development of cancer years before a tumor is apparent, a positive finding is a serious warning sign of a developing cancer. The CA Profile© test also can be used to monitor the response of cancer patients to various therapies: an increasing or decreasing value of a tumor marker may indicate the futility or benefits of a therapy.

Also, the CA Profile© can be combined with specific cancer tests, such as the PSA, CA 15.3 (to detect breast cancer), CA 125 (to detect ovarian cancer), and CA 19.9 (for pancreatic or gastric cancer) to provide the most complete picture of your risk and/or the status of almost every cancer.

Cancer may actually be the number-one killer of humans on the North American continent. Whereas there is no certain cure for cancer, it may be preventable. Fortunately, in most cases, treatments and therapies can successfully extend life for many years. It is essential for cancer patients and their physicians to know how a person is responding to therapy. Biochemical tests are the quickest and most sensitive heralds in this respect.

Persons who appear to be healthy may be harboring growing, developing cancer cells without any physical signs or symptoms. In other words, no diagnosis can be made by x-rays or other established methods. The importance of early diagnosis, made possible by biochemical tests, cannot be overemphasized.

The CA Profile©, together with a chemistry profile (SMAC or similar), CBC with differential and platelet count, PTH for the evaluation of calcium metabolism, PSA for men over 40, or CA 125 and CA 27.29 for women, and CA 19.9 for both genders, is the most comprehensive evaluation available for prevention, early detection, and therapeutic monitoring of metabolic disorders.

Dr. Schandl has tested thousands of patients. The results of these tests not only indicate whether or not cancer is present, but also measure the fluctuating conditions of the patient. Obviously this capacity is essential for assessing the effectiveness of the therapy instituted. This possible early diagnosis may add years of precious human life via prompt attention to the developing problem.

Even though our scientists consider the CA Profile© to be the most comprehensive of its kind, a negative score does not entirely rule out the presence of cancer. It does, however, provide a reasonable degree of confidence.

The blood usually carries messages of ill health before such a condition could be detected by any other method. However, it should be mentioned that the final, definitive diagnosis for cancer is tissue/cell examination by a pathologist. The CA profile is a very powerful tool as a part of a diagnostic workup. A positive value may suggest, sometimes strongly, the presence or the process of developing a cancer. The tests, in general, are not organ-specific.

The CA Profile© tests are the following:

Test	Description	Normal values
HCG	May be elevated in cancer, stress-related to cancer, a developing cancer, or pregnancy	Normal: less than 1 mIU/mL; gray up to 3.0
PHI	May be elevated above 42 in cancer; developing cancer; active AIDS; other viral disease; or acute heart, liver, or muscle disease	Normal: less than 42 U/L
GGTP	May be elevated above 41 U/L in females and 53 U/L in males in diseases of the liver, pancreas, and the biliary system	
TSH	Thyroid stimulating hormone, for thyroid and oxygen metabolism	Normals: 0.4–4.0 mcIU/mL
DHEA-S	Adrenal antistress, immunity, and longevity hormone; low or zero in most cancer patients	Normal: F 35–430 mcg/dL, M 80–560 mcg/dL. Results must be interpreted in reference to a person's age
CEA	Carcinoembryonic antigen is elevated in just about all malignancies	Normals: less than 3.0 ng/mL. Grave zone is 3.1–5.0

Tests also recommended:

Test	Description	Normal values
PSA	For men over the age of 40 to detect prostate cancer	Normals: less than 4.0 ng/mL. However, PSA values between 3.0 and 4.0 ng/mL or above should be verified by a free-PSA test.
PTH	Parathyroid hormone, for the detection of calcium depletion from the bones, e.g., osteoporosis	Normals: 12–72 pg/mL
CA 125	A sensitive marker for residual epithelial cancer of the ovary	Normals are less than 35 U/mL
CA 15.3	A sensitive breast cancer marker	Normals: less than 32 U/mL
CA 19.9	A sensitive test for gastric/pancreatic cancer	Normals are less than 37 U/mL

Somatomedin C (IGF 1) Human youth/longevity/growth hormone. Normals vary by age.

A Letter From Dr. Schandl

I designed the CA Profile© while in the nuclear medicine department of a large hospital. My work was to inject people with radioactive substances for the performance of various scans: brain, bone, liver, kidney, heart, lung, etc. I felt very uncomfortable making people radioactive for the tests, touching the radioactive materials, and having to be near the radiated, injected people.

The doses used were well within acceptable limits by all regulatory agencies. However, I have always maintained there is no such thing as safe radiation. So, having an excellent background in clinical chemistry, radiation biology, biochemistry, biology, genetics, and enzymology, I composed the CA Profile©. It is made up of various tests. It is not invasive or radioactive. It requires no radioactive substances nor any x-rays, CAT scan radiation, or even nuclear magnetic imaging (MRI). MRI involves speedy resonance of hydrogen atom protons due to an induced electromagnetic field, which is 3,000 to 25,000 times that of our Earth's own field.

No surgical manipulations are required or used. Most commonly used diagnostic modalities can potentially cause cancer themselves. A recent issue concerning mammograms is an example. There is also considerable information on the carcinogenic effects of high-energy, high-frequency magnetic (or any) radiation.

The CA Profile© is simply composed of blood tests. The only invasiveness is the prick of a needle. To assure specimen stability, samples must be handled strictly as instructed. Tests are performed weekly and results reported on Mondays. Thus, early detection and monitoring of cancers is reliably achieved. The CA Profile© is being used by many doctors in the U.S., as well as in Europe, Canada, South America, the Philippines, and the Atlantic island communities.

Many years of experience show the accuracy value can be as high as 92%. This means if there are 100 established cases with active cancer, 92 will yield positive results. Do not forget, however, the absolute final diagnosis is a biopsied specimen; that is, a tissue pathology. A positive test result may warrant a complete change of lifestyle through metabolic therapy. An M.D., D.O., chiropractor, podiatrist, or dentist can order the tests.

Sincerely yours in health,

Dr. Emil K. Schandl

How to Order Blood Tests

You can order blood tests by mail by calling (800) 208-3444. All tests must be prepaid unless the tests are covered by Medicare or other insurance, and you have submitted the Advanced Beneficiary Notice. As soon as you place your order, you will be sent a package with information regarding the location of the nearest blood-drawing stations, a Request for Phlebotomy form, a bullet tube (if required), and a postage-paid return envelope or overnight UPS label with envelope if you are ordering specialized tests.

You should take the Request for Phlebotomy form to any of the blood-drawing stations in your area (you are not limited to these facilities). There is a drawing fee, usually $5 to $10. A phlebotomist will draw the appropriate specimens of your blood; then you will ship your specimen(s) to the Foundation. We will send the specimen to the designated laboratory for testing. You (or your physician) will then be mailed your test results. These results will show if you have any abnormalities. If the results show abnormalities, you should make sure you show these results to your personal physician, who can determine if you have any serious problems and what you can do about them.

If longevity risk factors, such as glucose, iron, cholesterol, fibrinogen, or other tests such as the CA Profile© are abnormal–slightly elevated or below normal, for example—you can take nutritional steps to reverse the trend. You can repeat the test in 45 to 60 days, and then chart your progress in improving your health and your chances of living longer in good health.

For consultation, i.e., a professional test interpretation and a personal biochemical/nutritional program by Dr. Schandl, please call (800) 208-3444.

Important notes:

Remember, if you intend to bill your tests to an insurance company or to Medicare, you need to submit a completely filled-out insurance claim form and Advanced Beneficiary Notice form, your M.D. or D.O.'s UPIN number, the diagnostic code for each test ordered (medical necessity), your name, address, and phone number, and the prescription

M

for the tests. Other licensed practitioners of the healing arts who can order blood tests are chiropractors, podiatrists, and dentists. The Foundation cannot do mail-order blood testing paid by Medicare or other types of insurance without a healthcare practitioner first ordering the test and the Advanced Beneficiary Notice filled out.
Blood testing is an important and exacting science. Interpretations depend on the knowledge and expertise of trained clinical scientists. Therefore, it is recommended that you work closely with your physician or other qualified health professional for a satisfactory outcome.

Product availability. To order mail-order blood tests, phone (800) 208-3444 or ask your physician. Be sure to visit the Foundation's Web site www.lef.org.

MENINGITIS (VIRAL)

Meningitis means inflammation of the brain lining. Viral meningitis is the infection of the central nervous system by enteroviruses that can cause the infection. It is characterized by a severe headache, stiffness of the neck or back, fever, nausea, and malaise. The disease is typically severe and requires emergency medical care. It may occasionally progress to serious neurological confusion, particularly among infants infected before age 1 year.

According to the Meningitis Consensus Panel, Washington D.C., May, 1999, "The issue with viral meningitis is that there are no available treatments. As a consequence, patients suffer needlessly." Management of viral meningitis in the United States results in $1 billion in direct medical costs and an additional $200 million in indirect costs due to lost productivity. "Having meningitis once is a very scary thing, but to keep getting it and not even have a clue as to why, is a living nightmare!" These comments from a patient with recurrent viral meningitis were reported by the Meningitis Foundation in 1999.

Mollaret's (recurrent) meningitis is characterized by repeated episodes of fever (up to 104°F), meningismus, and severe headache separated by symptom-free intervals. Individual attacks are sudden, with signs and symptoms reaching maximum intensity within a few hours. Headache, neck pain, generalized muscle aches, and neck stiffness usually persist from 3 to 6 days, but may be present for up to 3 or more weeks. Following a number of recurrences, which can span a period of years, the disease suddenly disappears. The long-term health of the patient seems not to be adversely affected. Transient neurologic abnormalities (seizures, diplopia, pathologic reflexes, cranial nerve paresis, hallucinations, and coma) occur in as many as 50% of cases.

Current Therapy

Mollaret's meningitis is a syndrome rather than a disease. As such, the syndrome of Mollaret's meningitis appears to have multiple etiologies. Presently, herpes simplex type II, and to a lesser extent type I, appear to be etiologic in most cases. Because of the rarity of this syndrome, there are no large clinical trials comparing one therapy against another. However, acyclovir (intravenous or oral) or valacyclovir (oral only) are worthy of consideration for both therapy and prophylaxis. A pain killer is generally administered during the first several days of an attack to reduce patient suffering from the severe headaches, stiffness, and overall body aches produced by the onset of the disease.

There is currently no antiviral pharmaceutical for viral meningitis, although several are undergoing clinical trials and showing promise for use in treatment. ViroPharma Inc. is conducting a multicenter, double-blind, placebo-controlled phase IIIb clinical trial of an oral formulation of *pleconaril* for treatment in adults. Early endpoint research results indicate a significant shortening of disease duration by as much as 58%.

Possible Causes

Although there is no simple answer to what causes recurrence, there are some theories. Stress and depression, reduced immune function, and even prolonged sun exposure have been implicated in causing a recurrent meningitis attack. Additionally, the Meningitis Foundation (1999) has cited chromosome defect/FMF, intracranial epidermoid cysts, herpes virus reactivation (systemic), allergic reaction, and chemical reaction as other possible causes of attack.

Points to Remember

- Mollaret's meningitis is usually a benign (but painful) self-limited, recurrent, and often febrile meningitis.
- Transient neurologic deficits (seizures, cranial nerve paresis, pathologic reflexes) occur in 50% of cases.
- Mollaret's may be caused by herpes simplex type II; acyclovir may play a role in prophylaxis and therapy.
- Anecdotal patient information as well as scientific evidence suggests viral meningitis may be triggered by reduced immune system function, allergic response, stress and depression, as well as exposure to the sun. Recurrent meningitis sufferers should avoid becoming fatigued or stressed and should avoid excessive exposure to the sun.

Alternative Therapy

Nutritional and hormonal therapies to boost immune function, such as the recommended daily dose of Life Extension Mix, melatonin (500 mcg to 3 mg taken at bedtime), DHEA (25 to 50 mg a day), vitamin C (6000 mg a day), and Coenzyme Q_{10} (200 mg a day) are recommended. For associated pain consider *DL*-phenylalanine and tyrosine; refer to precautions before use. (*See the Immune Enhancement protocol for other suggestions.*)

Summary

Mollaret's meningitis is a poorly understood and rare disorder, the cause of which remains obscure. Typically, a physician's diagnosis of the disease is made by exclusion. The course of the disease, albeit protracted in some patients, is generally benign. Early recognition of this disorder and a patient's own self-care in maintaining optimum health may help reduce recurrence of the disease however, sudden onset of viral meningitis can occur in a seemingly healthy person with few warning symptoms. The following supplements are recommended to help boost overall immunity:

- Take Life Extension Mix, as directed, daily.
- Take 500 mcg of melatonin daily at bedtime.
- Take 25 to 50 mg of DHEA a day. (*See DHEA precautions in the DHEA Replacement Therapy protocol.*)
- Take 6000 mg of vitamin C a day.
- Take Coenzyme Q_{10}, 200 mg a day.
- Take *DL*-phenylalanine and tyrosine if needed for pain (*see Phenylalanine and Tyrosine Dosing and Precautions protocol*).

For more information. Contact the National Institute of Neurological Disorders and Stroke, (301) 496-5751.

Product availability. Life Extension Mix, melatonin, DHEA, vitamin C, Coenzyme Q_{10}, *DL*-phenylalanine, and tyrosine are available by phoning (800) 544-4440, or order on-line at www.lef.org.

M

MENOPAUSE

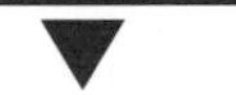

(See Female Hormone Modulation Therapy)

MENSTRUAL DISORDERS (PMS)

(See Female Hormone Modulation Therapy)

MIGRAINE

During Super Bowl XXXII, Terrell Davis, the physically powerful running back of the Denver Broncos and the eventual MVP, missed the second quarter of the game due to a migraine. Davis was suddenly incapacitated in the middle of the biggest game of his life—he was forced to the sideline because of severe headache pain and double vision. Fortunately for the Broncos, Davis was knowledgeable about his disease and he was able to return during the second half to help defeat the Green Bay Packers. Terrell Davis, a "migraineur," had learned through experience how to treat and manage his particular migraine disease. His detailed personal knowledge of the disease and effective treatment allowed him to overcome his migraine.

Migraine is pervasive throughout all human populations, and it affects the famous as well as our neighbors and family. Famous migraineurs include Julius Caesar, Napoleon, Vincent van Gogh, Robert E. Lee, Ulysses S. Grant, Lewis Carroll, Elvis Presley, Loretta Lynn, and Whoopi Goldberg. Migraine has affected a great many people throughout history and across society, with chronic sufferers accounting for as much as 5% of the American population. Approximately 75% of migraineurs are women of whom about 65% say they suffer their migraine headaches before, during, or immediately after their monthly period. Physicians report that on average, migraine patients suffer for 3.5 years before seeking treatment.

Migraine Is a Disease

Migraine is not just a bad headache. It is a disease that has a vast personal and medical impact on society. Migraine is a neurological and often a hereditary disease that affects between 18 and 26 million Americans overall—with 11 million migraineurs as chronic sufferers. According to the National Headache Foundation, migraine workplace losses amount to 157 million workdays (1200 million work hours) lost annually at a cost to the U.S. economy of $17.2 billion dollars. Each year about $4 billion is spent on over-the-counter pain medications for migraine. Further aggravating the plight of the migraineur is the personal cost due to being perceived as weak, a malingerer, a hypochondriac, or simply someone who is unproductive. Children may miss school, fall behind, be teased, and eventually become ostracized at school. Insurance companies may deny reimbursement for emergency room visits or hospitalizations.

Migraine headaches, sometimes referred to as "vascular headaches," can also be dangerous. Migraine headaches are not only disabling because of the severe head pain, they can also be life-threatening. To understand the magnitude of migraine to overall health in America and to gain a perspective, consider this: "more people died from migrainous stroke last year (1998) than were murdered with handguns." Migrainous strokes account for 27% of all strokes suffered by persons under the age of 45 and, according to the Mayo Clinic, 25% of all incidents of cerebral infarction are associated with migraines. Migraines are serious; physician intervention is recommended (*see also the Stroke protocol*).

Migraine is the disease and a *headache* is the symptom. During a migraine headache, blood vessels in the head go through a cycle of extreme constriction followed by rapid dilation. Nerve pathway changes and imbalances in brain chemistry may cause blood vessels to become inflamed. The actual interaction between the brain chemistry and blood vessel dilation is not clear, but scientists believe that migraine headaches are caused by alterations in the nerve pathways—specifically it is the trigeminal nerve system that is a major pathway in the brain. The trigeminal nerve pathway carries nerve signals from the head and face to the brain. When a migraine headache is triggered, the trigeminal nerve releases neuropeptides, causing inflammation and dilation of the blood vessels. Subsequently, trigeminal nerve endings stimulate the release of more neuropeptides, and a vicious cycle is begun.

Serotonin regulates pain messages via the trigeminal pathway. There is evidence that changed levels of serotonin (a neurotransmitter) may cause migraine headaches. Other common causes of migraine headaches include complicated combinations of "triggers" such as foods, food additives, medications, stress, flashing lights, loud sounds, changes in the weather, humidity, altitude, and hormonal changes including HRT (hormone replacement therapy). Three out of four migraineurs are women, and migraine is considered a hereditary disease. If both parents have migraine headaches, there is a 75% chance the child will be a migraineur; if only one parent suffers from the disease, the chance is a high 50% that the child will be affected.

Migraine headaches are generally of two types, known as classic and common. Typically, migraine headaches are biased to one side of the head and often the pain is localized. Classic migraine headache is characterized by an "aura" (light spots) or other sensations that are known by the migraineur to occur just prior to the migraine headache itself. A common migraine headache is considered any migraine headache not preceded by an aura or other symptomatic warning to the patient.

Migraine headaches often start in the teen years but are more likely to occur for the first time between 20 and 40 years of age. Frequency may be one a year or as often as once a week. The severity of the migraine may be aggravated by foods and food additives such as chocolates; meats preserved in nitrates (hams, etc.); pizza; aged cheese; alcohol, especially red wine and beer; caffeine (especially cutting back); nuts; fermented, pickled, or marinated foods; and foods prepared with monosodium glutamate (MSG). Medications such as birth control pills, certain blood pressure medications, certain antidepressants, and hormone replacement therapy can cause migraine headaches by their use, or by starting or stopping their use. Changes in drug therapy that may cause migraine headaches should be brought to the attention of a qualified physician.

In the past these migraineurs were often misdiagnosed or underdiagnosed. Migraineurs are commonly misdiagnosed with clinical depression, and therefore the drugs that are prescribed for the depression will leave the migraine unaffected. Follow-up may lead the physician to believe that the migraineur is still "depressed" and unable to cope, leading to continued unnecessary drug treatment. Dr. Fred D. Sheftell, M.D., Director and Founder for the New England Center for Headache, wrote in his letter of endorsement that "migraine is absolutely a biologically based disorder with the same validity as other medical disorders. . . . There have been many myths perpetrated in regard to this disorder, the most destructive of which are It is all in your head, You have to live with it, and Stress is the major cause." (From Migraine Awareness Group: A National Understanding for Migraineurs (M.A.G.N.U.M.) [http://www.migraines.org] magnumnonprofit@hotmail.com.

Not everyone in medicine has grasped the fact that migraine is a physiological (neurological) disease and not a psychological one. However, migraine as a disease, is about to be given the serious professional attention migraineurs have deserved. Intractable migraine may soon be included in the Code of Federal Regulations "Listing of Impairments" Parts A & B. This health-care reform law is being introduced by M.A.G.N.U.M. and U.S. Senator Charles Robb of Virginia.

During the last decade, a 60% increase in the prevalence of migraine has been noted due to better diagnoses and reporting, and, thankfully, success at identifying and managing the disease. Because symptoms vary among sufferers, making an accurate diagnosis is complicated. For those who suspect that they may suffer from migraine headaches or who may have been frustrated by the physicians they have seen, there is hope for a proper diagnosis, development of an effective treatment regimen, and overall migraine management.

Migraine Treatment and Management Begins with a Plan

Migraineurs should begin by seeking out a specialist in migraine, such as a neurologist or a physician with migraine experience, who is able to detect the specific symptoms of migraine. Migraine symptoms are easily understood even by the patient, and physicians knowledgeable about migraine will be able to help with a customized regimen of treatment. Migraine sufferers are so unique that their individual treatments are complex and varied—there is no single treatment method. Treatments for migraine include diet changes, stress management, proper sleep, hormone replacement therapy, supplements, and prescription drugs.

The first step is acknowledging that migraine is a disease and not "in your head." The next step is to see a knowledgeable physician (inquire about the physician's experience with diagnosis and treatment of migraine). Results of surveys indicate that 68% of women and 57% percent of men have never consulted a doctor for headache. Most successful migraineurs begin by keeping a daily diary, usually at the direction of their physicians. The diary is a written record to determine the kinds of foods eaten, the weather conditions prior to the migraine, medications being taken (when and how much), and any other trigger factors that may exist prior to or at the beginning of migraine headache onset. It is important to record the complete details of the symptoms such as the description and location of the pain, and treatment used. It is very important that all medications be brought to the attention of the physician. The daily diary is designed to identify and quantify possible migraine "triggers" that precede the head pain. The complexity of each individual migraineur's "triggers" can be extensive, so accurate entries in a diary must precede any therapeutic regimen. In many cases individual triggers may not cause migraine headaches; they may need to be in combination with other stimuli before a migraine headache will occur.

A comprehensive migraine therapy and management plan should consider the following:

Preventive therapy. Prescription medications such as calcium-channel blockers, methylsergide, some antidepressants, and cerebral vasoconstrictor abortive agents. A large selection of established and new nondrug alternatives to prevent migraine headaches is gaining in popularity. These alternatives are discussed in the next section.

Trigger management to prevent migraine attacks. Once triggering factors are recognized by the migraineur, a significant number of migraine headaches can be avoided altogether. Examples of triggers include bright sunlight, fluorescent lights, chemical fumes, menstrual cycles, and certain foods or food additives such as processed meats (nitrates), red wines (nitrites), fermented cheeses, MSG, and aspartame.

Attack aborting techniques to control migraine once it has begun. Generally attack-aborting medication should be taken as early as possible—for classic migraineurs this is more easily accomplished. Certain agents in the general class of drugs known as cerebral vasoconstrictors are specifically designed for migraine. Such examples are Imitrex, Migranal, and Zomig. Stadol NS (butorphanol tartrate)—a nonvasoconstrictive abortive agent—is available in a patient-administered injection and a nasal spray. There is also a class of drugs used for the relief of symptoms of nausea and vomiting associated with migraine, including metoclopramide (Reglan).

General pain management includes the use of drugs to control pain once the migraine headache has started. These are generally classed as narcotic, non-narcotic, and NSAIDs (non-steroidal anti-inflammatory drugs) such as naproxen, ketorolac, and ibuprofen. Simple analgesics such as aspirin and acetaminophen are also used.

Propranolol. Some people find that migraine headaches can be relieved by taking 10 to 40 mg of the beta-blocking drug propranolol. However, those with very low blood pressure, congestive heart failure, and asthma should avoid this class of drugs.

Preventive Therapy with Supplements

Nondrug alternative therapies offer effective methods to prevent migraine. For most migraineurs, prevention therapy is successful and easily managed. Physicians skilled in migraine therapy are more generally aware of the synergistic effects of nondrug therapies. Migraineurs are currently using the following supplements:

Feverfew (Chrysanthemum/*Tanacetum parthenium*) extracts are used widely in the UK and Germany. In a double-blind, placebo-controlled, crossover study conducted in Israel, 57 patients were selected at random and divided into two groups. Both groups were treated with feverfew in the initial phase lasting 2 months. During the second and third phases a double-blind crossover study was conducted. The results showed that feverfew caused a significant reduction in pain intensity compared with placebo. Symptoms such as vomiting, nausea, and sensitivity to noise and light were also dramatically reduced.

An earlier randomized double-blind placebo-controlled crossover study was conducted with 72 volunteers. At the completion of the trial, 59 patients remained; from their daily diaries and medical testing it was found that "treatment with feverfew was associated with a reduction in the mean number and severity of attacks [and a reduction in] . . . the degree of vomiting. . . . Scores also indicated a significant improvement with feverfew. There were no serious side effects" (*Lancet* [England], July 23, 1988; 2[8604]:189–92).

Magnesium supplementation. The role of magnesium in the pathogenesis of migraine has been studied extensively. The mechanism of action was presented in a Medline excerpted abstract. "Magnesium concentration has an effect on serotonin receptors, . . . NMDA receptors, and a variety of other migraine-related receptors and neurotransmitters. . . . Evidence suggests that up to 50% of patients . . . have lowered levels of ionized magnesium. Infusion of magnesium results in rapid and sustained relief of . . . acute migraine in such patients." The study also found through two double-blind studies that oral magnesium supplementation may also reduce the frequency of migraine attacks. The report concluded, "Because of an excellent safety profile and low cost, and despite the lack of definitive studies, we feel that . . . oral magnesium supplementation can be recommended to a majority of migraine sufferers" (*Clin. Neurosci.,* 1998; 5[1]:25–27).

Magnesium supplementation is used widely in Canada as a preventive regimen. At the Henry Ford Hospital, research on the pathogenesis of migraine found that these mechanisms include "aura mechanisms, . . . transient cerebral ischemia, and spreading depression . . . [and] headache involv[ing] trigeminovascular and brainstem mechanisms." The study concluded that "magnesium deficiency and abnormal presynaptic calcium channels may be responsible for neuronal hyperexcitability between attacks" (*Semin. Neurol.* [United States] 1997; 17[4]:335–41).

Decreased serum and intracellular levels of magnesium have been reported in patients with migraine. It was also found that platelet levels of ionized magnesium were significantly lower in patients who suffer from migraine headaches.

In juvenile migraine cases with low magnesium levels, it was found that a 20-day treatment with oral magnesium picolate seemed to normalize 90% of the patients. The data suggest that low brain magnesium may be related to migraine (University of L'Aquilla, Italy).

Riboflavin (vitamin B2) is used as a prophylactic treatment for migraine. In a study conducted at the University Department of Neurology in Liege, Belgium, it was postulated that, since the brains of migraineurs were characterized by reduced mitochondrial phosphorylation, riboflavin could be used because of its potential to increase mitochondrial energy efficiency, and that a prophylactic effect may be realized. A group of 49 patients were studied who suffered from migraine. Forty-five had common migraine and four with classic or "aura" migraine history. Patients were given 400 mg of riboflavin as a single oral dose for at least 3 months. Mean global improvement between the groups was 68.2%. It was concluded that high-dose riboflavin could be an effective, low-cost prophylactic treatment for migraine devoid of short-term side effects.

Butterbur root (*Petasites hybridus*) is the most recent nondrug preventive treatment to become available. In a double-blind test it was shown to be 77% effective as a migraine prophylaxis. Butterbur root has been available in Germany and is now available in the United States. The dose is one 50-mg capsule twice each day.

The hormone melatonin has been reported to reduce the incidence of migraine attacks and to treat active migraine. The suggested dose is 500 mcg to 10 mg a night for people over 40. Younger people may need only 500 mcg to 1 mg of melatonin every night. Those with acute migraine seeking to "sleep off" their pain may take melatonin to both facilitate sleep and provide relief from pain.

Summary

Migraine sufferers are finally receiving the attention they have deserved. This protocol was expanded because the number of people in the population affected by migraine is so large and because, until now, migraineurs were not being well served. Migraineurs now have more options open to them for the control and management of their disease. Those who suffer from migraine should begin by seeking a physician with the proper experience with migraine. Migraineurs should follow these guidelines to successful management of their disease.

1. Patients should write a detailed diary of all factors that pertain to migraine headaches. Include the types of foods eaten, the amount of sleep, and the weather conditions on each day. For women it is essential to keep a detailed accounting of menstrual periods and any hormonal therapy, including birth control pills. The more detail that is recorded, the more successful will be the treatment and management. Be aware of triggers and their role in migraine.
2. Consider a preventive protocol using supplements such as feverfew, magnesium, butterbur root, melatonin (before sleep), and riboflavin therapies as a second step to reduce the threshold of migraine onset. This kind of protocol should be used in combination with diet adjustments, trigger control, and, as necessary, drugs for severe attacks requiring attack-aborting techniques.
3. Because migraine headaches are also called "vascular headaches," some attention should be paid to the *Stroke protocols*. There may be useful supplements to overall vascular protection that may be appropriate to migraine preventive protocol and to prevent a migrainous stroke.

WARNING: The class of prescription drugs used for migraine treatment may have side effects. Consult your physician for an explanation of any side effects or interaction.

For more information. Contact the National Headache Foundation, (800) 843-2256.

Product availability. Mygracare (feverfew), Petadolex (butterbur root), magnesium, riboflavin, and melatonin can be ordered by phoning (800) 544-4440 or by ordering on-line at www.lef.org.

MULTIPLE SCLEROSIS

Multiple sclerosis (MS) is a chronic disabling disease of the central nervous system (CNS). MS usually appears between the ages of 20 and 40. Public service announcements have long called MS "The Great Crippler of Young Adults." Multiple sclerosis is now considered to be an autoimmune disease because of the heightened action of white blood cells that can attack the myelin of the central nervous system. The myelin is a fatty sheath that surrounds, insulates, and protects the nerve fibers. Myelin damage causes nerve signals to be slowed, shorted, or blocked, creating some of the classic symptoms of multiple sclerosis.

Symptoms

The many various symptoms of multiple sclerosis include difficulty in walking, numbness, paralysis, vision loss, pain, headache. Less common symptoms are coordination problems, slurred speech, tremors, a decline in cognitive function, and a sudden onset of paralysis (a symptom similar to stroke but without a cardiovascular connection).

Bladder dysfunction occurs in more that 80% of MS patients who can effectively manage their disease by using medications, diet, or mechanical help such as catheters. Bladder dysfunction occurs when the sphincter of muscles controlling the bladder does not receive a proper signal due to the demyelination of the nerve pathway, resulting in bladder incontinence. A similar condition occurs with MS patients who suffer from bowel dysfunction.

Cognitive dysfunction occurs in about half (50%) of patients with MS. Fortunately only about 10% of MS patients develop cognitive dysfunction severe enough to significantly impact daily life. Family members of MS patients are usually the first to notice changes in personality or changes in their daily routine. Cognitive dysfunction can range from not being able to find the right word in conversation, to impaired reasoning ability. Measuring cognitive dysfunction requires specially trained medical professionals known as neuropsychologists. Neuropsychologists conduct a series of tests used to determine the level of cognitive dysfunction present and the strengths still retained by the MS patient.

Depression is one of the most common symptoms of MS. Depression in MS, patients is commonly a reactive symptom of MS—the result of the impact of MS on the patient's life. MS depression episodes may exhibit sadness, changes in appetite or sleep, feelings of guilt, hopelessness, or worthlessness, violence and/or outburst of rage, and thoughts of death or suicide.

General symptoms such as dizziness and vertigo are common symptoms of MS, and these may include the more specific symptoms of feeling off balance, falling, or lightheadedness. Such symptoms are due to lesions or scarred areas in the pathways responsible for visual, spatial, and auditory signals reaching the brain and maintaining equilibrium. Vertigo or a sensation of spinning is much less common.

Other symptoms include dysphagia (difficulty swallowing), fatigue, headache (one third of MS patients report a history of migraine), difficulty with walking or gait, weakness, pain, numbness, and "spasticity" (muscle tightness that can interfere with normal either voluntary or involuntary muscular control). Sexual functional impairment is also common in MS patients, with symptoms ranging from loss of libido and sexual sensation to a difficulty or inability to ejaculate (63% of MS patients report some loss of sexual function).

Tremor or uncontrollable shaking is one of the most obvious MS symptoms because it can be seen so readily. Tremor in MS patients is termed intention tremor (the most common) where a patient exhibits no shaking while at rest; postural tremor where a limb may shake while sitting or standing but not while lying down; and nystagmus, which is tremor associated with jumpy eye movements. Tremor is an outward symptom of MS that can cause a patient to become embarrassed and depressed.

Optic neuritis (also known as retrobulbar neuritis), an inflammation of the optic nerve, is found in 55% of MS sufferers and often it is the first symptom of MS. Annette Funicello, the famous "Mouseketeer" of Disney fame, first became aware of her MS from her visual symptoms. Approximately 50 to 60% of people who have an inflammation of the optic nerve eventually develop MS.

For the purposes of classifying the symptoms of MS and for tracking the progress of the disease, MS patients fall into the following groups defined as primary, secondary, and tertiary symptoms.

Primary symptoms are those symptoms caused by the demyelination of the fatty nerve sheath (the myelin) that protects the nerve fibers of the central nervous system. These symptoms appear as weakness, numbness, pain, vision loss, bladder and bowel dysfunction, paralysis, tremor, and loss of balance. These symptoms are caused by nerve transmission or conduction problems to various organs and/or muscles.

Secondary symptoms are simply evolved symptoms that have resulted from primary symptoms; i.e., repeated urinary tract infections can be the result of bladder dysfunction. Physical atrophies (but not demyelination) may occur because of "disuse weaknesses," including decreased bone density, muscle imbalances, shallow breathing, and posture or alignment problems. In severe cases, problems such as bedsores could be the result of MS paralysis.

Tertiary symptoms are classified as the psychological, social, and vocational problems associated with either the primary or secondary symptoms above. Many with MS may not drive a personal car, operate heavy equipment (as an occupation), use a computer, or even walk. These limitations can have a profound psychological effect on people with MS.

Epidemiology

The causes of MS include environmental conditions and exposures, immune system factors, possibly viruses, and genetic factors. MS is more common among Caucasians than other races, especially those with connections to Northern Europeans, and some MS is very rare in groups such as Eskimos who live at high latitudes. Women are twice as likely to suffer from MS as men.

An unusual characteristic of multiple sclerosis worldwide is that MS occurs in the general population at roughly twice the rate for those living above approximately the 40° latitude than for those living below the 40° latitude. For the United States, this phenomenon shows that those people living above 37° latitude on a line from the North Carolina–Virginia border to mid-California will statistically have twice the occurrence of MS than those living in the warmer climes below 37° latitude. The total estimated MS population in the United States is approximately 300,000. Below the 37° latitude the MS occurrence is 62.5 per 100,000 population, while above the 37° latitude the occurrence is 125 patients per 100,000 population. This phenomenon is consistent and is exhibited by the statistics of those people who have moved from one area to another increasing or decreasing their risk for MS depending on the direction of their move and whether their move occurred before 15 years of age.

Etiology

The theories concerning the cause(s) of MS are not clearly known; however, scientific research seems to show that the causal factors of immunological, environmental, genetic and viral, in various combinations, are the most likely reason for MS.

Immunology

The theories concerning abnormal immune response as one of the causes for MS are now generally accepted even though the exact antigen has not been identified. Antigens stimulate a response from one or more of the protective immune system cells by sensitizing a specific target to destroy. In the case of MS, antigens target the myelin sheath for attack by the immune system. However, the types of immune cells that initiate cellular attacks and the receptors of the attacking cells have not been identified. The autoimmune system's destruction of the myelin sheath that protects and surrounds the nerve fibers produces the symptoms of MS. Some component of the myelin biochemistry is believed to be the immune target when some white blood cells or T cells become sensitized to myelin and attack the myelin sheath. Scientists are narrowing the receptor sites of T cells that bind to the myelin. With the exact identification of these receptor sites, an effective immunosuppressant therapy may soon be available.

Environment

The geographic location of a young person can have a significant factor (2X) in the probability of MS occurring. The environmental factor that demonstrates the geographic probability is the number of people who are exposed to the geographic factor before reaching puberty. These data suggest that an unknown environmental agent may predispose a person to develop MS later in life.

Genetics

MS is not a hereditary disease; however, the genetic component or marker for people who are predisposed to develop MS can be shown, and some probabilities can be calculated. The exact mechanism of action that causes this genetic marker to increase the probability factors to make the myelin of a patient sensitive to attack by immune system cells is not known. Scientists believe that certain "unlucky" combinations of genes may significantly increase a person's chance of developing MS. Genetic factors that are common among immediate family members such as parents, brothers, or sisters can increase the risk of developing MS by several-fold. Some neurologists experienced in working with MS patients have theorized that MS develops because a specific genetic predisposition makes the patient sensitive to an environmental stimulus which brings on the autoimmune response. New sophisticated techniques for identifying and tracking genes may solve questions concerning genetics and MS.

Statistical studies on the occurrence of MS have determined that in the general population of the United States, the average person has a 1 in 1000 chance of developing MS, but if that person has a close relative with MS, such as a parent or sibling, the occurrence of MS increases to 1 in 100 or even 1 in 50—a 20-fold increase in probability! Moreover, identical twins have a 1 in 3 chance of developing the disease if their brother or sister has MS!

Since 1991 the National MS Society has been collecting information on "multiplex" families to determine the extent and characteristics of genetic factors found in MS patients. This project is international in scope, and the hopes are that these "multiplex" families will provide the volume of data necessary to show complex patterns in genetic markers to help identify people likely to develop MS. In 1996, 20 genetic locations that were believed to be a factor in MS were identified.

Viruses

Some viruses are known to cause demyelination and inflammation, so the possibility of a viral factor as a trigger in the development of MS is considered by some researchers to be significant. Since the exposure to numerous viruses occurs frequently during the childhood years prior to puberty, some scientists believe that there is a mechanism yet to be discovered concerning the relationship between viruses that demyelinate and inflame the myelin sheath. Research into many viruses such as measles, canine distemper, and herpes have been studied to determine if these viruses play a role in MS. The number of viruses that are exposed to any patient may be a factor, especially considering the geographic component contributing to the number and severity of many bouts with the common cold and influenza.

Note: Trauma, long a controversial subject as a causal factor for MS, has been ruled out as a contributing factor for MS. In a study reported in 1991 (Sibley et al., *J. Neurology, Neurosurgery, and Psychiatry,* 54:584–89), it was found that with the exception of electrical injuries, no evidence was found of a direct link between trauma and MS. The Mayo Clinic concurred in 1993 when the records of 164 MS patients were examined for trauma history (Siva, et al., *Neurology,* 43:1878–82).

Diagnoses

MS is a complex disease with vague early symptoms. MS is not detected by a laboratory test or by positive physical findings. Doctors use two basic rules to determine if a patient has MS: (1) a patient must experience two separate attacks at least one month apart—an attack, also called a flare or relapse (exacerbation), is the sudden appearance (lasting at least 24 hours) of a classic MS symptom—and (2) there must be detectable damage to the myelin of the CNS. The myelin damage must have a history—it must have occurred more than one time with the patient and not have a causal connection with other demyelination diseases.

Magnetic Resonance Imaging (MRI) is better able to detect the plaque and scarring present in MS patients than other types of brain imaging such as CAT scans. However, an MRI examination by itself is not conclusive evidence because other disease may mimic MS lesions, and even healthy people can have "spots" that are not related to disease. Approximately 5% of patients with MS (confirmed by other methods) do not show any lesions in their MRI tests. MRI testing can be used to track and predict the progression of MS once the presence of the disease has been detected. MRI testing is sophisticated enough as a neuropsychologic tool to detect demyelination that is associated with cognitive function. Such cognitive impairment can be seen in certain areas of the brain using MRI.

Clinical examination is a critical tool for physicians to gather important information that will help in the proper diagnosis of MS. This type of examination includes a detailed review of the five senses, mental and cognitive function, language and speech function, family history, sex, emotional factors, geographic data, and the age when the symptoms first appeared. The medical history of MS patients should include information on the following: date and type of symptoms, medications, allergies, history of surgery or trauma, family history (MS positive), sexual function, bowel and bladder habits, exposure to environmental hazards such as chemicals, and foreign travel with the possibility of exposure to exotic diseases.

Other testing can be used to determine the presence of MS when other clinical data is not conclusive. These tests may include blood testing, evoked potential, and cerebrospinal fluid. Blood testing is used to determine the presence of a group of diseases known as collagen-vascular disease, Lyme disease, and AIDS.

Evoked potential testing is electrical diagnostic testing used to determine if there is a slowing of message transmission in various parts of the brain. These tests can often pinpoint nerve sheath (myelin) scarring not found in neurological examination.

Cerebrospinal fluid testing is used to detect the presence of immune system proteins known to be associated with MS and to detect the presence of oligoclonal bands. Oligoclonal bands are evidence of an autoimmune response caused by the CNS when the body is attacking itself. Oligoclonal bands are found in 90 to 95% of MS patients, but since these criteria are present in other diseases, by itself, the presence of oligoclonal bands does not conclusively indicate a diagnosis of MS.

Prognosis of Multiple Sclerosis

Many physicians are reluctant to predict the course of MS because the disease can vary widely from one person to another. Many neurologists predict the course of the disease using a "5-year rule" based on the medical evidence of the patient. Symptoms can be predicted using the 5-year rule, which will help in determining the likely condition of the patient at 10 or 15 years. According to the National MS Society, the disease of MS usually takes one of the following four courses:

- A *benign sensory* course of MS where attacks are limited to sensory symptoms or ON (optical neuritis)
- A *relapsing-remitting* course (1) that is characterized by total recovery after MS attacks, or flares
- A *relapsing-remitting* course (2) that becomes progressive as recovery from attacks is only partial (also known as *secondary progressive* MS)
- *Primary progressive* MS is progressive from the first onset of symptoms

Treatment of Multiple Sclerosis

The treatment of MS includes the use of mechanical devices such as canes, walkers, and catheters as well as a long list of prescription drugs to control, manage, or suppress the symptoms of the disease. Among the commonly used prescription drugs for MS are the following immunosuppressive drugs: azathioprine (Imuran), cladribine (Leustatin), and Clyclophosphamide (Cytoxan). The use of these drugs for the treatment of MS is controversial because the efficacy is not clearly established and the severe long-term side effects include mutations, sterility, and an increased risk of cancer. Other prescription drugs prescribed include a host of anticonvulsive drugs such as Dilantin, Tegretol, and Lioresal to control tremor and spasticity. Pain medications that are used for MS sufferers may include anti-inflammatory drugs such as ibuprofen.

Alternative therapies are very common among MS patients. In a study published in 1997, 64% of patients reported using alternative protocols to augment their conventional MS therapy. MS sufferers often use a variety of alternative methods to help with their disease because not much can be done to hold the line against this disease by using prescription drugs. Prescription drugs have a definite use, but these products have not been able to stop the progression of, or reverse the symptoms of, the disease.

The MacDougall Story

Dietary and nutritional supplements being used by MS patients have increased recently due to a significant history of success in improving MS symptoms. In 1953 a famous playwright, film writer, composer, and musician, Professor Roger MacDougall, was diagnosed with MS. His condition deteriorated rapidly until "he was a helpless invalid confined to a wheelchair." MacDougall was defiant in the face of his disease, and he took it upon himself to learn as much as he could about MS. He refused to accept that his condition was hopeless. MacDougall eventually came to the conclusion that a dietary approach could probably help him.

MacDougall began what was actually a protracted experiment on himself using diet and nutrition as his therapeutic protocols. This controversial approach, as claimed and documented by MacDougall himself, was successful to such an extent that MacDougall eventually returned to a normal life and lived well into his eighties without the symptoms of multiple sclerosis. MacDougall claimed his recovery was due to a self-induced, controlled remission. Critics might claim that MacDougall was lucky to have a simple remission of unknown cause. MacDougall himself does not claim his protocol will help everyone with MS, but he does say that many were helped using the information he provided. Recent studies point to the dietary approach as the likely reason MacDougall was able to control and eventually reverse his disease.

The dietary protocols used by MacDougall included the following assumptions: (1) a diet based on the "hunter-gatherer" concept that existed before man developed an agricultural community and before domesticated cattle, (2) the use of "live" foods whenever possible, (3) adding nutritional supplements as appropriate to known and observed MS deficiencies. This strict diet based on the hunter-gatherer model almost totally removed gluten, processed sugar, milk fat, and animal fats from the diet. (This concept has been around forever in natural health circles; however, it must be applied to each individual on a case-by-case basis.) MacDougall's adjusted diet was also based on extensive allergy testing conducted throughout his long recovery period.

Note: It must be pointed out that MacDougall did not see any improvement in his multiple sclerosis for more than 4 years! He kept the faith and never abandoned his diet regimen until eventually he was tested in 1975 by the same neurologist whom he visited in 1953. After testing MacDougall, the neurologist listened to MacDougall's explanation of his recovery and concluded, "I can't fault you." His reflexes, muscle control, gait, and movements were normal. The only measurable symptom remaining was a touch of nystagmus that was undetectable by the patient. This remarkable story is truly amazing given the fact that MacDougall maintained a positive attitude even though he did not see immediate results.

The MacDougall story is becoming more and more valuable as supporting scientific evidence is brought to bear on the question of improving the plight of MS patients. The popular Swank diet developed by Dr. Roy Swank of the clinic that bears his name has over 34 years of history in over 4000 patients. The data from the clinic were not conducted in a controlled environment nor was this data part of a classic double-blind test; however, the results realized by these MS patients is remarkable.

The Swank Diet

The Swank diet is very strict concerning the dietary intake of fats. It is referred to as a low-fat diet with a 90% reduction of fat intake as compared to the typical American diet. Included in the diet protocol is the use of rest and nutritional supplements—including highly unsaturated fish oils (EPA and DHA) and olive oils.

Dr. Swank gleaned the research used to develop the Swank diet during a 5-year study at the Montreal Neurological Institute. The research discovered that MS occurred only among those people living in countries where animal fat (including butter, milk, and cheese) were a substantial part of the diet—the United States, Canada, Argentina, and Western Europe. The study then focused on Norway, where two very interesting observation were made. High concentrations of animal fat (and high incidences of MS) were part of the regular diet inland, while the diet of the coastal population was low in fat (with a corresponding low incidence of MS). The difference between these geographic locations was eight fold—that is, inland people had 8 times the incidence of MS over the coastal people!

The diets of the coastal Norwegians consisted of a large amount of fish. Fish oils, known to be high in unsaturated fats, dovetailed with another study that found that southern Italians who consumed large amounts of olive oil, also known to be high in unsaturated fats, were very unlikely to develop MS.

Dr. Swank's clinical data were published in 1988 in the *American Journal of Clinical Nutrition*. He found that between 1949 and 1984, 150 MS patients were studied with the following results:

> All dietary factors were recorded, and because of the length of the study, progressive disabilities and deaths were also reported. For those patients who consumed less than 20.1 grams of fat per day, MS deterioration was slight (31% died, but remember that this study was for 35 years). For those who consumed more than 20 grams of fat per day, serious disability and a higher rate of death were observed, with 79% of patients dying who consumed an average of 25 grams of fat per day and 81% of patients dying whose fat intake was 45 grams per day.

Research Studies on Dietary Supplementation

Recent scientific research bears these studies out. A study in published in 1997 and conducted in Rome, Italy, found that essential fatty acids (EFA) deficiencies may cause hypomyelination in laboratory rats. The studies showed dietary fatty acids "can be positively involved in the control of central nervous system (CNS) myelogenesis." The study went on to say that "human brain myelogenesis can be affected by environmental factors. The study concluded that, "a diet which reduces the intake of saturated fatty acid and increases the quantity of polyunsaturates is suggested for multiple sclerosis patients."

Another study conducted in Montreal and published in the UK found that "a significant protective effect was observed with other nutrients—including vegetable protein, dietary fiber, cereal fiber, vitamin C, thiamin, riboflavin, calcium, and potassium." The study surveyed 197 incident cases on a 164-item frequency questionnaire with 202 frequency-matched controls between 1992 and 1995. The general conclusion of the study was that a protective role was found for common plant sources of food, and an increased risk was observed with high animal food intake.

Studies were conducted at the University of Wisconsin to examine the relationship between vitamin D and multiple sclerosis. Working with the basic research used to study the effects of vitamin D_3 on mouse models, it was found that vitamin D_3 could "completely prevent experimental autoimmune encephalomyelitis (EAE). EAE is the widely accepted mouse model of human multiple sclerosis. The working hypothesis used was that vitamin D produced in the skin was a selective immune system regulator capable of suppressing MS. The theory is supported by anecdotal evidence from Switzerland where a profound difference between MS rates exists between the high-altitude Swiss and the low-altitude coastal Norwegians. The study concluded that early intervention with a protocol of hormonally active vitamin D might prevent genetically susceptible people from developing MS.

The presence of toxic conditions due to a lack of trace metals essential to good health or due to the presence of high concentrations of mercury, or both, was studied in Germany in 1995 to determine a relationship to the development of MS. The trace metals selenium, copper, zinc, and mercury were measured in whole blood. The study was made of 64 MS patients and 62 control subjects generally equal in age and sex. Mean concentrations of zinc and copper were nearly equal between the two groups; however, mercury concentrations were significantly higher in MS patients, seven of whom had noxious levels of mercury. Selenium levels were found to be low in the MS patients, and the difference was deemed to be significant in those patients in the secondary progressive course of the disease. The report recommended that free-radical scavengers and antioxidants be taken with meals (selenium, vitamins C and E).

Research into the use of vitamin B_{12} has been conducted in Japan and England. In Japan, researchers found that massive doses of vitamin B_{12} (60 mg a day for 6 months) improved visual and auditory potentials over the pretreatment period. The study in England arrived at the conclusion that for those patients below the age of 18, early symptoms were associated with lower vitamin B_{12} levels, compared to those patients who were older than 18 when MS was first detected.

Several other studies present similar data concerning the presence of serum vitamin B_{12} and MS onset. Some studies were concerned with a causal relationship concerning the use of steroids, low folate count, poor vitamin B_{12} metabolism, and low serum vitamin B_{12}. A study published in the journal *Internal Medicine* (1994 Feb.; 33(2):82–86) investigated the daily administration of 60 mg of methylcobalamin to patients with chronic progressive MS. Although motor disability did not improve, there were clinical improvements in visual and auditory MS-related disabilities. The scientists stated that methylcobalamin might be an effective adjunct to immunosuppressive treatment for chronic progressive MS. Those with less serious forms of MS may consider adding methylcobalamin to their daily treatment regimen.

A Daily Supplement Protocol

The Life Extension Foundation's protocol for MS is based partially on the work of Dr. Hans Neiper of Germany, who has used for many years high-potency nutrient supplements to treat multiple sclerosis. The FDA has banned the importation of Dr. Neiper's MS nutrient formulas, but the Foundation has attempted to follow his recommendations.

To help correct autoimmune disorders and protect against free-radical injury to the myelin sheath, the 67-ingredient Life Extension Mix should be taken in doses of 4 tablets 3 times a day. In addition, 1 capsule of Life Extension Booster should be taken daily; men also should take 6 capsules of Mineral Formula For Men, and women should take 6 capsules of Bone Assure. These formulas contain important minerals that have helped both men and women MS patients.

To protect the myelin sheath against a deficiency of essential fatty acids, 8 capsules a day of Mega EPA fish oil and 5 capsules a day of Mega GLA borage oil should be taken. These oils help to suppress autoimmune reactions and provide the building blocks to help rebuild the myelin sheath.

Hydergine (5 to 20 mg a day), and/or acetyl-*L*-carnitine (1000 mg twice a day), and/or alpha-lipoic acid (500 mg twice a day) should be taken to provide myelin sheath protection and energy enhancement to the nerve fibers. Also, Coenzyme Q_{10} in doses of 100 mg 3 times a day can be especially important for MS patients. Coenzyme Q_{10} should be taken in oil-filled capsules for maximum assimilation. The addition of 30 to 60 mg of sublingual (taken under the tongue) vitamin B_{12} in the form of methylcobalamin could be beneficial. One tablespoon of soy lecithin should be taken every day to provide the phosphatides that are so important to maintaining the integrity of the cell membrane.

Summary

The amount of information researched for MS found that the following protocol measures are well represented by several research groups. The dietary and supplemental measures that may be taken to help anyone suffering from multiple sclerosis include the following:

1. Strict dietary measures should be taken to avoid animal fats, processed sugars, alcohol, glutens, and dairy products. These dietary constraints may be difficult for many MS sufferers to adopt.
2. Use allergy testing to determine if any food allergies exist, and then eliminate those foods that trigger an allergic response.
3. MacDougall's parting remark concerning diet was, "a diet must be tailor-made to suit a specific metabolism." Track and record dietary changes, and adjust based on nutritional needs and allergies.
4. Follow the Life Extension Supplement directions in the *Prevention protocol.* This supplement includes generous portions of fish and borage oils along with critical antioxidants.

For more information. Contact the National Multiple Sclerosis Society, (800) 344-4867.

Product availability. Life Extension Mix, Life Extension Booster, Mineral Formula for Men, Bone Assure, Mega EPA, Mega GLA, acetyl-*L*-carnitine, Coenzyme Q_{10}, alpha-lipoic acid, and methylcobalamin are available by calling (800) 544-4440, or order on-line at www.lef.org.

MUSCLE BUILDING

The Benefits of Muscle Building

Muscle building has several important health benefits other than looking good at the beach. Muscular fitness can be defined as the strength, muscular endurance, and flexibility that are needed to carry out daily tasks and avoid injury.

How you attain a certain degree of muscular development is dependent upon a number of factors. One thing is clear, however. A program that incorporates weight lifting along with weight-bearing aerobic activity is essential. Creatine and all the supplements in the world will make very little difference in terms of muscle building if resistance training is not included.

Even if you decide you don't need muscle building for injury prevention, performance, or even bodybuilding, you should still consider a minimum program throughout your life. A minimum program of muscle building will go a long way in the prevention of lower back and posture-related problems. In addition, research shows that a muscle-building program can help avoid the progressive decrease in the density of bones commonly known as osteoporosis.

Now that we realize the importance of resistance training in regard to muscle building, let's look at some of the things that may hinder the muscle-building process and what remedies or therapies are available to help.

Aging and Muscle Loss

Aging is characterized by a decline in protein synthesis that results in progressive weakening throughout the body as increasing numbers of cells fail to divide into fresh new cells. Aging causes a progressive catabolic (breaking down) effect on muscle tissue that results in muscle atrophy and a general weakening of the entire body. The underlying causes of muscle wasting are well-documented in the scientific literature. One cause of muscle atrophy is the age-associated breakdown of carbohydrate metabolism. This breakdown precludes the efficient use of insulin and glucose to rebuild muscle mass.

Carbohydrate Metabolism

Therapies that might restore youthful carbohydrate metabolism include 200 mcg of chromium 3 times a day, 3 to 6 grams of conjugated linoleic acid (CLA), and 250 to 500 mg a day of alpha-lipoic acid. All three supplements are effective in improving insulin efficiency and sensitivity. Alpha-lipoic acid is being touted as the "new insulin-mimicker" in many gyms. In several studies involving type II diabetics, alpha-lipoic acid was shown to increase the body's utilization of blood sugar. A greater uptake of blood sugar by muscles could lead to enhanced glycogen synthesis and ultimately greater gains in lean muscle.

Hormones

DHEA and growth hormone are two hormones that can restore aged muscles to a youthful anabolic state. Men with low levels of DHEA normally take 25 to 50 mg of the supplement per day. Women who test low for DHEA can usually restore the hormone to youthful levels with 15 to 25 mg a day. The dose of growth hormone replacement is based on serum levels of somatomedin C, a growth hormone metabolite. The normal dose to restore growth hormone to youthful levels is 2 to 4 IU injected subcutaneously 3 times per week. The so-called new testosterone boosters or prohormones, androstenedione and androstenediol, when taken orally, can be converted in the liver to the muscle-building hormone testosterone. In fact, these compounds have a higher conversion to testosterone than DHEA, and it appears that certain prohormones may be better than others for muscle building. Men should refer to the *Male Hormone Modulation Therapy protocol* for information about testosterone replacement therapy.

Estrogen is an important anabolic hormone in women. Some women find that DHEA provides benefits similar to estrogen, since DHEA favorably cascades down into estrogen in most women. Woman who are interested in estrogen therapy should refer to the Life Extension Foundation's *Female Hormone Modulation Therapy protocol* in this book.

Protein and Nitrogen Balance

Anyone interested in muscle building needs to be aware of the importance of maintaining a positive nitrogen balance. A positive nitrogen balance indicates that the body is receiving the optimum amount of protein that's required for muscle growth. Three to four scoops a day of the Enhanced Life Extension Protein will ensure one is obtaining a highly bioavailable and digestible source of protein. In addition, 6 to 10 grams of the amino acid glutamine can also help the muscle-building process. Research shows that levels of glutamine are closely associated with muscle protein synthesis.

Creatine is another amino acid that is phosphorylated in the muscles to store energy. Creatine is a natural by-product of liver, kidney, and pancreas metabolism. Over 70 years ago, it was found that creatine was associated with weight gain and improved nitrogen balance. The most stable and cost-effective form sold today is creatine monohydrate. It is one of the few supplements available to athletes that has legitimate research studies backing its benefits.

Recent studies reveal that combining creatine with high-glycemic carbohydrates such as grape juice will elicit an insulin response that will drive more creatine into muscle cells. This combination of creatine and carbohydrate appears to increase the rate of absorption. However, by loading the muscles with creatine more quickly, muscle cell threshold will be attained that much quicker. The fact is, human muscle appears to have a creatine ceiling, or limit. Once the saturation point is reached, only 2 to 3 grams of creatine per day will keep the cells supersaturated. Many athletes dissolve creatine in a warm beverage like tea. This method dissolves the creatine more efficiently and helps alleviate gastric problems sometimes associated with creatine.

Lately, there has been some concern about possible side effects from creatine use. Since creatine seems to act as an osmotic agent, that is, drawing fluid into the cells, it might cause occasional cramping. Therefore, an additional 4 to 6 glasses of water a day is recommended. Finally, although excess creatine is removed by the kidneys, those people with pre-existing kidney problems should use the supplement with caution.

Anti-Catabolics

Another supplement popular with bodybuilders is HMB. HMB, or beta-hydroxy beta-methyl butyrate, is a metabolite of the amino acid leucine. In addition to what our bodies make, HMB is present in small amounts in both plant and animal foods. In several studies involving HMB, participants gained both strength and lean body mass in as little as 3 weeks when 3 grams of HMB was added to their diets. Keep in mind, in these studies HMB was used in conjunction with resistance training. Although no one is exactly sure how HMB works, one hypothesis is that it appears to minimize the breakdown of muscle tissue, thus making it an effective anti-catabolic. Catabolism refers to the breakdown of muscle tissue and is not conducive to gains in lean muscle. Another supplement that may help with the muscle-building process is the brain nutrient phosphatidylserine. Several studies show that this nutrient, which is primarily known to accelerate brain function, may reduce cortisol levels as well. Cortisol is one of the primary catabolic hormones in the body and is typically secreted in response to physical trauma or prolonged stress. In one study, when 800 mg of phosphatidylserine was administered for 10 days, it significantly reduced cortisol levels in response to physical exercise.

Other Dietary Supplements

Many bodybuilders take a large number of supplements to generate an anabolic effect so as to build muscle mass. The most efficient way of taking most of the nutrients used by bodybuilders is to take 3 heaping scoops of Optifuel powder by Twinlab. Optifuel provides the full range of amino acids and other anabolic nutrients. It must be used in conjunction with an exercise program for maximum results.

A cell-energy enhancing program should include the daily intake of 1000 to 2000 mg of acetyl-*L*-carnitine, 100 to 300 mg of coenzyme Q_{10}, 1 tablespoon of Udo's Choice flax oil, and the standard dose of the 67-ingredient multinutrient Life Extension Mix. Essential fatty acids are also needed for hormones and energy production. Vitamin C is recommended to inhibit cortisol, which accelerates the loss of lean muscle.

Summary

The key to successful muscle building is to combine resistance training with proper nutrition and effective supplements so that an optimal anabolic environment is created.

1. To improve carbohydrate metabolism, take conjugated linoleic acid (CLA), 3 to 6 grams a day, chromium, 200 mg with each meal or 3 times a day, and alpha-lipoic acid, 250 to 500 mg a day.
2. To restore hormone levels, take DHEA, 25 to 50 mg a day (*refer to DHEA Replacement Therapy protocol for safety precautions*). To maintain a positive nitrogen balance, take Enhanced Life Extension Protein, 3 to 4 scoops, glutamine, 6 to 10 grams, creatine monohydrate, 2 to 3 grams a day.
3. To prevent catabolic breakdown, take HMB, 3 grams a day, phosphatidylserine, 800 mg a day.
4. To build body mass, take Optifuel powder, 3 heaping scoops a day.
5. To enhance cell energy, take acetyl-*L*-carnitine, 1000 to 2000 mg a day, Coenzyme Q_{10}, 100 to 300 mg a day, Udo's Choice flax oil, 1 tablespoon a day, and Life Extension Mix, at the standard dosage.

Men should also refer to the *Male Hormone Modulation Therapy protocol*.

Product availability. Chromium picolinate, alpha-lipoic acid, CLA, creatine monohydrate, HAB, DHEA, phosphatidylserine, glutamine, vitamin C, Udo's Choice Oil Blend, and testosterone boosters can be ordered by phoning (800) 544-4440, or order on-line at www.lef.org.

MUSCULAR DYSTROPHY

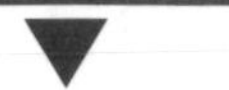

Description

Muscular dystrophy (MD) is a combination of over 40 different muscle diseases having three things in common: (1) the disease is inherited, (2) the disease gets progressively worse, and (3) there is a characteristic and selective pattern of weakness in the muscle groups. Even though muscular dystrophy can appear at any age through life, the disease is found most often in young people (male or female), from babies to young adults. Muscular dystrophy leads to the loss of muscle, weakness, and involuntary muscle contractions.

The earlier the clinical signs of muscular dystrophy occur, the more rapid the progression and more widespread and disabling the deterioration is. When the disease becomes more severe, the person cannot battle infections, and death will usually result from respiratory disease.

Cause

Muscular dystrophy is usually inherited from a parent, but it can also appear in a person with no history of the disease. There are three main types of MD inheritance: X-linked recessive, autosomal recessive, and autosomal dominant.

X-linked recessive is determined by the genes which are carried on one of the chromosomes that control the sex of the child. The result of this type of inheritance is that only boys are affected, and they inherit MD from their mothers, who are the carriers. The sons have a 50% chance of having muscular dystrophy, while the daughters have a 50% chance of being carriers. Duchenne, Becker, and scapuloperoneal muscular dystrophies are the three dystrophies that can occur due to the X-linked recessive gene.

Autosomal recessive occurs only if both parents carry a faulty gene, but do not have any evidence of the symptoms themselves. The son or daughter has a 25% chance of carrying both abnormal genes, and therefore becoming affected. Most types of spinal muscular atrophy, congenital MD, recessive childhood MD, and scapulohumeral MD are dystrophies that can occur due to the autosomal recessive gene.

The autosomal dominant condition becomes apparent even though the affected person has only one abnormal gene. Both the son and daughter can have the condition, and each child of the affected parent has a 50% chance of being affected, with the severity of the condition varying considerably in different individuals. Facioscapulohumoral MD, myotonic dystrophy, and oculopharyngeal or ocular MD are dystrophies that can occur due to this condition.

Symptoms

A parent should look for three things if they feel their child is suffering from muscular dystrophy: (1) a regression in gross motor development—the child will begin to waddle, will have difficulty climbing stairs, will fall more easily, and will have trouble picking him- or herself up after a fall; (2) in order to stand up from a sitting position, the child will push, walking up their legs with their hands; and (3) the calf muscles in the child's leg may appear enlarged, being caused by fatty deposits which are sometime misinterpreted as muscle tissue.

Progressive muscle weakness may lead to several disabilities depending on which muscle groups are affected. One of the first muscle groups affected are the muscles used for standing and walking. The facial muscles, if they are affected, may change the expression in a person's face. Muscular dystrophy can cause arrhythmias, an irregular heartbeat. Other problems can be drooping eyelids, drooling, bone deformities, mental impairment, clawfoot, and clawhand.

Duchenne's, along with Becker's muscular dystrophy, are the two most common forms of MD. The symptoms are almost identical, with muscle weakness affecting the pelvis, upper arms, and upper legs. These diseases will eventually affect all the voluntary muscles. Duchenne's MD usually occurs in boys between the ages of 2 to 6 years old. Boys with Duchenne's MD lack muscle protein, dystrophin, which is important for maintaining the structure of the muscle cells. Of every 100,000 boys born, 20 to 30 will have Duchenne's MD. They will tend to waddle, fall often, and have trouble climbing stairs. The muscles in their arms and legs will contract around the joints so they cannot be extended fully, and eventually their spines will become abnormally curved (called scoliosis). Most of these children will be wheelchair-bound by the age of 10 or 12. They are usually vulnerable to pneumonia and other illnesses, and most will die by the age of 20.

Becker's muscular dystrophy will occur in boys between the ages of 2 and 16 years old. The symptoms are almost the same as those of Duchenne's MD, but are less severe and progress more slowly. Becker's MD produces dystrophin that is oversized and does not properly function. Very few children are confined to wheelchairs at 16 years of age, and they tend to survive into middle age.

Some other forms of muscular dystrophy include

- Distal—symptoms include weakness and wasting away of the muscles of the hands, forearms, and lower legs and will eventually involve all the voluntary muscles. It starts to occur between the ages of 2 and 6. Survival rate beyond the 20s is rare.
- Facioscapulohumoral—symptoms include facial muscle weakness and some wasting of the shoulders and upper arms. It starts to occur in the teen years to early adulthood. Progress of the disease is slow with periods of accelerated deterioration. After the onset of the disease, the victim can survive for decades.
- Limb-girdle—symptoms include weakness and wasting and affects the shoulder and pelvic girdle. Progress of the disease is slow, and death is usually from cardiopulmonary complications.
- Amyotrophic lateral sclerosis (ALS; Lou Gehrig's disease)—symptoms first affect the legs, arms, and throat muscles, then waste away and weaken all the body muscles. Cramps and muscle twitches are common. Progression of the disease is relatively fast. People who get

this disease are usually between the ages of 35 and 65, and survival rarely exceeds 5 years.

Treatment

Because there is no cure for muscular dystrophy, treatment is based on controlling the symptoms of the disease, thereby allowing the person to lead the best quality life that is possible. The way to do this is through physical therapy or orthopedic devices to make the most of independence in day-to-day activities, and exercise. Physical therapy and exercise can help the muscles from contracting around the joints. Surgery can also be performed to release tight and painful muscles.

Those concerned about contracting muscular dystrophy can submit to genetic testing to find out whether they are carriers of the disease and whether or not there is a chance their child will inherit the disease. A blood sample is taken so the DNA can be analyzed. These tests can take up to months to complete and should preferably be done before the pregnancy is started so the parents can consider their options should they find out they are carriers.

Creatine kinase is normally found in healthy muscles. Large amounts of the creatine kinase will leak into the blood, and this leak can be measured to find out whether the person is a carrier of MD. This test should be done in conjunction with other tests because they are not reliable enough on their own.

Prenatal tests can be given during the pregnancy to try to find out if the fetus is affected. These tests are only conclusive for some muscular dystrophy disorders. Amniocentesis, used to identify the sex of the fetus, can also be used to discover whether or not the unborn child will get MD. In chorionic villus sampling, a sample of the tissue surrounding the fetus during early pregnancy is taken so DNA can be extracted and tested.

Alternative Treatment

A recent study showed significant benefits when muscular dystrophy patients were given high doses of Coenzyme Q_{10}. The recommended dose for muscular dystrophy patients of coenzyme Q_{10} is one 100-mg oil-filled capsule 3 times per day.

Vitamin E and selenium deficiencies have been shown to be a direct cause of muscular dystrophies in animal studies. Muscular dystrophy patients should consider taking 400 IU of vitamin E 3 times daily, and 200 mcg of selenium 2 to 3 times per day.

Subacute degeneration of the spinal cord can be caused by a vitamin B_{12} deficiency. Studies suggest that demyelination of the posterior part of the spinal cord and peripheral axonal degeneration might be related to vitamin B_{12} deficiency. The effects of methylcobalamin, the neurologically active form of vitamin B_{12}, were studied on an animal model of muscular dystrophy. This study, published in *Neuroscience Letters* (1994 Mar 28; 170[1]:195–97), looked at the degeneration of axon motor terminals. In mice receiving methylcobalamin, nerve sprouts were more frequently observed, and regeneration of motor nerve terminals occurred in sites that had previously been in a degenerating state. Muscular dystrophy patients should consider taking 5 to 30 mg of methylcobalamin a day under their tongue. There are many ancillary health benefits to vitamin-B_{12} supplementation.

The results of a controlled human study showed a significant increase of free radicals, nitric oxide, arginine, tryptophan, noradrenaline, and homocysteine in multiple sclerosis patients. This same study showed low levels of aspartate, glutamate, dopamine, and vitamin B_{12}.

Based on this study, muscular dystrophy patients should *avoid* arginine (which promotes nitric oxide formation) along with phenylalanine, tyrosine, and caffeine (which promotes noradrenaline). Muscular dystrophy patients should supplement with 2000 mg a day of *L*-glutamine, 250 mg a day of aspartic acid, along with the homocysteine-lowering nutrients folic acid, 800 mcg a day; vitamin B_6, 100 to 250 mg a day; and trimethylglycine (TMG), 500 to 2000 mg a day. Boosting dopamine levels could be accomplished with low doses of deprenyl (one 5-mg tablet twice per week), or high doses KH3 (2 to 3 tablets a day).

An interesting study showed that gamma-interferon could stimulate a calcium influx intracellular process that triggered muscular dystrophy activity. This study adds credence to the role played by autoimmunity in muscular dystrophy. Since melatonin may boost gamma-interferon production, those with muscular dystrophy may want to avoid melatonin. Muscular dystrophy patients may want to consider the calcium-channel blocking drug Nimotop (nimodipine). This FDA-approved prescription drug is specific to the central nervous system and significantly inhibits calcium infiltration into brain cells. The dose generally recommended is 30 mg 3 times a day.

S-adenosylmethionine (SAMe) is involved in numerous methylation reactions involving remyelination of nerves and neurotransmitter metabolism. For enhancing methylation, muscular dystrophy patients who can afford SAMe may consider taking 800 mg a day. The methylation-enhancing nutrients folic acid, vitamin B_{12}, and TMG may work as well as SAMe, and they cost a lot less.

Experimental autoimmune encephalomyelitis (EAE) in mice is an autoimmune disease believed to be a model for human muscular dystrophy. In one study, EAE was completely prevented by the administration of vitamin D_3. The researchers showed that vitamin D_3 also could prevent the progression of EAE when administered at the first appearance of the disability symptoms. Further, withdrawal of vitamin D_3 resulted in a resumption of the progression of EAE, and a deficiency of vitamin D_3 resulted in an increased susceptibility to EAE. The scientists concluded that vitamin D_3 or its analogues are potentially important for treatment of muscular dystrophy. Muscular dystrophy patients may consider taking around 1000 IU of vitamin D_3 once a day.

Summary

Muscular dystrophy, a combination of over 40 different muscle diseases, is a disease that has no cure. The disease is usually inherited from one or both parents. Muscular dystrophy can appear at any age during life, but usually occurs in young people anytime from babyhood to young adulthood. The two most common forms of muscular dystrophy are Duchenne's and Becker's MD.

A child suffering from muscular dystrophy will begin to waddle, will have a difficult time climbing stairs, will fall down easily and have a hard time picking himself or herself up, and to get up from a sitting position, will usually push then walk up their legs with their hands.

Treatment for the disease consists of controlling the symptoms, thereby allowing the person to lead as comfortable a life as possible under the circumstances. This involves physical therapy, exercise, and orthopedic devices such as wheelchairs to make the person as independent as possible.

Genetic tests, creatine kinase tests, and prenatal tests such as amniocentesis are tests given to the parent to find out if they are carrying a gene that could cause muscular dystrophy in their child.

Some supplements that can be beneficial to muscular dystrophy patients are

1. Coenzyme Q_{10}, one 100-mg oil-filled capsule, 3 times a day.
2. Vitamin E, 400 IU, 3 times a day.
3. Selenium, 200 mg, 2 to 3 times a day.
4. Vitamin B_{12}, 5 mg to 30 mg a day of the methylcobalamin form of vitamin B_{12}.
5. Vitamin B_6, 100 to 250 mg a day.
6. Vitamin D_3, 1000 IU a day.
7. *S*-adenosylmethionine (SAMe), 800 mg a day.
8. Trimethylglycine (TMG), 500 to 2000 mg a day.
9. Avoid melatonin supplements.

For more information. Muscular Dystrophy Association, 3300 E. Sunrise Dr., Tucson, AZ 85718-3208; (800) 572-1717; (520) 529-2000; FAX: (520) 529-5300; www.mdausa.org. The association is a voluntary health agency working to defeat muscular dystrophy through research, comprehensive service, and public health education. Muscular dystrophy patients also should refer to the *Muscle Building and Catabolic Wasting protocols* for additional suggestions.

Product availability. Coenzyme Q10, vitamin D_3, vitamin E, SAMe, TMG, methylcobalamin, and selenium are available by calling (800) 544-4440, or order on-line at www.lef.org.

MYASTHENIA GRAVIS

Description

Myasthenia gravis (MG) is an autoimmune disease that is characterized by impairment of motor nerve impulses causing episodic muscle weakness and fatigue, especially in the face, tongue, neck, and respiratory muscles. MG occurs at all ages, usually between the ages of 20 and 40, sometimes in association with a thymic tumor or thyrotoxicosis, as well as in rheumatoid arthritis and lupus erythematosus. It is commonest in young women with HLA-DR3; if thymoma is associated, older men are more commonly affected. Onset is usually insidious, but the disorder is sometimes unmasked by a coincidental infection that leads to exacerbation of symptoms. Exacerbations may also occur before the menstrual period and during or shortly after pregnancy.

Symptoms are due to a variable degree of neuromuscular transmission blockage caused by auto-antibodies binding to acetylcholine receptors. These auto-antibodies are found in most patients with the disease and have a primary role in reducing the number of functioning acetylcholine receptors. Additionally, cellular immune activity against the receptor is found. Clinically, this leads to weakness, and initially powerful movements fatigue readily. The external ocular muscles and certain other cranial muscles, including the masticatory, facial, and pharyngeal muscles, are especially likely to be affected, and the respiratory and limb muscles may also be involved. In the ocular variety, there is difficulty with movements of the lids and the eyeball itself. When the pharyngeal muscles are involved, difficulty in swallowing ensues.

Only voluntary (or striated) muscles are affected; involuntary heart muscle and smooth muscle of the gut, blood vessels, and uterus are not involved. Muscles of the limbs may also be affected in some MG patients. Asymmetrical weakness may occur, with one side of the body more affected than the other. Difficulty may be encountered with simple tasks such as combing one's hair, shaving, and putting on makeup. Climbing stairs or walking distances may cause the legs to easily tire. In 10% of the cases, people develop a weakness of the muscles needed for breathing, a condition known as myasthenia crisis. Hospitalization and mechanical breathing assistance may be necessary in such cases. The disease is painless but may become painful if the patient goes into spasm as a result of early fatigue. Skin sensation is preserved.

The effect of pregnancy on MG varies from patient to patient. Symptoms of the disease may disappear, worsen, or remain the same during the course of pregnancy. Obstetrical problems are usually not present because the smooth muscle of the uterus is unaffected by the disease. During second-stage labor, when voluntary striated abdominal muscles are used, weakness becomes noticeable. Pregnant women with MG may pass affected antibodies through the placenta to their unborn child. This results in temporary neonatal myasthenia, in which the infant has muscle weakness that disappears several days to a few weeks after birth.

Diagnosis

Doctors may suspect MG in anyone with generalized weakness that increases with the use of affected muscles and recovers with rest, or in anyone presenting with weakness in the muscles of the eye and face. Since acetylcholine receptors are blocked by MG, drugs that increase the amount of acetylcholine—such as edrophonium—can be used as a test drug, administered intravenously, to see if muscle strength will temporarily improve. Blood testing for antibodies to acetylcholine as well as diagnostic measurement of nerve and muscle function may also be administered. In equivocal cases, electrophysiological studies testing nerve transmission and muscle reaction may be helpful. A computerized axial tomographic (CAT) scan of the chest may reveal an associated thymoma.

Short-Term Conventional Treatment

Short-term treatment for MG includes medications to counteract the symptoms of weakness and muscle fatigue. Anticholinesterases, such as neostigmine and pyridostigmine, which boost the levels of acetylcholine by blocking the enzyme which breaks acetylcholine down, can provide temporary relief for a few hours. Some patients may show no response or even become weaker while taking the drug. Ephedrine sulfate may be used in conjunction with an anticholinesterase for added strength if patients are not bothered by possible side effects, such as nervousness and insomnia.

Plasmapheresis is an expensive short-term treatment in which several liters of blood are removed from the patient, centrifuged for removal of abnormal antibodies, and returned intravenously in artificial plasma. This treatment is considered when short-term improvement is crucial for the patient. However, the benefits of the procedure may last only weeks.

High-dose intravenous human immunoglobulin (IVIg) has emerged as a conventional therapy for various neurologic diseases. It may be considered the opposite of plasmapheresis. Rather than expunging the blood of abnormal antibodies, IVIg floods the body with pooled gamma globulin antibodies from several donors. Although expensive, IVIg has become a first-line or adjunctive therapy in the treatment of diverse autoimmune diseases, including MG. IVIg therapy has received Food and Drug Administration approval for use as a maintenance treatment of patients with primary humoral (blood-based) immunodeficiencies, and as therapy for acute or chronic autoimmune thrombocytopenic purpura. In controlled clinical trials, IVIg has been effective in treating chronic inflammatory demyelinating polyneuropathy. IVIg also has produced improvement in patients with MG, but has had a variable or unsubstantiated benefit in others.

Long-Term Conventional Treatment

Long-term treatment may include removal of the thymus gland. About 15% of patients with MG are found to have a tumor of the thymus gland, known as a thymoma. Most thymomas are benign. Thymectomy has become a common treatment modality for patients without thymoma. If most of the thymus is removed, symptoms usually lessen and, in some individuals, disappear completely. However, the thymus gland is the master gland of immunity, and removing this gland severely weakens the body's ability to fight infections and cancer.

Another long-term treatment approach is the use of immunosuppressive drugs. This group of drugs is used to suppress the body's immune system, although it is not known how they work in MG. Prednisone, azathioprine, cyclophosphamide, and cyclosporine are all immunosuppressive drugs. While patients may show significant improvement or drug-dependent remission of symptoms, they must be monitored closely for undesirable or serious side effects.

Alternative Treatments

A common sense approach can be very effective in coping with MG. Sufferers should get plenty of rest and pace their activities to avoid unnecessary fatigue. This may include resting frequently for a few minutes during the day. Emotional stress, excessive heat and cold, fever, and exposure to infections can worsen symptoms and should be avoided whenever possible.

A well-balanced diet can also reverse symptoms of weakness, especially those caused by too little potassium in the body. Oranges, tomatoes, apricots, bananas, broccoli, and the white meat of fowl, which are all high in potassium content, should be eaten regularly. In addition, there are nutritional therapies that appear to play an important role in the functioning and maintenance of muscle tissue.

Essential fatty acids have been shown to be effective in suppressing many autoimmune diseases. Since MG is caused by an autoimmune attack on the acetylcholine receptor affecting normal neuromuscular transmission, MG patients should consider taking 6 to 8 capsules a day of Mega EPA, a fish-oil concentrate that provides a potent dose of the omega-3 fatty acids, and 5 capsules a day of Mega GLA to provide the critical omega-6 fatty acid gamma-linolenic acid (GLA). Fish oil also may directly facilitate nerve conductivity. The lipotropic agent inositol is required to utilize the fatty acids; 1000 to 2000 mg per day could be helpful. Free-radical damage should be reduced by taking 3 tablets, 3 times a day, of Life Extension Mix.

To improve the transmission of nerve signals, 500 mg of alpha-lipoic acid should be taken twice a day. Vitamin D_3 at a dose of 1000 IU a day could help with calcium ion exchange, which is needed for nerve conduction. Also, Hydergine can be prescribed by your physician in the range of 5 to 20 mg a day, as can deprenyl, at a dose of 5 mg twice a week. To boost the levels of the neurotransmitter acetylcholine, 5 capsules a day of Cognitex (which includes choline and synergistic cofactors) is suggested.

Nerve-conduction failure can be caused by demyelinated nerve fibers. The role of demyelination of nerve fibers has not been fully established in MG, but some studies point to demyelinating diseases that have similarities to myasthenia gravis. Preliminary data show that drugs that prolong the action potentials of demyelinated and unmyelinated fibers can facilitate nerve conduction.

One such drug is called 4-aminopyridine, a potassium-channel blocking agent. 4-aminopyridine has been used in Britain with beneficial effects in the treatment of myasthenia gravis. The essential fatty acids (Mega EPA and Mega GLA) that have been shown to suppress autoimmune attacks also help to protect the myelin sheath, and therefore could provide additional benefit in the treatment of MG.

It is suggested that the reader review the *Autoimmune Diseases protocol* for general considerations and measures that may be of benefit for the treatment of MG as well.

Summary

1. Review the *Autoimmune Diseases protocol*.
2. Rest; avoid emotional stress.
3. Eat a well-balanced diet high in fresh vegetables, fruit, and grains.
4. Omega-3 fatty acids, 6 to 8 capsules a day of Mega EPA.
5. Omega-6 fatty acids, 5 capsules a day of Mega GLA.
6. Inositol, 1000 to 2000 mg a day.
7. Hydergine, 5 to 20 mg a day.
8. Deprenyl, 5 mg twice a week
9. Cognitex, 5 capsules per day.
10. Consider 4-aminopyridine.
11. Conventional therapies with plasmapheresis, immunoglobulin, immunosuppressive drugs, and removal of thymoma if present.

For more information. Contact the Myasthenia Gravis Foundation, (800) 541-5454.

Product availability. The essential fatty acids Mega EPA and Mega GLA, along with alpha-lipoic acid, vitamin D_3, vitamin E, choline, inositol, Cognitex, and Life Extension Mix can be ordered by calling (800) 544-4440, or order on-line at www.lef.org. Ask for a list of companies that ship medicines to Americans for personal use only. Your doctor can prescribe Hydergine and deprenyl. The conventional drugs used to treat myasthenia gravis are potentially toxic, and must be monitored by an experienced physician. Hydergine and deprenyl are available at Medical Center Pharmacy, (800) 723-PILL.

MYOFASCIAL SYNDROME

Myofascial syndrome (MS) has often been confused with fibromyalgia because they both involve muscle pain. MS is characterized by painful foci of muscle called trigger points. MS became better known based on the work of a well-known Washington, D.C. physician, the late Dr. Janet Travell. Dr. Travell had been the White House physician of a number of presidents.

Trigger points are different from tender points in that they may be just about anywhere. The tender points of fibromyalgia exist in a specified pattern. When a physician pushes on a tender point, the patient describes exactly that—tenderness. When a physician pushes a trigger point, it elicits an involuntary “twitch” response. Additionally, the patient may report pain which radiates away from the trigger point itself.

Patients with myofascial syndrome complain of one or more areas in muscles which are painful. The pain may be sharp, dull, burning, or aching. What is interesting about myofascial pain is the pattern in which it radiates. Most of the pain that people may have can usually be traced back to the nerve which serves that area of the body. This is called dermatomal pain, and most medical texts have figures that show these so-called dermatomes and the spinal nerve to which they are related. Myofascial pain does not follow the normal dermatomal pattern.

As an example, many people develop trigger points in the middle of the trapezius muscles on one or both sides. This point is usually exactly where the strap holding a bag would touch the shoulder, that is, right in the middle, between the tip of the shoulder and the base of the neck. If this area is pushed by an examining physician, the patient may not only have a twitch response and pain in this area, the response may refer from the top of the head just over the ear on the same side, down the back of the head, over the shoulder, and down the back to just under the armpit and around to the chest. This pain pattern cannot be described with a classical dermotomal distribution.

The region just described is a very common source of myofascial pain and may come from the continual wearing of a heavy bag with a strap, as described. Some people carry stress in this area, and a heavy bag and strap have nothing to do with it. Many patients complain of headaches or migraines and trace the origin to the trigger point described. The trigger point is pushed resulting in a twitch response followed by a headache or migraine.

Dr. Travell's work involved mapping out the myofascial pain regions and their associated trigger points. She developed a technique of either injecting a local anesthetic with mild anti-inflammatory steroid solution into the trigger point, or breaking up only the point with a needle. The exact pathology of the trigger point is not entirely understood. What is clear is that treating the trigger point is responsible for resolving many types of pain patterns.

Travell's work coincides with acupuncture points. The trigger points and associated pain radiation areas have been correlated by an acupuncture researcher. As it turns out, 87% of Dr. Travell's trigger points and their associated pain areas lie on acupuncture meridians and correlate with known acupuncture points. Additionally, acupuncturists describe a certain grabbing of the needle which is called taking Chi. This correlates with the twitch response described by Travell. When a trigger point is properly needled, there is a visible grab observed by the practitioner and a feeling of a grabbing or slight contraction around the needle experienced by the patient. Though new to Western medicine, Dr. Travell's work had already been discovered and utilized thousands of years before by the Chinese!

What distinguishes myofascial syndrome from fibromyalgia (FM) is that MS is not usually associated with poor sleep or chronic fatigue, although some patients may have a little bit of both. The trigger points of MS do not go away by getting the patient to sleep better. Since a patient can have both FM and MS, treating the FM may improve things. However, persistent painful areas may be the result of MS. For example, a patient may suffer from headaches and have classic FM. Following the FM protocol makes the patient feel much better, but the headache persists. Upon reexamination, the patient's physician finds the same mid-trapezoidal trigger points described above, greater on the right than the left. It turns out that the patient carries a heavy laptop every day on the right shoulder. When the trigger point is pressed upon very firmly, the patient develops neck pain, which evolves into a migraine. Treating the trigger point and having the patient stop carrying the laptop for a while results in resolution of the headaches. What has been described is, of course, the ideal diagnostic situation. Some patients may not develop the migraine right there in the office. However, any person who has unexplained headaches should have an evaluation for the presence of trigger points. The same is true for any persistent muscular pain which appears to be nondermatomal in origin.

In treating myofascial pain, traditional acupuncture can be coupled with electrical stimulation. Or, as developed by Dr. C. Chan Gunn, a physiotrist and acupuncturist who is Medical

Director of the Gunn Pain Clinic in Vancouver, B.C., Canada, and Visiting Scientist and Consultant to the University of Washington School of Medicine's Multidisciplinary Pain Center in Seattle, Washington, a Showa #6 Japanese needle plunger that holds one acupuncture needle is used to needle active trigger points. The plunger will allow for different needle lengths to treat varying muscle thicknesses.

For refractive cases, a homeopathic solution of traumeel and/or a mild narcotic called buprinorphine injected into the trigger point or points may be employed. The injection of corticosteroids and/or local anesthetics into trigger points as had been practiced by Dr. Travell many years ago is not often recommended. Trigger points may require multiple treatments that necessitate excessive amounts of steroid medication over time. Some physicians feel that local anesthetics may irritate the muscle tissue, and multiple injections into the same trigger point may aggravate the problem.

Buprinorphine, when diluted and injected into trigger points, may have a local pain-reducing action or in some way help to directly break up the trigger point. Additionally, buprinorphine is a mild narcotic analgesic that makes repetitive needling more tolerable for the patient. The dosage of traumeel is not critical since it is homeopathic. One to two amps per session may be adequate, depending upon the number of trigger points and the volume of the solution. The proportion works out to 1 amp per 10 cc of saline. Since buprinorphine has a systemic action and may produce drowsiness, no more than 2 amps are usually used per session, again depending upon the volume used. Some patients, especially those who are obese, may tolerate more than 2 amps per session. The dilution is ½ to 2 amps (0.15 to 0.6 mg) per 20 cc of saline depending upon patient response and number of trigger points treated per session. It is advised to begin with the lower concentrations. The injections are usually only 2 to 4 cc per trigger point. Someone must drive the patient home after treatment, because of the potential for sedation.

For really difficult-to-treat trigger points, the Edegawa technique involves taking a 60 cc syringe filled with saline (salt water) and injecting it rapidly through an 18-gauge (large!) needle. Anywhere from 20 cc up to the full 60 cc may be used for a particularly recalcitrant trigger point. It is believed that the rapid influx of saline pulls the muscle fibers apart where they cross the trigger point, resulting in a breakup of the trigger point itself.

If saline fails, traumeel and buprinorphine may be added to the saline. This combination is recommended at the outset due to the safety of the two preparations, the possible direct actions of both agents on the trigger point, and the systemic pain-killing properties of buprinorphine. After all, multiple injections of large volumes of fluid into muscle tissue are painful. The dilution is 6 amps of traumeel and 1 to 2 amps of buprinorphine per 60 cc of saline. Each trigger point may require anywhere from 10 to 60 cc of fluid as previously described. The amount must be found empirically. No matter how many trigger points are treated, it is suggested that no more than 3 amps per session of buprinorphine be used because of the potential for sedation. However, some patients, especially those who are obese, may require and tolerate more. Do not worry about addiction. (*See the Pain protocol for more information.*)

Many painful conditions—including headaches, migraines, and various muscle pains—improve when the trigger points associated with myofascial syndrome are identified and treated.

Patients with MS are encouraged to employ proper basic nutrition and supplementation.

Summary

1. Patients with unexplained persistent headaches or muscle pain should be examined for the presence of trigger points.
2. Follow good basic nutrition as for FM.
3. Take tryptophan or 5-hydroxytryptophan as for FM, but with smaller dosages.
4. Consider phenylalanine and/or tyrosine up to 1000 mg a day. (*See Phenylalanine and Tyrosine Dosing and Precautions protocol.*)
5. See a physician with experience in treating MS for proper treatment with dry needling (by definition, the pain will not go away until the trigger points have been located and treated).

6. Make sure that both you and your physician find the source of the trigger points and seek ways to prevent recurrence. Look for repetitive injury as the cause before deciding that stress is the etiology. If stress is the etiology, it is most important to find ways of relieving it, or the MS pain will recur.
7. For trigger points which do not respond to "dry needling," do not use steroids or local anesthetics.
8. Consider using traumeel and/or buprinorphine in small or large volume amounts as described above for resolving refractory trigger points.

Product availability. Phenylalanine and tyrosine supplements are available by phoning (800) 544-4440, or order on-line at www.lef.org.

NAILS

Nails are composed of a protein called keratin, woven together by sulfur containing the amino acid cysteine.

The fingernails protect the fingertips from injury, growing on average .05 to 1.2 millimeters a week. Fingernails grow faster than toenails, and also grow faster in the summer and during pregnancy. Certain environmental factors can damage the nail. These include exposure to strong cleaning fluids, excessive submersion in water, and dryness caused by indoor heat. Brittleness may occur as a result of frequent use of nail polish remover. Nail biting and picking can also damage the nail and surrounding skin.

There are various internal causes of nail abnormalities. Age, gender, the use of certain medications, and the presence of other physical symptoms determine whether a more serious medical condition exists.

Certain abnormalities can result from factors such as trauma due to injury, bacterial and fungal infections, skin diseases such as psoriasis, and internal disorders such as kidney, liver, and thyroid disease. It is important to consult a physician if abnormalities are unexplained, persist, or are associated with other symptoms.

One of the more common problems is that of fungal infection under the nail. This is common among diabetics, who are especially susceptible. A treatment that sometimes is effective and nonsystemic is a mixture of an antifungal, ketoconizol, in dimethylsulfoxide (DMSO). The DMSO carries the antifungal agent below the nail to do its work. Despite a lack of studies supporting this therapy, from an anecdotal, clinical perspective, it has proven useful in some cases. *Please see the Candida protocol.*

It is conceivable that some of the materials used in lengthening nails may cause a problem for some women, resulting in allergy or fatigue. The only advice one could give would be avoidance of these materials on a trial basis.

This brings us to the topic of nails from a cosmetic perspective. Aside from the nutritional supplementation given below, many women benefit from drinking a packet of plain Knox gelatin in a glass of water daily. The results are not seen for a few months.

M

Nutritional Considerations

When nails don't grow properly, or have other abnormalities, it is often caused by a nutritional deficiency stemming from an unbalanced diet, digestive problems, absorption problems, or eating disorders. The following list includes nutritional factors affecting the nails when there is a lack of vitamins, minerals, and trace elements in the diet.

- A lack of vitamin A and calcium causes dryness and brittleness.
- A vitamin B deficiency causes fragility of the horizontal and vertical ridges in the nail.
- A vitamin B_{12} deficiency leads to rounded and curved nails.
- A lack of protein, folic acid, and vitamin C causes hangnails.
- A lack of "friendly bacteria" (*lactobacillus*) leads to fungus under and around the nails.

- A deficiency in hydrochloric acid contributes to splitting nails.
- Low iron can cause "spoon" nails and/or vertical ridges (see below).

Iron deficiency anemia affects 20% of women, 50% of pregnant women, and 3% of men. It is caused by too little iron in the diet, poor bodily absorption of iron, and loss of blood including heavy menstrual bleeding. Pregnant or lactating women, and children in rapid growth stages have an increased requirement for iron. People with a diet consisting of little or no meat or eggs for a sustained period may also suffer from iron deficiency. Symptoms of anemia are pallor, fatigue, weakness, shortness of breath, low blood pressure, decreased appetite, and brittle nails. Iron deficiency anemia can also cause a condition called koilonychia in which the fingernail is abnormally shaped, is thin and concave, and has raised ridges. If these symptoms are present, dietary iron supplements should be taken.

The inability to absorb adequate amounts of zinc has been linked to several dermatological disorders, including alopecia (hair loss), dermatitis, and dystrophy of the nails. Oral administration of zinc compound appears to be effective in clearing up many of the dermatological manifestations associated with zinc deficiency.

Biotin, a B-complex vitamin, has been shown in several studies to improve firmness, hardness, and thickness in test subjects with frailty and brittleness of the fingernails. After a 6-month treatment regime consisting of oral administration of between 2.5 and 10 mg of biotin, most test subjects show a marked improvement in the condition of their nails, often with complete clearing of nail fragility.

In a placebo-controlled, double-blind clinical study, 60 patients with reduced nail quality, without biotin deficiency, were treated over a period of six months with a daily dose of 2500 mcg of oral biotin. The changes in nail quality were documented technically by measuring the swelling behavior of nail keratin after incubation with NaOH and the trans-onychial water loss, as well as by clinical judgment of the investigator and the patients themselves. All evaluation parameters showed improvement of nail quality.

Summary

Fingernails reflect our overall good health. Many factors contribute to the condition of nails, some of which are related to serious medical conditions. Studies repeatedly show that a diet that includes an adequate amount of essential nutrients is necessary to keep nails healthy.

1. Life Extension Mix 3 tablets, 3 times a day, with food.
2. Biosil, 6 drops orally a day (provides silica, a building block of nails).
3. Designer Protein, 2 servings a day.
4. *L*-cysteine, 1500 mg a day.
5. Biotin, 2500 mcg a day.
6. Knox gelatin, 1 packet mixed in water daily.

Product availability. Life Extension Mix, Biosil, Designer Protein, *L*-cysteine, and biotin can be ordered by calling (800) 544-4440, or order online at www.lef.org. DMSO/Ketoconizol mixture is available by prescription from the Medical Center Pharmacy, (800) 323-PILL.

NEUROPATHY

Neuropathy is the wasting and inflammation of nerve tissues. Peripheral neuropathy is a disease caused by damage to the nerves that extend from the brain and spinal cord to the rest of the body. Many of these nerves are involved with sensation and feeling things such as pain, touch, and temperature. The symptoms of chronic neuropathy include burning pain, numbness, and weakness of the extremities. Neuropathies are commonly caused by diabetes, fatty acid imbalance, restrictions of the blood supply to nerves, poisoning, drug side effects, and nutritional deficiencies, as well as infectious agents.

Up to 36% of people with HIV may have symptoms of peripheral neuropathy. Peripheral neuropathy is initially felt as tingling and numbness in the hands and feet. Symptoms have been described as burning, aching, shooting pain, throbbing, or "feeling like frostbite."

Drug-Induced Neuropathy

Peripheral neuropathy is often caused as a side effect of drugs. Diagnosis of peripheral neuropathy is done by a physical exam. If peripheral neuropathy is caused by a drug, the symptoms usually improve once the drug is stopped, although improvement can take 6 to 8 weeks, and the pain can actually worsen for a while before it gets better.

Diabetic Neuropathy

The majority of diabetics will eventually develop some degree of neuropathy. Conventional medicine offers little in the prevention or treatment of diabetic neuropathy, yet there is a great deal of published information showing that the proper use of dietary supplements can be of significant benefit.

Diabetes is associated with a fatty acid imbalance. In experimental models, essential fatty acid desaturation contributes to reductions in peripheral nerve-conduction velocity and blood flow. This fatty acid imbalance may be corrected by dietary supplements that contain gamma-linolenic acid (GLA), such as borage oil. In animal studies, significant improvements in blood flow and nerve-conduction velocity were observed in response to GLA supplementation.

Nerve conduction and perfusion deficits in diabetic rats have been corrected by a combination of antioxidant and gamma-linolenic acid (GLA) supplements. A deficit in sciatic nutritive endoneural blood flow was corrected by 34.8% with GLA therapy, and by 24.8% with free radical scavenger therapy. When both treatments were combined, a flow improvement of 72.5% was observed. This study showed a synergistic effect of antioxidant and omega-6 essential fatty acid (GLA) when used in combination against diabetic neuropathy.

A comparison was made of the benefits of a novel essential fatty acid derivative, ascorbyl gamma-linolenic acid, with that of gamma-linolenic acid in correcting diabetic neurovascular deficits. Conduction velocity was corrected by 39.8% with gamma-linolenic acid, 87.4% with ascorbyl gamma-linolenic acid, and 66.8% with a combination of gamma-linolenic acid plus ascorbate. Corresponding ameliorations of the nutritive blood flow deficit were 44% with gamma-linolenic acid, 87.4% with ascorbyl gamma-linolenic acid, and 65.7% with gamma-linolenic acid plus ascorbate.

Since ascorbyl gamma-linolenic acid is not commercially available, patients with neuropathy should take 1500 mg a day of GLA, along with 1000 mg a day of ascorbyl palmitate.

Fish oil concentrate (EPA) has been shown to improve the clinical symptoms (coldness, numbness) as well as the vibration perception threshold of the lower extremities. A significant decrease of serum triglycerides also was noted by EPA administration. The results of this study suggest that EPA has significant beneficial effects on diabetic neuropathy and serum lipids, as well as on other diabetic complications such as nephropathy and acroangiopathy.

A comparative study looked at the effect of dietary supplementation with fish oil on the sciatic nerve of diabetic rats. Nerve conduction velocity, as well as sodium-potassium ATPase activity, improved using the fish oil treatment. A preventive effect of fish oil was observed on nerve histological damage. An indicator of normal myelin fiber structure was absent in the olive oil group and was restored in the fish oil group. These data suggest that fish oil therapy may be effective in the prevention of diabetic neuropathy (*Journal of Nutrition*, 1999; 129 [1]:207–13).

Free Radical Involvement

In 1997 researchers reported in *Neuroscience Research Communications Journal* (United Kingdom) that oxidative stress is one of the factors contributing to the development of diabetic neuropathy. In this study, the doctors noted that nutrients such as alpha-lipoic acid, acetyl-*L*-carnitine (ALC), and vitamin E can prevent nerve dysfunction in diabetes. The Mayo Clinic also reported the role of oxidative stress in research disclosed in *Diabetes Journal*, September of 1997. The results of the study suggested the efficacy of antioxidants for the treatment of diabetic neuropathy.

N

Oxidative stress is present in the diabetic state. Antioxidant enzymes are reduced in peripheral nerves and are further reduced in diabetic nerves. The mechanism of oxidative stress appears primarily to be due to the processes of nerve ischemia (reduced blood flow) and hyperglycemia-induced oxidation.

Alpha-lipoic acid is a potent antioxidant that prevents lipid peroxidation *in vitro* and *in vivo*. Alpha-lipoic acid has been shown to prevent deficits in nerve conduction and nerve blood flow. Also, alpha-lipoic acid restores reduced glutathione levels in nerves, and reduces lipid peroxidation. Scientists believe that alpha-lipoic acid is potentially beneficial for human diabetic sensory neuropathy.

In Germany, alpha-lipoic acid is sold as a prescription drug for the treatment of various neuropathies. The benefits and safety of alpha-lipoic acid were studied in a 3-week double-blind placebo-controlled trial in 328 Type II diabetic patients with peripheral neuropathy and was reported in the September 1997 issue of *Diabetes Journal*. Patients were randomly assigned to treatment with intravenous infusion of alpha-lipoic acid, using three doses of either 100 mg, 600 mg, 1200 mg, or placebo. The response rates after 19 days on alpha-lipoic acid were 70.8% at 1200 mg of alpha-lipoic acid, 82.5% at 600 mg, and 65.2% at 100 mg. The response rate for the placebo group was 57.6%. These findings substantiate the benefits of intravenous treatment with alpha-lipoic acid using a dose of 600 mg a day for more than three weeks, benefits that are superior to the placebo in reducing symptoms of diabetic peripheral neuropathy without causing significant adverse reactions.

In another study, 28 out of 33 patients (84.8%) who were previously treated with alpha-lipoic acid for peripheral polyneuropathy showed further improvement after combination of alpha-lipoic acid with vitamin B_5 (pantothenic acid). The theoretical basis for this improvement is that both substances intervene at different sites and thus are more effective than each substance alone. In an overview, scientists pointed out that glutathione, the most important thiol antioxidant, cannot be directly administered, whereas alpha-lipoic acid, which boosts cellular glutathinone, can be administered. *In vitro*, animal and preliminary human studies indicate that alpha-lipoic acid may be effective in numerous neurodegenerative disorders, including neuropathies.

Additional research studies in the March 1997 *Diabetes Care Journal* suggest oral treatment with 800 to 1000 mg a day of alpha-lipoic acid for the treatment of peripheral neuropathy.

The effect of treatment with the glutathione precursor *N*-acetylcysteine on nerve conduction, blood flow, maturation, and regeneration was studied in diabetic mature rats. The deficits in sciatic motor conduction velocity and endoneural blood flow were largely corrected by *N*-acetylcysteine treatment during the second month.

Rats treated daily with acetyl-*L*-carnitine for 16 weeks showed an improvement in nerve conduction velocity. Treatment of hyperglycemic rats with acetyl-*L*-carnitine was associated with increased nerve conduction velocity, myelin width, and large myelinated fibers. In a prevention study with acetyl-*L*-carnitine, the nerve conduction defect was 73% prevented and structural abnormalities attenuated. Intervention with acetyl-*L*-carnitine resulted in a 76% recovery of the conduction defect, and corrected neuropathologic changes. Acetyl-*L*-carnitine treatment promoted nerve-fiber regeneration, which was increased twofold compared to nontreated diabetic rats.

A September 1997 study in Rome, Italy, indicates that acetyl-*L*-carnitine (ALC) may facilitate nerve regeneration after nerve injury (Fernandez et al., *Arch. Ital. Biol.*). Scientists surgically severed nerves and observed the typical motor neuron degeneration that occurred at the site of the injury. ALC was shown to have significant neuroprotective benefits against the degeneration of traumatized motor neurons. These observations prompted the scientists to postulate a better hypothesis concerning motor-neuron regeneration, and the possibility of inducing neuron proliferation. These findings have practical applications in patients who have suffered a loss of nerve function.

In two related studies of diabetic nerve degeneration and neuropathy, ALC was shown to accelerate nerve regeneration after experimental injury. In the first study conducted in 1997, doctors at the Hines V. A. Hospital in Illinois showed that diabetic rats treated with ALC maintained near-normal nerve conduction velocity without any adverse effects on glucose, insulin, or free fatty acid levels. These observations led the scientists to summarize that ALC can accelerate nerve regeneration after experimental injury (Soneru et al., *Endocr. Res.* [United States] 1997). In a 1998 study, doctors at the Nagoya University School of Medicine in Japan showed that carnitine deficiency was closely related to the pathogenesis of diabetic neuropathy. The doctors concluded that 66ALC has great potential for the treatment of this type of neuropathy (Nakamura et al., *J. Pharmacol. Exp. Ther.* [United States] 1998).

A December 1998 study by doctors in London noted that treatment with ALC may be one of the newer agents that could assist in the treatment of drug-induced peripheral neuropathy (Moyle et al., *Drug Safety* [New Zealand] 1998).

An interesting study in a 1998 issue of *Journal of Neurological Neuro-Psychiatry* discusses the underlying mechanisms and causes of neuropathy, and the role of oxidation on the methyl transfer cycle which causes a deficiency of *S*-adenosyl-methionine (SAMe). This report suggests that SAMe supplementation may be beneficial in the treatment of neuropathy. The suggested dosage is 400–1200 mg daily.

Nutrients used to treat neuropathies include alpha-lipoic (500 mg twice a day), acetyl-*L*-carnitine (1000 mg twice a day), and *N*-acetylcysteine (600 mg twice a day). The recommended dosage of essential fatty acid is five capsules a day of Mega GLA borage oil (provides 1500 mg of GLA) and five capsules a day of Mega EPA fish oil concentrate (provides 2000 mg of EPA/1500 mg of DHA).

To suppress free radical injury to nerve fibers, consider the 63-ingredient Life Extension Mix at a dose of 3 tablets 3 times a day. Life Extension Mix contains a relatively high level of pantothenic acid.

Vitamin Deficiency Neuropathy

In general, deficiency neuropathies can be corrected by dietary and nutritional therapies, however, the long-term presence of a severe deficiency can result in permanent damage. The degree of severity of this type of neuropathy can be measured accurately by the concentration of known nutrients such as vitamin B_{12}, vitamin C, and both high and low levels of protein in cerebral fluid.

Deficiencies are sometimes mistaken for disease or toxic forms of neuropathies. One report published showed that a vitamin B_{12} deficiency was responsible for neurologic and hematologic symptoms of a middle-aged man (*Arch. Fam. Med.* [United States] Jan Feb 1998; 7 [1]:85–87).

Vitamin B_{12} Deficiency

Over the last 10 years, a number of central and peripheral neurological disease states have been related to a deficiency of a specific form of vitamin B_{12}.

The most common form of vitamin B_{12} is cyanocobalamin. Although cyanocobalamin works well to prevent anemia, it is the methylcobalamin form of vitamin B_{12} that is required to protect against neurological disease. The liver naturally converts a small amount of cyanocobalamin into methylcobalamin, but to correct neurological defects, larger amounts of methylcobalamin are necessary. Published studies showed that high doses of methylcobalamin were needed to regenerate neurons and the myelin sheath which protects axons and peripheral nerves.

Few substances have been shown to regenerate nerves in humans with peripheral neuropathies. In a study published in the *Journal of Neurological Science* (April 1994; 122 [2]:140–43), scientists postulated that methylcobalamin could up-regulate protein synthesis and help regenerate nerves. The scientists showed that very high doses of methylcobalamin produced nerve regeneration in laboratory rats. The scientists stated that ultra high doses of methylcobalamin might be of clinical use for patients with peripheral neuropathies. The human equivalent dose to duplicate this study would be approximately 40 mg of sublingually administered methylcobalamin.

In humans, a subacute degeneration of the brain and spinal cord can occur by the demyelination of nerve sheaths caused by a folic acid or vitamin B_{12} deficiency. In a study published in the *Journal of Inherited Metabolic Diseases* (1993; 16

[4]:762–70), it was shown that some people have genetic defects which preclude them from naturally producing methylcobalamin. The scientists stated that a deficiency of methylcobalamin directly caused demyelination disease in people with the inborn defect.

An early study published in the Russian journal *Farmakol Toksikol* (Nov. 1983; 46 [6]:9–12) showed that the daily administration of methylcobalamin in rats markedly activated the regeneration of mechanically damaged axons of motor neurons. An even more pronounced effect was observed in laboratory rats whose sciatic nerves were mechanically crushed. Two studies published in the Japanese journal *Nippon Yakurigaku Zasshi* (March 1976; 72 [2]:269–78) showed that the administration of methylcobalamin caused significant increases in the *in vivo* incorporation of the amino acid leucine into the crushed sciatic nerve, resulting in a stimulating effect on protein synthesis repair and neural regeneration.

The effects of methylcobalamin were studied on an animal model of muscular dystrophy. This study, published in *Neuroscience Letters* (March 28 1994; 170 [1]:195–97), looked at the degeneration of axon motor terminals. In mice receiving methylcobalamin, nerve sprouts were more frequently observed, and regeneration of motor nerve terminals occurred at sites that had previously been in a degenerating state.

Those suffering from peripheral neuropathies often take alpha-lipoic acid. Based on new understandings about peripheral neuropathy, it is suggested that anyone using alpha-lipoic acid also take at least 5 mg a day of sublingually administered methylcobalamin to ensure that alpha-lipoic acid will be bioavailable to the peripheral nerves.

Deficiency in Vitamin E

A young man suffering since childhood from a progressive form of ataxia associated with peripheral neuropathy was found to be severely deficient in serum vitamin E. His symptoms included severe jerky movements of the limbs, disorientation and affected speech, and absence of any deep tendon reflexes. This patient received two years of high doses of vitamin E, and further progression of the disease was arrested. In fact, the neurophysiological characteristics of his neuropathy appeared clearly improved. An evaluation of serum vitamin E of the patient showed levels in the normal range after 13 months of therapy (*J. Neurol. Sci.* [Netherlands] April 1, 1998; 156 [2]:177–79).

The Cuban Experience

An epidemic of optic neuropathy and peripheral neuropathy occurred in Cuba from 1991 to 1993, affecting nearly 51,000 people. The optic symptoms observed were painless, symmetric vision loss with poor visual acuity, color vision loss, optic nerve pallor, and other factors. The neurologic symptoms included "stocking glove" sensory changes, hearing loss, sensory ataxia, and complaints of memory loss. The economic conditions in Cuba at the time were causing regular food shortages. It was also believed that the high use of tobacco as a toxic agent may have been a factor in both the optic and peripheral neuropathies. Investigators measured nutrient levels as well as querying subjects about toxic and dietary habits.

The number of new cases decreased immediately after vitamin supplements were made available to the general population. After investigators conducted a study to identify and characterize the risk factors associated with this syndrome, it was learned that subjects had increased risk for severe optic nerve neuropathy if positive for the following factors: tobacco use (specifically cigar smoking), a reduced total nutrient intake (not associated with supplements), and also sporadic food type and quantity availability. Most of the Cubans who exhibited optic neuropathy and peripheral neuropathy showed improvement after multivitamin therapy (*Neurology* [United States] Jan 1997; 48 1: 19–22), (*N. Engl. J. Med.* [United States] Nov. 2, 1995; 333 [18]:1176–82).

A related study focused on optic neuropathy in six patients with bilateral, progressive loss of vision and visual acuity, and poor color vision. All patients consumed tobacco and alcohol, and all were folate deficient, yet had normal levels of vitamin B_{12}. Patients were treated with oral folic acid at 1000 mcg a day. Visual acuity improved bilaterally in all patients in an average of two months. It was suggested that any patient with progressive bilateral neuropathy should be treated with folic acid, and that folic acid can result in significant improvement in visual function (*J. Neuroophthal.* [United States] Sept 1994; 14 [3]:163B9).

Toxin-Induced Neuropathies

Drinking alcohol and/or smoking tobacco are significant risk factors for developing neuropathy, as is the use of cocaine, methamphetamine, or heroin. In those vulnerable to neuropathy, even so-called recreational use of narcotics can precipitate neuropathy.

Forty-six chronic alcoholic men with peripheral neuropathy and encephalopathy were studied after two weeks of alcohol abstention. This complex study found that folate deficiency may contribute to the development of alcoholic polyneuropathy (*J. Nutr.* [United States] March 1998; 119 [3]:416–24).

A study in Canada investigating the role of tobacco smoking in 77 patients with toxic optic neuropathy found that, although folate levels were varied, the levels of serum vitamin B_{12} were significantly low (*Can. J. Ophthalmol.*, April 1978; 13 [2]:105–9).

A case reported in Florida found that peripheral neuropathy was exacerbated by several commonly used cholesterol-lowering "statin" drugs including lovastatin, simvastatin, pravastatin, and atorvastatin. This report included a review of literature where similar cases involving lipid-lowering drugs were documented (*South. Med. J.* [United States] July 1998; 91 [7]:667–68).

Some anti-HIV drugs can cause peripheral neuropathy. Not everyone taking these drugs will develop peripheral neuropathy, but it's something to watch out for. The risk of getting peripheral neuropathy can sometimes increase when the drugs listed here are taken in combination. The anti-HIV drugs Videx, Hivid, and Zerit are the most common drug-related causes of neuropathy. Other potentially harmful drugs causes are INH (isoniazid), ethambutol (Myambutol), vincristine (Oncovin), metronidazole (Flagyl), and dapsone.

Novel Treatment for Painful Neuropathy

A novel new therapy for pain was reported in the 1998 *Journal of Diabetes Research Clinical Practice* (Ireland). Forty-six diabetic patients with chronic, painful peripheral neuropathy were treated with acupuncture analgesia to determine its efficacy and long-term effectiveness. Twenty-nine (63%) patients were already on standard medical treatment for painful neuropathy. Patients initially received up to six courses of classical acupuncture analgesia over a period of 10 weeks, using traditional Chinese medicine acupuncture points. Seventy-seven percent showed significant improvement in their primary and/or secondary symptoms. These patients were followed up for a period of 18–52 weeks, and 67% were able to stop or reduce their medications significantly. This study strongly suggests that acupuncture is a possible new, safe, and effective therapy for the long-term management of painful diabetic neuropathy.

Summary

Deficient and toxic neuropathies can be alleviated by improving lifestyle and dietary factors. The following combinations of nutritional supplements might be particularly effective:

1. Gamma-linolenic acid (GLA), fish oil concentrate, and ascorbyl palmitate offer a potential synergistic approach to correcting a fatty acid imbalance by enhancing blood flow to the nerves, and protecting against free radicals. A suggested regimen would be to take 3 capsules of Mega GLA (gamma linolenic acid supplement), along with 3 capsules of Mega EPA (fish oil concentrate), and 500 mg of ascorbyl palmitate twice a day.

If symptoms alleviate or disappear, the dose of GLA and EPA could be reduced to 2 capsules twice a day.

2. Vitamin B_{12} in the form of methylcobalamin in the dose of 5 to 40 mg a day, taken in lozenge form under the tongue, along with 2000 to 5000 mcg of folic acid has been shown to correct many neurological diseases, including neuropathy.

3. Protect against free radicals and enhance neuronal energy metabolism by taking 250 mg of alpha-lipoic acid twice a day, 1000 mg of acetyl-*L*-carnitine twice a day, 600 mg of *N*-acetylcysteine twice a day, and 3000 mg of vitamin C twice a day.
4. Taking a broad-spectrum multinutrient formula can help suppress free radical injury to the nerves, while supplying supplemental amounts of folic acid and vitamin B_{12}. Life Extension Mix (3 tablets 3 times a day) is a 67-ingredient multivitamin, mineral, herbal, and amino acid supplement that provides a concentrated dose of nutrients. Life Extension Mix also has a high level of pantothenic acid, which has a synergistic benefit when used with alpha-lipoic acid (ALA) common in diabetic protocols. (*This relationship is discussed extensively in the diabetes protocol.*)

One or all of the above combination nutritional approaches may be considered by those suffering from optic, compression (induced by trauma), peripheral, or poly (multiple) neuropathies.

Sources of information relative to HIV drugs was taken from the AIDS treatment data network, 1999.

Product availability. Acetyl-*L* carnitine, alpha-lipoic acid, Mega EPA, Mega GLA, ascorbyl palmitate, vitamin E, folic acid, vitamin B_{12}, *N*-acetylcysteine, vitamin C, and Life Extension Mix can be ordered by calling (800) 544-4440, or order online at www.lef.org.

OBESITY

Being overweight and obese are underlying risk factors for the top causes of death, including hypertension, adult-onset diabetes, heart disease, cancer, and stroke. Obesity is a major cause of the overall loss of energy experienced by so many people.

According to the National Institutes of Health and the U.S. Surgeon General, most of "the top ten causes of death due to disease are attributable to health risks associated with excess body fat." The National Institutes of Health states it flatly: "Obesity is a leading cause of heart disease, hypertension, stroke, diabetes, and even cancer."

Sixty-eight percent of all Americans are overweight, and the percentage of adults who are obese has been rising for a decade. In 1998, the American Heart Association added obesity to its list of major risk factors for heart attack. Americans are obsessed with dieting, yet few are successful in attaining permanent weight loss. This "yo-yo" dieting can also contribute to health problems and chronic disease. It is estimated the ranks of diet-conscious adults will increase by 50% this year according to the National Center for Health Statistics in Washington, D.C.

More important is the fact that weight loss, or at least weight management, plays a significant role in our overall health. Scientific study after scientific study shows that being over the ideal body weight places us at a higher risk of disease.

Additionally, and of importance to all Americans, the *New England Journal of Medicine* reports that even a small amount of extra body weight increases our risk of disease and may affect longevity.

Body Fat and Life Span

We've learned in the last three decades that smoking reduces our life span. Likewise excess body fat also reduces our life span.

"Cardiovascular disease is the leading cause of mortality in women," according to the *Journal of Experimental Gerontology.* Obesity contributes to sudden death relative to heart disease, according to the *American Heart Journal*.

Those with existing disease, such as diabetics, already have a 2 to 3 times normal risk factor for cardiovascular disease. Add a little body fat and those risks increase dramatically. If you are suffering with a chronic disease, weight control is of utmost importance to your health and longevity. To attain optimal health and longevity, a person must be at or below their ideal body weight. Today's lifestyle and access to fast food makes that a hard goal to reach.

The risk of disease is not just confined to adults; recent studies have identified that children and young adults also face increased health risks if they are overweight or obese.

The *New England Journal of Medicine* article on women concluded that, "Body weight and mortality from all causes were directly related among . . . middle-aged women." Lean women did not have excess mortality. The lowest disease and mortality rate was observed among women who weighed at least 15% less than the U.S. average for women of similar age and among those whose weight had been stable since early adulthood.

While it may seem that the medical community has only recently become concerned about the health consequences of body fat distribution, the research goes back almost 100 years. Just after the turn of the century, insurance companies pooled data on the risk of body fat. They found increased weight and increased girth led to higher mortality.

Research, as we mentioned earlier, connects body weight, particularly being overweight, to many of the most deadly diseases. Researchers have found that, for example, obese patients have high rates of sudden, unexpected cardiac death.

The risk of cardiovascular disease is increased 7.7 times for those that are obese. Obesity is defined as those with body mass index of more than 30 kg/m^2 or higher. Many physicians become concerned when patients are over 19 kg/m^2 or higher according to a recent national survey conducted by Intelligent Health Research regarding preventive medicine and disease progression techniques used by general practitioners. Those concerns are validated by the recent *New England Journal of Medicine* article.

One study found that women who intentionally lose weight are much less likely to die prematurely. Another study found that obesity is associated not just with breast cancer, but also with a higher mortality in women with breast cancer. A study directed at men showed that men who are 100% over their ideal body weight (obese) face a minimum of a threefold increase in mortality.

Risks of Being Overweight and Dangers of Fat

It seems that nearly every health study done in the last decade mentions obesity and being overweight as a major health risk. The 1995 prevention index says less than one in five adults (18%) fall within their recommended weight range. "In the Surgeon General's Report on Nutrition and Health, of the ten leading causes of death in the United States, five are nutrition-related. Instead of nutritional deficiencies as seen in the 1940's, the national diet has shifted to dietary excesses and imbalances."

A 1995 study by the University of Texas Health Center at San Antonio states that "univariate analyses of many prospective studies have demonstrated that obesity increases the likelihood of developing cardiovascular disease."

Obesity and being overweight are major problems for Americans. "Severe obesity affects the health and quality of life of four million Americans," and "Americans suffer increased mortality and morbidity from being overweight and obese." If we could reduce our weight we could all live longer.

Obesity is not just a cosmetic problem. Being overweight is dangerous to our health. The danger isn't small. Nearly every serious disease we face is either brought on by or exacerbated by taking in too many calories and building up excess fat on our bodies.

"Forty million Americans have serum cholesterol levels that warrant medically supervised dietary intervention." "About one in four Americans have high blood pressure." Being overweight or obese contributes significantly to this health problem.

Costs of Fat

It's clear that America could reduce its massive health care bill if Americans would just lose weight. The average American has gained nearly 8 pounds in the past 10 years. Research shows that Americans would live longer and healthier if they were at their ideal body weight. Researchers at the Louisiana State University Medical Center recently estimated that "the direct costs of obesity in the United States are at $39.3 billion per year or more than 5% of all medical costs."

"Americans spent another $38 billion a year trying to lose weight," according to Market Data Enterprises, but without much permanent success.

How Much Does Long-Term Weight Loss Really Cost Americans?

Researchers reported after a four-and-a-half-year study involving 145 overweight patients that "the cost of long-term weight loss on a popular very-low-calorie diet program was $630 per kilogram" or $286.36 per pound!

Long-term weight loss is very expensive and hard to attain. At $286.36 per pound, times millions of people, "the problem represents hundreds of billions of dollars! These same researchers also pointed out the risks and adverse effects associated with low-calorie programs. They also stated, based on their limited success, "costs and adverse risks that such programs (offer) may not be outcome or cost justified."

Dieting

Forty-eight million people, or 25% of the U.S. adult population, is currently on a diet, according to the Atlanta-based Calorie Control Council's survey regarding dieting activities.

An earlier study by the Food and Drug Administration's Center for Food Safety and Applied Nutrition found that 62% of American men and 71% of women were trying to lose weight. The study found that the 1993 weight-loss attempt wasn't the first. As a matter of fact, researchers found that the respondents averaged a new diet attempt every year. These yearly failed attempts contribute significantly to the almost $40 billion spent every year on weight control. The federal study didn't offer any solutions, but did conclude that "policy efforts should be directed toward increasing the long-term effectiveness of individual weight-loss plans." Approaches were also recommended that involved behavioral changes, diet, and natural supplementation.

Weight and obesity aren't just of concern to the individual. These problems affect society as a whole since obesity and being overweight contribute to the overall incidences of chronic disease. Rising health care costs have become a major topic of debate in the political arena. Congress, the President, and American political leaders are struggling with health care, health insurance, and who will pay the costs.

The best way to avoid disease and the costs associated with disease is not to get sick in the first place. If we could all do a better job of controlling our weight, disease would drop significantly and cost of health would drop too.

According to the Surgeon General, "Obesity, with its rank among our top ten diseases, may be America's number-one contributor to health care costs."

Disease Preemption, Obesity, and Weight Loss

As early as 1987, researchers at a medical center in Fresno, California, used records of overweight and obese patients to predict and target health problems those patients would face in the future. The researchers and doctors at the St. Agnes Medical Center in Fresno were trying to plan for the type of clinical services they would need to provide in the future.

Some of the findings the same researchers later published (in 1990, 1993, and 1994) used the clinical knowledge and an early application of computer analysis to preempt disease. Once again the researchers focused some of their research on obese and overweight patients. Those researchers were some of the first to utilize the incidence of disease, disease risk, and disease progression in their protocols. They reported in their published reports high success rates using their analytical concepts. The science and treatment protocol often boiled down to simple weight control.

Since then medical centers, physicians, and physicians' groups have recognized the benefits of weight control for their patients. Many now use longitudinal treatment approaches developed in those clinical settings for weight control.

Mainstream medicine now seems to recognize the relationship between ideal body weight and health, and overweight and obesity and the increased incidence of disease. Maintaining the proper body weight as identified by total body mass index is becoming an accepted method of determining the risk potential for disease.

Many physicians are now turning to integrated medical treatments which include common-sense recommendations of moderate exercise, lifestyle and diet changes, combined with medically recommended supplementation.

Integrated and Alternative Therapies

Recently, "lite" versions of almost every processed food on the market have been consumed by Americans obsessed with losing weight. Yet, despite diet manipulation, vigorous exercise, and the use of diet drugs, the fat epidemic continues unabated.

The media blame high fat consumption for America's overweight problem, but the facts are that previous generations often consumed higher percentages of dietary fat than many overweight people today. Could a widespread deficiency of a specific nutrient be a major factor in causing the excess body fat in many people? Let's take a look at one hypothesis.

Conjugated Linoleic Acid and the Weight Connection

Conjugated linoleic acid (CLA) is a component of beef and milk that has been shown to reduce body fat in both animals and humans. CLA is essential for the transport of dietary fat into cells, where it is used to build muscle and produce energy. Fat that is not used for anabolic energy production is converted into newly stored fat cells. There are published research findings about how dietary CLA reduces body fat, but first let's take a look at why many Americans are now deficient in CLA compared with their parents.

The primary dietary sources of CLA are beef and milk, and Americans are eating less beef and drinking less whole milk in order to reduce their dietary intake of saturated fat. People often drink nonfat milk, but it's the fat content of the milk that contains CLA. Since skim milk contains virtually no CLA, those seeking to lose weight, those who use skim milk, are depriving themselves of a potential source of this fat-reducing nutrient.

Now, here's where the real problem occurs. In 1963, the CLA percentage in milk was as high as 2.81%. By 1992, the percentage of CLA in dairy products seldom exceeded 1%. The reason for the sharp reduction in milk CLA was because of changing feeding patterns. Cows that eat natural grass produce lots of CLA. Today's "efficient" feeding methods rely far less on natural grass. For example, grass-fed Australian cows have 3 to 4 times as much CLA in their meat as do American cows.

Researchers reported in June of 1999 in *Biosciences, Biotechnology, Biochemistry Journal* that animal studies demonstrated that "CLA has an obesity-preventing action."

Another study reported that CLA effects on glucose tolerance and glucose homeostasis indicate that dietary CLA may prove to be an important therapy for the prevention and treatment of obesity (*Biochem. Biophys. Res. Commun.*, 1998 [March]).

So health-conscious Americans are avoiding beef and whole milk because these foods are high in fat, and, when people do consume beef or milk, they are consuming very little CLA because of CLA-deficiency in today's cows. Thus, most Americans have inadequate amounts of CLA in their diet, and this CLA deficit may be at least partially responsible for the epidemic of overweight people of all ages that now exists.

Encouraging Results with CLA

How significant is CLA in preventing excess accumulation of body fat? The results to date are preliminary, but extremely encouraging.

Athletes are taking CLA to push glucose into their muscle cells and connective tissues instead of letting it turn into fat. CLA has been shown to reduce protein degradation in both humans and animals.

CLA is required to maintain optimal function of the phospholipid membranes of cells. Healthy cell membranes will allow fat, protein, and carbohydrates to flow into active cells such as muscle, connective tissue, and organ cells, instead of being stored passively in fat cells. A deficiency of CLA can inhibit fat from entering muscle cells, which can result in excessive accumulation of body fat.

CLA has been studied in different species of animals, and the results consistently show that CLA reduces the percentage of body fat. An abstract from the 1996 Environmental Biology Conference showed that rats, after 28 days of being supplemented with CLA, showed a 58% reduction in body fat, compared with the control animals which did not receive CLA. In addition, the percentage of muscle was greater in the CLA group; CLA did not induce weight loss, since muscle weighs more than fat.

In July 1997, the results of the first human study on CLA were released by the Medstat Research Ltd. group of Lillesterom, Norway. This 3-month preliminary study involved 20 healthy volunteers. Half the group was given six 500-mg CLA capsules a day, and the other half received identical-looking placebo capsules. The subjects were asked not to alter their diet or lifestyle; 18 of the 20 subjects completed the study protocol. The results showed that the people in the CLA group experienced a 15 to 20% reduction of average body fat, compared with the placebo group. In the CLA group, the initial body fat percentage was 21.3% at the beginning of the study, and only 17% body fat after 3 months on CLA capsules. In contrast, the placebo group started with an average of 22% body fat, and 3 months later recorded an average of 22.4% body fat.

CLA received widespread media attention in the early 1990s when it was identified as a component of red meat that helps prevent cancer. Further research showed that CLA is a potent anticancer agent, an anticatabolic agent and, through a unique mechanism, a fat metabolizing agent. CLA is one of the substances the FDA is investigating for disease prevention. New studies are appearing about the ability of CLA to prevent cancer, and possibly function as an adjuvant (assisting) cancer therapy. CLA appears to be especially effective in preventing breast cancer.

Using CLA to reduce body fat may reduce your risk of getting cancer. Compare this to FDA-approved diet drugs that were removed from the market after being linked to heart-valve degeneration.

A deficiency of CLA in our diet may be a major factor in causing Americans to gain so many fat pounds. CLA is a potent antioxidant, but appears to prevent cancer via other mechanisms of action.

A dose of three 1000-mg capsules of 70% CLA, taken in the morning on an empty stomach, may be an effective part of an overall weight-loss program. The studies indicate that it usually takes about 3 weeks before body fat loss occurs in response to CLA supplementation.

CLA inhibits fat storage by enhancing the ability of cell membranes (other than fat cells) to open up and allow the absorption of fats and other nutrients. CLA promotes the growth of muscles by letting nutrients into active muscle cells. That's why CLA has become such a popular supplement among body builders. The fat-reducing mechanism of CLA involves the rejuvenation of cell membranes in the muscles and connective tissues to allow fats to enter freely in order to generate energy and growth. This anabolic effect could provide anti-aging benefits in the elderly, but there have been no studies to date to investigate this.

Recent Findings on CLA

Several years ago, the discovery of conjugated linoleic acid (CLA) caused a scientific sensation. Here was a fatty acid found in red meat and cheese that showed strong anticancer properties, being particularly effective in inhibiting breast and prostate tumors, as well as colorectal, stomach, and skin cancer, including melanoma. On the whole, scientists found CLA to be more strongly anticarcinogenic than other fatty acids. What made CLA especially unique is that even low concentrations significantly inhibited cancer cell growth.

CLA supplementation was also shown to improve the ratio of lean mass to body fat, decreasing fat deposition, especially on the abdomen, and enhancing muscle growth. One way in which CLA reduces body fat is to enhance insulin sensitivity so that fatty acids and glucose can pass through muscle cell membranes and away from fat tissue. This results in an improved muscle-to-fat ratio.

CLA was also shown to have antioxidant properties and to prevent muscle wasting (an anticatabolic effect). It became popular with muscle builders because of its ability to improve the transport of glucose, fatty acids, and protein to the muscle tissue.

It is interesting that while it is chemically related to linolenic acid, conjugated linoleic acid (CLA) appears to have opposite effects in certain important areas. For instance, linolenic acid stimulates fat formation (lipogenesis) in adipose tissue, while CLA inhibits fat formation; linolenic acid tends to promote tumor growth, while CLA is an excellent inhibitor of tumor growth; linolenic acid makes cholesterol more susceptible to oxidation, while CLA makes cholesterol more stable.

One of the greatest problems with the Western diet during the last 50 years has been excessive consumption of linoleic acid, due to the introduction of margarine, seed oils, such as corn oil and safflower oil, and the modern artificial livestock feeding methods that have raised the linoleic-acid content of meat. At the same time, the consumption of beneficial fatty acids such as omega-3 fats (fish, flax, and perilla) and CLA has gone down. Because of the enormous impact that fatty acids have on our physiology, an excess of linoleic acid combined with a deficiency of CLA could have far-reaching effects on health and longevity. Let us now take a closer look at the current research findings about CLA.

CLA Reduces Body Fat in Mice by up to 88%

A study at Louisiana State University confirmed that feeding male mice a CLA-enriched diet (at 1% of the diet by weight, or 10 g/kg) for 6 weeks resulted in 43 to 88% lower body fat, especially in regard to abdominal fat. This occurred even if the mice were fed a high-fat diet. The effect was partly due to reduced calorie intake by CLA-supplemented mice, and partly to a shift in their metabolism, including a higher metabolic rate.

In another study, performed at the University of Wisconsin-Madison, mice supplemented with only 0.5% of CLA showed up to 60% lower body fat and up to 14% increased lean body mass compared to controls. The researchers discovered that CLA-fed animals showed greater activity of enzymes involved in the delivery of fatty acids to the muscle cells and the utilization of fat for energy, while the enzymes facilitating fat deposition were inhibited.

CLA Improves Insulin Sensitivity

A study using diabetic Zucker rats indicates that part of CLA's effectiveness in preventing obesity may lie in its ability to act as a potent insulin sensitizer, thus lowering insulin resistance and consequently insulin levels. Since elevated insulin is the chief pro-obesity agent, it is enormously important to keep insulin within the normal range. By activating certain enzymes and enhancing glucose transport into the cells, CLA acts to lower blood sugar levels and normalize insulin levels.

Thus, besides being antiatherogenic and anticarcinogenic, CLA is also antidiabetogenic: it helps prevent adult-onset diabetes, characterized by insulin resistance. If the current animal results are corroborated, CLA may prove to be important not only in the prevention of diabetes, but also as a new therapy for adult-onset diabetics, aimed at lowering insulin resistance.

CLA Inhibits the Growth of Prostate Cancer, While Linolenic Acid Promotes it

Immunodeficient mice inoculated with human prostate cancer cells were fed either a standard diet, a diet supplemented with 1% linolenic acid, or a diet supplemented with 1% CLA. Mice receiving linolenic acid showed significantly higher body weight and increased tumor load compared with the two other groups. CLA-supplemented mice, on the other hand, showed the lowest tumor load and a dramatic reduction in lung metastasis.

CLA Supplementation Helps Prevent the Initiation, Promotion, and Metastasis of Breast Cancer

In a study performed at Roswell Park Cancer Institute in Buffalo, 50-day-old rats were treated with a potent carcinogen and then supplemented with 1% CLA for 4, 8, or 20 weeks. Only rats receiving CLA for the full 20 weeks showed tumor inhibition. CLA lowered the total number of carcinomas by 70%. Interestingly, there was a much higher incorporation of CLA into the neutral lipids of the mammary tissue rather than into the phospholipids (cell membranes). While the physiological significance of this phenomenon is not understood, it seems that the presence of CLA in mammary tissue plays a highly protective role against the initiation of breast cancer.

In another study, immunodeficient mice were fed 1% CLA-enriched diet for 2 weeks prior to inoculation with human breast adenocarcinoma cells. Besides inhibiting tumor growth, CLA totally prevented the metastasis of breast cancer to lungs and bone marrow.

The preventive effect of CLA against breast cancer is independent of the amount of fat in the diet. Even when the tumor-promoting excess levels of linoleic acid reach 12% in the diet, CLA was still incorporated into the lipids of the mammary tissue and still provided protection against carcinogenesis. Anticarcinogenic effects of CLA did not increase with doses beyond 1% of CLA in the diet.

A recent *in vitro* study of breast cancer cells showed that CLA worked synergistically with nordihydroguaiaretic acid (NDGA), a potent antioxidant and lipoxygenase inhibitor found in the desert herb chaparral. This suggests that one mechanism of CLA's suppression of tumor growth is its ability to inhibit the production of leukotrienes, inflammatory compounds that may be even more harmful and difficult to control than series II prostaglandins. (Both series II prostaglandins and leukotrienes fuel tumor growth; both are metabolites of arachidonic fatty acid, itself a metabolite of linoleic acid.)

Yet another mechanism of CLA's anticancer action may be its interference with tumor-growth factors such as thymidine.

CLA is especially effective in inhibiting the proliferation of estrogen-receptor-positive breast cancer cells, arresting estrogen-dependent cell division.

Besides the oncostatic properties of CLA, it is also likely that CLA inhibits the enzymes that activate various carcinogens. Thus, CLA appears to protect against all three stages of cancer: initiation, promotion, and metastasis.

Early CLA Supplementation Lowers the Glandular Density in Mammary Tissue

Previous research showed that supplementation with CLA during the formative period in mammary-gland development confers a lasting protection against carcinogen-induced breast cancer. A new and more detailed study showed that female rats fed 1% CLA diet after weaning showed a 20% reduction in the density of the ductal-lobular tree, meaning that the glandular density of the mammaries was lower. High glandular density is a very significant breast cancer risk factor. This study implies that supplementing the diet of young girls with CLA might reduce the glandular density of their breast tissue, conferring a significant degree of life-long protection against breast cancer.

Immune-Enhancing Effects of CLA

CLA has been found to stimulate the production of lymphocytes and of interleukin-2, and to increase the levels of certain immunoglobulins, while lowering the release of immunoglobulin E, associated with allergies.

Improved immune function resulting from CLA supplementation can also be postulated on the basis of its ability to lower the production of immunosuppressive compounds such as leukotrienes and series II prostaglandins, and to improve insulin sensitivity (elevated insulin leads to immunosuppression).

The anti-obesity benefits of CLA do not necessarily manifest themselves as weight loss. Rather, CLA works through the process of "repartitioning," which results in improved muscle-to-fat ratio. Since CLA causes a loss of body fat, especially abdominal fat, while simultaneously stimulating muscle growth, the effect is a leaner, more muscular physique. This is much more beneficial than starvation diets, which cause a greater loss of muscle mass than of body fat, setting the stage for sluggish metabolism and even greater future obesity.

Anti-Atherogenic Effects of CLA

We have already mentioned that CLA improves insulin sensitivity. Since elevated insulin promotes atherosclerosis, any agent that lowers insulin levels by improving insulin sensitivity can be classified as anti-atherogenic. However, CLA has also been shown to have further anti-atherogenic benefits thanks to its ability to improve serum lipids and to its tocopherol (vitamin E)-sparing effect.

CLA Lowers Cholesterol and Triglycerides, Helps Keep Arteries Clean

A study at the University of Wisconsin–Madison found that rabbits supplemented with 0.5 g CLA per day showed markedly lower total and LDL cholesterol, lower LDL-to-HDL ratio, lower total cholesterol-to-HDL ratio, and lower serum triglycerides. On autopsy, the aortas of CLA-supplemented rabbits showed less atherosclerotic plaque.

A more recent study done at the University of Massachusetts confirmed that hamsters whose diets were supplemented with CLA showed significantly lower total cholesterol, LDL cholesterol, and triglycerides compared to controls. The serum of CLA-fed hamsters also showed higher tocopherol/cholesterol ratios, indicating that CLA has a tocopherol-sparing effect (that is, being less oxidizable than linoleic acid, it does not require as much vitamin E for antioxidant protection).

It is not cholesterol per se, but *oxidized* cholesterol that is harmful to the blood vessels. The oxidizability of cholesterol varies mainly in proportion to the percentage of linoleic acid that it contains; thus the more stable fatty acids, such as CLA, that can be incorporated into cholesterol serve to make it less vulnerable. CLA's antioxidant properties may also play a role in its ability to help keep the blood vessels clean.

As a side note, CLA tends to be incorporated more abundantly into the cell and mitochondrial membranes of the heart muscle. Since the heart relies on fatty acids rather than glucose as its energy source, greater abundance of CLA in the heart muscle may improve the efficiency of fat transport and fat metabolism in the cardiac mitochondria.

Possible Anti-Osteoporotic Effects of CLA

An *in vitro* study done at Purdue University showed that in various rat tissue cultures, including bone tissue, supplemental CLA (at 1% of diet) decreased the levels of omega-6 fatty acids and total monosaturated fatty acids, while increasing the concentrations of omega-3 fatty acids and saturated acids. The levels of inflammatory series II prostaglandins were also decreased by CLA feeding. Since inflammatory compounds lead to bone loss, CLA might potentially be of use in preventing osteoporosis.

We are gaining more and more understanding of the importance of beneficial fatty acids for bone health. Unfortunately, women aren't being told about the need to consume adequate amounts of healthy fats in order to prevent bone loss.

Recognizing the Importance of Essential Oils

Not long ago the low-fat diet gurus were trying to terrorize us into paring down all fat consumption. Now that we have witnessed the epidemic of obesity that followed, we know better. Healthy fats help keep us slender! They also help protect against atherosclerosis, cancer, diabetes, autoimmune diseases, and various other degenerative disorders.

Through their impact on important metabolic enzymes, healthy fats increase the synthesis of beneficial prostaglandins while decreasing the levels of inflammatory prostaglandins; they also modify cell membrane composition and fluidity. Hence, improved blood flow and tissue oxygenation, higher metabolic rate, improved insulin sensitivity, immune enhancement, more muscle and bone formation, better brain function and faster nerve impulse conductance result, to mention just a few of the major benefits.

Thus, while in the 70s and 80s dietary fat was demonized and presented as **the** problem, in the 90s we are beginning to see various kinds of healthy fat as part of the solution.

CLA is the collective name for a group of linoleic acid derivatives found chiefly in beef, lamb, and dairy fat. When ruminants such as cattle and sheep consume linoleic acid (an essential polyunsaturated fatty acid) in grass or feed, the bacteria in their stomachs convert some of that linoleic acid to its variant forms, or isomers (two isomers—cis-9, trans-11 and cis-12, trans-10—predominate; the 9,11 isomer is thought to be the most biologically active). Adding certain strains of starter culture bacteria to dairy products can also increase the content of conjugated linoleic acids—generally spoken of in the singular, much as we use the word "estrogen" to denote the whole family of various estrogens.

It turns out that the intestinal bacteria of rats are also capable of producing CLA out of linoleic acid. At this point, however, it is not known whether human intestinal flora can produce CLA.

The most studied and best understood mechanisms of CLA's benefits involve its modulation of eicosanoid (prostaglandin and leukotriene) synthesis and its cell-membrane effects.

A study of liver fatty acids in CLA-supplemented mice showed that CLA has powerful effects on the fatty-acid composition of neutral lipids and phospholipids (phospholipids are the building materials of cell membranes and membranes surrounding cellular organelles such as mitochondria). CLA lowers the levels of linoleic acid in phospholids; in neutral lipids, CLA lowers the levels of linoleic and arachidonic fatty acid, while increasing the more stable oleic acid. Other studies have found that CLA lowers the production of the inflammatory metabolites of arachidonic acid: leukotrienes and PGE2 (series II) prostaglandins.

CLA's ability to inhibit the production of leukotrienes is of particular interest. While various hormones and many other biochemical modulators inhibit the release of inflammatory prostaglandins, it is difficult to lower leukotriene levels—except by using cortisone and cortisone-like drugs, with their harmful side effects. CLA is a promising, nontoxic alternative.

Insofar as CLA is incorporated into phospholipids, it affects the transport properties of cell membranes and mitochondrial membranes. Apparently CLA facilitates the transport of glucose and fatty acids for energy, and of protein for muscle-building.

There is still much about CLA that needs further investigation. Part of its metabolism involves being desaturated into an as-yet unnamed fatty acid that may be analogous to gamma-linolenic acid (GLA). CLA and its metabolites seem to affect many important metabolic enzymes. A more detailed understanding of the mechanisms of CLA's action should help us develop ways of using it for maximum benefits. The common assumption is that we need to obtain CLA from diet or supplements. Commercial CLA supplements are manufactured by a special treatment (isomerization) of sunflower oil.

The Safety of CLA

In a study conducted by the Nutrition Department of Kraft Foods, male rats were fed a diet of 1.5% CLA, which is 50 times higher than the estimated upper-range human intake. The animals were examined weekly for any signs of toxicity; no toxicity was found. After the end of the 36-week study, the animals were sacrificed and autopsied. Again, no pathology was found. The study confirmed that CLA supplementation is safe even at high doses. Nevertheless, high doses are not necessary for obtaining the benefits of CLA.

Most people obtain their essential omega-3 fatty acids from flax, fish, or perilla oils. CLA appears to be in a class by itself as far as its unique mechanism of disease prevention and body-fat reduction. A deficiency of CLA in the diet may be a major factor in causing Americans to gain so many fat pounds. CLA is a potent antioxidant, but appears to prevent cancer via other mechanisms of action. A particularly rich source of CLA is melted cheddar cheese, yet most consumers prefer to obtain this fatty acid from low-cost CLA supplements that provide the exact isomers that have shown the greatest levels of protection against disease and obesity.

Chitosan—the Fat Magnet

Polysaccharides, including chitosan, are natural, but the substance in its current form hasn't been around for hundreds of years. Chitosan, from the exoskeleton of shellfish, has been synthesized by deacetylation only in the past few decades. Scientists, using research done over the last 17 years, have discovered that chitosan possesses valuable fat-blocking characteristics and could revolutionize weight control strategies for Americans.

Weight control, obesity, and of course dieting are major considerations for anyone concerned about health. Chitosan is a naturally occurring "fat inhibitor." Chitosan absorbs fat. Researchers are direct in their description: "chitosan inhibits fat digestion."

What is chitosan? Chemically, chitosan and chitin are nitrogenous polysaccharides. Chitosan's structure is similar to cellulose, but while cellulose comes from plant products, chitin comes from shellfish.

Chitosan Traps Fat

Crustacean polysaccharide as a product to control fat intake seems to offer major benefits. The fact that, as one scientist reports, "chitosan traps fat" is the bottom line for those trying to attain optimal health or to control their weight. One researcher says taking chitosan "reduces the calorie density of the diet."

Chitosan taken as a dietary supplement has been described as "dissolved in the stomach and then changed into a gelled form in the stomach, entrapping fat in the intestine." Chitosan binds to as much as 4 to 6 times its own weight in fat. Once the fat is bound, the body can't use it. As a matter of fact, the fat is eliminated from the body, tightly bound with the chitosan, and ends up in the sewer system. To quote a May 1995 study on laboratory animals, "The chitosan intake caused a higher level of fat to be excreted in the feces." That's the benefit of chitosan, and the key to its usefulness as a health-enhancement or weight-reduction approach.

Chitosan is more than just a simple sponge. As mentioned before, chitosan binds with 4 to 6 times its own weight of lipids, food, and blood fats.

Chitosan's binding activity isn't simply a mechanical bond, like a sponge holding water loosely in the holes in its fibrous body. The process is much more complicated. The chitosan/fat binding is actually chemical in nature. Chitosan particles in the human body release electrons and become positively charged groups of amino acids. The fatty acids and bile acids are negatively charged carboxylic groups. They link electrostatically in an extremely strong bond. Chitosan is also hydrophobicly linked to fat in a secondary bonding method. That link comes into play with neutrally charged but significant lipids in the body such as triglycerides, cholesterol, and other dietary sterols. As a matter of fact, one study shows that chitosan has a better lipid-binding capacity than some prescription cholesterol-fighting drugs.

A major study completed in Helsinki in late 1994 says chitosan is "polycationic (positively charged) and thus interacts with lipids orally as a solid formulation."

So what does that mean? It's definitely good news for those concerned and ready to take action to improve their health status.

Several studies show that chitosan binds with fats in the body. We've mentioned that before. (It's interesting to note that in the last 2 years scientists and medical researchers around the world have compiled more than 200 studies and research projects on chitosan.) The most recent clinical tests on human subjects confirmed animal studies that years ago showed a reduction in intestinal fat in laboratory animals. The human studies show real and useful weight loss.

Chitosan's Fat-Binding Capacity

So if the science is right, and it seems to be solidly documented, ingestion of 2 grams of chitosan (the typical intake of eight 250-mg capsules per day or four 500-mg capsules) will absorb and bind with 10 grams of fat, then shunt it right out of the body and down the toilet.

It's important to remember that even modest weight loss can reduce your risk to such diseases as heart disease and cancer.

That makes crustacean polysaccharide potentially a powerful new tool for someone trying to regulate fat intake into their body.

Chitosan and Your Health

Let's apply the science to real life. If an individual consumed a total of 40 fat grams during a given day, based on estimates of chitosan's fat absorption, four 500-mg chitosan caps would absorb 10 grams of fat. That would reduce that person's fat intake for the day to 30 grams, moving that person into a more acceptable level of fat consumption based on general health and nutrition recommendations. (Consumption of 8 caps would reduce the consumption to an estimated 20 grams of fat for the day).

The approach requires that people take the chitosan prior to consuming food. Therefore, consumption of chitosan before a meal would appear to be the best practice to receive the full benefit.

Weight Loss

Weight loss is the most dramatic result from pilot research conducted in Helsinki, Finland. The subjects lost an average of 8% of their body weight in a 4-week period. That was an average of more than 15 pounds per person.

Chitosan combined with a low-fat diet, moderate exercise, and appropriate supplementation can help people attain the long-term weight control and health everyone wants.

Researchers reported that their subjects "informed them that this (chitosan) was the best and most hygienic way to take a weight reducing substance." The researchers also praised the absence of side effects.

Chitosan's Effect on Cholesterol, Triglycerides, and HDL

The Helsinki research didn't study the effects of chitosan on cholesterol. Many other researchers have. Cholesterol is one of the leading suspects in heart attacks, so anything that reduces blood cholesterol is a prime subject for health researchers. The Food and Drug Administration stated the facts clearly in a final ruling: "on the basis of the totality of the publicly available scientific evidence, including recently available evidence, the agency has concluded that there is significant scientific agreement among qualified experts that a claim relating diets low in saturated fat and cholesterol . . . to reduced risk of coronary heart disease is supported." Chitosan's fat-trapping qualities put many foods in that category.

So many researchers have studied chitosan's effects on cholesterol that it's hard to know where to begin.

A 1991 study by Norwegian scientists lists the benefits like a prescribing doctor's checklist in favor of the use of chitosan as a medicine: "a marked lowering in serum cholesterol, a considerable lowering in triglyceride levels, tolerability judged to be good."

Chitosan had a positive effect on HDL cholesterol, the "good" cholesterol, according to the 1991 Norwegian study. "During the treatment period, a significant reduction was observed both in total cholesterol and triglycerides. An increase in the HDL-LDL ratio was also observed."

Researchers say, "chitosan, a natural product derived from chitin, possesses hypocholesterolemic properties similar to those of cholestyramine, but there has been no report concerning its effects on the equilibrium between dietary cholesterol and *de novo* cholesterol synthesis in the liver."

A study of laboratory animals in one research project showed that bile acids are trapped or bound at a higher rate with chitosan than with other dietary fibers such as guar gum and konjac mannan.

The same study reported that "cholestyramine and chitosan both significantly lowered serum cholesterol compared to the cellulose group." The study concludes that a series of experiments with male rats clearly demonstrated the hypocholesterolemic activity of dietary chitosan. Feeding the rats a high-cholesterol diet for 20 days and adding 2 to 5% chitosan resulted in a significant reduction, by 25 to 30%, of plasma cholesterol without influencing food intake and growth.

Another study reports that "cholesterol was reduced by 63 to 69% and absorption of oleic acid by 58 to 62%" with a 5% level of chitosan. Another reported "plasma and liver cholesterol . . . were lowered by 54% in plasma and 64% in liver by 5% chitosan." Yet another study says the effect was associated with normalization of direct bilirubin, cholesterol, and triglyceride levels. Once again, chitosan has been shown in study after study to reduce what some scientists call the cholesterol pool in the body.

Not all fibers are created equal relative to their abilities to absorb fat. Chitosan has one of the highest absorptions of fat-to-weight (or quantity consumed) ratios of any fiber tested, while remaining low in toxicity to the human body.

Therefore, chitosan should be more effective than any other currently known natural or synthetic substance in the binding and removing of fat from foods (after ingestion) prior to absorption by the human body.

Chitosan's Positive Effect on Blood Pressure

The 1994 Helsinki study researchers were surprised at chitosan's blood pressure–lowering effects; "another important finding is the excellent blood pressure decrease in the obese patients with hypertension, especially the diastolic blood pressure. Those patients who had normal blood pressure kept this over the study time, while the hypertensive reduced their pressure to normal levels."

The researchers go on to say that the results were equally as powerful as prescription blood-pressure medicine like beta-blockers and calcium-channel blockers. They pointed out that some of the blood-pressure benefits may be due to the weight loss.

Chitosan and Safety

But what about chitosan once a person takes it? Is it safe? Except for its fat-binding properties, chitosan seems almost inert in the human body. Research shows that "chitosan possess[es] low toxicity, allergize[s] only a little, and exert[s] moderate immunostimulating effects." One study even compared chitosan's toxicity to the toxicity of salt or sugar.

One clinical study done in Helsinki shows actual, direct weight loss in humans. That research is dramatic on several fronts. The study (along with other studies) shows that not only did the people taking chitosan lose weight, but their blood pressure dropped too.

Researchers divided the subjects into two groups: one which took chitosan and one which got placebo capsules. It's interesting to note that the placebo group reported some nausea and headaches, while the chitosan group reported none.

One side issue, which may mean little to some people but a lot to others, is that the chitosan group reported a change of consistency of the feces. Chitosan seemed to make the feces softer and smoother, which made defecation easier; a small thing, but important nonetheless to people with constipation.

It should be noted, however, that several researchers have observed that chitosan has the potential of absorbing some minerals, and/or fat-based vitamins. Chitosan is not selective in it's absorption of fat as it travels through the body. That effect could reduce availability of those substances to the body. No health issues are reported in the research regarding any adverse effect relative to this absorption.

It is not recommended within the context of good health practices that chitosan be utilized to offset abuses in fat consumption. In other words, a person who takes chitosan should not consume high quantities of fast foods or foods containing high fat content. The long-term effects of such a practice are currently unknown and have not been studied scientifically in humans.

Chitosan is not a magic pill. For the best long-term health results, the consumption of chitosan should be in combination with a balanced low-fat diet, appropriate dietary supplementation, moderate exercise, no smoking, and moderate consumption of alcohol.

Drink at least 8 ounces of water with the chitosan. The chitosan capsules will burst open in your stomach within 5 minutes and be available to absorb dietary fat in your stomach and intestine before the fat can be absorbed.

Chitosan is now available in 500-mg capsules, thus making it much easier to consume the optimal amount of chitosan needed to bind to the dietary fat contained in a typical high-fat meal. Those seeking to lose weight should take three to six 500-mg chitosan capsules before each fatty meal. This dose also should help to reduce LDL cholesterol by binding to bile acids secreted by the liver into the intestine, and preventing their reabsorption into the bloodstream.

In addition, studies show that ascorbic acid (vitamin C) helps dissolve the chitosan that is in the stomach and intestine into a fat-absorbing gel. When ascorbic acid was given with chitosan to rats, far more fat was trapped and excreted in the feces than when chitosan was given without ascorbic acid. It is important to take pure ascorbic acid to enhance the fat-absorbing effects of chitosan. Buffered ascorbate will not work.

Take three to six 500-mg chitosan capsules and one 1000-mg ascorbic acid capsule right before a high-fat meal.

CAUTION: Do not take chitosan and CLA together. The chitosan will absorb the CLA and prevent it from getting into the bloodstream. Do not take coenzyme Q_{10} rice bran oil capsules, Mega EPA, MEGA GLA, or flax oil with chitosan, since these important oils also will become trapped in the chitosan and be unavailable for absorption. It is best to take your essential fatty acid oil supplements all together first thing in the morning if you are going to use chitosan throughout the day to absorb dietary fat.

The Role of Thyroid Deficiency and Weight Loss

We tend to put on weight as we grow older in part because aging impairs our ability to metabolize carbohydrates. Since most food is eventually broken down into glucose (blood sugar), the age-related decline in our ability to metabolize glucose is a significant cause of degenerative disease and excessive weight gain associated with aging.

One cause of impaired carbohydrate metabolism is subclinical thyroid deficiency. Blood tests are not always reliable in diagnosing this condition. A study found that 18% of elderly people who were initially diagnosed as having normal thyroid levels were later found to have significant thyroid deficiency after undergoing extensive testing. Many physicians believe that most people over 40 suffer from a subclinical thyroid deficiency that contributes to their weight gain.

The thyroid gland secretes hormones involved in cellular energy expenditure. When you go on a diet, there is a decrease in thyroid-hormone secretion that causes your body's metabolic rate to slow down. This decrease occurs because your thyroid gland thinks you are starving and tries to conserve energy until you find more food to eat.

Everyone who has ever dieted knows about the rebound effect—your body resists losing weight while you "starve yourself," but then puts the weight back on with devastating quickness after you eat a little more. This is why dieting is such a miserable way to try to lose weight. Now you know why—it's because your thyroid gland fights you all the way by reducing your energy efficiency in order to keep you from losing weight.

This biological mechanism involving the thyroid gland, which evolved over hundreds of thousands of years to counter the very real risk of starvation, is what sabotages you in today's world of plenty when you deliberately eat less in an attempt to lose weight.

To give you an idea of how your thyroid gland dictates how much you weigh, consider the fact that, when the thyroid produces too much thyroid hormone, the most common clinical symptom is the significant loss of weight. The name for the disease caused by an overactive thyroid gland is hyperthyroidism, and in 76 to 83% of cases, patients' first complaint to their doctors is about how much weight they've been losing!

On the other hand, clinical studies have consistently shown that dieting produces a decline in thyroid output, resulting in a severe reduction in resting energy expenditure. This reduced metabolic rate prevents cells from burning calories to produce energy. If the cells do not take up glucose to produce energy, the sugar is stored as fat within the body. The only way dieting can produce significant long-term weight loss is for the cells to take up glucose for conversion into energy rather than into body fat.

One way of boosting thyroid function in order to lose weight and fight fatigue is to take supplemental thyroid hormone. People who have serious thyroid hormone deficiency should take it under the care of a doctor, but for most people the adverse side effects of supplementation with thyroid hormone outweigh the benefits.

While there are studies showing that thyroid supplementation promotes weight loss in some people, it also can kill you. Excessive thyroid hormone can cause rapid heart rate and atrial fibrillation—the abnormal, chaotic quivering of a heart chamber—that could lead to a heart attack or stroke. The problem is not thyroid deficiency per se, but that people become thyroid-deficient in response to dieting. In short, thyroid-hormone drugs don't always work and can be dangerous.

Later in this protocol, we're going to reveal a safe and effective, natural way of boosting your thyroid function without having to take thyroid hormone.

There are several reasons why thyroid hormone supplementation hasn't consistently produced weight loss in clinical studies:

- Commercially available thyroid supplements may not provide all the thyroid hormones needed to restore optimal carbohydrate metabolism. When safe doses of thyroid supplements are given to dieters, their resting energy expenditure still does not approach their prediet level, even though measurable serum levels of thyroid hormone are up to 130% higher than prediet levels.
- The thyroid supplements currently on the market have been tested only by themselves in clinical studies. When only one therapy is tested at a time without producing dramatic results, the therapy is considered useless. But thyroid deficiency is only one factor that works against successful weight loss in response to dieting.
- Normal diets do not provide optimal levels of minerals; dieting can cause severe deficiencies of chromium and magnesium, for example. These deficiencies cause insulin resistance, which is a major factor in carbohydrate metabolic disorders. Chromium and magnesium must be present if thyroid hormone is to work synergistically with insulin, in order to drive glucose into the cells for energy production.
- There are other hormones, such as DHEA and pregnenolone, that boost the effect of thyroid hormone on carbohydrate metabolism.

The scientific evidence shows that dieting induces a thyroid-deficient state that slows the body's metabolic rate. If body weight is to be controlled by diet, something must be done to safely boost thyroid hormone to near prediet levels.

Benefits of Soy Protein

There are more than 80 years of scientific research to document the ability of soy protein to lower blood fat levels. A study in the August 3, 1995, issue of the *New England Journal of Medicine* showed that soy protein lowered LDL cholesterol by 12.9% and triglycerides by 10.5%. One mechanism by which soy reduces blood fats is by boosting thyroid hormone levels. An added benefit: studies show that thyroid hormone burns up harmful LDL cholesterol globules in the blood.

Because of the many documented health benefits from soy intake, the Life Extension Foundation suggests that anyone seeking to lose weight safely through dieting should take 6 to 30 grams a day of soy protein concentrate. Soy protein not only boosts thyroid hormone levels to burn sugar calories, but it also contains an amino acid complex that helps spare the body's protein stores, which are often broken down in response to dieting. The phytoestrogens and essential fatty acids in soy further help to promote weight loss.

The Life Extension Foundation has recommended soy protein concentrates to cancer patients for many years. Soy protein extracts contain 8 to 10 times more of the active ingredients of soy than conventional soy extracts. Some of these ingredients are cancer-preventing phytoestrogens, such as genistein.

Soy protein powder has a light, pleasant-tasting nutty flavor. If you consume 6 to 30 grams of soy powder in water, you may be able to skip a meal because the soy protein—which contains essential fatty acids—and the soy fiber have a satiating effect.

The isoflavones (especially genistein) contained in soy protein extracts have potent cancer prevention effects, especially against breast and prostate cancer. Cancer patients often take high doses of soy protein extract as an adjuvant (assisting) therapy because of studies showing that the genistein inhibits cancer cell proliferation via several well-established mechanisms. And, as noted, soy protein also has been shown to lower cholesterol, possibly via its thyroid hormone–stimulating effect.

Soy intake is associated with significant reductions in the risk of many forms of cancer and in blood fat levels. Many Foundation members already are taking supplemental soy to reduce their risk of cancer, especially breast and prostate cancer.

The optimal method of taking soy protein extract is to take 1 to 2 heaping tablespoons (20 to 40 grams) of the powder each day. Soy extract capsules are available but may not provide the full spectrum of soy constituents needed to boost thyroid hormone output.

Benefits of Magnesium and Chromium

While thyroid hormone plays a definite role in weight management, the scientific literature makes it clear that both magnesium and chromium also are required to break down the cellular insulin resistance that causes higher-than-normal blood sugar levels.

A 1998 4-week, double-blind, weight-loss intervention study combining exercise and supplementation stated, "Results indicate that the addition of a natural dietary supplement during a 4-week diet-and-exercise weight-loss program accelerates the rate of body fat loss and helps maintain fat-free mass (lean tissue), thereby producing favorable changes in body composition" (*Adv. Ther.,* 1998 [Sept–Oct]; 15[5]:305–14).

Overweight people usually suffer from insulin impairment that prevents the proper cell uptake of carbohydrates (sugars). Excessive serum glucose is converted into body fat unless this insulin resistance is broken down and the cells are able to regain youthful carbohydrate metabolism. Chromium has received widespread publicity for its ability to lower serum glucose levels by potentiating insulin sensitivity. Studies have shown that chromium supplementation results in a slight reduction in body fat and an increase in lean body mass. Niacin has also been shown to improve the metabolic-enhancing effect of chromium.

In 1997, Austrian researchers conducted a study to assess the effects of chromium yeast and chromium picolinate on lean body mass during and after weight reduction with a very-low-calorie diet.

Thirty-six obese nondiabetic patients undergoing an 8-week very-low-calorie diet followed by an 18-week maintenance period were evaluated. During the 26-week treatment period, subjects received either placebo or chromium yeast (200 mcg/day) or chromium picolinate (200 mcg/day) in a double-blind manner. After 26 weeks, chromium picolinate–supplemented subjects showed increased lean body mass. Researchers reported chromium picolinate, but not chromium yeast, is able to increase lean body mass in obese patients in the maintenance period after a very-low-calorie diet without counteracting the weight loss achieved (*Acta Med. Austr.,* 1997; 24[5]:185–87).

To improve the fat-reducing effects of dieting, the Foundation now suggests that 1 capsule of this new chromium be taken with every meal to facilitate youthful carbohydrate metabolism. The importance of taking a chromium capsule with each meal is illustrated in animal studies in which chromium was given throughout the day in order to lower serum glucose levels. When you consume food, your serum glucose levels rise significantly unless your cells are sensitized to insulin. Chromium will help sensitize your cells to insulin by helping to lower your blood sugar levels.

You should not take more than three 200-mg chromium capsules a day. Always take antioxidant supplements like vitamin E when you take chromium, to protect against free-radical activity. At least 30 mg of niacin should be contained in each 200-mcg chromium capsule.

While chromium has received the most media attention, the scientific literature shows that magnesium plays an even more important role in regulating carbohydrate metabolism. Magnesium is involved in a number of enzymatic reactions required for cells to uptake and metabolize glucose. Magnesium deficiency causes insulin resistance and elevated blood sugar levels.

About 80% of Americans are magnesium-deficient. When they go on a diet, they become severely deficient in magnesium, which causes the insulin resistance that contributes to the failure of the diet. Life Extension Mix contains high amounts of magnesium. For those going on a calorie-restricted diet, it is suggested that at least one 500-mg magnesium capsule a day be taken in addition to the full dose Life Extension Mix.

Benefits of DHEA, the Anabolic Hormone

Hormone deficiencies are a cause of age-associated weight gain. DHEA has kept old animals remarkably thin, but has not worked well in humans. Nevertheless, many older people taking DHEA report anabolic muscle gain and fat loss. DHEA has been shown to boost insulin growth factor (IGF-1) in humans, and the increase in this youth factor may be responsible for the fat reduction and anabolic effects seen in some elderly people. The main benefits to people over 40 in restoring DHEA levels to a youthful state includes immune enhancement, protection against neurological disease and memory loss, reductions in risks of certain cancers, alleviation of depression, and protection against osteoporosis.

For people over 35 years of age, DHEA-replacement therapy is suggested as part of an overall weight management program. The average dose of DHEA for men should be 25 mg of DHEA, 3 times a day. Women need only 15 mg of DHEA, 3 times a day.

CAUTION: *Refer to the DHEA Replacement Therapy protocol before taking DHEA.*

Conclusion

Americans aren't overweight because they're bad; they're overweight because they don't always have the tools they need to maintain an ideal body weight. At the turn of the century a large percentage of our work was done on the farm. Most of our citizens performed strenuous physical labor.

We are no longer a nation of farmers, working at hard physical labor. We are now, in some ways, farmers and distributors of information and services. And, while the labor is mentally hard, it isn't physically demanding enough to burn off the calories we need to burn. We've known intuitively that our lifestyle hasn't been good for us, but our overindulgent lifestyle is actually dangerous. Medical researchers have only recently proved that our intuition has been right. So far though, the research has only been able to point out the dangers. It's only been in the last few years that we've been able to see some solutions.

We've gone from graham crackers as a health food (Dr. Graham developed his graham crackers as an early form of nutritional supplement) to scientifically developed, designed, and researched vitamin supplements, antioxidants, and nutrients.

Most dieters need help in taking off pounds. They need dietary aids to jump-start the weight-loss process to give them the encouragement they need to stay on the program long enough to succeed. That's why we recommend nutrients that fight diseases while taking off pounds. Nutrients make you look and feel better while you're losing weight, and it's easy to continue to take them year-after-year to stay healthy and fit.

Summary

Here are the disease-fighting nutrients we recommend for weight loss:

1. Chitosan B: take between 1500 and 3000 mg of chitosan immediately before a meal that contains fat. Drink at least 8 ounces of water with the chitosan. The recommended dosage also should help to reduce harmful LDL cholesterol by binding to bile acids secreted by the liver into the intestine and preventing their reabsorption into the bloodstream.

CAUTION: Do not take chitosan and CLA together. The chitosan will absorb the CLA and prevent it from entering the bloodstream. Do not take CoQ_{10} Rice Bran Oil capsules, Mega EPA, MEGA GLA, or flax oil with chitosan; they also will become trapped in the chitosan and be unavailable for absorption. Take your essential fatty acid oil supplements all together first thing in the morning if you are going to use chitosan throughout the day to absorb dietary fat.

2. Conjugated linoleic acid: take three 1000-mg capsules of CLA every day to duplicate successful fat-loss clinical studies.

   CLA inhibits fat storage by enhancing the ability of cell membranes (other than fat cells) to open up and allow the absorption of fats and other nutrients. CLA promotes the growth of

O

muscles by letting nutrients into active muscle cells. The fat-reducing mechanism of CLA involves the rejuvenation of cell membranes in the muscles and connective tissues to allow fats to enter freely in order to generate energy and growth. This anabolic effect could provide anti-aging benefits in the elderly.

Remember, do not take with chitosan, as the chitosan will absorb the CLA before it can get into your bloodstream.

3. Chromium and magnesium: take one 200-mcg capsule of chromium picolinate with each meal, and at least 500 mg of elemental magnesium daily.

   Insulin resistance prevents serum glucose from entering cells. If glucose cannot get into the cells to produce energy, it will be stored in the body as fat. Chromium and magnesium have been shown to help break down cellular insulin resistance. For chromium to be effective in the body, it needs to have niacin present. Many health-conscious people receive supplemental niacin with their B-complex formula, but Prolongevity's chromium supplement contains 30 mg of niacin in addition to 200 mcg of chromium in each capsule. This small amount of niacin does not usually produce a niacin "flush," but does ensure that niacin will be available to work with chromium to reduce serum glucose levels by breaking down insulin resistance. The published studies actually show that magnesium is more effective than chromium in breaking down insulin resistance.

   Magnesium deficiency is another cause of excess weight gain in Americans. Chromium can lower cholesterol levels as well as serum glucose levels. Magnesium can protect against heart attacks and stroke. Taking these supplements to help lose weight may provide significant life extension benefits in addition to weight loss.

4. Soy protein: take 20 to 40 grams of Soy Protein Extract Powder daily.

   A deficiency of thyroid hormone can slow down metabolic actions in the body and cause weight gain. Consumption of soy protein can boost the body's natural secretion of thyroid hormone, thereby increasing the body's metabolic rate. Thyroid hormone also is necessary to drive glucose into the cells. The isoflavones (especially genistein) contained in soy protein extracts have potent cancer-prevention effects, especially against breast and prostate cancer. Cancer patients often take high doses of soy protein extract as an adjuvant (assisting) therapy because of studies showing that the genistein inhibits cancer cell proliferation via several well-established mechanisms. Soy protein also has been shown to lower cholesterol, possibly via its thyroid hormone stimulating effect.

5. DHEA: men should take 25 mg of DHEA, 3 times a day. Women need only 15 mg of DHEA, 3 times a day. Take with an antioxidant formula such Life Extension Mix.

Almost everyone gains weight as he or she grows older. One cause of age-related weight gain is the progressive decline in the body's levels of the hormone DHEA. Many older people who take DHEA report muscle gain and fat loss. Other benefits to people over 40 in restoring DHEA to youthful levels include improved immune function, protection against memory loss, relief of depressive symptoms, protection against osteoporosis, and reduction in the risk of certain cancers. Refer to the *DHEA-Pregnenolone Precautions in the DHEA Replacement Therapy protocol* before taking DHEA.

The Weight-Loss Regimen

Those seeking significant fat-loss effects should commit to a 2- to 3-month program that would involve the following schedule:

First thing in the morning take:

1. Three 1000-mg CLA capsules.
2. One DHEA capsule (take with an antioxidant like Life Extension Mix).
3. One chromium-niacin capsule.
4. One heaping tablespoon of soy protein powder (soy can be taken at another time of the day if desired).

Five minutes before lunch take:

5. Six 500-mg chitosan capsules with an 8-ounce glass of water (some people need only three chitosan capsules).
6. One 1000-mg ascorbic acid capsule.
7. One 200-mcg chromium-niacin capsule.
8. One DHEA 15–25 mg capsule.

Five minutes before dinner take:

9. Six 500-mg chitosan capsules with an 8-ounce glass of water (some people need only three chitosan capsules).
10. One 1000-mg ascorbic acid capsule.
11. One chromium-niacin capsule.
12. One 500-mg magnesium capsule.

Product availability. Chromium with niacin, conjugated linoleic acid (CLA), Soy Protein Powder, magnesium, vitamin E, chitosan, and DHEA can be ordered by phoning 1-800-544-4440, or order on-line at www.lcf.org.

OBSESSIVE-COMPULSIVE DISORDER

Obsessive-compulsive disorder (OCD) is an anxiety disorder characterized by obsessions that cause marked anxiety or distress and/or by compulsions that serve to neutralize anxiety. Symptoms may be mild but merely annoying, or may disable a person throughout a lifetime.

Obsessions are persistent ideas, thoughts, impulses, or images that are experienced as intrusive and inappropriate, and that cause marked anxiety or distress. The most common obsessions are repeated thoughts about contamination (i.e., becoming contaminated by germs or by shaking hands); repeated doubts (wondering whether one has performed some act, such as having left a door unlocked or a coffee pot brewing on the stove); a need to have things in a particular order; aggressive or horrific impulses (which the person might never act on); or sexual imagery that is inappropriate or frightening.

Compulsions are repetitive behaviors (hand washing, checking) or mental acts (praying, counting, repeating words silently). The goal of compulsions is to prevent or reduce anxiety or distress. The person feels driven to perform the compulsion to reduce the distress caused by the obsessive thought.

Many people may consider themselves to be compulsive because they hold themselves to a high standard of performance and are perfectionist and highly organized in work and recreational activities. This type of compulsiveness often is an attribute that contributes to a person's self-esteem and success.

People who have been clinically diagnosed with OCD suffer from obsessive and compulsive behaviors that are extreme enough to interfere with their everyday lives. The obsessions and compulsions these people experience can wreck their lives.

Incidence of OCD

For a long time, mental health professionals considered OCD to be a rare condition. That may be because OCD often has gone unrecognized. Many people who suffer from OCD are ashamed of their irrational behaviors and try to keep their problem a secret. But in recent years, as science has confirmed that OCD is a potentially severe anxiety disorder, more people have begun to seek treatment.

OCD, in fact, affects more than 2% of the population, according to a survey conducted in the early 1980s by the National Institute of Mental Health (NIMH). That makes OCD more common than schizophrenia, bipolar disorder, or panic disorder. In addition, OCD is an "equal opportunity" illness, striking people of all ages, gender, and ethnic groups.

OCD's impact on society is devastating. In 1990, in the United States alone, OCD resulted in social and economic losses of more than $8 billion—nearly 6% of the nation's total mental health bill of $148 billion.

What Causes OCD?

Psychiatrists once thought that OCD was caused by traumatic past events in a person's life. A person with OCD, for example, might have learned as a child to overemphasize cleanliness or to develop a belief that certain thoughts were dangerous or unacceptable.

Now a growing body of research indicates that biological factors and/or cognitive processes may cause or contribute to the disorder. Many OCD patients, for example, respond well to medications that alter brain chemistry. Tendencies to develop OCD may be inherited: the condition has been known to run in families. And there is evidence that OCD involves abnormalities in brain chemistry.

To identify biological factors that may be relevant in onset or development of OCD, NIMH researchers used a device called a positron emission tomography (PET) scanner to study brains of OCD patients.

The investigators found that OCD patients exhibit brain activity that differs from that of people who do not suffer from mental illness, or who have mental problems other than OCD. Researchers found that OCD patients exhibited abnormal neurochemical activity in brain regions known to play a role in certain neurological disorders.

Other recent studies using magnetic resonance imaging (MRI) technology found that subjects with OCD had significantly less white brain matter than did normal control subjects.

Even if there is a biological basis for OCD, that doesn't mean that a person's environment, beliefs, and attitudes are not also linked to the disease. In addition, people with OCD may process information differently from those who do not have the illness.

How OCD Manifests

Traditionally, OCD was thought to show up during teenage years or in early adulthood. But new research indicates that some children develop the illness as early as preschool. In fact, a third of all OCD cases may begin in childhood.

The essential features of obsessive-compulsive disorder are recurrent obsessions or compulsions that are severe enough to be time-consuming (taking more than 1 hour a day) or that cause marked distress or significant impairment. Usually at some point during the course of the disorder, the person recognizes that the obsessions or compulsions are excessive or unreasonable, but is powerless to change behavior without intervention.

OCD is sometimes accompanied by other psychological problems, including depression, eating disorders, substance abuse disorder, personality disorder, attention deficit disorder, or another of the anxiety disorders. These co-existing conditions can make OCD difficult to diagnose and treat.

In addition, symptoms of OCD may be seen in conjunction with other neurological disorders. People with Tourette's syndrome, for example, may have an increased rate of OCD. Scientists now are investigating a hypothesis that a genetic relationship exists between OCD and such "tic" disorders, which are characterized by involuntary movements and vocalizations.

Other illnesses that may be linked to OCD are trichotillomania (a repeated urge to pull out scalp hair, eyelashes, eyebrows or other body hair); body dysmorphic disorder (excessive preoccupation with imaginary or exaggerated defects in appearance); and hypochondriasis (fear of having a serious disease, even though nothing is wrong with a person). In addition, NIMH researchers are looking at the possible link of OCD to some autoimmune diseases in which infection-fighting cells, or antibodies, turn against the body in an attempt to destroy it.

Most people with OCD know that their obsessions are unrealistic, but they may sometimes be uncertain about the validity of their fears or even believe that their fears are founded. In almost all cases, OCD victims struggle to banish their unwanted obsessive thoughts and to stop themselves from engaging in compulsive behaviors.

Many people seem to be able to keep their OCD symptoms under control at work or school, but resistance may weaken and then the condition can become so severe that compulsive rituals take over victims' lives, making it impossible for them to function normally.

People with OCD often try to hide the condition from friends and co-workers because they are ashamed of and confused by their seemingly senseless behaviors. Such feelings of inadequacy prevent many people from seeking treatment for the condition. This is regrettable, because science has developed many medications that can help people with OCD.

Pharmacological Treatment

Many persons with OCD benefit from pharmacological treatment. Others may be helped by medication in conjunction with behavioral therapy. Others begin with medication to gain control over symptoms and then switch to therapy.

In recent years several clinical trials have found that a number of drugs can affect the neurotransmitter serotonin and significantly decrease symptoms of OCD. The tricyclic antidepressant clomipramine (Anafranil) was the first of such serotonin reuptake inhibitors (SRIs) specifically approved to treat OCD.

Clomipramine was followed by other SRIs known as "selective serotonin reuptake inhibitors" (SSRIs). Those approved by the U.S. Food and Drug Administration to treat OCD include fluoxetine (Prozac), fluvoxamine (Luvoc), and paroxetine (Paxil). And several clinical trials suggest that OCD patients may be helped by sertraline (Zoloft).

Such medications have helped, to some degree, more than three quarters of patients who took them. In more than half of patients, the medications relieved OCD symptoms by diminishing frequency and intensity of obsessions and compulsions.

It may take 3 weeks or longer for the medicines to begin to work. If patients do not respond to a medication or develop side effects, doctors may try another SRI. Often, if medications are discontinued, patients relapse. If a medication works to alleviate symptoms, doctors may lower the dosage, but most patients take OCD medications indefinitely.

Psychotherapy

Most OCD patients have not responded well to traditional psychotherapy, the goal of which is to help people to gain insight into their problems. But one behavioral therapy that *has* worked for many people with OCD is called "exposure and response prevention." In this approach, the patient deliberately confronts a feared object or idea. The therapist then encourages the patient to refrain from ritualizing to obtain relief. A compulsive hand washer, for example, may be asked to touch an object believed to be "contaminated," and may then be urged to avoid washing for several hours, until the anxiety has decreased.

Most OCD patients who have completed behavioral therapy have reported a lessening of symptoms. Usually these patients are highly motivated and have a positive attitude about treatment. What's more, the therapy appears to have long-lasting effects. One recent study found that 76% of patients who underwent exposure and response prevention therapy still reported clinically significant relief from symptoms up to 6 months after treatment. Another study found that incorporating relapse-prevention components in a treatment program—including follow-up sessions after intensive therapy—contributed to maintenance of improvement.

Another type of psychological treatment, cognitive-behavioral therapy, may also help some people with OCD. This form of therapy attempts to change beliefs and thinking patterns of people with OCD. More studies are needed to evaluate the effects of cognitive-behavioral therapy.

Other Therapies

In addition, scientists are investigating the potential of neurosurgery, a new approach to treating OCD. In the few centers where neurosurgery has been performed, the treatment has been recommended only for people who have failed to respond to conventional medications or psychotherapy.

And over the past few years there have been several published anecdotal reports of the successful use of electroconvulsive therapy (ECT) in OCD patients. Most often, however, benefits of ECT have been short-lived. The treatment generally is restricted to people with treatment-resistant OCD accompanied by severe depression.

Natural Treatments

Some naturopathic physicians have reported success in treating OCD with a variety of natural therapies. These include the following:

Herbal therapy. Several herbs act directly on the nervous system, promoting relaxation and feelings of tranquillity. Other herbs may relax tense muscles, ease stress-related headaches, soothe stomachs upset by stress, and encourage restful sleep.

Kava kava *(Piper methysticum),* a South Pacific member of the pepper family, induces calm feelings, eases muscle tension, reduces emotional tension, and improves sleep. The safest and most effective way of using Kava is in liquid spray form that provides a standardized dose. Most people spray the Kava directly into their mouths 1 to 3 times a day. Each spray should be standardized to provide 60 mg of 30% kava lactones.

St. John's wort *(Hypericum perforatum),* an herb used extensively in Europe to treat depression, also may be of some benefit in treating OCD. Early laboratory research indicated that St. John's wort functions much as a monoamine oxidase (MAO) inhibitor, reducing anxiety and depression by reducing brain levels of the enzyme monoamine oxidase, which breaks down neurotransmitters such as serotonin. Newer studies, however, indicate that St. John's wort functions more like an SSRI, blocking reuptake of serotonin. If it does, then it may help OCD patients in the same way that SSRI medications do. The recommended dose of St. John's wort is 1 capsule, 3 times a day, of a 300-mg 0.3% hypericin extract. Hypericin is the primary active ingredient in St. John's wort. Avoid excessive sun exposure when using St. John's wort extract.

Other Therapies

Exercise. Canadian researchers report that regular exercise may help many people who suffer from psychiatric disorders, including phobias and OCD. Researchers Gregg A. Tkachuk and Garry L. Martin of the Department of Psychology at the University of Manitoba in Winnipeg examined studies of anxiety disorder and exercise dating back to 1981. They found that strength training, running, walking, and other forms of aerobic exercise help to alleviate mild to moderate depression, and may also help to treat other mental disorders including anxiety and substance abuse.

Nutritional supplements. Some studies indicate that niacinamide and calcium may be beneficial in reducing symptoms of anxiety and phobias.

Summary

New research indicates that biological factors and/or cognitive processes may cause or contribute to OCD. OCD sufferers, therefore, respond well to medications that alter brain chemistry. Success with natural therapies that act directly on the central nervous system has also been reported. These include

- Kava kava, to induce a feeling of calmness and ease muscle tension. One or two sprays, 1 to 3 times a day. Each spray should provide 60 mg of 30% kava lactones.
- Calcium, 1000 elemental milligrams, once or twice a day.
- Vitamin B_3 (niacinamide), 500 mg once or twice a day.
- St. John's wort, 300 mg, 3 times a day of a 0.3% hypericin extract.
- Regular exercise has been shown to relieve the symptoms of several psychiatric disorders, including phobias and OCD.
- Magnesium, 500 elemental milligrams a day.

For more information. Contact the National Mental Health Association, (800) 969-6642.

Product availability. Vitamin B_3 (niacin) and St. John's wort are available from the Life Extension Foundation by calling (800) 544-4440, or order online at www.lef.org. Ask the Foundation to provide you with a list of knowledgeable physicians in your area who will prescribe clomipramine and other drugs to treat OCD.

ORGANIC BRAIN SYNDROME

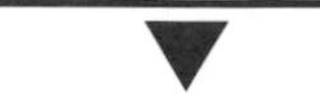

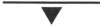

(See Alzheimer's Disease)

OSTEOPOROSIS

Normal aging causes a decline in bone density that occurs to varying degrees in otherwise healthy people. This decline does not induce bone fractures. Osteoporosis, on the other hand, causes a progressive marked reduction in bone mineral density that often results in pathological fractures, particularly of the vertebrae of the spine. It occurs more frequently in women than in men.

Many factors may cause osteoporotic bone loss that is not associated with aging. These include major surgery, glucocorticoid (anti-inflammatory steroid) drugs, liver cirrhosis, Crohn's inflammatory disease of the bowel, cystic fibrosis, and hormone deficiencies. This protocol confines itself to age-related osteoporosis.

Osteoporosis and Hormone Metabolism

The primary cause of osteoporosis is hormonal imbalances that interfere with the bone-forming cells. The osteoblasts are specialized bone cells that function to pull calcium, magnesium, and phosphorus from the blood in order to build bone mass. Osteoblasts require the hormone *progesterone* to maintain youthful bone-forming capability during and after menopause.

Provera is a drug frequently prescribed by conventional doctors that causes many side effects and problems in women. Provera (medroxyprogesterone) is an artificial molecule that should not be confused with natural progesterone. Natural progesterone provides the intended benefits with none of the side effects of the synthetic drug. A stark example of the safety of natural progesterone compared to synthetic progestin drugs can be seen by the labeling. Provera carries a warning that its use in early pregnancy may increase the risk of early abortion or inflict congenital deformities on the fetus. Natural progesterone, on the other hand, is necessary for the survival and development of the embryo throughout the pregnancy. In response to pregnancy, ovarian secretion of progesterone increases significantly. As a general rule, pregnant women should not use any hormone replacement therapy without consulting their obstetrician.

Natural progesterone may be obtained in several different forms. The safest route of progesterone administration is via a topically applied cream that absorbs directly through the skin and into fat cells. It is important to apply natural progesterone cream to different parts of the body (face, breasts, abdomen, and thighs) so as not to oversaturate the fat cells under the skin in any one particular area that are required to assimilate the hormone into the body. The topical application of progesterone enables it to enter the body without first going through the digestive system. If progesterone were to be taken orally, it would have to first pass through the liver, which degrades and excretes much of the hormone into the bile. Natural progesterone is available in topically applied creams that contain between 900 mg and 1400 mg of natural progesterone per 2-oz jar.

In using progesterone cream, pre- and postmenopausal women should start with ¼ to ½ of a teaspoon a day. Those with severe osteoporosis should use ½ teaspoon morning and night for the first jar followed by ¼ teaspoons a day for the second jar on. Premenopausal women who suffer from premenstrual syndrome (PMS) may consider taking ⅛ to ¼ teaspoons of progesterone on days 15 through 26 of their menstrual cycle.

It is advisable for women to ask their doctors to measure blood or saliva levels of the various hormones to best individualize the correct dosage, though natural progesterone has been safely used by millions of women by individually adjusting the dose to reflect alleviation of PMS or menopausal symptoms. In other words, if hot flashes, night sweats, headache, and depression are alleviated by using ¼ teaspoon of natural progesterone cream a day, then a woman may be able to safely stay at that dose. While it is prudent to consider progesterone blood or saliva testing, the safety of natural progesterone is such that a pregnant woman will naturally secrete the large amounts of progesterone without encountering toxicity. In an ideal setting, hormonal blood or saliva testing would be done routinely, but since most pre- and postmenopausal women produce very little progesterone, these women have historically safely self-administered topical progesterone cream according to how well it corrects their menopausal symptoms. With the advent of lower-cost saliva and blood testing, it should be possible for more women to target their ideal progesterone level.

Some women who do not respond well to progesterone creams may do very well with hormone implants. These are little pellets about 1/8 inch in diameter that are implanted under the skin every 6 to 12 months. The procedure is done in a physician's office, taking only 10 minutes.

In women whose doctors are prescribing excess amounts of supplemental estrogen, the administration of progesterone may enable the dose of estrogen to be reduced, since progesterone restores sensitivity to estrogen receptors on cell membranes. If the estrogen dose is not lowered, some women develop symptoms of "estrogen dominance" (such as water retention, headaches, weight gain, swollen breasts) when progesterone is first supplemented. The objective of the physician should be to gradually lower the dose of estrogen in relation to progesterone therapy. If estrogen is reduced too rapidly, hot flashes can occur.

Estrogen is used to prevent bone loss because it regulates the action of osteoclasts, which remove dead portions of demineralized bone. DHEA and/or soy extracts may provide enough estrogen to maintain youthful osteoclast activity. Based upon records of dietary soy consumption in Japan, the typical daily phytoestrogen intake from soy has been estimated at 50 mg a person. By contrast, the typical Western diet has been estimated to provide only 2 to 3 mg a day of the phytoestrogen genistein. Not only are certain cancer levels lower in those who consume soy, but menopausal symptoms and the incidence of osteoporosis are reduced. New studies are showing that soy isoflavones promote an anabolic effect on bone density in postmenopausal women by binding to an estrogen receptor in bone. The protective action of genistein seems to depend on stimulation of bone *formation* rather than estrogen's effect of suppressing bone resorption. Although both estrogen and genistein protect against bone loss after cessation of ovarian function, genistein has been shown to reduce both trabecular and compact bone loss.

A 6-month study on 66 postmenopausal women was conducted at the University of Illinois at Urbana-Champaign to investigate bone density and bone mineral content in response to soy therapy. In this study, postmenopausal women received on a daily basis either phytoestrogens derived from soy protein or milk-derived protein (that contained no phytoestrogens). The results showed significant increases in bone density and bone mineral content for the lumbar spine in the women receiving the phytoestrogens derived from soy protein diets compared to the control diet. Increases in other skeletal areas also were noted in the women on the soy diets. Dr. Erdman, the lead scientist, concluded that soy isoflavones show real potential for maintaining bone health. Kenneth D. Setchell, Ph.D. of Children's Hospital and Medical Center in Cincinnati, Ohio, confirmed the estrogenic activity of the principal soy isoflavones daidzein, genistein, and glycitein. Dr. Setchell conducted research on the chemical structure and metabolism of soy phytoestrogens and concluded that consuming modest amounts of soy protein results in relatively high blood concentrations of phytoestrogens and that this could have a significant hormonal effect in many individuals.

There are enough phytoestrogens in the newer soy extracts for many women to derive effective estrogen replacement therapy. A soy supplement called Mega Soy Extract provides 110 mg of soy phytoestrogens in just 2 capsules. This is more than twice the amount in the typical Japanese diet. Since the phytoestrogen genistein is water-soluble, it is suggested that 1 capsule of Mega Soy Extract be taken in the morning and 1 in the evening. While all women should benefit from Mega Soy Extract, some women may need to consider direct, natural hormone replacement depending upon family history, severity of osteoporosis if already present, and other considerations.

Estrogen is a general name for a group of similar compounds (estradiol, estrone, estriol, and their metabolites) with slightly different effects on the various tissues in a woman's body. A commonly prescribed drug is called Premarin because the estrogens it contains are an extraction from a pregnant mare's urine. As you might guess, the ratio of the various types of estrogens found in horse urine is different from that found in human females. So Premarin works fine if you are a horse. Women, however, should get their estrogens from another source. There are two main formulations which may be obtained by prescription from compounding pharmacies. One containing two types of estrogen is called Biest; the second containing three forms is Triest. Women seeking these prescription drugs (Biest and Triest) should see a physician familiar with natural hormone replacement in women.

Additionally, it is important for pre- and postmenopausal woman to consider testosterone. Women have less than men do, but it is just as important to them as it is to men. Why? It contributes to stamina, proper female muscle mass, sex drive, and preventing and treating osteoporosis.

Dosing of all the hormones is best done to mimic the normal menstrual cycle of the woman of childbearing age. To keep things simple, one physician recommends that pre- and postmenopausal women begin on the first day of the month taking their estrogen formulation from day 1 to day 25. The progesterone is used from day 1 to day 20.

One must bear in mind that while progesterone is protective in the sense that it protects against cancer, estrogens that are taken without progesterone, may increase a woman's risk of cancer of the breast and potentially the uterus. This is very easy to understand. Estrogens stimulate breast tissue and the lining of the uterus. During the menstrual cycle, progesterone production rapidly falls, resulting in the shedding of the uterine lining and menstrual flow. If estrogen is taken continually, building up the uterine lining without opposing progesterone, there is a theoretical increased cancer risk. This is why you must discuss this with a physician knowledgeable about the subject. The risk is minimized in a postmenopausal woman if hormone replacement results in monthly menstruation or if she undergoes yearly uterine tissue sampling or biopsy, which is a simple procedure done in the doctor's office.

Women over 30, particularly those with a family history of osteoporosis, should consider hormone level analysis in consultation with a physician to see if hormone supplementation should be undertaken prior to menopause.

Other hormones to consider are DHEA and melatonin. DHEA has been shown to stimulate osteoblast activity to help prevent bone loss. The recommended dose for most women is about 25 to 50 mg a day. (*Before taking DHEA, refer to the DHEA Precautions in the DHEA Replacement Therapy protocol*).

Women over the age of 35 or 40 should consider taking melatonin in the range of 500 mcg to 3 mg every night to help prevent osteoporosis and reduce the carcinogenic risks associated with estrogen-replacement therapy.

Nutrient and Supplement Considerations

A number of women take calcium tablets, but calcium is a strong binding agent that is often difficult to break down in the digestive tract. Calcium capsules, on the other hand, burst open in the stomach within 5 minutes for quick absorption into the bloodstream. Calcium supplementation is only one part of an osteoporosis prevention and treatment program.

For bone mineral maintenance and replacement, the Life Extension Foundation recommends that women take between 1000 and 2000 mg of elemental calcium along with 600 to 1000 mg of elemental magnesium every day. The addition of between 400 and 1000 IU of vitamin D_3 is mandatory to ensure optimal calcium absorption. The inability to absorb calcium is a major reason that calcium therapy fails to prevent or slow the progression of osteoporosis. Vitamin D_3 taken with calcium will normally promote absorption and assimilation of calcium into the bone matrix. Vitamin D_3 has also been shown to promote the production of IGF-1 and other growth factors in osteoporotic patients, which improves osteoblast (bone-building) function. Other minerals that are important for healthy bone metabolism include at least 30 mg a day of elemental zinc, 3 mg a day of elemental manganese, and 2 mg of elemental boron a day.

There are dietary supplements designed to prevent and treat osteoporosis. A product called Bone Assure provides the better-documented nutrients for the prevention and treatment of osteoporosis.

The daily dose of Bone Assure supplies the following nutrients in 6 capsules:

- Calcium (as *bis*-glycinate), 1000 mg (equals 1800 mg of elemental calcium citrate)
- Magnesium (oxide), 320 mg
- Zinc (citrate), 12 mg
- Manganese (citrate), 3 mg
- Boron (amino acid chelate), 2 mg
- Copper (sulfate), 1.5 mg (PIX)
- Oat straw (10:1) (silica source), 40 mg
- Vitamin D_3, 400 IU
- Folic acid, 200 IU
- TMG, 100 mg
- Vitamin B_6,15 mg

The recommended dose for women is 6 capsules a day. Healthy men should take 4 capsules a day. It is best to take calcium supplements with meals. While certain fibers such as wheat bran, psyllium, guar gum, and pectin can interfere with mineral absorption, calcium absorbs better with meals. The recommended dosage of a product like Bone Assure would be 2 capsules at lunch, dinner, and at bedtime.

Recent investigations and clinical studies suggest that essential fatty acids and antioxidant nutrients influence bone formation. In animals, bone modeling appears to be optimal when omega-3 and omega-6 fatty acids are supplied in the diet. These studies support the role that dietary fatty acids and antioxidants play in reducing the severity of diseases involving bone-density loss. Vitamin E was reported to increase bone-formation rate and to restore collagen synthesis. Daily supplementation with six 1000-mg capsules of perilla oil or 1 tablespoon of flax-seed oil a day will provide omega-3 fatty acids. Omega-6 can be obtained from borage or black currant–seed oils.

Vitamin K

One of the most scrutinized groups ever is the 85,000 female nurses who took part in "The Nurses Health Study." Researchers have been tracking the eating habits and health histories of these women since 1980. One of the things they've looked at is which participants are more likely to break a bone. Fractures are the classic symptom of osteoporosis.

Since eating animal protein has been linked to osteoporosis, an analysis was undertaken to determine whether meat-eating had an adverse effect on the nurses' bone density. In 1996, researchers reported the results. Nurses who ate 3 ounces of meat or more per day had a significantly increased risk of forearm fracture compared to those who ate less than 2 ounces.

Diets with more vegetables and less meat are higher in vitamin K. A different set of researchers wanted to know if there is a relationship between vitamin K intake and hip fracture in the same nurses. Using 10 years' worth of data on 72,000 participants, they came to the conclusion that the nurses who got the most vitamin K were about a third less likely to get a hip fracture. Those who ate lettuce every day slashed their risk of hip fracture in half compared to those who ate it once a day or less (lettuce is a source of vitamin K). The significance of taking vitamin K was greater than taking synthetic estrogen, which didn't protect the nurses' bone density in this study. Nor did vitamin D. In fact, women who took a lot of vitamin D, but had low intakes of vitamin K, had a doubled risk of hip fracture! While vitamin D increases the amount of bone-friendly osteocalcin, only vitamin K can make it work properly.

Most osteoporosis studies are done on postmenopausal women because this group experiences a dramatic decline of bone density. Vitamin K shows remarkable results against bone loss in this population. In a study from the Netherlands, 1 mg of vitamin K per day for 2 weeks increased a bone-building protein (carboxylated Gla) 70–80% in postmenopausal women, restoring it to premenopausal range. Another study shows that vitamin K slows calcium loss by one-third in people who have a tendency to lose it (including men). In Japan, drugs containing vitamins K_1 and K_2 are being used to treat osteoporosis. The doses used in Japan are 45 mg a day. For prevention, the suggested dose is to take a vitamin K supplement that provides 8 mg of K_1 and 2 mg of K_2, i.e., 10 mg of vitamin K a day. To treat osteoporosis, doses up to 45 mg a day of vitamin K_1-K_2 should be used only if a physician monitors blood coagulation factors to make sure that the vitamin K is not causing blood to over-coagulate.

The Importance of Exercise

Exercise is an effective therapy for preventing and treating osteoporosis. Its importance cannot be overstated. A study was performed to evaluate the effectiveness of certain exercises for the treatment of postmenopausal osteoporosis. Both back extension and posture exercises lasting for 1 hour were undertaken twice a week, as well as fast walking exercises for 1 hour 3 times a week. At the end of the study, women who added exercise to their medical therapy increased spinal bone density by 4.4%, while women receiving only bone-restoring medicines showed an increase in spinal bone density of just 1.6%.

Severe Osteoporosis and Conventional Treatment

Calcitriol and calcitonin are FDA-approved drugs that can facilitate calcium absorption if vitamin D_3 is not effective. One study showed that the addition of calcitonin (administered intramuscularly) to calcium supplementation not only inhibited bone loss but significantly increased bone mass in fractured forearm bones. Another study showed that the drug calcitriol corrects the malabsorption of calcium. Higher amounts of vitamin D_3 have also been shown to normalize the calcium malabsorption that occurs as a result of aging. Patients taking calcitriol should be monitored for serum and urine calcium response to the drug. As is common with most FDA-approved drugs, dangerous side effects are a significant risk. Prescription of calcitriol for the treatment of osteoporosis should be reserved for physicians and their patients with a special interest in the treatment of metabolic bone disease. The taking of high doses (over 1100 IU a day) of vitamin D_3 should also be under physician supervision.

Severe Osteoporosis and Alternative Treatment

Instead of using potentially toxic FDA-approved drugs such as calcitriol and calcitonin to treat severe bone loss, European doctors have found that the bisphosphonate drug *clodronate* safely protects and restores bone density. In one study, the effectiveness of different clodronate regimens in postmenopausal osteoporosis was evaluated. Sixty women were randomly assigned to one of three treatments: oral calcium, 1000 mg/day; oral calcium plus oral clodronate, 400 mg/day; oral calcium plus oral clodronate, 400 mg/day for 30 days, followed by a 60-day period of calcium supplement alone. This last regimen was repeated 4 times in the 12-month study period. The results showed that patients who received calcium alone showed a decline in spinal bone mass, both after 6 and 12 months; femoral density in this group also decreased after 6 and 12 months. On the other hand, both clodronate-treated groups had increased levels of lumbar bone mass compared with controls, both after 6 and 12 months of therapy. At the end of the study, it was found that patients treated with cyclical clodronate had higher spinal bone mass compared with those treated continuously. After 6 months, femoral bone density was significantly higher in subjects treated with clodronate, both cyclically and continuously, compared with controls who only received calcium. Continuous clodronate treatment resulted in a clear fall in biochemical indices of bone degradation. The doctors concluded that 1-year treatment with clodronate induces a gain in bone mass, especially in the spine.

Another study on 60 women with postmenopausal bone loss showed that just 400 mg a day of clodronate taken by mouth produced a progressive and significant increase in lumbar bone density at both 6 and 12 months. In contrast, there was a progressive and significant decline of bone mineral density in untreated patients. The doctors concluded that cyclical low-dose clodronate therapy induced a gain in lumbar spine bone mass in patients with postmenopausal osteoporosis.

While the FDA has approved expensive drugs such as Fosamax (alendronate) that work in a similar way to clodronate, the side effects of these drugs can be severe, to the point of requiring hospitalization. Clodronate, on the other hand, is virtually free of side effects. The dose used to treat osteoporosis is 400 mg a day (about ¼ the dose used to treat cancer patients with bone metastasis). Blood tests to measure serum calcium levels and kidney function should be done 10 days after initiating clodronate therapy and then every 1 to 2 months thereafter. The concern for a small minority of people is that clodronate will cause too much calcium to be pulled from the blood. Regular blood testing will detect a serum calcium deficit. One study warns against taking clodronate in those suffering from severe renal insufficiency. The kidneys normally remove excess clodronate, and dialysis may not efficiently remove clodronate from the blood. Another study encourages clodronate to be used in renal disease when hypercalcemia is present. Regular blood tests can detect kidney problems early, though clodronate does not appear to cause kidney disease in and of itself. Do not use clodronate if pregnant because it could adversely affect calcium metabolism in the fetus. Clodronate is banned by the FDA, despite its extraordinary 15-year track record for safety and efficacy.

For those with severe osteoporosis, higher amounts of calcium and vitamin D_3 may be required, along with a 6-month regimen of growth hormone–replacement therapy. A parathyroid hormone (PTH) test must be performed to see if calcium is leaving the bones—that is, if the process of bone demineralization is occurring. An elevated parathyroid hormone level indicates the possibility of osteoporosis, secondary to calcium deficiency.

Osteoporosis and Men

It is important for men to utilize the same nutritional guidelines as women. Attention to testosterone level is especially important. DHEA and melatonin may be helpful in men as well. In some cases a consideration for the use of some progesterone should be made. Lastly, the importance of exercise cannot be overemphasized. This should be done under the care of a physician, especially for men with a history of prostate cancer.

Chelation Therapy

Chelation therapy is a nonconventional treatment not yet approved by the FDA for treating atherosclerosis and a number of other diseases. Chelation therapy is available in the United States because the primary ingredient, EDTA, has been approved by the FDA for other uses. In an article by Rudolph, McDonagh, and Wussow, published in the *Journal of Advancement in Medicine* in 1988, chelation therapy was found to increase bone mineral density. The mechanism is believed to be the pulsing of the hormone, parathormone, which is made by the parathyroid glands and is essential in calcium metabolism. This pulsing probably results in deposition of calcium in the bones.

Toxins

There is ample evidence that fluoride found in drinking water and toothpaste may contribute to bone destruction. The use of properly filtered water and toothpaste without fluoride is recommended.

Summary

The prevention and treatment of osteoporosis depends largely upon several factors:

1. Proper nutritional supplementation with vitamins and minerals, in particular calcium. Six capsules a day of Bone Assure provide the ideal dosages and forms of calcium, magnesium, zinc, manganese, and vitamin D_3.
2. Exercise (weight bearing).
3. Supplemental DHEA (*see DHEA Replacement Therapy protocol*) and melatonin.
4. Consumption of soy extract, providing 110 mg of soy isoflavins.
5. Application of progesterone cream by women according to the dosage directions included in this protocol.

6. Consider hormone replacement for women: natural estrogens, progesterone, and testosterone (oral or implant).
7. Consider hormone replacement for men: testosterone and progesterone.
8. Consider chelation therapy.
9. Consider clodronate.
10. Consider taking 10 mg a day of vitamin K for prevention. Do not take vitamin K if you are taking coumadin or other anticoagulant medication. For treatment, take up to 45 mg a day under the care of a physician who monitors blood coagulation factors.

Conclusion

Osteoporosis is a progressive reduction in bone mineral density that can be corrected by the proper use of nutrients, hormones, and exercise that will promote overall health and reduce the risk of numerous other diseases. Bone loss resulting from causes other than aging is very often difficult to reverse without addressing the underlying cause. This is particularly true for patients who are on anti-inflammatory steroids for chronic conditions, because the bone loss is a side effect of the drug itself. Conventional medicine has for years emphasized the role of estrogen in preventing osteoporosis. Physicians were largely unaware of the fact that progesterone is more important than estrogen for preventing and treating osteoporosis. Our current knowledge is based largely on the work of Dr. John Lee. (*Readers are referred to the Female Hormone Replacement Therapy protocol or the Life Extension Web site at www.lef.org for more details regarding current thinking relating to both proper estrogen and progesterone therapy.*)

For more information. Contact the National Osteoporosis Foundation, (800) 223-9994.

Product availability. Progesterone cream, DHEA, pregnenolone, natural estrogen, Mineral Formula for Women, vitamin D_3, Life Extension Mix, and melatonin can be obtained by calling (800) 544-4440, or order online at www.lef.org. Ask for information on blood testing. If you need growth hormone–replacement therapy, ask for doctors who have expertise in this area.

PAIN

Pain is a major problem in this country, costing an annual $4 billion in pain medications, surgeries, and other treatments. More than 70 million Americans suffer from back pain; nearly 40 million are tortured by arthritis; and more than 20 million people struggle with the agony of migraine headaches.

But it's not just pain that's the problem. The side effects of chronic pain—illnesses caused by a sedentary lifestyle, seclusion, depression, and, in many cases, addiction to pain killers—can be just as devastating as the pain itself.

The Life Extension Foundation's fundamental protocol for pain management is to eradicate the underlying cause of chronic pain. You should, therefore, first consider the specific condition causing your pain (such as arthritis, for example) and refer to the protocol for that condition.

All pain, whether chronic or acute, physical or emotional, is recognized, interpreted, and acted on by the brain. We may "feel" the pain in our toes when we stub them, but the recognition, interpretation, and reaction to the pain occur in the brain.

Here's how it happens: Sensory neurons—special nerves throughout the body—react to pressure, mechanical trauma, heat, cold, and other stimuli. They also respond to prostaglandins, histamine, and other chemicals released by injured or inflamed body tissue. Whether sensory neurons are stimulated depends on how powerful, prolonged, and widespread the heat, pressure, or other stimuli are. When sensory neurons are stimulated, the nerves "fire," sending off messages that travel along the nervous system to the brain. There, the pain information is rapidly evaluated and orders are issued: "Yank the hand off the burning stove!" or "Stop smashing the hammer on your thumb!"

Acute Versus Chronic Pain

As a rule of thumb, doctors know how to treat acute pain well, but are not very good at helping people who suffer from chronic pain. That's because the cause of acute pain is often clear and easy to find, while the cause of chronic pain can baffle teams of specialists.

Acute pain is the pain that tells you something is harming, or about to harm, your body. Acute pain lets out a three-alarm warning when you accidentally put your hand on a hot stove, makes you rush to the hospital when your appendix is about to rupture, or forces you to leap to your feet when you sit on a thumbtack.

Chronic pain may be a dull ache that never goes away, a vise squeezing our heads, a sword piercing our abdomens every time we move a certain way, a sharp knife stabbing our backs, a hammer smashing our hips with every step. Chronic pain seems to have no reason for being, other than to vex us.

Sometimes we can determine the causes of chronic pain—cancer of the pancreas, for example, which has spread to the back. But often we're puzzled because the original condition has healed and the pain should have vanished.

Modern medicine has devised many methods of attacking pain. Doctors have pain-killing medicines, sedatives, antidepressants, muscle relaxants, and anticonvulsants. They can inject substances into the body to "block" the nerves and prevent transmission of pain signals to the brain, and they often perform surgery, especially on those with back pain. But none of those approaches is 100% successful and safe.

Pain Medicines

Practically every medicine chest in the country has at least one non-prescription drug for pain purchased over the counter in a drugstore supermarket. They're commonly taken without much regard for their possible side effects. But every medicine has potential side effects, which can appear even if you take it only once. Even those that don't cause an immediate reaction can slowly but surely harm the body if taken over a long time, or if mixed with the wrong medicines. Here are just a few of the most popular pain medicines:

Aspirin. This inexpensive drug has helped countless people with routine aches and pains, as well as others suffering from more serious ailments such as rheumatoid arthritis and osteoarthritis. But even this seemingly harmless pill has many potential side effects, including heartburn, nausea, vomiting, ringing in the ears, loss of hearing, hives, and itching. Other side effects include vomiting blood, blood in the urine or stool, drowsiness, confusion, loss of vision, and jaundice. Aspirin should be avoided by many people, including those with a bleeding disorder, ulcers, gout, asthma, liver or kidney disease, women who are pregnant or breast feeding, and anyone soon to undergo surgery. Neither should you take aspirin if you are taking blood-thinning medications for prevention or treatment of stroke, heart attack, atrial fibrillation, or blood clot. And if you are on long-term aspirin therapy, you must have your blood tested regularly by a physician to make sure the medicine is not harming your liver.

Aspirin can also cause trouble if mixed with other substances. For example, taking aspirin and alcohol increases the chances of bleeding from the gastrointestinal tract. Aspirin can also displace certain drugs from their binding sites on protein, making them less effective. Drugs that should not be taken with aspirin include tolbutamide/chlorpropamide for diabetes; commonly used nonsteroidal anti-inflammatory medicines; methotrexate, which is used to depress the immune systems of rheumatoid arthritis patients; phenytoin, which is used to control epileptic seizures; and heparin, which is used to thin the blood in the treatment of blood clots.

Acetaminophen. This is effective treatment for moderate pain and fever, but it does not act against inflammation, swelling, or redness. Potential side effects include trembling, light-headedness, fatigue, itching, fever, sore throat, unexplained bruises or bleeding, blood in the urine, and pain in the side or lower back. Long-term use may cause anemia, along with liver and kidney damage. Acetaminophen causes massive free radical damage to the liver that can be ameliorated with nutrients like *N*-acetyl-cysteine (NAC). Anyone taking acetaminophen should take 600 mg of NAC, along with 2000 mg of vitamin C, and 100 to 400 IU of vitamin E with each dose.

Nonsteroidal Anti-Inflammatory Drugs. Called NSAIDs, these are used for pain, stiffness, and swelling of the joints, and for painful menstrual periods. Potential side effects include stomach pains, gastritis, peptic ulcers, gastrointestinal bleeding, headaches, nausea, dizziness, depression, drowsiness, ringing in the ear, vomiting, diarrhea, cramps, convulsions, blood in the urine and stool, chest tightness, rapid heartbeat, fainting, and chills. Ironically, these medicines can actually cause pain, the very thing they are taken to eliminate.

NSAIDs should not be taken by anyone who has asthma, bleeding problems, heart failure, elevated blood pressure, peptic ulcer disease, ulcerative colitis, and a number of other diseases. Long-term use can damage the eyes and ears, and cause weight gain.

The more powerful pain medicines that you can only get with a doctor's prescription have worked well in blocking certain types of pain for limited periods. However, they also have their shortcomings and side effects.

Indocin. Used for arthritis and other ailments, this powerful drug quells pain and inflammation. But potential side effects include nausea, vomiting, diarrhea, constipation, pain in the abdomen, gas, ulcers, rectal bleeding, headaches, dizziness, depression, fatigue, anxiety, insomnia, confusion, fainting, blurred vision, deafness, vaginal bleeding, asthma, weight gain, irregular heartbeat, high blood pressure, chest pain, and even coma.

Talwin. A synthetic, addicting narcotic often prescribed for moderate pain, Talwin can cause nausea, vomiting, anorexia, diarrhea, dizziness, hallucinations, headaches, confusion, insomnia, fainting, sweating, chills, rash, lowered blood pressure, irregular heartbeat, and other problems.

Percodan. Doctors were handing out this pain medication freely in the 1950s. Then the government stepped in to discourage over-prescribing because too many patients were becoming addicted to the drug. Percodan's side effects include dizziness, nausea, vomiting, constipation, and sedation.

Limitations of Surgery

Surgery can be an excellent means of curing many types of pain. If the distress is caused by a tumor pressing down on a nerve or a broken bone, for example, surgery can often solve the problem by either removing the growth or helping to "knit" the bone. But surgery is not as effective as many surgeons claim.

Surgery is a questionable treatment for chronic pain because no one knows what the surgeon should do once the patient's body has been opened up on the operating table. If the patient has back pain, should you take out the disc with the slight bulge? Maybe/maybe not.

Surgical residents operate on the "3F" policy: Find it; fix it; forget it. Their motto is "When in doubt, cut it out."

As for surgery's side effects, any time a patient is cut into there is the risk of infection, excessive bleeding, shock, and even death. Every time people are put under general anesthetic for surgery, they run many risks, including allergic reactions to anesthetic drugs, coma, and death. There is no such thing as risk-free surgery.

Nerve Blocks

One of the most important tools for diagnosing and treating certain types of chronic pain is the nerve block (neural blockage). Doctors inject a local anesthetic or other drug to "block" nerve function in a specific area, thus temporarily stopping the pain message from flowing up to the brain.

However, after ascertaining that the procedure works, many doctors will make the nerve block permanent by injecting alcohol or another drug that destroys the nerve's ability to function.

Almost any nerve or nerve root can be found and blocked, producing at least temporary relief. But nerve blocks are not always the answer, because in blocking the pain, doctors also block the nerve's usefulness. If, for example, a nerve that helps us to move a finger is blocked, we can't use that finger.

Fighting Pain Naturally

Some people find that boosting brain levels of endorphins can provide natural pain suppression. This approach isn't an effective way of dealing with acute (short-term severe) pain but it is the safest method of alleviating chronic (long-lasting) pain.

Early in the 1970s, researchers at the Johns Hopkins University School of Medicine wrestled with a baffling puzzle. They had just proved that morphine, the powerful pain-killing drug, fits perfectly into special receptors in brain cells, just as a key slips into a lock. The brain receptors were just the right size and shape for the morphine "keys," suggesting that the human brain had been designed to work with morphine, allowing it to "unlock," enter, and control parts of the brain.

Why would the human brain have evolved receptors specifically designed for morphine? After all, morphine is made by plants, not by the human body. It's not supposed to be inside of humans, and rarely gets there. Most of us go through life without ever taking it.

The researchers theorized that if there were receptors for morphine in the brain, then there had to be morphine—or a morphine-like substance—somewhere in the body. But what was it? Where was it? And what did it do?

The puzzle was solved when the first components of the human body's natural, morphine-like substances were discovered. They were called endorphins (endogenous morphine) and, like the drug, they are powerful pain killers that can alter mood. In fact, studies have proved that an endorphin called beta-endorphin is up to 50 times better at quelling pain than morphine, which was the most powerful pain killer previously known.

Endorphins are part of the body's natural pain-control network. They work by interfering with pain messages traveling through the nervous system. Endorphins cut off the pain message, stopping it dead in its tracks. Unfortunately, we can't use the endorphins themselves as pain killers. Taking "endorphin pills" or injecting endorphins into the body is inefficient, costly, impractical, and potentially dangerous.

Supplements That Fight Pain

Fortunately, we don't have to take endorphins in order to enjoy their pain-killing benefits. Instead, we can use natural substances that protect or boost the endorphins in our bodies, allowing their levels to rise to higher, more powerful levels. Here are some of the supplements you may want to consider if you suffer from chronic pain:

Tyrosine. Tyrosine is a nonessential amino acid that is manufactured by the body or absorbed from food. The body uses tyrosine to make the neurotransmitters dopamine, norepinephrine, and epinephrine, all of which play a role in elevating mood and keeping us alert. Suggested dose: 500 mg, two to three times a day.

Phenylalanine. Like other amino acids, this one comes in "d" and "l" (right and left) forms. The difference between the forms is like the difference between your hands. They're identical but opposite, mirror images of each other. The "left-handed" form is known as l-phenylalanine, or LPA. This is the form in which phenylalanine is normally found in foods. The "right-handed" form is known as d-phenylalanine, or DPA. This is the form that protects endorphins in our bodies and helps us to fight pain and depression. A mixture of the two forms, which has been used to fight pain since 1978, is known as dl-phenylalanine, or DLPA.

Phenylalanine protects our endorphins. It has helped many people overcome pain, as well as the depression that often accompanies chronic pain. Three of the ten patients in the original study of phenylalanine's effects on pain reported significant relief. It has also proved effective against painful inflammation.

Phenylalanine is not a drug, and it does not work directly against pain. Instead, it acts as an "endorphin shield," battling pain indirectly by helping the body's built-in pain-control system grow more powerful.

Phenylalanine was first tested against pain in a 1978 study at the Chicago Medical School. Researchers began by timing how long laboratory mice would remain on a hot plate before jumping off. Then they injected hundreds of mice with phenylalanine and again watched to see how long the mice would remain on the heated surface before scurrying off.

The amino acid blocked pain in 70% of the mice, allowing them to stay on the hot surface longer. The pain-blocking action actually grew stronger with time. Standard medicines tend to become less effective over time, as the body grows accustomed to them, but phenylalanine was actually more effective on the ninth day than it was on the first. And there was more good news. Phenylalanine worked with other medicines, making them stronger, and did all this without any apparent side effects.

Excited by these surprisingly positive results, the Chicago scientists tested phenylalanine on humans. The results were astounding. Ten patients suffering from long-standing chronic pain—people who had not been helped by modern medicine—found relief with this simple amino acid. Phenylalanine relieved chronic pain that had not been helped by conventional methods. There were no harmful side effects, and no one became addicted (as can be the case with powerful pain medicines). Also, no one developed a tolerance to phenylalanine, requiring larger and larger doses to get the same effect, as is often the case with conventional pain drugs.

Further research supported the early promising results. In one landmark study, 43 patients suffering from various types of severe pain were given 250 mg of phenylalanine four times a day. Some of the patients reported marked relief within one week. But by the end of the fourth week, 75% of the patients said their pain had been relieved.

In Great Britain, a double-blind controlled study was undertaken to determine whether the amino acid really worked or whether the pain relief reported in other studies was caused by the so-called placebo effect. It's well known that the power of belief can act as a medicine. Thus, if you give people pills that contain no medicine but tell them that the pills are powerful drugs, many patients will get better.

The participants in this study were adults suffering from long-standing, intractable pain of varied causes that had not been cured by conventional drugs or physical therapy. Despite the fact that lower doses of the substance were given and a 50% reduction in pain was required to qualify as improvement, more than 30% of the participants enjoyed significant relief. Phenylalanine outperformed the placebo, showing that it is, indeed, a powerful medicine.

There are some people, however, who cannot use phenylalanine. This includes those born with a genetic deficiency called phenylketonuria (PKU) that prevents them from metabolizing phenylalanine; those with pre-existing high blood pressure (phenylalanine can elevate blood pressure in people who are already hypertensive); and people with cancer (phenylalanine can promote cancer-cell division).

Although phenylalanine is a powerful pain killer, it does not begin to work as rapidly as aspirin and other pain medications. This is because the amino acid helps to increase the body's supply of endorphins, rather than attacking pain directly. Strengthening the body's natural pain-control mechanisms is a very effective strategy, but it takes time to begin working. For headaches and other acute pain, people naturally prefer the instant pain relief they get from aspirin and other conventional medications.

What about chronic pain that does not respond to standard medicines, physical therapy, or surgery? Phenylalanine has ample time to begin working in such cases, so why isn't it used more? Because for drug companies, phenylalanine isn't profitable. It's a simple amino acid that cannot be patented. Thus, most doctors know that phenylalanine is an amino acid, but have never heard of its powerful antipain properties, because no drug companies promote it.

Suggested dose: 500 mg, 2 to 3 times a day.

Bovine cartilage. Connective tissue taken from cows contains several molecular biodirectors that help to repair cells and keep the body's chemistry properly balanced. Thanks to these and other properties, bovine cartilage is emerging as an exciting and effective treatment for pain caused by arthritis, psoriasis, cancer, and other ailments.

Bovine cartilage was used in a study on nine people whose symptoms were rated as "severe." Daily injections of bovine cartilage were given during the first phase of the study, then booster shots every several weeks thereafter. The results were

P

"astonishingly good." A third of the patients went from "severe" to "excellent," and the other two-thirds moved from "severe" to "good" ratings.

Bovine cartilage was also put to the test against osteoarthritis. In a double-blind study involving 194 patients, average pain scores fell by 50%. In another study, 28 patients suffering from osteoarthritis were given injections of bovine cartilage. Within 3 to 8 weeks, 19 reported excellent results, 6 had good results, and 2 experienced fair results. Only one failed to improve. Most impressively, the relief lasted for as long as 6 weeks to a year.

Although standard dosages have not yet been established, taking 9 g of bovine cartilage per day, in three divided doses, has helped many people.

SOD (Superoxide Dismutase). This enzyme produced by the body fights off dangerous oxidants and free radicals. Unfortunately, the body's ability to manufacture this important antioxidant decreases as we age, increasing the odds that oxidation and free radicals will attack the joints causing pain, stiffness, swelling, and other signs of arthritis. SOD has been available in supplement form for some time, but was not well absorbed by the body. Newer forms of SOD show promise of being absorbed and utilized by the body. For now, however, it may be best to eat a healthy diet, which contains all the building blocks the body needs to manufacture SOD.

Glucosamine. Found in fish, meat, and other foods, this amino acid is particularly helpful in treating arthritis pain because it stimulates connective tissue, encouraging it to repair itself. Glucosamine is chondroprotective, which means that it protects the chondrocytes, which are found in large quantities in the joints.

Glucosamine is made in the body from glucose (sugar) and an amino acid called glutamine. Glucosamine serves as a building block of MPS (mucopolysaccharides), which are important for the development of cartilage, bone, ligaments, nails, hair, and skin. We can also get glucosamine from supplements.

As we get older, or when we are injured, the body produces less glucosamine. This is odd, for you would think that the body would produce more in order to repair the injury. Unfortunately, small injuries that are not repaired can lead to greater damage and pain. Taking glucosamine gives the body the material it needs to help repair damaged cartilage. Some doctors have found that it works best when taken with GLA, DHA, EPA, chondroitin sulfate, manganese, vitamin C, and vitamin E.

Many studies have shown glucosamine to be a potent natural remedy for osteoarthritis, which seems to strike so many of us as we age. It also opposes the degeneration of the ground substance of the joints, which occurs in arthritis. Several studies conducted at research centers in Europe have shown that supplemental glucosamine reduces joint pain, tenderness, and swelling, making joints that had been "frozen" with pain and inflammation usable again.

Glucosamine did not work as fast as some standard pain medications, but it did so without the serious side effects associated with drugs. In fact, many European physicians are now giving glucosamine to their osteoarthritis patients as a first-line treatment, turning to drugs only in cases where the amino acid is not effective.

Glucosamine appears to be even more effective in the form of glucosamine sulfate. Like glucosamine, sulfate is a component of joint cartilage. The sulfate also appears to strengthen glucosamine's healing effects. Let's look at some of the studies on glucosamine sulfate.

Twenty-four patients with osteoarthritis of the knee were given either 500 mg of glucosamine sulfate 3 times a day, or a placebo. Within 6 to 8 weeks, those receiving the glucosamine sulfate enjoyed significant reductions in pain, joint tenderness, and swelling. There were no reported side effects.

Eighty osteoarthritis patients suffering from pain, movement restriction, and swelling were given either glucosamine sulfate or a placebo. Seventy-three percent of those receiving the glucosamine sulfate enjoyed an improvement in symptoms within 3 weeks. What's more, when those who received the glucosamine sulfate were biopsied and their cartilage was examined under an electron microscope, it looked much healthier than the cartilage taken from the placebo group.

Glucosamine sulfate was compared to ibuprofen in a double-blind study involving 40 patients with osteoarthritis of the knee. As expected, the drug worked faster. But, by the eighth week, those taking the glucosamine sulfate were doing better than those on the drug, with significantly fewer complaints. If you take glucosamine sulfate, follow label directions on the bottle.

Chondroitin sulfate. Chondroitin sulfate provides building materials for the cartilage, which is so often damaged in arthritis. Chondroitin sulfate slows the free radicals that attack the cartilage in joints. It also increases the flow of blood to joints, allowing antioxidants and other healing substances produced by the body to protect and repair body tissue. When arthritis patients were given injections of chondroitin sulfates, joint pain diminished significantly while mobility and function returned.

Chondroitin sulfate is found in shark cartilage. Shark cartilage made the headlines some years ago when researchers began reporting that it might be a new treatment for cancer. It seems that sharks rarely get cancer, even if exposed to tremendous doses of cancer-causing substances. Tumors force the body to create vast networks of new blood vessels to "feed" the hungry cancer cells. Shark cartilage appears to block cancer by preventing development of these new blood vessels. Because inappropriate growth of blood vessels into joint cartilage is thought to be a cause of arthritis symptoms, scientists wondered if shark cartilage would also be helpful for arthritis patients. Let's look at just two of the studies confirming their belief:

- Six osteoarthritis patients who had not found relief with conventional anti-inflammatory medications were given shark cartilage capsules. By the fourth week, they reported less pain and inflammation, and greater joint mobility.
- One hundred forty-seven patients suffering from osteoarthritis were given either cartilage extracts or a placebo in another long-term, double-blind study. Five years later, average pain scores had fallen by 85% in the cartilage group, compared with only 5% in those receiving the placebo. The cartilage group also had less joint deterioration and took significantly less time off work. If you try chondroitin sulfate, follow directions on the label.

Melatonin. This hormone is a potential therapy for treatment of diseases with pain and abnormal immune responses. The effects and mechanisms of melatonin on inflammation and immunoregulation have been studied systematically. Melatonin showed significant analgesic effects in animal studies. Melatonin was also shown to enhance the pain-suppressing effects of analgesics.

Further studies showed that melatonin could enhance the functions of T and B lymphocytes and macrophages *in vitro* and in adjuvant (assisting) arthritis treatment. In animal studies, melatonin was shown to inhibit swelling.

These factors suggest that melatonin possesses marked anti-inflammatory, immunoregulatory, and analgesic effects that may be related to the system of opiate modulation. Use melatonin cautiously when treating autoimmune diseases such as rheumatoid arthritis. Some scientists speculate that melatonin could worsen the severity of autoimmune diseases.

For night-time pain relief, 3 to10 mg of melatonin should be taken before bedtime. Melatonin should be used only at night before bedtime, not during the day.

Refer to the *Migraine protocol* for more information on melatonin's pain-relieving properties. Also refer to the *Arthritis* or *Fibromyalgia protocols* if these diseases are an underlying cause of your pain.

Vitamins That Fight Pain

Vitamins and antioxidants can help to reduce pain in many people. Like many things in life, the oxygen we breathe is both good and bad. On the one hand, oxygen is a nutrient gobbled up by every cell in the body. Without oxygen, we would quickly die. On the other hand, oxygen is a highly reactive substance that can do quite a bit of damage. We know what oxygen can do to metal: it causes it to rust. Uncontrolled, oxygen can do something equally dangerous to our body cells and tissues.

Oxygen appears in different "packets." The oxygen we breathe is composed of two oxygen molecules attached to each other. But other, highly toxic packets of single oxygen molecules called oxidants also appear in the body and can cause trouble. These are created as byproducts of bodily functions, but may also be inhaled, or taken in when we are exposed to drugs, pesticides, certain foods, cigarette smoke, and air pollution. If not carefully controlled by antioxidants, these oxidants would shove their way through the body, "rusting" substances in cells and tissues.

As more and more "rust spots" appear, the body's ability to function, heal itself, and fend off disease begins to falter. Little by little, the immune system, circulatory system, and nervous system weaken.

There are certain oxidants called free radicals, which are unstable molecules. Desperately seeking to "balance" themselves, free radicals steal electrons from other molecules. Setting up a chain reaction of electron stealing, free radicals can do irreparable damage to the body.

We have much to learn about oxidants; we haven't yet figured out all the ways they harm the body. But many researchers believe that oxidation is a major cause of many of the diseases associated with aging, including arthritis. And we know that oxidation can harm already damaged arthritic joints, as well as their surrounding tissue, making swelling and pain worse than ever.

The body maintains its own antioxidant "police force" to control oxidants. Superoxide dismutase (SOD), catalase, and glutathione peroxidase are three of our natural "oxidant cops." Unfortunately, our built-in antioxidant militia isn't always up to the task of protecting us, especially as we age or are subjected to various chemical substances. That's when antioxidant supplements, including vitamins, can be helpful.

One of the best antioxidant supplements is beta-carotene. Beta-carotene, which the body converts into vitamin A as necessary, is one of many carotenes found in carrots and other foods. Others are alpha-carotene, lycopene, zeaxanthin, lutein, and cryptoxanthin. The carotenes are useful in treating painful conditions, such as arthritis, that are associated with oxidation and free radicals. For chronic pain, some authorities recommend taking 25,000 IU (15 mg) of beta-carotene twice a day. Vitamins you may want to consider for treating pain include

Vitamin B_1 (riboflavin). This vitamin, also known as thiamin, is an overlooked source of pain relief. It is particularly helpful for patients with neuritis, shooting pains in the legs related to chronic liver disease or alcoholism, and diabetic neuropathy (nerve disease caused by diabetes), as well as nerve and joint pains associated with a B_1 deficiency.

In a study of B_1's efficacy, the vitamin was given to 133 people suffering from headaches, joint pain, nerve pain, or neuritis, which is pain caused by inflammation of the nerves. None of the patients had found relief with conventional pain pills or physical therapy. But when given 1 to 2 grams of B_1 once or twice daily, patients reported that 78% of headaches improved, and 71% of spine or joint pain improved; more than 62% of those with neuralgia reported relief.

Start with 25 mg of B_1 twice a day. Studies have shown that in order to get the best effect from water-soluble vitamins such as the B and C vitamins, they should be taken at least twice a day. You'll also find B_1 in almonds, whole grain wheat and oats, nuts, and beans.

Vitamin B_3. This vitamin contains niacinamide, a variation of niacin. It is a potent anti-arthritis supplement. In certain people, it may reduce pain and increase mobility in arthritic joints within 3 to 6 weeks. B_3's ability to make joints more mobile has been known for more than 40 years. In 1955, a study reported on 663 patients who, when given niacinamide, showed improved ability to move their joints (compared with 842 controls who did not receive the vitamin). Suggested dose: 500 mg taken three times a day.

Vitamin B_6 (pyridoxine). Although all vitamins are necessary for a fully functioning immune system, B_6 is the most important of the B vitamins. Vitamin B_6 has a special role to play in treating chronic pain. Pain patients tend to have lower pain thresholds, which means that they feel pain "sooner" than nonpain patients. In addition, they often have a smaller supply of the neurotransmitter serotonin.

Our body cells have special receptors, "parking spaces" where medicines "pull up" and interact with cells. But with long-term use of pain-killing medicines, the number of receptor sites for these drugs seems to diminish. This means that the medicines are less effective. Patients must take more and more pills, or else their pain will increase. And if they stop taking their medicines, they may suffer from severe "rebound" pain.

But if they are given B_6 as they are weaned from their medicines, they do much better. B_6 is also helpful in reducing the inflammatory component of arthritis. (In animals, B_6 deficiencies can even cause a version of human arthritis.) This vitamin has also been used successfully to treat the pain of carpal tunnel syndrome and unexplained, cyclical breast pain.

Although doses vary from person to person, many people find it helpful to take 20 mg of B_6 twice a day. The medical literature contains reports of neuritis and/or nerve damage caused by using large amounts (ranging from 1000 mg to 6000 mg per day) for long periods. There are also reports that certain susceptible people may develop neuritis from as little as 300 to 400 mg per day. Examine your vitamin and supplement combinations to ensure that you are not taking excessive doses. You can find B_6 in beans, brussels sprouts, cantaloupe, cauliflower, lentils, whole wheat, and rice.

Vitamin B_{12}. We normally associate the lack of B_{12} with pernicious anemia. It has shown powerful pain-killing abilities. In one study, 400 patients suffering from vertebral pain were given 5000 micrograms of B_{12} a day. Within 6 to 16 days, 50% of the patients were enjoying relief that they rated as "good" to "very good," and almost all of the remaining patients reported at least "satisfactory" results. Only 10 of the 400 said they felt no improvement at all. Larger doses of the vitamin have been used successfully to treat the pain of cancer and degenerative neuropathy. For chronic pain, some authorities recommend 500 micrograms of sublingual B_{12}, two or three times a day.

Vitamin C. This versatile immune-system booster and antioxidant is another natural shield against pain. When the pain becomes too strong for victims of breast cancer, and their usual medications aren't helping, giving vitamin C along with drugs sometimes quells the pain. The vitamin also has been used to treat gum and muscle pain. Start with 300 mg of supplemental vitamin C twice a day. Some people have taken as much as 1000 mg twice a day. Good food sources of vitamin C include broccoli, papaya, red peppers, oranges, cauliflower, and asparagus. In special cases, larger doses are suggested.

Vitamin E. Vitamin E has two possible ways of blocking pain: by working with endorphins, and as an antioxidant. A study of women with algomenorrhea (painful menstruation) found that E could reduce the discomfort and that endorphin levels rose. But when the women were given naloxone, a substance that blocks endorphins, the E lost its pain-killing power. This suggests that the vitamin and the morphine within are linked.

Vitamin E was put to the test in a double-blind study involving 50 patients with primary degenerative osteoarthrosis. The participants were given either vitamin E or a placebo (a sugar pill). Six weeks later, the vitamin E group reported less pain while moving or at rest, and less pain when their joints were subjected to pressure.

In another test of the vitamin's prowess against arthritis, 29 patients were given vitamin E for 10 days, and a placebo for another 10. (They didn't know which they were receiving at any given time.) Fifty-two percent reported relief from pain when they were on the vitamin, compared with only 4% on the placebo.

Some people take 200 to 400 IU of supplemental vitamin E, twice a day, in the form of *D*-alpha-tocopherol. This vitamin is also found in green leafy vegetables, green beans, seeds, broccoli, and nuts. Check all your supplements to make sure that your total vitamin E intake does not exceed 1200 IU per day, unless otherwise directed by your physician.

Minerals and Other Substances That Fight Pain

Studies show that a number of minerals also work to fight pain in many people. These include

Selenium. This antioxidant mineral works with vitamin E and other substances to control free-radical damage. It also has anti-inflammatory properties, which reduce pain. In combination with vitamin E, selenium works well against long-standing muscle pain, stiffness, and aching. Good sources of this mineral include whole grains, fish, and poultry. Selenium is also found in fruits and vegetables, but the amount varies, depending on how much of the mineral was present in the soil in which the food was grown. Up to 200 micrograms of supplemental selenium taken once a day can be helpful for controlling pain.

Magnesium. This mineral has been used to treat many painful states, especially headaches, with good results. When 3000 women who suffered from migraines were given 100 to 200 mg of magnesium, 80% reported a "good" response. The mineral is even more potent when mixed with B_6 and ascorbate (a form of vitamin C). Intravenous injections of the triple combination can substantially reduce or eliminate the pain of acute migraines in most cases.

Magnesium deficiencies have been linked to a variety of ailments. For example, a look at the blood of 26 women suffering from premenstrual tension found that they had less magnesium in their red blood cells than did control women.

You may take 250 mg of magnesium twice a day. Look on the label for elemental magnesium. Be sure to eat plenty of all-bran cereal, tofu, spinach, lima beans, and whole-grain pasta, which all contain magnesium.

Boron. Boron is a little-known mineral that plays an important role in bone health. We normally associate calcium with bones, and there is certainly more calcium in bones than boron. But boron acts as a "stop sign," helping to keep calcium in the body and in the bones. Studies comparing large populations in various countries have found that where there are higher amounts of boron in the soil (and thus presumably more of the mineral in foods), there is less osteoarthritis. And some clinicians have reported good results with boron supplements, which appear to relieve or almost completely eliminate the symptoms of osteoarthritis up to 90% of the time. You may take 3 mg a day, but don't exceed 9 to 10 mg a day.

Herbs That Fight Pain

Sometimes the best place to look for treatment is nature's pharmacy. Many plants have remarkable pain-reducing qualities. If you take herbs in supplement form, follow the directions on the label. To make herbal teas, steep 1 teaspoon of herb in 1 cup of hot water for 15 minutes. Here are some herbs that are useful for treating pain:

Ashwaganda has been used for many years to treat pain in Ayurvedic medicine. One to two cups of tea made from ashwaganda have been shown to reduce pain and inflammation. In a double-blind cross-over study, 42 patients with osteoarthritis who were given an herbal formula with ashwaganda and zinc showed a significant improvement in pain and stiffness.

CAUTION: In large doses, ashwaganda can be harmful. Discuss the use of ashwaganda with your physician, and do not drink more than the recommended doses.

Capsaicin, a chemical found in cayenne and other peppers, is a prime ingredient of over-the-counter and prescription antipain ointments. Rubbing it on the skin produces an immediate sensation of warmth. Capsaicin works by interfering with Substance P, a chemical messenger that transmits pain signals to the brain. Capsaicin can stop the pain of shingles, post-herpetic neuralgia, and diabetic nerve pain. Although mostly used as an ointment, it can be made into a tea or capsules. Drink one to two cups a day of tea.

Devil's claw comes from an African plant whose fruit bears a resemblance to a large, hooked claw. Tests conducted in 1958 at Germany's University of Jena found that devil's claw produces powerful anti-inflammatory effects. (At least two components of the plant, harpogoside and beta-sitosterol, have anti-inflammatory properties.) This makes devil's claw a pain killer, because reducing inflammation helps to relieve pain. More recent studies in Germany and France have found that the herb's ability to alleviate pain and inflammation compares well with that of the drugs cortisone and phenylbutazone. Although there is no official dosage for this herb, these amounts are usually helpful. Dried powdered root: 1 gram taken as a tea three times a day; tincture (1:5), 1 teaspoon three times a day; dry solid extract (3:1), 300 to 400 mg two to three times a day.

Feverfew is an herb that sprang to prominence in the late 1970s when newspapers in England carried reports of a woman whose headaches were cured by the herb. That anecdotal report was backed up by an article in a 1985 issue of the *British Medical Journal,* that described how eating feverfew leaves daily led to fewer and less severe migraine headaches in 70% of 270 cases. (Many of these were severe cases that had not responded to standard headache medications.) It's thought that feverfew counteracts headaches by inhibiting production of inflammation-causing substances in the body, and by helping to keep blood vessels supplying the head from being "squeezed down" on by vasoconstrictors. Take 25 mg twice a day. It is best to chew fresh leaves, if you can find them.

Ginger, commonly used to spice up foods, has anti-inflammatory and antipain effects. It has long been used to prevent and relieve migraine headaches. A versatile substance, ginger has also been used to treat headache, nausea, and vomiting. It is thought to have antioxidant and antidepressant properties as well. Add it to foods, brew it up in teas, or take capsules as directed.

Ginkgo biloba is an extract from the leaf of the ginkgo tree. It contains ginkgosides, which have anti-inflammatory and antipain properties. A good starting point for pain patients is to take 60 mg of ginkgo twice a day.

Green tea is a storehouse of beneficial, anti-inflammatory compounds called catechins. Because inflammation can cause pain, reducing inflammation often helps to reduce pain. Green tea also contains antioxidants that help the body to resist many diseases, including painful degenerative ailments associated with aging. Green tea suffers less processing than black tea, which means that it retains more of its catechins and possibly other beneficial compounds. It is worthwhile to drink 2 to 4 cups of green tea a day.

Horsetail is an ancient plant species containing silica alkaloids, saponins, flavonoids, phytosterols, tannins, and many minerals (including potassium, magnesium, and manganese). Horsetail has anti-inflammatory properties, making it effective against joint pain and stiffness. Take 1 to 2 capsules a day.

Licorice, which helps to reduce pain by controlling inflammation, has been used to treat arthritic pain and stiffness. Use caution when consuming this pleasant-tasting herb, which comes in capsules or as tea. Too much licorice can elevate your blood pressure. Those with high blood pressure or with a family history of high blood pressure, as well as pregnant women, should consult their physicians before taking licorice.

Primrose oil contains GLA (gamma linolenic acid), a substance capable of reducing inflammation. This helps to reduce the pain of active arthritis. Try taking a 250-mg capsule one to three times a day.

Pycnogenol is a compound of proanthocyanidins from the bark of the French maritime tree. Its extraordinary antioxidant properties are of value in reducing the inflammation associated with pain. For chronic pain, start with 100 mg, twice a day, for four to six months; then reduce the dosage by half.

Turmeric (curcumin) is a root that is used to add color and flavor to curry and other foods. Because it has anti-inflammatory properties, it has been used to combat the pain and swelling of arthritis. (Some researchers think that it is as powerful an anti-inflammatory as cortisone.) Turmeric may also help to lower cholesterol, reduce the risk of heart disease and stroke by "thinning" the blood to prevent unnecessary blood clots, lower blood sugar in diabetics, and help the body to counteract carcinogens. Doctors of Oriental Medicine also use the herb to treat colic, menstrual cramping, and shoulder pain. Many pain patients find it helpful to take 250 mg between breakfast and lunch, and an additional 250 mg between lunch and dinner.

Yucca. An average of 2 grams of yucca leaves in capsule form, taken three times a day, is helpful. Yucca has long been used by both traditional and modern healers to combat the symptoms of arthritis. In a study reported in the

Journal of Applied Nutrition, 149 arthritis patients were given either saponin (a substance extracted from yucca) or a placebo. Sixty-one percent of those who took the saponin reported less pain, swelling, and stiffness, compared with only 22% who took the placebo. This herb may be used in either tea or capsule form.

Foods That Fight Pain

Until recently, most people didn't think food had much to do with pain. Many physicians still don't see the connection, but little by little, doctors are realizing that there is often a connection between pain and what we eat.

We now know that certain foods and substances in foods can help to "heat up" or "cool down" inflammation. A good example is the link between high-protein diets and gouty arthritis.

The American diet is typically low in several nutrients. Deficiencies of many vitamins and minerals, including vitamins B_6, B_{12}, C, D, E, folic acid, selenium, magnesium, and zinc have been associated with arthritis. Even if the nutritional shortfalls don't cause the problem, they certainly don't help, and may make things worse.

The American diet is full of fat. When the very tiny blood vessels nourishing our joints fill with fat from our food, oxygen exchange is hampered and the body has difficulty removing waste products. As a result, body tissue may weaken or break down.

Certain foods, especially fats, can enhance or harm regulation of hormonal substances called eicosanoids. Eicosanoids are important to pain patients, because they help to control inflammation and pain, especially in the joints.

Certain foods may cause allergic reactions in some patients with rheumatoid arthritis, worsening their pain and other symptoms. Some forms of what we call rheumatoid arthritis may be what medical researchers call "allergic arthritis."

We react individually to foods, so it's impossible to issue blanket statements about which foods are "good" or "bad." Milk and other dairy products commonly cause problems for pain patients. Excessive fat seems to increase the levels of inflammatory substances in the body. Meat is also filled with substances that can trigger allergies. The chemicals given to animals bred for consumption tend to concentrate in fatty tissue. Bacon, hot dogs, ham, bologna, cold cuts, and other cured meats have preservatives and other chemicals that can trigger allergic reactions.

But there are foods that can reduce pain as well. Propolis, a substance found in honey, for example, blocks certain hormone-like substances called prostaglandins, which can cause pain and swelling.

Switching to a highly nutritious, low-fat, low-protein diet has helped many patients reduce or banish their pain. And it helps them to reduce or eliminate the need for their drugs as well. In general, pain patients should

- Eat a wide variety of foods—the more the better—because each food contains a unique formula of nutrients. Although there is no perfect food, a diet based on many fresh vegetables and fruits, plus a variety of whole grains, comes close to perfection.
- Think of the diet as a pyramid. The widest part of the pyramid, the foundation, is made up of fresh vegetables, fruits, and whole grains. On top of that, add smaller amounts of fish, low-fat dairy products, lean poultry, nuts, and seeds. At the top of the pyramid are the snack foods and desserts. Eat only tiny amounts of them.
- Eat as many "real" foods as possible. Take a look at your shopping cart as you roll it up to the checkout stand. Is it filled with boxes and cans, or do you see mostly fresh foods? Fresh foods should predominate.
- Avoid food additives, which are found mostly in packaged foods. And when you do select packaged foods, compare labels carefully, looking for those with the fewest additives.
- Keep your sugar consumption low. Nature has already packed inside its foods as much sugar as your body needs. Everything else that is added is debris that our bodies must remove. A little added sugar won't harm most of us. But a lot will hurt many of us.

- ▼ Don't add salt to your foods. Excess salt has a number of bad effects, and nature has already put plenty of salt in food. Extra salt, which is common in packaged foods, means extra work for your body.
- ▼ As much as possible, eat your meals at home, where you have control over your food intake.
- ▼ Snack frequently on low-fat foods to blunt your appetite so that you won't gorge yourself when you sit down at the dinner table. Snacking also helps to keep your blood sugar reasonably stable throughout the day. Carry a plastic bag filled with raw or cooked vegetables, and snack liberally on them throughout the day.
- ▼ Avoid large meals within several hours of going to sleep. It's not healthy, and more food will be stored as fat because you won't be burning the calories as quickly as you would if you were moving around.
- ▼ Eat slowly. Enjoy your food. Savor it. Give your appetite center time to tell you that you've had enough before you've had too much. Put down your fork or spoon while you are chewing. Don't overeat. Eat until you are comfortably full (but not stuffed), and then stop. If you're not hungry, don't eat. Let your stomach guide you, not the clock.
- ▼ Drink plenty of water, at least six to eight 8-ounce glasses of plain water a day.
- ▼ Keep fat consumption within healthful limits. Most vegetables, fruits, and whole grains are low in fat. It is only if you eat lots of processed and other high-fat foods that you're overloading your body with fat.

Go easy on snack foods, processed foods, and other foods with added fats. Excessive consumption of fat has been associated with heart disease, cancer, and many other deadly and disabling diseases. Fatty foods certainly can be tasty, but you'd be surprised how quickly you can lose your fat cravings once you set fatty foods aside.

Fatty Acids as Pain Fighters

There are, however, some types of fat that actually may help to reduce pain. Just as protein is built from amino acids, fats in the body are composed of smaller substances called fatty acids. You may have heard of the omega-3 fatty acids, which have generated a great deal of excitement in the scientific community. In the early 1970s, Danish scientists noted that Eskimos in Greenland ate a high-fat diet based on fatty fish, seal, and whale meat, but had relatively little heart disease. The researchers quickly surmised that something in the fatty fish warded off heart disease by thinning the Eskimos' blood, lowering blood fat (triglyceride) levels, reducing total cholesterol, and possibly even lowering LDL (the "bad" cholesterol that deposits fat along artery walls). That magical something was a fat (oil) in the fish they ate. Specifically, it was a type of fat composed of omega-3 fatty acids.

Since then we have learned that the omega-3 fatty acids not only protect against heart disease, but also may help to fight off arthritis and other painful diseases. In a 1985 study, patients with rheumatoid arthritis enjoyed a definite decrease in joint stiffness, and less tenderness of the joints after 3 months of treatment. And giving fish oil to laboratory mice as a dietary supplement suppressed lupus, a potentially fatal autoimmune disease that most often attacks young women.

Studies in humans have shown that enriching the diet with fish oil has an anti-inflammatory effect. Part of omega-3's effectiveness may come from its ability to act on the immune system, cutting by at least half the secretion of immune system substances called cytokines, which are involved in pain.

Three fatty acids found in fish and other foods have special value in fighting pain. GLA (gamma-linolenic acid), DHA (docosahexaenoic acid), and EPA (eicosapentaenoic acid) are extremely important fatty acids obtained from fish, as well as from the seed of the evening primrose, black currant seed oil, and borage oil. The body uses GLA, DHA, and EPA to manufacture PG1 and other prostaglandins, which help to reduce inflammation and pain.

In a study reported in the *Annals of Internal Medicine,* patients underwent a double-blind, placebo-controlled protocol lasting 24 weeks. Neither the patients nor the doctors knew until the test was over who was receiving the "real thing" and who was getting a placebo. The study was designed this way to rule out the placebo effect, the well-known tendency of some people to feel better simply because they believe in their medicine. When the study was completed and the code was broken, revealing who had received the GLA, the researchers discovered that those who took GLA experienced a 36% reduction in tender joints, and 41% fewer swollen joints. Those who had received the placebo reported no such benefits.

A later study reported in the *British Journal of Rheumatology* used oil taken from black currant seeds, which contains both GLA and alpha-lipoic acid. The rheumatoid arthritis patients in this double-blind, placebo-controlled study who got the black currant oil experienced relief, but those getting the placebo did not. There were no side effects noted.

An article in *Seminars in Arthritis and Rheumatism* looked at many studies on GLA and rheumatoid arthritis. It reported that GLA was proven effective in reducing the effects that autoimmune disease can have on joint linings. A second article, in the *Journal of Clinical Epidemiology*, also looked at a number of previously published studies on fish oil and reported that a 3-month course of treatment with fish oil led to a substantial improvement in joint tenderness and morning stiffness.

Now take a brief look at some of the studies demonstrating EPA's and DHA's effectiveness against rheumatoid arthritis. Forty-nine patients with rheumatoid arthritis were given capsules containing either high or low doses of EPA and DHA or olive oil. The high-dose group enjoyed significant reductions in the number of swollen joints by week 12, and the number of tender joints by week 18. The number of tender joints also fell in the low-dose group by week 12, but it took 24 weeks for them to enjoy the drop in swollen joints. Overall, those receiving the high or low doses of EPA and DHA did better than those who got the olive oil.

In another study, a double-blind cross-over, 12 people suffering from rheumatoid arthritis were begun on either EPA and DHA daily. Midway through the study, patients getting the DPA and DHA were switched to the placebo without their knowledge, while those who had been taking the placebo were given the EPA and DHA. (The secret switch was made to make sure the EPA/DHA pills really worked.) The study showed that the EPA/DHA combination led to a significant improvement in the clinical signs of the disease.

Thirty-three rheumatoid arthritis victims were given either EPA and DHA, or a placebo. Fourteen weeks later, those getting the EPA/DHA combination had fewer tender joints. The pain-killing effect lasted for more than 4 weeks once the EPA/DHA was discontinued. This was a double-blind, controlled, cross-over study, the most scientifically rigorous and valid form.

In an interesting study mixing diet and EPA, 17 participants were asked to eat a diet low in saturated fat, high in polyunsaturated fat, and supplemented with MaxEPA capsules. A control group of 20 was instructed to eat the typical American diet and take placebo capsules. Twelve weeks later, those on the special diet and EPA capsules reported significantly less morning stiffness—which had gotten worse in those on the standard American diet. Unfortunately, when those eating the special diet and taking EPA returned to their normal diet and gave up the EPA, their pain and stiffness returned rapidly.

For additional information on pain-relieving therapies, refer to the specific protocol that discusses the underlying cause of your pain (e.g., Arthritis, Fibromyalgia).

Summary

The Life Extension Foundation's recommendation for pain management is to eradicate the underlying cause of chronic pain. You should, therefore, first consider the specific condition causing your pain and refer to the protocol for that condition. Chronic pain is often more difficult to diagnose and treat than acute pain. Many times an original condition has healed but the pain remains, for no apparent reason. Chronic pain sufferers should adopt a high-nutrition, low-fat diet to reduce pain and potentially eliminate the need for harsh medications. Natural supplements are also recommended for chronic pain sufferers in providing gentle relief from pain, inflammation, and stiffness.

For more information. Contact the National Chronic Pain Outreach Association, (301) 652-4948.

Product availability. Most natural pain supplements are available by calling (800) 544-4440, or order on-line at www.lef.org.

PANCREATIC CANCER PROTOCOL AND REFERRAL

Overview

Pancreatic cancer is the fifth leading cause of cancer mortality in the United States. The American Cancer Society estimates that 29,000 Americans died of the disease in 1998. Conventional medicine's inability to effectively treat pancreatic cancer is evidenced by survival rates of only 18% at 1 year and 4% at 5 years—one of the poorest 5-year survival rates of any cancer. There is evidence in the scientific literature that the proper combination of cell-differentiating agents and cytotoxic chemotherapy may slow the progression of pancreatic cancer. In order to have a realistic chance of achieving a significant remission, the use of experimental therapies is highly recommended. This article succinctly describes some of the promising new therapies currently being studied. (*A more detailed description can be found in the Molecular Oncology section of the Cancer [Adjuvant] Treatment protocol.*)

Therapeutic Strategies

About 90 to 95% of pancreatic cancer cells possess a *ras oncogene* that makes them vulnerable to inhibition by a class of drugs known as "statins." These drugs are approved by the FDA to lower cholesterol, but they may also play a role in regulating the proliferation of ras oncogene-positive cancer cells. In order to determine whether your pancreatic cancer has a ras oncogene, it is usually necessary for the tumor to be biopsied and analyzed by a pathologist. Since almost all pancreatic cancer cells are regulated by the ras oncogenes, an appropriate adjuvant approach may be the administration of the drug **Lipotor** in the high dose of *80 mg a day.* Any doctor can prescribe Lipotor, as it is already approved by the FDA and sold in the United States. Depending on the pathology report of the pancreatic cell line, mutations to the p21 and p53 oncogenes may also play a role in determining the appropriate therapies to gain control of tumor growth.

Cancer cells often produce large amounts of COX-2 and use it as a biological fuel to cause rapid proliferation of cell division. An article in the journal *Cancer Research* (1999 Mar 1; 59 (5) shows that COX-2 levels in pancreatic cancer cells are 60 times greater than in adjacent normal tissue.

In the Sept 7, 1999, issue of *The Wall Street Journal,* an investigative report revealed that scientists are actively investigating COX-2 inhibitors as drugs that would be effective in the prevention and treatment of many cancers. When COX-2 drugs are given to patients with colon polyps (precancerous lesions), the lesions completely disappear. When a group of rats were given a potent carcinogen, there was a 90% reduction in those who developed cancer if they were on COX-2 inhibition therapy. In the few rats that did develop the tumors while taking COX-2 inhibition therapy, the tumors were 80% smaller and less numerous than the group not on COX-2 inhibition. *The Wall Street Journal* revealed that a handful of physicians knowledgeable about COX-2 and cancer are prescribing COX-2 inhibitors to their patients. (It was back in 1997 that The Life Extension Foundation recommended the European COX-2 inhibiting drug *nimesulide* to cancer patients.)

In a recent report published in *JAMA* (1999 Oct 6;282[13]), a 9.4-year epidemiological study showed that COX-2 expression in colorectal cancer was significantly related to survival. The doctors concluded that "these data add to the growing epidemiological and experimental evidence that COX-2 may play a role in colorectal tumorigenesis."

P

A novel treatment approach would be to combine a COX-2 inhibitor with a "statin" drug such as lovastatin. A study published in the journal *Gastroenterology* (1999; 116, [4], Supp A369) showed that lovastatin augmented, by up to fivefold, the cancer cell–killing effect of a drug with COX-2 inhibiting properties (Sulindac). In this study, three different colon cancer cell lines were killed (made to undergo programmed cell death) by depriving them of COX-2. When lovastatin was added to the COX-2 inhibitor, the kill rate was increased by up to fivefold.

We thus suggest that physicians consider prescribing a COX-2 inhibitor and a statin drug to pancreatic cancer patients (in addition to other therapies) for a period of 3 months. Here are 2 dosing schedules we suggest:

- **1000 mg** a day of **Lodine XL**, *and*
- **80 mg** a day of **Mevacor (lovastatin)** or **Lipotor**

Blood tests to assess liver and kidney function are critical in protecting against potential side effects. To ascertain efficacy, regular CA-19.9 serum tests and imagery testing are suggested.

Lodine XL is an arthritis drug approved by the FDA that interferes with COX-2 metabolic processes. The maximum dosage for Lodine is 1000 mg daily. The most convenient dosing schedule for the patient involves the prescribing of two Lodine XL 500-mg tablets in a single daily dose. As with any nonsteroidal anti-inflammatory drug (NSAID), extreme caution and physician supervision are necessary. The most common complaints associated with Lodine XL use relate to the gastrointestinal tract. Serious GI toxicity such as perforation, ulceration, and bleeding can occur in patients treated chronically with NSAID therapy. Serious renal and hepatic reactions have been reported rarely. Lodine XL should not be given to patients who have previously shown hypersensitivity to it or in whom aspirin or other NSAIDs induce asthma, rhinitis, urticaria, or other allergic reactions. Fatal asthmatic reactions have been reported in such patients receiving NSAIDs.

Nimesulide is a safer COX-2 inhibitor, but it is not approved by the FDA. It is available from Mexican pharmacies or can be ordered by mail from European pharmacies. The suggested dose for nimesulide is two 100-mg tablets a day. (The two newest COX-2 inhibitors are Celebrex and Vioxx, but we suggest that cancer patients consider older drugs that have a more predictable safety history.)

The Life Extension Foundation predicts that COX-2 inhibiting drugs will eventually be approved to treat cancer, but in the meantime we are asking physicians treating cancer patients to consider prescribing a COX-2–inhibiting drug, along with a "statin" drug as an adjuvant therapy.

Based on the need to inhibit the pancreatic cancer cell division at different stages of its growth and induce apoptosis of cancer cells (programmed cell death), multiple therapeutic modalities are probably required. One successful treatment modality is to combine the differentiation-inducing drug **Accutane** (13-*cis*-retinoic acid) with the cytotoxic chemotherapeutic drug, **5-fluorouracil** (5-FU). Both Accutane and 5-FU are toxic drugs that must be carefully administered by a medical oncologist.

In Europe, oncologists are combining 5-FU with **borage oil** (gamma-linolenic acid) to improve the cancer cell–killing effects of the 5-FU. Cancer patients using 5-FU might consider supplementing with the high dose of 2400 mg of gamma-linolenic acid from borage oil. Borage oil is available in health food stores and through the Life Extension Foundation.

Cyclooxygenase-2 (COX-2) and lipooxygenase inhibitors are being used to interfere with the growth of several different cell lines, including pancreatic cancer. One experimental approach is to use the 5-lipooxygenase inhibitor **MK886** along with borage oil. Other approaches to suppressing COX-2 could be the use of one of the new **COX-2 inhibiting** drugs used to treat rheumatoid arthritis; **fish oil** supplements providing at least 2400 mg of EPA (eicosapentaenoic acid) and 1800 mg DHA (docosahexaenoic acid) a day; or importing the drug **nimesulide** from Europe or Mexico for personal use.

If the pathology report shows the pancreatic cancer cells to have a mutated p53 oncogene, or if there is no p53 detected, then high-dose **genistein** therapy may be appropriate. The suggested dose is five capsules of the 700-mg **Mega-Soy Extract** supplement that provides over 2800 mg a day of genistein, 4 times a day. If the pathology report shows a functional p53, then genistein is far less effective in arresting cell growth.

To regulate the p21 oncogene, a combination of **sodium phenylbutyrate** and **Lipotor** and **Accutane** may be effective. Sodium phenylbutyrate is available as an experimental alternative cancer therapy, while Lipotor and Accutane must be prescribed by a knowledgeable physician.

Conventional Pancreatic Cancer Expertise

Some of the most advanced clinical application of the experimental therapies described so far to treat pancreatic cancer are being conducted at

University of Virginia
Dept of Medicine
Charlottesville, Virginia
Contact Dvorit Samid, M.D. at (804) 243-6747

Rush Presbyterian, St. Luke's Medical Center
Section of Medical Oncology
Chicago, Illinois
Contact K.N. Anderson, M.D. at (312) 942-5906

A Promising Experimental Cancer Therapy

A study appearing in the May 1999 issue of the *International Journal of Oncology* reported on a group of end-stage pancreatic cancer patients treated with an experimental drug called *rubitecan* (RFS-2000). The patients had failed all previous conventional therapies and were thus eligible to participate in this clinical study. Of the 60 patients who were able to complete the therapy, 31.7% responded favorably with a median survival of 18.6 months. Another 31.7% were stabilized with a 9.7 month median survival rate, while 36.6% were nonresponders with a 6.8 month median survival rate.

Considering how quickly pancreatic cancer kills (often 3 to 12 months after diagnosis), this new drug should be considered as a first-line therapy in the treatment of pancreatic and other cancers. These patients had already suffered through useless cytotoxic chemotherapy.

The company that makes rubitecan is SuperGen Inc. of San Ramon, California. On May 11, 1999, the company announced that it has more than doubled the number of cancer centers participating in its Phase III clinical trial of rubitecan (previously known as RFS 2000).

SuperGen has added 75 clinics operated by Dallas-based Physician Reliance Network (PRN), thus bringing the total number of centers participating in the trial to 132. Current enrollment is 255 patients, and this number is expected to increase rapidly.

Formed in 1993, Dallas-based PRN is the nation's largest oncology-focused physician practice management company. PRN manages the practices of some 340 physicians at 127 locations in 13 states, including 23 full-service cancer centers.

SuperGen expects to expand Phase II clinical trials of rubitecan in the United States to include four additional types: liver cancer, melanoma, glioma, and sarcoma. Thus, including recently announced European-based clinical studies of rubitecan in 7 solid tumors (colorectal, gastric, lung, breast, prostate, cervical, and head and neck cancers), rubitecan has been expanded to 11 tumor types beyond pancreatic cancer.

Finally, the company also announced that it has begun a study of rubitecan (RFS 2000)—combined with gemcitabine—to treat pancreatic cancer patients. This study is under way at a major cancer center in Philadelphia, PA.

"Rubitecan is the most important drug in our broad pipeline, as well as our most advanced and top-priority clinical project," said Dr. Joseph Rubinfeld, chairman and chief executive officer of SuperGen. "Due to the lack of effective treatment for pancreatic cancer patients, we are taking every step possible to accelerate our Phase III trial in order to be in position to submit a New Drug Application to the FDA as quickly as possible. We are confident that the addition of PRN's clinics will substantially increase enrollment of patients, thus leading to a rapid and successful conclusion of the Phase III study."

"Rubitecan has shown activity against a number of tumors, and we are very pleased to fast-forward our U.S.-based clinical development programs for rubitecan beyond pancreatic cancer," Dr. Rubinfeld added.

A significant advantage of rubitecan is that the drug can be given orally on an outpatient basis, thus providing convenience for patients. This is in contrast to other cancer drugs that have to be given intravenously either in a hospital or physician's office.

Rubitecan has also shown activity in hematologic tumors as well. A clinical study under way at the M.D. Anderson Cancer Center in Houston using rubitecan has shown efficacy in 50% of patients suffering from myelodysplastic syndrome (MDS)/chronic myelomonocytic leukemia (CMML), thus indicating a very broad spectrum of activity encompassing both solid tumors and hematologic malignancies.

"Several advantages distinguish rubitecan as a potential therapy for treating cancer. One advantage is its side-effect profile relative to other anticancer drugs. In studies to date, none of the cardiac, pulmonary, hepatic, neurological, or renal toxicities that limit the acute and/or chronic dosages of most chemotherapies have been observed and, in fact, studies suggest that rubitecan could be used to treat cancer on a chronic, rather than acute, basis," said Dr. Rubinfeld. "The side effects are manageable hematological toxicities, cystitis (bladder irritation), and some gastrointestinal disorder—in all, a relatively benign profile" (Stehlin, J.S. et al., A study of 9-nitrocamptothecin [RFS-2000] in patients with advanced pancreatic cancer, *International Journal of Oncology*, May 1999).

To inquire about entering a clinical study using rubitecan, call John Marinaro, Senior Director of Clinical Research at (925) 327-0200. SuperGen's Web address is www.suprgen.com

A Novel Herbal Approach

The September 17, 1998, issue of the *New England Journal of Medicine* published a study on a product called ***PC Spes*** that was 100% effective in reducing PSA levels in advanced prostate cancer patients. The company that makes *PC Spes* to treat prostate cancer also makes a herbal preparation to treat breast and certain other cancers called ***Spes***. The *Spes* preparation has been shown effective in the 2 years that Foundation members have been using it. The studies show that *Spes* works best against cancers with a mutated p53 oncogene and an over-expressed *N*-RAS gene. Cancer patients have been getting good results when combining *Spes* with high-dose genistein, soy extract, curcumin, and 83% green tea extract. What follows is a highly technical description of the molecular mechanisms of action of *Spes*. Please don't be intimidated if you can't understand all of this as it is written to inform the oncologist as well as the lay reader.

Spes has been shown to inhibit *prostaglandin E2* (PGE2) by about 50%. Cancer patients often develop high concentrations of PGE2 that can promote the proliferation of some cancer cell lines and also damage immune function. PGE2 inhibits the T-cell response, causes a decrease in natural killer (NK) cells, and inhibits lymphokine production. PGE2 enhances tumor survival by blocking the natural destruction via the lysis process of tumor cells. In addition, PGE2 promotes abnormal platelet aggregation, a common feature that enables cancer cells to enter the interstitial tissue through a blood vessel wall to establish metastatic sites. PGE2-induced endothelial cell damage attracts metastatic cancer cell colony formation. Many cancer patients succumb to acute death when an abnormal blood clot (thrombus) causes a heart attack or stroke. It is clearly desirable to suppress PGE2, and *Spes* does this by about 50%. The suppression of PGE2 by *Spes* has shown a dramatic increase in NK activity. While cancer drugs are in development that work by suppressing PGE2 formation, *Spes* is available as a dietary supplement for use today.

Nearly all cancer cells secrete a peptide hormone called *substance P* that promotes tumor growth. Substance P also functions as a neurotransmitter involved in pain pulse transmission through the nerves. *Spes* appears to lower the levels of substance P, thus potentially slowing tumor growth and alleviating pain.

Spes increases enkephalin production. Enkephalins are peptides produced in the brain that act as opiates, binding to receptor sites involved in pain perception. This could be a mechanism by which *Spes* alleviates pain. *Spes* may increase enkephalins between 30 to 50% in about 1 hour.

Beta-Endorphin levels are markedly depressed in the cerebrospinal fluid of cancer patients. Endorphins are polypeptides produced in the brain that also act as opiates producing an analgesic effect by binding to opiate receptor sites. The most active of the endorphins is beta-endorphin. *Spes* has been shown to normalize beta-endorphin levels. Another mechanism by which *Spes* provides analgesic action is lowering norepinephrine in relation to serotonin. *Spes* raises acetylcholine levels in the brain by an average of 60.4%. This also has a positive effect on pain reduction.

Spes increases cAMP (adenosine 3*N*,5*N*-cyclic monophosphate) by a dramatic 150%, but has only a modest effect on cGMP (cyclic guanosine monophosphate). This induces a hyperpolarization of the postsynaptic membranes, inducing an inhibition of the pain signal transmission, but not a blockage of the opium receptors. High levels of cAMP also normalize mitosis (cell division). Thus, *Spes* may promote cell differentiation and inhibit abnormal cell growth via its effects on cAMP and cGMP.

Spes reduces the afferent peripheral pain signals and increases the central pain-modulating function. This is a fancy way of saying *Spes* causes a reduction in internal organ pain or bone pain.

In the animal model, *Spes* was directly injected into the tumor site and caused an inhibition rate of 133% in tumor weight or volume. On hepatocarcinoma cell lines, *Spes* markedly reduced the number of survived cells in a total unit area, reversed the self-keeping system of the cancer cells, and caused the differentiation of the cancer cells to normal cells. By causing the cancer cells to differentiate normally, *Spes* may markedly inhibit the advancement of the tumor.

Alpha-Fetoprotein (AFP) is a specific marker for gene expression in hepatocellular carcinoma. AFP is a serum protein produced by the fetal liver and yolk sac during prenatal development and reaches its full expression at 15 weeks of gestation, falling rapidly thereafter until normal adult levels are reached. High levels in an adult is an indication of hepatocellular carcinoma. *Spes* was shown to block expression of AFP by 83.5%.

N-RAS gene is a "transforming" gene whose over-expression is required for the activation of hepatocellular carcinoma and approximately 30% of all other cancers. A mutation in the *N*-RAS gene tends to turn off the switch for cell cycle progression. *N*-RAS thus interacts with other proteins and stimulates cell growth. *Spes* was shown to block the over-expression of *N*-RAS gene.

Ribosomal RNA instructs specific ribosomes to join into a group called ribosomal complex. This is the production facility for making protein. A ribosome is a cell organelle. It is the site of amino acid assembly in the exact sequence ordered by messenger RNA (mRNA). mRNA receives instructions (the genetic code) in the nucleus for the exact sequence of the 22 different amino acids necessary to make a specific protein. This process is called transcription. It is at this point that over-expression often occurs and that the cell turns cancerous. IGF-II has a growth-promoting effect on cells, and *Spes* blocks the over-expression of mRNA for IGF-II synthesis.

Finally, *Spes* increases SOD production in the blood serum by 50% and suppresses free radical generation.

Dosage recommendations are based on body weight. Under 150 lbs., 2 capsules 2 hours prior to breakfast on an empty stomach and again two capsules 2 hours prior to dinner on an empty stomach. Over 150 lbs. of body weight, 3 capsules 2 hours prior to breakfast on an empty stomach and again 3 capsules 2 hours prior to dinner on an empty stomach. An empty stomach means no food or any other medication or supplement during the 2-hour period. *Spes* requires a noncompetitive stomach environment for proper absorption.

The pain-relieving effect should be felt within 2 hours. Also, mood and appetite should improve. Botaniclab, the manufacturer of the product, claims that *Spes* works as well as hydrazine sulfate in countering the cachexia that occurs in late-stage cancer. Testing for blood tumor markers and tumor volume should be done regularly to determine if *Spes* is effective against the individual's cancer.

Spes is available from the Life Extension Foundation as an adjuvant natural therapy by calling (800) 544-4440.

Tumor Marker Blood Tests

The three most important blood tumor markers to evaluate progression or regression of pancreatic cancer are

1. **CA-19-9**
2. **CEA** (carcinoembryonic antigen)
3. **GGTP** (liver enzyme)

In addition, when these tumor marker tests are done, a complete chemistry-CBC test should also be done to guard against toxicities from conventional and alternative therapies.

Additional Experimental Contacts

Pancreatic cancer cells often proliferate via the farnesyl transferase pathway. An experimental drug called *R115777* functions as a specific farnesyl transferase inhibitor. To find out about entering a clinical trial with R115777, call (301) 496-4891 and ask for information about *Protocol 97-C-0086.*

An experimental pancreatic cancer vaccine is being tested by a company called Antigenics. You can call them at (212) 332-4774 to find out about entering a clinical trial.

If your pancreatic cancer cells are deficient in cytochrome p53, a drug called *Onxy-015* might help restore normal cell division and differentiation to out-of-control cancer cells. This drug is made by Onyx Pharmaceuticals and is being tested at the University of California–San Francisco. Fax your request to Dr. Shawn Muldehill at (510)222-9758.

Another experimental drug that may be effective against pancreatic cancer is called *TNP-470* made by Tap Pharmaceuticals. You can call Tap Pharmaceuticals at (800) 621-1020 to see about entering a clinical trial using this experimental drug.

Complementary Therapies

Specific nutrients that have been shown to inhibit pancreatic cancer cell proliferation include green tea extract, soy genistein, DHEA, selenium, vitamin A, and D_3 analogs. (*Refer to the Cancer Treatment protocols for dosage information.*)

For further information. Call the Life Extension Foundation at (800) 544-4440. Please visit our Web site at www.lef.org.

Product availability. You can order Life Extension Mix, Life Extension Herbal Mix, selenium complex, Thymex, DHEA, melatonin, vitamin A emulsified drops, vitamin D_3, *Spes*, Mega Soy Extract, green tea caps, Coenzyme Q_{10}, garlic, vitamin C, and Phyto-Food, by calling (800) 544-4440, or order online at www.lef.org. Ask for the names of companies that will ship nimesulide and other cancer drugs to Americans for personal use. For some forms of cancer, you may be able to get into a free program utilizing experimental cancer therapies sponsored by the National Cancer Institute. For information about experimental cancer therapies, call (800) 4-CANCER. Make sure you do not enroll in a study where you may be part of a placebo group or where the potential toxicity of the drug may kill you before the cancer does.

PARATHYROID (HYPERPARATHYROIDISM)

The primary function of the parathyroid glands is to control calcium within the blood. The parathyroid glands also control how much calcium is in the bones, and therefore how strong and dense the bones are. Calcium is the primary element which causes muscles to contract. Calcium levels are also very important to the normal conduction of electrical currents along nerves.

Knowing the major functions of calcium helps explain why people can get a tingling sensation in their fingers or cramps in the muscles of their hands when calcium levels drop too low. Additionally, too high a calcium level can cause a person to feel run down and sleep poorly, and can make them more argumentative than usual. Too high a calcium blood level can even cause a decrease in memory. Over half of patients with this disease state that they feel just fine. However, after treatment more than 85% of these patients say they "feel much better"!

The parathyroid glands are sometimes confused with thyroid glands, but they have no related function. The thyroid gland regulates the body's metabolism and has no effect on calcium levels, while the parathyroid glands regulate calcium levels and have no effect on the metabolism.

Normal Parathyroid Activity

The four to six parathyroid glands are quite small, and are very vascular. This assists them in monitoring the calcium level in the blood 24 hours a day. As the blood flow filters through the parathyroid glands, the glands detect the amount of calcium in the blood. Depending on calcium levels, they react by making more or less parathyroid hormone (PTH).

If calcium levels in the blood are too low, the cells of the parathyroids sense it and make more parathyroid hormone. Once the parathyroid hormone is released into the blood, it circulates to act in a number of places to increase the amount of calcium in the blood (such as removing calcium from bones). When the calcium level in the blood is too high, the parathyroids make less parathyroid hormone, allowing calcium levels to naturally decrease.

Producing Calcium in the Blood

The parathyroids make a hormone, like all endocrine glands. Parathyroid hormone (PTH) has a strong effect on bone cells that causes them to release calcium into the bloodstream. Under the presence of too much parathyroid hormone, however, the bones will continue to release their calcium into the blood at a rate which is too high, resulting in bones which have too little calcium and in serum calcium overload. This results in conditions medically defined as osteopenia and osteoporosis. When bones are subjected to high levels of parathyroid hormones over several years, they become brittle and prone to fractures.

Additionally, parathyroid hormones can act to increase blood levels of calcium by their influence on the intestines. The presence of parathyroid hormone causes the lining of the intestine to become more efficient at absorbing calcium normally found in our diet.

Hyperparathyroidism: Overactivity

Too much parathyroid hormone secretion is the primary disease of parathyroid glands. This condition is called hyperparathyroidism. The condition occurs when one or more of the parathyroid glands function improperly, making excess hormones regardless of the level of calcium.

The most common cause of hyperparathyroidism (excess hormone production) is the development of a benign tumor in one or more of the parathyroid glands. Enlargement of one parathyroid gland is called a parathyroid adenoma, which accounts for about 90% of all primary hyperparathyroidism disease. Hyperparathyroidism causes damage to the body because it causes an abnormally high level of calcium in the blood, which slowly destroys the tissues of the body.

Parathyroid adenomas are typically much bigger than the normal pea-sized parathyroid (shown to scale) and will frequently be about the size of a walnut. Approximately 10% of all patients with primary hyperparathyroidism will have an enlargement of all parathyroid glands, called parathyroid hyperplasia. This condition is much less common than hyperparathyroidism, but the end results are identical on the tissues of the body.

Signs and Symptoms of Hyperparathyroidism

Although most people with hyperparathyroidism say they feel well when the diagnosis is made, the majority of these will actually say they feel better after the problem has been cured. This can only be known retrospectively when patients are allowed to comment on how they feel several months after the operation. Many patients who thought they were asymptomatic preoperatively will claim to sleep better at night, will be less irritable, and will find that they remember things much more easily than they could when their calcium levels were high (nervous system problems).

Patients with persistently elevated calcium levels due to overproduction of parathyroid hormones also can have complaints of bone pain. In the severe form, bones can give up so much of their calcium that the bones become brittle and break (osteoporosis and osteopenia). This problem is even more of a concern in older patients. Bones can also have small hemorrhages within their center that will cause "bone pain."

Other associated symptoms of hyperparathyroidism are the development of gastric ulcers and pancreatitis. High levels of calcium in the blood (hypercalcemia) can be dangerous to a number of cells, including the lining of the stomach and the pancreas, causing both of these organs to become inflamed and painful (ulcers and acute pancreatitis). The heart and vascular system may also be vulnerable to chronic calcium overload Another common presentation for persistently elevated calcium levels is the development of kidney stones. Since the major function of the kidneys is to filter and clean the blood, they will be constantly exposed to high levels of calcium in patients with hyperparathyroidism. The constant filtering of large amounts of calcium will cause the collection of calcium within the renal tubules, leading to kidney stones. In extreme cases the entire kidney can become calcified and even take on the characteristics of bone because of deposition of so much calcium within the tissues. Not only is this painful because of the presence of kidney stones; in severe cases it can cause kidney failure.

The incidence of these problems depends primarily on the duration of the disease and its severity. Everybody will lose bone density, which is progressive. Pancreatitis and ulcers are much more rare. After diagnosis, almost 80% of patients claim to feel better (sleep better, etc.) 3 months after the problem has been fixed.

Hyperparathyroidism is relatively easy to detect, as the parathyroid glands will be making an inappropriately large amount of parathyroid hormones in the presence of elevated serum calcium. Another way to confirm this diagnosis is by measuring the amount of calcium in the urine over a 24-hour period of time. If the kidneys are functioning normally, they will filter much of this calcium in an attempt to rid the body of calcium, leading to an abnormally large amount of calcium in the urine. Measuring calcium in the urine, however, is an indirect measure of parathyroid activity and is only accurate 25 to 35% of the time.

The most accurate and definitive way to diagnose primary hyperparathyroidism is by testing for an elevated parathyroid hormone (PTH) level in the face of an elevated serum calcium. A standard blood-chemistry test can reveal elevated calcium levels caused by hyperparathyroid disease. If your blood test is high in calcium and parathyroid hormones, it may be an indication of hyperparathyroidism. People who do not have regular blood tests usually find out they have hyperparathyroidism when a bone suddenly breaks, a kidney stone develops, or when their kidneys fail altogether.

Conventional Diagnosis and Treatment Options for Primary Hyperparathyroidism

There are diagnostic procedures (MRI, CT scans, sonography) to determine if the excess parathyroid hormone is caused by a tumor or by a vitamin D_3/calcium deficiency. Some physicians will elect not to refer their patients for an operation if they have a mild form of primary hyperparathyroidism.

Since the mid 1920s, the standard treatment for primary hyperparathyroidism has been to surgically remove the gland (or glands) overproducing hormones. Remember: this is a hormone problem, so the goal is to remove the source of the excess hormone. The patient is put to sleep under general anesthesia; an incision is made in the neck; and the thyroid gland is mobilized to allow the surgeon to identify the four to six parathyroid glands which reside moderately deep in the neck behind the thyroid. Patients are typically hospitalized overnight, and occasionally as long as a day or two. The incision must be of sufficient length to allow the surgeon adequate exposure of the numerous important structures in the neck, and thus it is typically 3 or 4 inches long. These wounds eventually heal.

Because of the numerous small nerves and other important structures within the neck, this operation can be technically challenging and is usually performed only by experienced endocrine surgeons or surgeons with extensive head and neck operative experience. During this operation, the surgeon identifies all four parathyroid glands and removes whichever ones are enlarged. As covered in the section describing hyperparathyroidism in detail, approximately 89% of the time there is one large gland (an adenoma) and three normal glands. In this situation the one large gland would be removed, leaving the three normal ones to function in a normal fashion indefinitely.

Interestingly, if the surgeon finds all four glands to be enlarged (hyperplasia), he or she typically takes out three or three and a half of these glands, leaving some parathyroid tissue behind to function normally in the future. In experienced hands, this operation has a cure rate of about 95%.

To complete this operation safely with a high rate of success, this standard bilateral neck exploration is almost always performed using general anesthesia. Because of the concern over general anesthesia, some physicians elect not to send patients for this operation until they develop symptoms or have a significant loss of bone density. This means of management may or may not always be in the best interest of the patient. You need to discuss the pros and cons of this operation with your endocrinologist and weigh the risks of surgery versus continued monitoring of your body calcium stores or trying the integrated medical approach profiled and recommended below.

CAUTION: A dangerous trend has emerged over the past several years! Some physicians have begun using a new drug (Fosomax) to increase bone calcium rather than referring a patient for surgery. This is an effective drug, but must be used appropriately. It is *not* a replacement for removal of the overactive parathyroid gland! This drug works through a mechanism different from that of the overproduced parathyroid hormone. Experts in the field feel that after a parathyroid is surgically removed, Fosomax may have a role in trying to build bone density and replace the calcium that the parathyroid hormone removed.

Integrated and Alternative Therapy

While primary hyperparathyroidism normally mandates surgery to remove one or more parathyroid glands that have developed benign tumors, secondary hyperparathyroidism can be caused by a dietary calcium/vitamin D deficiency. To rule out secondary hyperparathyroidism, a good first step is to supplement with 1000 IU of vitamin D_3 every day, along with 2000 mg of elemental calcium. This much calcium and vitamin D_3 will act as a signal to your parathyroid glands to stop producing so much parathyroid hormone. When your bloodstream is loaded with calcium, your parathyroid glands will no longer have to pull it from your bones to guarantee proper calcium metabolism. Many people undergo surgery to remove one or more parathyroid glands when, in fact, all they may need to do is take calcium and vitamin D_3. This amount of daily vitamin D_3 supplementation was confirmed to be safe in the *American Journal of Clinical Nutrition* in May 1999.

Numerous studies demonstrate and report that glucocorticoid-induced osteoporosis is associated with the development of secondary hyperparathyroidism. Alternate-day therapy with corticosteroid drugs can't prevent bone loss. Supplementation of calcium and vitamin D has been shown to be an effective method for prevention and treatment.

Estrogen-replacement therapy may potentially be an alternative form of therapy to surgery in elderly women with primary hyperparathyroidism. In one study, estrogen-replacement therapy (ERT) appeared as effective as parathyroidectomy (combined with either calcitriol or calcium supplements) for the treatment of osteoporosis in elderly postmenopausal women showing primary hyperparathyroidism symptoms as reported in the *Annals of Internal Medicine* (1996): "Although hormone replacement therapy has little effect on serum calcium levels, it suppresses bone turnover, reduces urinary calcium excretion, and increases bone mineral density throughout the skeleton in postmenopausal women with mild primary hyperparathyroidism. This therapy is thus an important management option for these patients."

Later that same year the Department of Endocrinology at St. George Hospital, Sydney, Australia, reported ERT appeared to be as effective as parathyroidectomy (combined with either calcitriol or calcium supplements) for the treatment of osteoporosis in elderly postmenopausal women presenting with PHPT (*Osteoporos. Int.*, 1996, 6 [4]:329–33).

In treating hemodialysis patients suffering from uremic hyperparathyroidism, the addition of the drug calcitonin to vitamin D_3 therapy may inhibit bone resorption and increase bone mineral density. Dialysis patients often suffer from uncontrolled serum phosphate levels that preclude successful treatment with vitamin D_3. Blood levels of phosphate should be carefully monitored in dialysis patients.

Calcium-alpha-ketoglutarate is known as a highly effective phosphate binder in hemodialysis patients. Also, alpha-ketoglutarate has been shown to improve metabolic alterations. A study investigated the effect of long-term phosphate-binding therapy with calcium-alpha-ketoglutarate to determine whether phosphate accumulation is the main reason for secondary hyperparathyroidism in kidney dialysis patients. Calcium ketoglutarate was prescribed to 14 patients in a mean dosage of 4.5 grams a day (which provided 975 mg of elemental calcium) for a period of 36 months. Serum phosphate levels continuously dropped, whereas serum calcium levels increased to normal levels. Intact parathyroid hormone continuously normalized in all patients. The present data show that long-term treatment with calcium-alpha-ketoglutarate normalizes secondary hyperparathyroidism by simultaneously binding phosphate and correcting the calcium/phosphate ratio in serum without vitamin D treatment (*Miner Electrolyte Metab.*, 1996, 22 [1–3]:196–99).

Summary

Too much parathyroid hormone is clinically defined as hyperparathyroidism. The excess parathyroid hormone pulls calcium from the bones, which overloads the blood system with excessive amounts of calcium. Many long-term degenerative diseases have been linked to this type of calcium imbalance.

A standard blood-chemistry test can reveal elevated calcium levels caused by hyperparathyroid disease. Only a PTH (parathyroid hormone) blood test can effectively diagnose hyperparathyroidism. If your blood test is high in calcium and parathyroid hormone, it may be an indication of hyperparathyroidism.

Surgery is necessary when there is a parathyroid tumor that causes the overproduction of parathyroid hormone. The first step in countering parathyroidism is to take 1000 IU of vitamin D_3 every day, along with 2000 mg of elemental calcium. This much calcium and vitamin D_3 will act as a signal to your parathyroid glands to stop producing so much parathyroid hormone. When your bloodstream is loaded with calcium, your parathyroid glands will no longer have to pull it from your bones to guarantee proper calcium metabolism. Many people undergo surgery to remove one or more parathyroid glands when, in fact, all they need to do is take calcium and vitamin D_3.

The life extension protocol for treating secondary hyperparathyroidism includes

1. Vitamin D_3, 1000 IU daily.
2. Encapsulated calcium, 2000 elemental mg daily.
3. Consider taking calcium ketoglutarate, 4.5 grams a day.
4. Elderly postmenopausal women showing primary hyperparathyroidism symptoms may consider estrogen-replacement therapy combined with either calcitriol or calcium supplements for the treatment of osteoporosis.

For treating primary hyperparathyroidism, surgery is often mandated. Refer to the *Osteoporosis protocol* for more information relative to the effects and treatment of hyperparathyroidism.

Product availability. Vitamin D_3 and an encapsulated calcium-mineral formula called Bone Assure can be ordered by phoning (800) 544-4440, or order on-line at www.lef.org.

PARKINSON'S DISEASE

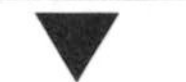

Parkinson's disease (PD) is a degenerative central nervous system (CNS) disorder characterized by uncontrolled body movements, rigidity, tremor, and gait difficulties. The American Parkinson Disease Association estimates that one million Americans are affected by the disease. The risk for developing PD increases with age, and onset usually occurs at around 50 years of age or older, although the disease is not unknown in people in their 30s and 40s. Parkinson's disease affects men and women equally. There are two types of Parkinson's disease: idiopathic PD and secondary PD. Idiopathic PD, also known as primary PD, has no known recognizable cause; secondary PD may result from trauma, tumor, or cerebrovascular disease, or may be drug induced. Patients with both types of PD are classified into stages (early, moderate, or advanced) based on the progression of disease. There is no known cure for the disease; rather, the treatment goal for patients with either form of PD is to control the symptoms and provide quality of life.

Parkinson's disease is actually a group of related CNS disorders caused by the destruction of the substantia nigra (pigmented brain cells), which produce dopamine (a neurotransmitter). The deficiency of dopamine results in the loss of muscle tone and voluntary muscle control seen in PD. Recent studies indicate that dopamine deficiencies in other areas of the brain and abnormalities of other neurotransmitters, such as norepinephrine and serotonin, may also contribute to the disease.

Signs and Symptoms

Although onset of PD can be rapid, it is generally insidious, with symptoms gradually progressing over a number of years until they interfere with daily activities. The four major symptoms of Parkinson's disease are

- Rigidity (stiffness when neck or extremities are moved).
- Resting tremor (involuntary movement of contracting muscles, especially when at rest).
- Bradykinesis (slowness in initiating movement).
- Poor posture and loss of balance.

Secondary symptoms of PD include

- Depression.
- Senility.
- Postural deformity.
- Speech difficulties.
- Emotional changes (patients become fearful or insecure).
- Memory loss and slowness of thought.
- Difficulty swallowing or chewing.
- Urinary dysfunction or constipation.
- Skin problems.
- Sleep disorders.

As PD progresses, patients develop a characteristic gait called *festination,* with which patients take small, hurried steps on tiptoe. Accidental falls occur frequently as a result of festination. As the disease progresses, it becomes more difficult for Parkinson's patients to manage daily activities, and full-time caregivers are often necessary.

Diagnosis of Parkinson's Disease

It is often difficult to diagnose the early stages of Parkinson's disease because the patient's symptoms may be vague. Often, diagnosis will be made only after the patient's tremors become readily apparent and one or more of the other classic symptoms appears. There is no specific test for the presence of the disease; rather, diagnosis is made on a thorough neurological examination. CT scans and MRIs may be ordered to rule out other diseases. There are multiple forms of PD, but the symptoms associated with all forms of the disease are similar. It is important to diagnose the specific form and the progression of PD because the treatment program will vary accordingly.

Conventional Treatment of PD

The treatment of PD patients is based on the type and stage of the disease, and is designed to alleviate symptoms. Some commonly used medications include anticholinergics (e.g., benztropine, biperiden, and orphenadine), dopamine receptor agonists (e.g., amantidine, bromocriptine, and pergolide), and monoamine oxidase (MAO) inhibitors, such as selegiline (deprenyl). Although deprenyl has been shown to be effective in the treatment of PD, recent research suggests that the effectiveness of this medication decreases over time. *L*-dopa, Sinemet, and Sinemet CR remain the most powerful medications for the treatment of PD, and are most often prescribed only during the advanced stage of the disease because their effectiveness decreases with time.

L-dopa can cross from the bloodstream to the brain and be converted to dopamine in the brain by the active form of vitamin B_6. Dopamine itself cannot enter the brain from the bloodstream. Sinemet is *L*-dopa in combination with the peripheral dopa-decarboxylase inhibitor Carbidopa. Without the Carbidopa, dopa decarboxylase enzymes in the intestine would convert *L*-dopa to dopamine, which cannot enter the brain. Ropinirole, a synthetic, nonergot dopamine agonist receptor, has been shown to improve motor function and delay disability in PD patients. Ropinirole may be used prior to treatment with *L*-dopa.

Patients on long-term dopamine therapy may experience the *on-off syndrome* associated with the medication. During the *on phase,* dopamine levels in the brain are high and symptoms are controlled; during the *off phase,* dopamine levels in the brain decrease and the patient's symptoms return. These changes may be sudden and dramatic as dopamine levels fluctuate. The syndrome is particularly frustrating to PD patients, because there are no warning signs prior to the onset of either phase of the syndrome.

Because PD patients may experience sleep disorders and depression, sedatives and antidepressant agents may be prescribed. These medications should be used with caution in elderly patients, because of the increased risk for unsteadiness, confusion, and delirium.

Surgical Interventions for PD

Stereotactic pallidotomy and thalamotomy are two surgical procedures that may relieve some of the symptoms of PD. Patients undergoing these procedures have MRI and CT scans done prior to surgery to pinpoint the specific brain structures to be targeted during the procedure. Because the goal of these procedures is to pinpoint those areas of the brain responsible for the patient's symptoms, local anesthesia is used so that the patient is able to respond verbally during surgery. During these procedures, a small incision is made into the cranium, and a small electrode is inserted. The surgeon positions the electrode, and a small electrical stimulation is given to the patient. If the patient feels symptomatic relief, the surgeon then increases the electrical charge to create a lesion that will permanently destroy that area of the brain. The goal of thalamotomy is to relieve tremors, and the goal of pallidotomy is to relieve dyskinesia, on-off syndrome, and rigidity. Not all PD patients are candidates for these procedures. Contraindications for the use of pallidotomy and thalamotomy include advanced age, dementia, speech disorders, and serious systemic disease.

Alternative Treatments for PD

For every decade we live past age 40, we lose an average of about 10% of our dopamine-producing brain cells. Once 80% of these brain cells have died, Parkinson's disease is often diagnosed. Studies have shown that if healthy people take antioxidants throughout most of their lives, their risk of acquiring Parkinson's disease is reduced considerably. When Parkinson's patients are given vitamin E by itself, however, there is no slowdown in disease progression. Since Parkinson's patients have already sustained massive damage to crucial brain cells, aggressive multiple therapies are required to have a chance of significantly slowing the natural progression of the disease.

The Life Extension Foundation's protocol for Parkinson's disease is based on studies showing that low doses of several drugs work better than high doses of a single drug. The many components that compose this protocol are suggested because of evidence of their safety and benefits in treating the multiple underlying neurological disorders linked to the disease.

Bromocriptine. Take the lowest effective dose to begin with, usually 1.25 mg a day. May be withheld until later in the disease phase.

Sinemet CR (controlled release) (*L*-dopa plus a dopa decarboxylase inhibitor). Take lowest effective dose to begin with. Some doctors withhold Sinemet until later in the progression of the disease in order to give the Parkinson's patient more time to benefit from Sinemet before its effects wear off.

Amantadine (anticholinergic). Take lowest effective dose to begin with, usually 300 mg a day.

Deprenyl (MAO B inhibitor). Take lowest effective dose to begin with, between 1.25 and 5 mg a day. Deprenyl dosing has been significantly reduced based on studies showing that high doses of Deprenyl may be detrimental to Parkinson's patients.

Hydergine. Take 10 to 20 mg a day.

Acetyl-L-carnitine. Take 1000 mg twice a day.

Phosphatidylserine. Take 200 mg twice a day.

NADH. Take 5 to 10 mg twice a day.

DHEA. Take 100 mg 3 times a day, and/or pregnenolone at 50 mg 3 times a day.

Pregnenolone is a DHEA precursor.

CAUTION: Refer to the DHEA-Pregnenolone Precautions in the *DHEA Replacement Therapy protocol* before taking DHEA or pregnenolone.

Coenzyme Q_{10}. Take 100 mg 3 times a day.

Life Extension Mix. Take 3 tablets, 3 times a day.

WARNING: May have to avoid if taking Sinemet because the vitamin B_6 in Life Extension Mix may prevent *L*-dopa from reaching the brain. Take other antioxidants that do not contain vitamin B_6 in place of Life Extension Mix.

Melatonin. Take 3 to 10 mg every night at bedtime.

Life Extension Booster. Take 1 capsule twice a day.

Human growth hormone. Take 2 IU daily, by injection.

Clinical research suggests that PD patients may derive some benefit from antioxidants and amino acids such as tyrosine. Antioxidants that may have some value in the treatment of PD include alpha-tocopherol (vitamin E) and Coenzyme Q_{10} (CoQ_{10}). The results of two studies suggest that alpha-tocopherol may have prophylactic value in the prevention of PD.

The beneficial effects of *L*-dopa decrease with time; many studies have shown that vitamin B_6 (pyridoxine) aggravates the loss of clinical effect of *L*-dopa by increasing decarboxylation. Patients taking *L*-dopa should not take more than 100 mg of pyridoxine a day, and should perhaps take much less. Clinical studies have suggested that *L*-tryptophan may help to ameliorate the motor complications sometimes seen in PD patients on long-term *L*-dopa therapy. *L*-tryptophan may also be helpful in the treatment of depression associated with this disease by increasing serotonin levels in the brain. A recent study of 23 patients with PD suggested that *L*-tyrosine may help to enhance dopamine synthesis.

Coenzyme Q_{10}, a naturally occurring substance, may help to curb the oxidative stress common in Parkinsonism. Other therapies that may provide some protection from the loss of cognitive function in certain PD patients include the chemical carnitine, Hydergine (a European medication), and phosphatidylserine (a phospholipid). Additional therapies that may be beneficial in treating the symptoms of PD include DHEA and NADH (hormones), and melatonin.

A report published in the *Annals of Neurology* (1997 August) identified a new mechanism that showed that CoQ_{10} might be effective in the prevention and treatment of Parkinson's disease.

The study showed that the brain cells of Parkinson's patients have a specific impairment that causes the disruption of healthy mitochondrial function. It is known that *mitochondrial disorder* causes cells in the substantia nigra region of the brain to malfunction and die, creating a shortage of dopamine. Another interesting finding was that CoQ_{10} levels in Parkinson's patients were 35% lower than in age-matched controls. This deficit of CoQ_{10} caused a significant reduction in the activity of enzyme complexes that are critical to the mitochondrial function of the brain cells affected by Parkinson's disease.

The ramifications of the study are significant. Parkinson's disease is becoming more prevalent as the human lifespan increases. The new study confirms previous studies that Parkinson's disease may be related to CoQ_{10} deficiency. The conclusion of the scientists was that

> The causes of Parkinson's disease are unknown. Evidence suggests that mitochondrial dysfunction and oxygen free radicals may be in involved in its pathogenesis. The dual function of CoQ_{10} as a constituent of the mitochondrial electron transport chain and a potent antioxidant suggest that it has the potential to slow the progression of Parkinson's disease.

CoQ_{10} levels decrease with aging. Depletion is caused by reduced synthesis of CoQ_{10} in the body along with increased oxidation of CoQ_{10} in the mitochondria. A CoQ_{10} deficiency results in the inactivation of enzymes needed for mitochondrial energy production, whereas supplementation with CoQ_{10} preserves mitochondrial function.

It is important to keep in mind that all therapies for Parkinson's disease are aimed at alleviating specific symptoms of the disease. A patient wishing to add new therapies to a treatment regimen should consult her physician regarding the potential risks and benefits.

Conclusion

Parkinson's disease is actually a number of related disorders affecting the central nervous system. Specifically, the disease affects the pigmented substantia nigra neurons responsible for producing dopamine. There are two types of Parkinson's disease: primary (or idiopathic) and secondary. Regardless of type, Parkinson's disease is divided into three stages (early, moderate, and advanced) based on symptoms and the progression of the disease. The onset of PD is insidious, with symptoms appearing over a number of years. The classic symptoms of PD are tremors, especially while at rest, rigidity of the neck and extremities, bradykinesis, and loss of postural reflexes. Secondary symptoms include sleep and skin disorders, difficulty swallowing, emotional changes, depression, and memory loss. Diagnosis of the disease consists of a thorough neurological examination; CT scans and MRIs may be done to rule out other causes for the patient's symptoms.

Treatment regimens are individualized according to the type and progression of PD. Commonly prescribed drug classes include anticholinergics, dopamine receptor agonists, and MAO inhibitors. The most effective treatment of PD is with *L*-dopa, which is usually not prescribed until the patient is in a more advanced stage of the disease. Recent clinical studies suggest that antioxidants, hormones, and amino acids such as tryptophan and tyrosine may be beneficial to the treatment of PD. Pallidotomy and thalamotomy are surgical procedures used to alleviate the major symptoms of PD. Patients may also wish to consider other therapies, including Hydergine, Coenzyme Q_{10} (ubiquinone), melatonin, and carnitine.

Summary

1. A thorough neurological examination is necessary to diagnosis Parkinson's disease. CT scans and MRIs may be ordered to rule out other causes for the patient's symptoms.
2. Conventional medications for the treatment of PD include anticholinergics, dopamine receptor agonists, and MAO inhibitors.
3. Anticholinergic medications commonly used for the treatment of PD include benztropine (1 to 2 mg daily, in separate doses), biperidon (2 mg, 3 to 4 times a day), and orphenadrine (50 mg 3 times daily, or 100 mg 2 times a day).
4. Dopamine receptor agonists include amantidine, bromocriptine, and pergolide. The recommended dosage for amantidine is 100 mg, 1

to 2 times a day; the recommended dosage for bromocriptine is 1.25 mg 1 to 2 times a day initially, gradually increased to 2.5 mg, 2 to 3 times a day.

5. Selegiline (Deprenyl) is a commonly prescribed MAO inhibitor for the treatment of PD. The recommended dosage is 5 mg, 2 times a day, taken with meals.

CAUTION: Selegiline should not be used if the patient is taking SSRI or tricyclic antidepressant drugs or meperidine or other opioid medications because of the risk of a serious, potentially fatal, reaction.

6. *L*-dopa, Sinemet, and Sinemet CR may be given to patients in the advanced stage of PD because the effectiveness of these medications decreases with time. The recommended dosage for *L*-dopa is 250 mg 2 to 4 times daily. The medication may be increased by 100 to 750 mg until the desired effect is achieved. The recommended dosage for Sinemet is 10/100 mg 3 to 4 times daily or 25/100 mg three times daily; the recommended dosage for Sinemet CR is 50/200 mg twice daily. (Note: Sinemet and Sinemet CR contain carbidopa and *L*-dopa; the notation 10/100 denotes the amount of each substance.)
7. Because PD patients often have sleep disorders and depression, sedatives and antidepressants may also be prescribed. These types of medications should be used with caution in elderly patients because of their side effects.
8. Antioxidants such as 200 mg a day of palm oil tocotrienols, 250 mg, twice a day of alpha-lipoic acid, 500 mg a day of ascorbyl palmitate, 120 mg a day of ginkgo extract, and 700 mg a day of green tea polyphenols.
9. Clinical studies have suggested that *L*-tryptophan may ameliorate motor complications associated with dopamine therapy, and may treat depression in PD patients. *L*-tyrosine may help to synthesize dopamine. Because these therapies are in the experimental stage for the treatment of this disease, a patient should consult her physician about them.
10. Coenzyme Q_{10} (ubiquinone) may help to curb the oxidative stress common in Parkinson's. The recommended dosage is 100 mg, 3 times daily.
11. Other beneficial therapies include Hydergine (10 to 20 mg daily), acetyl *L*-carnitine (1000 mg twice a day), DHEA (100 mg 3 times a day), NADH (5 to 10 mg twice daily), and melatonin (3 to 10 mg daily at bedtime).
12. PD patients should also consider human growth hormone (2 IUs injected daily) and testosterone replacement (Refer to *Male Hormone Modulation protocol*).

CAUTION: Life Extension Mix should be avoided by patients taking Sinemet, because the vitamin B_6 may prevent *L*-dopa from reaching the brain.

Because Parkinson's diseases involve a number of neurological problems, neurochemical imbalances, and hormonal imbalances, medications and hormonal therapies must be carefully monitored. Nutrient therapies can be used safely on a regular basis to protect and improve overall neurological functions.

For more information. Contact the American Parkinson Disease Association, (800) 223-2732, and Parkinson Support Groups of America, (301) 937-1545.

Product availability. Medications such as anticholinergics, dopamine receptor agonists, dopamine, and MAO inhibitors must be prescribed by a physician. Coenzyme Q_{10} (ubiquinone), Hydergine, carnitine, melatonin, phosphatidylserine, DHEA, NADH, Life Extension Mix, and Life Extension Booster, as well as other potentially beneficial products, such as Cognitex and pregnenolone, can be ordered by phoning (800) 544-1440, or order on-line at www.lef.org.

PHENYLALANINE AND TYROSINE DOSING AND PRECAUTIONS

Phenylalanine

- A precursor for neurotransmitter biosynthesis.
- One of 20 essential amino acids that the body cannot synthesize.

L-phenylalanine is an amino acid used in different biochemical processes to produce neurotransmitters, dopamine, norepinephrine, and epinephrine. It is claimed but not proven that phenylalanine can promote sexual arousal, and there is evidence that phenylalanine can increase mental alertness and release hormones affecting appetite. *D*-phenylalanine has been shown to inhibit the metabolism of opiate-like substances called enkephalins in the brain. It is claimed that *DL*-phenylalanine is effective in the treatment of chronic pain. There is some evidence that phenylalanine can help to overcome alcoholism and other drug addictions.

There have been reports that *L*-phenylalanine can promote high blood pressure in those predisposed to hypertension. Therefore, it is important to start off using moderate doses of phenylalanine, about 500 mg a day and slowly working up to 1500 mg a day. Monitoring in the first few months on phenylalanine can detect blood pressure increases in the minority of people who will present with this symptom.

Phenylalanine can promote the cell division of existing malignant melanoma cells. If you have melanoma, or any other form of cancer for that matter, avoid phenylalanine.

Those afflicted with PKU (phenylketonuria) cannot use phenylalanine. This includes those born with a genetic deficiency that prevents them from metabolizing phenylalanine.

Tyrosine

- A precursor for biosynthesis of neurotransmitters.
- A precursor for adrenaline and thyroid hormones.
- Used to treat depression, anxiety, and allergies.
- Combined with tryptophan to treat drug abuse.
- Suppresses appetite.
- Tyrosine deficiency will result in depression and mood disorders.
- As a dietary precursor, tryrosine is one of the major nutritional ingredients that affect neurotransmitter synthesis and brain functions.

Tyrosine is an amino acid synthesized in the body from phenylalanine. It is an important nutritional ingredient and factor for biosynthesis of the brain neurotransmitters epinephrine, norepinephrine, and dopamine. Tyrosine is also used to produce one of the major hormones, thyroxin, which plays an important role in controlling metabolic rate, skin health, mental health, and growth rate. Tyrosine is specifically used to treat depression because it is a precursor for those neurotransmitters that are responsible for transmitting nerve impulses and essential for preventing depression. It has been tested on humans for increasing their endurance to anxiety and stress under fatigue. It was proven in research studies that tyrosine supplementation results in increased performance over a control group. Tyrosine was also used with the amino acid tryptophan for treatment of cocaine abuse. Combined with imipramine, tyrosine has a greater than 74% success rate in the treatment of chronic cocaine abuse. Tyrosine is a mild antioxidant, reacting with free radicals that can cause damage to cells. It is also known that tyrosine promotes sexual drive. It may also be used as a mild appetite suppressant.

Summary

1. *L*-tyrosine may be effective as an adjuvant treatment in Parkinson's disease with more favorable clinical results and fewer side effects.

2. The family of neurotrophin proteins, including nerve growth factor (NGF), brain-derived nerve factor (BDNF), and neurotrophins (NT-3, NT-4/5, and 6) require tyrosine as precursors to synthesis.
3. Dietary precursors, especially in purified form, have been proven to promote the level of neurotransmitters in the brain. When taken orally or parenterally, they induce an increase of transmitter formation, further influencing a variety of brain functions.
4. Plasma levels of tyrosine can be elevated incrementally depending on dose, with concentrations raised more than three times that of the control group. No side effects were observed.
5. Dietary precursors, tyrosine, tryptophan, choline, and lecithin will affect brain neurotransmitter synthesis and brain function.

CAUTION: Tyrosine may also promote cancer cell division, especially malignant melanoma.

PHOBIAS

Phobias are fears that may seem irrational but which nonetheless produce disruptive symptoms of anxiety. Anxiety is the body's and mind's response to a dangerous or distressing situation, which may be real or imagined. Everyone experiences some degree of anxiety at some time. But anxiety can occur persistently, and may be triggered by vague notions of a threat. If anxiety interferes with normal activities, you are said to suffer from an anxiety disorder.

Phobias, which stem from or accompany anxiety disorders, may be simple in nature or debilitating, requiring extensive cognitive and pharmacological therapy, or even hospitalization.

Many people suffer from phobias, in one form or another. Surveys indicate that phobias are among the most common psychiatric disorders. More than half of psychiatric respondents, in fact, admit to having at least one phobia.

When we suffer from phobic fear, our bodies produce symptoms of anxiety. These symptoms may be fleeting or severe. They are caused when the adrenal glands release large amounts of adrenaline. At the same time, the brain releases its own form of adrenaline, a chemical called norepinephrine. This is an excitatory neurotransmitter that stimulates cells in the brain and other parts of the body. Norepinephrine initiates its effects by binding to beta-adrenergic sites on the cell membrane.

How Phobias Manifest

Phobias may result from or coexist with panic disorder, which is marked by intense, disabling feelings of tension or extreme fear for no apparent reason. People with panic disorder may experience panic attacks. These are periods in which there is a sudden onset of intense apprehension, fearfulness, or terror and, often, feelings of impending doom. Symptoms of panic attacks may include shortness of breath, palpitations, chest pain or discomfort, a sensation that you are choking or smothering, or a fear that you are losing control or even "going crazy."

Agoraphobia, often described as "a fear of open spaces," may be associated with panic disorder. Agoraphobia may be acute or chronic. The disorder produces anxiety about places or situations from which escape might be difficult or embarrassing. Often agoraphobics fear that if they leave the "safety" of their homes they may have a panic attack. Some agoraphobics have suffered symptoms so severe that they have confined themselves to their homes for years at a time.

Many people are plagued by specific phobias. These are characterized by anxiety provoked by exposure to a specific object or situation. A person may be severely afraid of snakes, for example, and experience extreme anxiety when confronted by the reptiles. People with severe specific phobias often go out of their way to avoid contact with the thing that frightens them.

Certain social situations as well may provoke anxiety in people who fear that they will become trapped or embarrassed. Such people may experience anxiety in groups, or suffer from performance anxiety, say, when taking a test.

Obsessive-compulsive disorder is characterized by obsessions that cause marked anxiety or distress and by compulsions that serve to neutralize anxiety. Obsessions are persistent ideas, thoughts, impulses, or images that are experienced as intrusive and inappropriate, and that cause marked anxiety or distress. The most common obsessions are repeated thoughts about contamination (i.e., becoming contaminated by germs, or by shaking hands); repeated doubts (wondering whether one has performed some act, such as having left a door unlocked or a coffee pot brewing on the stove); a need to have things in a particular order; aggressive or horrific impulses (which the person might never act on); or sexual imagery that is inappropriate or frightening.

Compulsions are repetitive behaviors (hand washing, checking) or mental acts (praying, counting, repeating words silently). The goal of compulsions is to prevent or reduce anxiety or distress. The person feels driven to perform the compulsion to reduce the distress caused by the obsessive thought.

The essential features of obsessive-compulsive disorder are recurrent obsessions or compulsions that are severe enough to be time consuming (taking more than one hour a day) or cause marked distress or significant impairment. Usually at some point during the course of the disorder, the person recognizes that the obsessions or compulsions are excessive or unreasonable, but is powerless to change his or her behavior without intervention.

Phobias and other anxiety disorders may cause anxiety, suspiciousness, affective instability, and other symptoms. Phobias also are linked with a number of other mental, addictive, and physical disorders, report researchers from the Division of Epidemiology and Services Research branch of the National Institute of Mental Health. The scientists studied more than 20,000 patients to determine prevalence of anxiety, mood, and addictive disorders and to identify the onset of those illnesses. Nearly half (47.2%) of patients diagnosed with major depression also met criteria for an anxiety disorder. The researchers concluded that anxiety disorders, especially social and simple phobias, appear to have an early onset with potentially severe consequences, predisposing those affected to greater vulnerability to major depression and addictive disorders.

Other studies also suggest that people develop phobias early in life, during or before adolescence. Researchers at the Department of Psychiatry and Behavioral Sciences at Stanford University School of Medicine in California concluded that people who develop phobias at an early age are more likely to develop major depression later in life.

Fears of heights and animals were the most commonly represented simple phobias experienced by 711 patients at Massachusetts Mental Health Center in Boston. In a multicenter, longitudinal study of anxiety disorders, 115 patients with simple phobias were compared with 596 anxiety disorder patients who did not also suffer from simple phobias. Researchers found that those with simple phobias reported more anxiety disorders than patients without phobias. The patients with phobias were also found to be more likely to suffer from post-traumatic stress disorder, which is marked by delayed response to a stressful or traumatic event.

Conventional Treatment

Allopathic medicine aims to relieve symptoms of anxiety disorders, including phobias, with drug therapy and to treat underlying disorders or conflicts with psychotherapy.

Some of the more commonly prescribed medicines used to treat phobias and anxiety disorders include

- ▼ *Benzodiazepine drugs*, such as diazepam and oxazepam, which limit brain activity, temporarily creating a state of relaxation. Because such tranquilizing drugs are potentially habit forming, they should be used only for short periods. Side effects may include daytime drowsiness, reduced concentration, and confusion.
- ▼ *Beta-blocking drugs.* These are taken before a phobia-inducing event (such as public speaking, flying in an airplane, or meeting new

people). Beta-blockers prevent excess adrenaline and norepinephrine from causing the anxiety, shaking, heart palpitations, sweating, and queasy stomach that often characterize a phobia.

The first beta-blocking drug was propranolol, which is also used to lower blood pressure in hypertensive patients. Propranolol has more than 30 years of clinical use to document its safety, and it is available in low-cost generic form. The suggested dose is 10 to 40 mg before a phobia-inducing event. People with very low blood pressure, certain forms of congestive heart failure, and asthma should not take propranolol or other beta-blocking drugs.

- *Anti-depressant drugs.* Some researchers think there may be a link between the brain chemical serotonin and nonpsychotic disorders, such as anxiety and affective and compulsive-obsessive disorders. Conventional doctors may prescribe selective serotonin reuptake inhibitor (SSRI) drugs, such as Prozac, Zoloft, or Paxil to treat anxiety, phobias, and obsessive-compulsive symptoms. While SSRIs are safer than such tranquilizers as Xanax and Valium, there are concerns in the life-extension community about long-term side effects, such as serotonin overload.

Recently, researchers have been working to develop a drug called befloxatone, which may be helpful in treating depression, social phobias, and panic disorders. Befloxatone is a long-acting selective and reversible monoamine oxidase A (MAO-A) inhibitor. The drug has been tested in clinical trials in France and the United States and has been found to be safe, causing no sedative, convulsant, or cardiovascular side effects. Initial results indicate that it is suitable to take befloxatone orally once a day.

In one trial, researchers gave 10 mg of befloxatone a day to 12 healthy elderly volunteers. The researchers then tested the subjects' psychomotor and cognitive function. They concluded that the drug did not produce any detrimental effects on performance, memory, or sleep patterns.

Psychotherapy

Doctors often recommend drug therapy in conjunction with psychotherapy. People with anxiety or phobias may be helped by talking with trained therapists about their symptoms, feelings, behavior, history, and concerns. This treatment approach may be simple, consisting of support and advice, or elaborate, involving extensive psychoanalysis. Options include one-on-one cognitive therapy and group therapy.

Often psychotherapy can be effective in helping patients who have not responded well to drug therapy. Researchers in The Netherlands, for example, found that cognitive therapy worked well for subjects plagued by paruresis, a fear of urinating in the proximity of others. After receiving cognitive therapy for 18 weeks, the patients reported a significant reduction of symptoms. Moreover, the researchers found that the patients maintained their psychiatric gains after 6 months.

Group therapy also may be effective in treating phobias. In Lyon, France, 55 patients with social phobias received cognitive and group therapy. The patients were evaluated after 6 and 12 months. Researchers found that the patients showed statistically significant improvement.

Natural Therapies

In addition, several natural therapies have been effective in treating phobias and other anxiety disorders. These alternative techniques may be employed individually or in conjunction with conventional treatments. They include

- Kava kava (*Piper methysticum*). A South Pacific member of the pepper family, Kava induces calm feelings, eases muscle tension, reduces emotional tension, and improves sleep. The safest and most effective way of using Kava is in liquid spray form that provides a standardized dose. Most people spray the Kava directly into their mouths 1 to 3 times a day. Each spray should be standardized to provide 60 mg of 30% kava lactones.
- Nutritional supplements. Some studies indicate that niacinamide (500 to 800 mg) and

calcium (1000 to 2000 elemental milligrams) may be beneficial in reducing symptoms of anxiety and phobias.

- Meditation. People who perform meditation exercises take an active role in their treatment, teaching themselves how to quiet or clear the mind. Several clinical studies have shown that during meditation the body is altered in ways that are beneficial for people who suffer from anxiety. For example, the rate of metabolism drops and blood pressure decreases. Meditation may be performed daily, several times a week, or just before a situation that might provoke anxiety.

In addition, Canadian researchers report that regular exercise may help many people who suffer from psychiatric disorders, including phobias. Researchers Gregg A. Tkachuk and Garry L. Martin of the Department of Psychology at the University of Manitoba examined studies of anxiety disorder and exercise dating back to 1981. They found that strength training, running, walking, and other forms of aerobic exercise help to alleviate mild to moderate depression, and also may help to treat other mental disorders, including anxiety and substance abuse. "There is now considerable evidence that regular exercise is a viable, cost-effective but underused treatment for mild to moderate depression that compares favorably to individual psychotherapy, group psychotherapy, and cognitive therapy," the researchers said in their study, which was published in *Professional Psychology*: *Research and Practice*.

In one study cited by the researchers, people who ran, walked, or performed strengthening exercises 3 times a week for 20 to 60 minutes were significantly less depressed after 5 weeks. What's more, their gains lasted for up to a year.

The Canadian researchers also reported that exercise is more effective than placebos at reducing symptoms of panic. In one study of 46 people with moderate to severe panic disorder, those who ran 3 times a week for 10 weeks and those who took anti-anxiety medications felt better than people who took placebo medicines. (The investigators noted, however, that treatment with the drug chlomipramine was a faster, more effective treatment than exercise in patients with panic disorder.)

Studies included in the Canadian review also showed that exercise may help to treat symptoms of schizophrenia, a psychiatric disorder marked by delusions, confusion, and emotional turmoil. However, more studies are needed to confirm these findings, the researchers noted.

In the meantime, the researchers said, exercise may be an important component of treatment for body image problems, substance abuse problems, and somatic disorders in which mental symptoms manifest as physical pain. And exercise, they said, is an affective short-term treatment for reduction of destructive behavior and for increasing work performance in people with developmental disabilities, such as attention deficit disorder, which is marked by an inability to concentrate, and hyperactivity.

Exactly how exercise helps to lessen depression and other psychiatric disorders is not fully understood. Improvements may result from a combination of factors, including release of brain chemicals called endorphins. Endorphins produce calming, soothing effects. In addition, exercise may provide a distraction from negative emotions such as sadness and hopelessness, two hallmarks of depression. And exercise may help to buffer the effects of stress.

Summary

Natural therapies for phobias and anxiety disorders may be employed individually or in conjunction with conventional treatments. They include

1. Kava kava, to induce a feeling of calmness and ease muscle tension, 1 or 2 sprays, 1 to 3 times a day. Each spray should provide 60 mg of 30% kava lactones.
2. Calcium, 1000 elemental milligrams, once to twice a day, along with 500 to 1000 elemental milligrams of magnesium.
3. Vitamin B_3 (niacinamide), 500 mg once or twice a day.
4. Exercise, to alleviate depression and reduce symptoms of panic and anxiety.
5. Meditation, to clear the mind of anxious or disturbing thoughts.

Refer to the *Anxiety and Stress protocol* for additional suggestions.

For more information. Contact the National Mental Health Association, (800) 969-6642.

Product availability. Kava kava liquid spray, niacinamide, and calcium supplements are available from the Life Extension Foundation by calling (800) 544-4440, or order on-line at www.lef.org. Ask for a list of knowledgeable physicians in your area who will prescribe propranolol to treat phobias.

POLYMYALGIA RHEUMATICA

Polymyalgia rheumatica is a systemic rheumatic inflammatory disease characterized by shoulder and hip girdle pain that in some patients can be associated with giant cell arteritis and other diseases. It appears that polymyalgia rheumatica can be an early symptom of a wide range of diseases, including rheumatoid arthritis, some cancers, and other degenerative diseases.

A recent study suggested that a thyroid hormone blood test be conducted to rule out hyperthyroidism (too much thyroid hormone). The tests most often used to evaluate thyroid output are TSH, T3, and T4. Correction of hyperthyroidism can reverse the disease.

Standard therapy is long-term, low-dose use of the corticosteroid drug *methylprednisolone*. This drug therapy has many side effects, including excessive loss of bone density and severe immune impairment. A careful prevention with calcium and vitamin D must be carried out systematically. The demineralization can be limited by the use of Deflazacort, a corticosteroid, which decreases the loss of calcium. One report suggested that high intramuscular doses of methylprednisolone were as effective as long-term oral intake of prednisolone and reduced the risk of bone fractures.

Here is one succinct description of the disease from a recent report:

> Polymyalgia rheumatica (PMR) is a disease of unknown etiology that occurs in elderly patients, predominantly affecting the Caucasian population. The disease has a slightly higher prevalence in women than in men. There is ongoing discussion regarding the relationship between PMR and giant cell arteritis; an increasing number of studies indicate that they are closely related. PMR has also been linked with rheumatoid arthritis, myopathy, and malignant disease. Oral corticosteroids remain the mainstay of drug therapy for PMR. These drugs usually induce prompt relief of symptoms, and some authors consider this dramatic response to be diagnostic for PMR. The ideal initial dosage, the duration of treatment, and the optimal tapering schedule, however, are much debated.
>
> Other drugs, such as methotrexate and azathioprine, have been suggested as corticosteroid-sparing agents. Nonsteroidal anti-inflammatory drugs are generally considered to be unsuitable for the long-term treatment of PMR.

Here is another description of the disease and various conventional treatments:

> There are no standardized diagnostic criteria for polymyalgia rheumatica. The combination of persistent pain (at least 1 month) with marked morning stiffness in at least two of the neck, shoulder, or pelvic girdle is characteristic of polymyalgia rheumatica. The other criteria are age >50 years, erythrocyte sedimentation rate (ESR) >40 mm/hour, rapid response to corticosteroids, and an absence of other diseases capable of causing the musculoskeletal symptoms. A normal ESR does not exclude a diagnosis of polymyalgia rheumatica. Diagnostic temporal artery biopsy is recommended in all patients suspected of having giant cell arteritis. The segment of temporal artery with abnormality on physical examination should be biopsied. The drugs of choice in the treatment of polymyalgia rheumatica/giant cell arteritis are corticosteroids. An initial prednisone dosage of 40 to 60 mg/day is adequate in almost all cases of giant cell arteritis. Higher dosages and/or intravenous pulse methylprednisolone can be tried on patients with partial response or with recent visual loss.
>
> Polymyalgia rheumatica in the absence of giant cell arteritis requires an initial dose of prednisone 10 to

20 mg/day. In some cases of mild polymyalgia rheumatica, a short course of nonsteroidal anti-inflammatory drugs may be tried. Long-term corticosteroid therapy in polymyalgia rheumatica and giant cell arteritis is complicated by serious adverse effects in between 48 and 65% of patients. Vertebral fractures and infections are among the most dangerous and frequent complications. Although there are limited data on the use of cytotoxic or immunosuppressive drugs, such as methotrexate, azathiopreine, and cyclosporine, in these indications, they might be effective either in sparing corticosteroids or in treating patients who do not respond to treatment with corticosteroids.

Here is another description of the disease:

> Polymyalgia rheumatica is a typical disease of the elderly. If vascular complications of giant cell arteritis have not developed before treatment starts, the prognosis is generally favorable. However, the course of the disease is often characterized by relapses requiring an increase in the corticosteroid dosage. This is associated with a higher rate of adverse reactions that modifies the otherwise favorable prognosis. We evaluated the course of the disease in 78 polymyalgia rheumatica patients who were observed for a mean of 28 plus or minus 20 months. Temporal arteritis was histologically confirmed in 20 out of 71 patients (28%). Of the 70 patients who were observed for more than 6 months, 18 (26%) suffered a relapse of corticosteroid dosages of 6.25 plus or minus 3.1 (0-12.5) mg. After 24 months 36% had been in remission without treatment for a period of 9.3 plus or minus 6.1 (3-18) months. Therapy-associated complications arose in 21 (34%) of 64 patients who were observed for more than 9 months. The most common were steroid-induced diabetes mellitus or aggravation of a known diabetic metabolic condition (33%).
>
> The most severe adverse reaction—osteoporotic vertebral fracture—was reported in three patients. Further complications of therapy were various frequencies of arterial hypertension, cataract, glaucoma, subjectively disturbing weight gain, and hypokalaemia. Overall, our data confirmed that the usually favorable course of polymyalgia rheumatica is modified by relapses and complications of therapy. Hence, we would tend to reduce steroids or use immunosuppressants at an early stage, especially in high-risk cases such as patients with inadequately controllable diabetes mellitus or manifest osteoporosis.

Since this disease is classified as an autoimmune disease, you may consider following the *Autoimmune Diseases protocol,* which includes DHEA and gamma-linolenic acid (GLA from borage oil) therapy. DHEA can also help to maintain bone density and immune function. Since autoimmune disease is poorly understood, there is some risk that DHEA could make the symptoms worse.

If *corticosteroid therapy* (prednisone-like) drugs are currently being administered, the patient should take 1000 to 2000 elemental mg of calcium a day along with other bone-protecting nutrients such as vitamin D_3. Most Foundation members use the product Bone Assure, which contains all the nutrients that have been shown to protect against bone loss due to aging and drug therapies. If corticosteroid therapy is effective, but a relapse occurs after the steroid therapy is discontinued, consider a course of *cyclosporine* therapy or low-dose chemotherapy with such drugs as *methotrexate.*

Protecting against the toxicities of conventional drugs is crucial, as the published literature clearly shows that the drugs used to treat this condition are especially toxic. The standard daily dose of Life Extension Mix may help protect against toxicity, while potentially correcting the underlying autoimmune disorder.

There may be some benefit in using cyclooxygenase II-inhibiting drugs such as Celebrex.

Methylcobalamin should be taken sublingually in the dose of 10 to 20 mg a day. This can help protect against nerve damage, but will do nothing to alleviate the underlying autoimmune disease that is causing the problem.

Summary

1. Corticosteroids such as methylprednisolone are effective in the treatment of polymyalgia rheumatica but may cause side effects such as loss of bone density and severe immune impairment.
2. Cyclosporine or low-dose chemotherapy with a drug such as methotrexate may be considered as an alternative to corticosteroids.
3. Protection from demineralization should include systematic supplementation with

calcium and vitamin D. Bone Assure contains nutrients that protect against bone loss due to aging and drug therapies.

4. DHEA can help maintain bone density and immune function.
5. Blood testing should be conducted to rule out hyperparathyroidism as a contributing factor.
6. Aspirin or other nonsteroidal anti-inflammatories may provide relief from pain and stiffness. Consider COX-2–inhibiting drug therapy.
7. Life Extension Mix may help protect against immunotoxicity.
8. Sublingual methylcobalamin can help protect against nerve damage but will not affect the underlying autoimmune disorder.

Product availability. Bone Assure, vitamin D, DHEA, Healthprin aspirin, and Life Extension Mix can be ordered by calling (800) 544-4440, or order on-line at www.lef.org.

PREGNENOLONE PRECAUTIONS

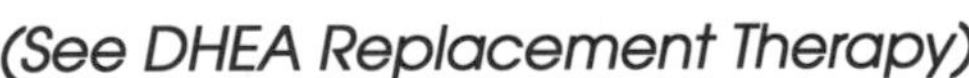

(See DHEA Replacement Therapy)

PREMENSTRUAL SYNDROME

(See Female Hormone Modulation Therapy)

PREVENTION PROTOCOLS

The concept of taking actions now to maintain youthful health is based on published scientific studies showing that the diseases of aging may be prevented, or can at least be postponed.

People who want to reduce their risk of disease are often overwhelmed by the volume of technical data on the subject. The Life Extension Foundation has reviewed more than 64 years' worth of published medical literature, and Foundation personnel have spent more than 35 years working with physicians and scientists in the anti-aging field.

Each year, the Foundation spends millions of dollars on research projects aimed at extending the healthy human lifespan. Since 1983, the Foundation has reviewed thousands of blood test results of members who have been following anti-aging supplement, drug, and hormone-replacement programs. Based on this vast accumulation of data, the Foundation has designed a practical disease prevention protocol that is based solely on scientific principles.

Before you embark on a program to reduce your risk of degenerative disease, it is important for you to know about scientific studies conducted on humans that show these therapies really work. If you are not aware of these published studies, you may be unlikely to methodically follow a long-term disease prevention program.

The Media Ignore Important Clinical Studies

Don't count on the new media or popular health publications to keep you fully informed about new medical findings. An article published in the December 25, 1996, issue of the *Journal of the American Medical Association* (*JAMA*) showed that 200 mcg of supplemental selenium a day reduced overall cancer mortality by 50% in humans compared to a placebo group not receiving supplemental selenium. This 9-year study, published in the American Medical Association's scientific journal (*JAMA*), demonstrated that a low-cost mineral supplement could cut the risk of dying from cancer in half.

In the prior week's issue of *JAMA* (December 18, 1996), an article was published indicating that folic acid could substantially reduce cardiovascular disease risk. The selenium-cancer study received some media attention, but the folic acid-cardiovascular study did not. The fact is that the news media have not been consistent in reporting on studies that substantiate the disease-preventing role of dietary supplements, even when these studies appear in the most prestigious medical journals in the world.

One of the most compelling reports that high-potency supplements extend lifespan in humans was published in the August 1996 issue of the *American Journal of Clinical Nutrition*. This study involved 11,178 elderly people, who participated in a trial to establish the effects of vitamin supplements on mortality. This study showed that the use of vitamin E reduced the risk of death from all causes by 34%. Effects were strongest for coronary artery disease, where vitamin E resulted in a 63% reduction in death from heart attack. In addition, the use of vitamin E resulted in a 59% reduction in cancer mortality. When the effects of vitamin C and E were combined, overall mortality was reduced by 42% (compared to 34% for vitamin E alone). These results are the most significant evidence yet presented about the value of vitamin supplementation, yet the media failed to report on it. What made this study so credible was that:

- It compared people who took low-potency "one-a-day" multiple vitamins to those who took higher-potency vitamin C and E supplements. Previous studies measuring the life expectancy of the "one-a-day" crowd did not show significant benefits, thereby causing most doctors to conclude there is no value in vitamin supplementation. In this new report, those taking "one-a-day" multivitamins did not do any better than people taking nothing at all, which supports the Life Extension Foundation's position that higher doses of antioxidants are required to reduce the risk of heart disease and cancer than those found in conventional supplements.
- It lasted 9 years! Most studies that attempt to evaluate the benefits of vitamin supplementation are for shorter time periods. It should be noted, however, that the famous Harvard *Nurses' Health Study* found that vitamin E reduced coronary artery disease mortality by over 40% after only 2 years!
- It included 11,178 people, a larger group than most previous studies.

The Suppression of Folic Acid

The Food and Drug Administration (FDA) has spent enormous resources trying to prevent people from supplementing with folic acid. The FDA argues against folic acid supplementation because the presence of folic acid in the blood could mask a serious vitamin B_{12} deficiency. *JAMA* (Dec. 18, 1996) addressed the FDA's concerns by recommending that folic acid supplements be fortified with vitamin B_{12} as a prudent way of gaining the cardiovascular benefits of folic acid without risking a B_{12} deficiency.

The April 9, 1998, issue of the *New England Journal of Medicine* endorsed the use of folic acid to reduce the incidence of heart attack and stroke, but the FDA still refuses to accept that folic acid has any benefit other than preventing a certain type of birth defect.

A study published in *Annals of Internal Medicine* (1998; 129:517–24) shows how fatally flawed the FDA's position is. Data from the famous *Nurses' Health Study* conducted at the Harvard Medical School showed that long-term supplementation with folic acid reduces the risk of colon cancer by an astounding 75% in women. The fact that there are 90,000 women participating in the *Nurses' Health Study* makes this finding especially significant. The authors of this study explained that folic acid obtained from supplements had a stronger protective effect against colon cancer than folic acid consumed in the diet. This new study helps to confirm the work of Dr. Bruce Ames, the famous molecular biologist who has authored numerous articles showing that folic acid is extremely effective in preventing the initial DNA mutations that can lead to cancer later in life. This Harvard report, showing a 75% reduction in colon cancer incidence, demonstrated that the degree of protection against cancer is correlated with how long a DNA-protecting substance (folic acid) is consumed. It was the women who took more than 400 mcg of folic acid a day for 15 years who experienced the 75% reduction in colon cancer, whereas short-term supplementation with folic acid produced only marginal protection.

There now exists a massive body of evidence that supplementation with folic acid can prevent both cardiovascular disease *and* cancer, yet the FDA has proposed rules that would prohibit the American public from even learning about these benefits. Colon cancer will kill 47,000 Americans this year. Too bad the FDA didn't "allow" these colon cancer victims to learn about folic acid in time.

The Vitamin C Controversy

Does vitamin C cause kidney stones? That's what some doctors still say, but a report from Harvard Medical School showed no increased risk of kidney stones when evaluating 85,557 women over a 14-year study period. This report, published in the April 1999 issue of the *Journal of the American Society of Nephrology*, showed that women who consumed 1500 mg a day or more of vitamin C were no more likely to develop kidney stones than women who consumed less than 250 mg of vitamin C a day. The study did reveal that women who consumed 40 mg or more of vitamin B_6 were 34% less likely to contract kidney stones compared to women taking fewer than 3 mg a day of B_6. So now that kidney stone risk has been ruled out, let's look at some of the human studies showing positive benefits to vitamin C supplementation.

In the early 1990s, several large population studies showed a reduction in cardiovascular disease in those who consumed vitamin C. The media reported on some of these findings and this favorable publicity helped push a bill through Congress that prevented the FDA from banning high-potency vitamin C and other supplements.

The most significant report emanated in 1992 from UCLA, where it was announced that men who took 800 mg a day of vitamin C lived 6 years longer than those who consumed the FDA's recommended daily allowance of 60 mg a day. The study, which evaluated 11,348 participants over a 10-year period of time, showed that high vitamin C intake extended average life span and reduced mortality from cardiovascular disease by 42%. This study was published in the journal *Epidemiology* (1992; 3 [3]:194–202).

A study published in the *British Medical Journal* (vol. 314, issue 708, 1997) evaluated 1605 randomly selected men in Finland aged 42–60 years between 1984 and 1989. None of these men had evidence of pre-existing heart disease. After adjusting for other confounding factors, men who were deficient in vitamin C had 3.5 times more heart attacks than men who were not deficient in vitamin C. The scientist's conclusion was, "Vitamin C deficiency, as assessed by low plasma ascorbate concentration, is a risk factor for coronary heart disease."

In the March 9, 1999, issue of the American Heart Association's journal *Circulation*, elevated homocysteine levels were shown to cause rapid onset of endothelial (arterial lining) dysfunction. This type of dysfunction reduces blood flow and can facilitate a lethal arterial spasm. Vitamin C inhibited arterial dysfunction by interfering with oxidative stress mechanisms. The doctors conducting the study stated that acute impairment of vascular endothelial function can be prevented by pretreatment with vitamin C.

A double-blind study published in the *Journal of the American College of Cardiology* (1998; 31[6]:1323–29) compared the effects of nitrate drugs in people receiving vitamin C to a placebo group not receiving vitamin C. The doctors administered nitrate drugs to healthy people and patients with coronary artery disease and then measured vasodilation response and cellular levels of cGMP, an energy substrate that is depleted by nitrate drugs. At day zero, all participants were measured to establish a baseline. After 3 days of vitamin C administration (2 grams/3 times daily), there was no change in either group. After 6 days of vitamin C therapy an impressive 42% improvement in vasodilation response was observed and a 60% improvement in cellular cGMP levels was measured in coronary artery disease patients receiving vitamin C compared to placebo. A similar improvement occurred in the healthy subjects taking vitamin C compared to the placebo group. The doctors concluded the study by stating that "these results indicate that combination therapy with vitamin C is potentially useful for preventing the development of nitrate tolerance."

Another study, published in the *Journal of Clinical Investigation* (July 1, 1998), looked at the effects of nitrate drug therapy on human patients. Tolerance development was monitored by changes in arterial pressure, pulse pressure, heart rate, and activity of isolated patients. All patients experienced the deleterious effects of nitrate tolerance. However, when vitamin C was co-administered with the nitrate drugs, the effects of nitrate tolerance were virtually eliminated. The most significant improvement was a 310% improvement in the arterial conductivity test. The nitrate drugs induced a dangerous upregulated activity of platelets, but this too was reversed with vitamin C supplementation. The doctors who conducted this study indicated that vitamin C may be of benefit during long-term, non-intermittent administration of nitrate drugs in humans.

Chronic heart failure is associated with reduced dilating capacity of the endothelial lining of the arterial system. Scientists tested heart failure patients by high-resolution ultrasound and Doppler to measure radial artery diameter and blood flow. Vitamin C restored arterial dilation response and blood flow velocity in patients with heart failure. The scientists determined that the mechanism of action was that vitamin C increased the availability of nitric oxide, an important precursor to cGMP. This study was published in the February 1998 issue of the journal *Circulation*.

Also in 1998, another aspect of vitamin C's effect on coronary artery disease was discovered. A study published in the *Journal of the American College of Cardiology* (1998; 41[5]:980–86) showed that low plasma ascorbic acid levels independently predict the presence of an unstable coronary syndrome in heart disease patients. According to the doctors, the study's results showed that the beneficial effects of vitamin C in treating coronary artery disease may result, in part, by an influence on arterial wall lesion activity rather than a reduction in the overall extent of fixed disease.

The published research findings suggest that vitamin C may reduce mortality in coronary artery disease patients, increase life span, and possibly eliminate the effects of nitrate tolerance in those taking nitrate drugs. While not recognized in the medical establishment as a therapy for coronary artery disease, there now exists an accumulated wealth of evidence that vitamin C has beneficial effects in the treatment of heart-related illnesses.

Mainstream medicine has historically ridiculed vitamin C supplementation. In today's modern world, conventional medicine says that only 200 mg a day of vitamin C is needed, despite findings showing that high doses of vitamin C are required to produce optimal benefit. Meanwhile, the FDA continues to stick with its position that no more than 60 to 100 mg a day of vitamin C is needed.

Saturating the Bladder

The most frequently voiced criticism about supplemental vitamin intake is that it produces "expensive urine," since water-soluble vitamins such as vitamin C and the B vitamins are rapidly excreted into the bladder within hours of ingestion. For years, the Life Extension Foundation has contended that these vitamins are beneficial in spite of their rapid excretion and that, moreover, it is desirable to have a bladder full of vitamins because certain vitamins inhibit chemicals that cause bladder cancer. In the September 1996 issue of the *American Journal of Epidemiology*, a study on the risk of bladder cancer in vitamin takers showed the following:

- High intake of vitamin A and beta-carotene was associated with a 48% reduction in bladder cancer incidence compared to the lowest levels of vitamin A and beta-carotene intake.
- People taking higher amounts of vitamin C had a 50% reduced rate of bladder cancer. Those who took 502 mg or more of vitamin C a day had a 60% reduction in bladder cancer compared to those who took no vitamin C.

- For those who took multivitamin supplements for at least 10 years, the reduction in bladder cancer was 61% compared to people who took no vitamin supplements.
- High intake of fried foods was associated with double the risk of bladder cancer.

It appears from this study that even low-potency "one-a-day" supplements (which do not protect against other types of cancer) can at least protect against bladder cancer.

Protecting Vision

Studies show that antioxidant supplements reduce the risk of cataracts. One study in the *American Journal of Epidemiology* (Sept. 1996) evaluated 410 men for 3 years to ascertain the association between serum vitamin E and the development of cortical lens opacities (cataracts). The men with the lowest level of serum vitamin E had a 3.7 times greater risk of this form of cataract compared to men with the highest serum level of vitamin E.

While cataracts are usually treatable, a disease called wet macular degeneration is not. Those who eat spinach and collard greens have low rates of macular degeneration, and extracts from these vegetables thought to protect against this blinding disease are now available in dietary supplements that contain lutein and zeaxanthin.

Keeping Arteries Clean

In a study reported in the *American Journal of Clinical Nutrition* (1997, 65 [1]), antioxidant status was assessed and carotid artery occlusion was measured in 1187 men and women 59–71 years of age without any history of coronary artery disease or stroke. The results showed that the higher the level of vitamin E in red blood cells, the lower the risk of carotid atherosclerosis. In men with the highest levels of carotid atherosclerotic plaques, the lowest levels of vitamin E, selenium, and carotenoids were found. The scientists concluded by stating, "Our findings give some epidemiological support to the hypothesis that lipid peroxidation and low antioxidant status are involved in the early stages of atherosclerosis."

A study published in the journal *Atherosclerosis* (1999; 144:237–49) showed that people who took a 900-mg garlic supplement every day for 4 years had 18% less plaque buildup in their carotid arteries compared to the placebo group. The women in the study group actually showed a 4.6% decrease in carotid plaque volume over a 4-year period, whereas the placebo group showed a 5.3% increase in artery-clogging plaque.

There are more studies showing that atherosclerosis can be prevented than for any other degenerative disease. Since more people die or become disabled from vascular diseases than any other cause, it would appear prudent to follow a program that would reduce one's risk of suffering a vascular-related heart attack or stroke.

Are You Concerned about Cancer?

Fear of cancer is a major reason why people take dietary supplements. As has already been shown, there is a compelling body of evidence that cancer risk can be reduced by taking the proper supplements over an extended period of time.

In the March 17, 1999, issue of the *Journal of the National Cancer Institute*, associations between intakes of specific nutrients and subsequent breast cancer risk were investigated in 83,234 women who were participating in the Nurses' Health Study. Breast cancer risks were significantly lower in women who consumed alpha-carotene, beta-carotene, lutein/zeaxanthin, and vitamins A and C. Among premenopausal women who consumed moderate amounts of alcohol (a known risk factor in breast cancer), beta-carotene lowered risk. Premenopausal women who consumed five or more servings per day of fruits and vegetables had modestly lower risk of breast cancer than those who had less than two servings per day.

A study published in the March 15, 1999, issue of *Cancer Research* showed that the tomato extract lycopene was the most effective nutrient shown to protect against the development of prostate cancer. This study, begun in 1982, followed 578 men for 13 years. Lycopene strongly reduced prostate cancer risk, and more importantly, lowered the risk for aggressive cancer. This study confirmed many previous studies showing that lycopene can help prevent pancreatic, prostate, and a host of other cancers. A surprising finding revealed at the April 12, 1999, meeting of the American Association of Cancer Research showed that 30 mg of lycopene supplements a day slowed the growth of existing prostate cancer and lowered serum PSA readings by 20%!

Men with high intake of vitamin E were 35% as likely to develop colorectal adenomas as men with low vitamin E intake (*American Journal of Epidemiology,* 1996; 144 [11]). (Adenomas are neoplastic lesions that are considered precursors to colon cancer.) In a related study published in the February 1999 issue of *Diseases of the Colon and Rectum,* the use of multivitamins, vitamin E, and calcium supplements was found to be associated with a lower incidence of recurrent adenomas in 448 patients with previous neoplasia who underwent follow-up colonoscopy. This study found a protective effect against the recurrence of pre-cancerous adenomas when any vitamin supplement was used. On this same subject, a report published in the *American Journal of Epidemiology* (1996; 144 [11]) showed that women with high folate intake were 40% less likely to develop adenomas of the colon than women with low folate intake.

But what if you already have cancer? Again, the research shows a prolongation of lifespan with proper supplementation.

In a study published in *Cancer Letters* (1997; 115 [1]), animals with malignant tumors given high doses of vitamins C and E and selenium manifested a significant prolongation of the mean survival time. Complete remission of tumors developed in 16.8% of the animals. Low-dose administration of these vitamins failed to exert any beneficial effect on mean survival time of the animals. Results indicated that high doses (mega doses) of vitamins C and E in combination with other carefully selected antioxidants are probably needed in order to achieve sufficient prevention and treatment of malignant diseases. This study indicated that low-potency supplements are of little value.

Vitamin E succinate was shown to inhibit growth and induced apoptotic cell death of estrogen receptor–negative human breast cancer cells in a study published in *Cancer Research* (1997; 57 [5]). These findings suggest that vitamin E succinate may be of clinical use in the treatment and possible prevention of human breast cancers.

The research clearly shows the risk of contracting cancer is reduced in those who supplement with adequate amounts of nutrients such as selenium, folate, carotenoids, vitamins, and other plant extracts.

Hormone Replacement

Proper hormone replacement can produce an immediate improvement in the quality of life and also prevent many diseases. DHEA is a hormone whose production in the body diminishes rapidly as people age past year 35. There now exists a wide body of evidence that supplementation with DHEA can prevent many degenerative diseases, while improving feelings of well-being and alleviating depression.

In the journal *Drugs and Aging* (Oct. 1996), an overview of published studies on DHEA revealed the following:

- In both humans and animals, the decline of DHEA production with aging is associated with immune depression, increased mortality, increased risk of several different cancers, loss of sleep, and decreased feelings of well-being.
- DHEA replacement in aged mice significantly normalized immune function to youthful levels.
- DHEA replacement has shown a favorable effect on osteoclasts and lymphoid cells, an effect that may delay osteoporosis.
- Low levels of DHEA inhibit energy metabolism, thus increasing the risk of heart disease and diabetes mellitus.
- Studies conducted on humans show essentially no toxicity at doses that restore DHEA to youthful levels.
- DHEA deficiency may expedite the development of some diseases that are common in the elderly.

Since this overview was published in 1996, hundreds of additional studies have substantiated DHEA's role as an anti-aging hormone-replacement supplement. In a study published in *Biological Psychiatry* (1997; 41 [3]:311–18), DHEA was tested on middle-aged and elderly patients with major depression. DHEA was administered for 4 weeks in doses ranging from 30 to 90 mg a day. This level of dosing elevated DHEA serum levels to those observed in younger people. Depression ratings as well as aspects of memory performance significantly improved. This data suggested that DHEA may have antidepressant and pro-memory effects and corresponded with previous human studies in which DHEA supplementation (50 mg a day) significantly elevated mood in elderly people.

For specific information on anti-aging hormone replacement, refer to the *Male Hormone Modulation Therapy protocol, Female Hormone Replacement Therapy protocol,* and *DHEA Replacement Therapy protocol.*

The Life Extension Foundation's Prevention Protocol

If you are healthy now, and want to stay that way, the Life Extension Foundation has designed protocols that incorporate the best-documented disease-preventing nutrients and hormones.

The Foundation's Prevention protocols consists of the 11 most important supplements for the average person to take every day to reduce risk of contracting the degenerative diseases of aging.

Remember, the Prevention protocol is for healthy people. Those seeking to treat an existing disease can refer to the many specific disease prevention protocols contained in this book.

The following recommendations are listed in order of importance:

Recommendation 1: Life Extension Mix

(Multivitamin-Mineral-Herbal-Amino Acid Formula)

Dosage: 3 tablets with breakfast; 3 tablets with lunch; 3 tablets with dinner

Life Extension Mix is a multi-ingredient formula containing 67 different vegetable, fruit, and herbal extracts along with amino acids, vitamins, minerals, and antioxidants that cannot be found on the commercial supplement market. Life Extension Mix has been designed according to the most recent research in order to prevent and minimize the negative effects of aging.

Hundreds of research studies have been published documenting the health benefits of antioxidants. Antioxidants protect the body against agents of disease called free radicals, which cause chemical reactions (oxidation) that destroy cells and damage tissues. Oxidation is thought to be not only one of the most common mechanisms of disease, but also a basis of the aging process. Free radicals cannot be avoided; ultraviolet light, for example, is a common source. Therefore, it is essential to take antioxidants in order to counteract this process and prevent the degenerative diseases of aging.

Life Extension Mix supplies potent doses of the most powerful antioxidants: vitamins C and E and vegetable extracts, which are known to repair the cellular damage that accumulates with age. Studies have shown a variety of health benefits for antioxidants. Research data have demonstrated consistently that cancer risk is decreased by antioxidants, especially vitamin C and lycopene. Beta-carotene helps offset the damage caused by environmental pollutants. Both vitamins C and E prevent the oxidation of "bad" LDL fat cells that leads to the buildup of fatty deposits inside arteries (atherosclerosis). The Cambridge Heart Antioxidant Study reported that those people with documented heart disease who took vitamin E significantly decreased their risk of heart attack. Another recent study found that vitamin E slows the loss of potency of the immune system that occurs with age. Vitamin E may also improve brain function. The Life Extension Mix makes it easy to ensure that you get the proper amounts of these compounds that from diet alone are impossible to obtain.

The Life Extension Mix saves time and money by combining the most popular nutrient supplements into one product, enabling most people to eliminate the need to buy and keep track of the many separate bottles of B-complex, vitamins C and E, mineral supplements, and so on that would be required to achieve the same effects. The Life Extension Mix is the cornerstone of a comprehensive supplement program because it provides so many different disease-preventing nutrients. If you are on a budget, the Life Extension Mix will provide you with more disease-preventing nutrients per dollar spent than any other product on earth.

The Life Extension Foundation mandates that the ingredients in the Life Extension Mix come only from pharmaceutical-grade suppliers such as Roche and Nutrition 21. These premium companies charge more for their vitamins and trace elements, but the pharmaceutical purity of these substances greatly exceeds that of the lower-cost generic versions that are so prevalent in the vitamin industry.

Recommendation 2: Life Extension Booster

Dosage: 1 capsule a day with a meal

The disease-prevention properties of some nutrients are so well-documented that many people want to take even higher amounts than provided by the Life Extension Mix. The Life Extension Booster contains many important nutrients that cannot fit into the tightly packed Life Extension Mix formula.

The Life Extension Booster is designed to be a convenient, low-cost method of obtaining the most critical disease-preventing nutrients such as lycopene, lutein, gamma-tocopherol, and selenium in just one capsule.

Recommendation 3: Coenzyme Q_{10} (CoQ_{10})

Dosage: 60 to 300 mg a day with a meal

CoQ_{10} is found in cellular organelles called mitochondria, which produce energy. High concentrations of CoQ_{10} are found in healthy heart muscles, helping to provide more energy to the heart and body. Supplementation of CoQ_{10} in patients with heart disease has shown improvement in exercise capacity, which in turn is linked to better overall health. Researchers are continuing to find short- and long-term benefits for heart patients taking regular dosages of CoQ_{10}. As an antioxidant, CoQ_{10} is known to act as a scavenger of free radicals, the molecular substances that damage healthy cells. In clinical trials, CoQ_{10} showed promising results in decreasing tumor spread in breast cancer patients.

The Life Extension Foundation was the first organization to introduce CoQ_{10} to the American public. Since that time, there have been many new studies on CoQ_{10} reported in the scientific literature documenting the multiple life-extension benefits of this versatile nutrient.

CoQ_{10} absorbs into the bloodstream much better when it is in an oil base: most dry powder CoQ_{10} supplements absorb into the bloodstream at about half the rate of oil-based CoQ_{10}. Since CoQ_{10} is a relatively expensive product, we recommend that it be taken as a separate oil-based supplement so that it is effectively absorbed. CoQ_{10} is available in 30- and 100-mg softgel capsules in which the CoQ_{10} is dissolved in tocotrienol-rich rice bran oil.

Recommendation 4: Restoring Youthful Hormone Balance

Youthful hormone balance is critical to maintaining health and preventing disease in all women and men over age 40.

Men should refer to the following separate protocols in this book:

- ▼ *Male Hormone Modulation Therapy protocol*
- ▼ *DHEA Replacement Therapy protocol*

Women should refer to the following separate protocols in this book:

- ▼ *Female Hormone Modulation Therapy protocol*
- ▼ *DHEA Replacement Therapy protocol*

Recommendation 5: Trimethylglycine (TMG)

Dosage: 1 to 8 tablets a day with meals, depending on what you need to keep homocysteine levels below 8 macromoles/L of blood (*see*

Homocysteine and Medical Testing protocols for more details).

TMG's unique biological effect makes it a critical component of a disease-prevention program: it is the most effective facilitator known of youthful methylation metabolism. Published research shows that methylation is related to a variety of diseases, including cardiovascular disease, cancer, liver disease, and neurological disorders. Enhancing methylation improves health and slows premature and, perhaps, normal aging. Published research shows three specific benefits:

1. Methylation lowers dangerous homocysteine levels, thus lowering the risk of heart disease and stroke.
2. Methylation produces SAMe, which may have potent anti-aging effects and has been shown to alleviate depression, remyelinate nerve cells, improve patients with Alzheimer's and Parkinson's diseases, and protect against alcohol-induced liver injury.
3. Methylation protects DNA, which may slow cellular aging.

TMG should be taken with cofactors vitamin B_{12} and folic acid. If you take the Life Extension Mix and the Life Extension Booster, you will get these cofactors.

Recommendation 6: Cognitex and Ginkgo

Dosage: 5 Cognitex capsules early in the day; one 120-milligram ginkgo capsule early in the day

Brain aging is a leading cause of disease, disability, and death in the elderly. The quest to slow brain aging—heralded by loss of ability in thinking, remembering, and reasoning—is the reason most people contact the Life Extension Foundation. The antioxidants found in the Life Extension Mix and the Life Extension Booster protect against free radical damage to brain cells. The Cognitex formula contains nutrients such as pregnenolone, phosphatidylserine (PS), and choline that may prevent other mechanisms of brain cell aging. For example, choline plays an important role in the construction of cell membranes and is a precursor molecule that the body uses to make the neurotransmitter acetylcholine, among other chemical messengers found in the brain.

The extract of the *Ginkgo biloba* has been used extensively in Europe and is approved in Europe for the treatment of dementia. It improves circulation by reducing blood platelet formation and enhances memory. A recent study reported in the *Journal of the American Medical Association* (*JAMA*) found it to be well tolerated and effective. Healthy people seeking to slow down brain aging often notice that Cognitex and ginkgo enhance their cognition. Ginkgo contains numerous antioxidants such as the proanthocyanidins, flavonoids that counteract free-radical activity. Flavonoids are also known to strengthen capillaries, which can improve blood flow to the brain. Gingko has been shown in numerous studies to improve attention span, memory, reaction time, perception, and learning ability.

The Life Extension Herbal Mix (*Recommendation 9*) contains ginkgo extract. If you take the Life Extension Herbal Mix, it is not necessary to take additional ginkgo.

Recommendation 7:

For Men: Saw Palmetto/ Nettle Extract

Dosage: 1 capsule with breakfast and 1 capsule with lunch

Prostate enlargement (BPH) is an inevitable consequence of aging for most men. An extract from the saw palmetto berry may prevent benign prostatic hypertrophy and possibly reduce the risk of prostate cancer. Saw palmetto is derived from the berries of a small bushy tree found in the southeast United States. Saw palmetto limits the production of DHT and inhibits binding at its receptor sites. Saw palmetto also acts as an alpha-adrenergic receptor inhibitor, reducing urinary urgency and having anti-inflammatory properties in the prostate gland. It has been used for decades in Europe for treating urogenital disorders, where researchers proved its effectiveness in treating benign prostate hypertrophy (BPH). Nettle extract (*Urtica dioica*) helps suppress the effects of estrogen and sex hormone–binding globulin by interfering with their attachment to prostate cells.

P

For Women: Bone Assure

Dosage: 6 capsules a day, 3 at dinner and 3 before bedtime

Osteoporosis, a common and costly condition that is a common consequence of aging for women, can cause disabling fractures (most commonly hip fractures) or even death. Since osteoporosis has no symptoms in its early stages, prevention with mineral supplementation is critical. Living bone is never at rest metabolically; its "walls," or matrix, and mineral stores are being remodeled constantly, and minerals such as calcium play crucial metabolic and structural roles.

For this reason, calcium supplements are often used, but osteoporosis is associated with deficiencies of a wide range of nutrients, including magnesium, vitamin D_3, and the hormones DHEA and progesterone. In order for calcium to prevent bone loss, adequate amounts of vitamin D_3 and progesterone must be available so that calcium, magnesium, and phosphorus will be incorporated into the bone matrix. The Bone Assure formula provides every single nutrient that has been shown to prevent bone loss and/or rebuild bone lost to osteoporosis.

Bone Assure is in capsule form to ensure that it breaks down fully in the digestive tract, unlike calcium tablets. The capsules burst open within 5 minutes of swallowing, making the minerals and vitamin D_3 immediately available for absorption into the bone.

The *Female Hormone Modulation Therapy protocol* provides dosage information about progesterone and DHEA.

Recommendation 8: Melatonin

Dosage: 500 mcg to 6 mg at bedtime

Melatonin has also been shown in published studies to reduce the risk of numerous degenerative diseases, boost immune function, inhibit cancer cell proliferation, and slow aging. Melatonin may be the most effective overall disease-preventing agent available for people over age 40, yet it is very inexpensive.

Surprisingly, over 15% of all adult Americans report sleep problems. Melatonin, a hormone produced in the brain's pineal gland, has become a popular sleep aid. Produced and excreted only at night, melatonin is part of the biological timekeeping mechanism of our bodies. As a modulator of the internal clock, it is recommended for sleep problems, such as a severe night owl pattern. Its mild sedative effect has been found useful for insomnia.

Many people take an average of 3 mg of melatonin each night to sleep better. If you are over 40 and sleep fine, we suggest taking only a 500-mcg capsule of melatonin at bedtime. People over age 50 may consider higher doses of melatonin for disease prevention.

Recommendation 9: Life Extension Herbal Mix

Dosage: 1 tablespoon early in the day, with or without food

Herbal extracts are among the world's best-studied medicines and have been researched for years in leading European universities and hospitals. Some have been in clinical use in Europe for over 10 years, with tens of millions of documented cases. Almost all of what we know as modern-day medicine has been derived either directly or indirectly from folk medicine, which relies on herbal treatments. Even today, 80% of the world (four billion people) use herbal treatments as part of their primary health care. Many of the drugs that are commonly used today are herbal in origin. In fact, the Office of Alternative Medicine of the National Institutes of Health reports that about one fourth of the prescription drugs dispensed in the United States have at least one active ingredient derived from plant material.

Numerous published studies show that specific herbal extracts can prevent a wide range of degenerative diseases and enhance cognitive function. The Life Extension Herbal Mix contains some of the best-documented herbals, including ginkgo extract (*see Recommendation 6*), grape-seed extract, green tea, ginseng extract, and bilberry extract, along with 21 other disease-fighting phytochemicals (*see Recommendation 8*) such as chlorella and soy.

The cost of taking these herbal extracts separately in capsule form would be around $100 a month, but Foundation members can save 60% by taking all of these herbals together in one good-tasting herbal drink mix. Herbal extracts are expensive because a large quantity of organic plant matter must be used to produce a minute quantity of pharmaceutical extract. Some members only take the Life Extension Herbal Mix several times a week in order to reduce the monthly cost.

Recommendation 10: Mega Soy Extract

Dosage: 1 capsule in the morning and 1 capsule in the evening.

Soy contains the phytoestrogen (plant estrogen) genistein and therefore can be used as an estrogen-replacement therapy for (post)menopausal women. It reduces hot flashes and other menopausal symptoms as well as decreasing the incidence of osteoporosis, which affects 30% of postmenopausal women. Hormones, including estrogen, encourage bone formation. One study shows that soy isoflavones promote an anabolic (building) effect on bone density by binding to an estrogen receptor in bone.

In addition, the isoflavones found in soy effectively lower cholesterol, according to a recent summary of 38 studies published in a major medical journal. Soy also blocks some hormonal activity in cells, lowering rates of hormone-related cancers such as breast, endometrial, and prostate cancer. In fact, the National Cancer Institute is studying genistein as a possible anti-cancer drug. Soy is also being investigated for its heart-protective, anti-atherogenic properties to prevent heart disease.

Based on records of dietary soy consumption in Japan, where breast and prostate cancer rates are very low, the typical daily phytoestrogen intake from soy has been estimated at 50 mg per person. In contrast, the typical Western diet has been estimated to provide only 2 to 3 mg a day. The supplement Mega Soy Extract provides 100 mg of soy phytoestrogens in just 2 capsules—more than twice the amount in the typical Japanese diet. Since the phytoestrogen genistein is water-soluble, we suggest that 1 capsule of Mega Soy Extract be taken in the morning and 1 in the evening.

Recommendation 11: Aspirin (Healthprin)

Dosage: 1 tablet a day with a heavy meal

The most common cause of disability and death in the United States is an abnormal clot that develops inside an artery to cause a heart attack (blocked blood vessel in the heart) or a stroke (blocked blood vessel in the brain). Aspirin has an immediate and lasting effect on blood platelets, making them less likely to clump together and form a catastrophic clot in arteries. The low dose of aspirin (81 mg) provided by the Healthprin tablet has been shown to be beneficial in the prevention of heart attacks, strokes, and transient ischemic attacks (little strokes).

More than 50 randomized trials have documented the safety and effectiveness of aspirin as a cardiovascular drug. Low-dose aspirin is advised by legions of physicians as well as a 70-member panel convened by the American College of Chest Physicians, which recommended aspirin for all people over 50 with one risk factor and no conditions that make aspirin use inadvisable. This translates into the majority of people over 50, since risk factors for heart disease include male gender, high blood pressure, elevated cholesterol, diabetes, cigarette smoking, lack of exercise, and family history of heart attack or stroke.

In fact, aspirin is commonly considered a "miracle" drug, and a recent report stated that it is expected to have many undiscovered health benefits. At this time aspirin is being studied as a way to lower the risk of colon cancer and to treat dementia.

While many of the nutrients included in the Prevention protocol will reduce the risk of an abnormal blood clot forming inside a blood vessel, it is still beneficial for most older people to take aspirin in the low dose provided by the Healthprin tablet, which minimizes stomach irritation. We also recommend that it be taken with a heavy meal to further decrease the possibility of stomach irritation.

Summary

The following supplements are the most important in preventing the common diseases of aging:

1. Life Extension Mix (available in tablets, capsules or powder)
2. Life Extension Booster
3. Coenzyme Q_{10}—oil-filled softgel caps
4. Restoring youthful hormone balance (Refer to specific *Male* or *Female Hormone Modulation protocol,* and the *DHEA Replacement protocol.*)
5. Trimethylglycine (TMG)
6. Cognitex and Ginkgo
7. Saw Palmetto/Nettle Extract for men; Bone Assure for women
8. Low-dose melatonin (for most people)
9. Life Extension Herbal Mix
10. Mega Soy Extract
11. Low-dose aspirin (for most people)

New members often write to the Foundation for evaluation lists of the supplements they are taking. Many of these health-conscious people are underdosing or overdosing on nutrient supplements. In many cases, people are missing just a few critical nutrients or hormones that would greatly enhance the effectiveness of their personal life extension program.

Foundation members are pleasantly surprised to find that they can drop many of the expensive supplements they are currently using and replace them with lower-priced and more complete disease-preventing formulations by following the step-by-step disease prevention program outlined above.

Product availability. Life Extension Mix, Life Extension Booster, Coenzyme Q_{10}, melatonin, trimethylglycine, Cognitex, ginkgo, saw palmetto extract, Life Extension Herbal Mix, Bone Assure, DHEA, Mega Soy Extract, and Healthprin can be ordered by phoning (800) 544-4440, or order online at www.lef.org.

PROSTATE CANCER: OVERVIEW

The Life Extension Foundation has developed an extensive array of integrated prostate cancer therapies based on published scientific findings and the clinical experience of practicing oncologists. After reading the following Overview, many lay people will require the assistance of their attending oncologist, as some of the protocols are technically challenging. This Overview should be read first by the patient and the physician, and then the appropriate protocol(s) referred to depending upon the stage of the disease and the therapies being considered. A complete listing of these specific prostate cancer protocols is printed at the end of this Overview.

Overview

Unlike most forms of cancer, early-stage prostate cancer is usually controllable with hormone (testosterone)-blocking therapy. The drugs used to contain early-stage prostate cancer are FDA-approved, yet only a small percentage of urologists are using hormone-blocking therapy properly in treating early-stage prostate cancer patients. The scientific literature indicates that radical prostatectomy (surgical removal of the prostate) and external beam radiation therapy fail to produce an acceptable percentage of long-term, disease-free survival. The severe long-term side effects of these conventional therapies (surgery and external-beam radiation) are well documented.

In lieu of radical surgery or external beam radiation, prostate cancer patients may want to consider the Life Extension Foundation's early-stage protocols that incorporate combined testosterone, 5-alpha-reductase, and prolactin inhibition for temporary control of most prostate cancers. Innovative natural therapies can be implemented upon the initiation of hormone-blocking drug therapies.

The goal is to give these natural therapies an opportunity to keep the PSA (prostate-specific antigen) measurement at a nondetectable level after the discontinuation of 3 to 12 months of combined hormone blockade.

Intermittent hormone-blockade drug therapy is advised for almost all prostate cancer patients, since this greatly enhances the time before prostate cancer cells become androgen-independent. Intermittent therapy involves a prostate cancer patient only using hormone blockade for 3 to 12 months, and then waiting until the PSA score approaches 20 before resuming. This of course is a general guideline for physicians and patients to consider.

If your PSA level is less than 11, the odds are that the cancer is confined to the prostate sack. Even if your PSA is greater than 11, there still is a good chance that the combination of FDA-approved hormone-blocking therapy, along with our innovative cancer-treatment protocols, can result in long-term remission. You should institute a 3- to 12-month course of complete hormone blockade by using the FDA-approved drug Casodex or Eulexin (flutamide), and then receive a pellet implant or injection of FDA-approved Lupron or Zoladex a week later. This combination therapy should reduce your PSA level to less than 1 after only a few months. Casodex or Eulexin is taken every day, and the Lupron or Zoladex is re-administered every 3 to 4 months.

Casodex or Eulexin should be taken orally for 1 week prior to an injection of Lupron or Zoladex. Many urologists do not know that Lupron causes a temporary prostate cancer cell flare-up if Casodex (or Eulexin) is not first given 1 week prior to Lupron's administration.

For many years, the Foundation has advocated that prostate cancer patients first try 3 to 9 months of complete hormone blockade before considering any permanent therapies. The rationale is to shrink the prostate-cancer volume by inhibiting testosterone production and blocking testosterone receptor sites on prostate cells. Testosterone is responsible for most prostate cancer-cell proliferation. Blocking testosterone will cause an elevated PSA blood reading to drop to virtually zero within 2 months in most cases. The reduced PSA is indicative of a significant drop in prostate cancer cell activity. The prostate-specific antigen test is an accurate measure of prostate cancer cell activity. Peer-reviewed studies show that hormone-blocking therapy instituted before aggressive therapy significantly increases your chances of a cure.

Studies have shown that prolactin also may be involved in prostate growth. A rising serum level of prolactin indicates progression in patients with advanced prostate cancer.

The presence of prolactin receptors in prostate cancer cells may facilitate the entry of testosterone into prostate cells. Since testosterone-blocking therapies do not completely eliminate testosterone from the blood, it is conceivable that prolactin could carry a small amount of residual testosterone into the prostate cells and cause cancer growth. Thus, suppressing prolactin secretion with relatively safe prescription drugs appears to be another method of slowing the progression of prostate cancer.

The Foundation has been recommending only a 3- to 12-month course of Casodex (or flutamide) and Lupron or Zoladex therapy. Prolactin suppression therapy may be continued longer. During this period, it is suggested that innovative natural cancer-control therapies be incorporated to see if long-term remission can be achieved.

In many cases, the PSA stays low after hormone-blocking therapy has been discontinued. If the PSA level does increase again to between 6 and 20, the prostate cancer patient is encouraged either to go on another 3- to 9-month hormone-blocking regimen and alter his natural cancer-control regimen, or seek out a permanent solution such as enhanced radioactive seed implantation, followed by conformal 3D radiation therapy.

Before a permanent remission therapy is sought (such as seed implantation followed by conformal 3D radiotherapy), it is critical that the prostate cancer patient have low or undetectable levels of PSA. This can be accomplished by a 3- to 12-month hormone blocking therapy regimen. An opposite view comes from doctors who perform enhanced radioactive seed implantation, who have said they do not want too much prostate-cancer shrinkage to occur in response to hormone-blocking therapy because they find they cannot find any tumor tissue to implant the seeds into.

If a person continuously stays on hormone-blocking therapy, after 2 to 4 years the prostate cancer cells will mutate to a new form of cancer cell that will not need testosterone to proliferate. Thus, once the cancer cells become androgen-independent, the prostate cancer is usually out of control and will freely metastasize throughout the body.

In a study published in the *Journal of Steroid Biochemistry and Molecular Biology* (May 1996), prostate cancer in mice was treated with either continuous hormone-blocking therapy or the intermittent hormone-blocking regimen recommended by the Life Extension Foundation. The results showed that five to six cycles of intermittent hormone blockade were possible before the prostate cancer cells mutated to a form that did not need testosterone to proliferate. There was an initial 66% greater time period of prostate cancer cell control in the intermittent group compared with the group receiving continuous hormone blockade. In the late term of the study, the mice on intermittent hormone-blocking therapy had an astounding 3.78-fold reduction in their PSA levels, compared with the mice receiving continuous hormone-blocking therapy.

This study showed that continuous hormone-blocking therapy accelerates the rate at which prostate cancer cells become resistant to testosterone-blocking therapy, and that intermittent hormone blockade significantly increases the length of effectiveness of hormone-blocking therapy in the long-term treatment of prostate cancer.

Cancer cells often produce large amounts of COX-2 and use it as a biological fuel to cause rapid proliferation of cell division. An article in the journal *Cancer Research* (1999 March 1;59 [5]) shows that COX-2 levels in **pancreatic cancer cells** are 60 times greater than in adjacent normal tissue.

According to a study in the *British Journal of Cancer* (1997;75 [8]), **human prostate cancer cells** sustain their growth by stimulating themselves to up-regulate their production of COX-2, which facilitates cell proliferation via several mechanisms. COX-2 inhibition results in a decrease in cell replication and a reduction in the synthesis of COX-2 and its metabolites (such as the dangerous prostaglandin E2). The authors of this study concluded that COX-2 is involved in the maintenance of growth and homeostasis of human prostate cancer cells.

In the Sept. 7, 1999, issue of *The Wall Street Journal*, an investigative report revealed that scientists are actively investigating COX-2 inhibitors as drugs that would be effective in the prevention and treatment of many cancers. When COX-2 drugs are given to patients with colon polyps (precancerous lesions), the lesions completely disappear. When a group of rats were given a potent carcinogen, there was a 90% reduction in those who developed cancer if they were on COX-2 inhibition therapy. In the few rats that did develop the tumors while taking COX-2 inhibition therapy, the tumors were 80% smaller and less numerous than the group not on COX-2 inhibition. *The Wall Street Journal* revealed that a handful of physicians knowledgeable about COX-2 and cancer are prescribing COX-2 inhibitors to their patients. (It was back in 1997 that the Life Extension Foundation recommended the European COX-2 inhibiting drug *nimesulide* to cancer patients.)

In the most recent report published in *JAMA* (1999 Oct. 6;282 [13]), a 9.4-year epidemiological study showed that COX-2 expression in colorectal cancer was significantly related to survival. The doctors concluded that these data add to the growing epidemiological and experimental evidence that COX-2 may play a role in colorectal tumorigenesis."

The Life Extension Foundation predicts that COX-2–inhibiting drugs will eventually be approved to treat cancer, but in the meantime, we are asking physicians treating cancer patients to consider prescribing a COX-2–inhibiting drug as an adjuvant therapy. The COX-2 drug of choice will be described later, but first we want to briefly discuss another prescription drug that may benefit cancer patients:

- The regulation of cancer cell growth is often governed by a family of proteins known as RAS oncogenes. The RAS family is responsible for modulating the regulatory signals that govern the cancer cell cycle and proliferation. Mutations in genes encoding RAS proteins have been intimately associated with unregulated cell proliferation (i.e., cancer).

- The "statin" class of cholesterol-lowering drugs has been shown to inhibit the activity of RAS oncogenes. Some of the "statin" drugs that have shown efficacy are lovastatin, simvastatin, and pravastatin.
- There are mechanisms other than inhibition of RAS oncogene activity that make the "statin" drugs attractive as adjuvant anticancer agents. According to a study in the *Journal of Biological Chemistry* (1998, Vol. 273, No.17), prostate cancer cells are very sensitive to the induction of growth arrest and cell death by lovastatin. This study showed that lovastatin was particularly effective in inducing prostate cancer cell G_1 arrest and cell death in human androgen–independent (hormone-refractory) lines. This study is confirmed by other studies showing that "statin" drugs interfere with critical growth pathways that enable cancer cells to proliferate out of control.

A suggested combination therapy to inhibit COX-2 and provide "statin" regulatory control of cell hyperproliferation is as follows:

- *Lodine XL* is an arthritis drug approved by the FDA that interferes with COX-2 metabolic processes. The maximum dosage for Lodine is 1000 mg daily. The most convenient dosing schedule for the patient involves the prescribing of two Lodine XL 500-mg tablets in a single daily dose. As with any nonsteroidal anti-inflammatory drug (NSAID), extreme caution and physician supervision is a must. The most common complaints associated with use of Lodine XL relate to the gastrointestinal tract. Serious GI toxicity such as perforation, ulceration, and bleeding can occur in patients treated chronically with NSAID therapy. Serious renal and hepatic reactions have been reported rarely. Lodine XL should not be given to patients who have previously shown hypersensitivity to it or in whom aspirin or other NSAIDs induce asthma, rhinitis, urticaria, or other allergic reactions. Fatal asthmatic reactions have been reported in such patients receiving NSAIDs.
- Nimesulide is a safer COX-2 inhibitor, but is not approved by the FDA. It is available from Mexican pharmacies, or can be ordered by mail from European pharmacies. The suggested dose for nimesulide is two 100-mg tablets a day.
- The two newest COX-2 inhibitors are Celebrex and Vioxx, but we suggest that cancer patients consider other drugs that have a more predictable safety history. Suppression of COX-1 is associated with the severe gastrointestinal complications induced by NSAIDs in humans, whereas selective inhibition of COX-2 reduces this side-effect risk. It is the COX-2 enzyme that fuels cancer cell proliferation, so the objective of choosing the proper NSAID in the treatment of cancer is to find one that suppresses the minimum percentage of COX-1 and the maximum percentage of COX-2. In other words, it is critical not to overly suppress COX-1 because the digestive tract needs COX-1 to maintain its structure, whereas it is important to suppress COX-2 because it is this enzyme that cancer cells use to proliferate.
- In a meticulous study published in the *Proceedings of the National Academy of Sciences* (1999;Vol. 96), Lodine (etodolac) was compared with other nonsteroidal antiinflammatory (NSAID) drugs (including Celebrex and Vioxx) to assess its effect on suppressing COX-1 and COX-2. This study showed that Lodine induced an 80% suppression of dangerous COX-2 while inhibiting only 25% of the important COX-1. This study showed that Lodine was slightly more effective than Celebrex in suppressing COX-2, and slightly less effective than Vioxx in suppressing COX-2.
- A novel treatment approach would be to combine a COX-2 inhibitor with a "statin" drug such as lovastatin. A study published in the journal *Gastroenterology* (1999, Vol.116, No. 4, Suppl. A369) showed that lovastatin augmented by up to fivefold, the cancer cell killing effect of a drug with COX-2 inhibiting properties (Sulindac). In this study, three different colon cancer cell lines were killed (made to undergo programmed cell death) by depriving them of COX-2. When lovastatin was added to the COX-2 inhibitor, the kill rate increased by up to fivefold.

P

We thus suggest that physicians consider prescribing a COX-2 inhibitor and a statin drug to prostate cancer patients (in addition to other therapies such as Lupron and Casodex) for a period of 3 months. Here are two dosing schedules we suggest

- **80 mg** a day of **Mevacor** (lovastatin) *and*
- **1000 mg** a day of **Lodine XL**

Blood tests to assess liver and kidney function are critical in protecting against potential side effects. To ascertain efficacy, regular PSA and other serum and imagery testing is suggested.

The Foundation has developed an integrated approach that involves the concomitant use of FDA-approved drugs combined with natural supplements. A brief description of these natural therapies follows, with a more extensive dissertation printed in the Prostate Cancer Adjuvant Therapy Protocol.

Prostate cancer patients usually take five 700-mg capsules of Mega Soy Extract 3 to 4 times a day. Mega Soy Extract provides pharmaceutical doses of soy isoflavones such as genistein. Cancer cells use the enzyme protein kinase as a growth factor. Soy genistein is a potent inhibitor of protein kinase activity. The effects of protein kinase inhibitors on human prostate cell growth have been extensively investigated.

These phytochemicals protect against cancer via several different mechanisms, including interacting with intracellular enzymes, regulating protein synthesis, controlling growth-factor action, inhibiting malignant cell proliferation, inducing differentiation, deterring cancer cell adhesion, and inhibiting angiogenesis. Animal experiments provide evidence suggesting that both lignins and isoflavonoids in soy may prevent the development of cancer.

Genistein may prevent the expression of metastasic capacity in hormone-dependent cancers. Studies have shown that genistein inhibits proliferation and expression of the invasive capacity of prostatic cancer cells with different invasive potentials. In a cell-culture system, genistein appears to be cytotoxic and inhibitory of prostate cancer cell proliferation.

Genistein's protein-tyrosine kinase inhibiting effects have been identified as a cancer-prevention mechanism. The consumption of soy is associated with a low incidence of clinical metastatic prostate cancer, even in the face of a sustained high incidence of organ-confined prostate cancer. A study examined genistein's effect upon cell adhesion as one possible mechanism by which it could be acting as an anti-metastatic agent. A morphogenic analysis revealed that genistein caused cell flattening in a way that prevented metastatic adhesion of prostate cancer cell lines.

CAUTION: Do not take any soy genistein product 10 days prior, during, or 3 weeks after any form of radiation therapy. Genistein may protect cancer cells against radiation-induced death.

Additional natural therapies include 1000 to 4000 IU of vitamin D_3, four saw palmetto/pygeum/nettle extract capsules, 40 mg a day of lycopene, and as much of the *Cancer (Adjuvant) Treatment protocol* in this book as possible. The Foundation especially recommends that prostate cancer patients take 4 to 10 capsules of 95% Green Tea Extract each day.

Epidemiological data suggest that vitamin D_3, obtained from dietary sources and sunlight exposure, may protect against mortality from prostate cancer. The most active vitamin D metabolite, vitamin D_3, inhibits the growth and differentiation of several human prostate cancer cell lines.

Permixon (saw palmetto extract) is a drug used in the treatment of benign prostatic hyperplasia. Men with prostate cancer often use it as a complementary therapy. Pygeum extract has been shown to specifically inhibit prostate-cell proliferation by inhibiting protein kinase C enzyme activity.

Prostate cancer patients should take a PSA test every 30 days, before and after hormone-blocking therapy is discontinued, to see if the innovative cancer therapies are keeping the prostate cancer under control. Serum calcium blood tests also are suggested to make sure that the relatively high daily doses of vitamin D_3 are not causing toxicity.

There are many prostate cancer patients following the Foundation's protocols with success. Individuals should become fully educated about their options in order to intelligently make decisions, based on a wide range of factors, regarding how they are going to deal with their prostate cancer in the long run. Every prostate cancer patient should consider 3 to 12 months of complete hormone blockade before attempting any form of permanent therapy, such as surgery, radiation, cryoablation, radioactive seeds, etc. For some prostate cancer patients, complete hormone-blocking therapy results in a long-term remission without the need of incorporating additional therapies.

For those seeking a permanent remission, the most effective and least likely therapy to produce complications (such as impotence, incontinence, pain) may be a combination of enhanced ultra-sound-guided radioactive seed implantation followed 3 weeks later by conformal external beam radiation aimed only at the implanted seeds in the prostate and seminal vesicle tissue. The seeds provide a greater amount of cancer cell–killing radiation directly to prostate cancer cells, while serving as an easy target for conformal external beam radiation therapy. Since the external radiation beam hits only the areas that have been "seeded," the long-term complication of rectal and bladder radiation damage is largely avoided, and the areas identified as having cancer cells are intensely irradiated.

As previously noted, during radiation therapy it is crucial that all soy supplements be discontinued since soy produces a specific mechanism that can protect cancer cells from radiation-induced death. Discontinue soy at least 10 days before radiation, during radiation, and for at least 3 weeks afterward.

During radiation therapy, the use of antioxidants will protect healthy cells from free-radical–induced radiation damage.

The combination of enhanced ultrasound radioactive seeding with followup by 3-D conformal beam radiation appears to offer the best hope for long-term remission in organ-confined disease.

Please see the following protocols in this book regarding the treatment of prostate cancer. We must warn the reader that some of these protocols are highly technical, and will often serve as a guideline for the medical oncologist, rather than the patient.

1. Prostate Cancer: Adjuvant Therapy
2. Prostate Cancer: Early-Stage
3. Prostate Cancer: Late-Stage
4. Prostate Cancer: PC Spes
5. Prostate Cancer: Chemotherapy
6. Prostate Cancer: PSA Parameters and Heredity
7. Prostate Enlargement: Benign Prostate Hypertrophy

Important Note. The Life Extension Foundation revises disease treatment protocols as new information becomes available. New information about treating prostate cancer can be obtained by accessing the Foundation's Web site [http:/ www.lef.org].

Product availability. Mega Soy extract, Green Tea 95% Extract, and Life Extension Mix, can be ordered by phoning (800) 544-4440, or order online at www.lef.org.

PROSTATE CANCER: ADJUVANT THERAPY (VITAMINS, MINERALS, TRACE ELEMENTS, AND HERBAL PREPARATIONS)

By Stephen B. Strum, M.D., and Jonathan E. McDermed, Pharm.D

Dr. Strum is on the Life Extension Medical Advisory Board, and Dr. McDermed is from the Prostate Cancer Research Institute (PCRI) in Los Angeles, California. Drs. Strum and McDermed are proponents of a holistic medical strategy that combines peer-reviewed conventional scientific publications with new findings in the areas of nutrition and supportive care of the patient. Dr. Strum and his partner, Mark C. Scholz, M.D., have a medical practice (Healing Touch Oncology) in Marina del Rey, California, that cares for patients with prostate cancer (PC) or who are at high risk of having PC.

We have routinely employed natural therapies in our holistic approach to oncology and internal medicine disorders for almost 30 years. Such therapies are based on published peer-reviewed literature and not hearsay from individuals or companies that appear to be in the business of medicine. The amount of literature in this area has grown exponentially. We are now at a phase in our acceptance of such approaches that medical studies are being conducted to verify the benefits of such "nutriceuticals" in pilot clinical trials with endpoints that are objectively evaluable. Most of the recommendations in this section are directed to one or more phases of prostate cancer (PC) management: prevention, early-stage treatment, late-stage treatment, and/or maintenance phase of active treatment. During radiation therapy, there is concern that the use of high doses of antioxidants will protect tumor cells from the cell-killing effects of radiation. This is a controversial issue. There is a randomized study indicating significant reduction in the radiation-induced side effects of cystitis and proctitis using SOD (Orgotein) in patients receiving radiation therapy (RT) for bladder cancer. This study involved 448 patients. It showed a dramatic lessening in the radiation therapy-induced side effects in the SOD treated arm (Sanchiz et al., *Anticancer Res.,* 1996). The differences in anticancer results in the treatment arm receiving Orgotein versus placebo are still not known. Orgotein is an injectable SOD drug approved in Europe, but not in the United States.

Nutritional Recommendations for Active PC

We use the nutritional approaches during the preventive phase in men at risk for developing PC. We employ the same strategy during the initial use of androgen deprivation therapy (ADT) and during the off-phase of ADT for the purpose of slowing the growth rate of PC as much as possible. In patients with active PC, we take a more aggressive stance on the dosing of these agents and also suggest the use of additional agents that appear promising in their activity against PC. However, it is important to indicate that the rationale for the use of many of these adjuncts is based on studies involving human cell lines of PC grown in animal models, usually mice. Clinical studies in humans have either not been started or are in progress but are too preliminary to report at this time.

Selenium

As noted above, we suggest the use of selenomethionine derived from yeast. We have seen no selenium toxicity at doses as high as 800 mcg a day. Larry Clark, at the University of Arizona, has recently initiated clinical trials using 800, 1600, and 3000 mcg a day of selenium in patients involved in watchful waiting. At 800 mcg a day, physician monitoring and consideration of selenium blood levels is advised. Please note that selenium blood levels will be elevated in most patients taking any selenium supplementation due to the fact that normal selenium levels were based on population sampling from men and women not taking selenium supplements. If selenium toxicity occurs, the most common signs are abnormalities in nail growth with loss of nails, hair loss, lack of appetite with weight loss, and a garlic-like odor to the breath. Personally, I have only seen hair loss, anorexia, and weight loss in one patient who received a dose of 300,000 mcg of selenium a day. That patient had a drop in his PSA and has had a slow recovery of PSA; he has been off therapy after ADT for 7 years. Carefully controlled trials with selenium such as at the University of Arizona are critically important to our understanding of how best to use selenium. We urge patients doing watchful waiting to join in such trials if this is possible. Call Trish Wilkens or Jennifer Hart at (520) 321-7798 (extension 19 or 23) for further information on this clinical trial.

Genistein

The use of soy and genistein in the prevention of PC was discussed above. Genistein has been proposed as an effective agent to prevent the expression of metastatic capacity in hormone-dependent cancers. In a cell-culture system, genistein appeared to be cytotoxic and inhibitory of PC cell proliferation (Geller et al., *Prostate,* 1998). Genistein and soy products therefore play a potential major role in established PC. Cancer cells use the enzyme tyrosine kinase as a growth factor. Soy genistein is a potent inhibitor of tyrosine kinase activity. The effects of protein kinase inhibitors on human prostate cell growth have been extensively investigated. Other biological activities of genistein have been demonstrated in animal models and include the following:

- ▼ Inhibition of DNA topoisomerase
- ▼ Inhibition of protein tyrosine kinase
- ▼ Anti-angiogenesis by modulation of FGF (fibroblast growth factor)
- ▼ Inhibition of EGF (epidermal growth factor)

In active PC patients, we are exploring higher doses of genistein using Life Extension Mega Soy Extract. Each 700-mg capsule of Mega Soy Extract contains 134 mg of genistein, 122 mg of daidzein, and 24 mg of glycetein. Currently, we are advising two of these capsules a day and are trying to arrange for serum genistein levels.

Synthetic Vitamin D, Bisphosphonates, Calcium Citrate

Other adjunctive therapies known to have an effect on PC include the use of vitamin D. Published studies using more potent synthetic vitamin D analogs such as Rocaltrol or Calcitriol have shown a slowing effect on PC growth (Gross et al., *J. Urol.,* 1998). These analogs affect the p27Kip1 oncogene that results in over-expression of enzymes that inhibit part of the tumor cell cycle (Koike et al., *Proc. Annu. Meet. Am. Assoc. Cancer Res.,* 1997). In short, synthetic vitamin D analogs cause a G_1 arrest in the cell cycle by over-expression of cyclin-dependent kinase inhibitors (CDKIs). We routinely use 0.5 mcg of Rocaltrol at bedtime. Rocaltrol requires a physician's prescription. When we employ Rocaltrol, we do so in a comprehensive setting of improving bone integrity. As mentioned earlier, the use of ADT results in an increase in bone resorption due to activation of bone-resorbing cells called osteoclasts. Excessive bone resorption leads to release of bone-derived growth factors that have been shown to play an important role in increasing PC growth. We block this bone resorption by using drugs in the bisphosphonate family. Examples of such drugs currently in use include alendronate (Fosamax), pamidronate (Aredia), and most recently Risedronate (Actonel). The proper use of these agents necessitates physician supervision. As bisphosphonates block excessive bone resorption, they favor bone growth that allows for calcium utilization. Therefore, we routinely combine calcium supplementation when employing bisphosphonate use. We enhance calcium absorption with Rocaltrol or Calcitriol and at the same time get a second benefit from these agents due to their effect on slowing the growth rate of PC cells. Our bone integrity approach therefore involves

1. **Bisphosphonate Compound(s).**
   - ▼ Actonel—30 mg 1 hour before breakfast taken with water *or*
   - ▼ Fosamax—10 mg 1 hour before breakfast taken with water *and/or*
   - ▼ Aredia—30 mg intravenously for the first dose (over 1.5 hours); followed every 2 weeks by 60 to 90 mg (over 1.5 hours). Patients unable to tolerate Fosamax or those whose insurance does not allow them to qualify for Aredia (bone metastases are currently an insurance requirement) may use Miacalcin nasal spray once a day to decrease bone resorption and enhance bone formation. Patients with severe bone resorption who are not responding to one of these agents may require the combination of two anti-osteoclastic agents. We monitor the effectiveness of the above therapies with the Pyrilinks-D urine test to quantitate bone resorption. Bone mineral density (BMD) evaluations every 6 to 12 months, as well as periodic serum calcium levels (part of a routine chemistry panel) are also part of the monitoring process.

You are encouraged to work with your physician(s) on these issues.

2. **Calcium citrate.** 500 mg with dinner and 500 mg at bedtime. Calcium citrate is much better absorbed than calcium carbonate. Utilization of calcium at night will lower excessive bone resorption by 20%. Calcium intake during the day has no such effect (Blomsohn et al., *J. Clin. Endocrinol. Metab.,* 1994).
3. **Synthetic vitamin D (1, 25-dihydroxycholecalciferol) as Rocaltrol.** 0.5 mcg at bedtime. The use of synthetic vitamin D at bedtime lowers the urinary calcium excretion. This suggests enhanced utilization of calcium and also diminishes the risk of calcium-based kidney stone formation. We are not concerned about the additional use of low doses of ordinary vitamin D (D_3) that is commonly added to most of the available calcium citrate products. However, we do recommend monitoring of the serum calcium levels to make sure that calcium balance is appropriate. In addition, the use of magnesium at a dose of at least half the daily intake of calcium will decrease the formation of calcium oxalate stones.
4. **Exercise.** We do encourage the use of exercise to decrease excessive bone resorption. This should be in the form of both aerobic and muscle-building exercises. We recommend reading Ken Cooper's *Anti-Oxidant Revolution* as well as Barry Sears's *Anti-Aging Zone* for detailed exercise programs and other important information.

Antimetastatic Agents

The inhibition of new blood vessel formation to block the growth and spread of PC is currently under investigation. Androgen deprivation therapy (ADT) is known to have this anti-angiogenesis effect as well as genistein. Other agents that have an effect on cancer cell invasiveness include green tea polyphenols. Green and black tea are derived from the same plant, *Camellia sinensis.* However, only green tea is rich in the flavonol group of polyphenols known as catechins. The fermentation process used in making black tea destroys the biologically active polyphenols of the fresh leaf. The catechins as a group have significant free-radical scavenging ability and are potent antioxidants. Four catechins are found in green tea leaves:

epicatechin (EC)
epigallocatechin (EGC)
epicatechin gallate (ECG)
epigallocatechin gallate (EGCG)

Of these four factions EGCG is the most important to the PC patient. Pharmacological activity extends beyond its actions as an antioxidant and free-radical scavenger. Epigallocatechin-3 gallate (EGCG) acts against urokinase, an enzyme often found in large amounts in human cancers (Jankun et al., *Nature*, 1997). Urokinase breaks down the basement membrane of cell junctions, which may be a key step in the process of tumor cell metastasis, as well as tumor growth (Ennis et al., *Proc. Annu. Meet. Am. Assoc. Cancer Res.*, 1997). EGCG attaches to urokinase and prevents these actions.

GTP also inhibits ornithine decarboxylase (ODC), resulting in a decrease in polyamine synthesis and cell growth (Carlin et al., *J. Urol.*, 1996). Inhibitors of 5-alpha-reductase (5AR) may be effective in the treatment of 5-alpha-dihydrotestosterone-dependent abnormalities, such as benign prostate hyperplasia, PC, and certain skin diseases. The green tea catechins are potent inhibitors of type-1 but not type-2 5AR (Liao and Hiipakka, *Biochem. Biophys. Res. Commun.,* 1995). They also inhibit accessory sex gland growth in rats. These results suggest the certain tea gallates can regulate androgen action in target organs. The 5AR inhibitor Proscar is predominantly a type-2 inhibitor.

Long-term consumption of tea catechins is common in China and Japan. The frequency of the latent, localized type of PC does not vary significantly between Eastern and Western cultures, but the clinical incidence of metastatic PC is generally lower in Japan and other Asian countries, in contrast to the common occurrence of metastatic PC in Europe and the United States. One possible explanation is that EGCG consumption in green tea in Asian countries prevents the progression and metastasis of PC cells. This explains the lower mortality rate due to PC and breast cancer in Asian countries as compared to Western countries.

In a study investigating the effect of intra-peritoneal injections of different catechins on the growth of the human PC cell lines PC-3 and LnCaP, and the human breast cancer cell line MCF-7 grown in nude mice, EGCG was found to play a key role (Figure 1). The injection of EGCG slowed the growth of tumors when administered to the control mice on day 14, while the growth of tumors accelerated when EGCG was stopped in the PC-3 line on day 14. Inhibition of PC-3 growth was EGCG specific; it was not seen with EC, EGC, or ECG (Liao et al., *Cancer Lett.,* 1995). The galloyl group of EGCG appears to be necessary for tumor growth inhibition since EGC is not active. EGCG accounts for about 50% of the solid matter in the hot water extract of green tea that is consumed as a beverage.

Figure 1: EGCG Effect on PC-3 Growth

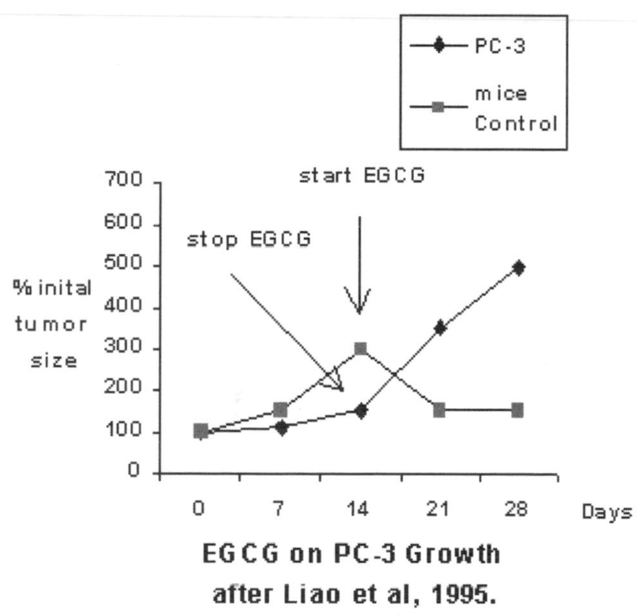

EGCG on PC-3 Growth after Liao et al, 1995.

Green tea is prepared from lightly steamed and dried leaves of the tea plant. The steaming process leaves the polyphenol activity intact. The polyphenol activity varies with climate, season, horticultural practices, and the position of the leaf on the harvested shoot. The Life Extension Foundation makes a 95% green tea extract that contains a high level of the active polyphenol EGCG. The polyphenolic profile of Green Tea 95% Extract is EGCG 35%. Each 350-mg capsule is an extract of green tea leaves containing 122.5 mg of EGCG. One 350-mg capsule of Green Tea 95% Extract is equivalent to 4 to 10 cups of Japanese green tea. Green Tea 95% Extract is available in decaffeinated form, or in a lightly caffeinated extract that contains 10 to 20 mg of caffeine. We suggest that GT 95% be used at a dose of 1 capsule 3 times a day in patients with active PC and perhaps once a day as prevention against PC. We would suggest that GT be taken with food to avoid stomach upset. GT should be kept in a dry, cool location and out of direct light.

Lycopene

Recent studies have shown a statistically significant inverse relationship between the ingestion of tomatoes, tomato sauce, and pizza with the development of prostate cancer. In a 6-year study by Giovannucci et al. (*J. Natl. Cancer. Inst.,* 1995) involving the intake of carotenoids and retinol in 47,894 men, lycopene-rich foods significantly lowered the risk of PC. Men who ingested 10 or more servings of tomatoes in several forms (sauce, juice, raw, or on pizza) had a 41% reduction in PC, while those who ate four to seven servings a week had a 22% reduction. Tomatoes and tomato sauce contain high amounts of lycopene, a carotenoid. Lycopene is the most predominant carotenoid in plasma and in various tissues, including the prostate gland. Lycopene is the most efficient scavenger of singlet oxygen among the common carotenoids. Lycopene is not converted to vitamin A. The major contributors to the specific carotenoids are shown below:

Carotenoid Class	Vegetable or Fruit
β-carotene	Carrots, yams, sweet potatoes, spinach
α-carotene	Carrots, mixed vegetables
Lutein	Spinach, broccoli, kale, mustard, chard
Lycopene	Tomatoes, tomato sauce, pizza, tomato juice
β-cryptoxanthin	Oranges

Another study evaluated the effect of lycopene on the development of mammary cancers in a mouse model. This showed a significant suppression of tumor growth in those mice receiving a diet supplemented with lycopene. Decreases in thymidylate synthetase within the breast tissue, lower levels of serum-free fatty acids, and decreased plasma prolactin levels by the pituitary were characteristic of the lycopene-supplemented group (Nagasawa et al., *Anticancer Res.,* 1995). Interestingly, the source of lycopene was a beta-carotene–rich algae called *Dunaliella bardawil.*

Recently, Kucuk et al. reported on 30 men with localized PC scheduled for radical prostatectomy. They were randomly assigned to receive either 15 mg of lycopene (Lyc-o-Mato, LycoRed, Beer Sheva, or Israel) orally twice daily, or no intervention for 3 weeks prior to surgery. Prostate specimens were step-sectioned, entirely embedded, and evaluated for pathological stage, Gleason score, the volume of PC, as well as the extent of PIN (a pathological finding often associated with PC) in the gland. The specimens were also examined for biomarkers of cell proliferation, differentiation, and apoptosis. Comparisons were made between intervention and control groups. Serum and tissue lycopene levels increased by 22% in the intervention group. At RP, within the treated group, 8 of 12 patients (67%) had organ-confined PC, and 84% had tumors ≤ 4 cc, compared to 44% and 55%, respectively, in the control group. Lesser glandular involvement by PIN was also observed in the intervention group. The expression of biomarkers of proliferation decreased, whereas the markers of differentiation and apoptosis increased in the intervention group. Serum PSA level also decreased significantly in the intervention group but not in the control group. The results suggest a role for lycopene in PC prevention. This is a very exciting study, and the full report should be published shortly. We currently advise patients with active PC to include 30 mg a day of lycopene in their diet.

Lifestyle Changes to Prevent and Treat Prostate Cancer

▼ Restrict Total Caloric Intake to 500 Calories a Meal

We believe that diet should be regarded as having serious biochemical relevance to the health of the individual. You are, for the most part, what you eat. Western society, and especially the United States, are over-consumers of calories. Excessive caloric consumption is a significant factor that adversely effects longevity. Caloric restriction has been shown to be an important factor in augmenting the immune system and improving longevity. We need to rethink how much food we need to eat. Our ideal body weight should be taken seriously. If we were to do this alone, we would virtually eliminate diabetes, hypertension, hypercholesterolemia, stroke, heart disease, and a significant amount of cancer from our lives. Patients should strive at a general figure of 500 calories a meal, and 100 calories per snack. Modifications of this are based on the level of activity, age, and body surface area. Nutritional software or nutritional counseling should be an integral part of our approach to good health.

▼ Eliminate Smoking, Reduce Alcohol Consumption, and Exercise Properly

If we were to eliminate major factors relating to oxidative damage such as cigarette smoking and excessive alcohol consumption, in conjunction with dietary restrictions, we would eliminate 80% of disease as we know it today. In the context of caloric excess, we have additional cofactors such as lack of routine exercise and over consumption of dietary fat. *The Anti-Oxidant Revolution*, 1994, by Kenneth Cooper, M.D., focuses on the causal association of over-exercise and the generation of injurious free-radicals with resultant increases in degenerative diseases and cancer. We agree with Cooper that exercise should be low impact and that we should routinely use free-radical scavengers, especially at times when we are more physically active, and certainly when we are exposed to excessive free-radical damage, i.e., sunlight, high altitude, and activities that generate tissue damage. It is ironic that we bring our automobiles in for a periodic oil change to remove the products of oxidative damage, but we do not attempt a similar maneuver for our own bodies to prevent oxidative damage due to the wear and tear of everyday life.

- ▼ Avoid Excessive Carbohydrate Intake to Prevent Hyperinsulinemia and the Generation of Unfavorable Eicosanoids

The dietary fat issue is significant. There are studies that show dietary fat to increase the growth rate of PC in animal models of human PC. However, the emphasis on dietary fat per se has taken attention away from caloric over-consumption. Fat excess, however, is linked to excessive calorie consumption, since fat contains twice as many calories, gram for gram, as protein or carbohydrate. In addition, the ratio of protein to carbohydrate in our meals is related to how our body reacts to the intake of food and how it handles calories that are ingested. The reader is advised to read Barry Sears's book *The Zone,* 1995, and *Anti-Aging Zone*, 1999, for an in-depth discussion of the dangers of over-consumption of carbohydrates and the ill effects of hyperinsulinemia that occur as a result. Our patients are advised to incorporate Sears's approach into their lives while consuming fewer calories a day and exercising moderately. The value of generating favorable eicosanoids is discussed in detail in both of these books. The free radical–generating fatty acid called arachidonic acid, an unfavorable eicosanoid, has been shown to stimulate PC cell growth. The molecular pathway of arachidonic stimulation involves the inflammatory enzyme 5-lipooxygenase. Recent papers show that inhibition of arachidonic acid leads to PC programmed cell death, or apoptosis (Ghosh and Myers, *Proc. Natl. Acad. Sci. USA*, 1998). Lipooxygenase also is involved in the formation of abnormal blood clots. Nutrients that specifically inhibit 5-lipooxygenase include garlic. Fish oil supplements (EPA), an omega-3 fatty acid, have been shown to suppress arachidonic acid formation.

Prostaglandins are synthesized from arachidonic acid by the enzyme cyclooxygenase. A particularly dangerous prostaglandin is PGE_2, which is involved in many chronic inflammatory diseases. The administration of PGE_2 to prostate, breast, and colon-cancer cells resulted in increased cellular proliferation. An ibuprofen derivative called Flurbiprofen inhibited PGE_2-induced PC cell growth (Tjandrawinata et al., *Br. J. Cancer,* 1997). Aspirin, ibuprofen, and fish oil are other available agents that inhibit PGE_2 synthesis. The eicosanoid pathways are shown in Figure 2 on the following page.

- ▼ Use Free-Radical Scavengers (Selenium and Vitamin E) to Prevent Oxidative Damage

In conjunction with dietary restriction of calories and alteration in the nature of the calories consumed as well as moderating our exercise, there is evidence that aging, degenerative disease, and cancer are all expressions of varying degrees of cellular oxidative damage. In fact, fat itself induces the generation of fatty acid peroxides that generate damaging free radicals. The concept here is that living organisms are subject to oxidation just as metal is subject to rusting. As part of aging, we see the sequelae of such oxidation manifested in the graying of hair, short-term memory loss, cataract formation, gum and jaw recession, vascular disease, cardiac disease, degenerative joint disease, and sun-induced skin changes ranging from wrinkling to skin cancer. The majority of items in health food stores today are antioxidants.

In regards to PC, there are now studies that show that vitamin E and selenium use will decrease the incidence as well as the mortality from PC. The ATBC study by Heinonen et al. (*J. Natl. Cancer Inst.*, 1998) demonstrated a 32% decrease in the incidence of PC and a 41% lower mortality rate from PC in men taking alpha-tocopherol (vitamin E). Another study by Fleshner et al. (*J. Urol.*, 1998) showed a reduction in growth rates of transplanted LNCaP cells in athymic mice induced by a high-fat diet (40.5%) by *dl*-alpha tocopherol (synthetic vitamin E). The landmark study by Clark et al. (*JAMA*, 1996) provided evidence that 200 mcg of selenium could reduce the incidence of PC by 63%. This is consistent with the observation that selenium inhibited the

Figure 2: The Eicosanoid Pathways and Their Metabolites

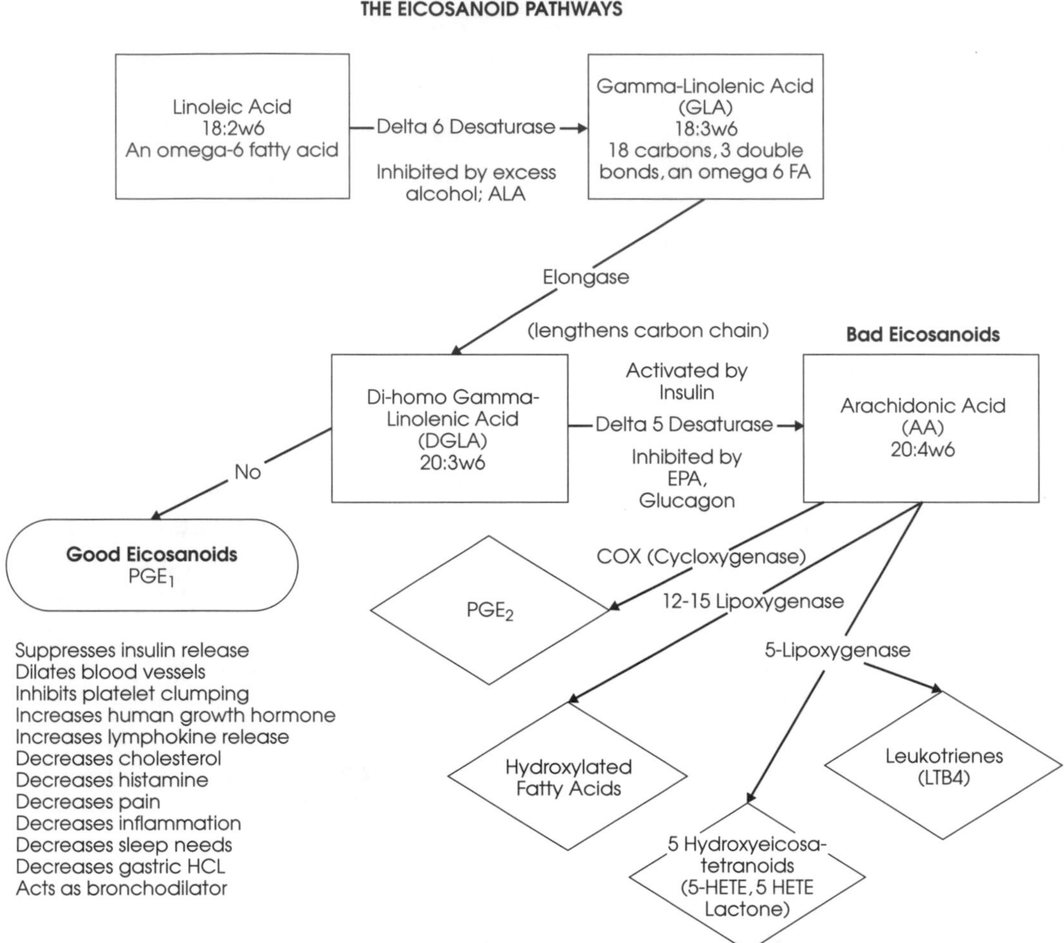

growth of DU-145—an androgen-independent human cell line of PC—by 50% at a selenium dose of 1×10^{-6} M and by 98% at a dose of 10^{-4} M. For comparison, selenium serum levels in humans living in high-selenium areas may be as high as 10^{-6} M (Webber et al., *Biochem. Biophys. Res. Commun.,* 1985). Our recommended vitamin E dose for prevention is 400 to 1000 IU a day as mixed tocopherols. Mixed tocopherols contain synthetic vitamin E (*d*-alpha-tocopherol and *dl*-alpha-tocopherol) as well as natural vitamin E. A study by Moyad et al. (in press, 1999) indicates gamma tocopherol has more anti-PC activity then conventional *d*-alpha-tocopherol.

The selenium dose recommended for prevention is 400 mcg a day. This is best given as selenomethionine, usually derived from yeast. Selenium works best in conjunction with vitamin E, which enhances its activity. Vitamin E works best in association with beta-carotene and vitamin C. We recommend 1000 mg of vitamin C to be taken after each meal to prevent fatty acid peroxide generation. In a likewise manner, Coenzyme Q_{10} has been shown to prevent the oxidation of LDL cholesterol. In fact, the prevention of fatty acid oxidation may be just as important as decreasing fat consumption. We suggest Coenzyme Q_{10} be taken at a dose of 200 mg a day. An added benefit of CoQ_{10} is the improvement in heart function and diabetic control as well as the treatment of periodontal disease. CoQ_{10} works best when given with vitamins E and C.

▼ Use Genistein to Decrease Cell Adhesion, Slow Proliferation, and Decrease Metastatic Potential

Incidences of PC are higher in the Western world than in Asia, where soy is consumed as part of the normal diet, producing higher levels of genistein in the blood, which in turn appear to prevent the expression of metastatic capacity in hormone-dependent cancers. Studies have shown that, in a cell-culture system, genistein appears to be cytotoxic and inhibitory of PC cell proliferation (Santibanez et al., *Anticancer Res.,* 1997; Peterson and Barnes, *Prostate*, 1993). Genistein's protein-tyrosine kinase-inhibiting effects have been identified as a cancer-prevention mechanism. One study examined genistein's effect upon cell adhesion as one possible mechanism by which it could be acting as an antimetastatic agent. A morphogenic analysis revealed that genistein caused cell flattening in a way that prevented metastatic adhesion of PC cell lines. We advise patients to eat a diet rich in soy products such as tofu, soy beans (edamame), soy milk, and miso. We recommend a breakfast and dinner drink that contains soy milk, isolated soy powder, many of the vitamins mentioned above, and strawberries. We use a Vita-Mix blender to pulverize the vitamins and add them to this drink. The protein-to-carbohydrate ratio of this drink is also close to the desired 3:4 ratio that Sears considers "zone" favorable. Life Extension makes a 700-mg Mega Soy product that contains 134 mg of genistein per capsule as well as the isoflavones daidzein, and glycitein. We would suggest that clinical trials be initiated that would determine the genistein oral intake associated with blood genistein levels similar to those found in Asian men. Currently, we recommend 100 to 200 mg of genistein a day in addition to a diet high in soy products. We also believe that the major source of protein in our diet should come from soy.

▼ Decrease Cell Proliferation with Pygeum and Silymarin

Pygeum extract also has been shown to specifically inhibit prostate-cell proliferation by inhibiting protein kinase C enzyme activity (Yablonsky et al., *J. Urol.*, 1993). Silymarin has been shown to have an anti-PC effect by virtue of increasing the levels of p27 (Zi et al., *Cancer Res.*, 1998; Gali et al., *Proc. Annu. Meet. Am. Assoc. Cancer Res.*, 1994). Silymarin also has protective effects against liver cell injury and skin cancer (Kropacova et al., *Radiat. Biol. Radioecol.*, 1998; Agarwal et al., *Proc. Annu. Meet. Am. Assoc. Cancer Res.*, 1995; Katiyar et al., *J. Natl. Cancer Inst.*, 1997).

Product availability. Mega Soy Extract, lycopene, silymarin, pygeum extracts, and selenium and vitamin E supplements are available by calling (800) 544-4440, or order online at www.lef.org.

PROSTATE CANCER: EARLY STAGE

CAUTION: Some readers will find this protocol technically challenging. It is written for both the patient and the attending oncologist.

Proper "Staging" and Use of Hormone Blocking Therapy

The sections below are written by Stephen B. Strum, M.D., and Jonathan E. McDermed, Pharm.D., of the Prostate Cancer Research Institute (PCRI) in Los Angeles, California. Dr. Strum is on the Life Extension Medical Advisory Board. Drs. Strum and McDermed are proponents of a holistic medical strategy that combines peer-reviewed conventional scientific publications with new findings in the areas of nutrition and supportive care of the patient. Dr. Strum and his partner Mark C. Scholz, M.D., have a medical practice (Healing Touch Oncology) in Marina del Rey, California, that cares for patients with prostate cancer (PC) or who are at high risk of having PC.

The Extent of Disease or Stage

Our current ability to assess disease is compromised by issues of resolution; what you see is *not* always what you have. The approach to "early stage" PC is confused by the fact that so-called "early stage" PC is frequently *not* early. In other words, what appears to be localized PC is often beyond the confines of the prostate gland. Our assessment of cancer extent (staging), in general, is often incorrect. That is, we underestimate the extent or stage of the cancer with the tools that we currently have available.

If we are to categorize PC as "early," we need to scrutinize men newly diagnosed with PC and optimally use the available staging tools. If PC is *not* confined to the prostate, then local therapies such as radical prostatectomy (RP) and radiation therapy (RT) will not eradicate or cure the disease. If PC is verified to be confined to the prostate (organ-confined) to the best of our ability, then a second important variable must be considered if local treatment is to be successful—the volume of the cancer. If the volume is too great, local RT—be it external beam RT, seed implantation, or cryosurgery—will not likely eradicate the disease. Therefore, two significant variables must be addressed for local therapy to optimally eradicate disease. These are

- Extent of disease: Organ-confined versus non-organ confined.
- Volume of disease: Minimal tumor burden versus moderate-large tumor burden.

These basic tenets are true for the vast majority of malignancies, not just for PC. Determination of the *extent* of disease is called "staging." The determination of the *volume* of cancer is often incorporated into staging. However, the volume of the disease plays a very important role in the ability of local therapies such as RT (external beam RT or brachytherapy) and cryosurgery to cure a patient with PC (Bostwick et al., *Urology,* 1993; Babaian et al., *J. Urol.,* 1995).

Basic Biological Principles

We believe staging involves a logical, stepwise approach that reflects an understanding of the important variables in the way a malignancy behaves. A malignancy expresses itself by virtue of a growth curve that is essentially logarithmic. This means that a tumor cell basically divides from one to two, from two to four, from four to eight, and so on. In reality, there are a certain number of tumor cells that are dying off during this process. Therefore, it is not exactly logarithmic, but close; the medical name for this growth curve is *Gompertzian*.

We measure proteins or antigens that are associated with malignant tumor cell growth. These proteins or antigens are called biomarkers, since they mark the biological activity of the tumor process. The most commonly used biomarker in PC is the prostate-specific antigen, or PSA. However, PSA is not the only marker of PC disease activity or aggressiveness.

PSADT, PSAV, and PSA

PSADT

PSA is currently the key antigen used in assessing PC. Measurements of PSA over time express a logarithmic pattern when PC is present. In this way, PC can be identified years before it may be suspected by an abnormal digital rectal exam (DRE). A calculated PSA doubling time (PSADT) provides the first clue to the presence of a malignant process. In cases of PC, the PSADT is shorter than 15 years (Stamey, *Quebec City,* 1995; Berry et al., *J. Urol.,* 1984). Most PC tumors have PSADTs in the 4- to 10-year range. When a PSADT in this range is documented, the physician's burden of proof is to exclude the presence of PC.

PSAV

PSA rates of increase (PSA velocity or PSAV) of 0.75 ng/ml/year or greater reflect production of a cell product consistent with malignancy (Carter et al., *JAMA,* 1992). Therefore, the rate of increase of PSA and its doubling time can indicate the presence of malignancy. A PSADT of less than 6 months most often represents a rapidly growing malignancy consistent with systemic spread of disease; i.e., it is not localized to the prostate and is likely to have spread to the lymph nodes and/or bone marrow (Fowler et al., *Surgery,* 1994; Fowler et al., *J. Urol.,* 1995). Software applications for determining the PSADT and PSAV are available for download at the PCRI Web site [http://www.prostate-cancer.org]. There are no charges for these and other programs.

Take-home Lesson 1

PC is often wider spread than believed at diagnosis. Is the PC organ-confined? Medical expertise currently underestimates the volume of cancer. Is the PC of low volume? The aggressiveness of cancer is significantly manifested in its growth rate. What are the PSAV and PSADT?

PSA

The amount of serum PSA is proportional to the tumor cell mass. There are modifying factors involved, however. These include PSA leak into the serum, which is related to Gleason score, and the contribution to the serum PSA from the benign component of the prostate. Therefore, additional ingredients to staging include the absolute PSA value, and the rapidity of PSA increase. PSA values at diagnosis of greater than 25 ng are more often associated with PC outside of the gland, involving seminal vesicle, lymph node, or bone. PSA values greater than 8 at diagnosis are associated with a lower percentage of cures using modalities such as RT or RP (Lattanzi et al., *Int. J. Radiat. Oncol. Biol. Phys.,* 1997). Therefore, the PSA absolute value becomes an important discriminant regarding likelihood of organ-confined disease, and hence cure, with a local therapy. This basic information has to be taken into account in any discussion on the value of RP and RT as well as any comparison studies of RP with RT. The story gets more complex, but it is rational and understandable.

The Gleason Score

There are other variables that relate to cell behavior that must also be taken into account. The most important of these is reflected in the microscopic appearance of the tumor and is called the Gleason score (GS). The higher the GS, the more aggressive the tumor. For a detailed description of the GS, please visit the PCRI Web site [http://www.prostate-cancer.org]. The GS should be read by an expert in the pathology of PC to be most valid. The above Web site also has listings of expert pathologists in the field of PC. Paradoxically, with a GS of 8 to 10, there is less PSA leakage from the tumor cell into the serum (Aihara et al., *J. Urol.,* 1994). This may result in a low serum PSA level despite a large volume of tumor. The table below relates the Gleason weighted grade to the PSA leak (Aihara et al., *J. Urol.,* 1994).

Table 1: PSA Leak vs Weighted Gleason Grade

Gleason grade (weighted)	PSA leak
5	1
4.5	1.5
4	2
3.5	3
3	4
2.5	6
2	10
1.5	15
1	20

To determine the weighted Gleason grade, you need to know the GS resulting from biopsies taken from areas of the gland that were positive for PC, assuming the GS from these areas was different.

If the GS was [3,2] from the right lobe, and 3 of 3 cores biopsied were positive, and if the GS was [3,3] for the left lobe, and 2 of 3 cores biopsied were positive, the weighted GS would = 5 (GS from right lobe) × 3 (# of cores positive) + 6 (GS from left lobe) × 2 (# of cores positive) divided by 5 (number of cores involved). Therefore, in this case the weighted GS would be $(5 \times 3 + 6 \times 2)/5$, or $27/5 = 5.4$. The weighted GG is half of the weighted GS, or 2.7. The paper relating GG to PSA leakage into the serum unfortunately does not give us exact values for intermediate GG. Therefore, we can only

P

estimate that the PSA leak for a weighted GG of 2.7 is halfway between that for 2.5 and 3.0, or 5. We use the gland volume determined at TRUSP to calculate benign-related PSA and cancer-specific (cs) PSA. This is shown below for a TRUSP volume of 60 cc and a PSA of 7.2 (D'Amico et al., *Int. J. Radiat. Oncol. Biol. Phys.*, 1996; D'Amico et al., *Urology*, 1997; Marks et al., *Urology*, 1994).

PSA_{cs} = cancer-specific PSA = $PSA_{total} - PSA_{benign}$

PSA_{benign} = epithelial fraction × PSA/cm^3 of epithelial tissue × TRUSP volume

Values for epithelial fraction are 0.2 (after Marks et al.) and 0.33 for PSA per cm^3 of benign tissue.

Therefore, if we have a TRUSP volume of 60 cm^3, we multiply this by 0.066 (product of 0.2 × 0.33) to get PSA_{benign} = 3.96. Benign PSA values per TRUSP volume are precalculated below for your convenience.

Table 2: Benign PSA per Gland Volume

TRUSP volume	PSA benign
Volume in cc or gm	ng/ml
20	1.32
25	1.65
30	1.98
35	2.31
40	2.64
45	2.97
50	3.3
55	3.63
60	3.96
65	4.29
70	4.62
75	4.95
80	5.28
85	5.61
90	5.94
95	6.27
100	6.6

The benign PSA is subtracted from the total PSA to give excess of PSA_{cs}. The PSA_{cs} = 7.2 – 3.96 or 3.2.

That is, for every 5 ng/ml of serum PSA for this particular patient with a weighted GG of 2.7, there is 1.0 cm^3 of tumor tissue that relates to producing this value in the serum. Therefore, we divide the PSA cs by 5 to get the cancer volume. In this case it would be 3.2/5, or 0.64 cm^3 of tumor.

Therefore, men with verified Gleason scores of 8 to 10 need to be aware that the PSA reading may be misleadingly low, and that, in some cases, there may be no PSA secretion of the tumor cell into the blood despite active disease of significant tumor volume. It is clearly essential in the evaluation and management of the man with PC that an accurate Gleason score be obtained. In most studies of PC, the GS is the most important of all clinical and pathologic variables relating to prognosis. A serious pitfall in our current evaluation of PC is a GS that is incorrectly read.

Take-home Lesson 2

The GS is the most important single variable in the natural history of PC. Always verify the GS by a second opinion with a PC pathology expert.

Clinical Stage (CS)

The other important variable, alluded to above, is the tumor volume or tumor burden. At diagnosis, the tumor burden is reflected in the PSA, the findings of digital rectal exam (DRE), the number of biopsy cores involved, and the extent of core involvement. The DRE findings are expressed in the clinical stage (CS). This is also discussed at the above Web site in the paper called "Treatment Options for Prostate Cancer Patients with Early Disease." We commonly see the patient and the physician confused when it comes to the CS. If the DRE does not reveal a palpable abnormality worrisome for PC, then the CS is T_{1c}. If the DRE is abnormal and consistent with PC confined to the prostate, the CS is T_2. Within the T_2 category, the subset designations of T_{2a}, T_{2b}, and T_{2c} reflect the extent of the abnormality palpated. If there is a palpable area of abnormality that is 50% or less of one lobe of the prostate, the CS is T_{2a}. If there is more than 50% of one lobe involved by PC, the CS is T_{2b}. If both lobes are involved, the CS is T_{2c}. If the DRE reflects disease that is outside the prostate, the designation T_3 is used. T_{3a} CS means unilateral (one-sided) extracapsular extension, whereas T_{3b} means bilateral extracapsular extension. T_{3c} means seminal vesicle(s) involvement. Finally, T_{4a} disease means that tumor invades the bladder neck, or external sphincter, or rectum, whereas T_{4b} indicates that PC invades the levator muscles and/or is fixed to the pelvic wall. The clinical stage, or CS, is used in the Partin and Bluestein algorithms for assessing extent of disease. What are algorithms?

Take-home Lesson 3

Understand the jargon used in PC medicine. It is your link to a higher communication with your medical coaches. Communication of critical issues is essential to patient empowerment.

Algorithms: Tools for Risk Assessment

Clinical and pathologic variables interact with one another to give us additional information. Such a process where combinations of 2 or more variables yield information more significant than any one variable is called an *algorithm*. The algorithms are important buoys to help us navigate through the confused seas encountered in the staging of PC. A description of the process of using the algorithms to derive a risk assessment in the newly diagnosed patient is found in the paper entitled "Predictive and Prognostic Counseling in the Newly Diagnosed Patient with Prostate Cancer" at the PCRI website [http://www.prostate-cancer.org]. It is important to realize that data derived from these algorithms result from almost 13,000 human clinical experiences—not from mouse models of PC or studies of PC cell lines grown in petri dishes. Algorithms may involve the newly diagnosed patient, or they may relate to the patient anywhere in the natural history of the disease. In the setting of newly diagnosed men with PC, these authors statistically analyzed preoperative variables that could predict for final pathologic stage. They concluded that the combinations of preoperative variables were of greater value than any single variable. Most of these studies employed a statistical maneuver called multivariate analysis. These algorithms are usually published with tables or graphs. Below is a listing of some of the studies employing this concept involving over 12,000 human experiences!

Table 3: Patients Enrolled in Various Studies Involving Predictive Algorithms

Senior Author: Institution	# of Pts	Reference
Partin: Hopkins, Baylor, Michigan	4,133*	JAMA 277: 1445–1451, 1997
Bluestein: Mayo	1,632*	J Urol 151: 1315–1320, 1994
Lerner: Mayo	904*	J Urol 156: 137–143, 1996
Narayan: U of Florida	813*	Urology 46: 205–21, 1995
Eastham: Baylor	766*	J Urol 157: 298, 1997
Partin (II): Hopkins	542	Urology 43: 649–659, 1994
Pisansky: Mayo	500	Cancer 79: 337–344, 1997
D'Amico: Harvard	480*	Cancer J Sci Am 2: 343, 1996
Dugan: Mayo	337*	JAMA 275: 288–294, 1996
Huncharek: Mass General	300	Cancer Invest 13: 31-35, 1995
Bostwick: Mayo, Baylor, Wash U, Laval	186*	Urology 48: 47–57, 1996
Oesterling: Mayo Clinic	852	JAMA 269: 57–60, 1993
Powell: Wayne St, Michigan	369*	Urology 49: 726–731, 1997
Kleer: Mayo Clinic	945*	Urology 41: 207–216, 1993
Total	12,759	

*Refer to studies involving 10,565 radical prostatectomy patients.

P

What does all of this lead to? It leads to a more accurate assessment of the patient's true status. Knowing where the PC may have spread gives direction to the patient-physician team to perform certain tests to exclude disease at those site(s). For example, if the algorithms show a high risk for lymph node disease, the staging process should include the monoclonal antibody scan called ProstaScint. If the risk is negligible for lymph node involvement, this study could be excluded. The same approach is used to evaluate disease at the different *stations of involvement*. Is there disease in the capsule of the prostate, the seminal vesicles, the lymph nodes, or the bones? If one finds a high probability of disease confined to the prostate, then local therapies such as RP, RT (external beam using 3D conformal techniques, or seed implantation or a combination of both), or cryosurgery can be used with a greater probability of success. However, there are caveats that relate to the successful use of these therapies as well.

Take-home Lesson 4

Algorithms involve human experiences of men who have gone before you. Take advantage of the information that others have provided you. Obtaining data from the algorithms is critical homework that must involve you and your medical coaches. Assessing your risk for PC spread to particular sites and evaluating those sites with special testing is an essential part of successful management of the man with PC.

Three Basic Ingredients of Successful Cancer Management

All treatments in cancer medicine are associated with a skill factor. In this respect, a treatment should be regarded as the "message," with the physician or technician performing them regarded as the "messenger" for that specific treatment or therapy. It is ignorant to believe that all urologists can do a radical prostatectomy with an equal degree of excellence, that all radiation oncologists have equivalent skills, or that all medical oncologists plan and execute chemotherapy treatments equally well. When we became superselective in our choice of consultants for RP, SI, and EBRT, the incidence of adverse side effects changed drastically. For example, the 40 to 50% significant incontinence rates that we had previously seen after RP became less than 1% when we directed patients to the very best urologists. Newer procedures such as cryosurgery have even fewer highly skilled physicians able to perform this treatment without a significant risk of leaving the patient with serious complications. I have heard physicians make derisive remarks about cryosurgery; in my experience with this modality, it is usually the ill-talented physician who has most of the complications as well as the poor anticancer results. Never get the message and the messenger confused.

The three basic ingredients that relate to the success of any treatment are (1) selection of the patient, (2) preparation of the patient, and (3) choice of a physician(s) to do the treatment(s).

It is important that the patient be aware of all these elements and that he network with support groups and his medical coaches to find the physicians involved in the therapy of PC. These physicians are needed to coordinate the selection, the preparation, and the definitive treatments of this disease. We need physicians to be graded according to skill and rewarded according to performance. Patient groups must push for societies of accredited physicians with credentialling at the highest levels.

Take-home Lesson 5

Not all men (or women) are created equal. Always look for the artist, be it the pathologist, the urologist, the radiation therapist, and/or the medical oncologist. Maintain a high level of communication among all health-care personnel involved with your life. Make sure you receive copies of all medical tests and consultations, and make copies for all your physicians. This is part of your mandate to optimize and maximize your chance for a healthy life.

Preparation of the Patient

We have not given details about item (2) above, the preparation of the patient. What is it all about?

Preparation of the patient refers to what we can do to increase the likelihood of success in any of the therapies of PC. Treatment with RT is limited by tumor volume. We can reduce tumor volume by using androgen deprivation therapy (ADT). ADT employs drugs that lower the testosterone (T) level as well as other androgens such as dihydrotestosterone (DHT) and adrenal androgen precursors such as DHEA-S and androstenedione. Most commonly, ADT involves the use of antiandrogens (AA) coupled with LHRH agonists (LHRH-A). Examples of AA include flutamide (Eulexin), bicalutamide (Casodex), and nilutamide (Nilandron). Examples of LHRH-A include leuprolide (Lupron) or goserelin (Zoladex). AAs are oral agents given on a daily basis, while LHRH-A are given intramuscularly or subcutaneously as long-acting depot injections on a monthly, or every 3 to 4 month, basis. It is critical to the proper use of the LHRH-A that the AA is given for at least one week before initiating the LHRH-A to prevent flare. Flare is a paradoxical reaction that occurs during initial exposure to the LHRH-A. It is characterized by an increased release of LH from the LHRH receptor that is interacting with the LHRH-A. This is described in detail in the paper "Hormone Therapy" on the PCRI Web site and also in issue number three of our newsletter *Insights*.

Monitoring of ADT

Patients receiving combination hormone blockade using the above couplets of drugs need to be monitored with chemistry panels, complete blood count (CBC), and PSA levels on a monthly basis to detect signs of possible toxicity resulting from this treatment. Both Eulexin and Casodex can cause elevations in the liver enzymes SGOT and SGPT. With monthly monitoring, the risk of significant liver toxicity is minimized. In addition, the avoidance of alcohol and the use of silymarin (100 to 200 mg 3 times a day) will prevent toxicity to the liver cell or hepatocyte (Dehmlow et al., *Hepatology,* 1996). The CBC checks the hematocrit to monitor the anemia of androgen deprivation that occurs in 80% of men on ADT (Strum et al., *J. Urol.,* 1997). In cases where the anemia is severe, the use of erythropoietin (Procrit) will correct this problem and alleviate symptoms of fatigue, shortness of breath, and possibly angina (Strum et al., *J. Urol.,* 1997).

Rationale for ADT

The rationale for the use of ADT is to reduce tumor volume to allow RT to be more effective. The efficacy of RT is compromised when the PC volume is too great to allow RT to effectively eradicate the total tumor cell population. ADT reduces the tumor volume, synergizes with RT, and decreases angiogenesis to allow for a better outcome with RT. This has already been reported in the landmark paper by Bolla et al., which employed RT with 3 years of LHRH agonist therapy to treat high-grade Gleason score lesions (GS 8–10) or locally advanced PC (CS T3–4) (Bolla et al., *N. Engl. J. Med.,* 1997). The literature on the use of ADT in patients with a lower clinical stage and lower GS is currently being written and appears to validate the use of ADT to allow RT to be more effective (Zelefsky et al., *J. Clin. Oncol.*, 1998). Studies are being published that now show the equivalence of RT approaches such as external beam RT or seed implantation when compared to similarly selected patients who undergo RP (Keyser et al., *Int. J. Radiat. Oncol. Biol. Phys.,* 1997). In such good-risk patients, the 10-year actuarial disease-free survival rates are about 80%. This means that there is no evidence of biochemical relapse as seen by a rising PSA in 80% of these patients at an actuarial time of 10 years. It is not surprising that this equivalence to RP is being seen with RT when the tumor volume is being controlled for by selecting patients with low levels of PSA and Gleason scores that reflect a lower tumor burden.

There are many fine points that relate to the above discussion. Limitations of space do not allow for all of these to be dealt with in this overview. We would suggest that the reader use the resources mentioned above along with those at the end of this section for a further understanding of the issues so far discussed. In addition, the PCRI newsletter *Insights* has examples of how a patient can proceed in a step-wise fashion in the evaluation of his disease; *Insights* can be printed off our homepage.

In lieu of RP, RT, or cryosurgery, PC patients may want to consider protocols that incorporate androgen deprivation therapy (ADT) for control of most prostate cancers. In essence, this is the primary use of hormone manipulations to control PC growth. Innovative natural adjunctive therapies are also implemented immediately upon the initiation of ADT or any anticancer therapy. Ideally, many of these adjunctive therapies should be utilized in a preventative fashion. This will be discussed in more detail later.

Take-home Lesson 6

PC is an endocrine-related malignancy. The growth of PC is highly dependent on the availability of male hormones or androgens. Androgen deprivation therapy (ADT) is an essential maneuver to kill PC cells. Despite controversial literature, it has become apparent that ADT is a key part of the strategy to reduce tumor volume. Future studies will show the successful use of ADT in the primary treatment of PC as well as in PC that is more advanced. Current studies are showing the value of ADT when used to reduce tumor volume in patients receiving EBRT and seed implantation.

What is involved in using androgen deprivation therapy (ADT)?

Combination Hormone Blockade (ADT2 or ADT3)

There is currently controversy as to the value of ADT using combined modalities of blockade versus one modality of blockade. A recent article, for example, showed no benefit of Eulexin when given with orchiectomy compared to orchiectomy alone in men with advanced PC involving the bone (D_2 disease) (Eisenberger et al., *N. Engl. J. Med.*, 1998). In this study, the patients with minimal bone disease had a 5-year survival of ~ 50%. In contrast, Labrie et al. reported a 66% 5-year survival in D_2 patients with 1 to 5 bone lesions receiving combination Eulexin and Lupron (Labrie et al., *Clin. Invest. Med.*, 1993). Moreover, EORTC study 30853 showed improved survival in the group receiving combination Zoladex + Flutamide versus orchiectomy. In this 327-patient study, there was a 39% decrease in the death rate in good-prognosis patients in the combination-arm versus the orchiectomy-only arm (Denis et al., *Eur. Urol.*, 1998). The different outcomes reported need to be resolved, since most men today are still receiving combined hormone blockade using an LHRH-A and an anti-androgen. In addition, clarification of other uses of hormone blockade remain relatively neglected. These include the use of ADT in earlier stages of PC, inhibition of dihydrotestosterone (DHT) production, and the use of prolactin inhibitors. These are discussed in the PCRI paper called "Hormone Therapy." In this paper, clinical detailed studies using agents that block additional areas in the hormonal axis are cited. Some of these issues are worth discussing here.

The use of finasteride (Proscar) to block 5-alpha-reductase, to prevent conversion of T into DHT (which is five to ten times as potent), appears reasonable. When we employ three drugs as part of ADT, we indicate this by the designation ADT3. We are striving for terminology that allows us to communicate more clearly. ADT3-LEP indicates three-drug ADT with Lupron, Eulexin, and Proscar. These are studies using Proscar in post-radical prostatectomy patients to delay the rise in PSA, as well as studies that have combined Proscar with an anti-androgen (AA) (Andriole et al., *Urology*, 1995; Brufsky et al., *Urology*, 1997). The latter approach is called sequential androgen blockade (SAB) since it involves blocking DHT production along with preventing both T and DHT from interacting with the nuclear androgen receptors. The SAB approach maintains a high level of T. In some men, this results in fewer problems with erectile dysfunction, muscle loss, and other signs and symptoms associated with androgen deficiency. We have used Proscar as part of ADT since 1990, employing a dose of 5 mg twice a day. To date, there are no randomized studies comparing two-drug ADT (ADT2) versus three-drug ADT (ADT3).

We have published preliminary findings using three-drug therapy in the setting of intermittent androgen deprivation (IAD). When such patients are taken off the LHRH-A and the anti-androgen, they are left on Proscar as maintenance therapy. Patients treated in this fashion had an extra 13 months "off time" from IAD compared to those who received ADT2 and no Proscar maintenance (Scholz et al., *J. Urol.*, 1999).

The use of prolactin inhibitors in PC patients is based on work showing that prolactin increases the number and sensitivity of androgen receptors. Rana et al. used the prolactin-suppressing drug bromocriptine along with orchiectomy and hydrocortisone (regimen A) in treating advanced PC. Regimen A was compared to orchiectomy plus Eulexin and to orchiectomy alone. Regimen A resulted in a 61% suppression of primary prostate growth, compared with only a 48% reduction with orchiectomy and Eulexin alone. After 36 months, 40% of the group receiving Regimen A experienced disease progression, compared with 60% in the orchiectomy-only group (Rana et al., *Eur. J. Cancer*, 1995).

PC patients should have their prolactin levels checked via a blood test drawn in the morning. If your prolactin levels are elevated, you should consider one of the following prescription drugs:

- Bromocriptine, 5 mg 1 to 2 times a day
- Pergolide, 0.25 mg to 0.5 mg twice a day
- Dostinex, 0.5 mg twice a week

Check your prolactin levels again in 30 days to make sure the drug you choose is, in fact, suppressing prolactin released into your blood from the pituitary gland. Dostinex is the newest and easiest drug to use since it has fewer side effects than the older drugs, is more effective in suppressing prolactin, and requires dosing only twice a week.

Many patients use ADT to prepare themselves for local therapies such as RP, RT, or cryosurgery. Others use ADT as a means to extend time before decisions on local therapy, hoping for a new breakthrough that preserves prostatic integrity. Still others are using ADT as primary therapy of PC. It is important that we inform patients that approaches like IAD are still considered investigational. When ADT is used in conjunction with local therapies such as RP, RT (including seed implantation), or cryosurgery, it is important to stress the need for baseline studies to assess the stage of disease before starting ADT, as well as to coordinate the goals of ADT with the team involved with the local prostate treatment. For example, the choice of external beam radiation therapy (EBRT) with seed implantation is based on evaluations that include Gleason score, PSA, local extent of disease, and gland volume. Studies that involve the latter two items should be done as baseline before ADT is begun. The gland volume should be monitored by digital rectal exam with the goal of lowering the prostate size for optimal implantation. For many brachytherapists, this is in the 15 to 30 cubic centimeter (cc) range.

Take-home Lesson 7

The hormonal axis in PC involves multiple areas that go beyond testosterone inhibition at the pituitary or testicular sites. These pathways involve the adrenal androgen precursors, prolactin, 5-alpha-reductase, ACTH, and serotonin, to name a few. We are most likely not optimally blocking the endocrine pathways with our current approaches to PC management. Further work is needed.

Biomarkers to Assess Tumor-cell Sensitivity

If tumor cells that make substances such as PSA and prolactin (as well as other biological markers such as PAP, NSE, CGA) are destroyed by anticancer therapy of any kind, then the biomarker levels drop to low or undetectable levels. The more sensitive the tumor cell population is to the therapy used, the more quickly and more sustained the biomarker(s) drop. It has been our practice to use ADT with the goal of achieving and maintaining an undetectable PSA (UD-PSA) level for at least 1 year in the setting of men using ADT as primary therapy for newly diagnosed PC. When we are able to achieve this, we feel comfortable that we are *not* dealing with other mutated tumor cell populations (clones). We believe that these mutated clones,

P

with continued growth, lead to the clinical expression of androgen-independent PC (AIPC). Therefore, our goal is to assess the tumor cell population comprehensively with various biomarkers, treat the tumor cell population with a combination approach to ADT, achieve a UD-PSA, and maintain it for approximately one year. We are routinely using the 3-drug combination of anti-androgen (Flutamide or Casodex), LHRH agonist (Lupron or Zoladex), and Proscar in our patients. In patients with elevated or high-normal prolactin levels, we suggest entry into a trial using Dostinex to see if this effects a change in PSA that correlates with prolactin suppression. Our results using Dostinex are too preliminary to report at this time. However, the results with our intermittent androgen deprivation (IAD) approach are mature enough to state that our average duration of time off therapy with an UD-PSA (ADT2 for approximately 13 months), achieved and maintained, is currently 19 months. We can also state that the use of Proscar during induction ADT and maintenance off ADT extends this time to an average of 32 months. Discontinuation of ADT allows normal T recovery and prevents the man on ADT from having chronic debilitation due to lack of male hormones. Work is needed to refine optimal drug combinations and duration of therapy.

Take-home Lesson 8

Biomarkers are the most sensitive indicators of successful treatment of cellular malignancy. The biomarker response to treatment provides clues to the nature of the PC and is an excellent prognostic indicator. Future studies should explore other biomarkers that may identify high-risk patients needing therapy that is more intensive.

The Androgen Deprivation Syndrome (ADS)

Signs and symptoms resulting from ADT are called the androgen deprivation syndrome, or ADS (Strum et al., *Proc. Amer. Soc. Clin. Oncol.*, 1998). Androgens are vital to the proper function of most organ systems. For example, blocking androgen in the nervous tissue of the brain may be associated with short-term memory loss, while blocking androgen receptors in the bone marrow often leads to the anemia of androgen deprivation. Many men on ADT report joint symptoms characterized by aches and pains in their feet, knees, and hips and stiffness in their hands. It is believed that the latter represents the effects of androgen deprivation leading to excessive bone resorption. If unchecked, this eventually leads to osteoporosis. How does this happen? Androgen receptors have been found on osteoblasts. Perhaps the androgen blockade that occurs as a result of ADT causes diminished osteoblast growth, leading to an uncoupling of osteoblast-osteoclast function with excessive osteoclastic activity and bone resorption. The signs and symptoms relating to the ADS are highly variable from man to man. Some men have few complaints from withdrawal of androgens, while others have multiple problems and are miserable. It is our goal to kill as many PC cells as possible while allowing a high quality of life. The second issue of *Insights* and the PCRI Web site have articles on ADS and how symptoms can be ameliorated to improve the quality of life of men experiencing such adverse effects from ADT.

Take-home Lesson 9

All of medicine is a two-edged sword. It is the goal of the physician to maximize benefits of therapy while minimizing or preventing adverse effects that are associated with therapy. We have learned a great deal about the natural history of PC and male menopause by understanding the signs and symptoms that may occur as part of the androgen deprivation syndrome or ADS.

Summary of Recommendations for Treatment of Apparent Early Prostate Cancer

The optimal treatment of apparently organ-confined PC requires the proper selection of the patient based on a careful risk assessment of known prognostic factors. This means that the patient should have an expert Gleason score obtained as well as a careful evaluation of all known factors that are involved in a thorough risk assessment of extent of disease. These include, at least, baseline PSA, PAP, clinical stage, gland volume, number of cores involved, ploidy, and pathological stage. Using this information and applying known algorithms to calculate PC risk outside the prostate, the clinician-patient team can exclude such extraprostatic involvement with appropriate tests and increase the chance of treating localized PC with a greater probability of cure. This approach to patient selection for localized treatment of PC is further enhanced by using ADT to reduce tumor and gland volume to increase the chances of cure with local therapy modalities such as external beam RT and/or seed implantation, or cryosurgery. To date, there is no data to suggest that ADT enhances the cure rate of RP. Perhaps the 3 months of neoadjuvant therapy used in most studies is insufficient time to achieve this goal. Finally, the choice of a physician(s) to deliver these therapies is critical to the successful treatment of PC.

Cancerfacts.com

Cancerfacts.com is a new Internet service that employs the philosophy and take-home lessons shown above. Patients are asked for essential data that are used to compile multiple algorithmic assessments. This is presented using a wizard to guide the patient while educating the patient with references, glossary, and abstracts. This leads to treatment options that are personalized to the patient depending on preferences that the patient has indicated and the results of the algorithmic assessment. The Internet URL for this service is [http://www.cancerfacts.com].

PROSTATE CANCER: LATE STAGE

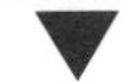

CAUTION: Some readers will find this protocol technically challenging. It is written for both the patient and the attending oncologist.

Introduction: Rationale to Diagnose PC Earlier

Not all PC is systemic, anymore than all breast cancer or other tumor types are systemic. If they were, we would never cure any man or woman of PC, breast cancer, or any other malignancy. Physicians claiming that every man with PC needs ADT as primary and sole therapy are blindly ignoring the growing numbers of men who present 8 to 15 years after RP or RT with a flat PSA graph. Emphasis on the use of routine PSA monitoring starting annually at the age of 40 with PSA velocity and doubling time determinations as a standard part of PSA reporting will increase the numbers of men diagnosed earlier, with a lower tumor burden, and cured with local modalities of treatment (Labrie et al., *J. Clin. Endocrinol. Metab.*, 1995; Labrie et al., *Urology*, 1996). PSA testing with these enhancements should start earlier, at age 35, in men with a familial history of PC.

In addition, the use of routine free/total PSA levels should increase our ability to diagnose PC earlier since fractionation of PSA allows us to monitor the malignant-associated portion of PSA called complexed PSA. Evaluation of risk of PC using neural net technology as per the ProstaSure blood test also will enable an earlier diagnosis of PC (Babaian et al., *Urology*, 1998). As our standard and hopefully routine approach to monitoring PSA and other biological expressions of tumor cell activity increases, the percentage of men cured with PC should increase as well.

This is borne out in a recent report in which PC was detected in 22% (73/332) of men 50 years or older whose PSA reading was between 2.6 and 4. All cancers detected in this setting were clinically localized. This study indicates that PSA readings greater than 2.6 and less than 4.0 may represent a 22% risk of PC (Catalona et al., *JAMA*, 1997). The use of a free PSA test would help determine which of these men whose PSA readings were greater than 2.6 but less than 4.0 have a high probability of PC versus a low probability of PC. Such a test could reduce the number of unnecessary biopsies in the low-risk subset and focus a need for more comprehensive biopsing in the high-risk subset.

Another study involved 760 men with an initial PSA of 4.0 ng/ml or less, plus a normal or suspicious DRE and a benign prostate biopsy. These men were monitored with PSA testing every 4 months. Of 559 men with an initial PSA of 2.0 ng/ml or less, only three (0.5%) had a persistently abnormal PSA for 3 years; in this group, one cancer was detected (0.2%). Of 201 men with a PSA of 2.1 to 4.0, 37 had PSA levels that became and remained abnormal (defined as > 4.0). Of this group, 23 biopsies were performed, and 8 (35%) revealed PC. The study indicated that in men with an initial PSA of 2.1 to 4, the cancer detection rate was 4.5%. This was approximately 15-fold greater ($p < 0.00001$) than the cancer detection rate in the men with an initial PSA of 2.0 or less (Harris et al., *J. Urol.*, 1997). Patients presenting with their first PSA at 2.1 or greater should therefore be the focus of more intense studies. This could include free/total PSA, PSA doubling time determination, and ProstaSure testing.

New biopsy techniques—such as 5-region biopsy of the prostate gland—have been shown to increase the diagnostic yield of PC by 35% (Eskew et al., 1997).

Despite these inroads, many men today are still being diagnosed with PC that is advanced, i.e., not organ-confined. What difference does this make?

The difference in treating early PC versus more advanced PC relates to the issue of cure as opposed to control. Early PC has the potential for cure via a local therapy combined with the use of ADT in situations where the tumor volume compromises the curative ability of local therapy such as RT (including seed implantation) or cryosurgery. This has been discussed in the section on Early PC.

The Biology of AIPC

When PC spreads to the capsular interface and leaves the prostate gland, it reflects a change in the biologic nature of the cancer. The PC now is expressing its more aggressive nature in its ability to spread and metastasize. Why?

The aggressiveness of these tumors appears to directly correlate with the proportion of higher Gleason grade cells. This frequently involves multiple clones of PC cells—some androgen-sensitive, but others androgen-insensitive, and/or possibly androgen-altered (Aihara et al., *Urology*, 1994; Brawn, *Cancer*, 1983). This heterogeneity appears related to tumor size or burden. As the tumor burden increases by cell division, the chances of gene mutation increase, which in turn may lead to androgen or drug-resistant tumors. Such mutations likely result from the activation of oncogenes or the inhibition of tumor suppressor genes.

In laboratory experiments, for example, expression of an activated H-ras oncogene in androgen-sensitive LNCaP PC cells allows these cells to grow *independent* of the presence of androgens. H-ras oncogene has also been shown to stimulate MDR-1, the multidrug resistance gene that is heavily implicated in chemotherapy drug resistance (Lehr et al., *Cell. Mol. Biol.*, 1998; Yamazaki, *Proc. Annu. Meet. Am. Assoc. Cancer. Res.*, 1993). Therefore, androgen independence and MDR-1 expression may go hand-in-hand. The sequence of events may be as follows:

Table 1: Hypothesis for Androgen Independence

Increasing tumor burden	⇒	gene mutation of an oncogene
Oncogene stimulation (e.g., H-ras)	⇒	stimulation of MDR gene
MDR expression	⇒	hormone independence

It is now clear that more than one genetic aberration can lead to androgen independence. Mechanisms that have been identified include expression of the proto-oncogene bcl-2 and mutation of the genetic biomarker p53, a tumor suppressor gene (McDonnell et al., *Cancer Res.*, 1992; Bookstein, *Cancer Res.*, 1993).

In essence, androgen independence is more likely to be present at the time patients are diagnosed with extensive disease, such as in the lymph nodes or bone, and possibly begins with the manifestation of capsular penetration. Since androgen deprivation therapy (ADT) primarily kills androgen-dependent and to a lesser extent androgen-sensitive cells, androgen-independent tumor cell populations will continue to grow and eventually emerge as the primary disease entity. It is therefore more likely that patients do not develop AIPC as a result of treatments such as ADT, but more likely that they already had AIPC at the time ADT was begun.

A mutation of the androgen receptor gene was hypothesized as one possible survival mechanism for AIPC during ADT. In an attempt to confirm the hypothesis that AIPC cell growth is mediated by gene mutation, Taplin et al. (*N. Engl. J. Med.*, 1995) examined the androgen receptor genes in 10 patients with AIPC. The authors noted high levels of androgen receptor gene expression in all of the patient samples, supporting the hypothesis that tumor progression requires a functional androgen receptor gene. In five patients, point mutations in the androgen receptor gene were found, and all were located on the androgen-binding domain. When functional studies were done, progesterone and estrogen were capable of activating mutant androgen receptors in two patients. The authors concluded ADT selects AIPC cells whose mutated androgen receptors stimulate growth without the presence of usual androgen levels.

One of the point mutations found by Taplin et al. had been previously reported by Veldscholte et al. (*Biochem. Biophys. Res. Commun.*, 1990) in LNCaP, a cell line used as an experimental model of androgen-sensitive human PC. This androgen receptor gene mutation resulted in an androgen receptor that could be activated by estrogen, progesterone, and the anti-androgen flutamide.

The critical issue for the patient with PC with evidence of disease progression is, Do I have AIPC or not? How can we logically explore this issue to more correctly guide such patients?

Defining AIPC and Excluding Other Causes of PSA Progression

The definition of AIPC is disease progression as evidenced by a progressively rising PSA (3 consecutive rises of at least 10% each, or 3 rises that involve an increase of 50% over the nadir PSA) or an increase in tumor mass on bone scan, x-ray, CT scan, or MRI despite a castrate level of testosterone (T < 20 ng/dL). There are further issues that must be addressed, however, before such a patient is categorized as having AIPC. Understanding the endocrinology of PC is essential to accurately define the patient's status.

Androgen Independent PC (AIPC) or Not?

- Is the Testosterone level <20 ng/dl or close to this?
  - If not, you may not have AIPC.
- Is the PSA showing a persistent rise, or is there some other evidence of biologic progression?
- Are the adrenal androgen levels low?

For example, if a patient's PSA stops falling and begins to rise on ADT2, the T level is castrate, and the adrenal androgen precursors are not low, then AIPC is presumed present until proven otherwise. If in the same setting above, the levels of the adrenal androgen precursors are suppressed, an androgen receptor mutation (ARM) should be excluded. The latter is confirmed by demonstrating a response to anti-androgen withdrawal with falling PSA levels.

If the testosterone is > 20 ng/dL, the patient's serum LH level should be checked. If LH is not completely suppressed (usually < 1.0), we believe

P

it is reasonable to increase the dosage of the LHRH-A. If the LH level is suppressed, we measure the levels of adrenal androgen precursors dehydroepiandrosterone sulfate (DHEA-S) and androstenedione. These hormones can be converted to T and may account for T levels of > 20 ng/dL. If such levels were found, we would prescribe drugs to suppress adrenal androgen precursor production such as Nizoral (high-dose ketoconazole, or HDK) and hydrocortisone. The analysis involved in a patient on ADT with a rising PSA is shown below.

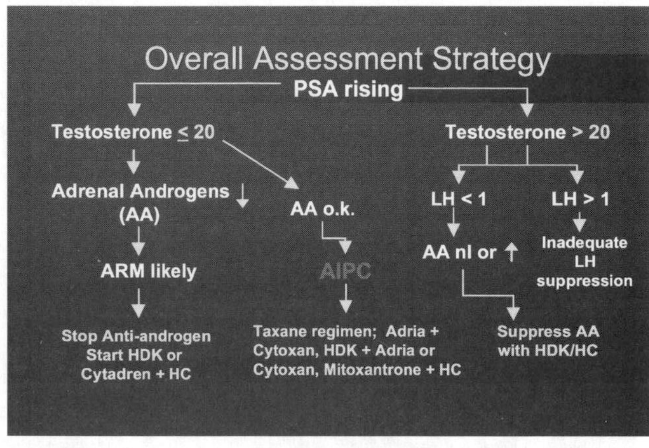

HDK = high-dose ketoconazole, HC = hydrocortisone, LH = luteinizing hormone, ARM = androgen receptor mutation.

There are studies to support the concern that adrenal androgen precursors can increase in the setting of PC treatment and that this increase leads to higher T levels, which in turn effects a poor clinical outcome, if unrecognized. The elevation in androstenedione and T shown below in 10 of 27 men undergoing orchiectomy for PC supports our concerns (Sciarra et al., *Clin. Endocrinol.*, 1993).

Take-home Lesson 1

In situations involving progressive disease as seen by a consistently rising PSA, stop and reassess the hormone status to determine whether AIPC is present.

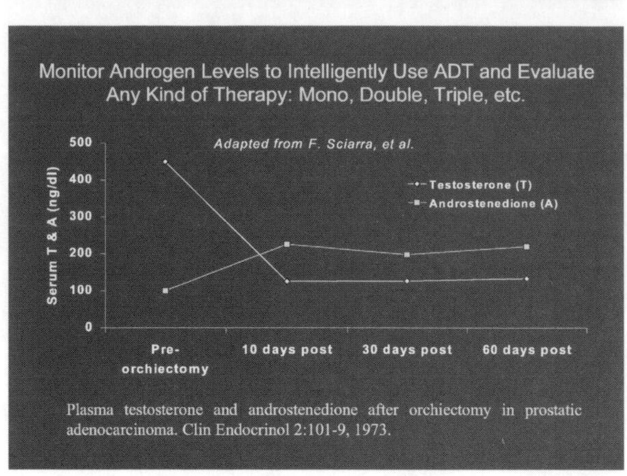

Plasma testosterone and androstenedione after orchiectomy in prostatic adenocarcinoma. Clin Endocrinol 2:101-9, 1973.

The Response to ADT as a Guide to the Presence of AIPC

The evaluation of the response of available biomarkers to ADT provides clues to the presence or absence of AIPC. In essence, it is an *in vivo* test of the tumor cell population. If the tumor cell population is predominantly that of ADPC (androgen-dependent PC), there is usually a brisk drop in PSA to very low levels that are maintained during the course of ADT. This assumes that an ARM has not developed over the course of time. The newly diagnosed patient with dramatic sensitivity to ADT, most likely has ADPC. We use an ultra-sensitive assay (3rd Generation Immulite from DPC International, Los Angeles) and define an undetectable PSA (UDPSA) as < 0.05. If the patient achieves and maintains this level, it has been our experience that the development of AIPC

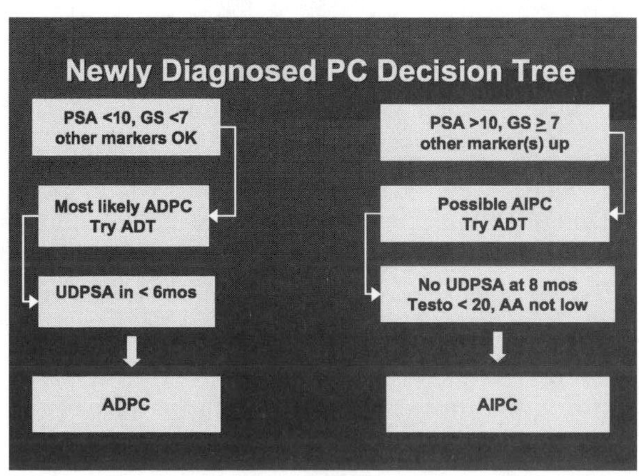

is rare. On the other hand, if a UDPSA is not achieved or is achieved after a prolonged period of time, we are concerned about the presence of AIPC. In our experience, the biology of the tumor is manifested in its response to ADT. It therefore becomes significant to use a sensitive assay to monitor the response to ADT to confirm suspicions to the presence of AIPC.

Take-home Lesson 2

The response to therapy using ADT is a clue to the nature of the tumor cell population. ADT and its response is an *in vivo* test of the tumor cell population. Understand the nature of the PC by its response to a treatment approach. If a UDPSA is not reached in a relatively short period of time, be more concerned about the presence of AIPC.

Androgen Receptor Mutation (ARM) and Anti-androgen Withdrawal (AAW)

We now know that an ARM can result in the anti-androgen paradoxically stimulating tumor growth. Antiandrogen withdrawal in such patients has been shown to result in tumor regression in approximately 20% of patients. This phenomenon is referred to as an anti-androgen withdrawal response (AAWR).

If androgen blockade included an anti-androgen— e.g. Eulexin, Casodex, or Nilandron— these agents must be stopped in order to monitor for a possible AAWR. Failure to recognize an AAWR is one of the problems encountered when we attempt to interpret results of studies of PC treatments published in the past. If a patient stopped anti-androgen therapy at the same time a different therapy was started, an AAWR, if it occurred, could affect the *assessment* of response to the second therapy. PC treatment studies should require withdrawal of anti-androgens for at least 2 to 6 weeks (the longer time in patients being withdrawn from Casodex) to assess whether or not the PSA decline is due to an AAWR.

Another reason for supporting measurement of adrenal androgen precursor levels was reported in a 1994 abstract. In that study, Herrada et al. (*Proc. Am. Soc. Clin. Oncol.*, 1994) measured serum levels of dehydroepiandrosterone (DHEA) in 10 patients with PSA progression on ADT. After anti-androgen therapy was stopped, patients were observed for an AAWR. None of the patients with DHEA levels > 75 ng/ml had an AAWR, while 3 of 5 patients (60%) with DHEA levels < 75 ng/ml achieved an AAWR. Therefore, DHEA levels at the time of PSA progression may be used to identify patients who may or may not benefit from anti-androgen withdrawal.

We have used the DHEA-S, a more stable blood level, to assess the presence of an AAWR. If the androgen receptor is regarding the anti-androgen as a growth stimulator (agonist), then the brain (hypothalamus) will sense adequate androgen levels and down-regulate the stimulatory hormones that are involved with T production. Such hormones would include LH and ACTH. LH stimulates the Leydig cells in the testicles to make T. This mechanism is already blocked by the LHRH-A. ACTH stimulates the adrenal cortex to make adrenal androgen precursors such as DHEA-S and androstenedione. Both of these are converted within prostate cells, be they benign or malignant, to T and then to DHT. If an ARM is operative, ACTH will be turned down and so will the levels of DHEA-S and androstenedione. Therefore, when we find suppressed levels of these two adrenal androgen precursors, we are suspicious of an ARM and proceed with anti-androgen withdrawal.

P

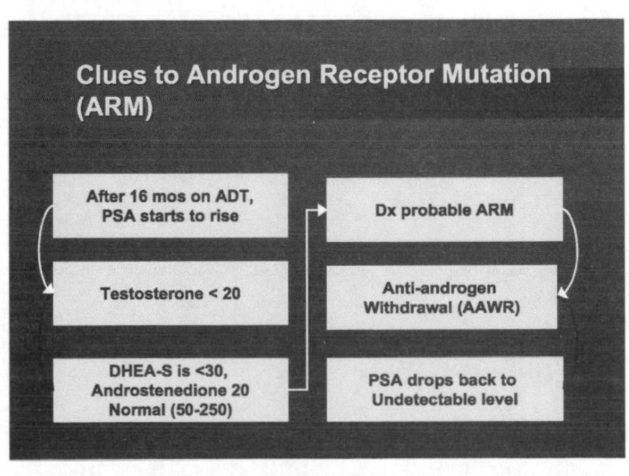
Clues to Androgen Receptor Mutation (ARM)
After 16 mos on ADT, PSA starts to rise
Testosterone < 20
DHEA-S is <30, Androstenedione 20 Normal (50-250)
Dx probable ARM
Anti-androgen Withdrawal (AAWR)
PSA drops back to Undetectable level

A PSA decline with flutamide withdrawal was first reported in 1993 by Scher and Kelly (*J. Clin. Oncol.*, 1993). Defining an AAWR by a greater than 50% decline from baseline PSA, the authors reported an AAWR in 10 of 36 (28%) patients after 3 months of Eulexin withdrawal. Twenty-five of these patients received ADT as initial treatment, of whom 10 (40%) had an AAWR. In this study, none of the 11 patients who received Eulexin after PSA relapse on "monotherapy" (orchiectomy or LHRH-A treatment alone) showed an AAWR.

Figg et al. (*Am. J. Med.*, 1995) and Small et al. (*Cancer*, 1995) subsequently published two other studies of Eulexin withdrawal responses, the latter of which evaluated a large cohort of advanced disease patients. In contrast to Scher et al., Small et al. showed similar rates of response regardless of when Eulexin was begun. Eight (14%) of 57 patients who received concomitant Eulexin with ADT had an AAWR, while 4 (16%) of 25 patients who received Eulexin after PSA progression on monotherapy had an AAWR. Patients who responded were treated with Eulexin for a longer time than nonresponding patients (median duration 21 months versus 12 months, respectively, $p = 0.2$).

Withdrawal of Casodex has also been reported to result in an AAWR (Small and Carroll, *Urology*, 1994; Small et al., *Proc. Am. Soc. Clin. Oncol.*, 1996). The time until PSA begins to decline after anti-androgen withdrawal is shorter with Eulexin than with Casodex, reflecting the longer half-life of elimination from the body with Casodex (7 days) versus Eulexin (5.2 hours) (Small et al., *Proc. Am. Soc. Clin. Oncol.*, 1996).

Withdrawal responses do not appear to be limited to nonsteroidal anti-androgens. A withdrawal response was reported in a patient receiving the progestin, megestrol acetate (Megace), which also binds to androgen receptors (Dawson and McLeod, *J. Urol.*, 1995) and in patients withdrawn from Diethylstilbestrol (Bissach and Kaczmaiek, *J. Urol.*, 1995).

High-dose Casodex after Eulexin Withdrawal

As described earlier, Veldscholte et al. (*Biochem. Biophys. Res. Commun.*, 1990) described an androgen receptor gene mutation in a LNCaP human PC cell line that could be activated by estrogen, progesterone, and Eulexin. This same point mutation and growth stimulating effect by Eulexin was noted by other investigators (Culig et al., *Mol. Endocrinol.*, 1993; Taplin, et al., *N. Engl. J. Med.*, 1995; Fenton et al., *Clin. Cancer Res.*, 1997). However, some mutant androgen receptors were found to be paradoxically antagonized by the structurally different anti-androgen, Casodex. Similarly, LNCaP cell growth was inhibited by Casodex (Olea et al., *Endocrinology*, 1990). Based upon these observations, Joyce et al. (*J. Urol.*, 1998) conducted a pilot study of high-dose Casodex (150 mg/day) in 30 patients who failed ADT that included Eulexin. Fourteen (48%) received Eulexin as part of the primary ADT, whereas the other 16 received Eulexin after PSA progression on monotherapy. Although 70% of patients had received at least one nonhormonal therapy prior to study entry, all patients had a rising PSA after Eulexin withdrawal and were progressing on their last treatment. Using a response criteria defined as a $\geq 50\%$ decline from baseline PSA maintained at least 2 months, 7 (23%) patients responded to high-dose Casodex. Six (43%) of the 14 patients receiving Eulexin as part of primary ADT were responders, whereas only 1 (6%) of 16 patients receiving Eulexin at PSA progression on monotherapy were responders ($p = 0.03$). There was no correlation between patients having a response to high-dose Casodex and those having had a prior anti-androgen response. Therefore, in this study, it appears that patients progressing on ADT that includes Eulexin as part of combination hormone blockade are candidates to receive high-dose Casodex at 150 mg a day, regardless of whether or not they had an AAWR upon discontinuing Eulexin. Treatment was generally well tolerated. The primary side effects reported included exacerbation of hot flushes (40%), nausea (10%), fatigue (10%) and gynecomastia (5%). There were no liver function abnormalities seen. The authors concluded that Casodex at this dose is modestly effective for patients with AIPC, particularly for those treated with long-term Eulexin.

In the setting of PSA progression, the above evaluations should be undertaken to properly diagnose the patient's situation. If such an analysis is not done, the patient may be inappropriately labeled as having "hormone refractory disease" when in fact he may have an ARM, or perhaps excessive production of adrenal androgen precursors, or perhaps insufficient suppression of LH. Once this analysis is complete and the above causes of PSA progression have been excluded, the physician and patient can focus on therapies used in the treatment of AIPC.

I have divided these therapies into two major categories that reflect ease of treatment administration. This is a separation based on quality of life issues and not on the magnitude of response to treatment. As we improve in our treatments of AIPC, this separation may disappear. The treatment strategy is shown below.

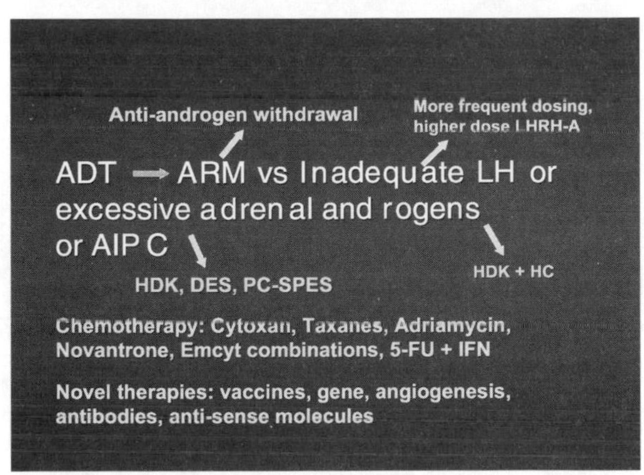

After Trachtenberg, et al. (*J. Urol.*, 1983)

Table 2

Hormone Blockade Regimen	Patient Number	High-Dose Casodex Response
Primary ADT including Eulexin	14	6/14 (43%)
Primary monotherapy without Eulexin. Eulexin added on PC progression	16	1/16 (6%)

After Joyce et al. (*J. Urol.*, 1998).

Nizoral blocks the production of testosterone produced by the testicles and blocks the production of androgen precursors (DHEA, DHEA-S, and androstenedione) that are metabolized to T and DHT within the prostate cell. Since Nizoral also may reduce cortisol production by approximately 25%, a small percentage of patients may develop symptoms consistent with adrenal mineralocorticoid deficiency. Patients therefore are usually given HC (hydrocortisone) along with Nizoral to prevent this potential side effect and also because of the known antitumor effect of HC against AIPC. The standard dose of HC advised is 20 mg with breakfast and 20 mg with dinner. Patients may have their dose of HC titrated down using the results of ACTH and cortisol levels.

The Treatment of AIPC

Nizoral or High-dose Ketoconazole (HDK) with Hydrocortisone (HC)

Nizoral plus hydrocortisone (HC) is an excellent treatment approach for men with AIPC. In fact, Nizoral has so many outstanding effects against both ADPC and AIPC that it is surprising not to see this agent as a mainstay in the initial treatment of PC. Nizoral rapidly lowers serum testosterone to castrate levels by 48 hours by mechanisms that are different than LHRH agonists and antiandrogens (see figure below after Trachtenberg et al.).

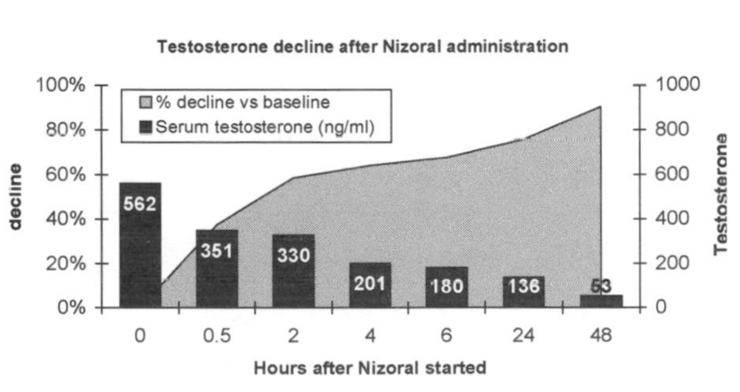

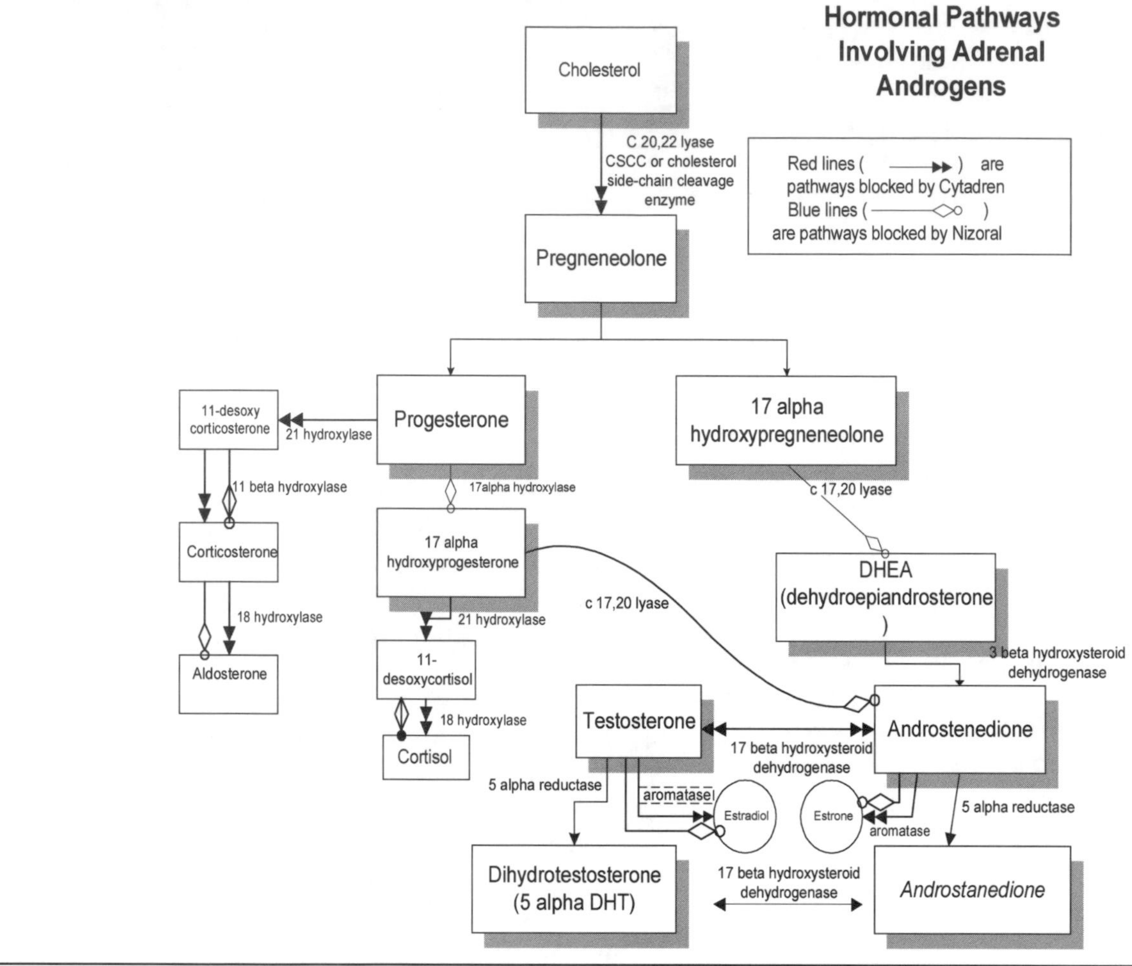

Other Anticancer Effects of Nizoral

Nizoral possesses other anti-cancer properties independent of its testosterone-lowering effects. In laboratory studies, Nizoral showed synergistic (more than additive) cell-killing effects when used with the chemotherapy drugs vinblastine (Velban) and etoposide (VePesid) in cancer cell cultures (Eichenberger et al., *Clin. Invest. Med.*, 1989).

Nizoral acts on cytochrome P-450-dependent 14-demethylation, and decreases conversion of lanosterol to cholesterol, and blocks 17,20-desmolase (or lyase), resulting in a decrease in serum T, androstenedione, and dehydroepiandrosterone (DHEA). Twenty-four-hour urinary free cortisol is reduced 25% but still remains within the range of normal, as mentioned above. Recent studies indicate that Nizoral also blocks 17a-hydroxylase.

Velban is an active agent in AIPC and is used with Nizoral, doxorubicin (Adriamycin), and estramustine (Emcyt) in the "Logothetis protocol." Nizoral also has a direct cytotoxic effect on the PC cell (see figure below). In two human cell lines of AIPC, PC-3, and DU-145, Nizoral had direct cell-killing effects at serum values that were attainable with oral doses used clinically, as shown on the following page (1.1 to 10.0 mcg/ml) (Eichenberger et al., *J. Urol.,* 1989).

Nizoral has additional anticancer effects. It has been proven to block the multidrug resistance (MDR) gene that is largely responsible for cancer cells developing resistance to many types of chemotherapy drugs. In a 1994 paper by Siegsmund et al., Nizoral added to *in vitro* cancer cell cultures was effective in overcoming MDR to Velban and Adriamycin (Siegsmund et al., *J. Urol.,* 1987).

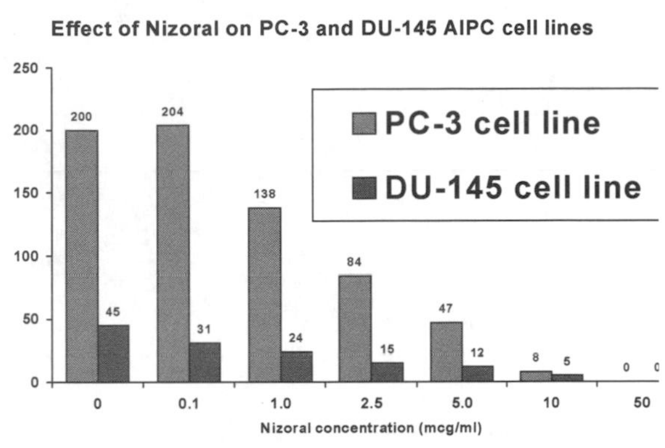

Nizoral and HC in AIPC

Published clinical trials of Nizoral involved studies in the pre-PSA era. In the current era, PSA is used as a surrogate biomarker of disease response. In the pre-PSA era, Pont et al. (*J. Urol.,* 1987) reported an 88% decrease or disappearance in pain in 17 previously untreated men with metastatic PC. Two of these patients remained in complete remission with no evidence of disease after 30 months of treatment.

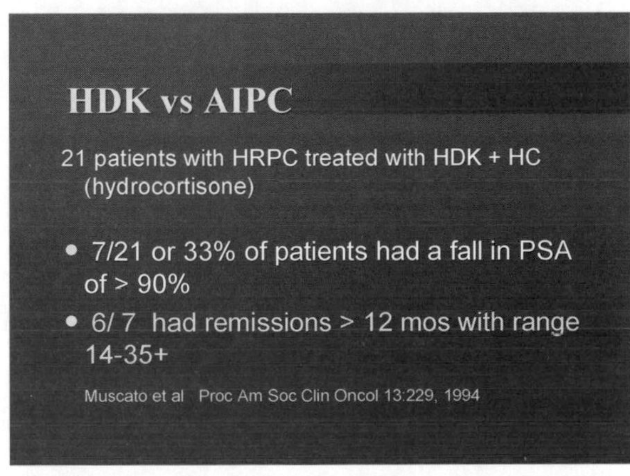

HDK vs AIPC
21 patients with HRPC treated with HDK + HC (hydrocortisone)
• 7/21 or 33% of patients had a fall in PSA of > 90%
• 6/ 7 had remissions > 12 mos with range 14-35+
Muscato et al Proc Am Soc Clin Oncol 13:229, 1994

Muscato et al. (*Proc. Am. Soc. Clin. Oncol.,* 1994) reported results with Nizoral + HC in 21 patients considered hormone-refractory. Seven (33%) of 21 patients had a greater than 90% fall in PSA, with six of these seven maintaining remissions lasting longer than 12 months (range 14 to 35+ months). Muscato et al. emphasized the importance of an acid environment for proper absorption, the avoidance of taking Nizoral with food, as well as the importance of making sure patients are not taking H2-blockers, Carafate, and/or antacids. Muscato et al. pointed out that H2-blockers (Zantac, Tagamet, Axid, Pepcid) or proton pump inhibitors (such as Prilosec or Prevacid) can decrease the absorption of Nizoral by as much as 75%. Therefore, Nizoral plus HC may be one of the most active regimens for AIPC.

In a recent paper, Small et al. (*J. Urol.,* 1997) reported the results of Nizoral plus HC therapy in men with progressive disease on ADT and after anti-androgen withdrawal. Of 48 evaluable patients, 30 (63%) had a PSA decrease of greater than 50% for at least 8 weeks, while 23 of these (48%) had a decrease in PSA of greater than 80% for at least 8 weeks. For all patients, the median PSA decrease was 79% (range 0 to 99%). The median duration of response was 3.5 months, with 23 of the 48patients having ongoing responses (range 3.3+ months to 12.8+ months). No difference was seen in response rates despite the presence or absence of an AAWR. The median survival of all patients had not been reached at 6+ months.

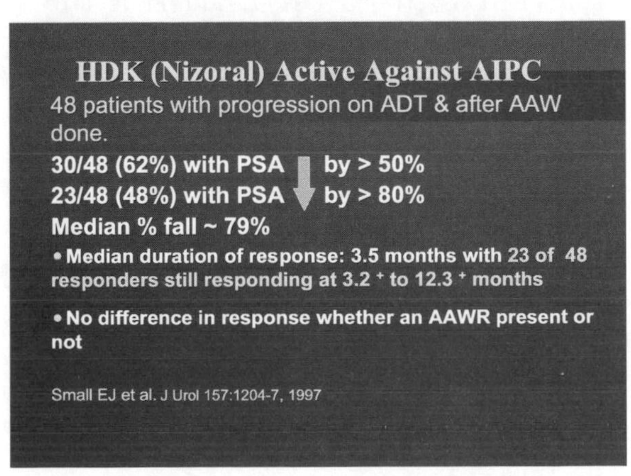

HDK (Nizoral) Active Against AIPC
48 patients with progression on ADT & after AAW done.
30/48 (62%) with PSA by > 50%
23/48 (48%) with PSA by > 80%
Median % fall ~ 79%
• Median duration of response: 3.5 months with 23 of 48 responders still responding at 3.2 + to 12.3 + months
• No difference in response whether an AAWR present or not
Small EJ et al. J Urol 157:1204-7, 1997

In another report, Small et al. (*Cancer,* 1997) treated 20 consecutive patients with simultaneous antiandrogen withdrawal and Nizoral + HC. The median PSA at entry was 13 ng/mL (range 1.9 to 1000 ng/mL). Eleven of 20 patients (55%) met their criteria for response, i.e., a greater than 50% decline from baseline PSA. The median duration of response was 8.5 months (95% confidence interval 7 to 17 months), and the median overall survival was 19 months. Due to its effects on the MDR gene, Nizoral has been studied in combination with chemotherapy.

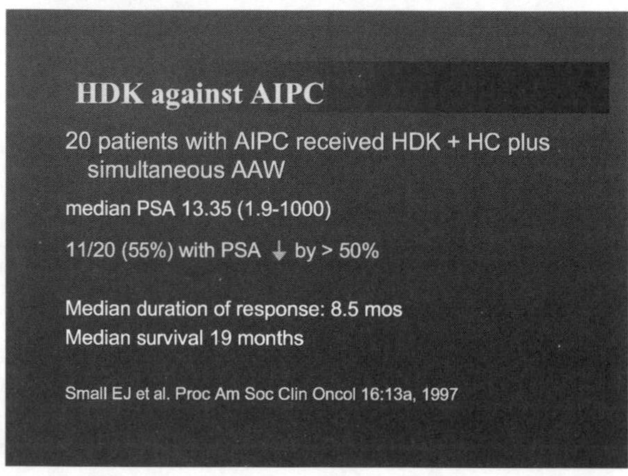

HDK in Regimens Combined with Chemotherapy

It is not clear whether HDK should be used in combination with HC versus a chemotherapy combination—in light of its synergism with Adriamycin and Velban—along with its ability to prevent MDR (multidrug resistance). There are two regimens that use HDK in combination with chemotherapy. The first regimen was a combination of Adriamycin and Ketoconazole (Sella et al., *J. Clin. Oncol.*, 1994).

The Sella regimen with its effectiveness was employed in a multidrug regimen that we have termed the Logothetis regimen (Ellerhorst et al., *Clin. Cancer Res.,* 1997). Dr. Christopher Logothetis has combined two most active chemotherapy regimens into one protocol of alternating regimens. Our modifications of this regimen are *italicized.*

HDK + Adriamycin vs AIPC

- HDK + Adria at 20 mg/m^2/24 hrs q wk studied in 38 consecutive men
- PSA levels decreased > 50% from baseline in 21/38 or 55%
- Median Survival in above pts 17.3$^+$ mos with MS of 20$^+$ mos if PSA decrease > 80%

Sella A, et al. JCO 12:683-688,1994

▼ ***Chemotherapy*** Cycle length = 56 days (8 weeks)

Adriamycin 20 mg/m^2 IV day 1, 15, 29
Ketoconazole 400 mg orally 3 times a day for days 1–7, 15–21, 29–35
Vinblastine 4 mg/m^2 IV day 8, 22, 36
Estramustine 140 mg orally 3 times a day for days 8–14, 22–28, 36–42
Rest period from day 43 to 56, then restart next cycle

▼ Supportive Medications

Hydrocortisone, 20 mg orally in A.M. and 10 mg in P.M. (take with food)

Coumadin dosed to maintain an INR between 1.75 and 2.25

Neupogen 300 mcg s.q. twice a week except during the rest period

Epogen, 10,000 units s.q. 3 times a week as needed to avert anemia

Kytril, 0.7 mg with each dose of Velban or Adriamycin

Decadron, 10 mg with each dose of Adriamycin

▼ Laboratory Tests

CBC blood test on the day of each injection and day #10 of the first cycle

Chemistry panel once a month and day #14 of the first cycle

PSA and PAP once a month

Prothrombin time weekly

▼ Information that We Also Discuss with the Patient

Nonspecific lassitude and tiredness may occur.

Hair loss to some degree is common.

Temporary mouth sores and/or diarrhea is unusual but can occur.

Adriamycin and Velban can cause low blood counts, which can increase the risk for serious infection. It is critical that weekly CBC tests are obtained to guide chemotherapy and Neupogen dosing.

Any fever greater than 100.5 should be called to your M.D. immediately, day or night.

Velban can cause numbness and tingling in the hands and feet.

Velban has caused temporary malfunction of the intestines, resulting in bloating (ileus). We recommend a small dose of milk of magnesia on the day of Velban therapy.

Ketoconazole and Estramustine can cause nausea and upset stomach, but with use of antinausea drugs this should *not* occur.

Estrogen in Estramustine can cause blood clots, thus the need for Coumadin.

Adriamycin, if it is used for more than 1 year, can occasionally cause weakening of the heart muscle.

Adriamycin and Velban, if they are improperly injected into the skin (outside of the vein), can cause severe skin reactions and ulcers.

Ketoconazole can cause hepatitis, thus the need to do monthly chemistry.

Hydrocortisone can cause adrenal atrophy, so when the protocol is stopped, the hydrocortisone must be tapered off over a 4 to 8 week period.

The results with the Logothetis regimen for AIPC indicate a median survival of 19 months. In responding patients, the median survival has not yet been reached.

Patient Guidelines for Nizoral and HC

We start Nizoral at a dose of 200 mg every 8 hours for 1 week, then increase the dose to 400 mg (2 tablets) every 8 hours thereafter. HC should be given at a dose of 20 mg with breakfast and 20 mg with dinner. If symptoms suggest HC excess (ankle swelling or diabetes in poor control), we decrease the dose to 20 mg with breakfast and 10 mg with dinner.

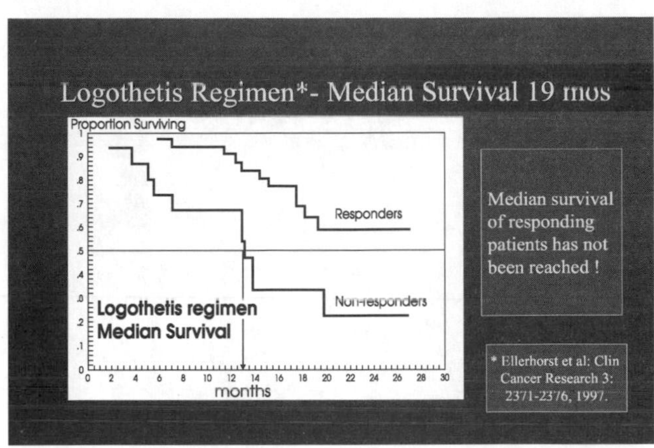

Stomach acid is needed to enhance Nizoral absorption. We advise patients to take Nizoral on an empty stomach since food reduces acid. As stated above, histamine-2 blockers (Zantac, Tagamet, Pepcid, and Axid) decrease Nizoral absorption by 75%. Prescription proton-pump inhibitors such as omeprazole (Prilosec) and lansoprazole (Prevacid) reduce stomach acid even more. Antacids and the prescription anti-ulcer agent sucralfate (Carafate) will also interfere with Nizoral absorption.

We recommend taking Nizoral with Coca-Cola, Pepsi, 1000 mg of chewable vitamin C, lemonade, or orange juice. In a recent study done in AIDS patients receiving acid-reducing drugs, the oral absorption (bioavailability) of Nizoral was increased by 50% by the concurrent intake of Coca-Cola or Pepsi (Chin et al., *Antimicrob. Agents Chemother.,* 1995).

It is now possible to measure Nizoral levels in the serum using a new assay method. We recommend monitoring serum drug levels at the onset and periodically on Nizoral therapy. A blood level between 3 and 5 mcg/mL is considered therapeutic when drawn 4 hours after the usual dose of Nizoral. Serum Nizoral values can also be obtained 1 hour post Nizoral ingestion (peak level) and just before the next dose of Nizoral (trough level).

HDK Administration Guidelines

- Acid pH in the stomach needed for absorption
  - Take HDK with Coke/ Pepsi (Diet OK), or chewable Vit C (1000 mg) or other acid beverage like orange juice; Do NOT take with food since food buffers the acid
- H-2 blockers decrease absorption by 75%
  - Avoid Zantac, Tagamet, Pepcid, Axid, Prilosec, Prevacid, Antacids, Carafate & food
- Monitor Ketoconazole blood levels
  - 4 hour post HDK blood levels are commercially available

Other drugs that have the potential to interfere with Nizoral absorption by decreasing stomach acid through anticholinergic mechanisms are listed below. Drugs commonly used in PC patients appear in **boldface** type.

Artane (trihexyphenidyl)	**Leversusin, Levbid, Leversusinex** (hyoscyamine)
Atrovent (ipratropium)	Transderm-V (scopolamine)
Beelith (magnesium + B1)	Librax (clindinium)
Bellergal (has belladonna)	Lomotil (atropine)
Bentyl (dicyclomine)	Pro-banthine (propantheline)
Cogentin (benztropine)	Robinul (glycopyrrolate)
Cystospaz (hyoscyamine)	**Urised** (hyoscyamine)
Ditropan (oxybutynin)	**Urispas** (hyoscyamine)
Donnatal (belladonna)	

The main side effects of Nizoral are nausea and loss of appetite in approximately 10% of patients. Concurrent administration of HC may reduce the frequency of this side effect. A number of skin changes—including rash; dry, cracked lips; and an unusual "sticky skin" syndrome—have also been reported in approximately 5% of patients. This can usually respond to topical application of vitamin E.

Side-effects of Nizoral + HC

Nausea 10%
Fatigue 6%
Leg swelling 6%
Skin rash or changes 4%
Abnormal liver function 4%

Small E, et al[103]

The peeling of the lips is very responsive to the use of Carmex topical ointment. Photophobia (sensitivity to light) is rarely seen in patients taking Nizoral for fungal infections, but may be more common with chronic use. Liver function tests (LFTs) include elevations in SGOT, SGPT, and/or alkaline phosphatase. These are generally mild and usually return to normal without intervention. Patients on Nizoral must have LFTs checked monthly. Although rare, a rise in serum bilirubin indicates that Nizoral must be discontinued. Intolerance of nausea, fatigue, or abnormal liver function tests is the most common reason patients stop Nizoral treatment.

Potential Drug Interactions with Nizoral

Interacting Drugs	Possible Drug Interaction
Claritin (loratadine) Hismanal (astemizole) Propulsid (cisapride)	Nizoral significantly increases blood levels of these drugs that can potentially cause a **severely irregular heartbeat.**
Glucotrol (glipizide) DiaBeta, Glynase, Micronase (glyburide) Glucophage (metformin) Diabinese (chlorpropamide)	Nizoral may increase the blood sugar-lowering effects of these drugs, which may result in **severe hypoglycemia (low blood sugar).**

Drugs That May Need Dose Changes If Nizoral Is Taken Concurrently

Drug with Dosage Affected	Precaution/Dosage Adjustment
Coumadin (warfarin)	Monitor prothrombin time — reduce dose if needed to prevent possible bleeding.
Dilantin (phenytoin)	Monitor blood levels and toxicity of both drugs— reduce doses if levels become elevated.
INH, Rifamate (isoniazid)	Both drugs may need to be stopped if liver function tests become abnormal.
Rimactane, Rifamate (rifampin)	Monitor Nizoral blood levels — if levels are below therapeutic range, increase dose.
Halcion (triazolam) Versed (midazolam)	Blood levels of both drugs may become increased and lead to excess sedative effects.
Medrol (methylprednisolone)	Blood levels are increased, but no adjustment in dosage is needed unless toxicity occurs.
Sandimmune (cyclosporin)	Monitor blood levels of both drugs and adjust doses if needed.

Warning: Nizoral should not be taken with alcohol. Concurrent use of Nizoral and alcohol-containing beverages may cause an "antabuse reaction" (skin flushing, rash, swollen legs, nausea, vomiting, and headache).

Corticosteroid Therapy in AIPC

Corticosteroids are a family of semisynthetic and synthetic compounds that mimic the anti-inflammatory effects of cortisol. Corticosteroids are produced naturally by the adrenal glands. The most commonly prescribed agents include cortisone acetate (Cortef), hydrocortisone (Hydrocortone), prednisone (Deltasone), and dexamethasone (Decadron or Hexadrol). It has been recognized for many years that corticosteroids have a definite palliative (symptom improving) and sometimes objectively beneficial effect on the clinical course of patients with AIPC.

Tannock et al. (*J. Clin. Oncol.,* 1989) studied the clinical benefit of Deltasone given at a dose of 7.5 to 10 mg a day in 13 patients with AIPC. Results of this study showed objective responses in 5 (38%) patients lasting a median of 3 months. The authors attempted to correlate patient response with suppression of the adrenal androgens DHEA-S and androstenedione. Twelve (92%) of 13 patients had significant suppression of either one or both hormones, with levels of < 1 mM/L and < 1 nM/L for DHEA-S and androstenedione, respectively. The authors concluded that low-dose Deltasone provided excellent suppression of adrenal androgen levels, which results in good palliative benefits for patients with AIPC. In a subsequent randomized trial by the same principal investigator, the response rate to Deltasone alone was lower, but still significant at 13.5%. The median duration of response to single, agent Deltasone in this trial was 4.5 months (Tannock et al., *J. Clin. Oncol.,* 1996).

Harvey et al. (*Proc. Am. Soc. Clin. Oncol.,* 1994) studied Decadron at a weekly dose of 10 mg intravenously in six patients with advanced-stage PC who had failed at least two prior hormone maneuvers and who also had received chemotherapy. Using a response criteria of a ≥ 50% decline of PSA from baseline, 5 of 6 (83%) of patients responded. They also demonstrated a decrease in pain and an improved performance status. The median duration of survival was 9 months (range of 4 to 20+ months) with 5 patients still responding at the time of the report.

Storlie et al. (*Proc. Am. Soc. Clin. Oncol.,* 1994) evaluated the effectiveness of oral Decadron in 38 patients with progressive disease after orchiectomy. The Decadron dose was 0.75 mg twice a day. Responses were seen in 23 of 38 (61%) of patients evidenced by a greater than 50% PSA decline. Thirteen of 38 (34%) of patients had a greater than 80% decline in PSA. In two of 23 responding patients, the possibility of an AAWR could not be excluded. However, 21 (55%) of 38 patients still had a greater than 50% decline in PSA if these two

P

patients are excluded from analysis. The authors unfortunately did not mention the duration of response in this abstract.

Kelly et al. (*Cancer,* 1973) conducted a prospective study in which patients with AIPC were initially treated with Hydrocortisone alone, and then were progressively given suramin. Patients treated with suramin require Hydrocortisone to replace the loss of adrenal cortisol production caused by suramin. In that report, only 10% of patients derived an independent benefit from suramin, suggesting that the use of Hydrocortisone may have accounted for the high rates of antitumor response previously reported in suramin trials for AIPC.

In our opinion, all of these studies should have measured DHEA-S and androstenedione levels at baseline and during steroid treatment. If the observations of Tannock et al. were correct in their initial study, the suppression of these hormone levels values may possibly identify which patients may respond best to corticosteroid therapy.

Estrogen Therapy for AIPC: Diethylstilbestrol (DES)

Estrogens have significant effects on the PC cell. Estradiol has been shown to localize irreversibly to the nuclear membrane of the tumor cell within 2 hours of exposure (Sinha et al., *Cancer,* 1973). Diethylstilbestrol, a nonsteroidal estrogen, has been shown to inhibit RNA polymerase activity in prostatic tissue and inhibit DNA synthesis in both benign and malignant prostate tissue (Davies and Griffiths, *J. Endocrinol.,* 1973; Lasnitzki, *J. Steroid Biochem.,* 1979). All estrogens also exert a competitive inhibitory effect on androgen-dependent cancers by suppressing LH secretion at the level of the pituitary-testicular axis.

Until the advent of LHRH agonists, estrogens and Diethylstilbestrol were extensively used in the treatment of advanced PC. In the initial Veterans Administration Cooperative Urologic Research Group (VACURG) studies, Diethylstilbestrol was found to be as effective as orchiectomy for PC, but at a dose of 5 mg/day, carried a significant risk of cardiovascular morbidity (Byer, *Cancer,* 1973).

More recently, single and cooperative group studies have evaluated the effectiveness of Diethylstilbestrol at dosages of 3 and 1 mg a day (Blackard, *Cancer Chemother. Rep.,* 1975; Pavone-Macaluso et al., *J. Urol.,* 1986; Emtage et al., *Eur. J. Cancer,* 1990).

Both dosages were found to be as effective as the 5 mg/day dosage with considerably fewer cardiovascular toxicities. Although serum T levels were not consistently suppressed to castrate levels using the 1 mg/day dose, this dosage showed an equivalent anticancer effect compared to the 5mg/day dosage (Byer and Corle, *NCI Monogr.,* 1988). It should be noted that the regression of metastatic disease can occur without maximal suppression of serum T levels (Scott et al., *Cancer,* 1990).

In a more recent study, Jazieh et al. (*Proc. Am. Assoc. Cancer Res.,* 1994) reported results using oral Diethylstilbestrol treatment in 14 patients with progressive AIPC. Diethylstilbestrol was given at a dose of 1 mg, 3 times a day along with routine anticoagulation with warfarin (Coumadin). In this study, 9 (64%) of 14 patients responded with a greater than 75% decline in baseline PSA. PSA levels normalized in 5 of 14 (36%) of patients. Two of these patients, however, may have had an anti-androgen withdrawal response. In patients with symptomatic disease, 50% showed improvement with Diethylstilbestrol treatment. The median duration of response was 8 months (range 2 to 24 months), and the median time to reach PSA nadir was 3 months (range 1 to 10 months). There were no cardiovascular or thrombotic (blood clotting) events reported.

DES in Post-Orchx Disease

- DES 3 mg per day orally + Coumadin to anticoagulate to an INR of ~ 1.8-2.0
- 9/14 patients (64%) with PSA decline of > 75% and 5 of 14 (36%) normalized the PSA
- 50% of patients with symptomatic improvement
- Median duration of response 8 months (range 2-24 mos)

Jazieh AR et al, Proc Am Assoc Ca Res 35:233, 1994

More recently, Smith et al. (*Urology,* 1998) reported results of a phase II study of Diethylstilbestrol at a dose of 1 mg/day in 21 patients failing ADT. All patients were withdrawn from antiandrogen therapy and started Diethylstilbestrol at PSA progression. LHRH agonist therapy was stopped simultaneously. Response in this study was defined as a ≥ 50% decline from baseline PSA. This was seen in 9 of 21 (43%) patients. In 13 patients who failed only one hormonal therapy, responses were seen in 8 (62%) patients. In the 13 patients who failed more than one prior hormone treatment, a response was seen in only 1 (13%) of 8 patients. Duration of response was not reported. Sixteen patients remained alive after a median follow-up of 82 weeks with a 2-year survival rate of 63%. Therapy was generally tolerated well. Nineteen (90%) patients complained of nipple tenderness, but none discontinued therapy because of this side effect. Three (14%) patients developed gynecomastia (breast enlargement), and one (5%) patient developed deep venous thrombosis.

DES

- 21 patients with "advanced PC" who had failed primary ADT
- 9/21 (43%) with PSA decline > 50%
- If only 1 prior hormone manipulation, then 8/13 or 62% PSA response
- Survival at 2 years is 63%

Smith DC, Redman BG, Flaherty LE: Urology 52:257-60, 1998.

Intravenous Estrogens (Fosfestrol or Stilbestrol Diphosphate)

Stilbestrol diphosphate (Stilphosterol) is a water-soluble formulation of nonsteroidal estrogen that can be injected intravenously. High-dose intravenous estrogens are thought to have a direct cytotoxic effect on the PC cell. In theory, Stilphosterol enters the cell, and free stilbestrol is liberated by an enzymatic action within the cancer. This enzyme, acid phosphatase, is abundant in malignant prostatic tissue and releases free stilbestrol via dephosphorylation. Within the cell, stilbestrol destroys the cell by inducing apoptosis (programmed cell suicide) (Colapino and Aberhart, *Br. J. Urol.,* 1961).

Selenomethionine is a radioactive isotope that is used as a marker for protein synthesis by the cell. At DES plasma levels of 1 mcg/ml, incorporation of this isotope into PC cells was inhibited 20%. At DES levels of 5 mcg/ml, isotope incorporation was inhibited by 69.6% (Ferro et al., *Br. J. Urol.,* 1988). DES blood levels of this magnitude can easily be achieved in the clinical setting. Using high-pressure liquid chromatography, a 1-gram intravenous injection of Stilphosterol resulted in a mean plasma DES level of 3.6 mcg/ml 30 minutes after injection (Abramson and Miller, *J. Urol.,* 1982).

Ferro et al. (*Urology,* 1989) conducted a prospective trial of high-dose intravenous Stilphosterol in 29 patients with symptomatic AIPC metastatic to bone. At baseline, all patients had elevated PSA levels, 24 (83%) had elevated PAP levels, and 28 (97%) had elevated alkaline phosphatase levels. Stilphosterol was administered as a dose of 1104 mg intravenously over 5 minutes daily for 7 days. A subjective response was seen in 22 (76%) patients as evidenced by improvement in bone pain, mobility, and/or decreased analgesic requirements. Significant decreases in serum PSA were noted in 13 (45%) patients, with PSA reductions ranging from 44 to 93%. Duration of patient response or survival were not reported. Side effects consisted of perineal discomfort, nausea, vomiting, and bone pain in some patients, with widespread bony metastases. No cardiovascular or thrombotic complications were reported.

Fosfestrol is a European formulation similar to stilbestrol diphosphate and is known by the names of Honvan, Fosfostilben, Honvol, and ST-52. In a study by Droz et al. (*Cancer,* 1993) 16 AIPC patients received fosfestrol, 4 grams a day intravenously over 3.5 hours for 5 consecutive days. For the remainder of the month, patients received an unspecified *oral* dose of fosfestrol, with intravenous therapy repeated once a month. Response, defined as a ≥ 50% decline in baseline PSA, was seen in seven (43%) patients. The median duration of survival was longer in responding patients (10 months versus 5 months, respectively). Cardiovascular complications occurred in 6% of patients.

Intravenous Estrogens in PC

- 16 patients given Fosfestrol at 4 grams per day over 3.5 hours for 5 consecutive days
- Regimen repeated every 4 weeks
- 7/16 (44%) with > 50% reduction in PSA
- Median survival responders 10 months
- Cardiovascular complications in 5% of pts

Droz et al. Cancer 71:1123-1130, 1993.

A slower rate of intravenous administration appears to reduce the risk for perineal discomfort, nausea, and vomiting. Intravenous Stilphosterol has not been reported to cause cardiovascular or thrombotic complications when the duration of treatment is limited to 7 days (Ferro, *Urol. Clin. N. Am.,* 1991). Since we use Stilphosterol over many weeks' duration, routine anticoagulation with Coumadin is advised.

Further studies with oral and intravenous estrogens are needed. The activity of both oral and high-dose intravenous therapy in AIPC patients who already have castrate testosterone levels clearly indicates their mechanism of action is different from simply effects upon the pituitary-testicular axis.

PROSTATE CANCER: ANTICANCER PROPERTIES AND ACTIVITY OF PC-SPES

Introduction

Herbal therapies have been part of traditional treatments for centuries. In the last few years they have emerged from the sidelines of alternative health care to be considered by mainstream medicine (Eisenberg et al., *JAMA*, 1998). Herbal therapies have important biological activities and are in wide use for numerous diseases. Ginkgo is used to protect neurological function, garlic to inhibit abnormal platelet aggregation, and saw palmetto is used to ease symptoms of noncancerous prostate enlargement. Among cancer patients, 5 to 60% use herbal therapies and other unconventional medicines (Risberg et al., *J. Clin Oncol.*, 1998; Eisenberg et al., *N. Engl. J. Med.*, 1993). An herbal mixture called PC-SPES (Fan and Wang, U.S. patent pending 08/697.920) has been used by men with prostate cancer to arrest the progression of the disease in cases not responsive to conventional treatment. The PC-SPES mixture (PC- for prostate cancer, SPES- the Latin word for hope) has been shown in laboratory studies to have multiple effects on lymphoma, leukemia, breast cancer, prostate cancer, and melanoma cell lines.

The Ingredients of PC-SPES

PC-SPES combines extracts of eight herbs: *Scutellaria baicalensis*, *Glycyrrhiza glabra*, *Ganoderma lucidium*, *Isatis indigotica, Panax pseudo-ginseng, Serenoa repens, Dendrantherma morifolium,* and *Rabdosia rubescens* (Borek, *Maximize Your Healthspan with Antioxidants*, 1995). All of these are Chinese herbs except *Serenoa repens*, an extract of the American dwarf palm, or saw palmetto. The combined mixture of herbs contains flavonoids that have antioxidant activity, anti-inflammatory and anticarcinogenic actions, and include isoflavones that have some estrogen-like activity (Lin and Shieh, *Am. J. Chin. Med.*, 1996). PC-SPES also contains compounds that may enhance immune cell action and components that interfere with testosterone metabolism and prevent testosterone from binding to prostate cells. Acting together in the PC-SPES mixture, individual components may team up to block prostate cancer progression, in part, by blocking androgen-supported prostate cell growth and by causing cell death.

Scutellaria contains baicalein and related compounds which are flavonoids with anti-inflammatory activity (Lin and Shieh, *Am. J. Chin. Med.*, 1996). Baicalein has been shown to have effects on the cell cycle similar to those of PC-SPES. Both cause an arrest of cell growth in the G_0/G_1 phase. Both are able to induce programmed cell death (apoptosis) in certain cancer cells in culture. Baicalein has antimutagenic (gene mutation–preventing) and anticarcinogenic biochemical effects that may indirectly be related to the activity of PC-SPES in treating prostate cancer (Huang et al., *Eur. J. Pharmacol.*, 1994; Motoo and Sawabu, *Cancer Lett.*, 1994; Okita et al., *Eur. J. Cancer Prev.*, 1993; Yano et al., *Cancer Res.*, 1994; Hamada et al., *Arch. Biochem Biophys.*, 1993; Hara et al., *Eur. J. Pharmacol.*, 1992). *Scutellaria* therefore seems to be an essential herb in the PC-SPES combination, probably due to the presence of baicalein.

Glycyrrhiza glabra (licorice) contains hundreds of phytochemicals (botanicals) with a wide range of activities. These include flavonoids with antimutagenic and anti-inflammatory effects, including isoflavones such as genistein, phytoestrogens (plant estrogens), saponins that experimentally have anticancer activity, and triterpenoids, which have been shown to increase cell toxicity of several antineoplastic compounds such as doxorubicin (Adriamycin) used in conventional cancer therapy.

Extracts of *Ganoderma lucidum*, a Chinese mushroom, contain glycans. These are polysaccharide substances with anticancer activity in animals that have shown ability to stimulate natural killer cell activity. *Ganoderma* therefore has potential activity as an immunomodulator.

Isatis, another component of PC-SPES, contains indirubin, which has antineoplastic activity and is used in China to treat leukemia. Isatis also contains polysaccharides with immune-enhancing activity, as mentioned above.

The lipido-sterol extract of *Serenoa repens* (LSESr) has been shown by Délos et al. and other investigators to have multiple sites of action. The efficacy of this herb, derived from the dwarf palm or saw palmetto, is unclear, the information being complicated by contradictory reports. Délos et al. studied the effects of three agents: LSESr, finasteride (Proscar), and 4-MA (an investigational 5AR inhibitor) on testosterone (T) metabolism of epithelial cells and fibroblasts from BPH and PC patients. Of the three agents, LSESr was the only one to decrease all T metabolites. In comparison, finasteride decreased 5a-androstanedione (5a-A) and dihydrotestosterone (DHT) in fibroblasts to a degree comparable to LSESr and 4-MA. 4-MA was the most potent inhibitor of 5a-A and DHT in BPH and PC epithelial cells and fibroblasts, followed by LSESr (Délos et al., *J. Steroid Biochem. Mol. Biol.*, 1995). What does all of this mean?

T and DHT are the two key androgens that drive the growth of PC. The adrenal androgen precursors—DHEA (and its sulfate DHEA-S) and androstenedione (A)—are converted within the prostate cell to T and to the more potent DHT (5 times as potent as T). T is reduced to DHT by 5a reductase (5AR) and oxidized to androstenedione by 17b-hydroxysteroid dehydrogenase (17-b HSD). The latter enzyme also oxidizes DHT to 5a-androstenedione (5a-A). The metabolism of testosterone is shown in the figure on the following page.

The metabolism of T involves precursors DHEA, androstenedione (D4), and 17-a hydroxyprogesterone. T can be oxidized to and reduced from androstenedione since the enzyme involved (17-b HSD) has bidirectional activity.

The amount of lowering of DHT by Serenoa in the above studies was relatively low in comparison to its effect on lowering the levels of androstenedione. Since DHT and T are the driving forces behind PC cell growth, it is unclear to us what value Serenoa has as an anticancer agent. These

P

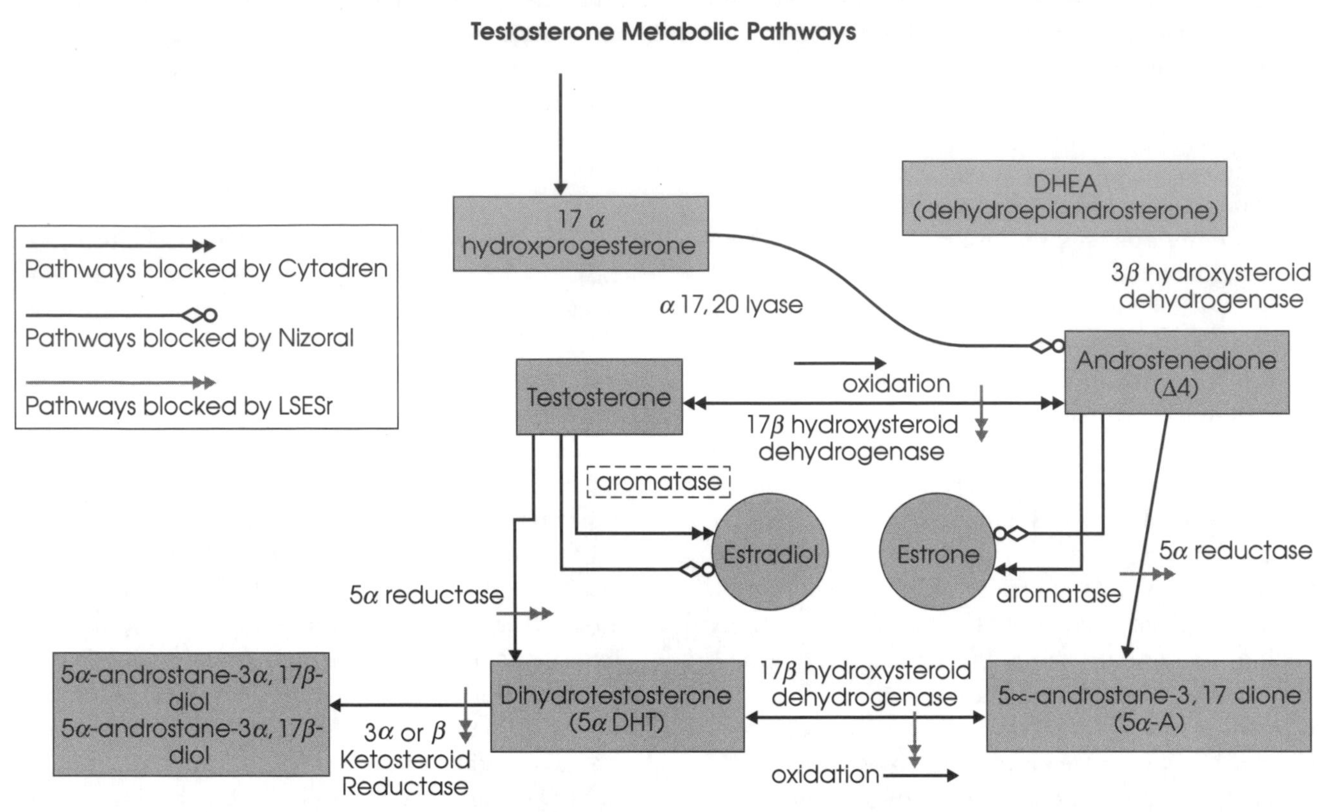

findings are confirmed by our clinical experience in that we have not seen lowering of DHT levels by Serenoa as compared to the profound lowering of DHT by finasteride (Proscar).

Ten Biological Actions of PC-SPES

Clinical studies in prostate cancer patients show that PC-SPES causes a reduction in the serum PSA level in most patients. Since this is usually associated with a lowering of T, PC-SPES should arrest prostate cancer growth and prevent further progression of androgen-dependent PC. Clinical trials are currently in progress to evaluate the efficacy of PC-SPES to reduce PSA, to determine the durability of such response, and to investigate the effect of PC-SPES on survival. Currently, men with prostate cancer who are consumers of PC-SPES but who were not enrolled in a formal clinical study have reported reductions in PSA. Some of these patients had advanced stages of prostate cancer and had progressed on conventional treatments such as surgery, radiation, and/or hormone ablation. In many such patients, there appeared to be inhibition of disease progression, improvement in quality of life, an improved sense of well being, and probably an extension of life span. We have data that show a decline in PSA in men previously treated, but we do not currently have evidence of significant durability of response or inhibition of progression of disease or improvement in survival. To corroborate all these reports and extend the data, the above-referenced studies are mandatory.

PC-SPES has at least ten biological actions involved in arresting the progression of prostate cancer according to the following reports.

1. PC-SPES Suppresses Cancer Cell Growth

Hsieh et al. (*Biochem. Mol. Biol. Int.*, 1997) from the New York Medical College studied the effects of PC-SPES on the human *androgen-dependent* prostate cancer cell line LNCaP. They demonstrated that extracts of PC-SPES suppressed the proliferation of the LNCaP cell line grown in cell culture. They showed that ethanolic extracts of

PC-SPES reduced cell growth in a time- and concentration-dependent manner. This decrease in cell proliferation was also correlated with a 50 to 65% decrease (down-regulation) in the expression of proliferating cell nuclear antigen (PCNA), a valuable biomarker used to quantitate cell proliferation.

2. & 3. PC-SPES Reduces Intracellular and Secreted PSA

After a 4- to 6-day treatment, LNCaP cell lines decreased their level of PSA secretion into the blood by 60 to 70%. They also decreased their intracellular PSA by 20 to 40%.

4. & 5. PC-SPES Decreases Quantity of the Androgen Receptor and the Intensity of Binding to the Androgen Receptor

Hsieh et al. (*Biochem. Mol. Biol. Int.*, 1997) also report that measurements of intranuclear androgen receptor (AR) indicated a down-regulation after exposure to PC-SPES associated with decreased expression of PSA. Not only was the quantity of AR down-regulated, but the binding to the AR was also decreased by about 2.5-fold. The latter measurement occurred after a 1-day treatment with PC-SPES.

The potential importance of decreasing the quantity of the AR and decreasing the intensity of binding to the AR is better understood in the context of the dependency of the prostate cell (both malignant and benign cells) on androgen. In the figure below of the endocrine axis, the sources of androgens from the testicles and from the adrenal glands are shown. Within the prostate cell (the largest rectangle in the figure), androgens and androgen precursors (DHEA-S, DHEA, and androstenedione) undergo conversion to T and DHT. T and DHT bind to the AR within the nucleus of the prostate cell. This is the site of PC-SPES effect on decreasing the quantity of AR and the affinity of T and DHT to the AR.

6. PC-SPES Decreases Clonogenicity

Growing cells go through a cell cycle during which the cell replicates its DNA and goes on to divide into two identical new cells, each containing the same DNA. In a landmark study at the Cancer Research Institute of New York Medical College, Halicka et al. (*Int. J. Oncol.*, 1997) showed that *PC-SPES treatment slowed down the cell cycle* and decreased growth of cultured cancer cells.

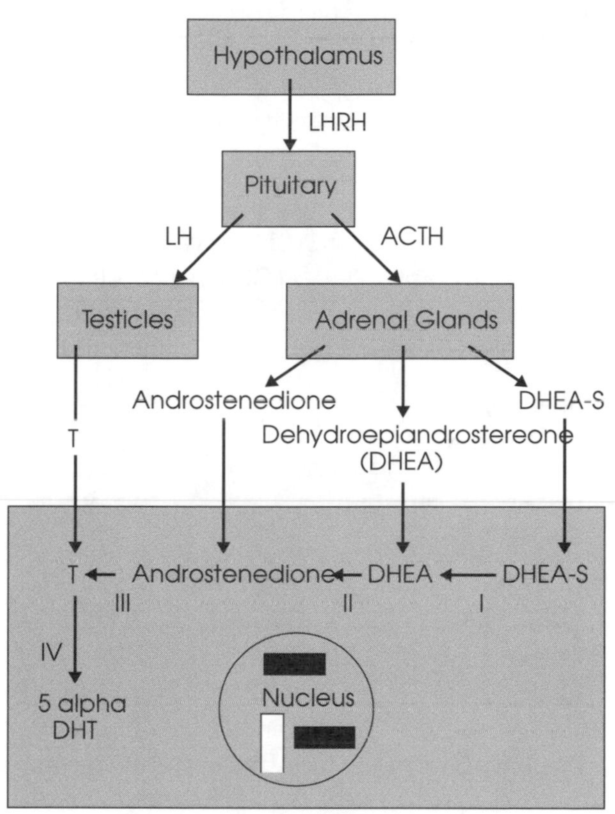

The Prostate Cell & Intra-Prostatic Synthesis of Androgens

Halicka et al. conducted *in vitro* studies of LNCaP and PC-3 cell lines vs. PC-SPES to explore clonogenicity. Clonogenicity refers to the suppressive effect of PC-SPES on the ability of the malignant cells to develop colonies. PC-SPES decreased clonogenicity the greatest in MCF-7 breast cancer cells followed by PC-3, SK-N-MC neuroepithelioma cells, LNCaP, and T47-D breast cancer cells. Colo 38 melanoma cells had the least decrease in clonogenicity to PC-SPES.

PC-SPES ethanolic extract concentrations needed to reduce tumor cell colony formation by 50% (IC_{50}) were determined and are shown in Table 1. PC-3 was the most sensitive prostate cell line at a PC-SPES concentration of 54 nL/mL.

PC-SPES decreases the quantity of androgen receptors within the nucleus and the affinity of binding of androgens to these receptor sites.

Table 1: Effect of PC-SPES on Tumor Cell Colony Formation (Clonogenicity)

Cell Line	Cell Type	PC-SPES IC_{50} in nL/mL
MCF-7	Breast	20
PC-3	Prostate	54
SK-N-MC	Neuroepithelioma	70
LNCaP	Prostate	120
T47-D	Breast	220
Colo 38	Melanoma	430

Legend: The lower the IC_{50}, the more sensitive the cell.

7. PC-SPES Slows the Cell Cycle and Prevents Tumor Cells from Going into S Phase

PC-SPES at a concentration of 2.0 ml/mL caused an arrest of cell growth at 48 hours as seen by an accumulation of cells in the G1 phase of the cell cycle. This increased accumulation of cells in G1 is associated with a concomitant decrease in the proportion of cells in S phase (DNA replication phase). This was most impressive for the MCF-7 breast cancer cell line (Halicka et al., *Int. J. Oncol.*, 1997).

8. & 9. PC-SPES Causes Programmed Cell Death (Apoptosis) and Down-regulates BCL-2

The herbal mixture within PC-SPES induces programmed cell death, or apoptosis. In essence, this is a cell suicide program that is regulated by specific genes. The cell tries to resist apoptosis by jump-starting a gene called bcl-2, which in turn produces an apoptosis-resistance protein. Apoptosis (pronounced "ay pop toe sis") can proceed if the bcl-2 protein is suppressed. PC-SPES treatment produced apoptosis in cancer cells, including the prostate cell line PC-3. PC-SPES decreased the bcl-2 protein by 36 to 43% in certain lymphoma and leukemia cells (Halicka et al., *Int. J. Oncol.*, 1997).

10. PC-SPES Is a Radiation Sensitizer

Radiation affects cells by damaging DNA, disrupting the cell growth cycle, and causing cell death. The effects of radiation depend on the doses used in treatment. PC-SPES can sensitize U937 lymphoma cells grown in culture to the effects of radiation. When cells were treated with PC-SPES alone, 22% of cells died by apoptosis. However, when treated with PC-SPES and then with radiation, apoptosis increased to 32% after a dose of 1.5 Gy of radiation and to 46% after 5.0 Gy (Halicka et al., *Int. J. Oncol.*, 1997). If similar effects are shown in animals and in human clinical trials, PC-SPES may be useful in combination therapy with radiation. Because of the potential synergistic effect of PC-SPES with radiation, patients should relate this information to their physician(s) if they are advised to have radiation therapy. Patients having had radiation therapy at the same time as being on PC-SPES should provide their medical records for review to the Prostate Cancer Research Institute.

Institute Clinical Studies: PC-SPES Reduces Serum PSA and Testosterone

A cooperative clinical study by DiPaola et al. was published as the lead article in the *New England Journal of Medicine,* 1998. This study involved eight prostate cancer patients, three of whom had no prior local treatment. Patients were required to take PC-SPES for at least 1 month and to have received a minimum of 4 capsules a day (320 mg a capsule) of PC-SPES for at least 2 weeks. No other treatment was allowed during the study period. Serum concentration of PSA and testosterone were measured during the study and 2 to 6 weeks after the patients stopped taking PC-SPES.

TABLE 2: Effects of Gamma Radiation +/– PC-SPES on U937 Lymphoma

Treatment	Apoptotic Cells (%)	G_1 Cells	S Phase cells	G2M Cells
Control	6	65	29	6
PC-SPES only	22	80	16	4
1500 cGy only	5	68	22	10
PC-SPES + 1500 cGy	32	83	2	15
5000 cGy only	11	62	11	27
PC-SPES + 5000 cGy	46	61	5	34

Legend: PC-SPES alone causes significant programmed cell death (apoptosis) and cell cycle arrest in G_1. Combined with radiation, there is further increase in apoptosis and a marked decrease in the number of cells going through the DNA synthesis phase of the cell cycle (S phase). This indicates a high probability of synergy between PC-SPES and radiation and mandates clinical trials to validate these findings.

PC-SPES produced clinically significant reductions in serum levels of both testosterone (T) and PSA during the period of use, suggesting that PC-SPES treatment could inhibit progression of the disease. However, at the dose of PC-SPES used in this study, T levels did not reach castrate levels (T < 20 ng/dL) in six of the eight patients. Four patients maintained T within the normal range, while two others had drops below normal but not to castrate levels. Only two of eight patients reached near-castrate T levels. In six patients who discontinued PC-SPES, PSA and testosterone increased within 3 weeks after stopping PC-SPES.

Side effects in the eight patients during treatment with PC-SPES involved loss of libido and breast tenderness. One patient had a superficial venous blood clot. The authors treated patients for a short time, i.e., at least 1 month, and used only 4 capsules a day (for at least 2 weeks) of PC-SPES rather than the usual starting dose of 3 capsules 3 times a day. DiPaola et al. did not comment on response rate or progression-free status in light of the short treatment period.

Recently, Kameda et al. (*Proc. Am Soc. Clin. Oncol.*, 1999) reported on 24 patients with PC receiving PC-SPES at a dose of 3 capsules 3 times a day. Twelve of these patients were completely untreated for PC, while the remaining 12 had evidence of androgen-independent PC (AIPC) and had gone through prior anti-androgen withdrawal. PSA declines of > 50% occurred in both groups. The period of follow-up for both groups was > 1 month of treatment. Toxicity consisted of tender gynecomastia in 71%, low-grade diarrhea in 33%, and low-grade nausea in 12%. One episode of thrombosis (pulmonary embolus) occurred in the 24 patients (4.2%).

In our practice, we have treated 21 AIPC patients with PC-SPES. Eighteen of these had castrate testosterone (T) levels, failed anti-androgen withdrawal, and second-line hormonal therapy. Twelve of these patients were chemotherapy-naive patients, and six were patients who had failed ≥ 1 chemotherapy regimen(s). All patients received 6 to 12 capsules a day of PC-SPES. Response was defined as a ≥ 50% fall from the baseline PSA. Response duration was measured from initiation of response until PSA rose to baseline. Our results appear in the following table.

PC-SPES in the Treatment of 18 Patients with AIPC

Response Parameter	Chemotherapy Naive	Prior Chemotherapy
Base PSA (median, ng/ml)	25.4	108
Nadir PSA (median, ng/mL)	4.54	34.9
Response # (%), duration	7 (58%), 6.3 month	2 (33%), 2.8 months

Chemotherapy-naive patients responded better than previously treated patients did. Six (50%) chemotherapy-naive patients continue to respond to PC-SPES (median 12+ months, range 3+ to 22.5+ months) while all six prior chemotherapy

P

patients failed PC-SPES. Side effects included nipple tenderness, gynecomastia, low T levels, and decreased libido. Two patients had thrombosis or embolic complications. We have prevented further thrombotic events by anticoagulating all patients with Warfarin (INR 1.5-2.5). Our study results suggest PC-SPES is an active treatment for chemotherapy-naive patients with AIPC. A major proportion of the anticancer activity of PC-SPES appears unrelated to T reduction (Strum et al., submitted for publication, 1999).

Overview Statement about PC-SPES

Rapid developments in medical science have made it possible to identify active substances in herbal medicines and test them for their effectiveness and safety as remedies. There may be an advantage to using a standardized herbal mixture of identified and relatively safe substances, such as PC-SPES, as opposed to using the individual components, because of possible synergistic interactions that produce anticancer effects. Standardization of the mixture and good quality control of its individual components are essential to assure purity, accurate dosing, and to maximize the avoidance of adverse side effects.

Cancer progression occurs partly because of an imbalance in the processes of growth, differentiation, and apoptosis. In prostate cells, these events are regulated in part by androgens, the male hormones such as testosterone, and DHT. Each of PC-SPES's eight herbs, in turn, contains many substances that may have multiple actions that have been shown experimentally in cancer cells to suppress growth, cause differentiation (reducing or reversing cancerous activity), and induce apoptosis. Clinically, PC-SPES has the potential to suppress prostate cancer progression, as measured by a dramatic reduction in the prostate marker PSA with a reduction in testosterone that may be the prime, but not sole, orchestrator of this effect. However, there are at least two important points to consider.

1. The statement that PC-SPES herbal mixture is an alternative treatment that is clinically effective in reducing PSA and arresting prostate cancer needs clarification. Precise studies of patients treated with PC-SPES alone with measurements of response, response duration, and effect of PC-SPES on objective measurements of tumor size are needed.

   With this proviso, it appears valid to state that PC-SPES appears to have an effect in patients with androgen-dependent prostate cancer and in patients whose prostate cancer is androgen independent.

   PC SPES in AIPC Promising Data

   - 12 patients with AIPC- Kameda et al, 1999
     - No prior chemotherapy
     - Anti-androgen withdrawal in all patients
     - 9/12 (75%) with PSA decline of ≥50%
     - Too early for data re: response duration
   - 12 patients with AIPC- Strum et al, 1999
     - 12 chemotherapy naïve, but had prior HDK, DES
     - 7/12 (58%) with PSA decline ≥50%
     - Median duration of response 6.3 months

   If PC-SPES has a significant and durable anticancer effect, it will do what other effective agents do and reduce pain in patients with advanced disease. We have heard and seen patient reports that are quite dramatic, but clear-cut studies are needed to show the effect of PC-SPES on increasing quality of life and extending survival.

2. Recommended doses should be followed to avoid unknown possible side effects. PC-SPES contains plant estrogenic compounds that contribute to its effectiveness. These may sometimes cause side effects similar to those produced in conventional hormone therapy. Such effects include decreased libido and breast tenderness, with possibilities of blood clot formation in the lower extremities. The estrogenic compounds identified in PC-SPES are different from estrogens used in conventional therapy.

   As a result of extensive experience using PC-SPES in our practice, we routinely use the anticoagulant Coumadin to guard against the formation of abnormal blood clots (thrombosis). We feel that this is in the best interest of patient safety until we have a clearer understanding of the risk of thrombo-embolic phenomena (thrombophlebitis, pulmonary embolism) resulting from PC-SPES. The incidence of thrombosis associated with PC-SPES is of the same order (5 to 8%) reported with other agents having estrogenic activity (Emcyt, DES, Premarin, and oral contraceptives). It is also important to point out that patients with advanced cancer also have a greater tendency towards thrombotic events. Coumadin, if monitored by a physician, is a safe and effective measure to prevent thrombosis. The side effects of decreased libido, gynecomastia (breast enlargement), and thrombo-embolic phenomena must be discussed frankly with the patient with options presented to prevent these side effects. However, PC-SPES offers a potentially important alternative treatment that may arrest the progression of the disease and may improve the quality of life of the patient. We have entered the age of herbal medicine in our country, and we should do so with a pioneering, yet scientific, spirit that will optimize progress against cancer.

PC-SPES Follow-Up

(by Carmia Borek, Ph.D.)

The following is a personal communication from Aaron Katz, M.D., of the Columbia Presbyterian Medical Center in New York. In a study of more than 80 prostate cancer patients, the use of PC-SPES resulted in PSA reductions within 7 months of treatment, occasionally reaching undetectable levels. The study showed that *hormone-responsive* patients whose PSA levels were reduced by prior hormone treatment with an anti-androgen (Casodex) and an LHRH-agonist (Lupron7), maintained stable levels of PSA that did not progress when employing a follow-up treatment using PC-SPES maintenance therapy alone. The patients were monitored for 3 years, with an average follow-up of 2 years. Four out of the 80 patients (5%) had blood clots (thrombophlebitis) involving the legs. According to Dr. Katz, PC-SPES treatment is best monitored by a physician to assure correct doses and to monitor any side effects.

Research results will be published by Dr. Katz and his group in the *British Journal of Urology* (De la Taille et al., in press 1999). The results presented in the article include the clinical effects of PC-SPES in treating 33 prostate cancer patients, as well as studies on the action of PC-SPES *in vitro*, on hormone-sensitive and hormone-resistant prostate cancer cells.

The in vitro studies show that both hormone-sensitive and hormone-insensitive prostate cancer cells showed a reduction in viability following exposure to PC-SPES. The effects of PC-SPES were dose-dependent. However, at the lowest dose of PC-SPES (2 mL/mL of medium), only the hormone-sensitive cells were affected by PC-SPES. This shows that in order to cause cell death in hormone-insensitive prostate cancer cells, higher doses of PC-SPES are required, compared to those needed to produce cell death in hormone-sensitive cells (De la Taille et al., *Br. J. Urol.*, in press, 1999).

The clinical studies reported in the *British Journal of Urology* are preliminary results of an ongoing study of over 80 patients (Dr. Katz, personal communication). The reported work (De la Taille et al., *Br. J. Urol.*, in press, 1999) describes a prospective study in 33 patients with proven prostate cancer, who have either refused conventional therapy (one patient) or who had failed with different forms of conventional therapy, including surgery. Twenty-eight patients had hormone therapy, five showed resistance to hormone treatment, and 23 stopped therapy. Four of the 23 patients interrupted hormone therapy 12 months before PC-SPES treatment, and the other patients stopped hormone therapy before starting treatment with PC-SPES. Patients received 320-mg capsules of PC-SPES (Botaniclabs, Brea, CA) 3 times a day. PSA was measured at 2 and 6 months initially, and every 6 months thereafter. Patients were also followed for signs of disease progression, including bone scans, bone pain, and urinary obstruction. At the time this report was submitted for publication, 33 of the patients had received a follow-up within

2 to 24 months of PC-SPES therapy (De la Taille et al., *Br. J. Urol.*, in press, 1999).

The overall results showed that patients receiving PC-SPES treatment showed no disease progression; there was no increased bone pain and no local recurrence of the cancer. Lack of recurrence was evident by the fact that there was no urinary obstruction and no positive bone scans that indicate metastases. The average PSA at the beginning of the study was 13.36 ng/mL (ranging from 0.1 to 110). After 2 months of treatment, 27 patients showed a decrease in serum by an average of 52%. In only one patient was there an increase in PSA levels to more than 50% of the initial PSA levels. Eighteen of the patients were evaluated 6 months after starting PC-SPES treatment. Of these, 78% showed a decrease in PSA, and 22% showed an increase in PSA by more than 50%, compared to initial PSA values. One patient stopped treatment because of an increased PSA at 6 months (De la Taille et al., *Br. J. Urol.*, in press, 1999).

Statistical analysis of the overall results showed that there was no PSA increase after PC-SPES treatment at 2 and 6 months. While there was a variability in responses, two of the patients showed dramatic response to PC-SPES. One patient had undergone surgery (orchiectomy) and had a PSA level of 110 ng/mL before PC-SPES treatment. After 2 months of PC-SPES treatment, PSA was reduced to 30 ng/mL. In another patient, initial PSA of 45 ng/mL was reduced to 24.3 after 2 months of PC-SPES treatment and stabilized at 24 ng/mL after 6 months, and at 25 ng/mL after 12 months.

Side effects in these patients were nipple tenderness in two patients and leg clots requiring treatment with heparin in two patients. Treatment was well tolerated and neither hot flashes nor breast enlargement were observed (De la Taille et al., *Br. J. Urol.*, in press, 1999).

Preliminary data from an ongoing clinical study on the efficacy of PC-SPES were reported from the University of California, San Francisco Cancer Center and the Memorial Sloan Kettering Institute in New York (Kamada et al., Am. Assoc. Clin. Oncol. Conf., 1999). The early results from a phase II trial were presented at the annual meeting of the American Association for Clinical Oncology, May 1999, in Atlanta. The study involved 66 patients with advanced prostate cancer who were given 9 capsules a day of PC-SPES. Two groups (cohorts) were treated: 32 patients were hormone-sensitive and had normal testosterone levels; 34 patients had prostate cancer that was androgen-independent and resistant to antiandrogen treatment.

Of the 32 hormone-sensitive patients, 27 are being evaluated after more than 1 month of treatment. By 1 month of PC-SPES treatment, all 27 patients had a PSA decline of more than 50%. Testosterone levels dropped to anorchid levels (levels in the absence of testes) in 22 out of 27 patients. Thirty-four hormone-resistant patients are being evaluated after more than 1 month of treatment with PC-SPES. Of these, 19 (56%) showed a PSA decline of more that 50%.

To date, side effects consisted of breast enlargement in 82% of patients and some nausea or diarrhea (grade 2) in 39%. One patient with advanced androgen-independent cancer had a blood clot event (pulmonary embolus). Of patients with previously normal testosterone levels, 52% have lost sexual drive (libido), and 33% have lost potency. The authors of the study state that PC-SPES is an active agent for treating hormone-sensitive PSA and also in treating patients with androgen-independent prostate cancer. Toxicity is manageable. Other responses: time to progression of the disease, overall survival, and long-term toxic effects remain under study (Kamada et al., Am. Assoc. Clin. Oncol. Conf., 1999).

Several publications in 1999 have addressed the use of PC-SPES in prostate cancer therapy. The important role that PC-SPES may play in treating prostate cancer as an alternative therapy is discussed by Moyad (*Urol. Clin. N. Am.*, 1999), who advocates that clinicians should objectively discuss the alternative treatment with their patients.

The 1998 article "Clinical and Biological Activity of Estrogenic Herbal Combinations (PC-SPES) in Prostate Cancer" by Dipole et al., (*New Engl. J. Med.,* 1998; 339:785–89), prompted a correspondence in the form of letters to the editor commenting on data and statements presented in the article (Small, *N. Engl. J. Med.*, 1999; Hsieh et al., *Biochem. Mol. Biol. Int.*, 1997; Geliebter et al., *N. Engl. J. Med.*, 1999). (Dr. EJ Small commented that there was an implication in the Dipole article that the estrogenic properties of PC-SPES, evaluated by the authors, are the only "active" component of PC-SPES. He does not agree and states that according to analyses by Hsieh et al., PC-SPES contains several "active" substances besides the identified estrogenic components.

Dr. J. Geliebter et al. from New York Medical College comments that doses of PC-SPES given to mice in the Dipole study resulting in estrogenic effects on the uterus correspond to a 60-kg man consuming 750 capsules (0.24 kg), which amounts to 83 times the conventional dose.

In reply, Dipole et al. (*N. Engl. J. Med.*, 1999) comment that their studies in mice were designed to investigate the estrogenic effects of PC-SPES in a classic animal model, and that the studies in yeast that depend on estrogen for growth suggest a potent estrogenic activity in PC-SPES.

Dr. Geliebter et al. critically question some of the data related to the effects of PC-SPES on testosterone and PSA. Dr. Geliebter et al. take issue with the lack of information in the study on testosterone levels before PC-SPES treatment and whether the values of PSA before PC-SPES treatment were obtained at diagnosis or after androgen ablation therapy. The paper by Dipole et al. states that "all eight patients had histologically proven prostate cancer, without progression, during previous androgen ablation therapy," and Dr. Geliebter states that "one patient had a PSA of 122 ng/mL, which is a high level for a patient without progression." The information in the Dipole article on the patients leads one to believe, states Dr. Geliebter, that values of testosterone and PSA were obtained before androgen ablation therapy (*N. Engl. J. Med.*, 1999). In the study by Dipole et al., the authors state that "serum testosterone concentrations decreased during the use of PC-SPES and increased within 3 weeks after PC-SPES was discontinued." Dr. Geliebter states that since no measurements of testosterone before PC-SPES treatment were provided in the Dipole study, "there is no initial testosterone concentration from which to assess whether there was a decrease." He further states that since all patients had received androgen ablation therapy before the PC-SPES therapy, it is possible that testosterone levels were low before PC-SPES treatment (as a result of androgen ablation) and rose after stopping androgen ablation therapy independent of PC-SPES treatment.

In reply to Dr. Geliebter, Dipole et al. (*N. Engl. J. Med.*, 1999) state that the "clinical results were not confounded by the recent use of standard androgen ablation therapy in our patients, contrary to suggestion of Geliebter et al.," and that seven of the eight patients studied had never received standard androgen ablation therapy. The one patient that did have androgen ablation therapy stopped treatment 22 months before the study with PC-SPES began (*N. Engl. J. Med.*, 1999). While the statement represents the authors' stand, Table 3 in their 1998 article indicates that five out of the eight patients studied had radiation therapy, surgery, or both prior to PC-SPES treatment.

In response to Dr. Small, Dipole et al. agree that when combining results from several types of analysis, PC-SPES shows multiple peaks that vary with the methods used. They state that PC-SPES has multiple organic compounds. Although non-estrogenic compounds with biological activity are present in PC-SPES, the authors comment that the androgen ablation effect is of a magnitude similar to that produced by known therapies (treatment with leuprolide, with pharmacological doses of estrogen, or following surgical removal of the testes). These treatments also have antitumor effects. Dipole et al. consider it likely that the clinical activity observed with PC-SPES is secondary to estrogenic activity, causing androgen ablation, and that further studies are in progress to identify other clinically active compounds.

Studies on the antitumor effects of PC-SPES were recently reported using a rat model of prostate cancer. The results showed that dietary PC-SPES at levels of 0.05 and 0.025 in the diet did not produce toxicity. When animals fed PC-SPES were injected with tumor cells, PC-SPES produced a dose-dependent reduction in tumor incidence and a suppression of tumor growth and metastases, suggesting a therapeutic benefit in this animal model that does not respond to other therapies (Tiwari, *Int. J. Oncol.*, 1999).

Extracts of *Ganoderma lucidum*, a Chinese mushroom, contain glycans that are polysaccharide substances. Three of these glycans have been shown to have anticancer activity in animals (Wang et al., *Biosci. Biotechnol. Biochem.*, 1993) that have shown ability to stimulate natural killer cell activity. *Ganoderma* therefore has the potential to act as an immunomodulator (Chen et al., *Am. Clin. Med.*, 1995). Isatis, another component of PC-SPES, contains indirubin, which has antineoplastic activity and is used in China to treat leukemia (Ma and Yao, *J. Trad. Clin. Med.*, 1983; Liu et al., *Sci. Sin. B,* 1982). Isatis also contains polysaccharides with immune-enhancing activity (Muon, *The Pharmacology of Chinese Herbs*, 1993).

The lipido-sterol extract of *Serenoa repens* (LSESr) has been shown by Delos et al. and other investigators to have multiple sites of action (Delos et al., *J. Steroid Biochem. Mol. Biol.* 1995). This herb, derived from the dwarf palm or saw palmetto (Wilt et al., *JAMA*, 1998), is used in treatment of benign prostate hypertrophy outside the United States, with efficacy comparable to finasteride (Proscar) (Strauch et al. *Eur. J. Urol.*, 1994; Champault et al., *Br. J. Clin. Pharmacol.,* 1984). However, the effect of LSESr is complicated by contradictory reports. For example, Delos et al. studied the effects of LSESr, finasteride (Proscar), and 4-MA, an investigational 5AR inhibitor, on testosterone metabolism of epithelial cells and fibroblasts from BPH and prostate cancer patients. Of the three agents, LSESr was the only one to decrease all testosterone metabolites. In comparison, finasteride decreased 5a-A and DHT in *fibroblasts* to a degree comparable to LSESr and 4-MA. 4-MA was the most potent inhibitor of 5a-A and DHT in BPH and PC *epithelial cells and fibroblasts*, followed by LSESr (Delos et al., *J. Steroid Biochem. Mol. Biol.*, 1995.

Product availability. PC-SPES can be ordered by calling (800) 544-4440, or order online at www.lef.org.

PROSTATE CANCER: CHEMOTHERAPY

(WRITTEN PRIMARILY FOR THE MEDICAL ONCOLOGIST)

By Stephen B. Strum, M.D., and Jonathan E. McDermed, Pharm.D

Dr. Strum is on the Life Extension Medical Advisory Board, and Dr. McDermed is from the Prostate Cancer Research Institute (PCRI) in Los Angeles, California. Drs. Strum and McDermed are proponents of a holistic medical strategy that combines peer-reviewed conventional scientific publications with new findings in the areas of nutrition and supportive care of the patient. Dr. Strum and his partner, Mark C. Scholz, M.D., have a medical practice (Healing Touch Oncology) in Marina del Rey, California, that cares for patients with prostate cancer (PC) or who are at high risk of having PC.

Many studies that evaluated the efficacy of various secondary treatments predated the days of PSA testing. In these studies, responses were evaluated by improvement in symptoms such as bone pain, or by reduction in tumor size on bone scans or CT scans. Based upon the limited sensitivity of scans to assess tumor response, older studies may have missed patient responses that might have been noted if PSA testing were available.

Past studies may have also underestimated the importance of drug *absorption*, proper drug *dosing* based on elimination half-life, *dose intensity,* and altered *drug metabolism*. Treatments that were labeled as ineffective in the past may conceivably turn out to be more effective when given to patients with less tumor volume and under better pharmacological conditions. In a thorough review of the literature, long-lasting responses to secondary therapies have been documented. What patient or treatment-related variables were present in such responding patients?

Dose Intensity

Dose intensity is a term used to compare relative amounts of a drug administered in a given unit of time. For example, compare the relative dose intensities of Regimens A and B. Regimen A delivers a dose intensity that averages 2000 mg a month. Regimen B delivers a dose intensity that averages 4000 mg a month.

Regimen A	Regimen B
Drug dose: 1000 mg	Drug dose: 3000 mg
Frequency: every 2 weeks	Frequency: every 3 weeks
Average: 2000 mg/ month	Average: 4000 mg/ month

Regimen A, with its lower, more frequently administered dose, may have less toxicity due to lower peak blood levels than Regimen B, with its higher but less frequently administered dosing. For example, Taxotere administered every 3 weeks at 70 mg/m^2 has a dose intensity of approximately 93 mg/m^2 a month. Taxotere administered weekly at 25 mg/m^2 has a dose intensity of 100 mg/m^2 a month. The latter regimen is associated with far less toxicity due to the lower but more frequent drug doses. The efficacies of these regimens have not been reported in a randomized trial. Low weekly doses of Taxotere are, in our experience, without question a more patient and friendly regimen compared to the standard, higher dose Taxotere protocol.

Exposure Time

Most chemotherapy agents kill cancer cells that are actively multiplying. PC cells generally grow slowly, which mandates that they receive a longer exposure time to the chemotherapy or other anticancer agent. Examples of ways to increase exposure time include daily oral therapy; a more frequent schedule of intravenous administration; or use of low-dose, continuous intravenous infusions administered by means of a computerized pump through a venous access device, such as a Port-a-Cath. Such protracted infusion delivery increases exposure time while decreasing the toxicity of chemotherapy. Drugs such as Cytoxan and Adriamycin have a much lower toxicity profile and a higher therapeutic index when given in this manner. We currently have a protocol in progress that employs Cytoxan, an active agent in PC, given as a continuous infusion over 120 hours. This is given in conjunction with another agent, 5-Fluorouracil, during the same period of time. This combination has shown high activity in advanced refractory breast cancer in a pilot trial. Since prostate and breast cancer are strikingly similar in so many ways, we have begun this program in advanced PC to utilize a long exposure time of drugs that are known to be active in PC. Moreover, the use of low-dose continuous chemotherapy has another advantage in lowering the toxicity of the drugs. Therefore, the therapeutic index, a measurement of efficacy and side effects, is greatly enhanced with protracted chemotherapy administration. Unfortunately, many oncologists are not familiar with the use of ambulatory infusion pumps or venous access devices such as the Port-A-Cath.

Bone Marrow Support

One of the essential factors in the successful management of the cancer patient is adequate supportive care. This involves multiple factors in the medical and surgical management of the patient, and includes psychological support as well. With the advent of agents that can stimulate the bone marrow, we now are able to give chemotherapy at higher doses by supporting and/or preventing toxicity such as low white blood cell counts, anemia, and low platelet counts.

Marrow Cell Stimulated	Trade Name	Generic Name
Granulocytes	Neupogen	Filgrastim
Granulocytes and macrophages	Leukine	Sargramostim
Erythrocytes	Procrit, Epogen	Erythropoietin alpha
Platelets	Numega	Oprelvekin

A low white blood cell count (also called *granulocytopenia* or *neutropenia*) is a major dose-limiting factor with chemotherapy and is the cause for the

P

most serious side effect of chemotherapy— infection. AIPC patients who receive agents that stimulate the bone marrow to produce white blood cells tolerate this chemotherapy side effect remarkably better. Neupogen or Leukine support reduces or eliminates the number of hospitalizations for infection associated with chemotherapy, and it reduces other problems such as mouth and throat sores.

A low red blood cell count, or *anemia,* can also be a significant source of concern for AIPC patients receiving chemotherapy. Anemia is usually already present to some degree in AIPC patients due to their ADT. Anemia, left untreated, can cause severe weakness, shortness of breath, dizziness, mental status changes, and chest pain. The availability of Procrit to stimulate bone marrow red blood cell production can help minimize the adverse effect severe anemia can have upon the AIPC patient. The use of Procrit has largely replaced the need for blood transfusions.

A low platelet count, also called *thrombocytopenia*, is another dose-limiting factor with chemotherapy and is the cause for a serious side effect of chemotherapy—bleeding. Until recently, thrombocytopenia could delay chemotherapy, cause dosage reductions, or even cause changes in drug therapy. Neumega has recently become available as a marrow stimulant specific for platelet production, and its use may treat patients for low platelet counts.

Other Supportive Care

A medical oncologist should offer the most effective medications or other approaches to maximize the level of supportive care for the AIPC patient receiving chemotherapy. Other chemotherapy side effects include the following

Potential Side Effect	Supportive Care Options
Loss of appetite	Megace (Megestrol acetate)
Nausea and/or vomiting	Zofran (Ondansetron), Kytril (Granisetron), Anzemet (Dolasetron), Reglan (Metoclopramide), Decadron (Dexamethasone)
Diarrhea	Imodium-AD (Loperamide), Lomotil
Constipation	Colace (Docusate sodium), milk of magnesia
Dry skin, hair loss	Emollients, vitamin E, zinc supplements
Heart injury	Zinecard (Dexrazoxane)
Bladder injury	Mesnex (Mesna)
Nerve injury	Ethyol (Amifostine)
Extravasation injury to soft tissue	DMSO topically (70% solution)
Kidney injury	Sodium thiosulfate injection

Unfortunately, there are no medications or approaches available that will prevent loss of hair from chemotherapy. However, hair will grow back in the weeks after therapy is stopped, and may actually begin to grow back during continued chemotherapy treatments.

Certain intravenous chemotherapy drugs, if they accidentally leak out of the vein and into surrounding tissues, can cause a significantly damaging *extravasation injury.* Drugs that can cause extravasation injuries are known as vesicant chemotherapy agents. To prevent potential extravasation injuries, vesicant chemotherapy should be given with caution to patients with poor-quality veins, or patients who are to receive drugs as a protracted infusion over several days. In most cases, it may be preferable in such patients for them to have a central venous catheter or access device, e.g., Port-A-Cath, placed before therapy is started. This not only avoids a potential extravasation injury, but also preserves access to a patient's veins to draw blood. If chemotherapy extravasation does occur, 70% DMSO applied topically prevents tissue injury and should be administered as soon as possible, and at least 4 to 6 times a day until the site of extravasation is fully healed. If stinging occurs with DMSO application, the patient should wipe off the remaining DMSO and apply aloe vera gel to the skin.

It is very important that a patient promptly report any unusual symptoms or side effects during chemotherapy treatment to his physician to be sure that it is not, or does not become, a major problem. Patients receiving vesicant chemotherapy through a peripheral (hand, arm, or leg) vein should inspect the chemotherapy injection site for several days after each treatment.

Concepts in AIPC Management

Due to our concern for the emergence of androgen independence in PC, the following principles are relevant until we have a better understanding of hormone sensitivity and independence.

Symptomatology Means Large Tumor Volume

There is an inverse correlation with diminished survival in patients who are more symptomatic from their PC than those with fewer symptoms. The symptom complex is a manifestation of tumor burden. It is also expressed in the stage of disease and may explain why patients with 1 to 5 bone metastases do so much better than those with greater numbers of bone lesions. Therefore, consider initiating treatment if there is a persistent increase in PSA. This can be confirmed by three consecutive increases of the PSA obtained in the same medical center or office using the same PSA methodology. Late treatment, when symptoms are prevalent, is more difficult. In such circumstances, the treatment is compromised by a debilitated patient who is less tolerant of the therapy and who has a large tumor burden that has had a chance to mutate to resistant clones. Earlier treatment, when the patient is asymptomatic, has a greater chance of a durable remission with a higher quality of survival. This is true of all cancer therapy. The relationship of tumor volume as seen in the number of bone lesions vs. survival in patients receiving ADT is shown below from the work of Labrie et al. (*Clin. Invest. Med., 1993*).

Use Multiple Biomarkers to More Clearly Define Response

Tumor biomarkers are the barometers that reflect the success or failure of therapy. A definite upward trend in the PSA level, for example, should dictate a treatment change, whereas a flat PSA graph or downward trend would suggest that the treatment remain unchanged. Other tumor markers, such as prostatic acid phosphatase (PAP), alkaline phosphatase, chromogranin A (CGA), neuron-specific enolase (NSE), or carcino-embryonic antigen (CEA), if initially abnormal, should be followed as well.

ADT2 (LF) vs # Bone Lesions: Median Survival

#bone lesions	# Pts	Median Survival (years) 3	5	8
11-40	50	45	18	10
6-10	45	59	30	17
1-5	105	82	66	58

after Labrie et al

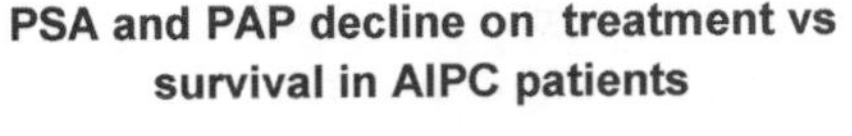

PSA and PAP decline on treatment vs
survival in AIPC patients

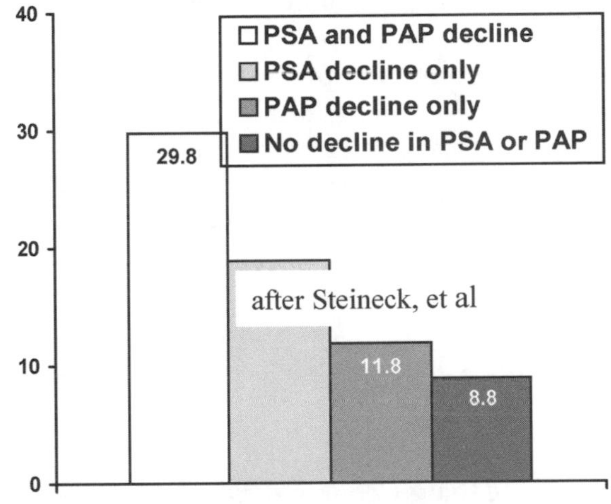

Steineck et al. showed the value of monitoring response to AIPC treatment by using more than one tumor marker. In a retrospective study, he demonstrated that the overall survival of AIPC patients was longer if both PSA and PAP levels declined on therapy than if only PSA or PAP declined. The shortest survival was seen in patients in whom neither marker declined.

Even if other tumor markers are not abnormal when a particular therapy is started, it is reasonable to monitor their levels periodically on treatment, especially if disease progression occurs. It is also better to follow trends in PSA in combination with other markers than to use the results from a single test.

Drug Absorption, Dosing, and Toxicity May Mean the Difference between Response and Progression

Many of the drugs currently in use do not have a long half-life in the body and are commonly given every 8 or 12 hours. Patient compliance to these dosing intervals is important to the success of such treatment. Nizoral and estramustine phosphate (Emcyt), for example, require an empty stomach for complete absorption. Nizoral also requires a sufficient amount of stomach acid to facilitate absorption. Many patients are not compliant and miss multiple doses of drug. This results in blood levels that are not therapeutic. Patients who understand the proper dosing and the toxicity of the medications they are taking will respond far better than those who are ignorant of this information. Nizoral blood levels are commercially available and are not expensive. It is recommended that patients on Nizoral obtain a blood level reading 4 hours after their last dose of drug to see if a therapeutic level is attained. This should be at least > 2.0 mcg/ml.

Synergistic Drug Combinations Are More Effective AntiCancer Therapies

Treatments employing synergistic combinations of more than one chemotherapy agent or chemotherapy combined with second-line hormonal therapy result in higher rates of anticancer response. It has been demonstrated that the duration of response and overall survival are significantly longer in patients who have ≥ 50% decrease in PSA with these therapies and even longer in patients who have ≥ 80% decrease in PSA. Combination treatments that fulfill these criteria for response, and that do so in at least 50% of the patients treated for a minimum average response time of 6 months, are considered "high-response regimens." These regimens will be discussed later. It is important for patients to understand the definitions of response, percentage of responders, and durability of response.

Additional Factors to Consider When Choosing a Treatment

The approach to the patient with PC that has progressed during ADT is complicated. A number of important variables in each patient history and previous pattern of response must be addressed. These include

- Age and general health of the patient.

  Patients with progressive disease after ADT who are elderly, frail, or have other significant medical problems do not tolerate many of the therapies for advanced PC compared to younger patients or patients in otherwise good health. This is not an absolute statement but a general observation.

- Amount of disease as reflected by PSA level.

  Patients who have extensive disease with large tumor burdens have a lower chance of a complete response. In addition, the duration of response, in general, is not as long in these patients. This is true for primary hormonal blockade and also secondary therapies. A high PSA does not preclude a major response to treatment, however.

- Potential response to "secondary" hormonal treatments.

  The term "secondary" hormone therapy includes nonchemotherapy treatments that may be effective in patients progressing after ADT as well as some patients with AIPC. Secondary "hormonal" treatments include antiandrogen withdrawal alone or coupled with high-dose ketoconazole (Nizoral) or aminoglutethimide (Cytadren) plus hydrocortisone, estrogens, or progestins. We are learning that the effectiveness of such therapies may relate to the nonhormonal effects of drugs such as Nizoral and estrogens. In other words, agents that previously were believed to work only via a hormonal mechanism are now being shown to have other biologic effects independent of the hormonal axis. Examples of such effects include direct cytotoxicity against the PC cell, cell differentiation, and down-regulation of oncogenes that protect the tumor cell from apoptosis (programmed cell death).

High-Response Regimens in the Treatment of AIPC in 1999–2000

The following table is a synopsis of the high-response regimens found in the peer-reviewed literature. PSA response criteria are generally the same, i.e., ≥ 50% drop in PSA from baseline is considered a PSA response. To be considered a high-response regimen, the required PSA response rate is approximately 50%. Following this table are specific comments about individual regimens. This section is constantly evolving and is by no means a definitive treatise on the chemotherapy of PC. Some of the regimens in the table have one diamond (♦). Two diamonds (♦♦) indicate longer median survival times than others. This is done with reluctance, since studies were not similarly stratified by extent of disease or prior treatment(s).

Regimen	Response Rate ≥ 50% ↓ in PSA	MDR-median duration of response MDS-median duration of survival	Reference and Year. See above listings for complete reference information.	Comments
Adriamycin + Cytoxan	46% (16/35)	MDS 11 months In responders it was 23 months	Small et al. *JCO* 1996	Adria 40/m^2 ; Cytoxan 800–2000 mg/m^2 q 21 days with G CSF support + dose escalation
Adria + 5-FU (CI)	61% (11/18)	MDR 7+ months with all pts still responding	Koch et al. *Proc Am Soc Clin Oncol* 1992	Adria 15 mg/m^2 q wk + 5-FU 250/m^2 daily by continuous infusion pump
Adriamycin + Ketoconazole ♦♦	55% (21/38)	MDS 17.3+ months if PSA ↓ > 80% then 20+ months MDR 7.1 months (3-26.9); 14 months if PSA decline ≥ 80%	Sella et al. *JCO* 12:683–688, 1994	Adria 20 mg/m^2 over 24 hours a week + Keto (1200/d) + HC
Logothetis (Adria, Nizoral, Emcyt, Velban) ♦♦	67% (31/46) 24/46 (52%) 80% or greater 12/16 soft tissue responses	MDR 8.4 months MDS 19 months MDS of PSA responders not reached; for nonresponders MDS 13 months	Ellerhorst et al. *Clin Ca Res* 1997	Adria HDK qo wk alt with Emcyt Vlb qo wk
Cytoxan, 5-FU, DES, Castration ♦	36 patients	Cumulative survival at 11 years is 56%	Servadio et al. *Urology* 1987	Orchx, breast RT, DES 3 mg/d, 5-FU + Cytx 10mg/kg/wk x 2 yrs, 5mg/kg/wk q 3 wks for yr 3–4; q 4 wks in yr 5
Cytoxan high dose ♦		Responders with MDS 18.6 months vs 8.1 in non-responders	Chlebowski et al. *Cancer* 1978	Cytx 800–1200mg/m^2 q 3 wks vs Cytx 150–200 mg/m^2 po 3–6 + 5-FU + Adria 30–50/m^2 day 1

P

Regimen	Response Rate ≥ 50% ↓ in PSA	MDR-median duration of response MDS-median duration of survival	Reference and Year. See above listings for complete reference information.	Comments
Cytoxan high dose i.v. ♦	75% (3/4) African Americans	MDS 12.5 months	Smith et al. *Proc Am Soc Clin Oncol* 1996	
Cytoxan + DPPE (histamine antagonist)	50% (10/20)	No data	Brandes LJ, et al. *JCO* 1995	DPPE 6 mg/kg i.v. over 80 minutes; Cytx 600–800 mg/m^2 over last 20 min of DPPE infusion q wk x 4, 1 week rest, then 2 out of every 3 weeks treatment
HDK, HC + Oral **Cytoxan**	78% (21/27)	MDR 9 months	Pavlick et al. *Proc Am Soc Clin Oncol* 1996	HDK 400 tid, HC 20/10, Cytx 100 mg/m^2 x 14 of 28 days; q 28 days
Keto + HC after AAWR	30/48 (62.5%)	MDR 3+ months (range 3.2–12.75+)	Small EJ, Baron AD. *J Urol* 1997	23/48 (48%) > 80% fall in PSA
Ketoconazole + Hydrocortisone + AAWR ♦	11/20 (55%)	MDR 8.5 months MS 19 months	Small EJ, Baron AD, Bok R. *Cancer* 1997	10/20 had > 80% fall in PSA
Emcyt + **Navelbine** vs NVB monoRx Chemo naïve ♦	NVB: 19/47 (40%) NVB + E 27/40 (68%) ≥ 50% PSA ↓	MDS 8 months MDS 12 months	Oudard et al. *Proc Am Soc Clin Oncol* 1999	NVB 25/m^2 days 1, 8, E 600 mg/m^2 qd every 21 days
Emcyt + **VP-16** ♦	53% (9/17) African American 53% (41/78) (Anglos)	MDS 12.8 months MDS 12 months	Smith DC, et al. *Proc Am Soc Clin Oncol* 1996	
Emcyt + **VP-16** ♦	58% (30/52)	MDS 13 months	Dimopoulos MA, et al. *Urology* 1997	
Emcyt + **VP-16** ♦♦	85.7% (30/35)	MDS (actuarial) 32 months	Cruciani, *Proc Am Soc Clin Oncol* 1998	
Emcyt + **VP16** + **Carbo**	61% 11/18	No data	Frank et al. *Proc Am Soc Clin Oncol* 1995	VP 100 × 14 or 120/m2 × 3; Carbo 5(CrCl + 25), emcyt 10/kg/d × 14
Emcyt + **velban**	54% (13/24)	MDR 7 months (4–10)	Seidman et al. *J Urol* 1992	emcyt 10 mg/kg velban 4 mg/m^2
Emcyt + **Taxol** (3 hour weekly)	9/14 (64%) ≥ 50% PSA↓ and 7/14 (50%) ≥ 80% PSA↓	No data	Haas et al. *Proc Am Soc Clin Oncol* 1999	Taxol weekly × 6 q 8 wks at 60 –107mg/m^2/wk; E 280 mg bid × 3 days of each week × 6 wks

Regimen	Response Rate ≥ 50% ↓ in PSA	MDR-median duration of response MDS-median duration of survival	Reference and Year. See above listings for complete reference information.	Comments
Emcyt + **Taxol** + **Carbo**	19/26 (73%) with ≥ 50% ↓PSA; 14/26 (54%) with ≥ 80% ↓PSA; 6/26 (23%) nl PSA	MDR 6+ months (5+–12+); measurable regression 9/14 (64%)	Kelly et al. *AUA* 1999; pts with AIPC had 2x as much DVT as second arm with ADPC (18% vs 9%) (166)	26 pts with AIPC; Taxol 100/m^2 weekly, E and C monthly
EMP + **Taxotere** + DXM after DXM failure	7/8 (88%) with ≥ 50% PSA ↓; 5/8 (63%) with ≥ 75% PSA ↓	No data	Shelton et al. *Proc Am Soc Clin Oncol* 1998	12 pts who rec'd DXM first, failed and then on EMP + Taxotere + Dex
Emcyt + **Taxol** ♦♦	53.1% (17/32)	MDR 9.25 months MDS 17.25 months	Hudes GR, et al. *JCO* 1997	Taxol 120/m^2 over 96 hrs q 3 wks + Emcyt at 600/m^2/d
Emcyt + **Taxotere** **Emcyt** + **Navelbine**	77%; 55%	No data	Natale et al. *Proc Am Soc Clin Oncol* 1998	Various dose regimens of weekly T or Navelbine
Emcyt + **Taxotere** weekly	14/18 (77.8%) for ≥ 50% PSA ↓; 9/18 (50%) for ≥ 75% PSA ↓	No data	Natale et al. *Proc Am Soc Clin Oncol* 1999	Weekly taxotere at doses ranging 20–35 mg/m^2 week for 6 of 8 weeks. EMP doses days 1–3 420 mg first 4 doses, 280 mg last 5 doses; DXM 4 bid day before, of and after T
Emcyt + **Taxotere** ♦♦	20/32 (63%) with ≥ 50% PSA ↓	MDS > 1 yr; not yet reached	Petrylak et al. *JCO* 1999	Multiple dose levels of Taxotere with optimal dose at 70 mg/m^2 on day 2 + emcyt 280 mg tid days 1–5, decadron 20 mg midnight, 6 am and just before Taxotere
Emcyt + **Taxotere** Emcyt 10mg/kg x 5 days + low dose HC Chemo naive	11/19 (57.9%) > 50% decline in PSA; 7/11 (63.6%) > 75% decline in PSA	No data; only 2 cycles of Rx	Savarese et al. *Proc Am Soc Clin Oncol* 1999	Taxotere at 70mg/m^2 q 3 weeks on day 2
Emcyt + **Taxotere** Chemo naïve	16/19 (84%) ≥ 50% PSA drop; 13/19 (68%) with ≥ 80% PSA drop	MDR if 50% drop 5.5 m(0.75 + –16 months); if 80% or more drop: 5 months (0.75–13 months)	Weitzman et al. *Proc Am Soc Clin Oncol* 1999	Taxotere 70 mg/m^2 Emcyt 280 tid × 5 days; DXM 20 po 12, 6 and just before chemo q 3 wks

Regimen	Response Rate ≥ 50% ↓ in PSA	MDR-median duration of response MDS-median duration of survival	Reference and Year. See above listings for complete reference information.	Comments
Taxotere Chemo naïve ♦	16/35 (45%) > 50% PSA decline; 7/35 > 80%	MDR 9 months MDS 12 months	Picus et al. *Proc Am Soc Clin Oncol* 1999	75 mg/m^2 q 3 wks No Emcyt
DES 3 mg a day + **Coumadin**	64% (9/14) with PSA ↓ of > 75%	MDR 8 months (2–24)	Jazieh et al. *Proc Ann Meet Am Ass Ca Res* 1994	Post-orchiectomy patients
DES 1 mg a day ♦♦	62% if only 1 prior hormone therapy	Median survival at 3 years not reached; survival rate at 2 years is 63%	Smith DC, et al. *Urology* 1998	Patients off LHRH and also had AAWR
DES + HC	54% (36/56)	MDR 8.5 months	Harland et al. *Proc Am Soc Clin Oncol* 1998	HC 20 bid, DES 1 mg qd, Coumadin 1 mg qd
5-FU + **IFN** ♦♦	43% (9/21)	MDS 18 months	Shinohara N, et al. *Prostate* 1998; 57% with partial or complete disappearance of bone pain (178)	5-FU 600 mg/m^2 × 5 days, bolus FU at 600/m^2 days 15, 22; IFN 3 m units days 1, 3, 5,15, 22 q 4 weeks

Adriamycin and Cytoxan Regimens

Adriamycin is definitely an active agent in PC. The Sella and Logothetis regimens have already been discussed. The combination of adriamycin plus 5-FU after Koch et al. involves a 24-hour infusion of adriamycin to lessen the cardiac toxicity from this agent. The Adriamycin + Cytoxan regimen after Small et al. is shown below. The use of Cytoxan, a high-response agent in PC, with dose escalation is used in this regimen to take advantage of the principle of dose intensity. Notice the similarity of responses of this regimen with that of Chlebowski et al., with median survivals of 23 months vs. 18.6 months.

Adriamycin + Cytoxan

- Dose-escalated Cytoxan (800-2,000 mg/m^2) along with Adriamycin (40mg/m^2) + growth factor (G-CSF) to support bone marrow
- 16/35 (46%) with > 50% decrease in PSA
- Median survival of above patients = 23 mos

Small E J et al., JCO 14:1617-25, 1996

Cytoxan: Dose Intensity

Single high dose Cytx (1000 mg/m^2) responders lived > 2 times longer vs Cytoxan combination responders given lower dose (720 mg/m^2) : 18.6 months vs 8.1 months

Chlebowski RT et al, Cytoxan vs Combination Adriamycin, 5-FU and Cytoxan in the treatment of metastatic prostatic cancer. Cancer 42:2546-2552,1978.

The PCRI has a protocol involving 5 days of continuous infusion Cytoxan at 600 mg/m^2 a day coupled with 5-FU at 300 mg/m^2 a day over 5 days. In addition, dexamethasone at 4 mg a day for 5 days is used as an anti-emetic and an anticancer agent in this regimen. The medications are given continuously using a Port-A-Cath and a computerized Cadd Pump with cycles repeated every 21 days. Neupogen and Procrit are used to protect the bone marrow. There is rationale for this based on outstanding responses in "refractory" breast cancer patients as well as responses to cytoxan shown here. The dose of 600 mg/m^2 a day for 5 days is equal to 3 grams per M^2, the same dose employed by Smith et al. Of 21 patients, 6 had a 90% reduction in PSA. Survival information is needed.

Cytoxan: Bone Marrow Support

- 21 patients: Cytoxan 3 grams/m^2
- GM-CSF 5 ug/kg on days 3-10
- Lower dose if prior pelvic radiation
- 6/21 (29%) with > 90% reduction in PSA
- No survival info in report

Smith DC et al. Hi-dose Cytoxan with GM-CSF in hormone-refractory prostatic carcinoma. 3rd Annual Pittsburgh Cancer Conference, November 19-20, 1992, p 12.

Cytoxan: Exposure Time

- Servadio et al: 36 D-2 pts treated with orchiectomy, DES 3 mg/d + weekly Cytoxan and 5-FU at 10 mg/kg x 2 years, then 5 mg/kg x 2 years but given every 3 weeks for 2 years, then every 4 weeks thereafter.
- 75% relief of bone pain
- Cumulative survival at 11 years 55.5%

Servadio C, Savion M, Mukamel E: Urology 30:352-355, 1987.

The Servadio regimen combines weekly Cytoxan with weekly 5-FU in combination with DES and orchiectomy. It has been used for 11 years in Israel, with an outstanding cumulative survival rate of 55.5%.

It would seem prudent to advise patients to consider such regimens using combinations rather than to employ single-agent therapy. This might lead to significantly longer response times than the results we are currently getting. The above regimen, however, is difficult to truly evaluate without knowing the extent of bone disease in the treated group. If you recall the Labrie et al. data on ADT2 in the 1 to 5 bone lesion group, they had an 8-year median survival rate of 58%.Therefore, if the patients receiving the Servadio regimen were heavily weighted in the 1 to 5 bone lesion category, their responses would be in keeping with those of Labrie et al. and would raise the issue of whether the chemotherapy portion of the Servadio regimen added to the response. Cytoxan has also been used in combination with HDK by Pavlick et al. (see chemotherapy table). Their response to this combination is shown below.

Cytoxan: synergy with HDK

27 patients treated with HDK + HC +
Cytoxan 100 mg/m^2 orally for 14 days.
New cycle every 28 days
21/27 or 78% with 50% or > decline PSA
Median PSA 68...median nadir PSA 5
Median duration of response 9 months

Pavlick AC et al. Treatment of hormone refractory PC with HDK, HC & Cytoxan. Proc Am Soc Clin Oncol: 15:A698, 1996.

Oral Cytoxan given for 14 out of each 28 days is an effective regimen, especially if combined with other active agents like Adriamycin (as shown above). The median duration of response (MDR) in this study was 8 months. Cytoxan has also been administered with a histamine antagonist, DPPE.

P

Cytoxan: Exposure Time

- Cytoxan orally at 100 mg per M^2 for 14 days of a 28 day cycle combined with Adriamycin intravenously at 30 mg per M^2 on 1st and 8th day of each 28 day cycle
- 32% partial response
- Median duration of response: 8 months (range 2-23)

Ihde DC et al. Effective treatment of hormonally unresponsive metastatic carcinoma of the prostate with Adriamcyin and cyclophosphamide, Cancer 45:1300-1310, 1980

The latter agent is under study. The preliminary findings are shown below.

Cytoxan: Bone Marrow Support

- DPPE (histamine antagonist)- potentiates chemotherapy cytotoxicity yet protects bone marrow, intestinal tract & hair.
- 20 patients with HRPC treated with Cytoxan at 600-800 mg/m^2 I.V. once a week x 4.
- 5/7(71%) PR in soft tissue tumor.
- 9/18 (50%) > 50% drop in PSA.
- 11/13 (85%) PR or CR of bone pain.

Brandes LJ et al, DPPE in combination with cytoxan: an active, low toxicity regimen for metastatic hormonally unresponsive PC. J Clin Onco 13:1398-403, 1995.

Emcyt Combinations: Emcyt + VP-16, Emcyt + Taxol, Emcyt + Taxotere

The use of Emcyt has been problematic for us due to the salt retention, increased risk of thrombosis necessitating routine anticoagulation, and the moderate frequent complaints of nausea and anorexia it causes. However, there are impressive response rates with various Emcyt combinations. A few are shown here.

Emcyt + VP16

- PSA ↓ > 50% in 30/35 (85.7%)
- 31 patients D-2
- Median age 70(range 55-81)
- Emcyt 2 capsules twice a day, VP-16 at 50-mg twice a day; Rx x 14 days out of 28
- Median survival (actuarial) 32 months
- Toxicity: hair loss in all, gastritis in others

Cruciani G: Proc Am Soc Clin Oncol 17:329a, 1998.

Emcyt + Taxol

- 17/32 (53%) with ≥50% PSA decline
- Median survival 17.25 months
- Taxol 120/m^2 (over 96 hrs) q 3 weeks
- Emcyt at 600 mg/m^2 per day

- Hudes GR et al: JCO 15:156-163, 1997.

Taxotere

Emcyt has also been combined with Taxotere (docetaxel). Taxotere is most often administered as an every-3-week regimen. The recent work of Natale using weekly Taxotere has led us to employ this patient-friendly regimen. Presented are the data from the work of Petrylak et al. on every 3-week Taxotere and that of Natale et al. using weekly Taxotere.

Taxotere is synergistic with Cytoxan, 5-FU, and Mitomycin C. There is virtually no bone marrow suppression using weekly Taxotere at the dose we employ (25 mg/m^2/week). We also are finding this regimen to have minimal, if any, tendency to cause nausea or vomiting and to cause only slight hair thinning (which is reversible). Taxotere's mechanism of action may involve inac-

Taxotere + Emcyt

- Emcyt 280 mg 3x/day x 5 days + Taxotere @ 40-70 mg/m^2 every 21 days. Decadron pretreatment to prevent side-effects
- Extensively Pretreated Pts 50% with > 50% decline in PSA
- Minimally Pretreated Pts 73% with > 50% decline in PSA
- 53% reduced pain meds by > 50%

Petrylak: Proc Am Soc Clin Oncol. 16:310A, 1997

tivation of BCL-2 via phosphorylation. Since 65% of AIPC specimens overexpress Bcl-2 (which inhibits apoptosis), this may be a critical area of Taxtotere action. *In vitro*, Taxotere has 100-fold greater potency than Taxol in inactivating Bcl-2 phosphorylation.

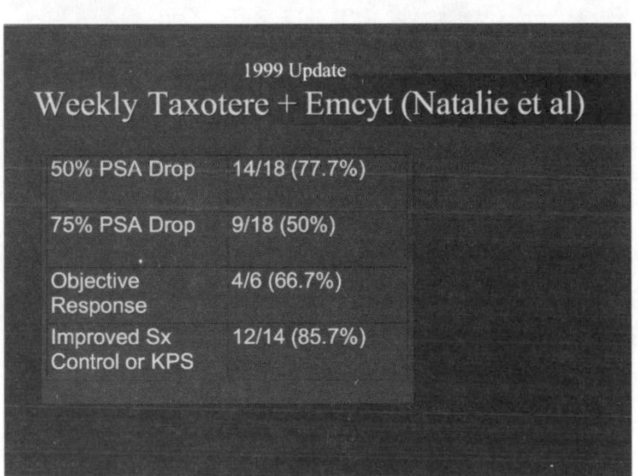

1999 Update

Weekly Taxotere + Emcyt (Natalie et al)

50% PSA Drop	14/18 (77.7%)
75% PSA Drop	9/18 (50%)
Objective Response	4/6 (66.7%)
Improved Sx Control or KPS	12/14 (85.7%)

5-FU + Interferon α-2a

5-FU—by continuous infusion given in combination with subcutaneously administered Interferon-alpha—resulted in a 43% response rate with a median survival time of 18 months. This is shown here.

5 FU + Interferon-α-2a

- 5 FU by continuous infusion @ 600 mg/m^2 per day x 5 days followed by bolus injection 5 FU on days 15,22.
- rIFN- -2a 3x10^6 on days 1,3,5,15,22
- Repeat cycle every 4 weeks
- 9/21(43%) with PSA response >50%
- Median survival 18 months

Shinohara N, Demura T, Matsumura K et al. The Prostate 35:56-62, 1998.

Mitoxantrone + Prednisone

The study of Tannock et al. indicated a median survival time of 12 months with or without the addition of prednisone. Patients receiving Mitoxantrone and Adriamycin need to have baseline ejection fractions done and interval ejection fractions to prevent the development of significant cardiomyopathy. The use of Coenzyme Q_{10}, selenium, and vitamin E in such patients may have some protective value. The data from the two major Mitoxantrone studies are shown below. There are many investigational trials using Mitoxantrone combinations.

Mitoxantrone (M) + Prednisone (P)

- M @ 12 mg/m^2 every 3 weeks + P 10 mg per day vs P alone
- Reduction in pain & analgesic use
- 38% response in M+P vs 21% with P alone
- ≥ 50% ↓ in PSA in 33% MP vs 22% P Duration of response 43 wks vs 18 wks
- Median survival 12 months: no difference

Tannock I, Osoba D, et al: JCO 14:1756-64, 1996.

Mitoxantrone(M) + Hydrocortisone (HC) vs HC only

101 patients with AIPC received either M + HC or HC alone. 50% decline in PSA seen in 33% of M + HC arm and 18% in HC only arm (p 0.035)

Time to failure 7.3 m in M + HC arm and 4 m in HC only (p value 0.065)

Survival 10.9 m vs 11.8 m (p 0.329)

Kantoff PW, Conaway M, Winer E, et al.Proc Amer Soc Clin Oncol 15:25a,1996.

Small Cell PC Regimen

Adriamycin + Cytoxan

- Infusion Adriamycin plus Cytoxan over 96 hrs
- Using Port-A-Cath
- Adriamycin at 10 mg/m^2 per day + Cytoxan at 200 mg/m^2 per day
- Cycle repeated every 22 days
- Neupogen used from days 5-10 at 600 ug qd
- Dose escalation of Cytoxan pending CBC

The above regimens are used to treat adenocarcinoma of the prostate. Two regimens that we have used successfully to treat small-cell prostate cancer (SCPC) are shown below. SCPC is characterized by elevations in neuroendocrine markers such as CGA, NSE, and, not uncommonly, CEA. The PSA may not be expressed significantly, bone lesions are often lytic and not blastic, and liver and lung lesions are not uncommonly detected by CT scanning.

Small Cell Clinical Vignette

- 77 yo with PC 7/91
- Failed RP, ADT
- CDE 4/93: baseline NSE 119
- response x 2 years, then infusion CDE 9/95 & response x 1 yr
- relapse 12/96 with rise in CGA to 99
- Infusion Cytoxan and Adria 3/97 with response to 9/97

Small Cell PC Regimens

CDE

- Cytoxan 50 mg bid x 14 days
- Doxorubicin(adriamycin) 20 mg q wk
- Etoposide(VP-16) 50 mg qd x 14-21days
- Neupogen support essential, Epo also

Conclusions

The chemotherapy of PC has changed significantly in the last 5 years. We are defining AIPC more precisely, detecting AIPC earlier, and treating patients at a lower tumor burden when the chance of a significant response is still possible. There remains, however, a need to educate patients and physicians about these and other fundamental issues in the care of the patient with AIPC. The coming years will see combinations of synergistic drugs, the employment of agents that affect angiogenesis, oncogenes, and growth factors as ways to eradicate the tumor cell population. The ability to control PC may be within our reach.

Further Information

Chemotherapy Options for Advanced Prostate Cancer

By Mark A. Moyad, M.P.H., and Kenneth J. Pienta, M.D., University of Michigan Comprehensive Cancer Center

Note: All of this information and in more detail is found in the upcoming book *The ABCs of*

Advanced Prostate Cancer (Sleeping Bear Press, (800) 487-2323). The percentages that are shown are the percent of individuals who respond or who are affected by the treatment.

The National Comprehensive Cancer Center Endorsed Chemotherapies

Estramustine and Etoposide
PSA response = 39–58%
Side effects: Nausea (decreases with decreasing estramustine dose), hair loss, decrease in white blood cells (about 25%), and blockage of the veins in the legs (less than 5%).

Paclitaxel (Taxol) and Extramustine
PSA response = 53%
Side effects: Nausea, breast enlargement, fluid buildup, and a decrease in white blood cells (21%).

Ketoconazule and Doxorubicin (Adriamycin)
Is also given with hydrocortisone
PSA response = 55%
Side effects: Remote possibility of sudden cardiac death—two patients have died— and inflammation of some areas of the body.

Mitroxantrone and Prednisone
PSA response = 33%
Side effects: A mild case of nausea.

Estramustine and Vinblastine
PSA response = 54–61%
Side effects: Nausea (20%), decrease in white blood cells (12%), constipation (20%), and temporary neuropathy (12%).

Newer Combinations and Options

Paclitaxel, Extramustine, and Etoposide
PSA response = 53%
Side effects: Nausea, hair loss, fatigue, and a decrease in one type of white blood cell

Doxorubicin/Ketoconazole alternating with Vinblastine/Estramustine
Is also used with hydrocortisone
PSA response = 67%
Side effects: Swelling or edema (49%), blockage of the veins in the legs (18%), cardiac problems (4%), and a decrease in one type of white blood cell (less than 2%)

Cytoxan, Diethylstilbestrol (DES), and Prednisone
PSA response = 39%
Side effects: Minimal

Secondary Hormonal Therapy (Newer Options)

Low-dose DES
PSA response = 43%
Side effects: Nipple sensitivity (90%), blockage of the veins in the legs (5%), and breast enlargement (14%)

High-dose Casodex
PSA response = 23%
Side effects: Hot flashes (40%), nipple sensitivity (5%), nausea (10%), itching (5%), and breast enlargement (5%)

PC-SPES in the Treatment of Prostate Cancer*

PC-SPES is a new herbal therapy for treating PC at various stages. PC-SPES consists of a combination of eight herbal extracts, and has been in development for 10 years. The minimum dose is one 320-mg capsule 3 times a day. Most PC patients take about 9 capsules a day. Up to 12 capsules a day for 1 to 2 months have been used by advanced PC patients.

(*Refer to the PC-SPES Prostate Cancer protocol for information about a natural herbal therapy.*)

A few statistically insignificant cases of thrombosis have been reported in users of PC-SPES. Anyone taking PC-SPES should carefully follow the Foundation's *Thrombosis Prevention protocol*. (*Refer to the Cancer: Early-Stage Prostate protocol for additional suggestions*).

For referrals to doctors experienced in using combined hormone blockade, cryo-ablation therapy, seed implantation, etc., call The Educational Center for Prostate Patients at (516) 997-1777 or PAACT at (616) 453-1477, or access the Web site of the Prostate Cancer Research Institute [http://www.prostate-cancer.org]. Hytrin, Cardura, Lupron, Zoladex, Casodex, and Eulexin are drugs that can be prescribed by your doctor.

PROSTATE CANCER: PSA PARAMETER AND HEREDITY FACTORS

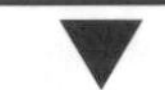

By Stephen B. Strum, M.D., and Jonathan E. McDermed, Pharm.D.

Dr. Strum is on the Life Extension Medical Advisory Board, and Dr. McDermed is from the Prostate Cancer Research Institute (PCRI) in Los Angeles, California. Drs. Strum and McDermed are proponents of a holistic medical strategy that combines peer-reviewed conventional scientific publications with new findings in the areas of nutrition and supportive care of the patient. Dr. Strum and his partner Mark C. Scholz, M.D., have a medical practice (Healing Touch Oncology) in Marina del Rey, California, that cares for patients with prostate cancer (PC) or who are at high risk of having PC.

Emphasis on the use of routine prostate-specific antigen (PSA) monitoring starting annually at the age of 40 with PSA velocity and doubling time determinations as a standard part of PSA reporting will increase the number of men diagnosed earlier, with a lower tumor burden and cured with local modalities of treatment (Labrie et al., *J. Clin. Endocrinol. Metab.*, 1995; Labrie et al., *Urology*, 1996). PSA testing with these enhancements should start earlier, at age 35, in men with a familial history of PC. In addition, the use of routine free/total PSA levels should increase our ability to diagnose PC earlier, since fractionation of PSA allows us to monitor the malignant-associated portion of PSA called complexed PSA. Evaluation of risk of PC using neural net technology as per the ProstaSure blood test will also enable an earlier diagnosis of PC (Babaian et al., *Urology*, 1998). As our standard, and ideally routine, approach to monitoring PSA and other biological expressions of tumor cell activity increases in use, the percentage of men cured with PC should increase as well. This is borne out in a recent report in which PC was detected in 22% (73/332) of men 50 years or older whose PSA reading was between 2.6 and 4. All cancers detected in this setting were clinically localized. This study indicates that PSA readings greater than 2.6 and less than 4.0 may represent a 22% risk of PC (Catalona et al., *JAMA*, 1997). The use of a free PSA test would help determine which of these men whose PSA readings were greater than 2.6 but less than 4.0 have a high probability of PC versus a low probability of PC. Such a test could reduce the number of unnecessary biopsies in the low-risk subset and focus a need for more comprehensive biopsing in the high-risk subset.

Another study involved 760 men with an initial PSA of 4.0 ng/mL or less, plus a normal or suspicious DRE, and a benign prostate biopsy. These men were monitored with PSA testing every 4 months. Of 559 men with an initial PSA of 2.0 ng/mL or less, only 3, or 0.5%, had a persistently abnormal PSA for 3 years; in this group, 1 cancer was detected (0.2%). Of 201 men with a PSA of 2.1 to 4.0, 37 had PSA levels that became and remained abnormal (defined as greater than 4.0). Of this group, 23 biopsies were performed, and 8 (35%) revealed PC. The study indicated that in men with an initial PSA of 2.1 to 4, the cancer detection rate was 4.5%. This was approximately 15-fold greater ($p < 0.00001$) than the cancer detection rate in the men with an initial PSA of 2.0 or less (Harris et al., *J. Urol.*, 1997). Patients presenting with their first PSA at 2.1 or greater should therefore be the focus of more intense studies. This could include free/total PSA, PSA doubling time determination, and ProstaSure testing.

New biopsy techniques such as 5-region biopsy of the prostate gland have been shown to increase the diagnostic yield of PC by 35% (Eskew et al., 1997).

Despite these inroads, many men today are still being diagnosed with PC that is advanced, i.e., not organ-confined. What difference does this make?

The difference in treating early PC versus more advanced PC relates to the issue of cure as opposed to control. Early PC has the potential for cure via a local therapy combined with the use of androgen deprivation therapy (ADT) in situations where the tumor volume compromises the curative ability of local therapy, such as radiation therapy (including seed implantation) or cryosurgery. (*Refer to the Prostate Cancer [Early-Stage] protocol for specific treatment information.*)

Heredity Factors in the Development of PC

PC is now being linked to genetic abnormalities that explain the familial occurrence of PC that we frequently see. An understanding of why PC affects certain populations of men more than others is now becoming better understood. We know that PC is equally as prevalent in Asian men as in Western men, but that the frequency of biologically aggressive PC is significantly greater in the non-Asian population. This finding is felt to be possibly related to the lower amount of dietary fat in the Asian diet as well as the frequent use of soy products and a higher intake of green tea polyphenols (Aldercreutz et al., *Proc. Annu. Meet. Cancer Res.*).

In the United States, 74% of men with PC are considered to have "sporadic" PC, while the remaining 26% demonstrate evidence of genetic clustering. Within the 26%, 19% are cases of hereditary PC (HPC) versus 81% designated as familial PC (FPC) (Bastacky et al., *J. Urol.,* 1995). Familial prostate cancer is defined as the simple clustering of the cancer in families, whereas hereditary prostate cancer requires any of the following three criteria: a family with three generations affected, three first-degree (brother[s] or father) relatives affected, or three relatives affected before the age of 55 years (Carter et al., *J. Urol.,* 1993). Men with either FPC or HPC are prime candidates for preventive approaches involving nutritional adjuncts.

HPC is a subtype of FPC with a Mendelian pattern of inheritance linked to a single gene that is transmitted as an autosomal dominant of high penetrance. In simpler terms, this gene is passed along from father to son, and from father to daughter and then to grandson. With HPC, due to the high penetrance of the gene, nearly half of the male offspring will have prostate cancer; many of these will develop PC at an early age, i.e., less than 55. Because the gene is passed along via female offspring, the family history should include questioning about maternal grandfather, maternal uncles, and maternal cousins. HPC accounts for 43% of early onset disease (age 55 years or younger) (Carter et al., *J. Urol.*, 1993; Carter et al., *Cancer Surv.*, 1991; Carter et al., *Proc. Natl. Acad. Sci. USA*, 1992). Extensive family studies of PC indicate that PC shows a stronger familial aggregation, even more than colon or breast cancer, but less than that of ovarian cancer (Cannon et al., *Cancer Surv.*, 1982).

Studies at Johns Hopkins indicated that HPC occurs in the general population at the rare frequency of 0.36% (Carter et al., *J. Urol.,* 1993). Men who carry this dominant gene will develop PC at the rate of 88% of the carriers that live to the age of 85 compared to 5% of the noncarriers (Carter et al., *J. Urol.*, 1993). The rarity of this gene will result in 9% of all PC occurrences by age 85 years being related to HPC (Carter et al., *J. Urol.*, 1993). Important aspects of HPC and FPC are shown in Table 1.

Early *detection* approaches have been recommended for men with a history of familial or hereditary PC (Spitz et al., *J. Urol.*, 1991). Such diagnostic measures could include yearly DRE, PSA, Free/Total PSA, ProstaSure, and tracking of PSA velocity and PSA doubling time. In my opinion, this should begin at age 35 to 40 in men with FPC or HPC. Men with a family history of breast cancer in the maternal line are also at greater risk for developing PC. Women with brothers and/or fathers with PC are also at higher risk for breast cancer, since breast cancer and PC share some common genes (Sellers et al., *Proc. Annu. Meet. Am. Assoc. Cancer. Res.*, 1994). Early nutritional intervention should be a major consideration to alter the natural history in such high-risk patients.

Table 1: Characteristics of Hereditary and Familial Prostate Cancer

Feature	HPC	FPC	Senior Authors
Definition	3 generations or 3 first degree relatives or 2 relatives with PC < 55 years of age	Clustering in families	Carter et al., *J. Urol.*, 1993
Frequency	~20% of clustered PC	~80% of clustered PC	Bastacky et al., *J. Urol.*, 1995
Early Onset PC	Accounts for 43% of early onset PC		Carter et al., *J. Urol.*, 1993 Carter et al., *Proc. Natl. Acad. Sci. USA*, 1992 Carter et al., *Cancer Surv.*, 1991
Number of 1st-Degree Affected Relatives vs. Risk	Increased Risk-Odds Ratio	95% Confidence Intervals	
1	2.2	1.4–3.5	Steinberg et al., *Prostate*, 1990
2	4.9	2.0–12.3	
3 or more	10.9	2.7–43.1	
Number 1st- or 2nd-Degree Affected Relatives vs. Risk[a]	Increased Risk-Odds Ratio	95% Confidence Interval	
1	1.5	1.3–1.8	Steinberg et al., *Prostate*, 1990
2	2.3	1.7–3.3	
3 or more	3.6	2.2–5.9	
Type of Relative with PC vs. Risk of Getting PC	Increased Risk-Odds Ratio	95% Confidence Intervals	
2nd degree: uncle or grandfather	1.7 (Steinberg) 2.1 (Spitz)	1.0–2.9 0.8–5.7	Steinberg et al., *Prostate*, 1990 Spitz et al., *J. Urol.*, 1991
1st degree: brother or father	2.0 (Steinberg) 2.4 (Spitz)	1.2–3.3 1.3–4.5	Steinberg et al., *Prostate*, 1990 Spitz et al., *J. Urol.*, 1991
1st and 2nd degree	8.8 (Steinberg)	2.8–28.1	Steinberg et al., *Prostate*, 1990
Age of PC Onset in Patient vs. Risk[b]	No Additional Relatives Affected	1 or More 1st Degree Relatives Affected	Carter et al., *J. Urol.*, 1993
50	1.9 (1.2–2.8)	7.1 (3.7–13.6)	
60	1.4 (1.1–1.7)	5.2 (3.1–8.7)	
70	1.0 (reference group)	3.8 (2.4–6.0)	

[a]This number does not include the patient.

[b]This relates to risk in first-degree relative(s) of the patient with PC; For example, a 50-year-old patient who has a father *or* brother(s) with PC would confer a 7.1-fold greater risk to an additional first-degree relative.

PROSTATE ENLARGEMENT: BENIGN PROSTATIC HYPERTROPHY

The benign enlargement of the prostate gland affects most men over the age of 60. The enlarged prostate interferes with the flow of urine from the bladder, which can produce mild to severe urinary obstruction. After age 60, the number of men who suffer urinary difficulties caused by prostate enlargement may exceed 70%. Autopsy studies show that 40% of men in their 50s are afflicted with benign prostate enlargement.

Those afflicted with benign prostate disease have trouble urinating and voiding, and are often overly sensitive to the presence of any residual urine in the bladder. Aged men are often forced to get up several times a night to urinate and still do not feel they have completely emptied their bladders. The relentless frustration of chronic urinary urgency is a major cause of sleep disturbance and loss of quality of life as men age.

The acronym used to describe prostate enlargement is "BPH," and this may stand for either benign prostatic "hyperplasia," which means an increase in the number of cells in the prostate, or benign prostatic "hypertrophy," which means an increase in the size of the prostate gland. In the medical literature, "hyperplasia" and "hypertrophy" are used interchangeably to define BPH.

The degree of benign prostate enlargement dictates the most practical therapeutic approach. Once prostate cancer has been ruled out, most men will find effective relief using natural plant extracts. These plant extracts, sold as dietary supplements in the United States, are approved as drugs in Europe for the primary treatment of the symptoms of BPH.

Those with severely enlarged prostate glands may want to add the prescription drug Proscar (finasteride) to a natural plant-extract program. Some studies indicate that Proscar is more effective in shrinking overgrown prostate glands, but less effective in alleviating actual symptoms of BPH compared to natural therapies.

The drug Proscar functions to suppress a testosterone metabolite called dihydrotestosterone (DHT). DHT partially causes age-related enlargement of the prostate gland. Estrogen is also involved in the development of BPH, and plant extracts block the binding of estrogen to prostate cells and possibly prevent testosterone from being excessively converted to estrogen in the blood. These natural plant extracts also have an inhibiting effect on DHT binding in the prostate gland.

The best documented plant extracts are obtained from saw palmetto berry, Pygeum africanum, and nettle root. These natural extracts are well substantiated in published human studies to alleviate the miseries of benign prostate enlargement. More recent research has shed light on the multiple mechanisms by which these herbal extracts function to prevent and treat the disease. One interesting study showed that saw palmetto functions similarly to drugs like Hytrin that are widely prescribed to alleviate urinary urgency.

A new drug therapy involves the use of aromatase-inhibiting drugs to suppress excess levels of estrogen in the blood. In many men, estrogen is the primary growth-stimulating agent that causes prostatic overgrowth.

For those with severe BPH, where phytoextracts and drug therapies fail, surgical procedures are often required to restore urine flow. The therapeutic objective therefore is to properly use nutrients and drugs so the prostate gland does not grow out of control to the point where transurethral resection becomes mandatory.

The Role of Hormones

According to the conventional view, benign prostatic hyperplasia (BPH) develops when the active form of testosterone, DHT, stimulates cell growth. Testosterone is converted to DHT systemically as well as within the prostate by an enzyme known as

5-alpha-reductase. DHT is far more active than testosterone in binding to sites in prostate cells that regulate prostate growth. When DHT binds to these sites, it activates growth factors that stimulate cell proliferation. Commonly used medications for BPH, such as saw palmetto and the drug finasteride (Proscar) inhibit 5-alpha-reductase in order to reduce DHT-stimulated growth in the prostate. While it is hardly surprising that prostate growth is under hormonal control, the above view of BPH is difficult to explain when we consider the effects of aging. BPH is, after all, a disease of aging, and testosterone production declines with age. Moreover, levels of free, physiologically active testosterone decline more sharply due to increased testosterone binding by a protein called sex hormone–binding globulin (SHBG). It is estimated that levels of free testosterone decline by about 1% per year from age 40 to age 70. So if testosterone production declines with age, could there be another mechanism contributing to prostrate enlargement?

The answer may be the growing imbalance in aging men between their levels of estrogen and testosterone. While levels of estrogen appear to be relatively stable in the aging male, the level of free testosterone precipitously declines. Thus with age, an imbalance develops between estrogens and androgens (female and male hormones). Compared to younger men, the ratio of free estradiol (the most potent form of estrogen) to free testosterone is up to 40% higher in older men. In the prostate itself, the contrast between rising estrogens and declining androgens is more sharply drawn. In the stroma of the prostate, the supporting tissue where BPH is thought to develop, estrogen levels increase significantly with age, while DHT levels remain stable. Estrogen levels in the stroma rise to even higher levels in BPH patients. In the epithelium of the prostate, DHT levels decline with age, while estrogen levels remain stable.

German researchers who have been studying this for more than 15 years describe a tremendous increase of the estrogen/androgen ratio in the human prostate with age. Their article in the *Journal of Clinical Endocrinology and Metabolism* concludes, "Our results indicate that the prostatic accumulation of DHT, estradiol, and estrone is in part intimately correlated with aging, leading with increasing age to a dramatic increase of the estrogen/androgen ratio particularly in stroma of BPH."

A study published in the journal *Prostate* bears out the concept of an elevated serum estrogen/androgen ratio as a risk factor for BPH. Analyzing frozen blood samples collected in the course of a large-scale health study, the researchers found that BPH risk increased with higher estradiol levels, and that the risk was concentrated in men with relatively low androgen levels.

A Japanese study came to a similar conclusion, finding that prostate size correlates with estradiol level and with the ratio of estradiol to free testosterone. They suggest that the endocrine environment tended to be estrogen-dominant with age—in particular, after middle age—and that patients with large prostates have more estrogen-dominant environments, concluding that estrogens are key hormones for the induction and the development of BPH.

Experimental attempts to induce BPH with hormones would answer many questions, but obviously cannot be carried out in humans. The only animals known to develop BPH with age are dogs and lions.

In experiments with dogs, it has been established than BPH cannot be induced without estrogen, but it should be noted that endocrine regulation and prostate structure are quite different in dog and man.

In men and postmenopausal women, most estrogens are produced from androgens; specifically, most estradiol is produced from testosterone. This conversion of androgens to estrogens is called aromatization, after the enzyme aromatase. In addition to receiving estrogen circulating through the bloodstream, the stroma of the prostate produces its own estrogen through aromatization.

It has long been suspected that estrogen, especially the estrogen/androgen imbalance associated with aging, plays a role in BPH, but until recent years no direct effect of estrogen on the prostate could be demonstrated. A key piece of this puzzle has now been supplied by a group of researchers at Columbia University, St. Luke's/Roosevelt Hospital in New York, and the pharmaceutical company Merck, Inc.

In a ground-breaking series of research papers culminating in articles published this past year in the journals *Endocrinology* and *Steroids,* they demonstrate the existence of a second hormonal pathway in the prostate whereby estrogens can mimic androgens. It may help to understand this breakthrough by thinking of hormones as chemical messengers. When a hormone attaches to its special binding site in a cell, it sends a signal to that cell. In the case of BPH, androgens signal cells to proliferate, causing prostate growth. These researchers have shown that messages sent to prostate cells by androgens can also be sent along an alternative signaling pathway, by estrogens. Even more surprisingly, the estrogens send this signal not by attaching to the usual cellular binding sites for estrogen, but instead to the sex hormone-binding globulin (SHBG) that is already bound to the cell membrane. As the authors put it, they have shown that in the prostate, estradiol is capable of activating pathways normally considered androgen responsive.

In a review article published in the journal *Prostate* in 1996, a pioneer of modern prostate research proposed a new model of prostate physiology and pathogenesis based in part upon this research. Wells Farnsworth, Professor of Urology at the Northwestern University Medical School, discovered the conversion of testosterone to DHT in the prostate in the early 1960s. In his article in *Prostate,* Professor Farnsworth proposes that estrogen, mediated by SHBG, participates with androgen in setting the pace of prostate growth and function. Farnsworth notes that, as explained above, SHBG increases with age and can act like an additional androgen receptor (binding site for androgen) in the prostate cell. He suggests that, when estrogen binds to SHBG in the cell membrane, a growth factor called IGF-I (insulin-like growth factor I) is synthesized, causing proliferation of epithelial cells in the prostate. This sets the stage for further proliferation when androgens activate binding sites for growth factors. In Farnsworth's language, estrogen not only directs stromal proliferation and secretion, but also, through IGF-I, conditions the response of epithelium to androgen.

Subsequent research suggests that IGF-II, which is less well understood than IGF-I, may also be involved. In addition to its possible role in BPH, recent research indicates that elevated IGF-I levels may be a key predictor of prostate cancer risk. IGF-I may also contribute to the age-related increase in SHBG. Farnsworth likens the protein SHBG to a hormone, concluding that (SHBG's) newfound capability to evoke BPH and its possible involvement in the transformation of normal cells to cancer cells by oncogenes calls for increased efforts to understand and manage SHBG and estrogen secretion.

The researchers who discovered the alternative signaling pathway concur—antagonism (inhibition) of the pathway by which SHBG leads to the induction of androgen-responsive genes may be a valuable therapeutic target for the treatment or prevention of BPH or prostate cancer. Accordingly, these researchers studied an agent thought to inhibit the binding of SHBG to the prostate cell membrane, an extract of the root of the stinging nettle plant, *Urtica dioica*.

In a paper published in 1995 in *Planta Medica* it was demonstrated that nettle root does indeed inhibit the binding of SHBG to the cell membrane.

In a subsequent series of articles, German researchers have identified a constituent of nettle root known as (-)-3,4-divanillyltetrahydrofuran, whose very high binding affinity to SHBG they describe as remarkable. These researchers suggest that the beneficial effects of plant lignins (such as found in flaxseed oil) on hormone-dependent cancers may be linked to their binding affinity to SHBG. The most potent known lignins in this respect are constituents of nettle root. In addition to inhibiting SHBG binding, at least six constituents of nettle root inhibit aromatase, reducing conversion of androgens to estrogens.

Combining nettle root with pygeum results in a stronger, synergistic inhibition. The studies on aromatase inhibition by nettle root used methanolic extracts.

A recent experimental study provides a dramatic demonstration of nettle root's effect on BPH tissue. This experiment was based upon the hypothesis that BPH is comparable to a reawakening of embryonic growth potential in the prostate.

A fetal urogenital sinus was implanted into a lobe of the prostate gland in adult mice. After 28 days, the implanted lobes of mice fed a nettle root

P

methanolic extract similar to an extract on the German pharmaceutical market showed 51.3% less growth than the lobes of mice in the control group. Nettle root is widely used as a first-line therapy for BPH in Germany, where there are 15 pharmaceutical drugs consisting solely of nettle root. Nettle root has been extensively studied in European clinical trials over the past 20 years.

Good study design is essential in evaluating BPH therapies, since sizable placebo effects are normal in BPH studies. A well-designed double-blind, placebo-controlled trial of nettle root was published in the German urological journal *Urologe* in 1996. This 3-month study involved 41 BPH patients with maximum urinary flow under 15 mL/sec and an average score of 18.2 on the IPSS (International Prostate Symptom Score) scale. An IPSS score of 0 to 7 is considered as slightly symptomatic, 8 to 19 as moderately symptomatic, and 20 to 35 as symptomatic. By the end of the trial, maximum urinary flow increased by an average of 66.1% (from 10.9 to 18.1 mL/sec) in the group treated with nettle root, compared to 36.6% (from 12.3 to 16.8 mL/sec) in the placebo group. Average IPSS scores dropped twice as much in the nettle root group (from 18.2 to 8.7) as in the placebo group (from 17.7 to 12.9).

By comparison, trials of the standard BPH drug finasteride (Proscar) show more modest improvements relative to placebo. Again, this study used the methanolic nettle extract. Eight previous trials of nettle root showed beneficial effects on approximately 15,000 BPH patients. These trials used daily doses of nettle extract ranging from 600 to 1200 mg and lasted from 3 weeks to 180 days.

In Europe, nettle root is also used in combination with saw palmetto. This combination is a logical one, since nettle root acts through the alternative signaling pathway in the prostate cell, while saw palmetto acts on the primary signaling pathway by limiting DHT activity. In effect, nettle root addresses the estrogen side of BPH, while saw palmetto addresses the androgen side. Additionally, both herbs have anti-inflammatory actions.

Since 1995, three clinical studies of a standard saw palmetto/nettle combination have been published in German medical journals. The studies used 2 capsules a day of 160 mg saw palmetto extract plus 120 mg nettle root extract.

A randomized double-blind study compared the saw palmetto/nettle combination to the standard BPH drug finasteride in 543 patients suffering from BPH stages I to II. The herbal therapy and drug therapy proved similarly effective in all measures: urinary flow rate, urination time, IPSS scores, and patients' quality of life assessments. Both therapies increased in effectiveness over a period of months. For example, the average IPSS score in the herbal therapy group declined from 11.3 to 8.2 after 24 weeks and to 6.5 after 48 weeks; in the finasteride group it declined from 11.8 to 8.0 after 24 weeks and to 6.2 after 48 weeks.

Patients tolerated herbal therapy better than finasteride, which causes diminished libido and sexual dysfunction, including impotence, in a small minority of patients. Another placebo-controlled study used a crossover design. Forty patients with BPH stage I or II and urinary flow below 20 mL/sec received either saw palmetto/nettle or placebo for 24 weeks.

Patients receiving the herbal combination showed significant improvement in maximum urine flow rate (3.3 mL/sec) compared to placebo, and there were similar improvements in average flow rate, total urination volume, urination time, and flow increase time. There was also a significant improvement on the American Urological Association symptom score compared to placebo. In the crossover phase of the trial, patients who had been on placebo for 24 weeks were switched to the herbal combination for another 24 weeks. These patients showed similar positive results.

A large observational study involving 419 urology practices followed 2030 patients with mild to moderate BPH. All patients received saw palmetto/nettle for 12 weeks. This study found the following average improvements: maximum urinary flow increased 25.8%, average urinary flow increased 29.0%, residual urine decreased 44.7%, nocturia declined 50.4%, dysuria declined 62.5%, and post-urination dribbling declined 53.6%. Eighty-six percent of patients reported symptom improvement. Fewer than 1% of the patients reported side effects, and these were mild. Thus far, there have been no clinical trials of a saw palmetto/nettle/pygeum combination.

As mentioned above, nettle root and pygeum synergize in inhibiting aromatase. In addition, these three herbs affect growth factors in ways that appear to be beneficial in the prevention and treatment of BPH. According to a 1997 article in the *Journal of Urology* pygeum inhibits cell proliferation induced by the growth factors EGF (epidermal growth factor), bFGF (basic fibroblast growth factor), and IGF-I (insulin-like growth factor I) in stromal cells from rat prostate.

A 1998 study in the journal *European Urology* found that saw palmetto inhibits bFGF-stimulated cell proliferation in human prostate cell cultures. Preliminary research suggests that a constituent of nettle root inhibits the binding of EGF to human prostate cells. As is the case for many medicinal herbs, the clinical efficacy of nettle root was demonstrated at a time when medical science had not yet made the basic advances needed to understand its mechanism of action. This may be one reason that nettle root is relatively unknown in the United States, whereas saw palmetto, with its relatively clear-cut mechanism of action based upon testosterone, is in common use. As was the case for saw palmetto, it will probably take years for the pharmaceutical companies to develop a synthetic drug to effectively address the mechanism of action of nettle root. Both of these extraordinarily well-tolerated herbal extracts are available now to BPH sufferers.

Research on Saw Palmetto Extract

Saw palmetto has multisite mechanisms of action, including binding inhibition of DHT to androgen receptors in prostatic cells. In the prostate gland, saw palmetto interferes with conversion of testosterone to the more potent cell-proliferating metabolite dihydrotestosterone (DHT). Saw palmetto decreases DHT concentrations in enlarged prostate tissues of treated patients. A marked decrease of epidermal growth factor, associated with DHT reduction, has also been observed. These biochemical effects, similar to those obtained with Proscar, are particularly evident in the periurethral region, where enlargement is responsible for much of the urinary obstruction seen in BPH.

Saw palmetto also reduces smooth-muscle contraction, thereby relaxing the bladder and sphincter muscles that cause urinary urgency. One study shows that saw palmetto alleviates urinary urgency by acting as an *alpha-1-receptor antagonist*. This is how the popular prescription drug Hytrin works.

A Belgian study involving 505 men with benign prostate disease showed that saw palmetto therapy improved urinary flow, reduced residual urinary volume and prostate size, and improved quality of life after only 45 days of treatment. After 90 days, 88% of the patients and their physicians considered the treatment effective. In addition, the study showed that saw palmetto does not mask the PSA (prostate-specific antigens) score as Proscar has been shown to do. The researchers concluded by stating, "The extract of saw palmetto appears to be an effective and well-tolerated pharmacologic agent in treating urinary problems accompanying benign prostatic hypertrophy."

Castrated animals treated with estradiol and testosterone showed a significant increase in the weight of the prostate gland compared with sham-operated rats. The increase of prostate total weight was inhibited by administration of saw palmetto extract. Indeed, the weight was significantly lower at day 60 and day 90 for the dorsal and lateral regions of the prostate. The weight of the ventral region of the prostate was significantly lower after day 30 and day 60 of treatment with saw palmetto extract. These results demonstrate that administering saw palmetto to hormone-treated castrated rats inhibits the increase in prostate wet weight. This effect may explain the beneficial effect of this extract in human benign prostatic hypertrophy. A double-blind placebo-controlled study performed on 35 BPH patients showed that saw palmetto interfered with the estrogen receptor on prostate cells.

Saw palmetto thus appears to have the following molecular mechanisms of action:

- Interferes with the binding of growth-stimulating estrogen and DHT to receptor sites on prostate cells

- Exhibits 5-alpha-reductase inhibition activity in the prostate gland (but not the blood), thereby reducing prostatic levels of DHT
- Acts as an alpha-1 receptor antagonist, thereby relieving urinary urgency by reducing sphincter smooth muscle contraction
- Decreases epidermal growth factor (EGF), another growth-promoting agent for prostate cells
- Inhibits the enzymes cyclooxygenase and 5-lipooxygenase in the prostate, thus inducing an anti-inflammatory effect

A study on 24 BPH patients treated with saw palmetto for 2 months showed a response rate of 66.7% judged by the patient's condition, quality of life, residual urine, and gland size. Anti-inflammatory actions were suggested as possible actions in addition to other documented mechanisms of effect.

The studies using saw palmetto extracts to treat prostate enlargement have shown the following clinical benefits:

- Reduction of nocturnal urinary urgency
- Increased urinary flow rate
- Reduced residual volume in the bladder
- Reduction in uncomfortable urination symptoms

Pygeum Research

For most men, saw palmetto extract by itself will provide considerable relief from benign prostate disease. The addition of *Pygeum africanum* may provide additional relief. Pygeum inhibits prostate-cell proliferation and produces an anti-edema effect.

Pygeum africanum extract is sold as a drug in many countries, including those in central and eastern Europe, for the treatment of mild to moderate BPH. Its efficacy and acceptability have been demonstrated in numerous open and placebo-controlled studies in large populations. A 1998 study sought to confirm the therapeutic profile of pygeum in conditions of daily practice using the IPSS and flowometry assessments. The changes after the 2-month treatment period were very statistically significant with mean improvements of 40% and 31%, respectively.

Nocturnal frequency was reduced by 32% and the mean reduction was again statistically significant. Mean maximum urinary flow, average urinary flow, and urine volume were also significantly improved, but the modest improvement in post-voiding volume did not reach statistical significance. No treatment-related adverse effects were observed. In conclusion, under conditions of daily practice, pygeum extract induces significant improvement in accepted scores of BPH treatment and uro-flowometry parameters. These positive effects are accompanied by a satisfactory safety profile with the overall result of a substantial improvement in quality of life.

A laboratory rat study found that *Pygeum africanum* is a potent inhibitor of rat prostatic fibroblast proliferation in response to direct activators of protein kinase C, another important prostate growth factor. This suggests that the therapeutic effect of pygeum may be due at least in part to the inhibition of growth factors responsible for the prostatic overgrowth in man.

Research on Nettle Extract

Although the majority of men report improvement after using saw palmetto or pygeum extracts, some prostate obstruction often remains that continues to interfere with urinary flow and bladder evacuation.

An herbal extract called *Urtica dioica* (nettle) has been shown to reduce the symptoms of benign prostatic hypertrophy by 86% in combination with saw palmetto after 3 months of use. Nettle extract is approved by the German government in combination with saw palmetto extract to treat the symptoms of benign prostate disease.

Another human study showed that, after 8 weeks of treatment with urtica extract, there was an 82% improvement or total elimination of disorders associated with prostate enlargement.

After learning the results of these European studies, researchers at St. Luke's/Roosevelt Hospital in New York conducted a study to discover the mechanism by which standardized urtica extract relieves the symptoms of benign prostate hyperplasia (excess cell proliferation). In their study, published in 1995, these scientists showed that urtica extract inhibits the binding of a testosterone-related protein to its receptor site on prostate cell membranes. Prostate cells grow out of control when DHT binds to prostate cell membranes, a process that induces the prostate cells to start dividing. If cell membrane receptors are blocked, the DHT cannot latch onto the cell. Urtica extract appears to work by preventing the binding of tes-tosterone metabolites to membrane receptor sites on prostate cells. It also inhibits the binding of growth-stimulating estrogen to prostate cells.

Saw palmetto, pygeum, and urtica (nettle) are approved drugs in Germany for the treatment of benign prostate enlargement. Urtica may be new to Americans, but it has been safely and successfully used throughout Europe for more than a decade.

Choosing the Right Supplements

Some companies sell saw palmetto "berry" capsules at very low prices. Saw palmetto berries do not provide the standardized extracts needed for therapeutic benefits. What's surprising is that there are major name-brand supplement companies that sell both standardized saw palmetto extract and saw palmetto berry capsules. These commercial companies know there are no prostate benefits from taking saw palmetto berry capsules, but they sell them anyway just to offer a lower-priced product. The Life Extension Foundation believes it is immoral to sell a supplement whose name ("saw palmetto") implies therapeutic benefit, but which doesn't actually deliver such benefit.

The Life Extension Foundation has expended significant resources to develop a better understanding of prostate cell proliferation and how to control it. In 1998, Foundation members were introduced to a supercritical fluid extraction from saw palmetto that delivers a purer, more effective extract of the classic herb for BPH. Supercritical fluid extraction is a nontoxic state-of-the-art technology originally commercialized for the food, fragrance, and environmental industries. It is prized for extraction since it preserves the light aromatic notes and nuances of smell and taste far better than steam distillation or solvent extraction. In addition, it is environmentally friendly and produces an extract of extraordinary purity while leaving behind no solvent residues on the product.

The first medicinal herb to benefit from large-scale supercritical fluid extraction is saw palmetto. Clinical and experimental studies of supercritical fluid extracts of saw palmetto demonstrate some remarkable advantages. Since saw palmetto is thought to interfere with testosterone-induced growth of the prostate, researchers tested the effect of saw palmetto extracts on prostate weight in castrated rats given testosterone. The rats were divided into control and treatment groups and given placebo, testosterone, or testosterone plus saw palmetto extract for 10 days. The rats were then sacrificed and their prostate glands weighed. In the control groups, normal rats had an average prostate weight of 20.6 mg at the end of the experiment, while castrated rats given testosterone had nearly normal prostate weights averaging 17.4 mg. Castrated rats given placebo instead of testosterone had an average prostate weight of 3.0 mg. When a conventional hexane extract of saw palmetto was given to castrated rats along with testosterone, average prostate weight was reduced to 11.7 mg. However, when a supercritical fluid extract of saw palmetto was given (in the same dosage as the conventional extract) along with testosterone, average prostate weight dropped to 6.5 mg. Furthermore, the supercritical fluid extract given at half dosage reduced average prostate weight as effectively (to 11.9 mg) as the hexane extract at full dosage. These data were presented in a review article on saw palmetto in the European journal *Fitoterapia,* one of the oldest and best European botanical medicine journals, with an international roster of contributors in each issue.

One mechanism by which saw palmetto is thought to work is by inhibiting an enzyme called 5-alpha-reductase in the prostate gland. This enzyme converts testosterone to an active form called DHT (dihydrotestosterone) that stimulates growth in prostatic tissue. A study published in a German urology journal tested the ability of the supercritical fluid extract of saw palmetto to inhibit this enzyme. The researchers concluded that the extract is a strong inhibitor of 5-alpha-reductase.

Saw palmetto also exerts an anti-inflammatory effect on prostate tissue. Research published in a German pharmaceutical journal demonstrates that the supercritical fluid extract of saw palmetto strongly inhibits the pro-inflammatory arachidonic acid cascade. They showed that the extract provides dual inhibition of the cyclooxygenase pathway and the 5-lipoxygenase pathway.

A large observational study in Germany followed 2000 BPH patients given a standard dosage of the supercritical fluid extract (160 mg capsules twice a day) for 3 to 6 months. Three fourths of the patients had stage II BPH, while the remainder had stage III disease. The main variable studied, residual urine, declined on average from 80 to 45 mL. Patients without severe symptoms of dysuria (painful or difficult urination) increased from 24.9 to 62.5%. Eighty-eight percent of patients subjectively evaluated the treatment as very good or good. Two to four percent of patients reported side effects, mostly mild gastrointestinal disturbances.

A well-designed European clinical trial compared two dose schedules for the supercritical fluid extract, the standard twice-a-day schedule, and a new once-a-day schedule. Eighty-four BPH patients with maximum urine flow between 5 and 15 mL/sec participated, with 67 patients completing the 1-year study. Patients were randomly assigned to a group given the standard 160-mg capsule twice a day, or to a group given one 320-mg capsule in the morning and a placebo capsule in the evening. The study found the two dose schedules to be equally safe and effective overall. In both groups, symptom scores on the IPSS scale dropped by about 60%, and maximum urinary flow rate increased by about 22%. Patients in each group reported adverse effects; in three quarters of these cases the physician judged the complaint to be a consequence of BPH itself rather than of the medication. Two patients in each group withdrew from the study due to side effects. The medication was well-tolerated by the remaining patients.

The supercritical fluid extract of saw palmetto is available in one-a-day capsules, giving men an equally convenient alternative to the drug finasteride (Proscar). Finasteride, a drug approved to treat for BPH, is normally taken once a day. Finasteride causes diminished libido and sexual dysfunctions in some patients; in particular, about 3 to 4% of patients experience impotence. Clinical physicians using Proscar have told the Foundation that libido normally returns within a few months in the small percentage of men whose sex drive is adversely affected by Proscar. By contrast, saw palmetto is very well tolerated and inexpensive. For men with especially large, overgrown prostate glands, Proscar may be considered in addition to phyto-extracts like saw palmetto.

Pygeum originally was shown to reduce prostate swelling (edema) and block dihydrotestosterone binding to prostate cells. New studies show that pygeum also interferes with protein kinase C activity to inhibit the proliferation of prostate cells. Rapidly growing benign and malignant cells both require the protein kinase C enzyme. Soy genistein is one of the most potent inhibitors of protein kinase C, a primary mechanism by which soy helps to prevent cancer and slows the growth of some existing cancers. Added to this herbal arsenal against enlarged prostate is the *Urtica dioica* (nettle) extract that interferes with the binding of estrogen to prostate cells.

In January 1998, the Life Extension Foundation introduced Americans to the identical *Urtica dioica* extract used in Germany to treat benign prostate enlargement. The urtica extract comes in an herbal formula that also contains pharmaceutical extracts of saw palmetto and pygeum.

This standardized herbal formula, called Natural Prostate Formula, is one of the most popular supplements used in the United States by BPH patients. Since it is not classified as a "drug," it costs far less than its European "drug" counterparts and is less expensive than FDA-approved drugs like Proscar.

Other Natural Therapies

Based upon records of dietary soy consumption in Japan, where prostate cancer rates are very low, the typical daily isoflavone intake has been estimated at 50 mg a person. By contrast, the typical Western diet has been estimated to provide only 2 to 3 mg a day of genistein. Soy phytoestrogens such as genistein may counteract some of the effects of dihydrotestosterone, and therefore may be helpful in treating benign prostate enlargement.

A soy supplement called Mega Soy Extract provides 110 mg of soy phytoestrogens in just 2 capsules, more than twice the amount in the typical Japanese diet. Since the phytoestrogen genistein is water-soluble, it is suggested that 1 capsule of Mega Soy Extract be taken in the morning and 1 in the evening.

Scientists have published papers indicating that the consumption of soy phytoestrogens may significantly reduce prostate cancer risk. Since men with benign prostate disease are at a greater risk for eventually developing prostate cancer, the use of high-potency soy supplements is highly recommended.

Using Aromatase-Inhibiting Drugs

A novel approach to treating severe BPH is to inhibit the amount of estrogen in a man's body by using an aromatase-inhibiting drug. As men age, they often produce too much aromatase enzyme that causes testosterone, DHEA, and other sex steroid hormones to be "aromatized" (converted) into estrogen. Estrogen can be a prime culprit leading to prostate cell proliferation in men, and preliminary studies show that suppressing estrogen levels by inhibiting the aromatase enzyme may be an effective therapy.

A study published in the Austrian journal *Wien Klin. Wochenschr.* (1998 Dec 11; 110(23): 817–23) is summarized as follows:

> Estrogen suppression has been introduced as a therapeutic strategy in the medical treatment of benign prostatic hyperplasia. Recent negative results obtained in placebo-controlled trials with the aromatase inhibitor atamestane raised doubts about the efficacy of estrogen reduction. However, inhibition of aromatase not only reduces estrogens but also increases androgens (DHT), which may promote prostatic growth. In order to reevaluate the therapeutic efficacy of estrogen suppression, we summarize clinical trials investigating the therapeutic effects of mepartricin in the treatment of uncomplicated benign prostatic hyperplasia. Mepartricin has been reported to lower the levels of circulating estrogens without causing changes in other hormones such as androgens. By applying stringent inclusion criteria, 23 studies (including 7 placebo-controlled trials, 3 post-marketing surveillance studies, and 13 open trials) published between 1982 and 1996 were selected to be included in this report. In 79.9% of 4635 patients treated with mepartricin, its therapeutic effect was rated "good" or "excellent." In 6 out of 7 placebo-controlled trials, the therapeutic efficacy of mepartricin was significantly superior to that of placebo. Comparison of these data with results obtained with alpha-1-adrenoceptor antagonists or with the 5-alpha-reductase inhibitor finasteride indicates that mepartricin is as efficient as these widely accepted medical treatments for benign prostatic hyperplasia. Since mepartricin acts selectively upon estrogens, the present results show that estrogen suppression may be considered an efficient pharmacotherapeutic strategy in the medical treatment of uncomplicated benign prostatic hyperplasia.

The drug mepartricin is not yet approved in the United States, but a rational strategy might be to use an approved aromatase inhibitor such as Arimidex in the low dose of 0.5 mg twice a week. In order to block the increase in DHT production that would most likely occur, 5 mg of Proscar taken every day or every other day should suppress excess formation of DHT, while enabling the Arimidex to eradicate over-production of estrogen. This dual effect of suppressing excess DHT and estrogen may result in significant clinical improvement and address the underlying cause of most cases of severe BPH. Side effects of Arimidex and Proscar are minimal if therapeutic results are obtained. The Male Hormone Modulation protocol provides a scientific rationale for a multitude of health benefits aging men can expect if they suppress excess estrogen and DHT levels.

Another study published in the *International Journal of Andrology* evaluated eight beagles with benign prostatic hypertrophy (BPH) treated by drugs that suppressed both estrogen and testosterone. The results showed that mean prostatic volume decreased to 56% of the pretreatment value. Histological examination of the prostate 1 week after treatment revealed reduction in diameter of the alveoli and in the height of the glandular epithelium. Degeneration and atrophy of the glands were marked 4 to 12 weeks after treatment. After treatment, levels of testosterone and estrogen were lower than before treatment. The results of this study indicate that suppression of estrogen and testosterone brings about resolution of the clinical signs and marked reduction in prostatic volume within 1 week of treatment. Since maintaining free testosterone is so important in maintaining the health and well-being in aging men, the rationale for using a drug to suppress estrogen and DHT (instead of testosterone) might be a more tolerable long-term treatment strategy. Remember, testosterone produces its most profound effect on prostate enlargement by converting to the far more potent prostate cell–proliferating metabolite DHT.

Clearly, more research is needed, but this relatively safe approach using an aromatase-inhibiting drug along with a potent DHT-blocking drug like Proscar may be considered in BPH patients who want to avoid mutilating surgery. (*Refer to the Male Hormone Modulation Therapy protocol for complete details on correcting estrogen and testosterone imbalance problems.*)

Recommended Blood Testing

Since men with benign prostate growth are at an increased risk of developing prostate cancer, the PSA and free-PSA blood tests should be considered every 6 months. The free-PSA test helps to determine if a moderately elevated PSA (with levels of 2.6 to 10) is indicative of early-stage prostate cancer. Testing for excess estrogen is also important in identifying the underlying cause of BPH. (*Again, please refer to the Male Hormone Modulation Therapy protocol for complete information on testing the blood for estrogen.*)

Summary

Enlargement of the prostate gland, which occurs in most men with advancing age, is accompanied by reduced urinary flow and increased residual urine volume. Hormonal imbalances are known to be a major cause of age-related prostate disorders.

Here is a step-by-step program to treat symptoms of BPH:

1. First of all, rule out prostate cancer by having a blood PSA test and a digital rectal exam.
2. Next, have your urologist evaluate the size of your prostate gland. A severely overgrown prostate gland may benefit from 5 mg of Proscar every day or every other day in addition to phytotherapies such as saw palmetto, pygeum, and nettle extracts.
3. Most men will experience significant alleviation of symptoms of BPH by using saw palmetto extract by itself, or in combination with pygeum or nettle extract. The precise doses used in the successful clinical studies have been combined into a single formula called Natural Prostate Formula. Suggested dose of Natural Prostate Formula is 1 capsule taken every 12 hours.
4. If severe symptoms of BPH persist, consider aromatase-inhibiting therapy to suppress excess serum estrogen that may be a primary factor in the development and progression of the disease. Arimidex in the low dose of just 0.5 mg, twice a week, usually produces a dramatic and immediate reduction in serum estrogen.
5. Mega Soy therapy in the dose of 135 mg, twice a day, is suggested to help block estrogen receptor sites in prostate cells.
6. If all else fails and urinary blockage manifests, BPH patients may have no choice but to undergo the transurethral resection procedure that involves the insertion of a "roto-rooter" device to literally grind away and remove excess prostate overgrowth. Some men undergo an outpatient procedure and experience little discomfort, while other men encounter pain and other long-term effects. Even after transurethral resection surgery, the proper use of phyto-extracts and/or drugs can help keep the prostate gland from over-growing again.

WARNING: *Men with early-stage prostate cancer manifesting a benign prostate disease should refer to the Foundation's Prostate Cancer: Early Stage protocol.*

Product availability. Saw palmetto extract, Mega Soy Extract, Natural Prostate Formula, and saw palmetto/pygeum extract are available by calling (800) 544-4440, or order online at www.lef.org. Arimidex and Proscar must be prescribed by your doctor.

PULMONARY INSUFFICIENCIES

(See Emphysema)

RAYNAUD'S SYNDROME

Raynaud's syndrome, first described in 1862 by French physician Maurice Raynaud, has no known cause or cure. The syndrome is a condition in which small arteries, most commonly in the fingers and toes, go into spasm and cause the skin to turn pale or a patchy red to blue. Estimates of its prevalence range from 5 to 30% of the population. It is 5 times more common in women, often striking females between the ages of 18 and 30. It is thought that 25 to 30% of cases occur in otherwise healthy women.

Treatments range widely, from behavioral changes to prescription drugs, but none is completely satisfactory. In fact, conventional medical therapies for this condition are characterized by their low efficacy and high incidence of unpleasant side effects. Although Raynaud's is usually a mild condition, it can have serious direct consequences, such as gangrene serious enough to warrant amputation, that can be avoided by controlling the condition as much as possible. In fact, a recent study from Johns Hopkins found that Raynaud's doubles the risk of coronary artery disease and stroke. For these reasons, the Life Extension Foundation has developed this protocol to offer helpful information, tips for preventing attacks, and alternative therapies.

Definitions

Raynaud's syndrome. Any form of Raynaud's.

Raynaud's disease. When Raynaud's symptoms appear alone without any other medical condition, it is called Raynaud's disease. This is also termed primary Raynaud's. In this condition, the blood vessels return to normal afterwards. Primary Raynaud's usually affects both hands and feet.

Raynaud's phenomenon. When Raynaud's symptoms have a specific cause or are accompanied by another disease, it is called Raynaud's phenomenon, or secondary Raynaud's. This condition, which more often affects either hands or feet, is often more serious and may result in blood vessel scarring and long-term consequences.

Occupational Raynaud's. Raynaud's symptoms may be caused by repetitive activities or using vibrating tools.

Symptoms

Diagnosis of Raynaud's requires no special tests, although tests such as nailfold capillaroscopy (examining the nailfold under magnification to see capillary changes indicative of connective tissue disease), cold stimulation (submerging the hands in ice and timing the return of normal color), or vascular laboratory assessment may be used to determine the severity of the disease. Although the severity, duration, and frequency of attacks vary both between individuals and over time, the primary symptoms of Raynaud's syndrome are:

Changes in skin color. Fingers and sometimes toes turn white, then blue, then red. The tip of the nose and the earlobes and, rarely, the cheeks or chin can also be affected. Sometimes the fingers perspire.

Pain. Numbness accompanies the white and blue phases. The red phase brings a burning, throbbing, or tingling sensation and sometimes swelling.

Sudden, brief attacks. The characteristic skin changes can occur in as little as 3 minutes; episodes usually last from 5 minutes to an hour.

These symptoms are caused by vasospasm, or spasm of the small vessels that supply blood to these areas of the body. Contraction of the blood vessels of the extremities (arms/hands and legs/feet) is a normal physiological response to low temperatures, helping the body conserve heat. In Raynaud's syndrome, nerve receptors in the extremities are overly sensitive to even the faint chill produced by opening a refrigerator door, causing a spasmodic constriction of the small arteries in the fingers and perhaps the toes. The white phase indicates total blood deprivation, progressing to the blue phase—limited blood flow—and finally the red phase, a sudden infusion of oxygenated blood. Damage to the tissue due to lack of oxygen during the cessation of blood flow can result in a vicious cycle of cause and effect. Attacks are precipitated by coldness and stress.

Frequently, Raynaud's syndrome is a mild but maddening condition. It may remain dormant for years, only to resurface suddenly in response to infection, fatigue, or stress. If the condition progresses, permanently decreased blood flow to the affected area can cause fingers to become thin and tapered, with smooth, shiny skin and slow-growing nails. Ordinarily its most serious consequence is a loss of sensitivity in the affected extremity. However, more severe cases can result in tissue death and possibly finger deformity, skin ulceration, or gangrene, a serious infection that occurs in tissue deprived of oxygen. Raynaud's can also affect the lungs. In this case, breathing cold air triggers a coughing attack. A recent review of knowledge about Raynaud's stated that the vasospasm found in the fingers can also affect the heart and kidneys.

In addition, Raynaud's syndrome is associated with problems with the nerves supplying muscles; pulmonary hypertension, which raises the blood pressure in the vessels of the lungs; diseases of the arteries, such as Buerger's disease and atherosclerosis (in people over 60); and autoimmune diseases, such as rheumatoid arthritis (a chronic inflammation and swelling of tissue in the joints), systemic lupus erythematosus (a chronic inflammation of the skin and organ systems), and scleroderma. Raynaud's can also be caused by hypothyroidism, whether isolated or affiliated with scleroderma. Treatment with supplemental thyroid hormones, sometimes used to treat hypothyroidism, has been shown in recent studies to resolve the Raynaud's. Because of the association of Raynaud's with other serious diseases, it is critical to consult a physician within the first year after developing the symptoms. A recent study found that 48% of patients with primary Raynaud's showed one or more clinical features indicating a fairly high risk of evolving into fully established systemic sclerosis (scleroderma).

Raynaud's is most frequently associated with scleroderma, a disease causing diffuse hardening of the skin and other tissues. One multicenter observational study found that 29% of patients with secondary Raynaud's had scleroderma, 7% lupus, and 5% rheumatoid arthritis. It is often the first symptom of scleroderma, and may precede onset of the disease by months or years. Over 95% of people with scleroderma have Raynaud's phenomenon, but only a small percentage of those with Raynaud's will develop scleroderma. Symptoms to watch for include gradual hardening and tightening of the skin, joint stiffness or pain, digestive difficulties, sores over the joints, and puffy hands and feet, particularly in the morning. Scleroderma is a serious disease that must be medically managed; early diagnosis is critical to postpone organ involvement (*please refer to the Scleroderma protocol*).

Preventing Attacks: Behavioral Strategies

Although Raynaud's cannot be cured, there are ways to minimize the number of attacks and protect the skin from lasting injury.

Keep warm. Remember that changes in temperature are worse than cold alone. Keeping your head and torso warm frees up blood that can be used to heat the extremities. Always dress in loose layers of blended fabrics, including a sweater. Silk long underwear is a good way to protect yourself against chills without overheating yourself. Wear socks (cotton over wool) and mittens to bed; use an electric blanket, and turn it on before you get into bed to warm your sheets. Be sure to wear a warm hat, and perhaps earmuffs, since most body heat escapes through the head. If you are going to be outside, try chemical "heaters" in your socks and mittens. Always cover exposed skin, including nose and cheeks if it is cold and windy; if you are in pain, consider it a warning signal from your body and go inside. Don't get wet, because water cools the skin as it evaporates (the same is true for sweat—wear an underlayer to wick away moisture). Be prepared for changes in your environment by carrying a bag of clothing with you, and keep one in your car and workplace. Ask friends and family for help, and modify your surroundings to minimize your exposure to cold. Have someone else defrost your refrigerator, or buy a frost-free model. Park your car in a protected area, and ask someone to start it and crank up the heater 15 minutes before you go out. Drink warm beverages. A hot-water bottle is useful, especially on car trips. Consider moving to a warmer climate.

Protect your hands from the cold. Mittens are far more effective at keeping your hands warm than gloves, since they pool the heat from the entire hand. Wear mittens whenever possible, especially when handling cold or frozen food, and carry them with you; also wear "wristlets", which close the gap between the sleeve and the mitten. Damp cold is the most likely to precipitate an attack. Never clean vegetables under cool running water. Use warm water or, better yet, take advantage of the prepared vegetables available in produce departments. Start running your bath or shower ahead of time so that you don't touch cold water. Make sure your hose doesn't leak. Use insulated cup holders for cold beverages, and use straws. Don't hang out wet clothes or shovel snow.

Avoid substances that make you vulnerable to chills. Smoking is a risk factor, since nicotine constricts blood vessels. If you smoke, quit. Avoid second-hand smoke. Caffeine is also a vasoconstrictor, and is found in many hidden sources, such as chocolate, some aspirin preparations, teas, and medications. Birth control pills, most over-the-counter decongestants, cold remedies, and diet pills should also be avoided. Some migraine headache and heart and blood medications may also cause Raynaud's symptoms.

Take good care of your skin. Use cream to keep your hands soft and protect them with gloves when using detergent or harsh chemicals or gardening. Keep fingers and toes dry with talcum powder. Be careful not to injure the skin in affected areas, and treat injuries without delay. Even minor cuts and scrapes take longer to heal and may be more susceptible to infection when circulation is impaired. Call your health care provider if the affected body part develops an infection or ulceration.

Find ways to reduce your stress levels. Since stress is a common precipitating factor, many people benefit from relaxation techniques, such as visual imaging, meditation, or massage. Find some time to relax every day, even if only for a few minutes. Avoid whatever stressors you can, and attempt to minimize stress on your job.

Avoid precipitating activities Episodes can also be brought on by operating vibrating equipment (chainsaw, jackhammer, drill), including the vacuum cleaner (wearing oven mitts can reduce the vibrations), or by repetitive hand motions (typing, playing the piano or guitar, sewing, chopping and dicing food). Don't carry heavy shopping bags with handles, which can restrict blood flow to your fingers.

Improve your circulation. Regular movement and exercise help to keep your skin flexible and maintain better circulation both by improving cardiovascular fitness and by stimulating blood flow. A warm bath for 20 minutes before bed each night can improve your circulation.

Specific Physical Therapies

Rewarming. When you have an attack, try to stay calm. Gently rewarm your fingers and toes as soon as you can using the following strategies. The sooner you respond, the easier it will be to restore circulation and the less chance of damage there will be. Just one prolonged instance of Raynaud's can lead to tissue death, gangrene, and possibly a need for amputation, so consider each attack an emergency and respond immediately. Try motion first (because you can do this instantly and perhaps avert the need for further measures), then moist heat. Always be prepared with a variety of rewarming strategies appropriate to the different environments you spend your time in.

- Place your hands under your armpits or between your legs. Cup your mouth and breathe into them. Have someone hold your hands (but not rub them, which can do damage).
- Wiggle your fingers or toes.
- Move or walk around to improve circulation.
- Do "windmills" by twirling your arms around in the air in large circles until circulation returns. If you're worried about causing a public scene, go into the restroom.

CAUTION: Do not do windmills if you have damaged vessels due to scleroderma.

- Run warm, not hot, water over the affected part until normal color returns—remember that moist heat is better than dry heat.
- Do not bang your hands or rub them vigorously, which might damage blood vessels.
- Do not overheat your hands, which will also shut down blood vessels and prolong the attack.

Biofeedback. Using biofeedback, people can "teach" their blood vessels to relax. One form of biofeedback is simply "thinking" your hands warm. Another is more specific. Starting in a warm room, place your hands in a warm bowl of water for 5 minutes, then move to a cold room or outdoors and again place your hands in warm water, this time for 10 minutes. Repeat the procedure several times a day for as many days as necessary to produce a conditioned reflex that is the opposite of the normal one: when exposed to cold, the blood vessels in the fingers will open up rather than close down, without the aid of warm water. The efficacy of biofeedback has been documented by many scientific studies. A recent study determined that biofeedback subjects showed significant elevations in finger blood flow, finger temperature, and skin conductance level, suggesting an active vasodilating mechanism that goes beyond generalized relaxation. Other studies have found that symptomatic improvement was maintained 9 weeks, 1 year, and even 3 years after the start of training. Biofeedback is generally not as effective for Raynaud's phenomenon as for primary Raynaud's and may not work as well for foot warming.

Heatsocks. Heatsocks are tubes of fabric filled with grain that can be warmed in the microwave and applied to affected areas. "Heat wheat" mitts are commercially available. You can make your own by filling a sock with heavy rice and heating it in the microwave for about 3 minutes. The heat will last around 3 hours.

Paraffin treatments. Regular paraffin (hot wax) treatments can be helpful, but caution must be exercised. Use only physician-prescribed hot wax units, since using wax that is too hot will damage already delicate blood vessels. Never heat wax on the stove or in crock pots. A physical or occupational hand therapist can train you in the proper procedure.

Pharmacological and Nutrient Therapies

Pharmacological treatments for Raynaud's syndrome have limited efficacy and unpleasant side effects.

Calcium channel blockers. Drugs that block the calcium channels found in blood vessels have traditionally been the first choice of prescription medications used to treat Raynaud's syndrome. Nifedipine is considered the standard. These drugs block the calcium channels in the smooth muscle of vessel walls, thereby preventing contraction. Side effects are frequent and include dizziness, headaches, nausea, feelings of warmth or flushing, ankle-swelling, constipation, and an increase in symptoms of heartburn, which may subside once the body becomes used to the drug. Long-acting preparations may minimize these side effects. Other blockers, such as diltiazem, have fewer side effects but are less effective.

Vasodilators and pentoxifylline. Drugs that work to dilate blood vessels (reserpine, guanethidine) would seem to be helpful in treating Raynaud's, but according to a recent review in a major American medical journal, they usually do not produce complete relief. In addition, the review reports that full benefit is often prevented by unpleasant and sometimes severe side effects. These drugs are considered second-tier choices. Both can enhance circulation: alpha-adrenergic blockers by dilating blood vessels, and pentoxifylline through an unclear mechanism that improves disorders in the circulation of the very small blood vessels such as capillaries where vasodilators have limited effect.

Antiplatelet agents. Platelets clump together to form clots, inhibiting circulation; antiplatelet agents prevent this. Dipyridamole is a prescription drug. Low-dose aspirin is also a highly effective antiplatelet agent. Take one Healthprin tablet (81 mg) a day.

New drugs. Recently, several new pharmacological therapies are being studied for effectiveness on Raynaud's syndrome, including Iloprost (stable prostacyclin), piracetam, Ketanserin (S2-serotonergic antagonist), and dazoxiben (thromboxane synthetase inhibitor). Although prostaglandin E1 and prostacyclin have been successfully used to treat Raynaud's, they are unstable and require intravenous administration (reserved for emergencies). Oral Iloprost was proven ineffective for Raynaud's phenomenon in scleroderma patients in a recent scientific study, although it has been reported as beneficial by patients, including those unresponsive to other treatments. Another route to increasing the levels of these beneficial molecules is to stimulate the body's own production using evening primrose oil (see below). Piracetam is a drug used in Europe whose therapeutic efficacy has been experimentally established. It has a unique dual mode of action: inhibition of platelet function by inhibition of thromboxane synthetase or antagonism of thromboxane and increasing cell membrane deformability and decreasing plasma concentrations of clotting factors. Piracetam appears to be devoid of adverse effects.

Nitroglycerine cream. Nitroglycerine dilates blood vessels, but must be used sparingly.

Nutrient Supplements

Nutrient supplements exert comparable preventive effects without side effects and at the same time improve overall health. Supplements important for Raynaud's sufferers include the following:

Vitamin E. Vitamin E (along with vitamin C) is the key antioxidant in the body, protecting polyunsaturated fatty acids from oxidation. Red blood cell membranes are especially rich in these fatty acids; therefore, vitamin E stabilizes red blood cells and maximizes their efficacy in carrying oxygen to the tissues. A recently published article argued that autoimmune diseases result from hydrolytic enzymes that escape from lysosomes (cellular organelles that digest waste) whose membranes have been damaged by oxidation. These enzymes denature (destroy) proteins to the point that they are viewed as foreign objects by the body's defenses. Vitamin E deficiency was proposed as the root cause of the damage to the lysosomal membranes. Vitamin E has also been found to have direct therapeutic effects. For example, a recent clinical trial stated that vitamin E was a "curative agent" for patients with occupational Raynaud's. Take 800 international units (IUs) of vitamin E a day as two divided doses.

Vitamin C. Vitamin C plays a key role in the synthesis of collagen, which is the key component in the walls of blood vessels. Vitamin C is therefore essential to ensure that the small arteries that supply the fingers do not become damaged during Raynaud's attacks. In addition, vitamin C is important in the synthesis of prostaglandin E1—a hormone-like unsaturated fatty acid that acts on the smooth muscle of small arteries and decreases platelet aggregation—which has been accepted as one of the most effective treatments for emergency cases of Raynaud's. Vitamin C deficiency was found to predispose toward irreversible injury in a recent study of Raynaud's patients. Research suggests that 500 mg of vitamin C a day is effective.

Other vitamins. The vitamins supplied by the Life Extension Mix, including vitamins B_6, D, and E and riboflavin and pantothenic acid, aid in the adrenal gland's ability to handle stress. This will positively impact Raynaud's, which is triggered by stress. Take three tablets of Life Extension Mix 3 times a day.

Inositol nicotinate or nicotinic acid. These are forms of niacin (vitamin B_3), which directly relaxes the smooth muscle in blood vessels. A recent experimental evaluation of the usefulness of inositol nicotinate in treating Raynaud's concluded that it produced beneficial therapeutic effects on the microcirculation not only through vasodilation, but also through mechanisms such as enhanced fibrinolysis (clot breakup) and lowering of lipids (fats) in the blood. Moreover, the researchers noted a lack of side effects and contrasted it with standard drug treatments. Another study agreed that long-term treatment with nicotinate acid derivatives may improve peripheral circulation through a different effect from the one detected by short-term studies. A variety of other research groups have documented statistically significant improvement in symptoms and reduction in frequency of Raynaud's attacks with inositol nicotinate. Depending on your sensitivity, nicotinic acid may cause flushing, the result of a harmless, temporary release of histamine, at doses as low as 50 to 75 mg. Some people like the sensation; others find it uncomfortable. It lasts 20 to 30 minutes. Doctors recommend staying at the lowest dose that relieves your symptoms and going no higher than 200 to 300 mg a day without medical supervision. Inositol nicotinate, at doses of 1500 to 4000 mg, which does not cause flushing, should be taken daily as three or four divided doses. Be aware that niacin is destroyed by excessive sugar, alcohol, sulfa drugs, and the antibiotic chloramphenicol.

CAUTION: Niacin has been known to cause liver damage in high doses. If you have liver disease, do not take high doses of niacin without medical supervision.

Magnesium and calcium. Adequate calcium and magnesium are essential to maintain relaxation of the smooth muscle of the small arteries affected by Raynaud's. In addition, the requirement for magnesium increases with psychological or physical stress, which in turn is associated with Raynaud's episodes. Take 500 mg of each a day. The Life Extension Foundation offers calcium citrate capsules (220 mg), Bone Assure (1000 mg calcium, 320 mg magnesium plus a host of other nutrients in 6 capsules), and Ultramag, which contains the different forms of magnesium (400 mg in 2 tablets).

Gamma-linolenic acid (GLA). GLA is an essential fatty acid found in primrose, borage, or black currant oils important for relaxing smooth muscles because it is the precursor for prostaglandin E1. A recent scientific study found that 12 capsules a day of primrose oil dramatically decreased the number of Raynaud's attacks, and blood tests showed some antiplatelet (blood thinning) activity. A typical daily dose of GLA is about 1500 mg. The Life Extension Foundation suggests that the optimal dose of GLA be obtained by taking five MEGA GLA (borage oil) capsules a day.

Omega-3 and omega-6 oils. Flax and fish oils contain essential polyunsaturated fatty acids, known as omega-3 and omega-6 fatty acids, that have been shown to lower serum triglycerides (fats) and decrease platelet aggregation (thin the blood). Research has demonstrated that fish oils inhibit arachidonic acid metabolism, which makes them useful in the treatment of autoimmune diseases like those associated with Raynaud's. One recent study found that a higher percentage of patients given fish oils reported clinical improvement in a variety of symptoms, including Raynaud's, in comparison to a control group. A significant decrease in laboratory values that reflect autoimmune disturbances (cryocrit and rheumatoid factor) was also observed. Another recent clinical study found that ingesting fish oil increased the median time (especially in those patients with primary Raynaud's) before the onset of Raynaud's after exposure to cold. Moreover, fish oil improved tolerance to cold exposure, as evidenced by significantly increased blood pressures in the fingers, and almost half of the patients in the fish oil group did not exhibit Raynaud's in response to cold water baths. The Foundation recommends that fish, flax, or perilla oil be taken in doses ranging from 4,000 to 8,000 mg a day.

Ginkgo biloba. This well-tolerated plant extract has been proven to stimulate circulation in the small blood vessels in addition to its other benefits. Take 120 mg once a day.

Summary

Raynaud's syndrome is a fairly common condition caused by spasms in the blood vessels supplying the fingers and toes. These spasms are brought on by cold or stress. Although maddening, it is usually mild but can have serious consequences, such as tissue death or gangrene, if not tended to. The best treatment for Raynaud's is prevention through behavioral strategies, including keeping yourself warm at all times, protecting your hands from any cold, and avoiding precipitating factors such as certain activities, substances, and stress.

1. Given the association of Raynaud's syndrome with serious diseases, consult a physician upon developing the symptoms.
2. Prevent attacks by adopting the behavioral strategies outlined above to keep yourself warm and protect your hands from the cold. Reduce stress and avoid precipitating substances and activities.
3. Respond immediately to every attack with motion and moist heat.
4. Use biofeedback to train your blood vessels to relax.
5. Take 800 IU of vitamin E a day as two divided doses.
    - Take 500 mg of vitamin C a day.
    - Take the lowest dose of nicotinic acid that relieves your symptoms, going no higher than 200 to 300 mg a day without medical supervision. 1500 to 4000 mg of inositol nicotinate, which does not cause flushing, should be taken daily as 3 or 4 divided doses.

CAUTION: Niacin has been known to damage liver in high doses. If you have liver disease, do not take high doses of niacin without medical supervision.

6. Take 500 mg of magnesium and calcium a day: calcium citrate (2 capsules a day) and Ultramag (1 to 2 tablets a day) or Bone Assure (6 capsules a day) plus extra magnesium.
7. Take 1500 mg of GLA a day from borage oil.
8. Take 4000 to 8000 mg of omega-3 fatty acids from fish, flax, or perilla oils.
9. Take 120 mg of ginkgo biloba extract once a day.
10. Take 1 Healthprin tablet (81 mg) a day with the heaviest meal.
11. Take 3 tablets of Life Extension Mix 3 times a day.

For unresponsive cases, consult your physician regarding pharmacological therapies.

Consult your physician regarding any progression in your condition, any alterations in your health, and any infections or injuries in affected areas to prevent serious consequences.

Product availability. Vitamin E, vitamin C, niacin tablets, inositol nicotinate, calcium citrate tablets, Bone Assure, Ultramag, borage oil, flax seed oil, fish oil, ginkgo biloba extract, Healthprin tablets, and Life Extension Mix are available from the Life Extension Buyers' Club by calling (800) 544-4440, or order on-line at www.lef.org.

RETINOPATHY

Diabetic retinopathy (DR), the leading cause of visual disability and blindness among adults in the developed world, may affect as many as 20 million people. Early detection and treatment are keys to preventing the vision loss and blindness associated with the disease. Unfortunately, only about half of those suffering from diabetes have proper eye examinations on a yearly basis. It is very important that diabetics have a dilated eye exam each year.

Retinopathy damages the retina by destroying the capillaries (minuscule blood vessels connecting arteries and veins) that provide blood to the retina, the light-sensitive nerve tissue that sends visual images to the brain. With the onset of retinopathy, these vessels weaken or bulge with microaneurysms that may hemorrhage, leaking blood or fluid into surrounding tissue. When new blood vessels grow on the retina (and into the vitreous), they can cause blurred vision and even temporary blindness. The real danger lies in the scar tissue that ultimately forms, detaching the retina from the back of the eye and often causing permanent loss of vision.

Chronic elevated blood glucose levels induce retinopathy. Unfortunately, even careful control of blood glucose does not always prevent the onset of the disease. There are additional precautions that can be taken to guard against the development of retinopathies. Deficiency of vitamin B_6, for instance, is a proven cause of the disease. In order to rule out a nutritional deficiency as the cause of retinopathy, a 10-week program is suggested that incorporates a high-potency B-complex vitamin formula along with other supplements that will be described in this protocol.

An Interesting Rat Study

A newborn rat model of retinopathy was used to test the hypothesis that a lack of the antioxidant superoxide dismutase (SOD) contributes to retinal damage. The study concluded that delivery of SOD to the retina via long-circulating liposomes was beneficial and suggested the potential value of the restoration or supplementation of antioxidants in retinal tissue as a therapeutic strategy. It is difficult to provide SOD directly to the retina, but adequate supplementation with nutrients such as zinc, copper, and manganese provide the minerals needed for the formation of SOD in the cells.

Antioxidant Lens and Vitreous Activity

Another study investigated antioxidant activity in the lens and vitreous of diabetic and nondiabetic subjects. Researchers found significantly decreased glutathione peroxidase activity and lower ascorbic acid levels in the lenses of diabetic patients, especially in the presence of retinal damage. (Ascorbic acid is known to exert important antioxidant functions in the eye compartment.) This study indicated that oxidative damage is involved in the onset of diabetic eye complications, in which the decrease in free radical scavengers was shown to be associated with the oxidation of vitreous and lens proteins.

Decreased Retinal Antioxidant Activity in Diabetics

Activities of enzymes that protect the retina from reactive oxygen species were investigated in diabetic rats known to have developed retinopathy. Diabetes significantly decreased the activities of glutathione reductase and glutathione peroxidase in the retina. Activities of two other important antioxidant defense enzymes—superoxide dismutase and catalase—were also decreased (by more than 25%) in the retinas of diabetic rats.

The study showed that diabetes is associated with significant impairment of the antioxidant defense system, and that antioxidant supplementation can help alleviate the subnormal activities of antioxidant defense enzymes. Administration of supplemental vitamins C and E for 2 months prevented the diabetes-induced impairment of the antioxidant defense system in the retina. Another study found no protective effect from antioxidant nutrients for diabetic retinopathy and concluded that further research is necessary to confirm associations of nutrient antioxidant intake and the disease.

Retinopathy of Prematurity

A recent study assessed retinopathy in 60 oxygen-treated premature infants and in their mothers. All 60 infants showed signs of acute oxidative stress. The concentrations of methionine-cysteine in the plasma, as well as blood selenium levels, were significantly lower in the premature infants suffering from moderate retinopathy than they were in the oxygen-treated premature infants without retinopathy. The mothers of the premature infants with retinopathy showed the same pattern of deficiencies as their babies. Vitamin E treatment of premature infants seemed to have a positive effect against the development of retinopathy of prematurity.

The close correlation between the antioxidant capacity of the mothers and babies suggests that supplementation with sulfur-containing amino acids (methionine, cysteine) and folic acid during pregnancy might improve the antioxidant capacity of premature infants. An antioxidant cocktail of selenium plus vitamin E given to high-risk mothers (high risk factors include advanced age, smoking, and pregnancy-induced hypertension) before delivery might be useful in the prevention of retinopathy in premature infants.

The Role of *L*-Carnitine

Other research examined the effect of propionyl-*L*-carnitine, an analogue of *L*-carnitine, on retinopathy in rats with laboratory-induced diabetes. Findings pointed to a potential therapeutic value of propionyl-*L*-carnitine for diabetic retinopathy. Until propionyl-*L*-carnitine becomes commercially available, taking 2000 mg a day of acetyl-*L*-carnitine should be considered by those with retinopathy. (*L*-carnitine is a natural substance which is found in meat. It is related to the B vitamins.)

Glycation

Glycation (glycation) of proteins has been shown to play a prominent role in the development of many diseases related to diabetes, including atherosclerosis, cataract formation, and retinopathy. Glycation also occurs as a result of general aging. Researchers have explored the possibility of preventing glycation by the use of pyruvate and alpha-ketoglutarate. Studies have shown that both compounds are effective in preventing the initial glycation reaction and in preventing the formation of eye disease.

Pyruvate and alpha-ketoglutarate can also inhibit the generation of high-molecular weight aggregates associated with cataract formation. Preventive effects appear to be due to competitive inhibition of glycation by the keto acids and antioxidant properties of these compounds. These agents might be useful in preventing glycation-related protein changes and consequent tissue-pathological manifestations associated with cataract, diabetes, and normal aging.

Diabetics should consider taking 650 mg of ornithine alpha-ketoglutarate 3 times a day. The best form of pyruvate for oral use is calcium pyruvate. A 500-mg capsule of calcium pyruvate provides 405 mg of elemental pyruvic acid. The suggested dose of calcium pyruvate is one to three capsules a day. The formation of advanced glycation products and free radicals has been implicated in the development of diabetic complications. Strategies for the prevention of diabetic complications, therefore, should aim to prevent both the effects of glycation and oxidative stress.

A drug called aminoguanidine has been used successfully to protect against glycation. Compounds produced through metabolism of sugars bind preferentially to aminoguanidine rather than to lysine proteins. Thus, aminoguanidine is able to inhibit advanced glycation end-product (AGE) formation, and can help prevent the harmful development of collagen cross-links and changes in the proliferation of mesangial cells.

Aminoguanidine used in the dose of 300 mg a day can specifically inhibit glycation, as can the nutrients keto-glutarate and pyruvate. Studies have shown aminoguanidine to be useful in slowing complications of diabetes, such as retinopathy. (It can also inhibit the formation of atherosclerotic plaques.)

The Importance of Adequate Vitamin Status

Vitamin B_{12} (cyanocobalamin, or hydroxycobalamin, a naturally occurring form) is critical for several functions such as folate metabolism, myelin synthesis, and the normal development of red blood cells. A lack of this vitamin may leave the optic nerve more susceptible to damage. Studies have suggested that marginal vitamin deficiency plays an indirect but important role in the development of diabetic complications.

Beta-carotene, a powerful antioxidant that helps prevent eye lesions and blindness, may not be indicated for diabetic retinopathy. (Some natural sources for beta-carotene are apricots, broccoli, carrots, kale, oranges, tomatoes, peaches, pumpkins, spinach, and squash. Some herbalists derive carotenes from marigolds.)

One study showed that reducing lipid peroxidation stress of the erythrocyte membrane using vitamin E (alpha-tocopherol nicotinate) therapy may be useful in slowing deterioration of microangiopathy in type II diabetes mellitus. The dose used in the study was 300 mg 3 times a day, after meals, for 3 months.

A convenient way of obtaining all of the nutrients that may protect against the development and progression of retinopathy is a multi-nutrient formula called Life Extension Mix. The suggested dose of Life Extension Mix is three tablets, 3 times a day. A supplement to Life Extension Mix called Life Extension Booster provides in one capsule additional potencies of lutein, vitamin E, selenium, and other important nutrients to protect against retinopathy.

Conclusion

Retinopathy is the primary cause of blindness among adults in the developed world. Risk factors are diabetes (especially with elevated blood glucose levels), vitamin deficiency, the use of growth hormone, and old age. In retinopathy, the retina of the eye is damaged when retinal capillaries bulge or burst, leaking blood or fluid into the surrounding tissue. New capillaries which grow on the retina (and into the vitreous) cause blurred vision or blindness. Permanent blindness can result from retinal detachment caused by scar tissue. The use of antioxidants to treat the condition has not been proven at present, with more research needed for the medical community to reach a consensus. Prevention requires annual dilated eye exams and proper vitamin and nutrient intake. Researchers conclude that improved levels of antioxidants in pregnant women could help prevent retinopathy in their premature infants.

Summary

1. Symptoms of retinopathy are blurred or dimmed vision and temporary blindness.
2. Retinopathy is generally diagnosed using a dilated eye exam.
3. If you are diabetic, such an exam should be conducted once a year, especially for those with high risk factors.
4. Diabetics should consider taking 650 mg of ornithine alpha-ketoglutarate 3 times a day.
5. One to three 500-mg capsules a day is the suggested dose of calcium pyruvate.
6. A dose of 300 mg a day of the drug aminoguanidine can specifically inhibit glycation, as can keto-glutarate and pyruvate.
7. Taking 2000 mg a day of acetyl-*L*-carnitine should be considered by those suffering from retinopathy, particularly if on a vegetarian diet.
8. Long-term antioxidant protection of the eyes can be provided by taking three tablets, 3 times a day of Life Extension Mix and one capsule a day of the Life Extension Booster formula. Minerals for the formation of superoxide dismutase (SOD) such as zinc and manganese, along with potent B complex vitamins, are included in Life Extension Mix. Some people may need supplemental copper in the dose of 1 to 2 mg a day. Some people may also want to take additional vitamin B_6 (up to 250 additional milligrams).

For more information. Contact the National Eye Health Education Program of the National Institutes of Health, (301) 496-5248.

Product availability. Life Extension Mix, Life Extension Booster, acetyl-*L*-carnitine and OptiZinc™ can be ordered by calling (800) 544-4440, or order on-line at www.lef.org. (Ornithine alpha-ketoglutarate and calcium pyruvate are contained at recommended levels in the Life Extension Mix.) Ask for a list of European suppliers of aminoguanidine.

SCLERODERMA (SYSTEMIC SCLEROSIS)

Scleroderma, also known as systemic sclerosis, is a chronic, progressive, disabling autoimmune connective tissue disorder with various complex symptoms. A highly individualized disease, its involvement may range from very mild symptoms to life-threatening complications. Fourteen million people worldwide, 150,000 in the United States, suffer from scleroderma. It affects four times more women than men, with symptoms usually occurring between the ages of 35 and 65. Scleroderma is not contagious, cancerous, or considered malignant in any way. The 5-year fatality rate of those with the severe form (about 60,000) has been estimated at 50 to 70%. The cause of scleroderma is unknown, although it is known that the disease process in scleroderma involves an overproduction of collagen. This protocol will briefly survey the most recent information regarding the symptoms, the hypothetical causes, and conventional and integrated medical treatments for scleroderma.

A potentially life-threatening condition, scleroderma must be managed by a knowledgeable physician. Because it is fairly rare, one should seek out specialists in the types of symptoms caused by scleroderma—that is, dermatologists (skin), rheumatologists (joints and connective tissue), and dentists—who have specific experience with the disease. Although there is no known treatment that can stop or slow the progression of scleroderma, many physicians feel that early medical intervention yields better results and positively affects the course of the disease. Given the ineffectiveness of conventional treatments, many physicians take the position that patients might as well try any alternative treatments that could be of benefit and won't hurt them. It is imperative that your physician knows all therapies you are using, and that you be an active self-advocate, asking for specific information, educating yourself about your disease, and seeking support.

Definitions

Localized scleroderma. Considered the mild form of scleroderma, localized disease predominantly affects the skin. Although it may affect muscles and joints, it does not affect organs. It is very rare for localized disease to become systemic; if this occurs, the initial diagnosis was likely mistaken. Two common types are:

- **Linear scleroderma** is characterized by a line of hardened skin affecting the underlying tissues (muscles, bones). It usually occurs on the arms, legs, and forehead on one side of the body and is common in children.
- **Morphea** is characterized by patches of yellowish or ivory-colored rigid, dry skin that become hard, slightly depressed oval plaques. It usually occurs on the trunk, although it may be widespread (generalized morphea).

Systemic scleroderma. The systemic disease occurs throughout the body, affecting internal organs. It is progressive and can be life-threatening because it affects the connective tissue of the lung, kidney, heart, and other organs as well as blood vessels, muscles, and joints. The skin thickening for which the disease is named is symmetrical on both sides of the body, usually beginning on the fingertips and moving up the arms. Legs and thighs also are affected. Some common medical terms associated with systemic scleroderma are:

- **CREST** stands for calcinosis (small, movable, non-tender calcium lumps under the skin). CREST may occur alone or in combination with any autoimmune disease. There is no way to predict if or when it will progress to diffuse scleroderma.
- **Limited scleroderma** occurs on the hands and possibly on the face and neck.
- **Diffuse scleroderma** is defined as skin tightening above the wrists or elbows. Early thickening and hardening of the skin, sometimes preceded by itching, are present in 95% of patients, although skin involvement may not be prominent. More widespread disease can lead to severe organ damage.

Disease Symptoms

The diagnosis of scleroderma is a clinical one based on symptoms rather than tests. However, skin or kidney biopsies can be done to look for signs of the disease, and other investigations can be carried out to evaluate the function of different organ systems. Blood tests commonly reveal certain antibodies, which may have informative value beyond simply confirming the diagnosis. For example, although antinuclear antibodies are some common findings in many autoimmune diseases

S

(90% in scleroderma), *anti-topoisomerase-I antibodies* and *anticentromere antibodies* are unique to scleroderma. Anti-topoisomerase-I antibodies are found in patients with predominant fibrotic (as opposed to vascular) changes who have diffuse scleroderma. Anticentromere antibodies are found in 90% of people with limited scleroderma, especially CREST, contrasted with 10% of people with diffuse scleroderma. Anti-Scl-70 antibodies, on the other hand, are found in up to 40% of people with diffuse scleroderma but are not found in other types of scleroderma.

Scleroderma's hallmark is inflammation and excessive *fibrosis* (the formation of fibrous connective tissue, like a scar). The basic disease process is excessive production of collagen, the most abundant connective tissue fiber in the body. Symptoms (with approximate percentages of patients in whom those organ systems are affected), may include the following:

- Thickening of the skin (90%)
- Swelling of the hands and feet
- Pain and stiffness of the joints (30–50%)
- Joint contractures (fingers curling up, difficulty of movement)
- Raynaud's phenomenon (70–90%)
- Gastrointestinal tract problems (90%)
- Sjogren's syndrome (dry mucus membranes)
- Facial problems (tightening of skin limiting mobility of mouth, eyelids; temporomandibular joint syndrome [TMJ], or pain in the joint of the jaw)
- Dental problems (change in bite, loosening of teeth because of collagen deposition increasing the size of the ligaments around the teeth, tooth sensitivity)
- Fatigue attributable to fibrosis in the heart muscle
- Generalized aching and weakness caused by fibrosis in the muscles (20%)
- Kidney (40–70%), heart (50–90%), and lung (40–90%) involvement

Many patients describe their path toward diagnosis as one of the most difficult periods of the illness, in part because the difficulty of the diagnosis can lead both physicians and patients to label the symptoms as psychosomatic, or caused by the mind. Scleroderma is often a difficult diagnosis for a variety of reasons. It is a rare disease that few physicians have experience with. The manifestations and progression of the disease vary, and its symptoms—especially initial symptoms such as fatigue, achiness, weight loss, and shortness of breath—are vague and could apply to many different diseases. In fact, scleroderma often overlaps with other autoimmune connective tissue diseases such as lupus erythematosus and rheumatoid arthritis, and scleroderma symptoms can be part of mixed connective tissue disorder or undifferentiated connective tissue disorder. Finally, doctors may be reluctant to name scleroderma because it has no treatment or because it would make a patient uninsurable.

The disease has three main components: vascular (blood vessels), fibrotic, and autoimmune.

Vascular. Scleroderma involves repeated constriction of small blood vessels that causes characteristic symptoms in certain areas of the body. (*See the Raynaud's Syndrome protocol for information on Raynaud's phenomenon, which is present in most people with scleroderma.*) Pulmonary arteries may also be subject to recurrent constriction, leading to a decrease in diameter that causes hypertension in the lung circulation. This may not cause any symptoms but is revealed on echocardiogram. Controlling Raynaud's and stopping smoking will help prevent pulmonary hypertension.

Small blood vessels also supply the nerves and muscles of the esophagus. When they are compromised, difficulty in swallowing, heartburn, aspiration pneumonia caused by breathing in stomach contents, and even blockage requiring mechanical dilation may occur. Antacids and diet are key to prevention. Eating small amounts of soft food divided into five meals a day while standing or sitting upright and waiting 3 to 4 hours before lying down afterward are critical. Avoid gas-producing foods, alcohol, and smoking. Use a cup of yogurt with acidophilus and live cultures to aid digestion. Rarely, the lower gastrointestinal tract may be affected, leading to slowed motility causing constipation and an overgrowth of bacteria, which in turn results in diarrhea that must be treated with antibiotics.

Fibrotic. Fibrosis is the accumulation of thick, rigid tissue in response to chronic inflammation. Scleroderma is named for its characteristic skin fibrosis, which usually begins in the fingers and progresses up the arms, sometimes within a few weeks, sometimes over years. By the time the arms are affected, so are the legs. During the first stages of skin tightening, occupational and physical therapy are crucial interventions to improve and prevent debilitating, irreversible contractures of the fingers. Skin fibrosis normally worsens during the first 2 to 5 years, and then improves. It may produce a sudden increase in the pressure under the skin, rubbing muscles and tendons and causing myositis (inflammatory muscle disease), evidenced by elevated muscle enzymes in the blood. If this occurs, exercise must be stopped and steroid therapy may be used.

Lung fibrosis is also common. Pulmonary function tests, chest x-rays, and high-resolution computerized tomography (CT) can detect pathologic changes. The general medical consensus is that if changes are detected, drug treatment (oral cyclophosphamide) should begin. Fibrosis of the heart can cause abnormalities in the heart rhythm, or heart failure.

Autoimmune. Autoimmune disease occurs when the immune system, which is geared to attack foreign particles such as viruses and bacteria, attacks the body's own cells. This abnormal reaction to the body's own cells can be seen in the antibodies (molecules produced by the B cells of the immune system) directed against bodily proteins that circulate in the blood of those with scleroderma.

Although both scleroderma and rheumatoid arthritis are autoimmune diseases and may overlap, joint pain in scleroderma, unlike that in rheumatoid arthritis, is thought to result primarily from contraction of the skin, which restricts motion. Exercise is the most important therapy.

Hypothetical Causes

The cause of scleroderma is not known. It is known, however, to arise in response to certain environmental exposures such as silica dust. Other causes have been suggested, including elevated levels of nitric oxide and impaired response to stresses on the skin.

One area of interest results from the finding that scleroderma patients tend to have a high number of foreign cells in their bodies. These cells most commonly arise from two-way transfer between a mother and her fetus, resulting in the appearance of fetal cells in the mother and maternal cells in the child. The mixing of these with the body's own cells may be what triggers the immune system to attack its own cells.

Another hypothesis seeks to explain why autoimmune diseases such as scleroderma are so much more common in women. Research has found elevations in certain estrogen metabolites in women with systemic lupus, and low levels of certain weak androgens including dehydroepiandrosterone (DHEA). This suggests that the interaction between hormones unique to women and the immune system is significant in the development of autoimmune diseases.

Conventional Treatments

Scleroderma therapy is guided by the specific clinical presentation of the patient; not all patients have the same symptoms. In general, conditions that may have been caused by scleroderma, such as heart or kidney failure, will be managed in much the same way as in any other patient. What follows is a short summary of conventional treatments organized according to symptoms.

General

D-penicillamine has been the treatment of choice for many years, but a recent multicenter research study found it ineffective in softening skin or preventing organ involvement. Recently an antibiotic, minocycline, was found to be beneficial, but the study has been severely criticized. Gamma-interferon may inhibit the proliferation of fibroblasts, the cells that produce collagen. Steroids such as prednisone are frequently used for their anti-inflammatory action, which includes alteration of white blood cell function. However, steroids have significant side effects: for instance, calcium supplements must be taken to counter a loss of bone density. Steroids also suppress the body's natural ability to handle stress, and are typically used for a short term. Relaxin is an experimental drug that shows much promise. It is a naturally occurring hormone that inhibits collagen formation and also stimulates collagenase, the enzyme that breaks down collagen.

Other treatments, with significant side effects, are being investigated for more serious disease. *Immunosuppressive drugs* that have been used for cancer chemotherapy and organ transplants may reduce the autoimmune response. These drugs are cytotoxic; that is, they kill cells that are extremely active, which in autoimmune disease are white blood cells. High-dose cyclophosphamide is the drug of choice; azathioprine has fewer side effects but is less potent. *Bone marrow transplants* can be used in conjunction with these drugs: the patient's bone marrow (where white blood cells are produced) is removed, treated, and then returned. Some physicians, however, argue that this is unnecessary since the stem cells that will produce new white blood cells will not be affected by the cytotoxic drugs. Cyclosporin, which blocks the activation and stimulation of a component of the immune system (T-cells), also is considered beneficial. *Photopheresis* is a procedure similar to dialysis. The patient's blood is removed, the white blood cells are treated to quell the autoimmune activity, and then the blood is returned to the body.

Skin Disease/Musculoskeletal and Joint Pain

Edema during the early stage of skin thickening may be controlled with steroids, but the side effects must be considered. Some physicians feel that colchicine can reduce skin thickening if used early. Calcinosis can be treated with low-dose warfarin, colchicine, or probenecid, but may not be treated at all because it causes no clinical problems. Musculoskeletal and joint pain are commonly treated with nonsteroidal anti-inflammatory drugs or with steroids. Topical pain relievers such as salicylate or capsaicin creams may be used.

Some specialist dermatology centers offer PUVA therapy, in which repeated sessions of exposure to ultraviolet light are coupled with psoralen, a drug that makes the skin more sensitive to light. This technique has been found to soften skin and reduce the diameter of plaques or even cure them. It is considered effective for localized disease.

A "wellness lifestyle" involves the use of thoughts and activities that will benefit your mind and body. Following your treatment plan is only one aspect. Physical therapy and regular, gentle stretching and exercise are critical to maintain range of motion. Exercise also keeps the heart, lungs, and bones strong and helps many people relieve stress (a trigger for autoimmune diseases), cope with pain, and achieve a feeling of well-being. Other pain relief and stress relief strategies include getting enough sleep and heat treatments (heating pads, electric blankets, or a 20-minute warm bath every night before bed).

In addition to exercise, you should practice "joint protection" procedures to protect painful, swollen joints from stresses and injuries. Avoid lifting objects more than 10 pounds; always bend with the legs rather than the back. Use your hands judiciously (*see the Raynaud's Syndrome protocol*) —for instance, buy precut vegetables, cheeses, and fruits, and install a jar-opener. Always listen to your body: if something is painful, stop doing it.

Maintaining a positive attitude and a sense of humor are considered just as important as physical therapies. Feeling helpless and depressed exacerbates symptoms and decreases your ability to cope. Some people find consulting a counselor or praying helpful. Relaxation techniques such as guided imagery (visualizing yourself in a favorite place), biofeedback training, and soothing audiotapes can help you manage pain before it becomes too severe.

Xerosis, or severe dry skin, is a common problem and can be treated with creams such as Eucerin or Vanicream, or with bag balm, which has antiseptic properties. Skin should be kept moist and protected from cold, injury, and infection by clothing, especially gloves. Avoid strong detergents and soaps, and use a humidifier.

Gastrointestinal

Metoclopramide and cisapride can aid esophageal contraction and stomach emptying. Acid reflux (heartburn) can be managed by diet, sleeping on the left side, and antacids, including omeprazole.

A balanced overall diet that includes nutritional supplements is considered vital to maintain body weight and health. Some literature advises avoiding caffeine, refined sugars, and food additives that have been implicated as carcinogens (BHA, BHT, aspartame, saccharin, sodium nitrite) or have side effects (caffeine, olestra, MSG).

Pulmonary

Fibrosis, or interstitial disease, of the lungs can be treated with steroids or immunosuppressants such as cyclophosphamide. Pulmonary hypertension will be treated with drugs that dilate the vessels, such as calcium channel blockers, or epoprostenol.

Renal

Kidney problems are thought to result not only from fibrosis, but also from overall hypertension or high blood pressure. It is critical, then, to control blood pressure carefully using ACE (angiotensin-converting enzyme) inhibitors.

Integrated and Alternative Treatment Therapies

The line between conventional and alternative treatments is often unclear. Whereas the above section centered on pharmaceutical treatments that are available only with a prescription, this section offers some supplemental therapies (to be used under the supervision of a physician in addition to other treatments) that do not require a prescription, do *not* have the significant side effects of drugs, and support general health.

Dimethyl sulfoxide (DMSO). DMSO is a solvent that readily penetrates the skin and is typically used to "carry" another substance. In scleroderma, it is used alone to soften the skin. In a study performed by the Departments of Rheumatic Diseases and Pathology of the Cleveland Clinic Foundation, DMSO was applied to the affected areas of 42 patients with varying degrees of systemic scleroderma. Initial concentrations ranged from 30 to 60% and were increased to 70 to 100% as tolerated (different parts of the body tolerated different concentrations). The DMSO was allowed to penetrate completely (about 30 minutes). A regimen of three treatments a day was continued for about 3 months until softness and range of motion returned to normal, and then the number of treatments was reduced to two and then one a day. Excellent (improvement in all initial disease manifestations) or good (improvement in more than half of the initial disease manifestations) results were achieved in 26 patients, 16 with mild disease, 8 with moderate, and 2 with severe. Three patients went into remission. Two patients showed decreased calcinosis. Ten patients who didn't respond to the topical application were treated with immersion of their hands in 50% DMSO for 1 minute a day; sessions were then increased up to 5 to 10 minutes twice a day. All patients responded satisfactorily, and all ischemic ulcers healed within 1 week. The only side effects observed were transient redness and a burning or sharp prickling sensation that subsided within about a week, after which time the intensity of the treatment was able to be increased without further reactions. The researchers concluded that long-term DMSO treatment slowly but definitely alleviated systemic scleroderma.

Another double-blind clinical study found that treatment with 50% DMSO led to decreases in the density of skin and edema, increased mobility of the fingers, and increased blood flow to the skin and muscles. The researchers also observed an intensification in the metabolism of the ground substance of the connective tissue, documented by increased excretion of glycosaminoglycans. The only side effects observed were transient skin irritation and a garlic odor to the breath. Another recent double-blind study showed that the therapeutic effect of DMSO in rheumatoid arthritis, Raynaud's, and scleroderma is linked to its normalizing action on the formation of fibrin (part of the connective tissue) and the microcirculation.

Gamma-linolenic acid (GLA). GLA is an essential fatty acid that is converted to the precursor for prostaglandin E1, a potent anti-inflammatory hormone-like fatty acid. The mechanism of Sjogren's syndrome, an overlapping condition with scleroderma, has been argued to be lack of adequate synthesis of prostaglandin E_1. Administration of essential fatty acid precursors and vitamin C, which plays a role in PGE1 biosynthesis, was successful in raising the rates of tear and saliva production in Sjogren's patients. GLA has also been shown to reduce autoimmune dysfunction in rheumatoid arthritis patients. A recent scientific study found that GLA dramatically decreased the number of Raynaud's attacks. GLA can be obtained from evening primrose oil, borage oil, or black currant seed oil. Borage oil is the most concentrated and economical source.

EPA and DHA. DHA (docosahexaenoic acid) and EPA (eicosapentaenoic acid) are essential long-chain fatty acids with anti-inflammatory effects found in flax seed oil and fish oil. Research has demonstrated that fish oils inhibit arachidonic acid metabolism, which plays a key role in autoimmune diseases. (See the Raynaud's Syndrome protocol for studies showing the beneficial effect of fish oil on Raynaud's.) Using a concentrated fish oil supplement can enable one to obtain optimal potencies of EPA and DHA by taking only five to eight capsules a day.

Antioxidants. Free radical damage (oxidation) has long been suspected as a major mechanism of autoimmune disease. One recent study found that low-density lipoproteins (LDL) from patients with scleroderma were more susceptible to oxidation than those from healthy subjects or patients with primary Raynaud's. Another study of micronutrient antioxidant status in patients with primary Raynaud's and scleroderma revealed reduced vitamin C and selenium, especially in those patients with diffuse scleroderma. Another journal article argued that autoimmune diseases are caused by a relative deficiency of vitamin E, a physiologic stabilizer of cellular membranes. This deficiency damages the membranes of lysosomes (cellular organelles that digest waste), allowing hydrolytic enzymes to escape that denature (destroy) proteins to the point at which they are no longer recognizable to the immune system and are attacked as if they were foreign particles.

Boswella. Boswella is an herb that inhibits the formation of leukotriene B_4, which causes inflammation and migration and adhesion of inflammatory cells as well as promoting free-radical damage. Although no research on boswella's effect on scleroderma has been performed, it has been shown to reduce joint swelling and stiffness—common scleroderma symptoms—in rheumatoid arthritis, another autoimmune condition. The recommended dose is two 150-mg capsules of standardized boswella, taken 3 times a day for a month, which can be reduced to three capsules a day after results have been achieved. A combination of high doses of fish oil (five to eight capsules of fish oil concentrate) and just one-fourth of a regular aspirin tablet a day can also suppress leukotriene B_4.

Conclusion

Scleroderma is a chronic, progressive, disabling autoimmune connective tissue disorder with no satisfactory treatment. Its complex, various symptoms are caused by chronic inflammation and fibrosis and include the characteristic thickening of the skin (typically beginning on the hands), Raynaud's phenomenon, difficulty in swallowing and heartburn, joint pain and stiffness, facial and dental problems, and generalized fatigue and weakness. It may be either localized to the skin and underlying tissues or systemic, affecting the organs as well. The gastrointestinal tract, especially the esophagus, the lungs, the heart, and the kidneys, are commonly affected. Scleroderma must be managed by a physician, but exercise, physical therapy, mental attitude and stress management, and a "wellness lifestyle" may be just as important as drug treatments. Supplemental, alternative therapies have been shown to be effective in softening the skin and reducing autoimmune dysfunction.

Summary

1. Seek out specialists in dermatology and rheumatology (as well as dentistry) with specific scleroderma experience.
2. The course of your medical treatment will depend on your individual symptoms; however, be certain that all major organ systems affected by scleroderma (lungs, heart, kidneys,

gastrointestinal tract) are evaluated initially and routinely.

3. Be your own advocate. Actively seek out information and support. Diligently follow your treatment program. Be sure to report any changes in your condition.
4. Incorporate physical or occupational therapy and regular exercise into your daily routine.
5. Manage stress and pain and practice relaxation techniques. Consult a counselor if you feel it would be helpful, or if you feel overwhelmed, helpless, or depressed.
6. If Raynaud's is present, aggressively control it (*see the Raynaud's Syndrome protocol*).
7. Protect your skin by keeping it moist and covered, and use your hands wisely.
8. Apply DMSO in concentrations as tolerated to affected areas for 30 minutes a day, or immerse your hands in 50% DMSO, gradually increasing the duration and frequency.
9. Take GLA: preferable in the form of borage oil (5 capsules a day each containing at least 300 mg of gamma linolenic acid).
10. Take EPA and DHA: flax seed oil (1 tbsp. a day), concentrated fish oil capsules (5 to 8 capsules daily with meals), or perilla oil (6 capsules a day).
11. Three tablets of Life Extension Mix 3 times a day will supply the necessary levels of antioxidants plus a variety of health-enhancing nutrients.
12. Take boswella, two 150-mg capsules three times a day for a month, then 3 capsules a day.

For more information. Contact the Scleroderma Foundation, (978) 750-4499.

Product availability. DMSO liquid, gel, spray, and roll-on; borage oil, black currant seed oil, and evening primrose oil; flax seed oil, fish oil, and EPA and DHA capsules; and boswella capsules are available from the Life Extension Buyers' Club by calling (800) 544-4440 or ordering online at www.lef.org. All other medications mentioned above require a prescription.

SEASONAL AFFECTIVE DISORDER (SAD)

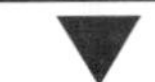

What Is Seasonal Affective Disorder?

Seasonal Affective Disorder (SAD) is a form of depression that begins in autumn or early winter and generally lasts from 5 to 7 months until spring. The early loss of sunlight in the winter appears to induce chemical changes in the brain that bring on depression. This lack of sunlight causes a reduction in serotonin production and an increase in the level of melatonin, which some research has shown to be responsible for producing the symptoms associated with SAD. When the days grow longer in the spring, symptoms disappear, not to reappear until the next autumn or winter.

SAD affects approximately 35 million Americans to some degree, although it occurs most often in children, adolescents, and women. Seventy-five to eighty percent of all SAD sufferers are women, with a higher incidence occurring past the age of 30.

Symptoms of SAD

Symptoms of SAD may vary in severity, but are characterized by their seasonal occurrence. Symptoms may include:

- Lack of energy
- Increased desire to sleep
- Depression
- Increased appetite leading to weight gain
- Anxiety
- Difficulty concentrating
- Irritability
- Withdrawal; difficulty with relationships; loss of sexual desire
- For women, increase in PMS-related symptoms

SAD is different from other forms of depression although it has similar symptoms. You should seek the advice of a physician rather than relying on self-diagnosis. It is important to distinguish SAD from other forms of depression as it is treated differently.

Treatment

Bright light therapy. Bright light therapy is an extremely effective treatment for seasonal affective disorder. Bright lights have also been used as adjuncts (assisting therapies) in the pharmacological treatment of other types of depressive illness. Standard morning light therapy regimen often consists of exposure of 10,000-lux cool-white fluorescent light for 30 minutes to 2 hours per day. This therapy requires special lamps that provide from 5 to 20 times the normal brightness of your home or office lighting.

Patients can take advantage of light therapy upon waking in the morning or during evening hours; however, research has shown early morning therapy to be more effective for most patients. Dawn simulation, where patients set a timer that turns on the lamp up to 2 hours before they wake up, simulating a natural sunrise, is also recommended. About 66% of SAD patients respond to light therapy. Significant improvement is usually noticed within 4 to 5 days following start of treatment. Light therapy appears to be an effective treatment for SAD sufferers of all ages, including pediatric SAD patients. Some side effects, such as headache or vision problems sometimes appear in early therapy, but are usually temporary.

Effect of melatonin. Although it cannot be established that SAD is caused by abnormal melatonin metabolism, in some people melatonin makes the symptoms of SAD worse. These people should stop melatonin or reduce its dosage during the times of the year when darkness appears early in the day.

Prescription medication. Some people take prescription antidepressants such as Prozac only during the time of the year they are affected by SAD. However, Prozac has a long half-life and it may take from 4 to 6 weeks to experience the full benefit of the treatment. It takes about the same amount of time to leave your system after the drug is discontinued. Prozac's mechanism of action is to selectively inhibit serotonin re-uptake. There is evidence that serotonergic dysregulation is involved in SAD and that the short-allele polymorphism for serotonin transporter is more common in patients with SAD than in healthy people.

Alternative Treatments

Tryptophan. A safer way than prescription medicine to boost serotonin levels is to ingest 2000 to 3000 mg of the amino acid tryptophan each night. Research has shown tryptophan to be equally effective to light therapy in treating SAD. The clinical use of L-tryptophan has also specifically been shown to improve response to light therapy. In clinical studies, SAD patients who were deprived of tryptophan were vulnerable to a relapse of SAD even in summer months.

St. John's wort. St. John's wort, or Hypericum extract, is one of the most popular herbal remedies for depression and is believed to alleviate the symptoms of SAD as well. Hypericum extract was found to be effective in a single-blind study with a dosage of 900 mg being given daily.

Vitamin D_3. Vitamin D_3 is believed to enhance positive affect in patients suffering from SAD. A dose of 400 to 800 IU per day is recommended.

Integrated "Common Sense" Treatment

One of the best ways to combat SAD is to maintain a healthy physical lifestyle. Take care of yourself by following these guidelines:

- Take a daily vitamin containing magnesium, B complex, and minerals.
- Get as much natural sunlight as possible.
- Stay physically active and enjoy outdoor exercise as frequently as possible.
- Follow a low-fat diet and avoid eating too much protein and red meat.
- Minimize your intake of caffeine.
- Take a winter vacation in a warm climate.

(*Refer to the Depression protocol.*) People with SAD should consider the Foundation's natural protocols before resorting to antidepressants drugs.

Summary

1. Bright light therapy with 10,000-lux cool-white fluorescent light for 30 minutes to 2 hours per day.
2. Stop melatonin or reduce its dosage during the times of the year when darkness appears early in the day.
3. Prescription antidepressants such as Prozac are effective for some patients.
4. Tryptophan, 2000 to 3000 mg each night.
5. St. John's wort, 900 mg per day.
6. Vitamin D_3, 400 to 800 IU per day.
7. Multivitamin containing magnesium, B-complex, and minerals daily.
8. Maintain proper nutrition and healthy physical lifestyle.

For more information. Contact the Mental Health Association of Colorado, Inc. 6795 East Tennessee Avenue, Suite 425, Denver, CO 80224; Phone: (303) 377-3040; FAX: (303) 377-4920 for a free brochure on SAD. Information regarding the support group NOSAD is available by writing: P.O. Box 40133, Washington D.C. 20016.

Product availability. Soy Power or Optifuel (for tryptophan), St. John's wort extract, vitamin D_3 capsules, and multivitamin supplements can be ordered by calling (800)544-4440 or by ordering online at www.lef.org.

SHINGLES AND POSTHERPETIC NEURALGIA

Shingles is a common, unpleasant condition characterized by localized rash and pain caused by the same virus that causes chickenpox. Shingles occurs in roughly 20% of the general population regardless of race, gender, or time of year. It is more common with age: 70% of cases occur in people over 50, and up to 50% of those who live to be 80 will experience shingles. Its most feared consequence is postherpetic neuralgia (PHN), pain that persists beyond the rash. This protocol will give suggestions to help minimize the risk of PHN, as well as explaining other complications, the cause of shingles and its symptoms, conventional medical treatments, and helpful nutritional supplements.

Cause

Shingles is caused by a reactivation of the varicella zoster virus (VZV), also known as human herpesvirus-3 (HHV-3). This virus is related to herpes simplex viruses types 1 and 2. It is a relatively fragile virus susceptible to disinfectants such as alcohol and hypochlorite. Initial infection with VZV results in chickenpox (varicella). Despite recovery from this illness, the virus lies dormant in the sensory nerve roots of the spinal cord for years or decades until it becomes active again and is then classified as herpes zoster and the condition is diagnosed as shingles. It is not known why the virus becomes active again but age-associated immune dysfunction or any other compromise of immune function is highly suspect.

Thus, all people who have ever had chickenpox (9 out of 10 adults) are at risk for developing shingles. Shingles arises from viruses that are already within the body and is not caught from someone else. Someone who has never had chickenpox has a low risk of contracting that illness from close contact with the shingles rash (vesicles containing virus). VZV infection typically occurs through inhalation of virus particles. Chickenpox is highly contagious because in that disease virus is shed from the throat into the air that others breathe. Since this does not occur in shingles, it is not very contagious and normal hand washing minimizes the risk. A second attack of shingles is very unusual and may signal an underlying immune disorder. Herpes simplex infection, which does recur, can also be misdiagnosed as shingles.

Symptoms

Shingles has two primary symptoms: rash and pain. More generalized symptoms include enlarged, tender lymph nodes draining the affected area and occasional mild malaise (fatigue).

Rash. The affected area is red, with small vesicles or blisters. Unlike the "dew drop on a rose petal" appearance of chickenpox, several blisters per area are common in shingles. New lesions may occur for up to one week, after which the rash shows signs of healing. In severe cases lesions may grow together, yielding a carpet of scabs and sometimes permanent scars. Overall, the rash usually lasts 2 to 5 weeks.

Pain. Pain in the area in which the rash will appear may precede the rash, known as *prodromal pain,* sometimes by a few days. The area often becomes flushed and unusually, sometimes unbearably, sensitive to pain. This is known as *allodynia.* The appearance of the rash often heralds a decrease in pain.

Shingles symptoms usually correspond to the skin area or dermatome supplied by the affected sensory nerve roots. The dermatome most commonly involved is the thoracic (trunk, palms, and inner arms, legs, and feet), followed by the trigeminal (face). Cervical (back of head, neck, shoulders, outer arms, and backs of hands), lumbar (waist, front of legs, and tops of feet), and sacral (buttocks, backs of legs, and soles of feet) dermatomes may also be affected. About 16% of shingles sufferers have more widespread rash.

Complications

Postherpetic Neuralgia (PHN). Pain that persists more than 30 days after the appearance of the rash is the most feared consequence of herpes zoster. The burning or stabbing pain of PHN is attributed to virus-induced damage to the nerve roots. General risk factors include anything that compromises the immune system such as age, illness, immune system disorders, certain cancers (especially those that affect the lymph or immune system), and medications that affect the immune system. More specifically, PHN has been linked to the following four factors:

- Age, which increases the likelihood and severity of PHN. People over 60 have about a 50% chance of having PHN.
- Prodromal (pre-rash) pain.
- Severe acute (with rash) pain.
- Failure to obtain adequate antiviral treatment within 3 days of the appearance of the rash.

Secondary infection. Shingles lesions usually dry quickly and heal well. However, secondary infection can occur, resulting in redness and swelling and often leading to scarring. Staphylococcus aureus is a common cause and may require consultation with a microbiologist because of problems with resistance.

Paralysis of the affected area. Some degree of motor paralysis is not uncommon but is not very evident on the trunk, as opposed to the face or limbs. It occurs from extension of the disease to the motor regions of the spinal cord or brainstem. Weakness follows the rash by a few days or weeks. About 55% of those affected make a complete recovery; 30% of those remaining show significant improvement.

Ramsay-Hunt syndrome. This syndrome has a well-known association with shingles. Its symptoms are pain in the middle ear; blistering of the external ear canal, pinna, and throat; and loss of taste (reflecting the involvement of the nerve supply to the tongue). Complete recovery is usual, although it may take months; in some cases a residual deficit may remain.

Meningoencephalitis. This very rare inflammation of the brain, despite the severity of symptoms such as coma, normally resolves completely.

Recurrent or Disseminated Herpes Zoster.

Shingles is 9 times more likely to develop in those infected with HIV. In the early stages of HIV infection, shingles symptoms are fairly typical. In more advanced infection, herpes zoster may take the form of repeated episodes of severe, prolonged, and sometimes atypical (VZV retinitis) disease. Shingles is also more common in immunocompromised children and adults (including organ recipients and chemotherapy patients). In these patients it may be recurrent and may disseminate or spread cutaneously (on the skin) or viscerally (among the organs), with life-threatening consequences necessitating intravenous antiviral drugs.

Standard Shingles Treatment

The standard treatment of shingles uses two types of drugs, analgesics (pain relievers), and antiviral agents, which reflect its two goals:

Resolve pain rapidly. Severe pain can predispose patients to PHN by permanently sensitizing nerves to even the mildest stimulation. Therefore, aggressive pain relief with paracetamol (codeine plus acetaminophen) is advised; some patients require opioids such as morphine. The goal is to reduce pain to a level compatible with daily activities and to have the patient confirm that the level of relief is satisfactory.

Stop virus replication. Antiviral drugs stop the virus from reproducing itself, thereby minimizing the damage it does to nerve cells. Three antiviral drugs are currently in use. Acyclovir is the standard, and has proven effective in accelerating pain resolution. Valaciclovir has been shown to be about one-third faster in resolving pain than acyclovir. Famciclovir does not appear to offer a significant advantage over acyclovir.

Older studies with a limited number of patients have indicated that oral corticosteroids (prednisone, triamcinolone) might decrease the likelihood of PHN. A 1994 article in the *New England Journal of Medicine* demonstrated a slight benefit of these drugs in decreasing the severity of acute herpes zoster but no long-term effects. A 1996 article by Whitley et al., in the *Annals of Internal Medicine* agreed, but found that oral corticosteroids may benefit quality of life. In general, the side effects of steroid therapy are felt to outweigh the benefits, although it may be considered in patients over 50 who have no contra-indications.

The rash may be treated with bland protective creams like zinc oxide. Calamine lotion may provide cooling comfort.

PHN Treatment

Tricyclics. The first line of PHN treatment is tricyclic antidepressants. In PHN, these drugs act as analgesics, not antidepressants. Therapy begins at doses lower than required for antidepressant activity, with stepwise increases. Their mechanism of action is unclear. They block reuptake of monoamine neurotransmitters (norepinephrine and/or serotonin) and may act on descending systems from the brainstem. Amitriptyline (Elavil), which affects both transmitters, is most effective, but nortriptyline, which works only on norepinephrine, has fewer side effects (dry mouth, constipation, drowsiness). Tricyclics are effective in 60–70% of patients. They decrease the intensity of pain but do not relieve it. Therapy should not end until 3–6 months after pain reduction, and then should be decreased gradually. Some shingles patients, however, may choose to end tricyclic drug therapy early because of unpleasant side effects.

Anticonvulsants and phenothiazines. Although these drugs have been used for certain types of PHN pain, no research evidence supports their effectiveness, and the risk of rendering elderly patients incompetent is high.

Opioids. Opioids can be used to manage PHN pain, although there is debate over whether PHN pain responds to opioids.

Topical therapies. Topical skin creams offer the benefit of massage as well as direct pain relief. Silvadene, Aspercreme, and capsaicin creams may supply some pain relief, although capsaicin must be used three to four times a day for several weeks to achieve relief and many complain of a burning after use. Wearing light cotton fabric or using plastic "artificial skin" sprays can minimize tactile allodynia caused by clothing. Cold packs applied over a cotton towel may also be helpful.

Psychological interventions. These therapies, which can be useful in any chronic pain syndrome, include counseling, cognitive behavior modification, relaxation training, biofeedback, and hypnosis.

Physical Therapies. Physical therapies such as ultrasound, laser therapy, and transcutaneous electrical nerve stimulation (TENS) can be helpful. Acupuncture reportedly has proven disappointing. A hand-held vibromassager may be just as effective and easier to manage than TENS, especially for elderly patients.

Surgery. A specialist may blockade peripheral nerves or use subcutaneous intravenous injection of a local anesthetic such as lidocaine to control PHN pain.

Nutrient supplements. Nutrient supplements and plant extracts helpful for shingles and PHN fall into four categories. The first two categories, those with antiviral and/or anti-inflammatory properties and those that enhance the immune system, have the same goal as conventional antiviral drugs: to stop the virus from replicating. Unlike antiviral drugs, however, many supplements have a number of health-optimizing actions and therefore also support recovery; these represent the third category of nutrient supplements helpful for shingles and PHN. Topical pain relievers comprise the fourth category.

Antiviral and/or anti-inflammatory supplements. A variety of plants are known for their virus-killing action, including garlic, oregano, and rosemary, which is also an antioxidant and anti-inflammatory. Olive leaves are an anti-inflammatory and have been used since ancient times to clean wounds. Flax seed oil and fish oil contain long-chain fatty acids with anti-inflammatory properties. Particularly helpful supplements include:

Monolaurin. Monolaurin is a fatty acid with antiviral properties that is found in coconut oil. It disrupts the lipid membranes of envelope viruses such as herpes, and has been proven effective against HSV-1. The Department of Health recently announced clinical trials testing its activity against HIV. The recommended dosage of lauric acid, the precursor to monolaurin, is 20 to 25 grams a day.

Sepium sebiferum. A potent anti-herpetic compound, methyl gallate (methyl-3,4,5-trihydroxybenzoate) has been scientifically purified from the leaves of this plant, also known as Chinese tallow tree or popcorn tree, which is a Chinese folk medicine for shingles.

Grapefruit seed extract. Grapefruit seed extract contains unstable polyphenolic compounds that are chemically converted into more stable substances that belong to a diverse class called quaternary ammonium compounds. These compounds exhibit broad-spectrum antimicrobial activity—the ability to kill a wide variety of bacteria and viruses—without the toxic side effects of the chemically derived quaternary ammonium compounds such as benzethonium chloride and benzalkonium chloride, which are used industrially as antimicrobials.

Green tea extract. Green tea exhibits antiviral, anti-inflammatory, and antioxidant powers. Research has demonstrated that green tea catechins can inhibit the viral enzymes reverse transcriptase and polymerases used in replication. They have been shown to be effective against herpes simplex 1 experimentally. In addition, various polymeric oxidation products of polyphenols contained in green tea have been found to inhibit the herpes simplex virus.

Immune-enhancing supplements. The healing properties of echinacea have long been known among American Indians. Studies have shown that it begins stimulating the immune tissue in the mouth as soon as it is taken. Echinacea enhances the body's ability to dispose of infected and damaged cells, it has interferon-like activity against viruses, and it stimulates the white blood cells that fight infection. Another supplement that enhances the immune system is HSOs, beneficial bacteria that will survive and grow in the intestine for a variety of health benefits, including stimulating the immune system. Scientific research has demonstrated that HSOs stimulate the body's production of alpha-interferon, used by the body to protect cells from invaders such as viruses. (See the Immune Enhancement protocol for more information.)

Supplements that support recovery. Almost all damage to the body occurs via molecules called free radicals, which oxidize molecules within cells. The remarkable health benefits of antioxidants, including vitamins C and E and beta-carotene, are supported by volumes of scientific research. Taking antioxidants in the course of shingles or PHN will support the body's recovery from the disease. A multi-nutrient formula like Life Extension Mix contains the key antioxidants in addition to a variety of other nutrients, such as the B vitamins, important for healing.

Topical pain relievers. A review of the actions of Chinese motherwort, *Leonurus sibericus,* published in the *American Journal of Chinese Medicine* (1976) reported that a bath prepared from the leafy shoot relieves the discomfort and itching of shingles. A 1998 article by Hijikata and Yamada in the same journal (accepted for publication, 1998) reported the findings of an experiment in which administration of hot water-soluble extracts of *Ganoderma lucidum* (36 to 72 grams dry weight a day) in a bath dramatically decreased pain in two patients with PHN unresponsive to standard treatment and two others with severe shingles pain. Also known as Ling Zhi, or "mushroom of immortality," this plant is a general tonic that stimulates the immune system with sedative and analgesic properties and is known especially for its benefits to the skin (ganoderma means smooth skin). Its active ingredients include polysaccharides, triterpenoids, adenosine and other amino acids, minerals, and organic germanium.

Ribavirin. A double-blind, placebo-controlled study using topically applied 5% ribavirin in ointment base against herpes zoster in cancer patients indicated definite efficacy as reported in the *Annals of the NY Academy of Sciences* (1977 [March]; 284:284–88). Ribavirin is approved in the United States only as a secondary therapy against the hepatitis C virus and a primary therapy against respiratory syncytial virus (RSV) in infants. This drug has been politically suppressed by the FDA, and no further studies to substantiate the role of ribavirin in treating shingles can be found. Offshore pharmacies might offer topical ribavirin ointment.

Conclusion

Since almost all adults have been infected with the varicella zoster virus that causes chickenpox, almost everyone is at risk of developing shingles, an unpleasant condition characterized by rash and pain. Symptoms are usually localized in a particular area of the body supplied by the sensory nerve root in which the virus has lain dormant. It is not known why the virus becomes active again, although age and any compromise of the immune system are factors. Normally, with prompt antiviral and pain-relieving therapy, shingles resolves within about 1 month, never to return. However, herpes zoster infection can have serious complications, including secondary infection leading to scarring, paralysis of the affected area, and pain that persists beyond 30 days after rash onset, known as postherpetic neuralgia (PHN). Most risk factors for PHN—age, pain before rash, and severe pain with rash—cannot be controlled. However, rapid and sufficient therapies that stop virus replication, which damages the nerve root and leads to PHN, and pain, which sensitizes the nerve root, can minimize the risk. For this reason, complementing conventional drugs with nutrient supplements and plant extracts is recommended by the Life Extension Foundation. These supplements do not have the side effects of conventional treatments, and they offer a variety of actions that optimize health and support recovery from the infection.

(*Refer to the Foundation's Immune Enhancement protocol for more specific information on what can be done to boost immune function, which appears to be an important adjuvant therapy in the prevention and treatment of shingles.*)

Summary

Acute Herpes Zoster

1. Within 3 days after the onset of the shingles rash, see a physician to begin a program of antiviral drugs and aggressive pain relief therapy. If you are over 50 and have no contra-indications, steroid therapy may hold benefits for quality of life.
2. At the same time, begin a regimen of nutrient supplements with antiviral and/or anti-inflammatory actions—garlic extract, oregano and rosemary oil, olive leaf extract, flax seed oil or fish oil, monolaurin, Chinese tallow tree extract, grapefruit seed extract, or green tea extract—to help minimize the replication of the virus and therefore complications like PHN.
3. Also use immune-enhancing supplements such as echinacea or HSOs to stimulate the body's natural ability to fight the virus.

4. Extracts of Chinese motherwort and Ling Zhi can be used in a bath to relieve the itching and discomfort of the shingles rash.
5. Use zinc oxide or calamine lotion on the rash, and watch for signs of secondary infection such as redness or swelling. If these signs are present, consult a physician immediately to help prevent scarring.

Postherpetic Neuralgia

6. If pain persists for 30 days after the onset of rash, consult a physician for tricyclic therapy and pain relievers.
7. Try topical therapies as well to reduce pain. Ling Zhi extract can be used in a bath. Creams such as Silvadene, Aspercreme, or capsaicin may provide relief. Cold packs applied over cotton may be helpful. Wear light cotton clothing or use an "artificial skin" spray to minimize allodynia.
8. Nutrient supplements with anti-inflammatory actions may provide some benefit by soothing inflammation of the irritated nerve roots.
9. Consider physical therapies such as ultrasound, laser therapy, transcutaneous electrical stimulation, and acupuncture. Use a hand-held vibromassager.
10. Consider psychological interventions such as counseling, cognitive behavior modification, relaxation training, biofeedback, and hypnosis to aid in coping with chronic pain.
11. If pain is unresponsive to these therapies, consult a specialist regarding surgical treatments such as peripheral nerve blockade or subcutaneous injection of local anesthetic.
12. Take three tablets of Life Extension Mix 3 times a day to provide the antioxidants and other nutrients necessary to support recovery.

For more information. Contact the American Academy of Dermatology, (708) 330-0230.

Product availability. Green tea extract, Life Extension Mix, and echinacea can be ordered by phoning (800) 544-4440, or order online at www.lef.org.

SKIN AGING

by Professor Carmen Fusco

Skin does not seem like the most exciting part of the body, but it's actually a dynamic, complex organ. So much hormone activity occurs in skin that it has been called another endocrine gland. Skin has its own immune system and specialized enzymes that no other part of the body has. According to research, skin cannot function without hormones.

DHEA, Melatonin, and Skin

The sleep hormone (melatonin) and the anti-stress hormone (DHEA) are both found in human skin. Both are converted to other entities with important jobs to do. DHEA is converted into estrogen and androgen-type metabolites found only in skin. Melatonin is synthesized in skin. In low concentrations it can stimulate cell growth. This type of on-site, organ-specific production of hormones is called *intracrine biosynthesis*. Intracrine biosynthesis allows different organs to manufacture the substances they need without flooding the entire body with growth factors.

Estrogen's skin-enhancing effects are well-known. It provokes collagen and a moisture factor known as *hyaluronic acid*. Aging decreases both estrogen and collagen. Enzymes that convert DHEA to estrogen also decline. Not surprisingly, women who take synthetic estrogen have scientifically proven thicker skin. Women who take both estrogen and testosterone have really thick skin–48% thicker than women who don't take either hormone. DHEA is converted to both estrogen and testosterone, providing the benefits of both hormones.

While the exact roles of DHEA and melatonin in human skin are still under scrutiny, researchers have identified several mechanisms through which these hormones protect against aging, maintain the health of skin, and affect how sunlight reacts with skin cells. All three are connected. For example, sunlight and aging suppress immunity, immunity affects health, and melatonin and DHEA affect them all.

Skin is such a specialized organ that it has its own immune system. It has been proposed that faulty skin immunity affects the entire immune system. Sunlight can penetrate deep into skin and alter immunity directly, or it can cause changes in dermis and epidermis that provoke immune changes. Sunlight affects hormones. It decreases melatonin, norepinephrine, and acetylcholine and increases cortisol, serotonin, GABA, and dopamine.

Studies show that both DHEA and melatonin are absorbed by skin when applied topically. A study from CHUL Research Center (in Canada) shows that the activity of DHEA applied topically is 85–90% greater than when taken orally (at least in rodents). No special carriers are needed to get DHEA and melatonin into skin. A properly formulated topical preparation of melatonin and DHEA will contain just enough hormone to benefit skin without providing enough to escape into circulation. It makes sense to apply the hormones directly to the skin if skin protection is the goal, since ingested hormones may end up everywhere *but* the skin.

DHEA Saves Skin

DHEA has beneficial effects beyond its conversion to skin-friendly hormones. DHEA itself has powerful skin protective effects. A study published in the *Journal of Surgical Research* demonstrates the extraordinary ability of topically-applied DHEA to protect skin's delicate blood vessels. Researchers found that if DHEA was applied after a serious burn, the blood vessels underlying the burned area are protected. Protecting the blood vessels saves the skin. Skin and blood vessels that would otherwise die and peel off can be saved by DHEA. No one knows for sure how DHEA saves skin this way, but its anti-inflammatory action no doubt has something to do with it. DHEA prevents destructive white blood cells and their biochemical cousins from gearing up. In particular, DHEA affects a blood vessel killer known as "tumor necrosis factor." At the same time it's inhibiting the destructive process, it appears to be prolonging the healing process: DHEA causes edema (swelling) to last longer. This apparently helps save tissue.

Antioxidant Action

DHEA has action against everyday insults as well. By maintaining skin immunity, DHEA preserves the ability of skin to react to cancer-causing, skin-destroying pollutants in air, food, and water. DHEA also has antioxidant action against peroxyl and superoxide free radicals.

Superoxide defense may have a lot to do with DHEA's ability to prevent skin cancer and papillomas (benign tumors). According to a mouse study, topically applied DHEA keeps oxidant-loving enzymes at bay. Chemicals with carcinogenic potential depend on oxidases for transformation. DHEA's antioxidant action stops them. DHEA has another important defense: it keeps chemical carcinogens from binding to DNA. According to some very interesting rodent studies conducted at Fels Research Institute and Temple University, cancers simply can't get started if enough DHEA is present. If this research holds up in humans, topically applied DHEA is an exciting prospect for skin cancer. Another interesting finding is that cancer-causing chemicals are more likely to cause carcinogenesis at certain times of the day, indicating that certain hormones which are only active at certain times of the day give cancer protection. But this research is in its infancy.

Melatonin Protects

Melatonin is another antioxidant that protects against UV radiation. A group at the University of Zurich has shown that topical melatonin gives excellent protection against sunburn if applied *before* sun exposure. Melatonin also appears to have a role in repairing burned skin. In a study published in *Brain Research Bulletin*, melatonin levels rose 6 hours after burn injury, then fell to normal.

In small amounts, melatonin causes skin cells to proliferate. (In large amounts, it stops proliferation). People with psoriasis and atopic eczema do not have normal melatonin secretion. Instead of peaks, they have valleys. With psoriasis, melatonin peaks in the day when it shouldn't, and patients have little at night. It's surprising that a hormone connected to sleep has a lot to do with skin health, but maybe not to those researchers who consider it another endocrine gland.

Other Factors in Skin Aging

There are many causes for the accumulated cellular damage in the skin that we call aging. Among these are the oxidative processes and related free radical damage that result from UV sunlight, smog, toxins, cigarette smoke, X-rays, drugs, and other stressors.

Young skins are also exposed to these potentially damaging changes, but when we are young, there is sufficient cellular energy (ATP) for DNA repair and cell renewal. Enzymes that provide antioxidant activity such as SOD and catalase are readily available. As we age, there is increased wear and tear, while at the same time the energy for cell repair and renewal is diminished, and the antioxidant enzymes are less available.

How to Improve Cell Energy and Antioxidant Activity

Foods rich in nucleic acids (RNA) such as sardines, salmon, tuna, shell fish, lentils, and beans help improve cell energy through a "salvage pathway" (see *Life Extension Magazine*, Aug. 1997, 5–8).

Foods rich in antioxidants and other phytochemicals such as fruits, vegetables, and green tea help protect against oxidative damage and free radical attack of all body cells including the skin.

The oral intake of supplements, particularly the antioxidants, vitamins E and C and the mineral selenium, and vitamin A, the "skin vitamin,"—together with supplements of RNA and B vitamins (for coenzymes) and the minerals zinc, copper, and manganese, provide even more intensive protection against damaging free radicals. The increased cellular energy helps the skin repair, renew, and revitalize itself.

Keeping the Skin Well Oiled

Aging causes a progressive decline in our ability to internally synthesize the essential fatty acids (EFAs) required by the skin to maintain a youthful, moist appearance. The most important oils to supplement are the omega-3s that can make the skin smoother, softer, and look more radiant. When skin is properly nourished, it shows less of the effects of aging. The oral ingestion of fish, flax, or perilla oil provides abundant quantities of the omega-3 fatty acids that are so beneficial to the health and appearance of the skin.

Additional Measures for Keeping the Skin Young

Avoidance of more than modest exposure to the sun's ultraviolet light is critically important to protect the skin against the oxidizing effects of solar radiation. Ultraviolet rays are categorized by wavelengths: UVA, UVB, and UVC.

The ozone layer filters out the UVC and much of UVB rays, but the ozone layer is not what it used to be, and it seems to have little or no effect on UVA rays which make up 90% or more of the sun's radiation that reaches the earth. Indeed it is exposure to UVA that causes most of the photoaging damage: the premature wrinkles, loss of elasticity, hyperpigmentation, and dry and leathery dull texture.

UVB, which is most intense between the hours of 10:00 A.M. and 2:00 P.M., can cause sunburns and basal-cell cancers of the skin as well as increase the risk of melanomas. Yet sunscreens, which are geared to filter out UVB, seem to have no effect on the incidence of melanoma, and according to some studies may even increase its risk. Whether the increased risk is from the greater exposure to the sun by people who use sunscreen is not yet known. Of interest are studies showing that people who are continuously exposed to the sun, such as farmers and fisherman, seem to be at less at risk for melanoma than a vacationer, especially a fair-skinned sunbather who exposes their skin to intense sun for a few days or a week.

To Prevent Skin Aging and Cancer

It seams reasonable to avoid midday sun when possible, and avoid tanning salons. Use protective clothing, hats, and umbrellas during prolonged sun exposure. Apply and reapply sunscreen or use preparations that contain micronized zinc oxide or titanium oxide for more complete protection.

Published research (*Med. Pregl.*) indicates that both children and adults are still spending considerable time in the sun during peak UV exposure periods. A survey conducted on 51 physician volunteers of various specialties showed that 33% spent over 2 peak UV hours outdoors every day and another 33.33% are regularly sun exposed for at least 5 hours. Only 39% of the survey group regularly used sunscreen and those that did used an inadequate amount for full body protection. A majority of the respondents did not believe that sunscreens protected against skin cancer, but they did believe that sunscreens could slow the aging process. Common reasons for not using sunscreen were the amount of time involved in application and the relative high cost. The researchers concluded that participants lacked well-formed sun protection habits and that there continues to be a poor understanding of the need for sun protection despite worldwide campaigns warning of the dangers.

SolarMax 17 is a sun protection formula containing antioxidant vitamins and sun protection factor (SPF) 17. Vitamins A, C, E, contained in SolarMax 17, protect skin cells from free radical damage caused by UV light exposure. The formula is moisture-proof, sweat-resistant, and can be worn under makeup.

The *new* Rejuvenex Body Lotion contains some titanium oxide, but more importantly it was formulated with precise amounts of glycolic acid, vitamin C, and melatonin which, according to recent studies, protect against photoaging of the skin epidermis.

Rejuvenex with Advanced Vitamin C contains minimal sunscreen protection (SPF-12), but ingredients such as vitamin C complex, vitamin E, ceraphyl GA-D, vitamin A, and RNA do more to prevent and repair DNA damage than even the strongest sunscreen.

The Dream Cream, also known as *Rejuve-Night,* contains all the anti-aging ingredients (including DHEA and melatonin) to help the skin repair, renew, and revitalize itself. Although it was intended as an intensive night recovery cream, it can be used any time. The precise DHEA amounts and melatonin, together with associated factors, work specifically in the epidermis of the skin, not transdermally. There is no sunscreen in the Dream Cream, so if using it during the day in the sunlight, the user should wear makeup that contains zinc oxide or a sunscreen (and most of them do), or use a sunscreen.

A Word about Thyroid Function

Like most hormones in our body, as we age less and less thyroid hormone is available. Glands, which produce these hormones, become sluggish or irregular. The thyroid gland is no exception. Often physicians will see patients who are not only overweight but who also have dry, flaky, sluggish skin. A thyroid profile in the blood will often show a low or borderline-low thyroid function. Nutrients and foods which support the thyroid such as sea vegetables, seafood, fish, iodized sea salt, and natural thyroid preparations, or prescription Synthroid, when necessary, reverse this form of skin aging.

Summary

1. RNA-rich foods such as sardines, salmon, tuna, shell fish, lentils, and beans help improve cell energy through a "salvage pathway."
2. Antioxidant- and phytochemical-rich foods such as fruits, vegetables, and green tea help protect against oxidative damage and free radical attack of all body cells including the skin.
3. Antioxidant vitamins E and C, the "skin vitamin," A, B vitamins and their coenzymes, and the minerals selenium, zinc, copper, and manganese provide protection against damaging free radicals and help to repair, renew, and revitalize skin.
4. Take 6000–7000 mg a day of perilla or flax oils or 3000–4000 mg of fish oil highly concentrated with EPA and DHEA. Please note that fish oil produces gastro-intestinal upset in some people, whereas perilla and flax oils are usually well tolerated.
5. Rejuvenex Body Lotion, containing titanium oxide, glycolic acid, vitamin C, and melatonin, protects against photoaging of the epidermis.

6. Rejuvenex with Advanced Vitamin C contains SPF-12 and vitamin C complex, vitamin E, ceraphyl GA-D, vitamin A, and RNA. These ingredients are more effective than the strongest sunscreen in prevention and repair of DNA damage.
7. The Dream Cream contains anti-aging ingredients (such as DHEA and melatonin) and can be used as a day or night cream. The ingredients in Dream Cream work specifically in the epidermis of the skin, not transdermally.
8. SolarMax 17 is a sun protection formula containing antioxidant vitamins and sun protection factor (SPF) 17. The spray bottle makes it easy to apply to all body parts.
9. If skin is dry and flaky, consider a thyroid profile to determine if the thyroid gland is producing an adequate amount of hormone.
10. Use protective clothing, hats, and umbrellas during prolonged sun exposure.
11. Apply and reapply sunscreen or use preparations that contain micronized zinc oxide or titanium oxide for more complete protection.

Product availability. Vitamins A, B complex, C, E, selenium, essential fatty acids, Rejuvenex Body Lotion, Rejuvenex with Advanced Vitamin C, and Dream Cream can be ordered by phoning (800) 544-4440, or order online at www.lef.org.

STRESS

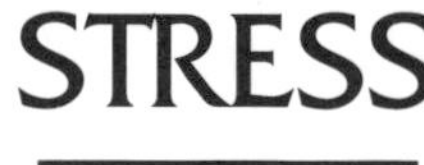

(See Anxiety and Stress)

STROKE (HEMORRHAGIC)

Stroke is the third leading cause of hospitalization in the United States. A stroke is defined as the sudden reduction of blood flow to a portion of the brain. There are two main types of strokes: ischemic (also known as thrombotic) and hemorrhagic. A stroke of any type is an extreme medical emergency, and prompt treatment is imperative. Although hemorrhagic strokes account for only 15% of all strokes, they have a much higher mortality rate. There are two subcategories of hemorrhagic stroke: intracerebral hemorrhage (ICH) and subarachnoid hemorrhage (SAH). Although ICH and SAH are very similar, they generally result from different causes.

Intracerebral Hemorrhage (ICH)

Intracerebral hemorrhage is defined as the rupturing of cranial blood vessels, resulting in the leakage of blood into brain tissues. The most common risk factor for ICH is chronic hypertension; hypertension causes arteries and arterioles to become weakened, resulting in leakage. A Chinese study noted that there was considerable increased risk for ICH in hypertensive patients who did not regularly take their medications. Additional risk factors for ICH include drug and alcohol abuse, anticoagulant medications, age, gender, and race. Excessive alcohol consumption and drug use, particularly of cocaine and amphetamines, are the most common causes of ICH for people in their 20s and 30s. Anticoagulants, such as Coumadin or Heparin, are prescribed for a variety of conditions, including ischemic stroke, myocardial infarction, and deep vein thrombosis. Proper monitoring of these medications is essential because they increase the risk of ICH. Aspirin has also been shown to increase the risk of ICH in elderly patients. ICH rarely occurs in people under the age of 45, and the risk for developing ICH doubles every 10 years thereafter. Intracerebral hemorrhage occurs more frequently in men, and African-Americans are more likely to be affected than are Caucasians.

Symptoms of ICH include the following:

- Partial or total loss of consciousness
- Vomiting or severe nausea
- Weakness, numbness, or paralysis, especially on one side of the body
- Sudden, severe headache

If these symptoms occur, it is essential to receive immediate medical attention.

Subarachnoid Hemorrhage (SAH)

A subarachnoid hemorrhage occurs when blood leaks into the membranes that surround the brain; the underlying causes for SAH include ruptured aneurysm (a ballooning of the arterial wall) and vascular malformations. Risk factors for SAH are more difficult to define than those for ICH but include age, gender, race, use of cigarettes and alcohol, and family history. The incidence of SAH increases throughout middle age, and peaks between the ages of 40 and 60. SAH affects women in 60% of all cases. African-Americans have nearly twice the risk as Caucasians. Cigarettes and alcohol abuse have been shown to increase aneurysm rupture. People with a family history of aneurysm-induced SAH are at higher risk because certain types of aneurysms appear to run in families. Symptoms of SAH include

- Sudden onset of severe headache
- Nausea or vomiting
- Stiff neck
- Light intolerance
- Total or partial loss of consciousness

After an aneurysm ruptures, a blood clot forms over the affected area. If the clot is disturbed, rebleeding occurs; rebleeding is the leading cause of death among SAH patients. It is critical that patients with the symptoms of SAH seek immediate medical attention.

Diagnosis of Hemorrhagic Stroke

The most common diagnostic procedures for determining the cause of hemorrhagic stroke are CT scan, MRI, and cerebral angiogram. These procedures are used to determine the type of stroke and the specific area of the brain that has been affected. Treatment of the stroke is based on the findings of these procedures.

Conventional Treatment of Hemorrhagic Stroke

Treatment of hemorrhagic stroke is based on the underlying cause of the hemorrhage and the extent of damage to the brain: treatment includes medication and surgical intervention. In patients with hypertension-induced ICH, initial treatment involves the use of antihypertensive agents. If the hemorrhage results from the use of anticoagulants, such as Coumadin or Heparin, these medications are discontinued immediately. Protamine and vitamin K may be given to reduce bleeding in patients with anticoagulant-induced bleeding.

In patients with ruptured aneurysms, surgical intervention is the method of treatment and includes placing a clip across the aneurysm or embolization if the damaged area is difficult to approach. During embolization, a wire-packed catheter is threaded through the blood vessels until it reaches the damaged area; the wires are then detached so that they form coils that attract blood cells to promote clot formation. Patients with ICH may benefit from a surgical evacuation of the hematoma. Surgical intervention is contra-indicated in patients who are 75 years old or older, who have significant pre-existing disease, or who arrive at the hospital in very poor condition.

Other Beneficial Treatments for Hemorrhagic Stroke

Hydergine, an antioxidant medication that helps to protect brain cells, may be beneficial for the treatment of hemorrhagic shock. In Europe, Hydergine is administered on an acute-care basis for the prevention of brain damage following stroke. The recommended dosage of Hydergine in an acute situation is 10 mg administered sublingually (under the tongue) and 10 mg given orally. Because the FDA has not approved Hydergine for use in the treatment of stroke, emergency room physicians may not be willing to administer this medication. Patients or their surrogates can, however, request that this medication be used. Hydergine has been approved in the treatment of other diseases, so it is available through the hospital pharmacy.

Piracetam, a nootropic medication similar to pyroglutamate (an amino acid), may be useful in the treatment of hemorrhagic stroke. Piracetam appears to protect brain cells from injury and death during stroke, thereby lessening the potential for permanent neurological damage. The recommended dosage for piracetam is 4800 mg a day taken orally. A recent Belgian study indicated that piracetam may be very beneficial if administered within 7 hours after the onset of stroke. Piracetam is not currently available in the United States.

Any disruption of blood flow to the brain causes massive free radical damage that induces much of the re-perfusion injury to brain cells characteristic of stroke. When blood flow is interrupted and subsequently restored (re-perfused), tissues release iron that provides a catalyst for the formation of free radicals that often permanently damage brain cells. The Life Extension Foundation has spent millions of dollars conducting research that involves developing methods of protecting the brain cells from injury caused by blood-flow disruption. The use of antioxidant nutrients, drugs and hormones, along with specific calcium-channel blockers and cell membrane stabilizing agents provide enormous protection to brain cells.

To learn about therapies that may strengthen arteries in the brain prior to hemorrhagic stroke, refer to the Life Extension Foundation's protocol on treating Cerebrovascular Disease. (*To learn more about therapies that may restore neurological function following hemorrhagic stroke, refer to the Foundation's protocol for Age-Associated Mental Impairment [Brain Aging].*)

Can Cholesterol Levels Be Too Low?

Cholesterol has obtained such a bad reputation, that some people may be inadvertently killing themselves by intentionally keeping their serum cholesterol too low. At the American Heart Association's annual stroke conference (February 1999), a report was presented showing that people with cholesterol levels under 180 doubled their risk of hemorrhagic stroke compared to those with cholesterol levels of 230. Hemorrhagic stroke occurs when a blood vessel in the brain breaks open and is different than the more common thrombotic stroke caused by an abnormal blood clot. This study also showed that the risk of thrombotic stroke was twice as likely in those with cholesterol levels over 280 compared to those at 230. The report concluded that the optimal cholesterol level for overall stroke prevention was around 200.

Some Foundation members have been pushing their cholesterol levels way below 180. In the few reports of hemorrhagic stroke suffered by Foundation members, their cholesterol levels have all been far below 180 mg/dL.

Mid-Life Blood Pressure a New Risk Factor

A 30-year study of male twins showed that elevated blood pressure in mid-life predisposed men to accelerated brain aging and an increase in stroke later in life. Men with even mildly elevated blood pressure 25 years before showed smaller brain volumes and more strokes compared to their twin brothers who did not have the elevation in blood pressure. This study, published in the journal *Stroke* (1999;30), emphasized the importance of aggressively treating elevated blood pressure even if it is not grossly abnormal. (*Refer to the Foundations Hypertension protocol for information about blood pressure control therapies and diets.*)

Conclusion

Hemorrhagic stroke is a medical emergency. The two types of hemorrhages involved are ICH and SAH. The primary risk factor for ICH is hypertension because chronic hypertension weakens blood vessels. Other risk factors include drug and alcohol abuse, anticoagulant medications, age, gender, and race. The underlying cause for SAH is cerebral aneurysm. Risk factors for SAH include family history of aneurysm, age, gender, and race. Symptoms for both types of hemorrhagic stroke are similar and include sudden onset of severe headache, loss of consciousness, nausea and vomiting, and partial or total paralysis. Diagnosis of the underlying cause of hemorrhagic stroke is by CT scan, MRI, and angiography. Treatment for hemorrhagic stroke depends on the underlying cause. For ICH resulting from hypertension, the initial treatment is blood pressure control. If anticoagulants are the cause of ICH, these medications are immediately discontinued. Surgical evacuation of the hematoma may be necessary. For SAH, treatment includes clipping or embolization of the aneurysm.

The medications Hydergine and piracetam may be beneficial to patients with hemorrhagic shock. The FDA has not approved Hydergine for the treatment of stroke, but it should be available through the hospital pharmacy, and patients or their surrogates should request its use. Piracetam may be beneficial in preventing permanent neurological damage following stroke. Piracetam is not currently available in the United States.

Summary

1. The symptoms of intracerebral hemorrhage (ICH) include nausea and vomiting; sudden, severe headache; weakness, numbness; paralysis, particularly to one side of the body; and partial or total loss of consciousness. The symptoms of subarachnoid hemorrhage (SAH) include sudden, severe headache; nausea and vomiting; stiff neck; light intolerance; and partial or total loss of consciousness.
2. Diagnostic procedures for hemorrhagic stroke include CT scan, MRI, and cerebral angiogram.
3. Treatment of hemorrhagic stroke consists of medication and surgical interventions, based on the underlying cause of the hemorrhage. Controlling high blood pressure is essential to preventing further strokes.
4. Hydergine, an antioxidant medication that protects brain cells, may be given in an acute situation. The recommended dosage is 10 mg given sublingually and 10 mg administered orally. Because the FDA has not approved Hydergine for this purpose, the patient or patient's advocate should request that the medication be given.
5. Piracetam, a nootropic medication, may be useful in the prevention of hemorrhagic stroke because it appears to protect brain cells from injury during the stroke event. The recommended dosage for piracetam is 4800 mg a day, administered orally.
6. Consider taking 500 mcg to 10 mg of melatonin (at night) and 100–200 mg of palm-oil tocotrienols a day to protect against further free-radical–induced brain cell injury.

For more information. Contact the National Institute of Neurological Disorders and Stroke, (800) 352-9424.

Product availability. Hydergine tablets and piracetam can be ordered from off-shore suppliers who will ship to the United States for personal use. For a list of offshore suppliers of these medications, phone (800) 544-4440.

STROKE (THROMBOTIC)

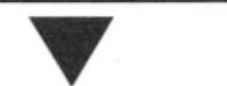

(Ischemic, Thrombotic, Embolic, and Transient Ischemic Attack)

Amazingly, 42% of stroke patients wait as long as 24 hours before presenting for medical treatment. That's 21 hours too late! The delay in presenting at the emergency room results in a missed opportunity to effectively treat, and possibly reverse, the damage caused by thrombotic stroke. According to one published study, "Patients with milder symptoms, for whom treatment might be more effective, were less likely to arrive in time for therapy" (*Stroke* [USA], May 1997; 28[5]:1092).

Stroke is the third leading cause of death in developed countries. About 25% of sufferers die as a result of the stroke or its complications, and almost 50% have moderate to severe health impairments and long-term disabilities. Only 26% recover most or all normal health and function.

We often consider "heart attack" as a "life or death" health event. Strokes have been given less attention, but the new realization that the disease is an acute event has now led to stroke being referred to as a "brain attack." Thrombotic strokes are a major cause of brain attacks, and are caused in part by atherosclerosis, hypertension, and diseases that cause abnormal arterial blood clot formation (thrombosis) such as atrial fibrillation and heart valve replacement.

The time it takes to receive treatment is as important to stroke victims as it is for those suffering a heart attack! Not recognizing the symptoms of a stroke, or believing that stroke is untreatable, too many people fail to respond to the warning symptoms of stroke by seeking immediate medical attention.

Further contributing to stroke deaths is the belief by many health care providers that stroke is untreatable, leading to an attitude of "watchful waiting" with an onset of a stroke, instead of being focused on treating the stroke as a medical emergency. The National Stroke Association succinctly described this problem in 1999 as follows: "These outdated attitudes serve as the largest obstacle to the effective prevention and emergency treatment of strokes."

The Underlying Causes

As with almost all cardiovascular disease, strokes are generally the result of several underlying diseases which work to stop or reduce the flow of blood to the brain, causing disability or death.

The majority of strokes occur when a blood clot blocks the flow of oxygenated blood to a portion of the brain. This type of stroke, caused by a blood clot blocking, or "plugging," a blood vessel, is called *ischemic stroke.* An ischemic stroke can be caused by a blood clot that forms inside the artery of the brain (*thrombotic stroke*), or by a clot that forms somewhere else in the body and travels to the brain (*embolic stroke*). In healthy individuals, blood clotting is beneficial. When you are bleeding from a wound, blood clots work to stop the bleeding. In the case of ischemic stroke, abnormal blood clotting blocks large as well as small arteries in the brain, cutting off blood flow, resulting in a clinical diagnosis of ischemic, thrombotic, or embolic stroke.

Ischemic strokes account for 83% of all strokes, and occur as either an embolic or thrombotic stroke. Thrombotic strokes represent 52% of all ischemic strokes. Thrombotic stroke is caused by unhealthy blood vessels becoming clogged with a buildup of fatty deposits, calcium, and blood clotting factors such as fibrinogen and cholesterol. We generally refer to this as atherosclerotic disease. Simplistically, what happens with a thrombotic stroke is that our bodies regard these "buildups" as multiple, infinitesimal, repeated injuries to the blood vessel wall. Our own bodies react to these injuries, and just as they would if we were bleeding from a small wound, respond by forming blood clots. Unfortunately, in the case of thrombotic strokes, these blood clots get caught on the plaque on the vessel walls and reduce or stop blood flow to the brain. That's when we suffer a brain attack.

Two types of thrombosis can cause a stroke: large vessel thrombosis and small vessel disease. Thrombotic stroke occurs most often in the large arteries, magnifying the impact and devastation of disease. Most large vessel thrombosis is caused by a combination of long-term atherosclerosis followed by rapid blood clot formation. Many thrombotic stroke patients have coronary artery disease, and heart attacks are a frequent cause of death in patients who have suffered this type of brain attack.

The second type of thrombotic stroke is small vessel disease, which occurs when blood flow is blocked to a very small arterial vessel. Little is known about the specific causes of small vessel disease, but it is often closely linked to hypertension and is an indicator of atherosclerotic disease.

In an embolic stroke, a blood clot forms somewhere in the body (usually the heart) and travels through the bloodstream to the brain. Once in the brain, the clot eventually travels to a blood vessel small enough to block its passage. The clot lodges there, blocking the blood vessel and causing a stroke.

The other type of stroke is called hemorrhagic stroke and is not caused by a blood clot. A hemorrhagic stroke, also known as a cerebral hemorrhage, occurs when a blood vessel in the brain breaks or ruptures. This type of stroke occurs less frequently than ischemic stroke.

Risk Factors for Strokes

The top risk factors for thrombotic strokes are the presence of hypertension, atherosclerosis, excessive blood-clotting factors (such as homocysteine, fibrinogen, and LDL cholesterol), heart valve defects, diabetes, and aging.

High blood pressure. High blood pressure is the most prominent risk factor for stroke. In fact, stroke risk varies directly with blood pressure. Many people believe the effective treatment of high blood pressure is a key reason for the accelerated decline in the death rates for strokes.

Increasing age. The chance of having a stroke more than doubles for each decade of life after age 55. While strokes are common among the elderly, substantial numbers of people less than 65 also have strokes.

Gender. Overall, men have about a 19% greater chance of a stroke than women. Among people under age 65, the risk for men is even greater when compared to that of women.

Heredity (family history) and race. The chance of a stroke is greater in people who have a family history of strokes. African-Americans have a much higher risk of death and disability from a stroke than Caucasians, in part because African-Americans have a greater incidence of high blood pressure.

Prior stroke. The risk of a stroke for someone who has already had one is several times that of a person who has not.

Cigarette smoking. In recent years studies have shown cigarette smoking to be an important risk factor for stroke. The nicotine and carbon monoxide in cigarette smoke damage the cardiovascular system in many ways. The use of oral contraceptives combined with cigarette smoking also greatly increases stroke risk.

Diabetes mellitus. Diabetes is an independent risk factor for stroke and is strongly correlated with high blood pressure. While diabetes is treatable, having it still increases a person's risk of a stroke. People with diabetes often also have high cholesterol and are overweight, increasing their risk even more.

Carotid artery disease. The carotid arteries in your neck supply blood to your brain. A carotid artery damaged by atherosclerosis (a fatty buildup of plaque in the artery wall) may become blocked by a blood clot, which may result in a stroke. If you have a diseased carotid artery, your health care provider may hear an abnormal sound in your neck, called a bruit, when listening with a stethoscope.

Heart disease. A diseased heart increases the risk of a stroke. In fact, people with heart problems have more than twice the risk of a stroke as those with hearts that work normally. Atrial fibrillation (the rapid, uncoordinated beating of the heart's upper chambers), in particular, raises the risk for stroke. Heart attack is also the major cause of death among survivors of a stroke.

Transient ischemic attacks (TIAs). TIAs are "mini-strokes" that produce stroke-like symptoms, but no lasting damage. They are strong predictors of a stroke. A person who has had one or more TIAs is almost 10 times more likely to have a stroke than someone of the same age and sex who hasn't.

WARNING: TIAs are extremely important stroke warning signs. Don't ignore them!

High red blood cell count. A moderate or marked increase in the red blood cell count is a risk factor for stroke. The reason is that more red blood cells thicken the blood and make clots more likely.

Heart disease risk factors related to stroke. Other secondary risk factors for a stroke are caused by increasing the risk of heart disease. These indirect factors include high blood cholesterol and lipids, physical inactivity, and obesity.

Other potential risk factors for stroke are

Geographic location. Stroke is more common in the southeastern United States than in other areas. These are the so-called "stroke belt" states. The age-adjusted death rates from a stroke are much higher in these states than in the rest of the country.

Season and climate. Stroke deaths occur more often during periods of extremely hot or cold temperatures.

Socioeconomic factors. There is some evidence that people of lower income and educational levels have a higher risk for stroke.

Excessive alcohol intake. Excessive drinking (an average of more than 1 drink per day for women and more than 2 drinks per day for men) and binge drinking can raise blood pressure; contribute to obesity, high triglycerides, cancer, and other diseases; and cause heart failure, leading to stroke.

Certain kinds of drug abuse. Intravenous drug abuse carries a high risk of stroke from cerebral embolisms. Cocaine use has been closely related to strokes, heart attacks, and a variety of other cardiovascular complications. Some of them have been fatal even in first-time cocaine users.

Source of risk factors: National Stroke Association, 1999.

WARNING: Recognizing stroke symptoms and realizing that the symptoms require immediate emergency treatment can save your life!

Symptoms of Stroke

- Sudden trouble standing or walking, dizziness, loss of balance or coordination.
- Sudden numbness of the face or weakness of arm or leg, especially on one side of the body.
- Sudden confusion, trouble speaking or understanding.
- Sudden trouble seeing in one or both eyes.
- Sudden, very severe headaches with no known cause.

WARNING: Any of the above signs may be only temporary and may last only a few minutes.

Stroke Symptoms Source: Mayo Medical Clinic, 1999 and The National Stroke Association, 1999.

Aggressive Stroke Therapy

A revolutionary improvement has occurred in the treatment of ischemic strokes, yet health care providers still do not treat stroke as aggressively as they do heart attack. Many therapies that are proven to work are not made available to the acute stroke patient presenting in the emergency room.

Development of computerized tomography (CT) and Doppler ultrasonography has made radical changes in early diagnosis of ischemic and hemorrhagic strokes. These advances have resulted in declines in stroke mortality. In the 1980s, the development of MRI imaging further improved evaluation of persons with cerebrovascular disease.

Then in the 1990s came conclusive evidence that specialized stroke centers for more immediate and intensive treatment, combined with educating the public that *time to treatment* decreases mortality and improves outcome for stroke, further decreased the incidence of death associated with all types of strokes. Oral anticoagulants and aspirin, as well as natural supplements, are demonstrated to be very effective in diminishing the risk of a stroke.

The FDA approved the use of a tissue plasminogen activator (t-PA) in June 1996 to treat strokes. t-PA had already been approved to dissolve clots that occurred in the coronary arteries (acute heart attack), but the FDA delayed approving t-PA to treat ischemic stroke for many years. Millions of cases of death and permanent paralysis occurred because of the FDA's delay in approving t-PA in treating stroke caused by abnormal blood clotting in the brain's arteries. Physicians affiliated with the Life Extension Foundation were using t-PA in emergency rooms to treat ischemic stroke years before the FDA gave its official seal of approval.

Insist That t-PA Be Administered upon Diagnosis of Ischemic Stroke

t-PA (sold under the brand name Activase) should be administered immediately (or within 3 hours) after a stroke in order to dissolve the clot that is preventing blood from reaching a portion of your brain. t-PA stands for tissue plasminogen activators. It is a natural clot-dissolving substance produced by the body and can literally blow open a blood clot in the brain that causes the acute ischemic brain damage characteristic of a stroke.

In the latest study, 30% more stroke victims were able to regain full use of their faculties after receiving t-PA. Even today, patients may encounter severe resistance from emergency room physicians who are reluctant to administer it, even if a patient's life is at stake. In some cases, surgery may be needed to remove any blockage of blood vessels going to the brain since it is important to get the blood circulating to the brain.

While t-PA can dissolve the blood clot that causes a blood-vessel blockage, there are other complications that occur during ischemic stroke that have to be addressed if permanent brain damage is to be prevented. Any interruption in blood flow causes an oxygen imbalance that results in massive free radical damage. It is critically important to have antioxidants in your bloodstream when t-PA is administered to reduce the free radical damage that will occur when blood flow is restored.

The most potent antioxidant that a hospital pharmacy normally stocks for the treatment of strokes is Hydergine. You should insist that the emergency room doctor administer 10 mg of Hydergine sublingually, and another 10 mg of Hydergine orally in liquid form. Hydergine is a powerful antioxidant that reduces free radical damage. Hydergine will increase the amount of oxygen delivered to the brain, enhance the energy metabolism of brain cells, and protect brain cells against both the low- and high-oxygen environments that ischemic stroke victims often encounter.

Hydergine is used routinely in Europe and the rest of the world as a treatment for stroke, but most emergency room physicians in the United States are reluctant to prescribe it because the FDA does not recognize its value in preventing brain-cell death. Paralyzed stroke victims consume billions of health care dollars every year, and the reason most *ischemic* stroke victims are permanently paralyzed is that the FDA has stopped patients from being treated with medications to prevent brain-cell death.

Conventional Therapies to Prevent Another Stroke

There are conventional drugs that can be prescribed to reduce the risk of a second stroke: (1) anti-platelet drugs such as Trental (pentoxifylline) and Ticlid (ticlopidine) inhibit abnormal platelet aggregation, thereby reducing the risk of a new blood clot forming in the brain; (2) anticoagulant drugs such as heparin or Coumadin interfere with the initiation of the coagulation cascade, and significantly reduce the risk that a blood clot will form. The use of anticoagulant drugs involves frequent blood testing and adjusting of dose since the anti-coagulating response to these drugs varies between individuals. These drugs DON'T do anything to the clots that may already have been formed. The side effects of anticoagulant drugs mandates careful monitoring, and some people avoid these drugs because of the risk of serious side effects.

For those who have high or borderline high blood pressure, precise management of anti-hypertensive drug therapy is critical. (*Refer to the Hypertension protocol for further information.*)

Integrated or Alternative Treatment Therapies

In the 1960s hypertension was identified as a treatable risk factor for stroke, and the decline in the incidence of and mortality from a stroke began when doctors began implementing aggressive anti-hypertensive therapies. In the 1970s aspirin was first demonstrated effective in preventing strokes, though few doctors prescribe aspirin even to this day to reduce the risk of ischemic stroke. Cigarette smoking has been proven conclusively as a major risk factor for stroke, and smoking cessation produces a significant risk reduction within 2 years.

Researchers now believe there are an immense number of mechanisms at work causing brain cell damage and death following a stroke. Each of these mechanisms represents a potential route for intervention, as well as prevention. Given the multidimensional nature of ischemic brain cell injury, stroke experts predict that no single drug will be able to completely protect the brain during a stroke. More likely, a combination of agents will be necessary for full recovery potential.

Most strokes culminate in a core area of cell death (infarction) in which blood flow is so drastically reduced that the cells usually cannot recover. This threshold seems to occur when cerebral blood flow is 20% of normal or less. Brain cells ultimately die as a result of the actions of calcium-activated proteases (enzymes which digest cell proteins), lipases (enzymes which digest cell membranes), and free radicals formed as a result of the ischemic cascade.

Without neuroprotective agents, nerve and brain cells may be irreversibly damaged within several minutes. This knowledge is leading to unprecedented therapy development. Expanding knowledge regarding the nature of ischemic brain cell injury is leading researchers to focus on the development of calcium antagonists, glutamate antagonists, antioxidants, and other types of neuroprotective agents. As discussed above, the use of Hydergine to treat acute stroke may be the most effective therapy to combine with t-PA to prevent permanent brain damage.

Piracetam, a nootropic medication similar to pyroglutamate (an amino acid), would be useful in the treatment of ischemic stroke if it were approved in the United States for acute use. Piracetam appears to protect brain cells from injury and death during a stroke, thereby lessening the potential for permanent neurological damage. The recommended dosage for piracetam is 4800 mg taken orally. A recent Belgian study indicated that piracetam may be very beneficial if administered within seven hours after the onset of a stroke. Piracetam is not currently available in the United States, but has been successfully used in Europe for 25 years as reported in the *Journal of Pharmacopsychiatry*, March 1999.

Any disruption of blood flow to the brain causes massive free radical damage that induces much of the re-perfusion injury to brain cells characteristic of strokes. When blood flow is interrupted and subsequently restored (re-perfused), tissues release iron that provides a catalyst for the formation of free radicals that often permanently damage brain cells. The Life Extension Foundation has spent millions of dollars conducting research that involves developing methods of protecting the brain cells from injury caused by blood-flow disruption. The use of antioxidant nutrients, drugs, and hormones, along with specific calcium-channel blockers and cell membrane–stabilizing agents, provides enormous protection to brain cells.

If you know an ischemic stroke is occurring, large quantities of antioxidant vitamins and herbs such as ginkgo biloba would be of benefit. Magnesium in an oral dose of 1500 mg is a safe nutrient to relieve an arterial spasm, a common problem in thrombotic strokes. If you take high-potency antioxidant nutrients at least 3 times a day, your chances of fully recovering from an ischemic stroke may be significantly improved.

An analysis of 18 trials documented a 23% reduction in stroke risk with anti-platelet agents. The drug ticlopidine was found to be the most effective anti-platelet agent, but its adverse side effects frequently restrict its long-term use. A more benign approach such as use of aspirin or nutrients like ginkgo biloba, melatonin, fish oil, and garlic, as well as green tea extract, may be as effective and are free of side effects.

Benefits of Low-Dose Aspirin

Low-dose aspirin is the anti-platelet agent of choice for stroke prevention. The Second European Stroke Prevention Study reported risk reductions for aspirin treatment, when compared with a placebo, to be as high as 27.6% (*Acta Neurol. Scand.*, 1999, [Jan] 99[1]:54–60).

Aspirin has shown such a potent effect in preventing strokes that the use of anticoagulants such as heparin to treat ischemic strokes decreased from 1985 to 1990, whereas the use of aspirin increased by more than 50% as reported in the Minnesota Stroke Survey published in the *Journal of Stroke and Cerebral Diseases*, 1998.

A study on patients who had survived a stroke or transient ischemic attacks (TIAs) showed that the use of a low-dose aspirin (50 mg) reduced the incidence of stroke by 18 to 28% when study participants consumed aspirin over a period of time. This study was reported in *Thrombosis Research* (1998,15; 92 [1 Suppl. 1]:S1–6).

Benefits of Ginkgo Biloba

The conclusions of a January 1999 report of 40 clinical trials published in the journal *Neuroreport* stated that "positive results have been reported for ginkgo biloba extracts in the treatment of cerebral insufficiency."

Earlier 1995 double-blind placebo-controlled trials of ginkgo biloba extract involving 55 patients with acute cerebral ischemia showed a significant improvement in cognitive function–based Mathews scale cognitive assessment (*J. Assoc. Physicians India*, [Nov] 1995; 43 [11]:760–63).

Gingko biloba was used with heart patients in a treadmill test in France, and the doctors concluded "In a comparison of the differences before and after treatment, the areas of ischemia decreased by 38%" after its use (*Angiology* [USA], 1994, 45 [6]:413–17).

A French study of mice at the Universite de la Mediterranee, Marseille, France in 1998 says that "neuroprotective drugs such as ginkgo biloba extract could prevent the ischemia-induced impairment."

Ginkgo appears not only to protect against free radicals and abnormal blood clotting, but also to enhance neuronal metabolic rates that are severely impaired as a result of ischemic insult.

Benefits of Melatonin

Consideration should be given to the use of melatonin as part of an integrated treatment for thrombotic stroke. According to a 1998 report, "Melatonin is one of the most powerful scavengers of free radicals. Because it easily penetrates the blood-brain barrier, this antioxidant may, in the future, be used for the treatment of Alzheimer's and Parkinson's diseases, stroke, nitric oxide, neurotoxicity and hyperbaric oxygen exposure" (*Biol. Signals Recept.*, 1998 [July] 7 [4]:195–219).

Another study, at the University of Texas Health Sciences Center in San Antonio, Texas, reporting in the November 1998 *Journal of Neuroscience Research,* indicates that "Considering melatonin's relative lack of toxicity and ability to enter the brain, these [study] results along with previous evidence suggest that melatonin, which is a natural substance, may be useful in combating free radical–induced neuronal injury in acute situations such as strokes."

In laboratory experiments funded by the Life Extension Foundation, where severe brain ischemia is artificially induced, the addition of melatonin to a "cocktail" of antioxidants, calcium-channel antagonists, and cell membrane–stabilizing agents provides significant protection against brain damage. It is unfortunate that conventional emergency rooms may not incorporate melatonin into the treatment of stroke for many years to come.

Mid-Life Blood Pressure: A New Risk Factor for Stroke

A 30-year study of male twins showed that elevated blood pressure in mid-life predisposed men to accelerated brain aging and an increase in strokes later in life. Men with even mildly elevated blood pressure 25 years before showed smaller brain volumes and more strokes compared to their twin brothers who did not have the elevation in blood pressure. This study, published in the 1999 *Journal of Stroke,* emphasized the importance of aggressively treating elevated blood pressure even if it is not grossly abnormal. Refer to the *Hypertension protocol* for information about blood pressure control therapies and diets.

Conclusion

Ischemic stroke is a medical emergency. Time to treatment of this "brain attack" is important, as what is done once in the emergency room. Request t-PA and Hydergine therapy as suggested in this protocol.

The risk factors for ischemic strokes are hypertension, arteriosclerosis, and blood that has a propensity to clot abnormally inside vessels. Blood components that increase the risk of abnormal arterial clotting include elevated levels of LDL cholesterol, homocysteine, or fibrinogen. Drug and alcohol abuse, age, gender, and race are also factors.

Some indications of ischemic stroke risk are transient ischemic attacks (TIAs)—"mini-strokes" that produce stroke-like symptoms, but no lasting damage.

Symptoms for thrombotic stroke are (1) sudden trouble standing or walking, dizziness, loss of balance or coordination; (2) sudden numbness of the face or weakness of the arm or leg, especially on one side of the body; (3) sudden confusion, trouble speaking or understanding; (4) sudden trouble seeing in one or both eyes; (5) sudden, very severe headaches with no known cause. Diagnosis of thrombotic strokes is by Doppler ultrasonography, CT scan, and MRI.

Treatment for thrombotic strokes depends on the underlying cause. Treatment of early-stage ischemic stroke should include t-PA and Hydergine. Surgery may be needed in some cases to remove any blockage of blood vessels going to the brain. Doctors may prescribe anti-coagulation and platelet aggregation inhibitor drugs to reduce the risk of a first or secondary stroke in high-risk individuals. Additionally, aspirin, ginkgo biloba, melatonin, fish oil, garlic, and green tea extract may be taken to reduce the damage from, or recurrence of, ischemic strokes.

Hydergine and piracetam may be beneficial to stroke patients. The FDA has not approved Hydergine for the treatment of strokes, but it should be available through the hospital pharmacy, and patients or their family should request its use. Piracetam may be beneficial in preventing permanent neurological damage following a stroke. Piracetam is not currently available in the United States.

Promise of a New Protein Therapy for Stroke

Researchers at Columbia University in New York have discovered that nerve cells surrounding the area of the brain affected by a stroke display a certain protein on their surface after a stroke occurs. Results of a study in mice show that in a response known as the complement cascade, the protein basically calls the body's own immune system in to destroy its own cells. If activation of this immune mechanism can be prevented, these neurons and the brain can be protected from the body's own immune systems normally damaging response.

In their July 1999 study reported in *Science* magazine, the researchers found that injecting a protein called sCR1 into mice 45 minutes after a stroke reduced the impact of the complement cascade. The researchers were not only able to impede even more brain damage; by modifying the protein, they also were able to reduce potentially damaging blood clots by stopping white blood cells and platelets from accumulating in arteries.

We will continue to follow this important research, and report to you on new research or on this protein's availability for use.

Summary

1. The symptoms of thrombotic strokes include nausea and dizziness; sudden, severe headaches; weakness, numbness; paralysis, particularly to one side of the body; partial or total loss of sight in one eye.
2. Diagnostic procedures for thrombotic strokes include ultrasound, CT scan, and MRI.
3. Treatment of thrombotic strokes consists of medication, natural supplements, and surgical interventions, based on the underlying cause. Controlling hypertension is essential prevention in the occurrence of ischemic strokes.
4. Hydergine, an antioxidant medication that protects brain cells, may be given in an acute situation. The recommended dosage is 10 mg given sublingually and 10 mg administered orally. Because the FDA has not approved Hydergine for this purpose, the patient or patient's advocate should request that the medication be given.
5. Piracetam, a nootropic medication, may be useful in the prevention of thrombotic strokes because it appears to protect brain cells from injury during the stroke event. The recommended dosage for piracetam is 4800 mg a day, administered orally.
6. Consider low-dose aspirin, ¼ tablet a day with a heavy meal.
7. Consider 120 mg daily of ginkgo biloba extract.
8. Consider garlic extract, 1500 to 6000 mg daily.
9. Consider fish oil concentrate, 4 to 10 capsules of a highly concentrated supplement.
10. Consider 350 mg daily of a 95% green tea extract.
11. Consider taking 500 mcg to 3 mg of melatonin (at night) and 100–200 mg of palm-oil

tocotrienols a day to protect against further free radical–induced brain cell injury.

(To learn about therapies that may protect arteries prior to a thrombotic stroke, or to reduce the risk of further disease or stroke attacks, refer to the protocols on treating Atherosclerosis, Hypertension, and Thrombosis Prevention. To learn more about therapies that may restore neurological function following thrombotic stroke, refer to the protocol for Age-Associated Mental Impairment.)

For more information. Contact the National Institute of Neurological Disorders and Stroke, (800) 352-9424.

Product availability. Low-dose aspirin, ginkgo biloba, garlic extract, fish oil concentrate, green tea extract, and melatonin can be ordered by calling (800) 544-4440, or order on-line at www.lef.org. Ask for a list of offshore suppliers of Hydergine tablets and piracetam.

SURGICAL PRECAUTIONS

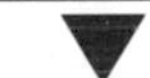

(See Anesthesia and Surgical Precautions protocol.)

THROMBOSIS PREVENTION

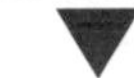

by Calin V. Pop, M.D.

Definition

An abnormal blood clot inside a blood vessel is defined as thrombosis. Thrombosis has been described as coagulation occurring in the wrong place or at the wrong time. The end result of thrombosis is an obstruction of the blood flow. Since the leading cause of death in the Western world is the formation of an abnormal blood clot inside a blood vessel, it is important for healthy people to take steps to prevent thrombosis. For those with risk factors for developing thrombosis, aggressive actions must be taken to protect against stroke, heart attack, kidney failure, and pulmonary embolus.

General Considerations

Preventing thrombosis is essential for living. All of us need to prevent clots inside the circulatory system every single minute. Coagulation-anticoagulation is a perfect "mechanism" that our body has to maintain. If this process of keeping an optimal balance between coagulation and anticoagulation fails, our lives can be in danger in a matter of minutes.

What we need for optimal function is to keep blood flowing well in all our vessels, whether small or big. When a leak (or damage) occurs in a vessel, we need to encourage the coagulation aspect of this balance in order to seal the leakage.

On the other hand, whenever there is a significant disturbance in the blood flow, the consequences are often lethal.

Symptoms

The symptoms depend on where the clot is formed. Heart attacks, stroke, or pulmonary embolism are examples of localized clots that may have various symptoms. If a clot occurs in a coronary artery, a person can have a heart attack. If the clot occurs in an artery in the brain, a person can have a stroke. Clots that form anywhere inside the vascular system can travel elsewhere in the body, causing lethal damage to the lungs (pulmonary emboli), kidneys, or other parts of the body. Cancer patients are especially vulnerable to disability and death from abnormal clot formation inside the blood vessels, particularly in the veins. Symptoms may be totally different, strictly depending on the position of the clot.

Clotting can be localized, but it can also be generalized, such as in a condition called Disseminated Intravascular Coagulation, which also occurs when we die. Up to a point, aggressive medical management can reverse this condition.

Clots can stay where they form or travel to a different location. Whether the clot forms on the spot or travels, the size of the clot is secondary in importance to the location of the clot and the specifics of the area occluded. In general, clots in areas with less collateral circulation are more serious and may be life threatening.

Causes

There are hundreds of possible factors that can precipitate blood clots. Our body is so designed that *any* circulatory disturbance in the blood flow from any cause can result in blood clots. This multiplicity of possible causes is a reason that circulatory problems and thrombosis are a major medical problem today.

In general, for the same location, larger clots are more dangerous than smaller ones. Because the clot formation can have numerous causes, the most obvious correlations are called "risk factors." Some of them are

- Atrial fibrillation
- Heart valve replacement
- Heart failure
- Postsurgery
- Cigarette smoking
- Atherosclerosis
- Cancer
- Lupus
- Oral contraceptives
- Nephrotic syndrome
- Heart attack
- Carotid stenosis
- Diabetes
- Cold weather
- Aging
- Pregnancy
- Artificial hormones (e.g., "estrogens")

How it Happens

A blood clot is formed in a framework of a fibrin mesh on which specific blood components called platelets stick. Later, red blood cells become trapped in the fibrin mesh. Either fibrin or platelets can trigger a clot. Clotting usually proceeds in a step-by-step fashion, called a coagulation cascade, that can develop very quickly. This cascade is extremely complex and has a vast number of factors that can influence it.

The process of clot formation is not uniform and does not proceed with the same speed throughout the body. The composition of the blood clot varies with the site of injury. For example, vein clots (red color) have more fibrin and are friable (easily crumbled), while arterial clots (white color) have more platelets and dislodge easily.

Prevention and Treatment

Because so many factors can contribute to coagulation and therefore should be considered for prevention, it is very difficult to control them all. In medicine we can exert control on some crucial steps in the coagulation cascade, but it is almost impossible to influence them all.

Conventional medicine prescribes drugs like Coumadin and heparin to reduce the risk of abnormal blood clotting cascade (thrombosis), but these drugs block merely a third of the coagulation cascade. As a result, many who are taking prescription anticoagulants often die from a heart attack or stroke caused directly by the formation of a blood vessel clot, even though they properly took their medicine. Prescription anticoagulation drugs do not effectively deal with all the factors that have been identified as directly causing blood clots to form inside of blood vessels.

The modern arsenal for anticoagulation/clot prevention is not vast. There are drugs that will either work on the fibrin formation or drugs that work on platelet aggregation. All these drugs are to be monitored extremely carefully as they may easily be overdosed or cause adverse reactions. It is noticeable that some of these reactions or secondary bleedings may be worse than the clots they tried to prevent in the first place.

People who take vitamin supplements are getting some protection against thrombosis. Published studies show that people taking vitamin supplements have reduced incidence of heart disease, stroke, and a host of other diseases related to thrombosis. Enumerated below are some of the elements that contribute to thrombosis as well as some of their "nutritional antidotes":

Causes of Thrombosis	Nutritional Prophylaxis
Elevated homocysteine	Vitamins B_{12}, B_6, folate, trimethylglycine (TMG)
Oxidized LDL	Antioxidants (such as vitamin E)
Elevated fibrinogen	Enzymes, bromelain
Excess platelet free-radical activity	Antioxidants, EDTA
Elevated thromboxane A_2 prostaglandin E_2, lipoxygenase, and/or cyclooxygenase	Aspirin; gingko; green tea; fish, flax, or perilla oil
Thrombin activating factor	Licorice extract
Platelet activating factor	Antiplatelet drugs (aspirin, Plavix, Ticlid); green tea
Deficiency of TPA	Enzymes: one glass of wine nightly
Hyperaggregation of red blood cells and loss of red blood cell fluidity	Essential fatty acids: fish, flax, or perilla oil
Increased blood viscosity	Hydration: drink water (not fluids)
Increased thrombocyte count	Hydration: treat underlying cause
Inflammation of arterial wall	Enzymes, anti-inflammatories
Atherosclerotic plaque	EDTA, garlic
Elevated triglycerides	Fish oil, niacin
Increased platelet adhesion	Garlic
Collagen-induced platelet aggregation	Vitamin C, *L*-lysine, *L*-proline
Epinephrine-induced platelet aggregation	Avoid stress, coffee, and smoking

From the above list of "natural" solutions to clot-forming risk factors, we can infer that there are dietary supplements that can prevent thrombosis. They have to be taken in the right dose and the right combination. Studies about nutritional supplements in medicine are being performed in great numbers nowadays, and more and more are being performed every day.

Interactions

There are specific nutrients that have been identified to lower the risk of thrombosis. These nutrients provide many other health benefits, and many people already take these supplements to maintain overall good health.

What is not fully understood is how these nutrients interact with prescription anticoagulant drugs such as heparin and Coumadin (warfarin). For example, there are no published studies in which these nutrients have been combined with anticoagulant drugs to ascertain whether the blood loses too much of its proper coagulation characteristics. For those taking Coumadin or heparin who also want to follow some or all of this Thrombosis Prevention protocol, weekly or biweekly prothrombin (PT) blood tests are recommended. In addition to prothrombin, the following blood tests taken every 30 to 60 days to help precisely measure thrombotic risk are

- Partial thromboplastin time (PTT)
- Fibrinogen
- *D*-dimer of fibrin

There is much debate and confusion about the interactions between dietary nutrients and prescription antithrombotic medications regarding clot formation. For quite some time, there has been concern that certain supplements negatively affect the coagulation process, i.e., the nutrients could cause too much suppression of blood clotting factors and increase the risk of blood vessel bleeding.

However, my clinical experience shows that this concept is not a great concern. When we have any prescription drugs that affect coagulation (heparin, Coumadin) as well as over-the-counter anti-inflammatories (such as aspirin and ibuprofen), corticosteroids, or anti-malarials, close supervision of the clinical condition as well as supervision of the clotting balance by blood tests is needed.

When supplements such as aspirin, vitamins, herbs, and oils are used as the primary antithrombotic therapy, the risk of undesirable side effects is mitigated. In other words, if you are taking anticoagulant drugs such as Coumadin or heparin, you need to be careful and check the blood regularly. This is even more necessary if there is a combination of drugs or over-the-counter medication. With the use of natural therapies and aspirin, the need for weekly or biweekly blood monitoring is reduced, but those with thrombotic risk factors such as atrial fibrillation, valve replacement, or cancer should still consider testing their blood for the following coagulation factors every 14 to 90 days:

- Prothrombin (PT)
- Partial thromboplastin time (PTT)
- Fibrinogen
- *D*-dimer of fibrin

Cancer Patients

In patients affected with different tumors, disorders concerning blood clotting are frequently observed. The biological processes leading to coagulation are probably involved in the mechanisms of metastasis. About 50% of all cancer patients, and up to 95% of those with metastatic disease, show some abnormalities—a prethrombotic state—in the coagulation-fibrinolytic system. Thromboembolic complications are seen in up to 11% of cancer patients, and hemorrhage occurs in about 10%. Thromboembolism and hemorrhage, as a whole, are the second most common cause of death after infection.

In one study, subclinical changes in the coagulation-fibrinolytic system were frequently detected in lung cancer patients. Five conventional tests and one new test of blood coagulation—that is, platelet count (P), prothrombin time (PT), partial thromboplastin time (PTT), fibrinogen (F), and *D*-dimer of fibrin (DD)—were prospectively recorded in a series of 286 patients with new primary lung cancer. A prethrombotic state (depicted by a prolongation of PT, PTT, and increase of *D*-dimer of fibrin) was significantly associated with an adverse outcome.

Anticoagulant treatment of cancer patients, particularly those with lung cancer, has been reported to improve survival. These interesting, although preliminary, results of controlled trials lent some support to the argument that activation of blood coagulation plays a role in the natural history of tumor growth. Recently, two studies compared the effectiveness of standard heparin with low molecular weight heparin (LMWH) in the treatment of deep vein thrombosis (DVT). In both studies, mortality rates were lower in the patients randomized to LMWH. The analysis of these deaths reveals a striking difference in cancer-related mortality.

Cancer-related mortality with standard heparin was 31%, versus 11% with low molecular weight heparin. This difference cannot solely be attributed to thrombotic or bleeding events. Since large numbers of cancer patients were included in the studies, it seems unlikely that ones with more advanced tumors were present in the standard heparin group. While it also is possible that standard heparin increases cancer mortality, such an adverse effect has not been previously reported. These considerations suggest that low molecular weight heparin might exert an inhibitory effect on tumor growth. If your oncologist will not test for thrombotic risk factors, contact the Life Extension Foundation at (800) 544-4440.

Thrombosis Prevention Protocol — General Instructions

- Avoid inactivity, junk food, coffee, smoking, refined sugar, carbonated beverages, and stress as much as possible.
- Drink at least 8 to 10 glasses of water a day, and exercise regularly.
- Eat plenty of raw, fresh fruits and vegetables or fresh juices, fiber, and pectin with alkaline components.
- Use olive oil as main dietary fat.

Nutrients

- Vitamin C, 3000 to 5000 mg daily. Aids in healthy collagen formation, platelet function, as well many other important activities.
- Vitamin E, 800 IU daily. Decreases platelet aggregation and has strong antioxidant function.

- Vitamin B complex, at least 50 mg of the B vitamins. Decreases homocysteine involved in metabolic reactions of the platelets and vessel wall.
- Aspirin, ¼ tablet with the heaviest meal of the day. Some patients are prescribed 1 aspirin tablet 5 days a week and ¼ tablet the other 2 days.
- Bromelain, 1000 to 2000 mg a day on an empty stomach once or twice daily. Excellent enzyme activity; it reduces fibrin formation and platelet reactivity.
- Rutin, 100 to 200 mg. Helps in healthy collagen formation and maintains good elasticity of the vessel wall.
- Omega 3 fatty acids (fish, flax, or perilla). About 4000 mg of EPA/DHA (from fish) or alpha-linolenic acid (from flax or perilla oils). Helps reduce aggregation of red blood cells and red blood cell fluidity.
- Garlic. Excellent platelet adhesion and aggregation inhibitor.
- EDTA. Chelates heavy metals and prevents free-radical reactions. Chelates excess calcium and reduces atherosclerotic plaque. Intravenous EDTA is about 20 times stronger than the oral form.
- Gingko biloba. Maintains capillary elasticity and inhibits thromboxane A_2.
- Flavonoids, bilberry, pycnogenol. Maintains capillary integrity, resistance to oxidative stress of the capillary wall, keeps capillaries elastic, and protects against abnormal platelet aggregation.
- Licorice extract (Glycyrrhizin). Works on thrombin-activating factor and increases resistance to stress.
- Wheat germ oil. Contains natural tocopherols (vitamin E), antioxidants, and is a platelet aggregation inhibitor.
- White oak bark tea, 1 to 2 cups daily. Helps prevent clots.
- Enzymes, pineapple, papaya, and alfalfa. Ingesting plenty of enzymes found in these plants and in fresh fruits and vegetables is an important factor in preventing blood clots.
- Green tea. Drink 1 to 10 cups a day or consume 300 to 600 mg of the polyphenol extract from green tea in supplement form. Some studies show drinking just one cup a day of black tea to be highly effective.
- Folic acid, 800 mcg; vitamin B_{12}, 1000 mcg; and vitamin B_6, 100 to 250 mg to keep serum homocysteine levels in the safe range.
- Betaine (TMG), 1000 mg 3 times daily if homocysteine levels are high despite the use of folic acid and vitamins B_{12} and B_6.

Check the ratio of testosterone to estrogens. The more estrogens present relative to testosterone, the higher the risk is in both men and women. Especially risky are the contraceptives or the so-called "hormone replacement therapies." These are artificial substances with a similar (but not exact) structure to human hormones. They are also imbalanced megadoses of only one of the three or four needed hormones usually derived from the urine of pregnant mares. Testosterone has a somewhat protective action against thrombosis formation.

Summary

Prevention of blood clots is a complex task that involves keeping a fine balance in place between the process of coagulation and anticoagulation. Patients on prescription medication as well as any combination of these with over-the-counter anti-inflammatories or aspirin need close monitoring by periodic laboratory testing of their blood. Patients on supplements (such as vitamins, herbs, or oils) need their risk factors (fibrinogen and homocysteine) evaluated in the same way. However, a close monitoring of the coagulation balance is not usually necessary in otherwise healthy people.

WARNING: Never change anticoagulation medication without physician approval, because thrombosis, bleeding, and sudden death may occur.

Product availability. Low-dose aspirin (Healthprin), Life Extension Booster, Life Extension Mix, garlic with EDTA, gingko biloba, vitamin C, vitamin B complex, vitamin E, and highly concentrated fish oil capsules are available by calling (800) 544-4440, or order online at www.lef.org.

THYROID DEFICIENCY

The Function of the Thyroid Gland

The thyroid gland lies in the neck, just below the Adam's apple. It measures about 2 inches across and normally can't be seen. It can barely be felt upon palpation. An enlarged thyroid, known as a goiter, can easily be detected by a physician upon examination. The thyroid gland secretes hormones which control the body's metabolic rate in two primary ways: by stimulating tissue response in the body to produce proteins, and by increasing cell oxygenation. To produce these vital hormones, the thyroid needs the element iodine, which is ingested from food and water.

The regulation of thyroid hormone levels is controlled by several mechanisms. The hypothalamus, located in the brain just above the pituitary gland, secretes thyrotropin-releasing hormone, which triggers the pituitary to release thyroid-stimulating hormone (TSH). When the amount of thyroid hormone in the blood reaches a certain level, the pituitary will produce less thyroid-stimulating hormone; conversely, when the amount of thyroid hormone in the blood decreases to a certain level, the pituitary produces more thyroid-stimulating hormone.

There are two forms of thyroid hormone. Thyroxine (T4), produced in the thyroid, has only a slight impact on speeding up the body's metabolic rate. Thyroxine is converted by the liver and other organs to triiodothyronine (T3), which is the metabolically active form. Most of the T4 and T3 remains tightly bound to certain proteins in the blood in an inactive form. The body's continually changing need for more or less thyroid hormone will determine the rate of T4 to T3 conversion and the release of bound T3 and T4 in blood protein. In this way, the body will maintain the proper levels of thyroid hormone to regulate normal metabolic rate.

Thyroid Deficiency

A thyroid deficiency (hypothyroidism) means that the thyroid gland is producing too little thyroid hormone. The symptoms of hypothyroidism are gradual and are sometimes mistaken for depression. Facial expressions become dull, the voice becomes hoarse, eyelids droop, and the face and eyes become puffy and swollen. Thyroid deficiency generally affects women who are over the age of 40, but it can also affect men and teenagers, especially if it runs in the family. Hypothyroidism can cause a number of other conditions, such as allergies, skin problems, fatigue, nervousness, gaining or losing weight, brittle nails, dry skin, gastrointestinal problems (constipation), infertility, mental sluggishness, low immune function, depression, and intolerance to cold. Carpal tunnel syndrome has also been associated with thyroid deficiency.

Hashemite's thyroiditis is the most common form of hypothyroidism presenting with an enlarged thyroid gland that becomes nonfunctional, with the active parts of the gland deteriorating after several years. Treatment for hyperthyroidism, which includes administering radioactive iodine and surgical removal, may also result in hypothyroidism. In many undeveloped countries where there is a chronic lack of iodine in the diet, goitrous hypothyroidism resulting from an underactive thyroid gland is common. Hypothyroidism resulting from a lack of dietary iodine has disappeared in the United States Severe hypothyroidism is known as myxedema.

Diagnosis

Overt hypothyroidism is easy to diagnose by a simple blood test. Low levels of T3 and T4 are signs that you do not have enough thyroid hormones. Also, an elevated TSH is a sign of thyroid deficiency. When your TSH is high, it means the pituitary gland is trying to make the thyroid gland produce more hormones.

If, however, someone is suffering from the classic symptoms of thyroid deficiency but has normal test results, the thyroid slowdown could be slight or age related and is not easily detected by a blood test. Thyroid deficiency often mimics many symptoms associated with old age. One way to determine a thyroid deficiency is to have your physician test for a substance called transthyretrin (also known as prealbumin). Thyroid hormone is carried through the bloodstream and brain by transthyretrin. Even when all other hormones are normal, a low level of transthyretrin could mean that you are not producing enough thyroid hormones and that it is not being delivered to the cells. Another way of detecting a possible thyroid deficiency is to take your basal body temperature.

The Basal Body Temperature Test

Broda O. Barnes, M.D., developed the basal body temperature test. Barnes recommends the following procedure:

1. Shake down an oral glass thermometer and leave it on the night table before going to bed.
2. Upon awakening, with as little movement as possible, place the thermometer firmly in your armpit or under your tongue. (Menstruating women should do this test only on the second and third days of their menstrual flow.)
3. Keep the thermometer there for 10 minutes.
4. Record the readings on three consecutive days.

A normal functioning thyroid should have a reading of 97.8 to 98.2. A reading of 97.8 or lower, according to Dr. Barnes, may indicate low thyroid function.

Treatment

If left untreated, hypothyroidism can cause anemia, low body temperature, and heart failure. A life-threatening condition known as myxedema coma may ensue in which respiration slows, seizures occur, and blood flow to the brain decreases. Exposure to cold, infections, tranquilizing drugs, and trauma can trigger myxedema coma.

Conventional treatment calls for the oral replacement of deficient thyroid hormones. A synthetic form of T4 (Synthroid and Levothroid) is most often administered. Treatment, especially in older people, begins with low doses of thyroid hormone, since serious side effects may occur with too large a dose. The dose is gradually increased until TSH levels in the blood return to normal. The medication must usually be taken for life.

Dietary Supplementation for Thyroid Deficiency

Proper supplementation along with natural glandular concentrates may help return the TSH to the normal range. There are natural glandular concentrates that can be prescribed by a physician to treat thyroid deficiencies. These include Armour Desiccated Thyroid Hormone, Nathroid, and Westhroid, all of which are derived from the thyroid gland of the pig. They contain T4 and T3 and most closely resemble natural human thyroid hormone. Most conventional physicians prefer synthetic products, like Synthroid and Levothroid, which are widely promoted by pharmaceutical companies, but these synthetic products consist mostly of T4, and the body must convert T4 to T3 and other metabolites. This could be a problem for the patient whose thyroid does not properly convert T4 to T3. This may be the reason many people who are on Synthroid still claim that they "don't feel right." Some doctors recognize Synthroid's limitations and prescribe the drug Cytomel to directly provide the metabolically active T3 form of thyroid hormone.

Most physicians are reluctant to prescribe natural glandulars because they are told that they are impure and inconsistent from dose to dose. Armour Thyroid and most other natural glandular preparations are made to standards approved by the United States Pharmacopoeia (U.S.P.), which assures that its potency is accurately stated on the label. If your physician requires more information on natural glandulars, contact the Broda O. Barnes foundation listed below.

Supplementation includes vitamin A; vitamin B complex; and vitamins A, B_{12}, C, and E; as well as Coenzyme Q_{10}; and especially the minerals magnesium, manganese, selenium, and zinc, all of which can be found in ample amounts in the Life Extension Mix. Deficiencies of any of these minerals can prevent the conversion of T4 to T3 and should be corrected. Sufficient protein iodine and especially the amino acid tyrosine are necessary to make T4 in the thyroid gland. Soy supplements are known to boost thyroid output.

The amino acid tyrosine is converted into thyroxine, or T4. This is the same substance that doctors give as medication. Enzymatic Therapy makes Thyroid & *L*-Tyrosine Complex which contains added essential minerals along with L-tyrosine, multiglandular complex, and kelp, which is a rich source of iodine.

DHEA, a hormone that enhances the body's metabolic functioning, may also be deficient in individuals with hypothyroidism. A DHEA blood test should be administered to achieve optimal dosing. (*See the DHEA-Pregnenolone Precautions in the DHEA Replacement Therapy protocol* for more detailed information.)

Summary

Thyroid deficiency occurs when the thyroid gland underproduces the hormones thyroxine (T4) and triiodothyronine (T3) needed to regulate the body's metabolic rate. In some individuals, the thyroid does not properly convert T4 to T3, the metabolically active form. Supplementation with synthetic or animal-derived thyroid hormone is necessary to return hormone levels to normal. Suggested supplements and their dosages follow:

1. Synthetic hormone supplementation, prescribed by a physician, includes Synthroid and Levothroid (synthetic T4) and/or Cyotmel (synthetic T3).
2. Natural glandulars (by prescription) such as Armour Desiccated Thyroid Hormone, Nathroid, and Westhroid, derived from the thyroid gland of the pig, contain T4 and T3, and most closely resemble natural human thyroid hormone.
3. Iodine, 1 mg per day.
4. Tyrosine, 500 to 1000 mg per day.
5. Melatonin, 3 mg at bedtime.
6. Mega Soy Extract, 1 capsule, 2 times a day.
7. DHEA, 25 mg 1 to 3 times a day (*Refer to DHEA Replacement Therapy protocol*).
8. Life Extension Mix for vitamin A, vitamin B complex, magnesium, manganese, selenium, and zinc, to be taken as directed.

For more information. Contact the Thyroid Foundation of America, (800) 832-8321. For more information on natural glandulars or the basal body temperature test, contact the Broda O. Barnes, M.D., Research Foundation at P.O. Box 98, Trembly, CT 06611, (203) 261-2101.

Product availability. Life Extension Mix, Coenzyme Q_{10}, and Thyroid & *L*-Tyrosine Complex by Enzymatic Therapy are available by calling (800) 544-4440, or order online at www.lef.org.

TINNITUS

Tinnitus is diagnosed as chronic ringing, roaring, buzzing, humming, or hissing in the ears. The symptoms of tinnitus are frequently found in the elderly. Although the cause of tinnitus is unknown, it can be a symptom of almost any ear disorder such as infection, blocked ear canal or eustachian tube, otosclerosis (overgrowth of bone in the middle ear), and Meuniere's disease. Blast injury from explosions has also been known to cause symptoms of tinnitus, as have adverse effects from drugs such as aspirin or antibiotics.

Tinnitus currently affects about 50 million adults in the United States. It may disappear on its own or when the underlying problem is successfully treated. In cases of chronic tinnitus for which there is no treatable underlying problem, a variety of therapies and steps may provide substantial relief for the sufferer.

Lifestyle Changes

- Recordings of soothing music or sounds may help cover the unwanted noise, especially while sleeping.

- Regular exercise may provide relief by increasing blood circulation to the head.
- A small electronic device worn in the ear, called a tinnitus masker, produces a pleasant sound that will compete with the tinnitus.
- Avoid alcohol, smoking, and caffeine, all of which may aggravate the condition.
- Cut down on salt, which may increase fluid buildup in the ear.
- Practice relaxation techniques.

Gingko Biloba

Gingko biloba is a plant extract used to reduce symptoms of various cognitive deficits such as decreased memory function, lack of concentration, and lack of alertness. Positive results in the treatment of tinnitus and dizziness have also been reported in the literature. Published studies have shown that 120 to 240 mg a day of pharmaceutical-grade gingko biloba extract can alleviate tinnitus, though some earlier studies failed to show benefits. The therapeutic effect of gingko is attributed to several active constituents with vasoactive and free radical–scavenging properties.

In a recent study conducted in Denmark, tinnitus and dizziness were reduced after a 4- to 6-week treatment regimen with gingko biloba. Researchers also noted minimal side effects in patients following the recommended dosage.

Another controlled study showed that gingko extract caused a statistically significant decrease in behavioral manifestation in the animal model of tinnitus. In human studies, it was shown that in patients suffering from cerebrovascular insufficiency (a common problem associated with normal aging), gingko extract produced a significant improvement in the symptoms of vertigo, tinnitus, headache, and forgetfulness.

Melatonin

Rosenberg et al. evaluated melatonin as a treatment for subjective tinnitus at the Ear Research Foundation in Sarasota, Florida. Patients were given 3 mg of melatonin nightly for 30 days. In patients with difficulty sleeping due to symptoms of tinnitus, an overall improvement was seen in 46% of the study group as opposed to 20% for the group given placebo. The researchers also concluded that patients with bilateral (two-sided) tinnitus showed significant improvement over those with unilateral (one-sided) tinnitus. Because of the minimal side effects associated with melatonin, it is considered a safe alternative treatment for chronic tinnitus.

Other Dietary Supplements

The ergot derivative, Hydergine, at a dosage level of 10 to 15 mg per day, has been shown to alleviate tinnitus in some people. The cerebral vasodilator, vinpocetine, can also be effective at a dosage of 20 to 40 mg per day. Additionally, vitamin A, 50,000 IU/day, should be taken, tapering as the condition improves; watch for signs of toxicity. Some patients may respond to vitamin B_{12} (1 mg, intramuscularly) 2 times per week. Carmen Fusco notes she has had excellent results with niacin/niacinamide in relatively high doses, along with 25 mg of zinc gluconate twice a day.

If the tinnitus is of recent duration, complete improvement is possible. If of long duration, the symptoms can be lessened with the nutrients described above in most people.

Summary

1. Medical workup to rule out underlying disease.
2. Lifestyle changes, as above.
3. Gingko biloba, 120 to 240 mg a day.
4. Melatonin, 3 mg a night.
5. Consider Hydergine, 10 to 15 mg a day.
6. Consider vinpocetine, 20 to 40 mg a day.
7. Consider piracetam, 1600 to 4800 a day.
8. Consider high doses of niacin/niacinamide with 25 mg zinc gluconate 2 times a day. Balance with 2 mg of copper a day.
9. Vitamin A, 50,000 IU per day with tapering as condition improves, watching for toxicity.
10. Vitamin B_{12}, 1 mg intramuscularly 2 times a week.

T

For more information. Contact the American Tinnitus Association, P.O. Box 5, Portland, OR 97207; (503) 248-9985.

Product availability. To order pharmaceutical gingko biloba extract, melatonin, or vinpocetin, phone (800) 544-4440, or order on-line at www.lef.org. Ask for a list of offshore suppliers who will ship high-potency Hydergine and vinpocetin to Americans for personal use.

TRAUMA

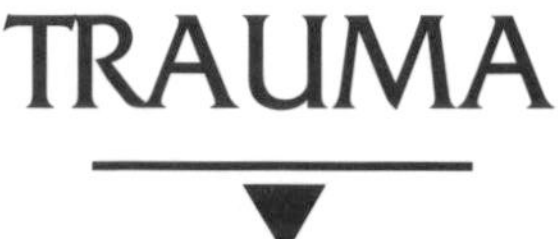

Trauma may be described as a body wound or shock due to accident or injury. Permanent injury or death due to trauma is often caused by free radicals generated when the tissues of the body are physically disrupted. This is well-documented in spinal cord injury cases where the free-radical damage that occurs immediately after the injury causes permanent paralysis.

Antioxidants such as vitamin E, glutathione, and palm-oil tocotrienols should immediately be administered to most victims of trauma to protect against free-radical injury. Trauma involving massive bleeding may preclude the use of antioxidants such as gingko that could accelerate hemorrhaging.

Protecting Brain Cells

To protect brain cells against oxygen deprivation or permanent damage from direct trauma to the head, 10 mg of sublingual Hydergine should be immediately administered along with 10 mg of Hydergine LC capsules. If piracetam is available, 4800 mg of piracetam should be administered to further protect against brain damage.

Vitamin E administration has been shown to reverse free-radical damage induced by trauma and to reverse the effects of lipid peroxidation after trauma. The administration of vitamin E has been shown to therapeutically protect against reduced T-cell membrane fluidity and suppressed T-cell functions. A vitamin E–enriched diet has been shown to protect the brains of mice against brain-circulatory injury. Also, diabetic rats experience a delay in corneal healing when deficient in vitamin E. Trauma patients should consider supplementing with 800 IU a day of vitamin E.

Protecting against Paralysis

In laboratory studies where two groups of animals were exposed to the same traumatic force, animals given high doses of vitamin C died less frequently than animals not given vitamin C. Antioxidants appear to protect against many forms of permanent damage inflicted by trauma.

The hormone pregnenolone has been shown to protect against paralysis from spinal cord injury in laboratory animals. The immediate administration of 400 mg of pregnenolone, along with 800 IU of vitamin E, to a spinal injury patient might be advisable. Vitamin E could speed the bleeding process, so do not use Vitamin E if excessive bleeding is occurring.

Dietary Supplementation in Trauma Patients

Nutritional supplementation, both enteric and intravenous, has been shown to impede further physical degeneration and accelerate the healing process in immunocompromised trauma patients. In recent studies, the administration of arginine, glutamine, and fish oil (omega 3 fatty acids) has been shown to reduce the incidence of systemic inflammatory response syndrome (SIRS) and multiple organ failure (MOF) due to severe trauma including burn wounds. In the same studies, an improvement in total lymphocyte count was seen.

In immunosuppressed burn patients with massive cutaneous trace element losses, large intravenous intake of copper (Cu), selenium (Se), and zinc (Zn) can aid in tissue repair and boost antioxidative defense mechanisms. Other research has shown that on animals treated postburn, intra-peritoneal injections of 3000 IU vitamin A improved immunosuppression response rate to 52% of unburned controls versus 21% for the postburn saline-treated test group. The study suggests that in humans, vitamin A may be an effective agent in the reversal of cellular immunosuppression.

DHEA and Immune Function

Researchers know that a depression in immune function occurs following injury but are uncertain as to the mechanism responsible. Steroid hormones are important mediators in the regulation of immune function. Dehydroepiandrosterone (DHEA) was recently studied on male mice to determine whether it has positive or negative effects on immune responses after trauma and hemorrhage. The mice were subjected to trauma, hemorrhage, and resuscitation, after which they received either DHEA or placebo subcutaneously. DHEA administration restored the normally depressed splenocyte proliferation as well as interleukin 2, interleukin 3, and interferon-gamma elaboration following trauma and hemorrhage.

The researchers then studied the mechanisms mediating this effect and found that T-cells were stimulated *in vitro* in the presence of DHEA and a variety of hormone antagonists. The stimulatory effect of DHEA on splenocyte proliferation was unaltered by the testosterone receptor antagonist flutamide, while the estrogen antagonist tamoxifen completely canceled its effect. In addition, DHEA administration normalized the elevated serum corticosterone level typically seen following injury. The researchers concluded, "These results indicate, therefore, that DHEA improves splenocyte function after trauma and hemorrhage by directly stimulating T cells and also by preventing a rise in serum corticosterone."

Summary

1. To prevent permanent injury due to free-radical damage, antioxidants should be administered immediately.

CAUTION: Injury involving massive bleeding may preclude the use of certain antioxidants such as gingko that might accelerate hemorrhaging.

2. To protect brain cells against oxygen deprivation resulting from trauma to the head, Hydergine and piracetam should be administered immediately.
3. The hormone pregnenolone has protected against paralysis in spinal cord–injured laboratory animals.
4. DHEA has been shown in laboratory experiments to improve splenocyte function, stimulate T cells, and prevent a rise in serum corticosterone.
5. Omega 3 fatty acids (fish oil), arginine, and glutamine may protect against multiple organ failure and systemic inflammatory response syndrome.

CAUTION: Any serious wound or injury must be examined and treated immediately by a medical professional.

Product availability. Vitamin E, DHEA, Mega EPA fish-oil concentrate, zinc, selenium, tocotrienols, and pregnenolone can be ordered by calling (800) 544-4440, or order online at www.lef.org. Call for a list of offshore companies that sell high-dose Hydergine and piracetam to Americans for personal use.

URINARY TRACT INFECTION

Urinary tract infections (UTIs) may be caused by bacteria, viruses (herpes simplex type 2), fungi (*Candida*), and a variety of parasites (worms and protozoa). Lower UTIs occur in the urethra or bladder and are more common in women than in men because the female urethra is much shorter and offers less of a barrier to bacterial invasion. The bacteria (85% of the time) come from normal intestinal flora that pass into the bladder. Urine found in the bladder should be sterile. The large bowel is not sterile in healthy adults. However, when large bowel bacteria colonize the bladder, the result is cystitis or bladder infection. Cystitis, though rare in young men, can occur as a result of urethral obstruction from prior infections of sexually transmitted disease or from congenital defect of the urethra which requires surgical correction.

Upper UTIs are infections involving kidneys (pyelonephritis), ureters (ureteritis), or both. They may occur in both men and women as a complication of a lower UTI or arise without lower urinary tract involvement. The latter may occur in younger women or men as a result of obstruction somewhere in the urinary tract. Examples are a kidney stone or abdominal tumor which obstructs the ureter. Symptoms of upper UTI include fever, chills, lower back pain, nausea, and vomiting. The most common bacteria causing the infection is *E. coli.*

Men, though generally not prone to lower UTIs, may develop upper UTIs as they become older and cannot fully empty their bladders as a result of prostatic enlargement. Urine cannot remain sterile when it sits in the bladder for a long period of time. In elderly men this evolves into full-blown urinary retention where a liter or more may have to be drained by catheter. This problem is potentially very serious and can result in urosepsis, where overwhelming disseminated infection invades the bloodstream and can be fatal.

One of the more common predisposing factors of UTIs is diabetes mellitus; the spillage of glucose in the urine makes a good culture medium for bacteria. Other causes include improper bladder emptying from neurological diseases such as paraplegia, valve leakage between the ureter and the bladder, and in-dwelling urinary catheters left unchanged for too long a period of time. The underlying cause must be found and treated.

Bacterial UTIs and Interstitial Cystitis

Bacterial UTIs

Bacterial infections are the most common type of infection occurring in the bladder in women of reproductive age. It is often the result of a bruised urethra during intercourse, although the exact mechanism is not entirely clear. Symptoms of cystitis include a frequent, urgent desire to urinate, and pain above the pelvic bone and often in the lower back. Urine may be cloudy and contain visible blood. What is most significant is that many women have recurrent bouts of cystitis and no underlying cause, including sexual intercourse, can be found. How do we know? Recurrent cystitis is found in nuns. What is clear is that the infection is caused by bacteria; the reason for the recurrence is not clear.

Interstitial Cystitis

Cystitis is caused by an incestuous organism. This distinguishes cystitis from another disease called interstitial cystitis. Interstitial cystitis is more common in women than men. Often a person who has it can tell you the exact moment the symptoms began. It is often characterized by severe superpubic pain which is relieved by urinating. However, time after time when these patients go to the doctor, *bacteria are not grown from a culture of their urine.*

Interstitial cystitis is not widely recognized by most primary care physicians. As a result, the average time until diagnosis is *seven years!* The pain associated with this disease rivals that of cancer. Eventually, the diagnosis is made when a urologist finally decides to perform cystoscopy and look in the bladder. The appearance may be totally normal. However, when the urologist attempts to fill the bladder up with water, he finds that the bladder capacity is markedly diminished. Additionally, when the water is released, the bladder wall oozes blood in a manner causing a characteristic appearance called glomeration. If a biopsy is taken, mast cells, not normally present in the bladder, are seen. This is a diagnostic finding.

In worst-case scenarios, the condition progresses with ever-increasing replacement of normal bladder tissue with fibrosis or scar tissue. The bladder capacity lessens. The person with the disease cannot go anywhere or maintain employment because they must urinate constantly. Sufferers can't sleep because they must continually get up at night to urinate. Some patients end up having to replace the bladder dome with part of their own colon to increase capacity. Others end up with removal of their bladders and creation of a urinary diversion to an exterior bag.

The disease has no known cure. Treatment has consisted of bladder installations of DMSO and other agents, hydrostatic dilatation of the bladder under pressure, and a newer drug called Elmiron, which is effective in 30% of cases. Changes in diet may also be helpful. Relief of symptoms is variable. Presently, there are some who think there is an incestuous agent responsible which has not been identified. Research trials, including those with antibiotics, are presently being conducted.

Urinary Tract Infection Prevention

Because UTIs may be the result of a more serious medical condition, it is important to seek prompt medical advice for proper diagnosis and treatment. Most UTIs are painful and bothersome, but can usually be treated successfully with antibiotics. Sufferers of chronic UTIs can take certain steps to lower the likelihood of recurrence:

- ▼ Avoid caffeine, alcohol, and spicy foods which may further irritate the bladder.
- ▼ Drink eight to ten glasses of water or other fluids per day to dilute the bacteria in your urine.
- ▼ Eat plain yogurt to help control yeast infection after taking antibiotics for UTI.
- ▼ Wash before and after sex; ask your partner to do the same.
- ▼ Take showers instead of baths.
- ▼ Wear cotton underwear and loose-fitting clothes.
- ▼ For women: if using a diaphragm, wash, rinse, and carefully dry after each use. After using the toilet, always wipe from front to back.

What Causes UTIs?

The organism most often responsible for UTIs is *Escherichia coli* (*E. coli*), a bacterium normally found in the digestive tract and present on the skin around the rectal area. Other bacteria can also be involved, but E. coli is by far the most prevalent cause (over 80% of UTIs).

Female anatomy predisposes women to infection because the urethra opening is located very close to the anus, a common source of bacteria. These bacteria can migrate across the perineum (the narrow band of flesh between the anus and the vagina) to the urethra. This bacterial invasion can result in acute cystitis, the most common urinary tract infection. A more rare condition is called urethritis, in which only the urethra is inflamed. When bacteria from the bladder ascend to the kidneys via the ureters, they can cause a more serious infection called pyelonephritis. Although men do get UTIs, their physical anatomy makes infection less likely. The male urethra is much longer, and secretions from the prostate gland present a better barrier to this type of infection.

Treatments

Alternative Treatments For Recurrent Urinary Tract Infections

Cranberry Juice

Cranberry juice can be an effective deterrent to the recurrence of simple urinary tract infections. It has developed into a nondrug means to reduce or treat UTIs. Studies document that drinking eight glasses of cranberry juice twice a day can eradicate most simple UTIs. As long as the cranberry juice consumption is continued, the infections are not likely to return. One way that cranberry juice works is to prevent bacteria from adhering to the linings of the urinary tract. Studies suggest that bacterial infections (bacteriuria) and the associated influx of white blood cells into the urine (pyuria) can be reduced by nearly 50% in elderly women who drink 300 mL of cranberry juice cocktail each day.

In urostomy patients, urinary wall skin problems are common and may stem from alkaline urine. Cranberry juice appears to acidify urine and has bacteriostatic properties, and is thus widely recommended for the reduction of urinary tract infections. A recent study showed that drinking cranberry juice could help to prevent and/or improve skin complications for urostomy patients. It also showed that cranberry juice resulted in improvements of skin conditions and a reduction in skin complications in patients with severe urinary wall disease.

Most people would find it difficult to drink 16 8-ounce glasses of cranberry juice a day, but there are dietary supplements that provide the equivalent of eight to sixteen 8-ounce glasses of cranberry juice in just one capsule.

Cranberries under the Microscope

In a body of work undertaken separately and in parallel in both the United States and Israel, studies have now established that:

- ▼ Bacterial adherence to the walls of the urinary tract is an important prerequisite for the colonization of *E. coli*. The bacteria adhere to these cells using hair-like fimbriae (or pili) that protrude from their surfaces. These fimbriae attach to specific monosaccharide or oligosaccharide receptors on urothelial cells. The fimbriae are designated either Type1 (mannose sensitive) or Type P (mannose resistant).
- ▼ Through adherence to cells in the urinary tract, *E. coli* can withstand cleaning mechanisms and overcome nutrient deprivation, leading to infection and toxicity.
- ▼ Cranberry contains a potent factor which affects and disables the very cell structure of *E. coli*, thus inhibiting the ability of these bacteria to adhere to the wall of the urinary tract.
- ▼ This factor in cranberry is composed of certain condensed tannins, or proanthocyanidins, which collectively prevent *E. coli* from colonizing in the urinary tract.

In 1994, a landmark study at Harvard Medical School demonstrated that regular use of cranberry juice significantly reduced bacterial growth in the urinary tract, as well as the body's response to infection in the form of white blood cells. This study added impetus to the familiar woman's lore about cranberries and their benefits against UTIs.

Self-medication with cranberry juice cocktail is a common approach to dealing with a UTI—and has often been recommended by physicians as an adjunct to antibiotic treatments. But this could certainly be termed the old-fashioned route.

First of all, cranberry juice cocktail contains only 27% cranberry juice (the remainder is sweetened water). While it may be somewhat effective against UTIs, drinking large amounts of this super-sweetened cocktail has many drawbacks in our health-conscious society—too much sugar, all those calories. This isn't the preference of most women. For diabetics, this becomes an impossible prescription.

An obvious alternative would be a cranberry supplement. The most potent cranberry supplements to date have provided the equivalent of sixteen 8-oz glasses of cranberry juice in two capsules. The recommended dose is one capsule every 12 hours. These highly concentrated cranberry supplements have shown efficacy in preventing and facilitating treatment in those suffering UTI.

The ultimate way of treating UTIs is to prevent bacterial adherence to the urinary wall. The development of a low-cost, one-a-day cranberry extract supplement makes an ideal supplement for women who are at risk for developing a urinary tract infection. For most people, it's far easier to remember to take one pill a day, rather than to take one pill every 12 hours.

Acupuncture

In a recently published study in Norway, researchers conducted a 6-month clinical trial to evaluate the effect of acupuncture on 67 women with recurrent cystitis. The trial was divided into three arms: the acupuncture group, a sham-acupuncture group, and an untreated control group. In the 6-month trial period, 85% of subjects in the acupuncture group were free of cystitis, compared to 58% in the sham group and 36% in the control group. The results of the study suggest that acupuncture treatment may be a viable alternative in the prevention of chronic cystitis.

Summary

Recurrent UTIs

1. Have a thorough evaluation by a urologist.
2. Take one Cran-Max cranberry juice concentrate capsule per day.
3. Consider potassium, magnesium, or calcium citrate at a dose of 125 to 250 mg, 3 or 4 times a day.

Interstitial Cystitis

1. Have a thorough evaluation by a urologist with experience in interstitial cystitis.
2. For pain management consider buprinorphine (1 to 5 mg sublingual troche every 6 to 8 hours). *See Pain protocol.*

3. Consider intravenous vitamin C, 50 mg 3 times a week.
4. Consider intravenous DMSO.

WARNING: DMSO should not be used during pregnancy.

For a physician familiar with orthomolecular medicine, contact the American College for Advancement in Medicine: (800) 532-3688.

For more information. Contact the Bladder Health Council, 300 W. Pratt St., Suite 401, Baltimore, MD 21201. For more information about interstitial cystitis, contact the Interstitial Cystitis Association of America, P.O. Box 1553, Madison Square Station, New York, NY 10159.

Product availability. You can order Cran-Max by calling (800) 544-4440, or order online at www.lef.org. Buprinorphine is available as a sublingual troche at Medical Center Pharmacy, (800) 723-PILL.

VALVULAR INSUFFICIENCY/ HEART VALVE DEFECTS

There are numerous causes of heart valve defects and deterioration, including inherited defects, bacterial infections, reaction to drugs, and age-associated aortic valve stenosis (narrowing). Rheumatic heart disease can also cause valvular heart problems. Although rheumatic heart disease has greatly diminished since the advent of antibiotics to treat streptococcal infections, it still affects more than 1 million Americans and causes about 6000 deaths per year. Since heart valve diseases are anatomical in nature, it is challenging to address an existing valve defect from a nutritional or drug standpoint.

The most common serious heart valve defect is called aortic stenosis. Aortic stenosis is normally an age-related disease that consists of the aortic valve progressively narrowing and reducing the amount of blood that is able to be pumped to the body by the ventricle. The result is often ventricular enlargement, as the heart muscle has to grow to allow it to pump harder to force blood through the narrowing aortic valve.

In valvular stenosis, a valve that fails to open properly impairs the forward flow of blood to the body. In either case, the heart has to work harder to pump enough blood to the body, eventually leading to heart muscle damage. Congestive heart failure, syncope (fainting), and arrhythmias are common signs of valve disease.

Diagnosis

Valvular heart disease is most easily diagnosed by Doppler echocardiography. This noninvasive diagnostic technique makes it possible to measure blood flow and to evaluate the extent of valve defects. The color Doppler echocardiography gives the physician a better survey of the severity of valve disease, and the spectral Doppler provides an exact analysis and quantification of the valve defect and the degree of stenosis. The most precise diagnosis is made by cardiac catheterization and angiocardiography carried out in the vascular lab, generally by an invasive cardiologist, allowing immediate intervention to take place.

Cardiac disability and death from congestive heart failure will result if the aortic valve cannot be reopened or replaced. Valve-replacement surgical procedures currently are the only effective long-term therapy. Regrettably, this surgical procedure also has numerous potential long-term side effects, especially in elderly people who often need an aortic-valve replacement. The potential development of nonsurgical therapies to correct aortic-valve stenosis offers some hope of an alternative to valve-replacement surgery.

Treatment

Conventional Treatment

Depending on the type of valvular problem, patients often can go for many years without any special treatment. A common example is a mitral valve prolapse. Up to 7% of the population has mitral valve prolapse, which for unknown reasons are most common in women. In most people, it is not medically serious. Conventional therapies now available are as follows.

Drug Therapy

Drugs to treat heart valve disease are used to relieve symptoms and prevent complications. They do not provide a cure. For example, in mitral valve prolapse, a beta-blocking drug may be prescribed to treat troublesome symptoms such as palpitations and chest pain, even though the condition itself is not serious.

In other forms of valvular disease, digitalis or other drugs to slow the heartbeat and increase its output may be prescribed. A diuretic may be added to prevent retention of salt and water; a salt-restricted diet may be recommended for the same reason. Anticoagulant drugs may be prescribed to prevent blood clots, and anti-arrhythmic drugs may be used to maintain a normal heart rate and rhythm.

Diseased heart valves are highly susceptible to a serious infection called bacterial endocarditis, so it is important to take antibiotics before any dental or surgical procedure that may release bacteria into the bloodstream. Depending on the severity of the disease, a doctor may also recommend avoiding strenuous activities and taking frequent rest periods during the day to minimize the workload on the heart. Supplements that strengthen the immune system may also be helpful.

Immediate and careful treatment of streptococcal throat infections with antibiotics can prevent most cases of rheumatic fever, one of the leading causes of heart valve disease.

(*See the Immune Enhancement protocol for more information on strengthening your immune system.*)

Surgical Treatment

When the heart valves are seriously damaged and impairing blood flow to the rest of the body or causing heart muscle damage, surgery to replace the defective valve may be recommended. For example, in rare cases of a mitral valve prolapse, the valve may become so weakened that there is excessive backflow of blood or a danger of the valve's rupturing, which can lead to death. In such unusual circumstances, replacement of the defective valve is necessary. A number of durable and highly efficient artificial valves have been developed from animal parts, plastic, and metal.

Novel surgery to fix leaking aortic valves—pulmonary valve transplants

Surgeons at UCSF Stanford go to an unlikely source for a new heart valve in those patients suffering from aortic valvular disease—the other side of a patient's own heart. They use the pulmonary valve from the right side of a patient's heart to replace the defective aortic valve on the left side of the heart.

The pulmonary valve makes an ideal substitute because it is about the same size and shape as the aortic valve, and is able to close tightly, even under high pressure. And the valve is not rejected by the immune system because it is the patient's own tissue.

The aortic valve must form a solid seal to prevent blood from reversing into the heart during contraction. Leakage can occur if the flaps of the valve are congenitally malformed or are corroded by infections or diseases like rheumatoid arthritis. For the patient, a faulty aortic valve causes shortness of breath and fatigue because the heart begins to fail due to the extra work load.

This novel procedure is better than the current alternatives, such as implantation of a mechanical valve or one taken from a pig's heart, which give inferior results over time. Pig valves eventually may be rejected by the body's own immune system, which attacks the animal implants, and blood clots may form on the mechanical valves. A pulmonary human valve transplant, however, can last the lifetime of the patient.

Surgeons can also implant a pulmonary valve taken from the hospital's tissue bank from donated human valves which match the recipient's tissue. If you are facing an aortic valve problem, you may want to ask your physician about this surgical approach.

Integrated and Alternative Prevention

Because of the anatomical nature of valvular disease, prevention may be the best approach to avoid this disorder. For example, there is evidence that the deposition of apolipoprotein A, B, and E (protein variations of the LDL cholesterol) on the aortic valve creates a binding site for calcium. Aortic valve stenosis is often described as a calcification process. Fibrinogen may also contribute to this process by depositing on aortic valves, further adding to deposit buildup by binding with calcium deposits already present on valves. Studies also implicate a chronic inflammatory process that promotes calcium infiltration into the aortic valve.

Preventing or curbing the progression of aortic-valve disease may involve lowering homocysteine, fibrinogen, and apolipoproteins A, B, and E in the blood. Consider regular blood tests to guard against hypercalcemia (too much calcium in the blood) and supplementing with magnesium (500 elemental mg a day) to possibly inhibit excess calcification of the aortic valve. Supplementing with 10 mg a day of vitamin K_1 may be especially effective in preventing aortic valve calcification. Long-term anti-inflammatory therapy with nonsteroidal anti-inflammatory drugs (aspirin, ibuprofen, or prescription drugs) may be considered under the supervision of a physician. Nutrients that safely inhibit many chronic inflammatory reactions include fish oil, borage oil, curcumin, and ginger. *(See the Fibrinogen, Homocysteine, and Atherosclerosis protocols for suggestions on lowering homocysteine, fibrinogen, and apolipoprotein levels.)*

Since narrowed and/or leaky heart valves keep blood from being efficiently pumped, and thus place a strain on the heart muscle, we suggest you follow the *Congestive Heart Failure and Cardiomyopathy protocol.* The nutrients in this protocol will help strengthen the contractility of the heart muscle, but will do nothing to alleviate or correct the underlying anatomical valvular defect.

Summary

Valve-replacement surgical procedures currently are the only effective long-term therapy for valvular insufficiency. Beta-blockers, digitalis, and anticoagulants may be prescribed, depending on the underlying condition, to relieve symptoms and prevent complications, although they do not provide a cure.

Preventing or curbing the progression of aortic-valve disease may involve lowering of homocysteine, fibrinogen, and apolipoproteins A, B, and E in the blood. Natural nonsteroidal anti-inflammatory supplements—including aspirin, fish oil, borage oil, curcumin, and ginger—may be considered under physician supervision. Vitamin K_1 and magnesium may prevent calcification of the aortic valve. Readers should refer to specific heart disease–related protocols for detailed suggestions regarding nutritional supplementation.

For more information. Contact the National Heart, Lung, & Blood Institute, (301) 251-1222.

VERTIGO

Vertigo is a sensation of moving or spinning within stable surroundings, and it may be accompanied by loss of balance and nausea. These symptoms distinguish vertigo from dizziness, which is more of a feeling of lightheadedness, as though a person were going to pass out. Vertigo may last for a few moments, several hours, or even days. The most common cases of vertigo are caused by abnormalities in the semicircular canals in the inner ear, the vestibulocochlear nerve, which connects the ear to the brain, or by abnormalities in the brain itself.

The inner ear contains a set of what could best be described as two tiny, circular tubes at right angles to each other. The tubes are lines with little hair-like objects that connect ultimately to the vestibulocochlear nerve, which leads to the brain. The cerebellum is the part of the brain where most of this information is processed. The tubes are filled with a fluid called endolymph. When we move about, the fluid in the tubes moves, stimulating the little "hairs," which send signals to the brain. There the signals are processed with other sensory information that tells us our orientation in space so we can maintain our balance. That is why conditions affecting the inner ear—such as viral or bacterial infections, tumors, nerve inflammation, or Meuniere's syndrome (abnormal fluid buildup)—may cause vertigo. In fact, problems of the inner ear are the most common cause of vertigo. Motion sickness, which affects people who are sensitive to certain movements such as swaying or sudden starts and stops, may also cause vertigo.

Vertigo occurs most often in relationship to an infection, particularly if the ear is involved. This condition is called labarynthitis and is usually self-limiting. Vertigo that persists warrants a medical workup. Most often this workup will fail to disclose a cause. This is usually benign positional vertigo and is treated with certain head exercises.

Certain neurological disorders such as multiple sclerosis, skull fractures, and tumors may also cause vertigo by acting on either the vestibulocochlear nerve or the brain itself. Symptoms such as headaches, slurred speech, double vision, and weakness in an arm or leg will also be apparent. Prescription drugs for treating high blood pressure or heart disease may cause dizziness due to rapid lowering of blood pressure in certain individuals when they stand up too quickly. This is not the same as vertigo and is best described as a feeling of lightheadedness. The medical term is *orthostatic hypotension.*

The workup for persistent vertigo includes tests to determine abnormal eye movements, balance, and hearing loss. Additional tests such as CAT scans and MRIs can show tumors pressing on the vestibulocochlear nerve.

Treatment

Vertigo is treated by diagnosing its nature and treating the underlying cause. The conventional medication is Antivert, which may cause drowsiness. If conventional medicine is unable to treat vertigo successfully, you may want to consider taking medications that can correct a neurological deficit that may be causing your vertigo. Some people have found that 5 to 10 mg a day of Hydergine can be an effective therapy for vertigo. Other people have successfully used 2400 to 4800 mg of piracetam a day for this condition. A third option is to take 20 to 40 mg of vinpocetine a day.

In the most recent human study, ginkgo extract was shown to improve the symptoms of vertigo, tinnitus, headache, and forgetfulness in people suffering from a cerebral circulatory deficit. The reduction of blood circulation to the brain is a common problem in aging humans, and this circulatory deficit can cause many neurological disease states, including vertigo.

Piracetam has been shown in several published studies to alleviate vertigo through diverse effects in the brain. In a recent multicenter, double-blind, placebo-controlled study, piracetam was administered in a dose of 800 mg 3 times a day for 8 weeks. The study group consisted of 143 middle-aged and elderly outpatients who had suffered from vertigo for at least 3 months, had experienced at least three episodes a month, and experienced vertigo severe enough to disrupt daily life. Tolerance to piracetam was good, with few drug-related adverse events occurring. The findings showed that piracetam alleviated vertigo by reducing the frequency of episodes, the severity of malaise, imbalance between episodes, and the duration of vertigo-induced incapacity.

Summary

For treatment of persistent vertigo,

1. Consider Hydergine, 5 to 10 mg a day.
2. Consider piracetam, 2400 to 4800 mg a day.
3. Consider vinpocetine, 20 to 40 mg a day.

For more information. Contact Meuniere's Network, EAR Foundation, (800) 545-HEAR.

Product availability. To obtain high-potency Hydergine, piracetam, or vinpocetine, phone (800) 544-4440 for a list of offshore suppliers who ship these products to Americans for personal use. Piracetam is available by prescription from the Medical Center Pharmacy, (800) 723-PILL.

WEIGHT LOSS

(See Obesity)

WOUND HEALING (SURGICAL WOUNDS, TRAUMA, BURNS)

Wound healing consists of an orderly progression of events that reestablish the integrity of the damaged tissue. The initial wound touches off a series of programmed, separate yet interdependent responses to the injury, including inflammation, epithelialization (growth of new skin), angiogenesis (blood vessel regeneration), and the accumulation of matrix, the cells necessary to heal the tissue. Many wounds pose no challenge to the body's innate ability to heal; some wounds, however, may not heal easily, either because of the severity of the wounds themselves, or because of the poor state of health of the body. The Life Extension Foundation has designed this protocol to support and enhance the healing of internal and external wounds that fall into this category (*for related information on how to support the body's ability to heal and rebuild itself, refer to the Catabolic Wasting and Muscle Building protocols*). Any wound that does not heal should be examined by a healthcare professional, as it might be infected, might reflect an underlying disease such as diabetes, or might be a serious wound requiring medical treatment. Always inform your healthcare provider of all supplements and treatments you are using.

Types of Wounds

Although all wounds follow roughly the same healing process, there are many different causes of wounds. One medical term for a wound is an ulcer. Partial-thickness wounds penetrate the outer layers of the skin, the epidermis and the superficial dermis, and heal by regeneration of epithelial tissue (skin). Full-thickness wounds involve a loss of dermis (deeper layers of skin and fat) and of deep tissue, as well as disruption of the blood vessels; they heal by producing a scar. Wounds are classified by stage. Stage 1 wounds are characterized by redness or discoloration, warmth, and swelling or hardness. Stage 2 wounds partially penetrate the skin. Stage 3 describes full-thickness wounds that do not penetrate the tough white membrane (fascia) separating the skin and fat from the deeper tissues. Stage 4 wounds involve damage to muscle or bone and undermining of adjacent tissue. They may also involve sinus tracts (red streaks indicating infected lymph vessels).

Traumatic ulcers. An injury caused by any kind of accident, or trauma, can result in a wound that affects the skin, blood vessels, bones, muscles, soft tissue, or organs.

Burns. Most burns occur in the home. They can be caused by scalding hot liquids, grease fires, car accidents, chemical explosions, frayed electrical cords, house fires, hot objects (stoves, irons, tailpipes), or even the sun. A first-degree burn results in a superficial reddened area like that caused by a mild sunburn. A second-degree burn results in a blistered injury that heals spontaneously after the blister fluid has been removed. A third-degree burn penetrates the layers of the skin and will usually require surgical intervention in order to heal. Immediate care of a burn consists of cooling the affected area. Superficial burns heal on their own within 2 weeks with routine wound care and protection from infection. Deeper burns require medical attention, including nutritional support and assessment of lung function, and may require skin grafts and vascular or reconstructive surgery.

Arterial ulcers. The arteries supply blood, which carries the oxygen that cells need to live. If arterial circulation is partially or completely blocked, the tissue will begin to die, resulting in a painful wound. Impaired circulation of this type usually occurs in the extremities (arms and legs), especially on the top of the foot, and is signaled by lack of pulse; cool or cold skin; skin that appears shiny, thin, and dry; loss of skin hair; and delayed capillary return time. (To test capillary return time, briefly push on an area and then release: normal color should return in 3 seconds or less). Treatment of arterial ulcers has two goals: reestablishing circulation with medical treatment and healing the wound(s).

Venous ulcers. Veins carry deoxygenated blood back to the lungs. Veins contain valves that prevent backflow, but when these valves become incompetent, too much blood remains in the tissues. This condition is called congestion. Venous congestion commonly affects the legs, causing swelling (edema) and a brownish discoloration from the hemoglobin of the immobile red blood cells that leak out. Venous ulcers are the most common wounds affecting the legs, and are frequently found on the ankles. They are shallow, not too painful, and may have a weeping discharge. Although venous valves cannot be repaired, the return of blood through the veins can be improved by physical activity and by compression, which can be supplied by compression stockings, dressings, or mechanical pumping devices.

Diabetic foot ulcers. Diabetes results in a narrowing of the small arteries, which can cause ulcers. This narrowing cannot be resolved, but can be prevented by careful glucose control. Diabetes also causes peripheral neuropathy and the loss of sensation, especially sharp-dull discrimination, in the legs and feet. For this reason, injuries to the feet may go unnoticed and can progress into serious wounds. In addition, peripheral neuropathy can cause deformity of the foot (Charcot foot deformity) because of inappropriate stresses being placed on the bones, resulting in microfractures; this deformity in turn results in bony prominences and swelling that contributes to ulceration. Neuropathy cannot be cured, but careful glucose control slows its progress. Diabetics must be extremely vigilant about foot care, and should seek immediate medical attention for any wounds. Special shoes can help relieve pressure.

Pressure ulcers. Also known as bedsores, pressure ulcers are very common in older and immobile persons. When too much pressure is placed on them, cells do not get enough oxygen. Such pressure occurs when cells are sandwiched between a bony prominence (elbow, heel, or tailbone) and a hard surface (bed or wheelchair). Those cells closest to the bone begin to die, and the wound spreads toward the skin surface. Thus, a pressure ulcer indicates not only a surface wound, but also a deep tissue wound. The risk of pressure ulcers can be reduced by enhancing mobility, maintaining skin and general health, ensuring good nutrition, and monitoring weight (patient should be neither too heavy nor too light).

Stages of Wound Healing

Wounds with even edges that come together spontaneously (minor cuts) or can be brought together with stitches often heal well with routine wound care. Wounds with rough edges and tissue deficit (a crater) may take longer to heal. All wounds heal in three stages.

Inflammatory stage. This stage occurs during the first few days. The wounded area attempts to restore its normal state (homeostasis) by constricting blood vessels to control bleeding; platelets and thromboplastin make a clot. Inflammation—redness, heat, swelling—also occurs and is a visible indicator of the immune response. White blood cells clean the wound of debris and bacteria.

Proliferative stage. After the inflammatory stage, the proliferative stage lasts about 3 weeks. Granulation occurs, which means that special cells called fibroblasts make collagen to fill in the wound. New blood vessels form. The wound contracts and is covered by a layer of skin.

Maturation and remodeling stage. This stage may last up to 2 years. New collagen forms, changing the shape and increasing the strength of the area; scar tissue, however, is only about 80% as strong as the original tissue. The body's ability to heal during this stage is diminished in the elderly.

Wound Care

There are four basic steps to follow in caring for any wound. Perhaps the most important factor in wound healing is compliance, in other words, caring for the wound consistently and correctly.

Debride and cleanse. Debridement means the removal of dead tissue. It can be accomplished in an autolytic manner, in which the wound itself is encouraged to do this task by the use of dressings. A medical professional may also use biochemical enzymes, wet-to-dry dressings (in which a wet dressing is allowed to dry, trapping material in it, and is then carefully removed), or mechanical implements such as scalpel or scissors to remove dead tissue from more serious wounds. Cleansing refers to the removal from the wound of any foreign debris (such as residuum from previous dressings) and any bacteria. Cleansing is usually accomplished by irrigating the wound with fluid from a disposable syringe. Many previously accepted wound-cleansing solutions have been found to be toxic to fibroblasts and lymphocytes, the cells required to heal wounds. These solutions include povidone-iodine, acetic acid, iodophor, hydrogen peroxide, and Dakin's solution (sodium hypochlorite). Commercially prepared solutions are not regulated by the FDA, and many have been found to be cytotoxic. The only acceptable wound-cleansing solution is normal saline solution (0.9% sodium chloride [salt] in water). Normal saline solution effectively removes contaminants and has the same salt concentration as the fluid in cells, so it doesn't damage cells by pulling water out of them. It is also inexpensive and readily available.

Maintain a moist environment. During wound healing, cells and fluid are slowly exuded, or discharged. The exudate provides an environment that stimulates healing because it contains white blood cells, growth factors, and other special enzymes and hormones. A moist environment preserves this exudate, speeding wound healing and promoting skin growth. It also prevents dressings from adhering to the wound and damaging the fragile tissue when they are removed. A moist environment can easily be maintained using gauze moistened with normal saline solution. The solution will support autolytic debridement, absorb discharge, and trap bacteria. For partial thickness wounds with no infection, polyvinyl dressings, which are semipermeable to oxygen and impermeable to bacteria, can also be used. They have the advantage of concentrating the cells responsible for healing in the wound bed, but the disadvantage is that they are adhesive and may therefore damage the fragile skin surrounding the wound. Hydrocolloid dressings are not adhesive and are impermeable to oxygen and bacteria, but may leave a residue in the wound, which must then be removed. Absorptive dressings are used on wounds with a lot of discharge.

CAUTION: It is critical that the first two steps of wound care be performed regularly and gently. Dislodging the fragile granulation tissue or skin that is forming in the wound bed will delay healing. For most wounds, the first two steps can be accomplished easily and effectively by using gauze that is kept moist with normal saline solution.

Prevent further injury. In order to prevent further injury, the cause of the wound must be determined and addressed, as described above.

Provide materials for healing. Proteins, made up of amino acids, are necessary for all phases of wound healing, including angiogenesis, fibroblast proliferation, collagen synthesis, and scar remodeling. Proteins also support the immune system, which will prevent infection. One recent study found that protein depletion before surgery is a risk factor in wound infection. Fats and carbohydrates are also needed to supply the extra energy used in healing and to prevent proteins from being used for energy. Water is necessary to replace losses through vomiting, bleeding, discharge, and fever. Vitamins and minerals also play key roles in the healing process, as will be discussed below.

The Danger of Infection

Infection of a wound with a large number of bacteria, a process known as colonization, will slow the healing process. All wounds, however, contain some bacteria. This is called contamination and does not affect the healing process. The difference between contamination and colonization is the concentration of bacteria. Signs of infection include red skin around the wound, discharge containing pus, swelling, warmth, foul odor, and fever.

Health care providers can also conduct laboratory tests to investigate for signs of infection. The routine wound care outlined above is usually sufficient to prevent infection. Since all wounds are contaminated, sterile materials and technique are not necessary. The best way to prevent infection is to carefully wash your hands. Antibiotic creams should be used only if signs of infection are present, and then only sparingly to prevent bacterial resistance (bacteria develop the ability to live in the presence of the medication). If a wound is infected and does not respond immediately to over-the-counter antibacterial creams, it must be evaluated by a health care professional, who may prescribe antibiotics.

Alternative Treatments

Many alternative treatments are available to help heal wounds that do not respond to the conventional methods described above. These treatments should be undertaken in coordination with your health care provider.

Hyperbaric oxygen therapy. In this therapy, used to treat very serious wounds, the patient breathes 100% oxygen in a pressurized chamber for 90 to 120 minutes. The oxygen dissolves into the blood and is distributed throughout the body, providing extra oxygen to the cells attempting to heal the wound. Hyperbaric oxygen treatments have been found to increase the rate of collagen deposition, angiogenesis, and bacterial clearance. Another benefit is that, if the wound environment has more oxygen, certain types of bacteria that cause serious infections cannot grow.

Whirlpool therapy. Physical therapists use whirlpool therapy once or twice daily for about 20 minutes during the inflammatory stage of healing to enhance circulation and bring more oxygen into the wound area. The whirlpool also softens and loosens dead tissue and cleanses the wound. Some patients find that whirlpool therapy relieves wound pain. Whirlpool therapy should not be used on wounds that are in the proliferative stage of healing because it will damage the fragile skin cells, nor should it be used on venous ulcers, which result from too much blood in the area.

Ultrasound treatment. Ultrasound treatment uses mechanical vibration delivered at a frequency above the range of human hearing. Physical therapists report that covering the wound area with a hydrogel sheet and applying ultrasound during the inflammatory and proliferative stages stimulates the cells involved in wound healing and also heats the tissue, enhancing healing by improving circulation.

Electrical stimulation. The body has its own bioelectric system, which influences wound healing by attracting repair cells, changing the permeability of cell membranes, and therefore affecting secretions and orienting cell structures. A current of energy is generated between the skin and inner tissues when a break in the skin occurs. This current is enhanced by a moist wound environment and can be mimicked by electrical stimulation, which is believed to accelerate the healing process. Electrical stimulation uses electrodes that are positioned around the wound area. It can be used on most wounds during all three stages to support, speed, and even improve wound healing. Use of this therapy results in a smoother, thinner scar. In 1994, the Agency for Health Care Policy and Research endorsed the therapy for treating Stage 3 and 4 pressure ulcers, based on data from five clinical trials involving 147 patients.

Magnetic therapy. Magnetic therapy has a rationale similar to that for electrical stimulation, since the body's magnetic field is related to its bioelectric system. The use of magnets has been reported to increase blood flow and enhance cell growth by transferring energy. Magnets also affect nerve signals in ways that may relieve pain. A recent, published case study describes the complete healing of an abdominal wound by using magnet therapy for 1 month. Despite traditional approaches to wound care, the wound had been present for over a year.

Therapeutic touch. Biofield therapy, the laying on of hands, is a very old form of healing. Underlying rationales fall into two categories: one, that the practitioner modifies, directs, or amplifies the human biofield; and two, that the healing force comes through the practitioner from a supernatural source, such as God or the cosmos. Biofield practitioners use a variety of approaches, but have a holistic focus that incorporates mental, emotional, and physical health. Massage therapy is thought to enhance healing, both by relieving stress and by stimulating the nervous and circulatory systems. One recent study found that massage therapy improved activity, vocalizations, and behavior ratings of state, and also decreased anxiety in burn patients. Long-term effects were significantly better for the massage-therapy group in comparison with a control. Benefits of therapeutic touch included decreased depression, anger, and pain.

Nutritional Supplements

Research has shown that certain nutrients such as aloe vera, arginine, glutamine, zinc, copper, and vitamin C play key roles in wound healing. The typical Western diet is deficient in these nutrients. Under normal conditions, the 5 grams a day of arginine found in the typical Western diet would be marginally sufficient to maintain tissue health. Research has demonstrated, however, that in patients undergoing gall bladder surgery, supplementing 15 grams of arginine for 3 days prior to surgery significantly reduced nitrogen excretion (evidence that the patients were using, not excreting, amino acids in order to heal) when compared with patients receiving conventional nutritional support. In patients undergoing surgery for gastrointestinal cancer, supplementation with 25 grams of arginine a day for 7 days improved their nitrogen balance as measured 5 to 7 days after surgery and led to more rapid recovery and discharge from the hospital. One recent study revealed that dietary intake of energy and of such key wound-healing nutrients as vitamin C and zinc were not optimal despite well-organized food habits in women being treated for venous leg ulcers.

Aloe vera. The healing properties of aloe vera are well known and have been scientifically documented, and the *aloe barbadensis* plant has been used in healing for over 2000 years. Major universities and research groups have published volumes of reports documenting its enhancement of general cell growth and the immune system. Although it is not known how aloe vera works, it has been proven more effective than placebo in research trials. What is known is that aloe vera contains up to 200 different substances beneficial to the human body. These substances include enzymes, glycoproteins, growth factors, vitamins, and minerals. Long-chain sugars, or mucopolysaccharides (especially acemannan), have been of particular interest for their remarkable properties. Aloe vera is commonly considered a general tonic for increasing well-being and longevity. It provides the micronutrients required for protein synthesis. In ways not yet fully understood, its components work together to reduce inflammation and pain, to promote healing, and to stop infection. Some of these components cause cells to divide and multiply; some stimulate the growth of white blood cells. Aloe vera also enhances cell-wall permeability, increasing cell access to nutrients and facilitating the removal of toxins from the cells. Aloe vera can be used on the skin and can also be taken internally as a juice (2 ounces of concentrate in a 6-ounce beverage).

Arginine. Injury significantly increases the need for the amino acid arginine, which is essential for a variety of metabolic functions. Animal studies have demonstrated that, following surgical trauma, dietary supplementation with arginine results in an increase in nitrogen retention and increased body weight, both of which are essential for successful recovery. In a clinical study published in a major medical journal, arginine supplementation significantly increased the amount of reparative collagen synthesized at the site of a "standard wound" (an incision 5 centimeters long and 1 millimeter in diameter, into which a catheter was inserted) made in healthy volunteers. The same study found marked enhancement of the activity and efficacy of peripheral T-lymphocytes (white blood cells in the bloodstream).

Other animal and human studies have demonstrated that arginine stimulates the cell-mediated immune response and protects against bacterial challenges. In animals, dietary supplementation with arginine increases the weight of the thymus, the master gland of the immune system, and reduces shrinkage of the thymus following trauma and in normally aging animals. The benefits of arginine for thymic function have also been demonstrated. Its ability to restore thymic endocrine function is evidenced by increased blood levels of thymulin, one of the hormones secreted by the thymus gland. Clinical studies have shown improved immune function in cancer patients fed arginine. Arginine's ability to improve wound healing and immune-system function is thought to be related to its stimulation of the release of growth hormone. Growth hormone plays a critical role in modulating the immune system and is essential for muscle growth and development. That growth hormone secretion diminishes progressively with advancing age is one of the primary reasons for the decline in immune-system function and muscular strength as we grow older. To accelerate wound healing, the Life Extension Foundation recommends 10 to 22 grams of supplemental arginine a day.

Glutamine. The amino acid glutamine is an important substrate for rapidly proliferating cells, including lymphocytes (white blood cells). It is also the major amino acid lost during muscle protein catabolism in the initial response to injury. A recent article documented beneficial effects from supplying burn patients with glutamine and arginine in amounts two to seven times those found in the normal diet of healthy persons. The Foundation recommends 2000 mg of glutamine a day.

Zinc. Zinc plays a well-documented role in wound healing. Although it is present in the body in only a small quantity, it is found in many tissues, including bone, skin, muscle, and organs. It is a component of DNA, RNA, and numerous enzyme systems that participate in tissue growth and healing. It is crucial for protein synthesis and is a key part of the thymulin molecule, which enables T-lymphocytes to mature. The Foundation recommends 90 mg of zinc a day.

CAUTION: Zinc should be taken at least 2 hours after copper or the antibiotic tetracycline.

Copper. A German physician first observed the role of copper in healing. He noted that broken bones seemed to heal faster when patients were given a copper salt during convalescence. Since then, the role of copper in the biosynthesis of bone and connective tissue has been well established. Copper supplementation has enhanced bone healing. It works with vitamin C to create strong collagen, and it creates cross links in collagen and elastin that give strength to proteins.

Note: the Life Extension Foundation does not recommend copper as a long-term dietary supplement because of the preponderance of evidence that long-term copper supplementation generates too much free-radical activity throughout the body. On the other hand, therapeutic, short-term supplementation of copper (8 mg a day) to enhance wound healing at localized injury sites is appropriate. Copper supplementation as early as possible after serious burns has been demonstrated to replenish the copper depletion that is so typical of burn victims.

Superoxide dismutase (SOD). Copper also plays a critical role in the synthesis of a natural antioxidant called copper/zinc superoxide dismutase (SOD). In the initial phase of wound healing, immune cells are rushed to the wound site to protect against harmful invaders. They actually use free radicals to fight bacteria and to dispose of dead tissue. Once the free radicals have accomplished their job, however, they must be neutralized so the actual healing process can begin. SOD and other antioxidants such as vitamins C and D stop the free-radical oxidation process and promote the healing and repair process itself. Injury can deplete SOD and other antioxidants; antioxidant depletion levels as high as 70% have been reported following injury. SOD should be supplemented to encourage new tissue to grow, and to enhance collagen and reduce swelling. Wounds treated with SOD have been shown to heal better and more quickly. Current research consistently demonstrates that SOD taken orally is totally destroyed in the digestive tract. A lipid encapsulated (LIPSOD) injectable form of SOD and a sublingually administered form currently show the most promise for direct supplementation.

Vitamin C. Vitamin C is crucial for the proper function of the enzyme protocollagen hydroxylase, which produces collagen, the primary constituent of the granulation tissue that heals a wound and the key component in blood vessel walls. A recently published review stated that vitamin C plays a variety of roles in the prevention and treatment of cancer, including stimulating the immune system and enhancing wound healing. Wound healing requires more vitamin C than diet alone can easily provide. It must be replenished daily because it is water-soluble, and any excess is excreted rather than stored. Three tablets of Life Extension Mix 3 times a day provides the vitamin C and other nutrients needed for wound healing. For instance, vitamin A is important for tissue synthesis and enhances resistance to infection; iron is lost through bleeding; B vitamins are needed for cell proliferation and for the replacement and maturation of red blood cells lost through bleeding. One response to a wound is a higher rate of metabolism. This leads to higher energy-level requirements in order to heal a wound, and to increased requirements for thiamine, niacin, and riboflavin. Life Extension Mix will also improve overall health, assisting wound healing now and in the future (*see Prevention protocols*).

Vitamin B_5. Research published in the *International Journal of Vitamin and Nutrition Research* showed startling results in skin cells treated with pantothenic acid, or vitamin B_5. Cameras captured long, narrow skin cells (instead of the usual clumped, short and fat cells) racing toward an artificial wound to establish epithelialization. Vitamin B_5 has been demonstrated to speed up wound healing, increase protein synthesis, and multiply the number of repair cells available at the wound site. Vitamin B_5 seems to have the most benefit early on in wound repair, actually increasing the distance that repair cells can travel. Life Extension Mix contains 5 mg of Pantothene, a pantothenic acid analogue that may produce superior effects in the body, compared with regular B_5. Vitamin B_5 is also available from the Life Extension Foundation as a powder and as vitamin caps.

Vitamins B_5 and C in combination. French research examined combined supplementation with vitamins B_5 and C before the removal of tattoos. One week prior to surgery, some patients were administered 200 mg of vitamin B_5 and 1 gram of vitamin C. Scars of all patients were measured 75 days after surgery. The scars of those who had been supplemented with vitamins B_5 and C were stronger and thicker, and had more color. Researchers concluded that the vitamins had "recruited" more minerals to the wound areas. These "recruited" minerals included copper, magnesium, and manganese, all proven to enhance wound repair. Vitamins B_5 and C also kept iron from the wound areas, thus enhancing the healing process. The same group of researchers found that supplementation of vitamins B_5 and C strengthens the healing of wounds incidental to colon surgery.

Human Research Needed

Research has been done on the cellular-level benefits of vitamin supplementation on wound repair, but little research has been done in live human patients. The potential benefits are so great that more human research should be encouraged. Benefits could range from shorter hospital stays following surgery to the prevention of bone loss following serious surgery.

Summary

Determine the type of wound, its cause, and its severity. Serious wounds must be evaluated and treated by health care professionals to prevent infection and serious complications. Identify the stage of healing that the wound is in. Follow the four principles of basic wound care: debride and cleanse, maintain a moist environment, prevent further injury, and provide materials for healing. If the wound becomes infected, consult a health care professional.

1. Use aloe vera topically, and take it internally as a juice (2 ounces concentrate in a 6-ounce beverage).
2. Take arginine, 10 to 22 grams a day.
3. Take glutamine, 2000 mg a day.
4. Zinc, 90 mg a day, must be taken at least 2 hours after copper, as they antagonize each other.
5. Take 8 mg of copper a day, only for a limited time during healing.

6. Take 3 tablets of Life Extension Mix 3 times a day to provide the necessary vitamin C, Pantothene, and other essential nutrients to support and enhance wound healing.
7. Additional vitamin C may be supplemented up to several times the daily recommended dosage when given under the direction of a health care provider.
8. Take LIPSOD, an injectable form of SOD and a sublingually administered form, to stop free-radical oxidation and promote healing.
9. For chronic or serious wounds, consider alternative treatments such as hyperbaric oxygen therapy, whirlpool therapy, ultrasound treatment, electrical stimulation, magnetic therapy, and therapeutic touch.

To learn what you can do to reduce the risk of medically-induced complications, refer to the Foundation's *Anesthesia and Surgical Precautions protocol.*

Product availability. You can obtain premium-grade, cold-pressed, whole-leaf aloe vera juice concentrate; topical aloe vera ointment; arginine powder, tablets, and capsules; glutamine powder and capsules; vitamin B_5 powder and capsules; zinc; copper; and Life Extension Mix by phoning (800) 544-4440, or order on-line at www.lef.org.

YEAST INFECTIONS

(See Candida (Fungal, Yeast) Infections)

APPENDIX A: AVOIDING VITAMIN A TOXICITY

Based upon hundreds of published studies, the Life Extension Foundation has recommended vitamin A analogs drugs to cancer patients. For the many cancer patients who cannot gain access to vitamin A analogs because the FDA classifies them as "unapproved new drugs," the Foundation has recommended the use of water-soluble vitamin A liquid drops.

The dosage range of vitamin A liquid drops that cancer patients have been using is 100,000 to 300,000 IU a day. The Foundation has cautioned that these high doses could produce toxicity if taken over extended periods of time, yet cancer patients often are forced to risk some degree of toxicity to obtain an effective dose of vitamin A.

Anyone taking very high doses of vitamin A for cancer or any other reason should do so under the care of a physician, and should be on the lookout for symptoms of vitamin A toxicity. The following are common symptoms of vitamin A overdose that should be watched for in cancer patients taking high doses of any vitamin A product:

- Headache
- Dizziness
- Blurred vision
- Joint pain
- Dry lips
- Scaly, dry skin
- Excessive hair loss

Blood tests showing elevated liver enzymes may be a sign of a vitamin A overdose. If any of these symptoms appear, discontinue using vitamin A until the symptoms disappear, and then resume vitamin A therapy at a much lower dosage. The cancer patient faces a dilemma in attempting to use the maximum dose of vitamin A to fight his or her cancer, while trying to avoid vitamin A toxicity. *Those with thyroid cancer should avoid vitamin A.*

APPENDIX B: HOW TO DO AN ASCORBATE (VITAMIN C) FLUSH

Dissolve the proper amount (see instructions below) of buffered ascorbate (a potassium-calcium-magnesium-zinc combination is preferred) in 1 to 2 ounces of water or juice. Use the buffered ascorbate your practitioner recommends for your situation.

After dissolving the ascorbate and allowing any effervescence to abate (typically about 2 minutes), drink the beverage until watery diarrhea occurs. A flush should be reached before going to bed. The protocol to follow depends on the individual's health status.

- A *healthy* person begins with ½ teaspoon every 15 minutes.
- A *moderately healthy* person begins with 1 teaspoon every 15 minutes.
- A *person in ill health* begins with 2 teaspoons every 15 minutes.

Many people find that dissolving ascorbate in a number of ounces of liquid (e.g., 40 grams in 10 to 20 ounces of liquid) allows for easier, more timely consumption of the beverage than making up a new batch at each time interval. If you make up a batch of liquid ascorbate, we recommend a sealed bottle, such as a "jogger's bottle," to avoid air oxidation of the ascorbate. Dissolved ascorbate is stable for a day if kept tightly sealed and cool or cold. Press on to an enema-like release of a pint to a quart of liquid. Do not stop at loose stool. After watery diarrhea occurs, stop consuming the ascorbate.

Next, calculate the total ascorbate consumed [g = grams].

$$2\text{ g} \times 12\text{ doses} = 24\text{ g or } 4\text{ g} \times 22\text{ doses} = 88\text{ g}$$

Seventy-five percent (three-fourths) of this total is your approximate daily need ("bowel tolerance"). If this total is greater than 50 g, you are welcome to mix the buffered ascorbate with equal amounts of pure ascorbic acid. Consume as liquid, tablet, or capsule in four or more doses per day. The goal for ascorbate consumption, in a state of good health, is 2 to 10 grams per day.

As you become healthier, the useful lifespan of ascorbate inside your body will increase and less ascorbate will be needed to achieve the desired effect. As your need for ascorbate decreases, you may notice loosening of the stool, indicating that your body is using up ascorbate more slowly. Repeat the flush to determine what your current need is for ascorbate.

By following this approach you will be well-hydrated. The buffered ascorbate contains more minerals than the fluid you lose from the flush. The risk of fluid or electrolyte loss from the diarrhea is minimized by this scientifically designed approach.

- Some people report gas or fullness while doing the vitamin C flush, but that is almost always due to dissolving the vitamin C in too much water or rushing the procedure.
- Room temperature liquid is best for absorption.
- Occasionally, cramps occur—usually because too little fluid is used to dissolve the ascorbate. The procedure can mobilize metabolic toxic "refuse." It is important to complete the flush briskly to help eliminate these effectively.

Many people report a sense of improved well-being after the completion of a vitamin C flush. This may be of short duration initially but is a promising sign for long-term improvement. As toxins are eliminated from the body through the action of ascorbate, you should feel better for longer periods of time.

For most rapid progress, repeat the flush weekly. Discuss with your practitioner the right frequency for you. Many people find that their need for ascorbate increases as active repair is accelerated and toxic matter eliminated more efficiently. Once repair deficits have been overcome and toxic residue eliminated, the life of ascorbate in the body lengthens and less is needed to energize the system. Use the frequency that meets your needs. Repair deficits increase needs over time until a consistent dose of vitamin C is maintained.

To reduce the biochemical tax imposed by steroid medications, those taking steroid medications should include, at least on the days the "C flush" is done (and preferably during the time of high need for ascorbate),

- ▼ Choline citrate (half teaspoon = 1300 mg twice daily in juice or water).
- ▼ Magnesium (88 mg elemental magnesium twice daily).
- ▼ *L*-glutamine (either 1500 mg of *L*-glutamine PAK [the PAK recycles and potentiates the glutamine so less is needed] twice daily *or* 10 grams of *L*-glutamine free-form amino acid twice daily).

References

Anderson, R. Ascorbic acid and immune functions. In *Vitamin C: Ascorbic Acid*, J. N. Counsel, D. H. Horned, Eds., London: Applied Science, 1984: pp. 249–72.

Anderson, R. The immunostimulatory, anti-inflammatory and anti-allergic properties of ascorbic. *Add. Enter. Res.*, 1984; 6:19–45.

Delafuente, J. C., Panush, R. S. Modulation of certain immunologic responses by vitamin C. *Int. J. Vitamin Nutr. Res.*, 1980; 50:44–51.

Seib, P. A., Delbert, B. M., Eds., *Ascorbic Acid: Chemistry, Metabolism and Uses,* Advanced Chem. User. 200. Washington DC: Am. Chem. Soc. 1982: 604 pp.

Thomas, W. R., Holt, P. G. Vitamin C and immunity: An assessment of the evidence. *Clin. Exp. Immunol.*, 1978; 32:370–79.

Banhegyi, G., Braun, L., Csala, M., Puskas, F. and Mandl, J. Ascorbate metabolism and its regulation in animals. *Free Radical Biol. Med.*, 1997; 23 (5):793 –803.

Meister, A. Glutathione-ascorbic acid antioxidant system in animals. *J. Biol. Chem.,* 1994; 269:9397 – 9400.

Winkler, B. S., Orselli, S. M., Rex, T. S. The redox couple between dilatation and ascorbic acid: A chemical and physiological perspective. *Free Radical Biol. Med.,* 1994; 17:333–49.

Smirnoff, N., Pallanca, J. E. Ascorbate metabolism in relation to oxidative stress. *Biochem. Soc. Trans.,* 1994; 24:472–78.

Bode, A. M, Yavarow, C. R., Fry, D. A., Vargas, T. Enzymatic basis for altered ascorbic acid and dehydroascorbic acid levels in diabetes. *Biochem. Biophys. Res. Commun.,* 1993; 191:1347–1353.

Frei, B., England, L., and Ames, B. N. Ascorbate is an outstanding antioxidant in human blood plasma. *Proc. Natl. Acad. Sci. USA*, 1989; 86:6377–6381.

Chatterjee, I. B. Ascorbic acid metabolism. *World Rev. Nutr. Diet,* 1978; 30:69–87.

Johnson, F. C. The antioxidant vitamins. *CRC Crit. Rev. Food Sci. Nutr.,* 1979; 11:217–309.

Levine, M., Morita, K. Ascorbic acid in endocrine systems. *Vit. Horm.,* 1985; 42:1–64.

Lewin, S. *Vitamin C: Its Molecular Biology and Medical Potential*. New York/London: Academic Press, 1976.

May, J. M., Qu, Z. C., Whitesell, R. R. Ascorbic acid recycling enhances the antioxidant reserve of human erythrocytes. *Biochemistry,* 1995; 34:12721–2728.

APPENDIX C: DIETARY SUPPLEMENT SUPPLIERS—WHOM CAN YOU TRUST?

There are thousands of commercial supplement companies in the United States. Some of these companies sell only pharmaceutical-grade supplements, while others sell products that have zero efficacy because there are no active ingredients in them.

The FDA stopped regulating dietary supplements in 1994, and for the most part this has been great news for the consumer. Prices have come down for many supplements, and there is now a greater selection of safe and proven effective dietary supplements sold in the United States than in any other country.

The Life Extension Buyers Club was created to provide only pharmaceutical-grade supplements at near wholesale prices to Foundation members. The Buyers Club offers supplements from a wide range of premium supplement companies and mandates that all of its products meet the strictest quality control standards.

Most consumers do not understand the importance of using pharmaceutical-grade nutrients. The purity of supplements is critical if you plan to take them for the rest of your life. For example, many discount products use low-grade vitamin C imported from China, which contains traces of toxic arsenic, lead, and iron. Since the Food and Drug Administration (FDA) does not believe anyone should take more than 100 mg a day of vitamin C, the agency permits the importation of this contaminated vitamin C. However, health-conscious people often take 3000 to 10,000 mg of vitamin C every day, so it is crucial that they use a pharmaceutical-grade vitamin C that has gone through 18 purification steps to remove all possible contaminants. The Buyers Club uses only this pharmaceutical-grade vitamin C.

Since the FDA does not properly regulate dietary supplement manufacturing, the Foundation employs an independent quality-control expert to verify that only good manufacturing procedures are followed for its products. The Buyers Club also has access to a state-of-the-art laboratory, where trained chemists conduct assays of the nutrients in its products and develop new assays to guarantee quality control in even the most advanced formulas.

The Foundation has gained such a solid reputation for its quality control standards that the news media have asked us to assay commercial dietary supplements to verify that the products meet label potency. When we tell the media that we are not an independent testing laboratory, we are told that the independent labs do not have the technical competence or confidence to assay for unusual ingredients such as SAMe, lycopene, and lutein.

Although the primary goal of the Life Extension Foundation is to support research aimed at extending the healthy human life span, we have also assumed the obligation to help our members prevent and treat today's degenerative diseases. In taking on this enormous responsibility, it's hard to ignore the fact that some unscrupulous companies sell bogus products.

In April, 1999, we were asked to analyze seven different brands of SAMe. The results were as follows. Two of the seven had no SAMe present whatsoever, one brand used the wrong form of SAMe, and two other brands had less than 100% potency. Only Life Extension (our brand) and Nature's Made products had 100% of the right form of SAMe. Many consumers who trusted the reputations of some very well-known companies were clearly not getting what they paid for.

Life Extension Mix is a 67-ingredient, high-potency, multinutrient formula that most Foundation members use as the cornerstone of their disease-prevention program. For several years, a mail-order company promoted an old version of Life Extension Mix at the price of the current Life Extension Mix formula. The old, pirated formula was identical to the formula the Buyers Club sold 5 years ago. (There have been many improvements since.) Foundation members who saw this old formula promoted were outraged when the doctor claimed that *he* had done the research to formulate this product. In reality, he had merely copied the formula from an old bottle of Life Extension Mix.

After enough members inquired about the old formula being promoted by this doctor, we decided to buy several bottles ourselves and assay it to see if what was on the label was in the product. For the most part, the regular vitamins were present in their proper amounts, though we question whether this company used expensive pharmaceutical-grade nutrients from suppliers such as Roche, BASF, Nutrition 21, and Masquelier. When it came to the expensive unique ingredients, however, we found that the old formula contained only 2.6% of the lutein and 9.7% of the lycopene it was supposed to have. Consumers were thus being defrauded of their money *and* their health when buying this counterfeit product.

An equally disturbing problem exists with companies that promote products with grossly exaggerated health claims. Increasing numbers of solicitations are being made for products whose efficacy has *not* been substantiated in the peer-reviewed scientific literature. One of the founders of the Life Extension Foundation, Saul Kent, has spent the last 37 years investigating scientific methods to gain control over aging. Saul jokingly comments that all he has to do these days is go to his mailbox to find a "new cure for aging." This kind of unvarnished lying is an insult to the dedicated scientists who are working around the clock to develop authentic antiaging therapies.

So the question begs, what can consumers do to protect themselves against fraud? The answer is not much, but we would like to think that the Foundation's track record of innovation and unsurpassed quality control gives LEF members peace of mind that they are getting what they pay for.

As far as verifying health claims is concerned, anyone who has access to the Web can check out MEDLINE to help verify the accuracy of a health claim a company is making. This becomes difficult when deceitful companies come up with fancy trade names for their products—tradenames that do not reveal their alleged "breakthrough" ingredients. Don't think that even the government is capable of deciphering all of this. "Regulated" products kill over 125,000 Americans every year and are often as worthless as the products being sold with fraudulent health claims.

Foundation members know the difference between buying products from a company seeking only financial success and buying from an organization dedicated to achieving an *indefinitely* extended life span—no matter what costs or legal risks are involved. At the Life Extension Foundation, we've been battling the federal government for the last 15 years to protect the freedom in health care that will enable revolutionary medical breakthroughs to occur in our lifetimes. The struggle has been slow and arduous, but the controversial predictions we made years ago are increasingly becoming part of mainstream science and medicine.

Foundation members are an elite group of people who are willing to take extraordinary steps to stave off aging and death. When members buy products from the Life Extension Buyers Club, they know that the quality of the products is backed up by the organization's commitment to achieving an indefinitely extended life span, free from the ravages of disease. Members of the Life Extension Foundation receive large discounts that enable them to purchase premium-grade nutrient supplements at discounts that are substantially below the prices charged by commercial companies.

Be sure to visit our web site at www.lef.org. For a free catalog from the Life Extension Buyers Club, call (800) 544-4440, or write to

Life Extension Buyers Club
PO Box 229120
Hollywood, FL 33022

APPENDIX D: THERAPY CAVEATS

Remember that the information in this book is not intended to replace the attention or advice of a physician or other health care professional. Anyone who wishes to embark on any dietary, drug, exercise, or other lifestyle change intended to prevent or treat a specific disease or condition should consult with, and seek clearance and guidance from, a qualified health care professional.

The book offers general suggestions based on scientific evidence, not specific advice or recommendations. Patients need to be treated in an individual manner by their own personal physicians, and the information in this book must not be considered a substitute for the individual attention of a personal physician.

Individuals should be aware of a number of caveats when considering certain therapies, or when they are suffering from specific problems. These include, but are not limited to, the following.

Adrenal diseases. Some adrenal diseases, such as Addison's disease, involve underproduction of cortisol. This is a potentially acute, life-threatening condition that requires expert physician intervention.

Arginine. For a minority of Type II diabetics, arginine can elevate blood sugar by neutralizing insulin. Therefore, any diabetics who are contemplating using arginine or Powermaker II (sugar-free) should check their blood sugar with a glucometer every time they take an arginine supplement during the first three weeks of treatment.

Also, some nutritionists are concerned about using of high doses of arginine in cancer patients. Arginine promotes cellular growth, and the concern is that this amino acid could cause cancer cells to grow faster. Scientific studies show, however, that arginine provides beneficial effects to cancer patients. Only one study—of breast cancer patients—hinted at a risk from arginine supplementation.

Bee products. Bee products should not be administered to children under the age of three.

Beta-carotene. A patient suffering from a damaged liver should avoid niacin, vitamin A, and beta-carotene, because these nutrients can be harmful to patients with this condition. Also, the Life Extension Foundation recommends against high doses of beta-carotene in AIDS patients who have hepatitis.

Caffeine. Patients with cardiac arrhythmias should avoid caffeine, which promotes noradrenalin hypersecretion.

Coumadin. It is not known how nutrients recommended by the Foundation to avoid thrombosis interact with anticoagulation prescription drugs such as Coumadin and heparin. It is suggested that patients on physician-prescribed anticoagulation drugs introduce these nutrients very slowly. Weekly blood tests are suggested to make sure the blood is not becoming too thin.

Curcumin. Do not use curcumin if you have biliary tract obstruction, because curcumin could eliminate the flow of bile excreted through the bile duct. High doses of curcumin on an empty stomach can cause stomach ulceration.

Deprenyl. High doses of deprenyl may be detrimental to a Parkinson's disease patient, especially when the patient is taking *L*-dopa.

Depression. Anyone suffering from clinical depression of any type should be under the care of a physician.

DHEA. Men with prostate cancer should avoid DHEA. Generally, it is a good idea to use any hormone with caution and under the direction of a competent physician.

Fish oil concentrates. Extreme caution should be exercised by patients with leaky blood vessels when taking essential fatty acids in the form of fish oil concentrates such as Mega-EPA, because they inhibit blood clotting. There is a chance that a cerebral hemorrhage could occur because of the blood-thinning effects these nutrients can produce. Blood tests that measure clotting time can be used to ensure these nutrients are not reducing the clotting factors in your blood too much.

Forskolin. Do not use forskolin if you have prostate cancer or low blood pressure. If you are going to use forskolin or any other alternative therapy to replace drugs that strengthen heart muscle contraction, extreme caution is mandatory and physician cooperation is essential. Tests should be conducted to ensure forskolin and other nutrients are maintaining sufficient cardiac output.

If you'd like to see whether forskolin can replace your antihypertensive drugs, extreme caution is mandatory and physician cooperation is essential. Reduce the dosage of your antihypertensive drug very slowly while increasing your intake of forskolin, and monitor your blood pressure on a daily basis. If you do not exercise caution, an acute hypertensive event could occur, resulting in a stroke.

Garlic. Garlic taken in high doses—for example, 6000 to 8000 mg to lower cholesterol—can cause stomach irritation if taken on an empty stomach.

Genistein. Do not take soy extract when undergoing radiation therapy because the genistein in soy can interfere with the ability of radiation to kill cancer cells.

Glutamine. Some nutritionists are concerned about the use of high doses of glutamine in cancer patients. Glutamine promotes cellular growth, and the concern is that this amino acid could cause cancer cells to grow faster. Scientific studies show, however, that glutamine provides beneficial effects to cancer patients.

Ginkgo. Trauma involving massive bleeding may preclude the use of antioxidants such as ginkgo that could accelerate hemorrhaging.

Heparin. It is not known how nutrients recommended by the Foundation to avoid thrombosis interact with anticoagulation prescription drugs such as Coumadin and heparin. It is suggested that patients who are on physician-prescribed anticoagulation drugs introduce these nutrients very slowly. Weekly blood tests are suggested to make sure the blood is not becoming too thin.

Hodgkin's disease. See *Melatonin.*

Hops. See *Valerian.*

Hydergine. Liquid hydergine should be avoided in treating hemorrhagic stroke because of its high alcohol content.

Hypertension. The Foundation's general precaution is that attempting to use any of the nutrients the Foundation recommends to replace antihypertensive drugs must be with the cooperation of your physician. You cannot assume that any nutrients will be able to replace a drug that is effectively controlling your blood pressure. Daily blood pressure monitoring is mandatory to ensure that the nutrient regimen you are following is keeping your blood pressure under control.

Imitrex. Imitrex, a drug used to block migraine headaches, may have dangerous side effects in the middle-aged and the elderly.

Interleukin-2. Although melatonin is strongly recommended for breast cancer patients, interleukin-2, which is often combined with melatonin, should be avoided by breast cancer patients. Interleukin-2 may promote breast cancer cell division.

Leukemia. Alternative cancer therapies should be used with caution when treating leukemia or lymphoma. Most alternative therapies boost immune cell function, which could speed the proliferation of leukemia and lymphoma cancer cells. See also, *Melatonin.*

Lupus. Lupus patients should exercise extreme caution when attempting any new medical therapy, because there is a chance the condition could worsen.

Lymphoma. Alternative cancer therapies should be used with caution when treating leukemia or lymphoma. Most alternative therapies boost immune cell function, which could speed the proliferation of leukemia and lymphoma cancer cells. See also, *Melatonin.*

KH3. People allergic to procaine (the active ingredient in KH3) or taking sulfa drugs should not take KH3.

Melatonin. Some doctors are under the impression that leukemia, Hodgkin's disease, and lymphoma patients should avoid melatonin until more is known about its effects on these forms of cancer. If melatonin is tried in these types of cancer, tumor blood markers should be closely monitored for signs that melatonin is promoting tumor growth.

Use melatonin cautiously when treating autoimmune diseases such as rheumatoid arthritis. Some scientists have speculated that melatonin could increase the severity of an autoimmune disease.

Niacin. Patients suffering from a severely damaged liver should avoid niacin, vitamin A, and beta-carotene, because these nutrients can be harmful to patients with such conditions.

Pain. Before starting on a pain management program, please refer to the *Phenylalanine and Tyrosine Dosing and Precautions protocol.*

Passion flower. See *Valerian.*

Phenylalanine or tyrosine. There are some people who are genetically sensitive to phenylalanine and cannot take it. Hypertensive people should use phenylalanine with caution because it can elevate blood pressure in people who already have high blood pressure. Cancer patients should avoid taking extra phenylalanine and tyrosine because these amino acids can contribute to cancer cell proliferation. Muscular dystrophy patients should avoid phenylalanine and tyrosine.

Pregnenolone. See DHEA Dosing and Safety Precautions in the *DHEA Replacement Therapy protocol.*

Procaine. People allergic to procaine (the active ingredient in KH3) or taking sulfa drugs should not take KH3.

Propranolol. Those with very low blood pressure or certain forms of congestive heart failure and asthma should not take propanolol or other beta-blocking drugs.

St. John's wort. When using St. John's wort, avoid prolonged sunlight exposure. The active ingredient, hypericin, may make the skin more sensitive to UV light.

Shark liver oil. Do not take shark liver oil for more than 30 days, because it may cause the overproduction of blood platelets.

Soy extract. Do not take soy extract when undergoing radiation therapy. The genistein in soy can interfere with the ability of the radiation to kill cancer cells.

Sulfa drugs. People allergic to procaine (the active ingredient in KH3) or taking sulfa drugs should not take KH3.

Thalidomide. Users are cautioned that thalidomide—which may be useful in treating wet macular degeneration—causes severe birth defects and must never be used by pregnant women, or by women who may become pregnant.

Thyroid hormone therapy. You must be careful not to overdose on thyroid hormones. The advice of a knowledgeable physician is important when considering thyroid hormone therapy.

Valerian. Some people use the herb valerian to fall asleep. Valerian produces a druglike, hypnotic effect within the central nervous system, similar to that of benzodiazepine drugs such as Valium and Halcion. Because valerian-containing products are often promoted as natural herbal remedies, the public mistakenly believes they are safe to take on a regular basis. Studies indicate, however, that there is a significant toxicity risk when valerian is taken over an extended period of time. A tolerance effect occurs with valerian because of its Valium-like properties, and people often need to take increasing amounts of it as time goes by to continue to obtain the desired hypnotic effect. The chronic use of valerian could result in permanent liver damage and potential central nervous system impairment. The Life Extension Foundation has thoroughly investigated the use of herbal insomnia remedies such as valerian, hops, and passion flower and has found that they have an unacceptable risk of toxicity with long-term use.

Vitamin A liquid drops. The dosage of vitamin A liquid drops used by cancer patients ranges between 100,000 and 200,000 IU a day. The Foundation has cautioned that such high doses could produce toxicity if taken over extended periods of time. See *Appendix A: Avoiding Vitamin A Toxicity* for details.

Vitamin B_6. Because high doses of vitamin B_6 taken over a long period of time may cause peripheral nerve damage, high doses (500 mg a day and higher) should be used only when a blood test documents the failure of folic acid, vitamin B_{12}, and TMG to lower homocysteine levels. Never take high doses of vitamin B_6 without also taking the other B complex vitamins.

Vitamin D_3. Monthly blood tests to monitor serum calcium and parathyroid hormone levels should be done to protect against vitamin D_3 toxicity. Underlying kidney disease precludes high-dose vitamin D_3 supplementation.

Vitamin E. Because vitamin E inhibits blood clotting, it should not be used if excessive bleeding is occurring.

REFERENCES

The Life Extension Foundation's protocols are based on sound scientific research. Here are pertinent references from studies worldwide that support the protocols in this book. Readers who are interested in particular protocols, and wish to know more about the Foundation's protocol recommendations and the original science on which they are based, can use these references to find the original abstracts on-line through a computer database such as MEDLINE. The articles and papers can also be found at a medical library. The abstracts for these references can be accessed at the Foundation's Web site, **www.lef.org.**

Acetaminophen Poisoning (Analgesic Toxicity)

Mechanism of action and value of *N*-acetylcysteine in the treatment of early and late acetaminophen poisoning: a critical review. *J Toxicol Clin Toxicol* 1998, 36 (4) p277-85

Efficacy of oral versus intravenous *N*-acetylcysteine in acetaminophen overdose: Results of an open-label, clinical trial. *Journal of Pediatrics*, 1998, 132/1 (149-152)

Pearls, pitfalls, and updates in toxicology. *Emergency Medicine Clinics of North America*, 1997, 15/2 (427-450)

Refining the level for anticipated hepatotoxicity in acetaminophen poisoning. *Journal of Emergency Medicine*, 1996, 14/6 (691-695)

Outpatient *N*-acetylcysteine treatment for acetaminophen poisoning: An ethical dilemma or a new financial mandate? *Veterinary and Human Toxicology*, 1996, 38/3 (222-224)

Management of acetaminophen toxicity. *American Family Physician*, 1996, 53/1 (185-190)

[Recommendations for treatment of paracetamol poisoning. Danish Medical Society, Study of the Liver]. *Ugeskr Laeger* (Denmark) Nov 25 1996, 158 (48) p6892-5

Factors responsible for continuing morbidity after paracetamol poisoning in Chinese patients in Hong Kong. *Singapore Med J* (Singapore) Jun 1996, 37 (3) p275-7

[Clinical-toxicological case (1). Dosage of *N*-acetylcysteine in acute paracetamol poisoning]. *Schweiz Rundsch Med Prax* (Switzerland) Aug 2 1996, 85 (31-32) p935-8

Acute renal failure due to acetaminophen ingestion: a case report and review of the literature. *J Am Soc Nephrol* Jul 1995

Acute hepatic and renal toxicity from low doses of acetaminophen in the absence of alcohol abuse or malnutrition: evidence for increased susceptibility to drug toxicity due to cardiopulmonary and renal insufficiency. *Hepatology* May 1994

Protective effect of oral acetylcysteine against the hepatorenal toxicity of carbon tetrachloride potentiated by ethyl alcohol. *Alcohol Clin Exp Res* Aug 1992

Cholestyramine as an antidote against paracetamol-induced hepato- and nephrotoxicity in the rat. *Toxicol Lett* (Netherlands) May 1989

Relation of analgesic use to renal cancer: population-based findings. *Natl Cancer Inst Monogr* Dec 1985

Acetaminophen-induced depletion of glutathione and cysteine in the aging mouse kidney. *Biochem Pharmacol* (England) Jul 7 1992

Cysteine isopropylester protects against paracetamol-induced toxicity. *Biochem Pharmacol* (England) Feb 4 1992

Fatal acetaminophen poisoning with evidence of subendocardial necrosis of the heart. *J Forensic Sci* May 1991

Intrinsic susceptibility of the kidney to acetaminophen toxicity in middle-aged rats. *Toxicol Lett* (Netherlands) Jun 1990

Glutathione enhancement in various mouse organs and protection by glutathione isopropyl ester against liver injury. *Biochem Pharmacol* (England) Jun 15 1990

A comparison of the protective effects of *N*-acetyl-cysteine and *S*-carboxymethylcysteine against paracetamol (acetaminophen)-induced hepatotoxicity. *Toxicology* (Netherlands) Nov 1983

Acetaminophen hepatotoxicity. An alternative mechanism. *Biochem Pharmacol* (England) Jul 1 1983, 32 (13) p2053-9

Glutathione Metabolism and Its Role in Hepatotoxicity. *Pharmacologic Therapy*, 1991;52:287-305

Overdose of Extended-Release Acetaminophen. *New England Journal of Medicine*, July 20, 1995;196

Acute renal failure due to acetaminophen ingestion: a case report and review of the literature. *J Am Soc Nephrol* Jul 1995

Acute hepatic and renal toxicity from low doses of acetaminophen in the absence of alcohol abuse or malnutrition: evidence for increased susceptibility to drug toxicity due to cardiopulmonary and renal insufficiency. *Hepatology* May 1994

Protective effect of oral acetylcysteine against the hepatorenal toxicity of carbon tetrachloride potentiated by ethyl alcohol. *Alcohol Clin Exp Res* Aug 1992

Cholestyramine as an antidote against paracetamol-induced hepato- and nephrotoxicity in the rat. *Toxicol Lett* (Netherlands) May 1989

Relation of analgesic use to renal cancer: population-based findings. *Natl Cancer Inst Monogr* Dec 1985

Acetaminophen-induced depletion of glutathione and cysteine in the aging mouse kidney. *Biochem Pharmacol* (England) Jul 7 1992

Cysteine isopropylester protects against paracetamol-induced toxicity. *Biochem Pharmacol* (England) Feb 4 1992

Fatal acetaminophen poisoning with evidence of subendocardial necrosis of the heart. *J Forensic Sci* May 1991

Intrinsic susceptibility of the kidney to acetaminophen toxicity in middle-aged rats. *Toxicol Lett* (Netherlands) Jun 1990

Glutathione enhancement in various mouse organs and protection by glutathione isopropyl ester against liver injury. *Biochem Pharmacol* (England) Jun 15 1990

A comparison of the protective effects of *N*-acetyl-cysteine and *S*-carboxymethylcysteine against paracetamol (acetaminophen)-induced hepatotoxicity. *Toxicology* (Netherlands) Nov 1983

Acetaminophen hepatotoxicity. An alternative mechanism. *Biochem Pharmacol* (England) Jul 1 1983, 32 (13) p2053-9

Glutathione Metabolism and Its Role in Hepatotoxicity. *Pharmacologic Therapy*, 1991;52:287-305

Overdose of Extended-Release Acetaminophen. *New England Journal of Medicine*, July 20, 1995;196

Acne

Acne: Endrocrinological aspects, *Cutis* 30:212-22, 1982

Elevated free testosterone levels in women with acne. *Arch Dermatol* 119:799-802. 1983

Androgen status in women with late onsete or pserisistent acne vulgaris. *Clin Exp Dermatol* 9:28-35, 1984

Activity of testosterone 5-alpha-reductase in various tissues of human skin. *J Invest Dermatol* 74:187-91, 1980

Differential rates of conversion of testosterone to dihydrotestosterone in acne and normal human skin B A possible pathogenic factor in acne. *J Invest Dermatol* 56:366-72, 1971

Nutrition-endocrine interations: Induction of reciprocal changes in the delta-5-alpha-reduction of testosterone and the cytochrome P-450-dependent oxidation of estradiol by dietary macronutrients in man. *Proc Natl Acad Sci* USA 80:7646-9, 1983

Acne vulgaris: Therapy directed at pathophysiological defects. *Cutis* 28:41-2, 1981

Serum zinc and retinol-binding protein in acne. *Br J Dermatol* 96:283-6, 1977

The effect of zinc on the 5-alpha-reduction of testosterone by the hyperplastic human prostatic gland. *J Steroid Biochem* 20:651-5, 1984

Effects of oral zinc and vitamin A on acne. *Arch Dermatol* 113:31-6, 1977

A double blind study of the effect of zinc and oxytetracycline in acne vulgaris. *Br J Dermatol* 97:561-5, 1977

Zinc sulphate in acne vulgaris. *Arch Dermatol* 114:1776-8, 1978

Oral vitamin A in acne vulgaris. *Int J Dermatol* 20:278-85, 1981

High-dose vitamin A therapy in Darier=s disease. *Arch Dermatol* 118-891-4, 1982

Toxic doses of vitamin A for pityriasis rubra pilaris. *Arch Dermatol* 116:888-92, 1980

Local therapy of oral leukoplakia with vitamin A. *Arch Dermatol* 78:637-8, 1958

Vitamin A studies in cases of keratosis folliculitis (Darier=s disease). *Arch Dermatol Syph* 48:17-31

Erythrocyte glutathione peroxidase activity in acne vulgaris and the effect of selenium and vitamin E treatment. *Acta Derm Venerol* (StockH) 64:9-14, 1984

Fibrin microclot formation in patients with acne. *Acta Derm Venerol* (StockH) 63:538-40, 1983

Endotoxin-induced changes in copper and zinc metabolism in the syrian hamster. *J Nutr* 112:2363-73, 1982

Pyridoxine therapy for premenstrual acne flare. *Arch Dermatol* 110:103-1, 1974

Increased target tissue uptake of, and sensitivity to, testosterone in the vitamin B6 deficient rat. *J Steroid Biochem* 20:1089-93, 1984

Scientific American Medicine. Scientific American Inc, New York, NY, 1984. P2:1:3.

Thyroid therapy in dermatology. *Cutis* 8:581-3, 1971

Impaired handling of orally administered zinc in pancreatic insufficiency. *Am J. Clin Nutr* 37:268-71, 1983

Some observations on the sugar metabolism in acne vulgaris, and its treatment by insulin. *Br J Derm* 52:123-8, 1940

The effect of intralesional insulin and glucagon in acne vulgaris. *L Invest Derm* 40:259-61, 1963

Glucose tolerance in blood and skin of patients with acne vulgaris. *Ind J Derm* 22:139-49, 1977

Pustular acne staphyloderma and its treatment with tolbutamide. *Can Med Assoc J* 80:629-32, 1959

Beneficial effect of chromium-rich yeast on glucose tolerance and blood lipids in elderly patients. *Diabetes* 29:919-25, 1980

High chromium yeast for acne? *Med Hypoth* 14:307-10, 1984

The use of retinoids in the pediatric patient *Dermatol Clin* Jul 1998, 16(3) p553-69

Polymorphisms in the human cytochrome P-450 1A1 gene (CYP1A1) as a factor for developing acne. *Dermatology* (Switzerland) 1998, 196 (1) p171-5

A double-blind controlled evaluation of the sebosuppressive activity of topical erythromycin- zinc complex. *Eur J Clin Pharmacol* (Germany) 1995, 49 (1-2) p57-60

Inhibition of erythromycin-resistant propionibacteria on the skin of acne patients by topical erythromycin with and without zinc. *Br J Dermatol* (England) Mar 1994, 130 (3) p329-36

"Retinotherapy of skin diseases (editorial)" *La retinotherapie des maladies de la peau. Presse Med* (France) Nov 5 1994, 23 (34) p1551-3

Historical aspects of the oral use of retinoids in acne. *J Dermatol* (Japan) Nov 1993, 20 (11) p674-8

G. v. Preyer'sches Kinderspital, Wien, Osterreich.Recommendations for treatment of acne vulgaris; *Padiatr Padol* (Austria) 1993, 28 (3) pA33-5

Current aspects about the role of zinc in nutrition] Actualites sur la place du zinc en nutrition. *Rev Prat* (France) Jan 15 1993, 43 (2) p146-51

Adrenal Disease

Transcriptional regulation of Na/K-ATPase by corticosteroids, glycyrrhetinic acid and second messenger pathways in rat kidney epithelial cells. *J Mol Endocrinol* 1995 Aug;15(1):93-103

Licorice ingestion and blood pressure regulating hormones. *Steroids* 1994 Feb;59(2):127-30

Licorice raises urinary cortisol in man. *J Clin Endocrinol Metab* 1978 Aug;47(2):397-400

Assessment of thyroid and adrenal function in patients with familial amyloidotic polyneuropathy. *J Intern Med* 1989 May;225(5):337-41

Adrenocortical insufficiency. *Clinical Endocrinology Metab* (England) Nov 1995, 14 (4) p947-76

Changes in serum concentrations of conjugated and unconjugated steroids. *J Clin Endocrinol Metab* Oct 1994, 79 (4) p1086–90

Ovarian suppression with triptorelin and adrenal stimulation with adrenocorticotropin in functional hyperadrogenism: role of adrenal and ovarian cytochrome P450c17 alpha. *Fertil Steril* Sep 1994, 62 (3) p521–30

Pattern of plasma dehydroepiandrosterone sulfate levels in humans from birth to adulthood: evidence for testicular production. *J Clin Endocrinol Metab* Sep 1978, 47 (3) p572–7

Adrenal function and ascorbic acid concentrations in elderly women. *Gerontology* (Switzerland) 1978, 24 (6) p473–6

Age-Associated Mental Impairment (Brain Aging)

Dietary intake and cognitive function in a group of elderly people. *Am J Clin Nutr* Oct 1997, 66 (4) p803–9

The relation between antioxidants and memory performance in the old and very old. *J Am Geriatr Soc* Jun 1997, 45 (6) p718–24

Nutritional status and cognitive functioning in a normally aging sample: a 6-year reassessment [see comments]. *Am J Clin Nutr* Jan 1997, 65 (1) p20–9

Low folate levels in the cognitive decline of elderly patients and the efficacy of folate as a treatment for improving memory deficits. *Archives of Gerontology and Geriatrics (Arch. Gerontol. Geriatr.)* (Ireland) 1997, 26/1 (1–13)

Polyunsaturated fatty acids, antioxidants, and cognitive function in very old men. *American Journal of Epidemiology (Am. J. Epidemiol.)* 1997, 145/1 (33–41)

Effect of docosahexaenoic acid on the synthesis of phosphatidylserine in rat brain microsomes and C6 glioma cells. *Journal of Neurochemistry*, 1998, 70/1 (24-30)

Enhancement of brain choline levels by nicotinamide: Mechanism of action. *Neuroscience Letters* (Ireland), 1998, 249/2-3 (111-114)

Egg phosphatidylcholine combined with vitamin B_{12} improved memory impairment following lesioning of nucleus basalis in rats. *Life Sciences*, 1998, 62/9 (813-822)

The cognitive, subjective, and physical effects of a ginkgo biloba/panax ginseng combination in healthy volunteers with neurasthenic complaints. *Psychopharmacol Bull* 1997, 33 (4) p677–83

Ginkgo biloba L. *Fitoterapia* (Italy), 1998, 69/3 (195-244)

The effect of an extract of Ginkgo biloba, EGb 761, on cognitive behavior and longevity in the rat. *Physiology and Behavior*, 1998, 63/3 (425-433)

A ginkgo biloba extract (EGb 761) prevents mitochondrial aging by protecting against oxidative stress. *Free Radical Biology and Medicine*, 1998, 24/2 (298-304)

[Combined therapies in family practice and hospitals. A controlled clinical study of a population of 162 patients with criteria of age-related memory disorders]. *Presse Med* (France) Sep 6 1997, 26 (25) p1186–91

The effect of meclofenoxate with ginkgo biloba extract or zinc on lipid peroxide, some free radical scavengers and the cardiovascular system of aged rats. *Pharmacological Research* (UK), 1998, 38/1 (65-72)

Acetyl-*L*-carnitine modulates glucose metabolism and stimulates glycogen synthesis in rat brain. *Brain Research* (Netherlands), 1998, 796/1-2 (75-81)

Low folate levels in the cognitive decline of elderly patients and the efficacy of folate as a treatment for improving memory deficits. *Archives of Gerontology and Geriatrics (Arch. Gerontol. Geriatr.)* (Ireland) 1997, 26/1 (1–13)

Multicenter study with standardized extract of Ginko-Biloba EGB 761 in the treatment of memory alteration, vertigo and tinnitus. *Investigacion Medica Internacional* (Mexico) 1997, 24/2 (31–39)

Effects of EGb 761 on fatty acid reincorporation during reperfusion following ischemia in the brain of the awake gerbil. *Molecular and Chemical Neuropathology*, 1998, 34/1 (79-101)

Piracetam: A review of its clinical potential in the management of patients with stroke. *CNS Drugs* (New Zealand), 1998, 9/6 (497-511)

Piracetam treatment in post-stroke aphasia. *CNS Drugs* (New Zealand), 1998, 9/Suppl. 1 (51-56)

Piracetam in the treatment of acute stroke. *CNS Drugs* (New Zealand), 1998, 9/Suppl. 1 (41-49)

Pharmacological properties of piracetam: Rationale for use in stroke patients. *CNS Drugs* (New Zealand), 1998, 9/Suppl. 1 (19-27)

Piracetam facilitates long-term memory for a passive avoidance task in chicks through a mechanism that requires a brain corticosteroid action. *European Journal of Neuroscience* (UK), 1998, 10/7 (2238–2243)

Abnormal content of n-6 and n-3 long-chain unsaturated fatty acids in the phosphoglycerides and cholesterol esters of parahippocampal cortex from Alzheimer's disease patients and its relationship to acetyl CoA content. *International Journal of Biochemistry and Cell Biology* (UK), 1998, 30/2 (197-207)

Regional membrane phospholipid alterations in Alzheimer's disease. *Neurochemical Research*, 1998, 23/1 (81-88)

Acetyl-*L*-carnitine slows decline in younger patients with Alzheimer's disease: A reanalysis of a double-blind, placebo-controlled study using the trilinear approach. *International Psychogeriatrics*, 1998, 10/2 (193-203)

Cognition enhancers in age-related cognitive decline. *Drugs Aging* (New Zealand) Apr 1996, 8 (4) p245–74

Ginkgo biloba extract (EGb 761) independently improves changes in passive avoidance learning and brain membrane fluidity in the aging mouse. *Pharmacopsychiatry* (Germany) Jul 1996, 29 (4) p144–9

Neuronal actions of dehydroepiandrosterone. Possible roles in brain development, aging, memory, and affect. *Ann N Y Acad Sci* Dec 29 1995, 774 p111–20

Effects of CDP-choline treatment on neurobehavioral deficits after TBI and on hippocampal and neocortical acetylcholine release. *J Neurotrauma* Mar 1997, 14 (3) p161–9

Potentiation by DSP-4 of EEG slowing and memory impairment in basal forebrain-lesioned rats. *Eur J Pharmacol* (Netherlands) Feb 26 1997, 321 (2) p149–55

Cholinergic neurotransmission and synaptic plasticity concerning memory processing. *Neurochem Res* Apr 1997, 22 (4) p507–15

Nutritional status and cognitive functioning in a normally aging sample: a 6-y reassessment. *Am J Clin Nutr* Jan 1997, 65 (1) p20–9

The neurosteroid dehydroepiandrosterone sulfate (DHEAS) enhances hippocampal primed burst, but not long-term, potentiation. *Neurosci Lett* (Ireland) Jan 5 1996, 202 (3) p204–8

The neuroprotective properties of the Ginkgo biloba leaf: a review of the possible relationship to platelet-activating factor (PAF). *J Ethnopharmacol* (Ireland) Mar 1996, 50 (3) p131–9

Relations of vitamin B_{12}, vitamin B_6, folate, and homocysteine to cognitive performance in the Normative Aging Study. *Am J Clin Nutr* Mar 1996, 63 (3) p306–14

Piracetam and fipexide prevent PTZ-kindling-provoked amnesia in rats. *Eur Neuropsychopharmacol* (Netherlands) Nov 1996, 6 (4) p285–90

Nootropics: preclinical results in the light of clinical effects; comparison with tacrine. *Crit Rev Neurobiol* 1996, 10 (3-4) p357–70

Piracetam and aniracetam antagonism of centrally active drug-induced antinociception. *Pharmacol Biochem Behav* Apr 1996, 53 (4) p943–50

Effects of nicotinamide on central cholinergic transmission and on spatial learning in rats. *Pharmacol Biochem Behav* Apr 1996, 53 (4) p783–90

Piracetam. An overview of its pharmacological properties and a review of its therapeutic use in senile cognitive disorders. *Drugs Aging* (New Zealand) Jan 1991, 1 (1) p17–35

Memory-enhancing effects in male mice of pregnenolone and steroids metabolically derived from it. *Proc Natl Acad Sci U S A* Mar 1 1992, 89 (5) p156–71

Piracetam elevates muscarinic cholinergic receptor density in the frontal cortex of aged but not of young mice. *Psychopharmacology* (Berl) (Germany, West) 1988, 94 (1) p74–8

Habituation of exploratory activity in mice: effects of combinations of piracetam and choline on memory processes. *Pharmacol Biochem Behav* Aug 1984, 21 (2) p209–12

Profound effects of combining choline and piracetam on memory enhancement and cholinergic function in aged rats. *Neurobiol Aging* Summer 1981, 2 (2) p105–11

Interaction between psychological and pharmacological treatment in cognitive impairment. *Life Sci* (England) 1994, 55 (25–26) p2057–66

Impairment of learning and memory in shuttle box-trained rats neonatally injected with 6-hydroxydopamine. Effects of nootropic drugs. *Acta Physiol Pharmacol Bulg* (Bulgaria) 1993, 19 (3) p77–82

Latency of memory consolidation induced in mice by piracetam, a nootropic agent. *Indian J Exp Biol* (India) Nov 1993, 31 (11) p898–901

Elevated corticosteroid levels block the memory-improving effects of nootropics and cholinomimetics. *Psychopharmacology* (Berl) (Germany) 1992, 108 (1–2) p11–5

A trial of piracetam in two subgroups of students with dyslexia enrolled in summer tutoring. *J Learn Disabil* Nov 1991, 24 (9) p542–9

Aldosterone receptors are involved in the mediation of the memory-enhancing effects of piracetam. *Brain Res* (Netherlands) Aug 6 1990, 524 (2) p203–7

Pharmacological restoration of scopolamine-impaired memory. *Acta Physiol Pharmacol Bulg* (Bulgaria) 1985, 11 (3) p37–43

Gerontopsychological studies using NAI ('Nurnberger Alters-Inventar') on patients with organic psychosyndrome (DSM III, Category 1) treated with centrophenoxine in a double blind, comparative, randomized clinical trial. *Arch Gerontol Geriatr* (Netherlands) Jul 1989, 9 (1) p17–30

[Characteristics of the action of psychostimulants on learning and memory in rats]. *Biull Eksp Biol Med* (USSR) Aug 1988, 106 (8) p161–3

Centrophenoxine: effects on aging mammalian brain. *J Am Geriatr Soc* Feb 1978, 26 (2) p74–81

Centrophenoxine activates acetylcholinesterase activity in hippocampus of aged rats. *Indian J Exp Biol* (India) May 1995, 33 (5) p365–8

On the role of intracellular physicochemistry in quantitative gene expression during aging and the effect of centrophenoxine. A review. *Arch Gerontol Geriatr* (Netherlands) Nov–Dec 1989, 9 (3) p215–29

Neuronal lipopigment: a marker for cognitive impairment and long-term effects of psychotropic drugs [see comments]. *Br J Psychiatry* (England) Jul 1989, 155 p1–11

Age-related change in the multiple unit activity of the rat brain parietal cortex and the effect of centrophenoxine. *Exp Gerontol* (England) 1988, 23 (3) p161–74

[Effect of centrophenoxine, piracetam and aniracetam on the monoamine oxidase activity in different brain structures of rats]. *Farmakol Toksikol* (USSR) May–Jun 1988, 51 (3) p16–8

[Comparative neurophysiological study of the nootropic drugs piracetam and centrophenoxine]. *Farmakol Toksikol* (USSR) Nov–Dec 1987, 50 (6) p17–20

Fluidizing effects of centrophenoxine in vitro on brain and liver membranes from different age groups of mice. *Life Sci* (England) Dec 1 1986, 39 (22) p2089–95

Studies on the effect of iron overload on rat cortex synaptosomal membranes. *Biochim Biophys Acta* (Netherlands) Nov 7 1985, 820 (2) p216–22

Alterations of the intracellular water and ion concentrations in brain and liver cells during aging as revealed by energy dispersive X-ray microanalysis of bulk specimens. *Scan Electron Microsc* 1985, (Pt 1) p323–37

Alterations in the molecular weight distribution of proteins in rat brain synaptosomes during aging and centrophenoxine treatment of old rats. *Mech Ageing Dev* (Switzerland) Dec 1984, 28 (2–3) p171–6

Study on the anti-hypoxic effect of some drugs used in the pharmacotherapy of cerebrovascular disease. *Methods Find Exp Clin Pharmacol* (Spain) Nov 1983, 5 (9) p607–12

Inability to deactivate the sympathetic nervous system in patients with brainstem infarction; correction of the disorder by centrophenoxine administration. *Neurol Psychiatr* (Bucur) (Romania) Oct-Dec 1983, 21 (4) p425–39

Participation of adrenergic mechanisms in brain acetylcholine release produced by centrophenoxine. *Acta Physiol Pharmacol Bulg* (Bulgaria) 1979, 5 (4) p21–6

Acetyl-*L*-Carnitine: chronic treatment improves spatial acquisition in a new environment in aged rats. *J Gerontol A Biol Sci Med Sci* Jul 1995, 50 (4) pB232–36

[Effects of *L*-acetylcarnitine on mental deterioration in the aged: initial results]. *Clin Ter* (Italy) Mar 31 1990, 132 (6 Suppl) p479–510

Effect of acetyl-L-carnitine on conditioned reflex learning rate and retention in laboratory animals. *Drugs Exp Clin Res* (Switzerland) 1986, 12 (11) p911–6

The effects of acetyl-*L*-carnitine on experimental models of learning and memory deficits in the old rat. *Funct Neurol* (Italy) Oct-Dec 1989, 4 (4) p387–90

Alzheimer dementia and reduced nicotinamide adenine dinucleotide (NADH)-diaphorase activity in senile plaques and the basal forebrain. *Neurosci Lett* (Netherlands) Jan 7 1985, 53 (1) p39–44

Effects of phosphatidylserine in Alzheimer's disease. *Psychopharmacol Bull* 1992, 28 (1) p61–6

Nootropic drugs and brain cholinergic mechanisms. *Prog Neuropsychopharmacol Biol Psychiatry* (England) 1989, 13 Suppl pS77–88

Effects of phosphatidylserine in age-associated memory impairment. *Neurology* (United States) May 1991, 41 (5) p644–9

Memory effects of standardized extracts of Panax ginseng (G115), Ginkgo biloba (GK 501) and their combination Gincosan (PHL-00701). *Planta Med* (Germany) Apr 1993, 59 (2) p106–14

[Activity of Ginkgo biloba extract on short-term memory]. *Presse Med* (France) Sep 25 1986, 15 (31) p1592–4

Piracetam. An overview of its pharmacological properties and a review of its therapeutic use in senile cognitive disorders. *Drugs Aging* (New Zealand) Jan 1991, 1 (1) p17–35

Memory-enhancing effects in male mice of pregnenolone and steroids metabolically derived from it. *Proc Natl Acad Sci U S A* Mar 1 1992, 89 (5) p1567–71

[Characteristics of the action of psychostimulants on learning and memory in rats] *Biull Eksp Biol Med* (USSR) Aug 1988, 106 (8) p161–3

Centrophenoxine: effects on aging mammalian brain. *J Am Geriatr Soc* Feb 1978, 26 (2) p74–81

Centrophenoxine activates acetylcholinesterase activity in hippocampus of aged rats. *Indian J Exp Biol* (India) May 1995, 33 (5) p365–8

On the role of intracellular physicochemistry in quantitative gene expression during aging and the effect of centrophenoxine. A review. *Arch Gerontol Geriatr* (Netherlands) Nov–Dec 1989, 9 (3) p215–29

Neuronal lipopigment: a marker for cognitive impairment and long-term effects of psychotropic drugs [see comments]. *Br J Psychiatry* (England) Jul 1989, 155 p1–11

Age-related change in the multiple unit activity of the rat brain parietal cortex and the effect of centrophenoxine. *Exp Gerontol* (England) 1988, 23 (3) p161–74

[Effect of centrophenoxine, piracetam and aniracetam on the monoamine oxidase activity in different brain structures of rats]. *Farmakol Toksikol* (USSR) May–Jun 1988, 51 (3) p16–8

[Comparative neurophysiological study of the nootropic drugs piracetam and centrophenoxine]. *Farmakol Toksikol* (USSR) Nov–Dec 1987, 50 (6) p17–20

Fluidizing effects of centrophenoxine in vitro on brain and liver membranes from different age groups of mice. *Life Sci* (England) Dec 1 1986, 39 (22) p2089–95

Studies on the effect of iron overload on rat cortex synaptosomal. *Biochim Biophys Acta* (Netherlands) Nov 7 1985, 820 (2) p216–22

Alterations of the intracellular water and ion concentrations in brain and liver cells during aging as revealed by energy dispersive X-ray microanalysis of bulk specimens. *Scan Electron Microsc* 1985, (Pt 1) p323–37

Alterations in the molecular weight distribution of proteins in rat brain synaptosomes during aging and centrophenoxine treatment of old rats. *Mech Ageing Dev* (Switzerland) Dec 1984, 28 (2–3) p171–6

Study on the anti-hypoxic effect of some drugs used in the pharmacotherapy of cerebrovascular disease. *Methods Find Exp Clin Pharmacol* (Spain) Nov 1983, 5 (9) p607–12

Inability to deactivate the sympathetic nervous system in patients with brainstem infarction; correction of the disorder by centrophenoxine administration. *Neurol Psychiatr* (Bucur) (Romania) Oct-Dec 1983, 21 (4) p425–39

Participation of adrenergic mechanisms in brain acetylcholine release produced by centrophenoxine. *Acta Physiol Pharmacol Bulg* (Bulgaria) 1979, 5 (4) p21–6

Acetyl-*L*-Carnitine: chronic treatment improves spatial acquisition in a new environment in aged rats. *J Gerontol A Biol Sci Med Sci* Jul 1995, 50 (4) pB232–36

[Effects of *L*-acetylcarnitine on mental deterioration in the aged: initial results]. *Clin Ter* (Italy) Mar 31 1990, 132 (6 Suppl) p479–510

Effect of acetyl-L-carnitine on conditioned reflex learning rate and retention in laboratory animals. *Drugs Exp Clin Res* (Switzerland) 1986, 12 (11) p911–6

The effects of acetyl-l-carnitine on experimental models of learning and memory deficits in the old rat. *Funct Neurol* (Italy) Oct-Dec 1989, 4 (4) p387–90

Alzheimer dementia and reduced nicotinamide adenine dinucleotide (NADH)- diaphorase activity in senile plaques and the basal forebrain. *Neurosci Lett* (Netherlands) Jan 7 1985, 53 (1) p39–44

Effects of phosphatidylserine in Alzheimer's disease. *Psychopharmacol Bull* 1992, 28 (1) p61–6

Nootropic drugs and brain cholinergic mechanisms. *Prog Neuropsychopharmacol Biol Psychiatry* (England) 1989, 13 Suppl pS77–88

Effects of phosphatidylserine in age-associated memory impairment. *Neurology* May 1991, 41 (5) p644–9

Memory effects of standardized extracts of Panax ginseng (G115), Ginkgo biloba (GK 501) and their combination Gincosan (PHL-00701). *Planta Med* (Germany) Apr 1993, 59 (2) p106–14

[Activity of Ginkgo biloba extract on short-term memory]. *Presse Med* (France) Sep 25 1986, 15 (31) p1592–4

Alcohol-Induced Hangover: Prevention

Reduction of lower motor neuron degeneration in wobbler mice by *N*-acetyl-*L*-cysteine. *Journal of Neuroscience*, 1996, 16/23 (7574–7582)

Role of oxidative stress and antioxidant therapy in alcoholic and nonalcoholic liver diseases. *Adv Pharmacol* 1997, 38 p601–28

Protective action of ascorbic acid and sulfur compounds against acetaldehyde toxicity: implications in alcoholism and smoking. *Agents Actions* (Switzerland) May 1975, 5 (2) p164–73

Sulfur amino acid metabolism in hepatobiliary disorders. *Scand J Gastroenterol* (Norway) May 1992, 27 (5) p405–11

[Severe somatic complications of acute alcoholic intoxication]. *Rev Prat* (France) Oct 15 1993, 43 (16) p2047–51

[The therapeutic approach in optic neuropathy due to methyl alcohol]. *Oftalmologia* (Romania) Jan-Mar 1991, 35 (1) p39–42

Alcohol and brain damage. *Hum Toxicol* (England) Sep 1988, 7 (5) p455–63

Acute ethanol poisoning and the ethanol withdrawal syndrome. *Med Toxicol Adverse Drug Exp* (New Zealand) May-Jun 1988, 3 (3) p172–96

Clinical signs in the Wernicke-Korsakoff complex: a retrospective analysis of 131 cases diagnosed at necropsy. *J Neurol Neurosurg Psychiatry* (England) Apr 1986, 49 (4) p341–5

Thiamine status of institutionalised and non-institutionalised aged. *Int J Vitam Nutr Res* (Switzerland) 1977, 47 (4) p325–35

[Vitamin B_1 deficiency in chronic alcoholics and its clinical correlation *J. Schweiz Med Wochenschr* (Switzerland) Oct 23 1976, 106 (43) p1466–70

Glutathione prevents ethanol induced gastric mucosal damage and depletion of sulfhydryl compounds in humans. *Gut* (England) Feb 1993, 34 (2) p161–5

Effects of amino acids on acute alcohol intoxication in mice—concentrations of ethanol, acetaldehyde, acetate and acetone in blood and tissues. *Arukoru Kenkyuto Yakubutsu Ison* (Japan) Oct 1990, 25 (5) p429–40

A possible protective role for sulphydryl compounds in acute alcoholic liver injury. *Biochem Pharmacol* Aug 15 1977, 26 (16) p1529–31

Protection against toxic effects of formaldehyde in vitro, and of methanol or formaldehyde in vivo, by subsequent administration of SH reagents Ph. *Physiol Chem ys* 1976, 8 (6) p543–50

N-Acetylcysteine for Lung Cancer Prevention. *Nico Chest* May 1995;107(5):1437–41

S-Adenosylmethionine and the Liver. *The Liver: Biology and Pathobiology, 3rd Edition*, 1994; 27:461–470

Allergies

Byssinosis: airway responses in textile dust exposure. *J.Occup.Med.*, 1975, 17/6 (357-359)

Intracellular (polymorphonuclear) magnesium content in patients with bronchial asthma between attacks. *Journal of the Royal Society of Medicine* (UK), 1995, 88/8 (441-445)

Consequences of magnesium deficiency on the enhancement of stress reactions; Preventive and therapeutic implications (A review). *J. Am. Coll. Nutr.*, 1994, 13/5 (429-446)

A hypothesis: The role of magnesium and possibly copper deficiency in the pathogenesis of the adult or acute respiratory distress syndrome (ARDS) as it occurs in infants, children, and adults. *Pediatr. Asthma Allergy Immunol.*, 1993, 7/4 (195–206)

Cytokines, neuropeptides, and reperfusion injury during magnesium deficiency. *Ann. New York Acad. Sci.*, 1994, 723/(246–257)

Downbeat nystagmus with magnesium depletion. *Arch. Neurol. (Chicago)*, 1981, 38/10 (650–652)

Regulation and function of pyridoxal phosphate in CNS. *Neurochem. Int.* (England), 1981, 3/3-4 (181-206)

The action of aspirin in preventing the niacin flush and its relevance to the antischizophrenic action of megadose niacin. *J. Orthomolec. Psychiat.* (Canada), 1976, 5/2 (89-100)

Copper, zinc, manganese, niacin and pyridoxine in the schizophrenias. *J. Appl. Nutr.*, 1975, 27/2-3 (9-39)

Nutrition in the prevention and treatment of nervous and mental diseases. *J. Appl. Nutr.*, 1974, 26/3 (27-35)

Effect of long-term gastric acid suppressive therapy on serum vitamin B_{12} levels in patients with Zollinger-Ellison syndrome. *American Journal of Medicine*, 1998, 104/5 (422-430)

Pernicious anaemia in a Chinese man; a medical experience from the Indonesian period. *Nederlands Tijdschrift voor Geneeskunde* (Netherlands), 1996, 140/10 (561-563)

Effect of histamine H2-receptor antagonists on vitamin B12 absorption. *Ann. Pharmacother.*, 1992, 26/10 (1283-1286)

The present state of controlled hypotension. *Anaesthesist* (Berl.) (Germany, West), 1977, 26/5 (212-219)

Vitamin B_{12} depletion in obese patients treated with jejunoileal shunt. *Scand. J. Gastroent.* (Norway), 1974, 9/6 (543-547)

The pill, hormone replacement therapy, vascular and mood over-reactivity, and mineral imbalance. *Journal of Nutritional and Environmental Medicine* (UK), 1998 8/2 (105-116)

Bronchial reactivity and dietary antioxidants. *Thorax* (UK), 1997, 52/2 (166-170)

Diet and nutritional status in children with cow's milk allergy. *European Journal of Clinical Nutrition* (UK), 1995, 49/8 (605-612)

Food for the weanling: The next priority in infant nutrition. *Acta Paediatr. Scand* (Sweden), 1986, 75/Suppl. 323 (96-102)

Potential toxicity due to dolomite and bonemeal. *South. Med. J.*, 1983, 76/5 (556-559)

Biotin deficiency in an infant fed with amino acid formula and hypoallergenic rice. *Acta Paediatrica, International Journal of Paediatrics* (Norway), 1996, 85/7 (872-874)

Atopic dermatitis and essential fatty acids: A biochemical basis for atopy? *Acta Derm.-Venereol.* (Sweden), 1985, 65/Suppl. 114 (143-145)

Biochemical evidence for a deficiency of vitamin B_6 in subjects reacting to monosodium *L*-glutamate by the Chinese restaurant syndrome. *Biochem. Biophys. Res. Commun.*, 1981, 100/3 (972-977)

Biochemical correlations of a deficiency of vitamin B_6, the carpal tunnel syndrome and the. *Ircs Med. Sci.* (England), 1981, 9/5 (444)

Precipitating factors in asthma. Aspirin, sulfites, and other drugs and chemicals. *Chest*, 1985, 87/1 Suppl. (50S-54S)

Chemoprevention of colorectal cancer. *Gut* (UK), 1998, 43/4 (578-585)

Effect of vitamin C on histamine bronchial responsiveness of patients with allergic rhinitis. *Ann. Allergy*, 1990, 65/4 (311-314)

Colds and vitamin C. *Irish Med.J.* (Ireland), 1975, 68/20 (511-516)

Colds, ascorbic acid metabolism, and vitamin C. *J. Clin. Pharmacol.*, 1975, 15/8-9 (570-578)

Vitamin C metabolism and the common cold. *Eur. J. Clin. Pharmacol.* (Germany, West), 1974, 7/6 (421-428)

Pretreatment of skin with a Ginkgo biloba extract/sodium carboxymethylbeta-1,3-glucan formulation appears to inhibit the elicitation of allergic contact dermatitis in man. *Contact Dermatitis* (Denmark), 1998, 38/3 (123-126)

Chemistry and biology of alkylphenols from Ginkgo biloba L. *Pharmazie* (Germany), 1997, 52/10 (735-738)

Special therapy for allergic rhinitis. Hay fever without antihistaminics. *Therapiewoche* (Germany), 1994, 44/6 (344-346)

Anatomical, phytochemical and immunochemical studies on Ligaria cuneifolia (R. et P.) Tiegh (Loranthaceae). *Pharmaceutical Biology* (Netherlands), 1998, 36/2 (131-139)

Biologically active constituents of the crude drug of Hypericum perforatum L. *Psychopharmakotherapie, Supplement* (Germany), 1998, 5/8 (34-39)

Pharmacological actions of proanthocyanidins. *Revista Portuguesa de Farmacia* (Portugal), 1998, 48/1 (9-12)

Proanthocyanidins from the bark of Hamamelis virginiana exhibit antimutagenic properties against nitroaromatic compounds. *Planta Medica* (Germany), 1998, 64/4 (324-327)

Study of the extraction of proanthocyanidins from grape seeds. *Food Chemistry* (UK), 1998, 61/1-2 (201-206)

Separations of flavan-3-ols and dimeric proanthocyanidins by capillary electrophoresis. *Planta Medica* (Germany), 1998, 64/1 (63-67)

Characterization of monomeric and oligomeric flavan-3-ols from unripe almond fruits. *Phytochemical Analysis* (UK), 1998, 9/1 (21-27)

The steroid hormone dehydroepiandrosterone (DHEA) breaks intranasally induced tolerance, when administered at time of systemic immunization. *Journal of Neuroimmunology* (Netherlands), 1998, 89/1-2 (19-25)

Serum levels of phospholipid fatty acids in mothers and their babies in relation to allergic disease. *European Journal of Pediatrics* (Germany), 1998, 157/4 (298-303)

Comparative nutrition of pantothenic acid. *Journal of Nutritional Biochemistry* 7 (6):p312–321 1996

Pantothenic acid derivatives: Modulators of adrenal function. *Vyestsi Akademii Navuk Byelarusi Syeryya Biyalahichnykh Navuk* 0 (3):p48-51, 124 1993

Evidence for an Increased Secretory Capacity for Dehydroepiandrosterone Sulfate in the Pantothenic Acid-Deficient Rat Associated with an Impaired Adrenal Cholesterol Deposition. *J Clin Biochem Nutr* 7 (2). 1989. 115–132

Effects of Pantothenate Deficiency on Steroid Hormone Secretion In Rats I. Assessment of the State of Function of the Adrenal Cortex . *J Clin Biochem Nutr* 6 (1). 1989. 1–14

Functional Activity of the Adrenal Cortex in Ethanol Intake and in Additional Use of Riboflavin and Pantothenate. *Vyestsi Akademii Navuk Bssr Syeryya Biyalahichnykh Navuk* (5). 1986 (Recd. 1987). 88–91

Adrenocortical Function under Pantothenate Deficiency and During Administration of This Vitamin Or Its Derivatives. *Voprosy Pitaniya* 0 (4). 1985. 51–54

The Influence of Microorganisms and of Stress on the Chicks Requirement for Pantothenic-Acid. *British Journal of Nutrition* 45 (2). 1981. 441–450

Hypo Glycemia in Mice Exposed to an Environment of High Temperature and Humidity. *Research Communications in Chemical Pathology and Pharmacology (Res Commun Chem Pathol Pharmacol)* 32 (2). 1981. 261–280

Distribution Of 1 Carbon-14 Labeled Pantothenic-Acid in Rats. *International Journal for Vitamin and Nutrition Research* 50 (3). 1980. 283–293

Influence of High Doses of Sodium Pantothenate on the Production of Cortico Steroids. *Bollettino della Societa Italiana di Biologia Sperimentale* 54 (22). 1978 (Recd. 1979). 2248 2250

Modifying Acetylation Capability And Cortico Sterone Biosynthesis By Means Of Pantothenic-Acid Deficiency In Long-Term Experiments With Rats. *International Journal for Vitamin and Nutrition Research (Int J Vitam Nutr Res)* 45 (3). 1975 251-261

Effect Of Pantothenic-Acid On Cholesterol And Ascorbic-Acid Of Adrenals In Normal And Scorbutic Guinea-Pigs. *Indian Sci Cong Assoc Proc* 59 Part. 1972 621–622

Thymic Weight In Pantothenic-Acid Deficiency. *Nutrition and Metabolism* 20 (4). 1976 (Recd 1977) 272–277

Study of the effect of Lactobacillus paracasei and fructooligosaccharides on the faecal microflora in weanling piglets. *Berl Munch Tierarztl Wochenschr* 1999 Jun-Jul;112(6–7):225–8

Continuous culture selection of bifidobacteria and lactobacilli from human faecal samples using fructooligosaccharide as selective substrate. *J Appl Microbiol* 1998 Oct;85(4):769–77

Health benefits of non-digestible oligosaccharides. *Adv Exp Med Biol* 1997;427:211–9

Bacterial fermentation of fructooligosaccharides and resistant starch in patients with an ileal pouch-anal anastomosis. *Am J Clin Nutr* 1997 Nov;66(5):1286–92

Therapeutic considerations of *L*-Glutamine: a review of the literature. *Altern Med Rev* 1999 Aug;4(4):239–248

Reduction of chemotherapy-induced side-effects by parenteral glutamine supplementation in patients with metastatic colorectal cancer. *Eur J Cancer* 1999 Feb;35(2):202–7

Early Gastrointestinal Regulatory Peptide Response to Intestinal Resection in the Rat Is Stimulated by Enteral Glutamine Supplementation. *Dig Surg* 1999;16(3):197–203

Interventional nutrition for gastrointestinal disease. *Clin Tech Small Anim Pract* 1998 Nov;13(4):211-6

Inhibition of antigen-induced lung anaphylaxis in the guinea-pig by BN 52021 a new specific paf-acether receptor antagonist isolated from Ginkgo biloba. *Agents Actions* 1986 Jan;17(3-4):371–2

A modified determination of Coenzyme Q_{10} in human blood and CoQ_{10} blood levels in diverse patients with allergies. *Biofactors* 1988 Dec;1(4):303–6

The effect of gamma-linolenic acid on clinical status, red cell fatty acid composition and membrane microviscosity in infants with atopic dermatitis. *Drugs Exp Clin Res*. 1994. 20(2). p77–84.

Fatty acid compositions of plasma lipids in atopic dermatitis/ asthma patients. *Arerugi*. 1994 Jan. 43(1). p37–43

Autoimmune disease and allergy are controlled by vitamin C treatment. *In Vivo* (Greece), 1994, 8/2 (251–258)

Immune senescence and adrenal steroids: Immune dysregulation and the action of dehydroepiandrosterone (DHEA) in old animals. *Eur. J. Clin. Pharmacol*. (Germany), 1993, 45/Suppl. 1 (S21–S23)

Omega-3 fatty acids in respiratory diseases: A review. *J. Am. Coll. Nutr.*, 1995, 14/1 (18–23)

Vitamin C and the genesis of autoimmune disease and allergy (Review). *In Vivo* (Greece), 1995, 9/3 (231–238)

Is Linus Pauling, a vitamin C advocate, just making much ado about nothing? *In Vivo* (Greece), 1994, 8/3 (391–400)

Asthma and vitamin C. *Ann. Allergy*, 1994, 73/2 (89–99)

The effect of vitamin C infusion treatment on immune disorders: An invitation to a trial in AIDS patients (Review). *Int. J. Oncol*. (Greece), 1994, 4/4 (831–838)

Chromium dermatitis and ascorbic acid. *Contact Dermatitis* (Denmark), 1984, 10/4 (252–253)

Colds and vitamin C. *Irish Med.J.* (Ireland), 1975 *Clin.Allergy* (England), 68/20 (511–516)

Vitamin C metabolism and atopic allergy.), 1975, 5/3 (317–324)

Alzheimer's Disease

Cognitive enhancement therapy for Alzheimer's disease. The way forward. *Drugs* (New Zealand), 1997, 53/5 (752-768)

Alzheimer's disease: Fundamental and therapeutic aspects. *Experientia* (Switzerland) 1995, 51/2 (99–105)

Newer and older monoamine oxidase inhibitors. A comparative profile. *CNS Drugs* (New Zealand), 1995, 3/2 (145-158)

The possible role of peroxynitrite in Alzheimer's disease: a simple hypothesis that could be tested more thoroughly. *Med Hypotheses* (England) May 1997, 48 (5) p375-80

A new model for the pathophysiology of Alzheimer's disease. Aluminium toxicity is exacerbated by hydrogen peroxide and attenuated by an amyloid protein fragment and melatonin. *South African Medical Journal* (South Africa), 1997, 87/9 (1111–1115)

Cerebrospinal fluid levels of alpha-tocopherol (vitamin E) in Alzheimer's disease. *J Neural Transm* (Austria) 1997, 104 (6–7) p703–10

Plastic neuronal remodeling is impaired in patients with Alzheimer's disease carrying apolipoprotein epsilon 4 allele. *J Neurosci* Jan 15 1997, 17 (2) p516–29

Hemodynamic consequences of deformed microvessels in the brain in Alzheimer's disease. *Ann N Y Acad Sci* Sep 26 1997, 826 p75–91

The cholinergic system in Alzheimer's disease. *Prog Neurobiol* (England) Aug 1997, 52 (6) p511–35

The choline-leakage hypothesis for the loss of acetylcholine in Alzheimer's disease. *Biophys J* Sep 1997, 73 (3) p1276-80

Increased susceptibility of Alzheimer's disease temporal cortex to oxygen free radical-mediated processes. *Free Radic Biol Med* 1997, 23 (2) p183-90

A controlled trial of selegiline, alpha-tocopherol, or both as treatment for Alzheimer's disease. The Alzheimer's Disease Cooperative Study [see comments]. *N Engl J Med* Apr 24 1997, 336 (17) p1216-22; Comment in *N Engl J Med* 1997 Apr 24;336(17):1245-7; Comment in: *N Engl J Med* 1997 Aug 21;337(8):572; discussion 573; Comment in: *N Engl J Med* 1997 Aug 21;337(8):572-3

Is metabolic evidence for vitamin B-12 and folate deficiency more frequent in elderly patients with Alzheimer's disease? *J Gerontol A Biol Sci Med Sci* Mar 1997, 52 (2)

Antiamyloid strategies for the treatment of Alzheimer's disease. *Drugs of Today* (Spain), 1998, 34/8 (673-689)

Oxidative damage in the central nervous system: Protection by melatonin. *Progress in Neurobiology* (UK), 1998, 56/3 (359-384)

Inhibition of Alzheimer beta-fibrillogenesis by melatonin. *Journal of Biological Chemistry*, 1998, 273/13 (7185-7188)

Melatonin prevents beta-amyloid-induced lipid peroxidation. *Journal of Pineal Research* (Denmark), 1998, 24/2 (78-82)

The interaction of melatonin and its precursors with aluminium, cadmium, copper, iron, lead, and zinc: An adsorptive voltammetric study. *Journal of Pineal Research* (Denmark), 1998, 24/1 (15-21)

N-acetyl-serotonin (normelatonin) and melatonin protect neurons against oxidative challenges and suppress the activity of the transcription factor *NF*-kappaB Lezoualc'h F.; Sparapani M.; Behl C. *Journal of Pineal Research* (Denmark), 1998, 24/3 (168-178)

'Amyloid is not a tombstone'—A summation. The primary role for cerebrovascular and CSF dynamics as factors in Alzheimer's disease (AD): DMSO, fluorocarbon oxygen carriers, thyroid hormonal, and other suggested therapeutic measures. *Annals of the New York Academy of Sciences*, 1997, 826/- (348-374)

Drugs for the prevention and treatment of Alzheimer's disease. *Medical Journal of Australia* (Australia), 1997, 167/8 (447-449,452)

Melatonin prevents death of neuroblastoma cells exposed to the Alzheimer amyloid peptide. *Journal of Neuroscience*, 1997, 17/5 (1683-1690)

Loss of intraventricular fluid melatonin can explain the neuropathology of Alzheimer's disease. *Medical Hypotheses* (UK), 1997, 49/2 (153-158)

Acetyl *L*-carnitine slows decline in younger patients with Alzheimer's disease: A reanalysis of a double-blind, placebo-controlled study using the trilinear approach. *International Psychogeriatrics*, 1998, 10/2 (193-203)

Advances in the treatment of Alzheimer's disease. *Pharmaceutical Journal* (UK), 1997, 259/6966 (693-696)

Deprenyl monotherapy improves visuo-motor control in early parkinsonism. *Journal of Neural Transmission*, Supplement (Austria), 1998, -/52 (63-69)

A randomized, double-blind, placebo-controlled trial of deprenyl and thioctic acid in human immunodeficiency virus-associated cognitive impairment. *Neurology*, 1998, 50/3 (645-651)

The clinical potential of Deprenyl in neurologic and psychiatric disorders. *Journal of Neural Transmission, Supplement* (Austria), 1996, -/48 (85-93)

Monoaminooxidase (MAO)B-Hemmer. *Neuropsychiatrie* (Germany), 1995, 9/Suppl. 1 (S20-S22)

Selegiline: A review of its clinical efficacy in Parkinson's disease and its clinical potential in Alzheimer's disease. *CNS Drugs* (New Zealand), 1995, 4/3 (230-246)

Therapy with *L*-deprenyl (selegiline) and relation to abuse liability. *Clin. Pharmacol. Ther.*, 1994, 56/6 II Suppl. (750-756)

Biochemical actions of *L*-deprenyl (selegiline). *Clin. Pharmacol. Ther.*, 1994, 56/6 II Suppl. (734-741)

Neuroprotection by dopamine agonists. *J. Neural Transm. Suppl.* (Austria), 1994, -/43 (183-201)

Slow recovery of human brain MAO B after *L*-deprenyl (selegeline) withdrawal. *SYNAPSE*, 1994, 18/2 (86-93)

Emerging drugs for Alzheimer's disease: Mechanisms of action and prospects for cognitive enhancing medications. *Med. Clin. North Am.*, 1994, 78/4 (911-934)

A double-blind crossover pilot study of *L*-deprenyl (selegiline) combined with cholinesterase inhibitor in Alzheimer's disease. *Am. J. Psychiatry*, 1993, 150/2 (321-323)

Neurotoxicity of levodopa on catecholamine-rich neurons. *Mov. Disord.*, 1992, 7/1 (23-31)

Effects of a MAO-B inhibitor in the treatment of Alzheimer disease. *Eur. Neurol.* (Switzerland), 1991, 31/2 (100-107)

A controlled study of the antidepressant efficacy and side effects of (-)-deprenyl. A selective monoamine oxidase inhibitor. *Arch. Gen. Psychiatry*, 1989, 46/1 (45-50)

Brief information on an early phase-II-study with deprenyl in demented patients. *Pharmacopsychiatry* (Germany, Federal Republic of), 1987, 20/6 (256-257)

Abnormal content of n-6 and n-3 long-chain unsaturated fatty acids in the phosphoglycerides and cholesterol esters of parahippocampal cortex from Alzheimer's disease patients and its relationship to acetyl CoA content. *International Journal of Biochemistry and Cell Biology* (UK), 1998, 30/2 (197-207)

Pharmacological treatment of Alzheimer's disease: Achievements and perspectives. *Revista Espanola de Geriatria y Gerontologia* (Spain), 1998, 33/1 (27-41)

Treatment of cognitive deficits in Alzheimer's disease. *Primary Care Psychiatry* (UK), 1997, 3/4 (151-162)

Modulating excitatory synaptic neurotransmission: Potential treatment for neurological disease? *Neurobiology of Disease*, 1998, 5/2 (67-80)

Experimental approaches to cognitive disturbance in Alzheimer's disease. *Harvard Review of Psychiatry*, 1998, 6/1 (11-22)

Advances in the drug treatment of Alzheimer's disease. *Human Psychopharmacology* (UK), 1998, 13/2 (83-90)

Receptors of the low density lipoprotein (LDL) receptor family in man. Multiple functions of the large family members via interaction with complex ligands. *Biological Chemistry* (Germany), 1998, 379/8-9 (951-964)

Predictors of longitudinal changes in memory, visuospatial, and verbal functioning in very old demented adults. *Dementia and Geriatric Cognitive Disorders* (Switzerland), 1998, 9/5 (258-266)

Apolipoprotein E genotyping and cerebrospinal fluid tau protein: Implications for the clinical diagnosis of Alzheimer's disease. *Gerontology* (Switzerland), 1997, 43/Suppl. 1 (2-10)

Alzheimer's disease: Cognitive and behavioral pharmacotherapy. *Connecticut Medicine*, 1997, 61/9 (543-552)

Diagnosis and treatment of Alzheimer's disease. *Munchener Medizinische Wochenschrift* (Germany), 1997, 139/36 (35-41)

Assessment of nootropic and amnestic activity of centrally acting agents. *Indian Journal of Pharmacology* (India), 1997, 29/4 (208-221)

Prostaglandins as putative neurotoxins in Alzheimer's disease. *Proceedings of the Society for Experimental Biology and Medicine*, 1998, 219/2 (120-125)

Vitamin E and other endogenous antioxidants in the central nervous system. *Geriatrics*, 1998, 53/9 Suppl. 1 (S25-S27)

Medical costs preceding diagnosis of probable Alzheimer disease. *Archives of Gerontology and Geriatrics* (Ireland), 1998, 27/Suppl. 6 (247-254)

A review on the relations between the vitamin status and cognitive performances. *Archives of Gerontology and Geriatrics* (Ireland), 1998, 27/Suppl. 6 (207-214)

Pharmacological treatments for Alzheimer disease. *Giornale di Gerontologia* (Italy), 1997, 45/9 (613-623)

In vitro kinetic studies of formation of antigenic advanced glycation end products (AGEs). Novel inhibition of post-Amadori glycation pathways. *Journal of Biological Chemistry*, 1997, 272/9 (5430-5437)

Low folate levels in the cognitive decline of elderly patients and the efficacy of folate as a treatment for improving memory deficits. *Archives of Gerontology and Geriatrics* (Ireland), 1997, 26/1 (1-13)

Intravenous methotrexate for primary central nervous system non-Hodgkin's lymphoma in AIDS. *AIDS* (UK), 1997, 11/14 (1725-1730)

Folate deficiency, anticonvulsant drugs, and psychiatric morbidity. *Clinical Neuropharmacology*, 1995, 18/2 (165-182)

SA4503: A novel sigma1 receptor agonist. *CNS Drug Reviews*, 1998, 4/1 (1-24)

Cognitive and noncognitive symptoms in dementia patients: Relationship to cortisol and dehydroepiandrosterone. *International Psychogeriatrics*, 1998, 10/1 (85-96)

Dehydroepiandrosterone (DHEA) in aging, disease modification, and symptom control. *Journal of Pharmaceutical Care in Pain and Symptom Control*, 1998, 6/2 (5-41)

Increased total 7alpha-hydroxy-dehydroepiandrosterone in serum of patients with Alzheimer's disease. *Journals of Gerontology—Series A Biological Sciences and Medical Sciences*, 1998, 53/2 (B125-B132)

Neuroprotection by dehydroepiandrosteronesulfate: Role of an NF-similar B-like factor. *NeuroReport* (UK), 1998, 9/4 (759-763)

Effects of hormone replacement therapy on serum amyloid P component in postmenopausal women. *Maturitas* (Ireland), 1997, 26/2 (113-119)

Free radicals, oxidants, antioxidants and the degenerative disease of aging. *Romanian Journal of Gerontology and Geriatrics* (Romania), 1997, 19/1 (3-17)

Pharmacotherapy in Alzheimer's dementia: Treatment of cognitive symptoms—Results of new studies. *Fortschritte der Neurologie Psychiatrie* (Germany), 1997, 65/3 (108-121)

Combination therapy for early Alzheimer's disease: What are we waiting for? *Journal of the American Geriatrics Society*, 1998, 46/10 (1322-1324)

Treatment of Alzheimer's disease: Current approaches and promising developments. *American Journal of Medicine*, 1998, 104/4 A (32S-38S)

Epidemiology of dementia and Alzheimer's disease. *American Journal of Geriatric Psychiatry*, 1998, 6/2 Suppl. (S3-S18)

Oxidative stress during the pathogenesis of Alzheimer's disease and antioxidant neuroprotection. *Fortschritte der Neurologie Psychiatrie* (Germany), 1998, 66/3 (113-121)

Current therapeutic strategies in Alzheimer's disease. *Lege Artis Medicine* (Hungary), 1997, 7/12 (778-788)

Selective modulation of GABA(A) receptors by aluminum. *Journal of Neurophysiology*, 1998, 80/2 (755-761)

Occupational exposures to solvents and aluminium and estimated risk of Alzheimer's disease. *Occupational and Environmental Medicine* (UK), 1998, 55/9 (627-633)

Promotion of transition metal-induced reactive oxygen species formation by beta-amyloid. *Brain Research* (Netherlands), 1998, 799/1 (91-96)

Chronic exposure to aluminum impairs neuronal glutamate-nitric oxide-cyclic GMP pathway. *Journal of Neurochemistry*, 1998, 70/4 (1609-1614)

Absence of aluminium in neurofibrillary tangles in Alzheimer's disease. *Neuroscience Letters* (Ireland), 1998, 240/3 (123-126)

Do aluminium and/or glutamate induce Alzheimer PHF-like formation? An electron microscopic study. *Journal of Neurocytology* (UK), 1998, 27/1 (59-68)

Molecular neurobiology of Alzheimer's disease (syndrome?). *Harvard Review of Psychiatry*, 1997, 5/4 (177-213)

Alzheimer's disease risk factors as related to cerebral blood flow: Additional evidence. *Medical Hypotheses* (UK), 1998, 50/1 (25-36)

Cerebrospinal fluid levels of transition metals in patients with Alzheimer's disease. *Journal of Neural Transmission* (Germany), 1998, 105/4-5 (479-488)

Nitric oxide generators produce accumulation of chelatable zinc in hippocampal neuronal perikarya. *Brain Research* (Netherlands), 1998, 799/1 (118-129)

Trace elements in Alzheimer's disease pituitary glands. *Biological Trace Element Research*, 1998, 62/1-2 (107-114)

Imbalances of trace elements related to oxidative damage in Alzheimer's disease brain. *NeuroToxicology*, 1998, 19/3 (339-346)

Zinc and platelet membrane microviscosity in Alzheimer's disease. The in vivo effect of zinc on platelet membranes and cognition. *South African Medical Journal* (South Africa), 1997, 87/9 (1116-1119)

Zinc metabolism in the brain: Relevance to human neurodegenerative disorders. *Neurobiology of Disease*, 1997, 4/3-4 (137-169)

Selective aggregation of endogenous beta-amyloid peptide and soluble amyloid precursor protein in cerebrospinal fluid by zinc. *Journal of Neurochemistry*, 1997, 69/3 (1204-1212)

Zinc alters conformation and inhibits biological activities of nerve growth factor and related neurotrophins. *Nature Medicine*, 1997, 3/8 (872-878)

Zinc and Alzheimer's disease: Is there a direct link?. *Brain Research Reviews* (Netherlands), 1997, 23/3 (219-236)

Progress in the management of alzheimer's disease. *Hospital Practice*, 1998, 33/3 (151-166)

A placebo-controlled, double-blind, randomized trial of an extract of Ginkgo biloba for dementia. *Journal of the American Medical Association,* 1997, 278/16 (1327-1332)

Cognition-enhancing drugs in dementia: A guide to the near future. *Canadian Journal of Psychiatry* (Canada), 1997, 42/ Suppl. 1 (35S-50S)

Systemic administration of defined extracts from Withania somnifera (Indian Ginseng) and Shilajit differentially affects cholinergic but not glutamatergic and gabaergic markers in rat brain. *Neurochemistry International* (UK), 1997, 30/2 (181-190)

Alzheimer's disease patients and its relationship to acetyl CoA content. *International Journal of Biochemistry and Cell Biology* (UK), 1998, 30/2 (197-207)

Regional membrane phospholipid alterations in Alzheimer's disease. *Neurochemical Research*, 1998, 23/1 (81-88)

Reduced cholinergic function in normal and Alzheimer's disease brain is associated with apolipoprotein E4 genotype. *Neurosci Lett* 1997 Dec 12;239(1):33-6

Brain aging and Alzheimer's disease, 'Wear and tear' versus 'Use it or lose it'. Swaab D.F., *Neurobiol. Aging,* 1991, 12/4 (317-324), Netherlands Institute for Brain Research, Meibergdreef 33, 1105 AZ Amsterdam, Netherlands

Immunohistochemical localization of advanced glycation end products, pentosidine, and carboxymethyllysine in lipofuscin pigments of Alzheimer's disease and aged neurons. Horie K.; Miyata T.; Yasuda T.; Takeda A.; Yasuda Y.; Maeda K.; Sobue G.; Kurokawa K., *Biochemical and Biophysical Research Communications*, 1997, 236/2 (327-332), K. Kurokawa, Institute of Medical Sciences, Tokai University School of Medicine, Isehara, Kanagawa 259-11 Japan

Neuroanatomical aspects of neurotransmitters affected in Alzheimer's disease. Emson P.C.; Lindvall O., *Br. Med. Bull.*(England), 1986, 42/1 (57-62), MRC Neurochemical Pharmacology Unit, Cambridge United Kingdom

Non-cholinergic neurotransmitter abnormalities in Alzheimer's disease. Rossor M.; Iversen L.L., *Br. Med. Bull.*(England), 1986, 42/1 (70-74), Institute of Neurology, London United Kingdom

Changes in nerve cells of the nucleus basalis of Meynert in Alzheimer's disease and their relationship to ageing and to the accumulation of lipofuscin pigment. Mann D.M.A.; Yates P.O.; Marcyniuk *B., Mech. Ageing Dev.* (Ireland), 1984, 25/1-2 (189-204), Department of Pathology, University of Manchester, Manchester M13 9PT United Kingdom

Physical basis of cognitive alterations in Alzheimer's disease: synapse loss is the major correlate of cognitive impairment. Terry RD; Masliah E; Salmon DP; Butters N; DeTeresa R; Hill R; Hansen LA; Katzman R, *Ann Neurol* Oct 1991, 30 (4) p572-80, Department of Neurosciences, University of California-San Diego, La Jolla 92093-0624

Synapse loss in frontal cortex biopsies in Alzheimer's disease: correlation with cognitive severity. DeKosky ST; Scheff SW, *Ann Neurol* May 1990, 27 (5) p457-64, Department of Neurology, Lexington Veterans Administration, Medical Center, KY

Neurofibrillary tangles but not senile plaques parallel duration and severity of Alzheimer's disease. Arriagada PV; Growdon JH; Hedley-Whyte ET; Hyman BT, *Neurology* Mar 1992, 42 (3 Pt 1) p631-9, Department of Pathology, Massachusetts General Hospital, Harvard Medical School, Boston 02114

Biochemical and anatomical redistribution of tau protein in Alzheimer's disease. Mukaetova-Ladinska EB; Harrington CR; Roth M; Wischik CM, Cambridge Brain Bank Laboratory, University of Cambridge Department of Psychiatry, England, *Am J Pathol* Aug 1993, 143 (2) p565-78

Functional studies of Alzheimer's disease tau protein. Lu Q; Wood JG, Department of Anatomy and Cell Biology, Emory University School of Medicine, Atlanta, Georgia 30322, *J Neurosci* Feb 1993, 13 (2) p508-15

Tau protein and the neurofibrillary pathology of Alzheimer's disease. Goedert M, Medical Research Council, Laboratory of Molecular Biology, Cambridge, UK, *Trends Neurosci* (England) Nov 1993, 16 (11) p460-5

Dorothy Russell Memorial Lecture. The molecular pathology of Alzheimer's disease: are we any closer to understanding the neurodegenerative process? Smith C; Anderton BH, Department of Neuroscience, Institute of Psychiatry, London, UK, *Neuropathol Appl Neurobiol* (England) Aug 1994, 20 (4) p322-38

Gene dose of apolipoprotein E type 4 allele and the risk of Alzheimer's disease in late onset families. Corder EH; Saunders AM; Strittmatter WJ; Schmechel DE; Gaskell PC; Small, GW; Roses AD; Haines JL; Pericak-Vance MA, Department of Medicine, Joseph and Kathleen Bryan Alzheimer's Disease Research Center, Duke University Medical Center, Durham, NC 27710, *Science* Aug 13 1993, 261 (5123) p921-3

Immunodetection of the amyloid P component in Alzheimer's disease. Duong T.; Pommier E.C.; Scheibel A.B., Department of Anatomy and Cell Biology, UCLA Medical School, Los Angeles, CA 90024-1763 USA, *Acta Neuropathol.* (Germany, Federal Republic of), 1989, 78/4 (429-437)

Blood brain barrier dysfunction in acute lead encephalopathy: a reappraisal. Bouldin T.W.; Mushak P.; O'Tuama L.A.; Krigman M.R., Dept. Pathol., Univ. North Carolina Sch. Med., Chapel Hill, N.C. 27514 USA, *Environm.Hlth Perspect.*, 1975, Vol.12 (81-88)

Can blood-brain barrier play a role in the development of cerebral amyloidosis and Alzheimer's disease pathology [editorial; comment]. Zlokovic B, *Neurobiol Dis* 1997, 4 (1) p23-6

Development and in vitro characterization of a cationized monoclonal antibody against beta A4 protein: a potential probe for Alzheimer's disease. Bickel U; Lee VM; Trojanowski JQ; Pardridge WM, Department of Medicine, UCLA School of Medicine 90024, *Bioconjug Chem* Mar-Apr 1994, 5 (2) p119-25

Beta-Amyloid precursor protein gene in squirrel monkeys with cerebral amyloid angiopathy. Levy E; Amorim A; Frangione B; Walker LC, Department of Pharmacology, New York University Medical Center, NY 10016, USA, *Neurobiol Aging* Sep-Oct 1995, 16 (5) p805-8

Therapeutic approaches related to amyloid-beta peptide and Alzheimer's disease. Schenk DB; Rydel RE; May P; Little S; Panetta J; Lieberburg I; Sinha S, Athena Neurosciences, Inc., South San Francisco, California 94080, USA, *J Med Chem* Oct 13 1995, 38 (21) p4141-54

Molecular mechanisms of Alzheimer's disease. Simons M., Monchgasse 9, D-69117 Heidelberg Germany, *Fortschritte der Medizin* (Germany), 1995, 113/31 (31-32)

Neuropathy in Waldenstrom's macroglobulinemia. Coimbra J.; Costa A.P.; Pita F.; Rosado P.; Bigotte De Almeida L., Servico de Neurologia, Hospital Garcia de Orta, Almada Portugal, *Acta Medica Portuguesa* (Portugal), 1995, 8/4 (253-257)

Advanced glycation endproducts in ageing and Alzheimer's disease. Munch G.; Thome J.; Foley P.; Schinzel R.; Riederer P., Germany, *Brain Research Reviews* (Netherlands), 1997, 23/1-2 (134-143)

Changes in biomechanical properties, composition of collagen and elastin, and advanced glycation endproducts of the rat aorta in relation to age. Bruel A.; Oxlund H., A. Bruel, Dept. of Connective Tissue Biology, Institute of Anatomy, University of Aarhus, DK-8000 Aarhus C Denmark, *Atherosclerosis* (Ireland), 1996, 127/2 (155-165)

Physiological production of the beta-amyloid protein and the mechanism of Alzheimer's disease. Selkoe D.J., Center for Neurological Diseases, Harvard Medical School, Brigham and Women's Hospital, Boston, MA 02115 USA, *Trends Neurosci.* (UK), 1993, 16/10 (403-409)

Aluminum, iron, and zinc ions promote aggregation of physiological concentrations of beta-amyloid peptide. Mantyh P.W.; Ghilardi J.R.; Rogers S.; DeMaster E.; Allen C.J.; Stimson E.R.; Maggio J.E., Molecular Neurobiology Laboratory, Veterans Administration Medical Ctr., Minneapolis, MN 55417 USA, *J. Neurochem.*, 1993, 61/3 (1171-1174)

Acetyl-L-carnitine: A drug able to slow the progress of Alzheimer's disease? Carta A.; Calvani M., Department of Neurological Research, Sigma-Tau, Pomezia, Rome 00040 Italy, *Ann. New York Acad. Sci.*, 1991, 640/- (228-232)

Clinical and neurochemical effects of acetyl-*L*-carnitine in Alzheimer's disease. Pettegrew J.W.; Klunk W.E.; Panchalingam K.; Kanfer J.N.; McClure R.J., University of Pittsburgh, Western Psychiatric Institute/Clinic, A710 Crabtree Hall/GSPH, 130 DeSoto Street, Pittsburgh, PA 15261 USA, *Neurobiol. Aging*, 1995, 16/1 (1-4)

Vitamin E protects nerve cells from amyloid beta protein toxicity. Behl C; Davis J; Cole GM; Schubert D, Salk Institute for Biological Studies, San Diego, CA 92186-5800, *Biochem Biophys Res Commun* Jul 31 1992, 186 (2) p944-50

The lipid peroxidation product, 4-hydroxy-2-trans-nonenal, alters the conformation of cortical synaptosomal membrane proteins. Subramaniam R; Roediger F; Jordan B; Mattson MP; Keller JN; Waeg G; Butterfield DA, Department of Chemistry, Center of Membrane Science, University of Kentucky, Lexington 40506, U.S.A., *J Neurochem* Sep 1997, 69 (3) p1161-9

Deleterious network: a testable pathogenetic concept of Alzheimer's disease. Department of Physiology, School of Medicine, University of New Mexico, Albuquerque, USA. *Gerontology* (Switzerland) 1997, 43 (4) p242-53

Oxidative stress hypothesis in Alzheimer's disease. Markesbery WR, Sanders-Brown Center on Aging, Lexington, KY 40536-0230, USA, *Free Radic Biol Med* 1997, 23 (1) p134-47

Amyloid precursor protein, copper and Alzheimer's disease. ZMBH Center for Molecular Biology, University of Heidelberg, Germany, *Biomed Pharmacother* (France) 1997, 51 (3) p105-11

Oxidative-stress associated parameters (lactoferrin, superoxide dismutases) in serum of patients with Alzheimer's disease. Thome J; Gsell W; Rosler M; Kornhuber J; Frolich L; Hashimoto E; Zielke B; Wiesbeck GA; Riederer P, Department of Psychiatry, University of Wurzburg, Germany, *Life Sci* (England) 1997, 60 (1) p13-9

Methodologic aspects of a population pharmacodynamic model for cognitive effects in Alzheimer patients treated with tacrine. Holford NH; Peace KE, Department of Pharmacology and Clinical Pharmacology, University of Auckland, New Zealand, *Proc Natl Acad Sci U S A* Dec 1 1992, 89 (23) p11466-70

Implications of the study population in the early evaluation of anticholinesterase inhibitors for Alzheimer's disease. Cutler NR; Sramek JJ; Murphy MF; Nash RJ, California Clinical Trials, Beverly Hills 90211, *Ann Pharmacother* Sep 1992, 26 (9) p1118-22

A double-blind, placebo-controlled multicenter study of tacrine for Alzheimer's disease. The Tacrine Collaborative Study Group [see comments]. Davis KL; Thal LJ; Gamzu ER; Davis CS; Woolson RF; Gracon SI; Drachman DA; Schneider LS; Whitehouse PJ; Hoover TM; et al, Mount Sinai Medical Center, New York, NY 10029-6574, *N Engl J Med* Oct 29 1992, 327 (18) p1253-9

A controlled trial of tacrine in Alzheimer's disease. The Tacrine Study Group [see comments]. Farlow M; Gracon SI; Hershey LA; Lewis KW; Sadowsky CH; Dolan-Ureno J, Center for Alzheimer's Disease and Related Disorders, Indiana University Medical Center, Indianapolis, *Jama* Nov 11 1992, 268 (18) p2523-9

Effect of oestrogen during menopause on risk and age at onset of Alzheimer's disease [see comments]. Tang MX; Jacobs D; Stern Y; Marder K; Schofield P; Gurland B; Andrews H; Mayeux R, Gertrude H Serglevsky Center, Columbia University, New York, NY 10032, USA, *Lancet* (England) Aug 17 1996, 348 (9025) p429-32

Use of phosphatidylserine in Alzheimer's disease. Amaducci L.; Crook T.H.; Lippi A.; Bracco L.; Baldereschi M.; Latorraca S.; Piersanti P.; Tesco G.; Sorbi S., Dept. of Neurologic/Psychiatric Sci., S.M.I.D. Center, University of Florence, 50123 Florence Italy, *Ann. New York Acad. Sci.*, 1991, 640/- (245-249)

Abnormalities of energy metabolism in Alzheimer's disease studied with PET. Heiss W.-D.; Szelies B.; Kessler J.; Herholz K., Max-Planck-Inst. Neurol. Forschung, Universitatsklinik für Neurologie, Joseph-Stelzmann-Str. 9, D-5000 Koln 41 Germany, *Ann. New York Acad. Sci.*, 1991, 640/- (65-71)

Contrasting patterns of protein phosphorylation in human normal and Alzheimer brain: Focus on protein kinase C and protein F1/GAP-43. Florez J.C.; Nelson R.B.; Routtenberg A., Department of Neurobiology and Physiology, Northwestern University, Evanston, IL 60208 USA, *Exp. Neurol.*, 1991, 112/3 (264-272)

Drug treatment of Alzheimer's disease. Cooper J.K., University of California Davis Medical Center, 2221 Stockton Blvd, Sacramento, CA 95817 USA, *Arch. Intern. Med.*, 1991, 151/2 (245-249)

Clinical trial of indomethacin in Alzheimer's disease. Rogers J.; Kirby L.C.; Hempelman S.R.; Berry D.L.; McGeer P.L.; Kaszniak A.W.; Zalinski J.; Cofield M.; Mansukhani L.; Willson P.; Kogan F., Sun Health Research Institute, P.O. Box 1278, Sun City, AZ 85372 USA, *Neurology*, 1993, 43/8 (1609-1611)

Inflammatory mechanisms in Alzheimer's disease. Eikelenboom P.; Zhan S.-S.; Van Gool W.A.; Allsop D., Department of Psychiatry, PCA Valeriuskliniek, Valeriusplein 9, 1075 BG Amsterdam Netherlands, *Trends Pharmacol. Sci.* (UK), 1994, 15/12 (447-450)

Inflammatory mechanisms in Alzheimer's disease: Implications for therapy. Aisen P.S.; Davis K.L., Department of Psychiatry, Mount Sinai School of Medicine, Box 1230, One Gustave L. Levy Place, New York, NY 10029 USA, *Am. J. Psychiatry,* 1994, 151/8 (1105-1113)

Brain interleukin-1beta in Alzheimer's disease and vascular dementia. Cacabelos R.; Alvarez X.A.; Fernandez-Novoa L.; Franco A.; Mangues R.; Pellicer A.; Nishimura T., Institute for CNS Disorders, P.O. Box 733, 15080 La Coruna Spain, *Methods Find. Exp. Clin. Pharmacol.* (Spain), 1994, 16/2 (141-151)

The role of estrogen in the treatment of Alzheimer's disease. *Neurology,* 1997, 48/5 Suppl. 7 (S36-S41)

Pharmacotherapy in Alzheimer's dementia: Treatment of cognitive symptoms. Results of new studies. *Fortschritte der Neurologie Psychiatrie* (Germany), 1997, 65/3 (108-121)

Therapy of dementia—Neurologic and psychiatric aspects. *Wiener Medizinische Wochenschrift* (Austria), 1996, 146/21-22 (546-548)

The clinical potential of Deprenyl in neurologic and psychiatric disorders. (Austria), 1996, -/48 (85-93)

Modulation of gene expression rather than monoamine oxidase inhibition: (-)-Deprenyl-related compounds in controlling neurodegeneration. *Neurology,* 1996, 47/6 Suppl. 3 (S171-S183)

Neuroendocrine aspects of the menopause and hormone replacement therapy. *Journal of Cardiovascular Pharmacology,* 1996, 28/Suppl. 5

A 1-year multicenter placebo-controlled study of acetyl-L-carnitine in patients with Alzheimer's disease. *Neurology,* 1996, 47/3 (705-711)

Monoamine oxidase B inhibitors. Current status and future potential. *CNS Drugs* (New Zealand), 1996, 6/3 (217-236)

Drug treatment of Alzheimer's disease. Effects on caregiver burden and patient quality of life. *Drugs Aging* (New Zealand) Jan 1996, 8 (1) p47-55

Orally active NGF synthesis stimulators: potential therapeutic agents in Alzheimer's disease. *Behav Brain Res* (Netherlands) Feb 1997, 83 (1-2) p117-22

Calcium homeostasis and reactive oxygen species production in cells transformed by mitochondria from individuals with sporadic Alzheimer's disease. *J Neurosci* Jun 15 1997, 17 (12) p4612-22

The search for disease-modifying treatment for Alzheimer's disease. *Neurology* May 1997, 48 (5 Suppl 6) pS35-41

Molecular basis of Alzheimer's disease. *Am J Health Syst Pharm* Jul 1 1996, 53 (13) p1545-57; quiz 1603-4

Functional studies of new drugs for the treatment of Alzheimer's disease. *Acta Neurol Scand Suppl* (Denmark) 1996, 165 p137-44

Treatment of Alzheimer's disease: future directions. *Acta Neurol Scand Suppl* (Denmark) 1996, 165 p128-36

Acetyl-L-carnitine restores choline acetyltransferase activity in the hippocampus of rats with partial unilateral fimbria-fornix transection. *Int J Dev Neurosci* (England) Feb 1995, 13 (1) p13-9

Acetyl-L-carnitine arginyl amide (ST857) increases calcium channel density in rat pheochromocytoma (PC12) cells. *J Neurosci Res* Feb 15 1995, 40 (3) p371-8

Neurite outgrowth in PC12 cells stimulated by acetyl-L-carnitine arginine amide *Neurochem Res* Jan 1995, 20 (1) p1-9

Effects of acetyl-L-carnitine treatment and stress exposure on the nerve growth factor receptor (p75NGFR) mRNA level in the central nervous system of aged rats. *Prog Neuropsychopharmacol Biol Psychiatry* (England) Jan 1995, 19 (1) p117-33

Acetyl-L-carnitine treatment increases nerve growth factor levels and choline acetyltransferase activity in the central nervous system of aged rats. *Exp Gerontol* (England) Jan-Feb 1994, 29 (1) p55-66

Acetyl-L-carnitine affects aged brain receptorial system in rodents. *Life Sci* (England) 1994, 54 (17) p1205-14

Stimulation of nerve growth factor receptors in PC12 by acetyl-L-carnitine. *Biochem Pharmacol* (England) Aug 4 1992, 44 (3) p577-85

Culture of dorsal root ganglion neurons from aged rats: effects of acetyl-L-carnitine and NGF. *Int J Dev Neurosci* (England) Aug 1992, 10 (4) p321-9

Acetyl-L-carnitine enhances the response of PC12 cells to nerve growth factor. *Brain Res Dev Brain Res* (Netherlands) Apr 24 1991, 59 (2) p221-30

Effect of acetyl-L-carnitine on forebrain cholinergic neurons of developing rats. *Int J Dev Neurosci* (England) 1991, 9 (1) p39-46

Nerve growth factor binding in aged rat central nervous system: effect of acetyl-*L*-carnitine. *J Neurosci Res* Aug 1988, 20 (4) p491-6

Nootropics: preclinical results in the light of clinical effects; comparison with tacrine. *Crit Rev Neurobiol* 1996, 10 (3-4) p357-70

[Neuroprotective therapy of Alzheimer's disease?]. *Dtsch Med Wochenschr* (Germany) Nov 29 1996, 121 (48) p1515

Prescribing practice with cognition enhancers in outpatient care: are there differences regarding type of dementia?—Results of a representative survey in lower Saxony, Germany. *Pharmacopsychiatry* (Germany) Jul 1996, 29 (4) p150-5

Coenzyme nicotinamide adenine dinucleotide: new therapeutic approach for improving dementia of the Alzheimer type. *Ann Clin Lab Sci* Jan-Feb 1996, 26 (1) p1-9

Deprenyl reduces neuronal apoptosis and facilitates neuronal outgrowth by altering protein synthesis without inhibiting monoamine oxidase. *J Neural Transm Suppl* (Austria) 1996, 48 p45-59

Protection of the aged substantia nigra of the rat against oxidative damage by (-)-deprenyl. *Br J Pharmacol* (England) Apr 1996, 117 (8) p1756-60

Different mechanisms regulate phosphatidylserine synthesis in rat cerebral cortex. *Mol Cell Biochem* (Netherlands) Mar 1997, 168 (1-2) p41-9

Relationships between phosphatidylcholine, phosphatidylethanolamine, and sphingomyelin metabolism in cultured oligodendrocytes. *J Neurochem* Mar 1997, 68 (3) p1252-60

Effect of phosphatidylserine on the binding properties of glutamate receptors in brain sections from adult and neonatal rats. *Brain Res* (Netherlands) Nov 18 1996, 740 (1-2) p337-45

Pharmacological effects of phosphatidylserine enzymatically synthesized from soybean lecithin on brain functions in rodents. *J Nutr Sci Vitaminol* (Tokyo) (Japan) Feb 1996, 42 (1) p47-54

Aluminum facilitation of iron-mediated lipid peroxidation is dependent on substrate, pH and aluminum and iron concentrations. *Arch Biochem Biophys* Mar 15 1996, 327 (2) p222-6

Influence of vitamin B12 on brain methionine adenosyltransferase activity in senile dementia of the Alzheimer's type. *J Neural Transm Gen Sect* (Austria) 1996, 103 (7) p861-72

Dementia and subnormal levels of vitamin B_{12}: effects of replacement therapy on dementia. *J Neurol* (Germany) Jul 1996, 243 (7) p522-9

Is metabolic evidence for vitamin B-12 and folate deficiency more frequent in elderly patients with Alzheimer's disease? *J Gerontol A Biol Sci Med Sci* Mar 1997, 52 (2) pM76-9

Effects of hormone replacement therapy on serum amyloid P component in postmenopausal women. *Maturitas* (Ireland) Mar 1997, 26 (2) p113-9

Dehydroepiandrosterone and diseases of aging. *Drugs Aging* (New Zealand) Oct 1996, 9 (4) p274-91

Dehydroepiandrosterone (DHEA) increases production and release of Alzheimer's amyloid precursor protein. *Life Sci* (England) 1996, 59 (19) p1651-7

[Change of serum amyloid P component concentrations in women]. *Nippon Sanka Fujinka Gakkai Zasshi* (Japan) Jul 1996, 48 (7) p481-7

Serum dehydroepiandrosterone (DHEA) and DHEA-sulfate (DHEA-S) in Alzheimer's disease and in cerebrovascular dementia. *Endocr J* (Japan) Feb 1996, 43 (1) p119-23

Melatonin prevents death of neuroblastoma cells exposed to the Alzheimer amyloid peptide. *J Neurosci* Mar 1 1997, 17 (5) p1683-90

[Melatonin. Hormone or wonder drug?]. *Med Monatsschr Pharm* (Germany) Mar 1996, 19 (3) p69-75

Daily rhythm of serum melatonin in patients with dementia of the degenerate type. *Brain Res* (Netherlands) Apr 22 1996, 717 (1-2) p154-9

Alzheimer's disease: new horizons in diagnosis and treatment. *Iowa Med* May-Jun 1997, 87 (5) p199-201

Cognitive enhancers in theory and practice: studies of the cholinergic hypothesis of cognitive deficits in Alzheimer's disease. *Behav Brain Res* (Netherlands) Feb 1997, 83 (1-2) p15-23

The presence of leuko-araiosis in patients with Alzheimer's disease predicts poor tolerance to tacrine, but does not discriminate responders from non-responders. *Age Ageing* (England) Jan 1997, 26 (1) p25-9

Characteristics of the binding of tacrine to acidic phospholipids. *Biophys J* May 1996, 70 (5) p2185-2194

A risk-benefit assessment of tacrine in the treatment of Alzheimer's disease. *Drug Saf* (New Zealand) Jan 1997, 16 (1) p66-77

[A clinic for the study of dementia—110 consecutive patients]. *Ugeskr Laeger* (Denmark) Feb 24 1997, 159 (9) p1246-51

Developing treatment guidelines for Alzheimer's disease and other dementias. *J Clin Psychiatry* 1996, 57 Suppl 14 p37-8

New therapeutic approaches to Alzheimer's disease. *J Clin Psychiatry* 1996, 57 Suppl 14 p30-6

Novel anticholinesterase and antiamnesic activities of dehydroevodiamine, a constituent of Evodia rutaecarpa. *Planta Med* (Germany) Oct 1996, 62 (5) p405-9

An enriched-population, double-blind, placebo-controlled, crossover study of tacrine and lecithin in Alzheimer's disease. The Tacrine 970-6 Study Group. *Dementia* (Switzerland) Sep-Oct 1996, 7 (5) p260-6

Amnesia induced in mice by centrally administered beta-amyloid peptides involves cholinergic dysfunction. *Brain Res* (Netherlands) Jan 15 1996, 706 (2) p181-93

Evaluation of tacrine hydrochloride (Cognex) in two parallel-group studies. *Acta Neurol Scand Suppl* (Denmark) 1996, 165 p114-22

[Should Alzheimer disease be treated with tacrine? Review of the literature]. *Tidsskr Nor Laegeforen* (Norway) Sep 30 1996, 116 (23) p2791-4

Maximizing function in Alzheimer's disease: what role for tacrine? *Am Fam Physician* Aug 1996, 54 (2) p645-52

Effects of estrogen replacement therapy on response to tacrine in patients with Alzheimer's disease. *Neurology* Jun 1996, 46 (6) p1580-4

Determination of aluminium in samples from bone and liver of elderly Norwegians. *J Trace Elem Med Biol* (Germany) Apr 1996, 10 (1) p6-11

[Therapy approaches in cerebral cognitive deficits—neuropsychiatric aspects]. *Wien Med Wochenschr* (Austria) 1996, 146 (21-22) p546-8

[Effectiveness of brief infusions with Ginkgo biloba Special Extract EGb 761 in dementia of the vascular and Alzheimer type]. *Z Gerontol Geriatr* (Germany) Jul-Aug 1996, 29 (4) p302-9

Proof of efficacy of the ginkgo biloba special extract EGb 761 in outpatients suffering from mild to moderate primary degenerative dementia of the Alzheimer type or multi-infarct dementia. *Pharmacopsychiatry* (Germany) Mar 1996, 29 (2) p47-56

Isolated cerebral and cerebellar mitochondria produce free radicals when exposed to elevated CA2+ and Na+: implications for neurodegeneration. *J Neurochem* Aug 1994, 63 (2)

Isoprenoids (CoQ_{10}) in aging and neurodegeneration. *Neurochem Int* (England) Jul 1994, 25 (1) p35-8

Therapy for Alzheimer's disease. Symptomatic or neuroprotective? *Mol Neurobiol* Aug-Dec 1994, 9 (1-3)

The mystery of Alzheimer's disease and its prevention by melatonin. *Med Hypotheses* (England) Oct 1995, 45 (4) p339-40

Chrono-neuroendocrinological aspects of physiological aging and senile dementia. *Chronobiologia* (Italy) Jan-Jun 1994, 21 (1-2) p121-6

Overview of clinical trials of hydergine in dementia. *Arch. Neurol.*, 1994, 51/8 (787-798)

Combined cholinergic precursor treatment and dihydroergotoxine mesylate in Alzheimer's disease. *Ircs Med. Sci.* (England), 1983, 11/12 (1048-1049)

Hydergine treatment and brain functioning (CNV rebound) in Alzheimer's patients: Preliminary findings. *Psychopharmacol. Bull.* (Usa), 1981, 17/3 (202-206)

Single-case study of clinical response to high-dose ergot alkaloid treatment for dementia. Preliminary report. *Gerontology* (Switzerland), 1981, 27/1-2 (76-78)

Analyses of energy metabolism and mitochondrial genome in post-mortem brain from patients with Alzheimer's disease. *J. Neurol.* (Germany), 1993, 240/6 (377-380)

Muscle biopsy in Alzheimer's disease: Morphological and biochemical findings. *Clin. Neuropathol.* (Germany), 1991, 10/4 (171-176)

Growth hormone secretion in Alzheimer's disease: Studies with growth hormone-releasing hormone alone and combined with pyridostigmine or arginine. *Dementia* (Switzerland), 1993, 4/6 (315-320)

Selegiline: A review of its clinical efficacy in Parkinson's disease and its clinical potential in Alzheimer's disease. *CNS Drugs* (New Zealand), 1995, 4/3 (230-246)

Age-related memory decline and longevity under treatment with selegiline. *Life Sci.*, 1994, 55/25-26

Long-term effects of phosphatidylserine, pyritinol, and cognitive training in Alzheimer's disease. A neuropsychological, EEG, and PET investigation. *Dementia* (Switzerland), 1994, 5/2 (88-98)

Abnormalities of energy metabolism in Alzheimer's disease studied with PET. *Ann. New York Acad. Sci.*, 1991, 640/- (65-71)

Effects of phosphatidylserine in Alzheimer's disease. *Usa Psychopharmacol. Bull.*, 1992, 28/1 (61-66)

Effect of phosphatidylserine on cerebral glucose metabolism in Alzheimer's disease. *Dementia* (Switzerland), 1990, (197-201)

Decreased methionine adenosyltransferase activity in erythrocytes of patients with dementia disorders. *Sweden European Neuropsychopharmacology* (Netherlands), 1995, 5/2 (107-114)

Folate, vitamin B12 and cognitive impairment in patients with Alzheimer's disease. *Acta Psychiatr. Scand.* (Denmark), 1992, 86/4 (301-305)

Alzheimer's Disease: A 'cobalaminergic' hypothesis. *Med. Hypotheses* (UK), 1992, 37/3 (161-165)

Vitamin B12 and folate concentrations in serum and cerebrospinal fluid of neurological patients with special reference to multiple sclerosis and dementia. *J. Neurol. Neurosurg. Psychiatry* (UK), 1990, 53/11 (951-954)

Vitamin B12 levels in serum and cerebrospinal fluid of people with Alzheimer's disease. *Acta Psychiatr. Scand.* (Denmark), 1990, 82/4 (327-329)

Alzheimers disease/alcohol dementia: Association with zinc deficiency and cerebral vitamin B12 deficiency. *J. Orthomol. Psychiatry* (Canada), 1984, 13/2 (97-104)

Carnitine and acetyl-L-carnitine content of human hippocampus and erythrocytes in Alzheimer's disease. *Journal of Nutritional and Environmental Medicine* (UK), 1995, 5/1 (35-39)

Advances in the pharmacotherapy of Alzheimer's disease. *Eur. Arch. Psychiatry Clin. Neurosci.* (Germany), 1994, 244/5 (261-271)

Clinical and neurochemical effects of acetyl-L-carnitine in Alzheimer's disease. *Neurobiol. Aging*, 1995, 16/1 (1-4)

Neuroprotective activity of acetyl-L-carnitine: Studies in vitro. *Neurosci. Res.*, 1994, 37/1 (92-96)

Acetyl-L-carnitine and Alzheimer's disease: Pharmacological beyond the cholinergic sphere. *Ann. New York Acad. Sci.*, 1993, 695/- (324-326)

Acetyl-L-carnitine: A drug able to slow the progress of Alzheimer's disease? *Ann. New York Acad. Sci.*, 1991, 640/- (228-232)

Pharmacokinetics of IV and oral acetyl-L-carnitine in a multiple dose regimen in patients with senile dementia of Alzheimer Type. *Eur. J. Clin. Pharmacol.* (Germany), 1992, 42/1 (89-93)

Double-blind, placebo-controlled study of acetyl-l-carnitine in patients with Alzheimer's disease. *Curr. Med. Res. Opin.* (UK), 1989, 11/10 (638-647)

The pharmacotherapy of Alzheimer's disease based on the cholinergic hypothesis: An update. *Neurodegeneration* (UK),1995, 4/4 (349-356)

Aniracetam: A new nootropic drug with excellent tolerance for mild to moderate cognitive impairment in elderly people. *Drugs Today* (Spain), 1994, 30/1 (9-24)

Auditory and visual event-related potentials in patients suffering from Alzheimer's dementia and multiinfarct dementia, before and after treatment with piracetam. *Funct. Neurol.* (Italy), 1993, 8/5 (335-345)

Isolated cerebral and cerebellar mitochondria produce free radicals when exposed to elevated CA2+ and Na+: implications for neurodegeneration. *J Neurochem* Aug 1994, 63 (2)

Isoprenoids (CoQ_{10}) in aging and neurodegeneration. *Neurochem Int* (England) Jul 1994, 25 (1) p35-8

Therapy for Alzheimer's disease. Symptomatic or neuroprotective? *Mol Neurobiol* Aug-Dec 1994, 9 (1-3)

The mystery of Alzheimer's disease and its prevention by melatonin. *Med Hypotheses* (England) Oct 1995, 45 (4) p339-40

Advances in the pharmacotherapy of Alzheimer's disease. *Eur Arch Psychiatry Clin Neurosci* (Germany) 1994, 244 (5)

Chrono-neuroendocrinological aspects of physiological aging and senile dementia. *Chronobiologia* (Italy) Jan-Jun 1994, 21 (1-2) p121-6

Overview of clinical trials of hydergine in dementia. *Arch. Neurol.*, 1994, 51/8 (787 798)

Combined cholinergic precursor treatment and dihydroergotoxine mesylate in Alzheimer's disease. *Ircs Med. Sci.* (England), 1983, 11/12 (1048-1049)

Hydergine treatment and brain functioning (CNV rebound) in Alzheimer's patients: Preliminary findings. *Psychopharmacol. Bull.*, 1981, 17/3 (202-206)

Single-case study of clinical response to high-dose ergot alkaloid treatment for dementia. Preliminary report. *Gerontology* (Switzerland), 1981, 27/1-2 (76-78)

Isoprenoids (coQ10) in aging and neurodegeneration. *Neurochem. Int.* (UK), 1994, 25/1 (35-38)

Analyses of energy metabolism and mitochondrial genome in post-mortem brain from patients with Alzheimer's disease. *J. Neurol.* (Germany), 1993, 240/6 (377-380)

Muscle biopsy in Alzheimer's disease: Morphological and biochemical findings. *Clin. Neuropathol.* (Germany), 1991, 10/4 (171-176)

Growth hormone secretion in Alzheimer's disease: Studies with growth hormone-releasing hormone alone and combined with pyridostigmine or arginine. *Dementia* (Switzerland), 1993, 4/6 (315-320)

Selegiline: A review of its clinical efficacy in Parkinson's disease and its clinical potential in Alzheimer's disease. *CNS Drugs* (New Zealand), 1995, 4/3 (230-246)

Age-related memory decline and longevity under treatment with selegiline. *Life Sci.*, 1994, 55/25-26

Long-term effects of phosphatidylserine, pyritinol, and cognitive training in Alzheimer's disease. A neuropsychological, EEG, and PET investigation. *Dementia* (Switzerland), 1994, 5/2 (88-98)

Abnormalities of energy metabolism in Alzheimer's disease studied with PET. *Ann. New York Acad. Sci.,* 1991, 640/- (65-71)

Effects of phosphatidylserine in Alzheimer's disease. *Usa Psychopharmacol. Bull.*, 1992, 28/1 (61-66)

Effect of phosphatidylserine on cerebral glucose metabolism in Alzheimer's disease. *Dementia* (Switzerland), 1990, (197-201)

Decreased methionine adenosyltransferase activity in erythrocytes of patients with dementia disorders. *Sweden European Neuropsychopharmacology* (Netherlands), 1995, 5/2 (107-114)

Folate, vitamin B12 and cognitive impairment in patients with Alzheimer's disease. *Acta Psychiatr. Scand.* (Denmark), 1992, 86/4 (301-305)

Alzheimer's Disease: A 'cobalaminergic' hypothesis. *Med. Hypotheses* (UK), 1992, 37/3 (161-165)

Vitamin B12 and folate concentrations in serum and cerebrospinal fluid of neurological patients with special reference to multiple sclerosis and dementia. *J. Neurol. Neurosurg. Psychiatry* (UK), 1990, 53/11 (951-954)

Vitamin B12 levels in serum and cerebrospinal fluid of people with Alzheimer's disease. *Acta Psychiatr. Scand.* (Denmark), 1990, 82/4 (327-329)

Alzheimers disease/alcohol dementia: Association with zinc deficiency and cerebral vitamin B12 deficiency. *J. Orthomol. Psychiatry* (Canada), 1984, 13/2 (97-104)

Carnitine and acetyl-L-carnitine content of human hippocampus and erythrocytes in Alzheimer's disease. *Journal of Nutritional and Environmental Medicine* (UK), 1995, 5/1 (35-39)

Advances in the pharmacotherapy of Alzheimer's disease. *Eur. Arch. Psychiatry Clin. Neurosci.* (Germany), 1994, 244/5 (261-271)

Clinical and neurochemical effects of acetyl-L-carnitine in Alzheimer's disease. *Neurobiol. Aging*, 1995, 16/1 (1-4)

Neuroprotective activity of acetyl-L-carnitine: Studies in vitro. *Neurosci. Res.*, 1994, 37/1 (92-96)

Acetyl-L-carnitine and Alzheimer's disease: Pharmacological beyond the cholinergic sphere. *Ann. New York Acad. Sci.*, 1993, 695/- (324-326)

Acetyl-L-carnitine: A drug able to slow the progress of Alzheimer's disease? *Ann. New York Acad. Sci.*, 1991, 640/- (228-232)

Pharmacokinetics of IV and oral acetyl-L-carnitine in a multiple dose regimen in patients with senile dementia of Alzheimer Type. *Eur. J. Clin. Pharmacol.* (Germany), 1992, 42/1 (89-93)

Double-blind, placebo-controlled study of acetyl-L-carnitine in patients with Alzheimer's disease. *Curr. Med. Res. Opin.* (UK), 1989, 11/10 (638-647)

The pharmacotherapy of Alzheimer's disease based on the cholinergic hypothesis: An update. *Neurodegeneration* (UK),1995, 4/4 (349-356)

Aniracetam: A new nootropic drug with excellent tolerance for mild to moderate cognitive impairment in elderly people. *Drugs Today* (Spain), 1994, 30/1 (9-24)

Auditory and visual event-related potentials in patients suffering from Alzheimer's dementia and multiinfarct dementia, before and after treatment with piracetam. *Funct. Neurol.* (Italy), 1993, 8/5 (335-345)

Amnesia

[Antagonism of piracetam with proline in relation to amnestic effects]. *Biull Eksp Biol Med* (USSR) Mar 1985, 99 (3) p311-4

[Effect of mental stimulants on electroconvulsive shock-induced retrograde amnesia]. *Pharmazie* (Germany, East) Dec 1983, 38 (12) p869-71

Hypoxia-induced amnesia in one-trial learning and pharmacological protection by piracetam. *Psychopharmacologia* (Germany, West) 1972, 25 (1) p32-40

Pre-clinical evaluation of cognition enhancing drugs. *Prog Neuropsychopharmacol Biol Psychiatry* (England) 1989, 13 Suppl pS99-115

Nootropic drugs and brain cholinergic mechanisms. *Prog Neuropsychopharmacol Biol Psychiatry* (England) 1989, 13 Suppl pS77-88

Specificity of piracetam's anti-amnesic activity in three models of amnesia in the mouse. *Pharmacol Biochem Behav* Mar 1988, 29 (3) p625-9

[Effects of piracetam during prolonged use in an experiment] Effekty piratsetama pri dlitel'nom primenenii v eksperimente. *Farmakol Toksikol* (USSR) Jul-Aug 1985, 48 (4) p42-6

Amyotrophic Lateral Sclerosis (ALS) (Lou Gehrig's Disease)

Hypovitaminosis D and decreased bone mineral density in amyotrophic lateral sclerosis. *Eur Neurol* (Switzerland) 1997, 37 (4) p225-9

Increased mitochondrial superoxide dismutase activity in Parkinson's disease but not amyotrophic lateral sclerosis motor cortex. *Neurosci Lett* (Ireland) Dec 19 1997, 239 (2-3) p105-8

A summary of mechanistic hypotheses of gabapentin pharmacology. *Epilepsy Research* (Netherlands), 1998, 29/3 (233-249)

Effects of branched-chain amino acids on plasma amino acids in amyotrophic lateral sclerosis. *Amino Acids* (Austria), 1996, 11/1 (37-42)

Superoxide dismutase 1: Identification of a novel mutation in a case of familial amyotrophic lateral sclerosis. *Human Genetics* (Germany), 1996, 98/1 (48-50)

Clinical characteristics of familial amyotrophic lateral sclerosis with Cu/Zn superoxide dismutase gene mutations. *Journal of the Neurological Sciences* (Netherlands), 1996, 136/1-2 (108-116)

SOD1 mutation is associated with accumulation of neurofilaments in amyotrophic lateral sclerosis. *Annals of Neurology,* 1996, 39/1 (128-131)

Potential treatment of amyotrophic lateral sclerosis with gabapentin: A hypothesis. *Annals of Pharmacotherapy,* 1995, 29/11 (1164-1167)

The imbalance of brain large-chain aminoacid availability in amyotrophic lateral sclerosis patients treated with high doses of branched-chain aminoacids. *Neurochemistry International* (UK), 1995, 27/6 (467-472)

Familial amyotrophic lateral sclerosis with a point mutation of SOD-1: Intrafamilial heterogeneity of disease duration associated with neurofrbrillary tangles. *Journal of Neurology Neurosurgery and Psychiatry* (UK), 1995, 59/3 (266-270)

Branched-chain amino acids and amyotrophic lateral sclerosis: A treatment failure? *Neurology,* 1993, 43/12 I (2466-2470)

Fasting plasma and CSF amino acid levels in amyotrophic lateral sclerosis: A subtype analysis. *Acta Neurol. Scand.* (Denmark), 1993, 88/1 (51-55)

Branched-chain amino acids in the treatment of amyotrophic latera sclerosis. *J. Neurol.* (Germany, Federal Republic of), 1989, 236/8 (445-447)

Pilot trial of branched-chain aminoacids in amyotrophic lateral sclerosis. *Lancet* (UK), 1988, 1/8593 (1015-1018)

Oxidative chemistry of nitric oxide: The roles of superoxide, peroxynitrite, and carbon dioxide. *Free Radical Biology and Medicine,* 1998, 25/4-5 (392-403)

Elevated 'hydroxyl radical' generation in vivo in an animal model of amyotrophic lateral sclerosis. *Journal of Neurochemistry,* 1998, 71/3 (1321-1324)

Oxidative damage to nucleic acids in motor neurons containing mercury. *Journal of the Neurological Sciences* (Netherlands), 1998, 159/2 (121-126)

Neural injury, repair, and adaptation in the GI tract I. New insights into neuronal injury: A cautionary tale. American Journal of Physiology—*Gastrointestinal and Liver Physiology,* 1998, 274/6 37-6 (G978-G983)

Chaperone-facilitated copper binding is a property common to several classes of familial amyotrophic lateral sclerosis-linked superoxide dismutase mutants. *Proceedings of the National Academy of Sciences of the United States of America,* 1998, 95/11 (6361-6366)

Reduced fertility in female mice lacking copper-zinc superoxide dismutase. *Journal of Biological Chemistry,* 1998, 273/13 (7765-7769)

A novel neurological phenotype in mice lacking mitochondrial manganese superoxide dismutase. *Nature Genetics,* 1998, 18/2 (159-163)

Aluminum potentiates glutamate-induced calcium accumulation and iron- induced oxygen free radical formation in primary neuronal cultures. *Molecular and Chemical Neuropathology,* 1997, 32/1-3 (41-57)

Zinc metabolism in the brain: Relevance to human neurodegenerative disorders. *Neurobiology of Disease,* 1997, 4/3-4 (137-169)

Reactive oxygen species and Alzheimer's disease. *Biochemical Pharmacology,* 1997, 54/5 (533-539)

A novel glycosylphosphatidylinositol-anchored form of ceruloplasmin is expressed by mammalian astrocytes. *Journal of Biological Chemistry,* 1997, 272/32 (20185-20190)

Bromocriptine prevents neuron damage following inhibition of superoxide dismutase in cultured ventral spinal cord neurons. *Neurological Research,* 1997, 19/4 (389-392)

High affinity glutamate transporters: Regulation of expression and activity. *Molecular Pharmacology,* 1997, 52/1 (6-15)

Effects of wild-type and mutated copper/zinc superoxide dismutase on neuronal survival and *L*-DOPA-induced toxicity in postnatal midbrain culture. *Journal of Neurochemistry,* 1997, 69/1 (21-33)

Transgenic animal models of familial amyotrophic lateral sclerosis. *Journal of Neurology, Supplement* (Germany), 1997, 244/2 (S15-S20)

Amyloid precursor protein, copper and Alzheimer's disease. *Biomedicine and Pharmacotherapy* (France), 1997, 51/3 (105-111)

Reactive oxygen species and the neurodegenerative disorders. *Annals of Clinical and Laboratory Science,* 1997, 27/1 (11-25)

Effect of ultrahigh-dose methylcobalamin on compound muscle action potentials in amyotrophic lateral sclerosis: a double-blind controlled study. *Muscle Nerve* Dec 1998, 21 (12) p1775-8

Pigment epithelium-derived factor (PEDF) protects motor neurons from chronic glutamate-mediated neurodegeneration. *J Neuropathol Exp Neurol* 1999 Jul;58(7):719-28

Neuroprotective effects of creatine in a transgenic animal model of amyotrophic lateral sclerosis., *Nat Med* 1999 Mar;5(3):347-50

Neuroprotective utility and neurotrophic action of neurturin in postnatal motor neurons: comparison with GDNF and persephin. *Mol Cell Neurosci* 1999 May;13(5):326-36

Genistein is neuroprotective in murine models of familial amyotrophic lateral sclerosis and stroke. *Biochem Biophys Res Commun* 1999 May 19;258(3):685-8

Coenzyme Q_{10} administration increases brain mitochondrial concentrations and exerts neuroprotective effects. *Proc Natl Acad Sci U S A* 1998 Jul 21;95(15):8892-7

Evaluation of antioxidants, protein, and lipid oxidation products in blood from sporadic amyotrophic lateral sclerosis patients. *Neurochem Res* 1997 Apr;22(4):535-9

Protective effects of a vitamin B12 analog, methylcobalamin, against glutamate cytotoxicity in cultured cortical neurons. *Eur J Pharmacol* 1993 Sep 7;241(1):1-6

Protective effects of methylcobalamin, a vitamin B12 analog, against glutamate-induced neurotoxicity in retinal cell culture. *Invest Ophthalmol Vis Sci* 1997 Apr;38(5):848-54

Vitamin B_{12} metabolism and massive-dose methyl vitamin B_{12} therapy in Japanese patients with multiple sclerosis. *Intern Med* 1994 Feb;33(2):82-6

Methylcobalamin (methyl-B12) promotes regeneration of motor nerve terminals degenerating in anterior gracile muscle of gracile axonal dystrophy (GAD) mutant mouse. *Neurosci Lett* 1994 Mar 28;170(1):195-7

Ultra-high dose methylcobalamin promotes nerve regeneration in experimental acrylamide neuropathy. *J Neurol Sci* 1994 Apr;122(2):140-3

Biochemical pathogenesis of subacute combined degeneration of the spinal cord and brain. *J Inherit Metab Dis* 1993;16(4):762-70

[Mechanism of the effect of methylcobalamin on the recovery of neuromuscular functions in mechanical and toxin denervation]. *Farmakol Toksikol* 1983 Nov-Dec;46(6):9-12

[Pharmacological studies on degeneration and regeneration of the peripheral nerves. (2) Effects of methylcobalamin on mitosis of Schwann cells and incorporation of labeled amino acid into protein fractions of crushed sciatic nerve in rats]. *Nippon Yakurigaku Zasshi* 1976 Mar;72(2):269-78

Preliminary results of proton magnetic resonance spectroscopy in motor neurone disease (amytrophic lateral sclerosis). *J Neurol Sci* 1995 May;129 Suppl:85-9

The copper chelator d-penicillamine delays onset of disease and extends survival in a transgenic mouse model of familial amyotrophic lateral sclerosis. *Eur J Neurosci* 1997 Jul;9(7):1548-51

Coenzyme Q_{10} administration and its potential for treatment of neurodegenerative diseases. *Biofactors* 1999;9(2-4):261-6

Possible involvement of folate cycle in the pathogenesis of amyotrophic lateral sclerosis. *Neurochem Res* Mar 1984, 9 (3) p387-91

Inhibition of terminal axonal sprouting by serum from patients with amyotrophic lateral sclerosis. *N Engl J Med* Oct 11 1984, 311 (15) p933-9

Cerebrospinal fluid (CSF) findings in amyotrophic lateral sclerosis. *J Neurol* (Germany, West) 1984, 231 (2) p75-8

Increased fragility of erythrocytes from amyotrophic lateral sclerosis (ALS) patients provoked by mechanical stress. *Acta Neurol Scand* (Denmark) Jan 1984, 69 (1) p20-6

Passive transfer experiments in amyotrophic lateral sclerosis. *Arch Neurol* Feb 1984, 41 (2) p161-3

Neuroprotective effects of creatine in a transgenic animal model of amyotrophic lateral sclerosis. *Nat Med* 1999 Mar;5(3):347-50

[Untitled] *Journal of Neural Transmission* (Suppl 1999;55: 79-95)

Free Radicals Appear to Fuel Lou Gehrig's Disease. *Family Practice News,* Rockville, MD

In vivo generation of hydroxyl radicals and MPTP-induced dopaminergic toxicity in the basal ganglia. *Ann N Y Acad Sci* Nov 17, 1994, 738 p25-36

Detection of point mutations in codon 331 of mitochondrial NADH dehydrogenase subunit 2 in Alzheimer's brains. *Biochem Biophys Res Commun* Jan 15 1992, 182 (1) p238-46

Deprenyl enhances neurite outgrowth in cultured rat spinal ventral horn neurons. *J Neurol Sci* (Netherlands) Aug 1994, 125 (1) p11-3

Therapeutic trial with *N*-acetylcysteine in amyotrophic lateral sclerosis. *Adv Exp Med Biol* 1987, 209 p281-4

Attempted treatment of motor neuron disease with *N*-acetylcysteine and dithiothreitol. *Adv Exp Med Biol* 1987, 209 p277-80

Anti-Glutamate Therapy in Amyotrophic Lateral Sclerosis: A Trial Using Lamotrigine. *Canadian Journal of Neurological Sciences,* 1993; 20:297-301

A Controlled Trial of Riluzole in Amyotrophic Lateral Sclerosis. *New England Journal of Medicine*, March 3, 1994; 330(9):585-591

Aluminum Deposition in Central Nervous System of Patients with Amyotrophic Lateral Sclerosis From the Kii Peninsula of Japan. *Neurotoxicology,* 1991; 615-620

Free Radicals and Neuroprotection. By B, J. Wilder, M. D., Professor Emeritus of Neurology University of Florida College of Medicine and Consultant in Neurology Department of Veterans Affairs Medical Center

Anemia-Thrombocytopenia-Leukopenia

Vitamin B12 levels in pregnancy influence erythropoietin response to anemia. *Eur J Obstet Gynecol Reprod Biol* (Ireland) Sep 1998, 80 (1) p63-6

Supplemental iron: A key to optimizing the response of cancer-related anemia to rHuEPO? *Oncologist*, 1998, 3/4 (275-278)

Effects of *L*-carnitine on anemia in aged hemodialysis patients treated with recombinant human erythropoietin: A pilot study. *Dialysis and Transplantation*, 1998, 27/8 (498-506)

The cytotoxic effect of the vitamin B12 inhibitor cyanocobalamin [c-lactam], and a review of other vitamin B12 antagonists. *Leukemia and Lymphoma* (UK), 1998, 31/1-2 (21-37)

Retardation of myelination due to dietary vitamin B12 deficiency: Cranial MRI findings. *Pediatric Radiology* (Germany), 1997, 27/2 (155-158)

More than 10 years'follow-up of total colonic aganglionosis—Severe iron deficiency anemia and growth retardation. *Journal of Pediatric Surgery,* 1997, 32/1 (25-27)

The role of prophylactic iron supplementation in pregnancy. *International Journal of Food Sciences and Nutrition* (UK), 1998, 49/5 (383-389)

Prevalence and etiology of nutritional anaemias in early childhood in an urban slum. *Indian Journal of Medical Research* (India), 1998, 107/June (269-273)

Biliopancreatic diversion. *World Journal of Surgery,* 1998, 22/9 (936-946)

Prophylactic iron supplementation after Roux-en-Y gastric bypass. A prospective, double-blind, randomized study. *Archives of Surgery,* 1998, 133/7 (740-744)

Human immunodeficiency virus-related wasting: Malabsorption syndromes. *Seminars in Oncology,* 1998, 25/2 Suppl.6 (70-75)

Evaluation of hemoglobin and hematocrit in pregnant women receiving folate and iron supplements. *Minerva Ginecologica* (Italy), 1997, 49/12 (571-576)

Micronutrient status in patients receiving home parenteral nutrition. *Nutrition,* 1997, 13/11-12 (941-944)

Folate-responsive homocystinuria and megaloblastic anaemia in a female patient with functional methionine synthase deficiency (cblE disease). *Journal of Inherited Metabolic Disease* (Netherlands), 1997, 20/6 (731-741)

Biochemical monitoring of vitamin B12 substitution therapy. *Klinicka Biochemie a Metabolismus* (Czech Republic), 1997, 5/3 (180-184)

Definition and prevalence of anemia in Bolivian women of childbearing age living at high altitudes: The effect of iron-folate supplementation. *Nutrition Reviews,* 1997, 55/6 (247-256)

Iron supplementation for the control of iron deficiency in populations at risk. *Nutrition Reviews,* 1997, 55/6 (195-209)

Iron, folate and vitamin B12 status of an elderly South African population. *European Journal of Clinical Nutrition* (UK), 1997, 51/7 (424-430)

Anemias in Thai patients with cirrhosis. *International Journal of Hematology* (Ireland), 1997, 65/4 (365-373)

Infantile megaloblastosis secondary to maternal vitamin B12 deficiency. *Clinical and Laboratory Haematology* (UK), 1997, 19/1 (23-25)

Mechanism for reduction of serum folate by antiepileptic drugs during prolonged therapy. *Journal of the Neurological Sciences* (Netherlands), 1997, 145/1 (109-112)

Is metabolic evidence for vitamin B-12 and folate deficiency more frequent in elderly patients with. *Journals of Gerontology—Series A Biological Sciences & Medical Sciences,*1997,52/2 (M76-M79)

The role of folic acid in deficiency states and prevention of disease. *Journal of Family Practice,* 1997, 44/2 (138-144)

Platelet defects in liver diseases. *Hamostaseologie* (Germany), 1998, 18/2 (56-60)

Folic acid deficiency anaemia resembling onset of a HELLP syndrome in twin pregnancy after maximal sterility therapy and innovative hormonal stimulation. *Geburtshilfe und Frauenheilkunde* (Germany), 1998, 58/3 (155-158)

Treatment of cancer chemotherapy-induced toxicity with the pineal hormone melatonin. *Supportive Care in Cancer* (Germany), 1997, 5/2 (126-129)

Methotrexate in rheumatoid arthritis: An update with focus on mechanisms involved in toxicity. *Seminars in Arthritis and Rheumatism,* 1998, 27/5 (277-292)

Seizure disorders in pregnancy. *International Journal of Gynecology and Obstetrics* (Ireland), 1997, 56/3 (279-286)

Thiamine-responsive myelodysplasia. *British Journal of Haematology* (UK), 1998, 102/4 (1098-1100)

Vitamin B12 replacement. To B12 or not to B12? *Canadian Family Physician* (Canada), 1997, 43/MAY (917-922)

Myelopathy due to vitamin B12 deficiency presenting only sensory disturbances in upper extremities: A case report. *Clinical Neurology* (Japan), 1997, 37/2 (135-138)

Folic acid supplementation improves erythropoietin response. *Nephron* (Switzerland) 1995, 71 (4) p395-400

Partial amelioration of AZT-induced macrocytic anemia in the mouse by folic acid. *Stem Cells (Dayt)* Sep 1993, 11 (5) p393-7

Megaloblastic anemia in patients receiving total parenteral nutrition without folic acid or vitamin B12 supplementation. *Can Med Assoc J* (Canada) Jul 23 1977, 117 (2) p144-6

Modulation of tumor necrosis factor-alpha (TNF-alpha) toxicity by the pineal hormone melatonin (MLT) in metastatic solid tumor patients. *Annals of the New York Academy of Sciences,* 1995, 768 (334-336)

[Anemias due to disorder of folate, vitamin B12 and transcobalamin metabolism]. *Rev Prat* (France) Jun 1 1993, 43 (11) p1358-63

[Is it necessary to supplement with folic acid patients in chronic dialysis treated with erythropoietin?]. *Rev Med Chil* (Chile) Jan 1993, 121 (1) p30-5

Ineffective hematopoiesis in folate-deficient mice. *Blood* May 1 1992, 79 (9) p2273-80

[Primary prophylaxis against cerebral toxoplasmosis. Efficacy of folinic acid in the prevention of hematologic toxicity of pyrimethamine]. *Presse Med* (France) Apr 2 1994, 23 (13) p613-5

Nutritional status of an institutionalized aged population. *J Am Coll Nutr* 1984, 3 (1) p13-25

[Acquired, vitamin B6-responsive, primary sideroblastic anemia, an enzyme deficiency in heme synthesis]. *Schweiz Med Wochenschr* (Switzerland) Oct 10 1981, 111 (41) p1533-5

Intakes of vitamins and minerals by pregnant women with selected clinical symptoms. *J Am Diet Assoc* May 1981, 78 (5) p477-82

[Anemia with hypersideroblastosis during anti-tuberculosis therapy. Cure with vitamin therapy]. *Nouv Rev Fr Hematol* (France) Apr 14 1978, 20 (1) p99-110

[Myelopathy and macrocytic anemia associated with a folate deficiency. Cure by folic acid]. *Ann Med Interne* (Paris) (France) May 1975, 126 (5) p339-48

[Vitamin B 6 deficiency anemia]. *Schweiz Med Wochenschr* (Switzerland) Oct 11 1975, 105 (41) p1319-24

Premature infants require additional folate and vitamin B-12 to reduce the severity of the anemia of prematurity. *Am J Clin Nutr* Dec 1994, 60 (6) p930-5

Apoptosis mediates and thymidine prevents erythroblast destruction in folate deficiency anemia. *Proc Natl Acad Sci U S A* Apr 26 1994, 91 (9) p4067-71

Acute folate deficiency associated with intravenous nutrition with aminoacid-sorbitol-ethanol: prophylaxis with intravenous folic acid. *Br J Haematol* (England) Dec 1977, 37 (4) p521-6

Interactions between folate and ascorbic acid in the guinea pig. *J Nutr* Apr 1982, 112 (4) p673-80

Modulation of human lymphoblastoid interferon activity by melatonin in metastatic renal cell carcinoma. *A phase II study. Cancer* Jun 15 1994, 73 (12) p3015-9

A biological study on the efficacy of low-dose subcutaneous interleukin-2 plus melatonin in the treatment of cancer-related thrombocytopenia. *Oncology* (Switzerland) Sep-Oct 1995, 52 (5) p360-2

A new class of antihypertensive neutral lipid: 1-alkyl-2-acetyl-sn-glycerols, a precursor of platelet activating factor. *Biochem. Biophys. Res. Commun.*, 1984, 118/1 (344-350)

Metabolism of 1-O-alkyl-2-acetyl-sn-glycerol by washed rabbit platelets: Formation of platelet activating factor. *Arch. Biochem. Biophys.*, 1984, 234/1 (318-321)

Conversion of 1-alkyl-2-acetyl-sn-glycerols to platelet activating factor and related phospholipids by rabbit platelets. *Biochem. Biophys. Res. Commun.*, 1984, 124/1 (156-163)

Anti-neoplastic action of peritoneal macrophages after oral admin. of ether analogueues of lysophospholipids. *Eur. J. Cancer Part A Gen. Top.* 1992, 28/10 (1637-1642)

Anesthesia and Surgery Precautions

Low-dose and high-dose acetylsalicylic acid for patients undergoing carotid endarterectomy: a randomised controlled trial. ASA and Carotid Endarterectomy (ACE) Trial Collaborators. *Lancet* 1999 Jun 26;353(9171):2179-84

Glutamine metabolism and transport in skeletal muscle and heart and their clinical relevance. *J Nutr* Apr 1996, 126 (4 Suppl) p1142S-9S

Lung glutamine flux following open heart surgery. *J Surg Res* Jul 1991, 51 (1) p82-6

Glutamine: Effects on the immune system, protein metabolism and intestinal function. *Wiener Klinische Wochenschrift* (Austria)1996,108/21 (669-676)

Integrative cardiac revitalization: bypass surgery, angioplasty, and chelation. Benefits, risks, and limitations. *Altern Med Rev* Feb 1998, 3 (1) p4-17

Growth hormone treatment prevents the decrease in insulin-like growth factor I gene expression in patients undergoing abdominal surgery. *J Clin Endocrinol Metab* May 1998, 83 (5) p1566-72

The estimation of efficacy of oral iron supplementation during treatment with epoetin beta (recombinant human erythropoietin) in patients undergoing cardiac surgery. *Eur J Haematol* (Denmark) Apr 1998, 60 (4) p252-9

Total parenteral nutrition with glutamine dipeptide after major abdominal surgery: a randomized, double-blind, controlled study. *Ann Surg* Feb 1998, 227 (2) p302-8

Nutrition in spinal surgery. *Current Opinion in Orthopaedics* (UK), 1998, 9/2 (39-42)

A case of vitamin A deficiency after small-intestinal bypass surgery for leiomyosarcoma. *Folia Ophthalmologica Japonica* (Japan), 1998, 49/3 (272-275)

Preoperative nutrition in elective abdominal surgery: Audit of nutritional support in a university hospital. *Nutrition Clinique et Metabolisme* (France), 1998, 12/1 (13-20)

Changes in the defense against free radicals in the liver and plasma of the dog during hypoxia and/or halothane anaesthesia. *Toxicology* (Ireland), 1998, 128/1 (25-34)

Plasma catalase and glutathione levels are decreased in response to inhalation injury. *Journal of Burn Care and Rehabilitation*, 1997, 18/6 (515-519)

Effect of chronic anesthesia on the drug-metabolizing enzyme system and heme pathway regulation. *General Pharmacology*, 1997, 28/4 (577-582)

No beneficial effects of taurine application on oxygen free radical production after hemorrhagic shock in rats. *Advances in Experimental Medicine and Biology*, 1998, 442/- (193-200)

Free radicals in the cerebrospinal fluid are associated with neurological disorders including mitochondrial encephalomyopathy. *Biochemistry and Molecular Biology International* (Australia), 1997, 42/5 (937-947)

Deformability and oxidant stress in red blood cells under the influence of halothane and isoflurane anesthesia. *General Pharmacology*, 1998, 31/1 (33-36)

Oxygen free radical activity in the second stage of labor. *Acta Obstetricia et Gynecologica Scandinavica* (Denmark), 1997, 76/8 (765-768)

Myocardial preservation by therapy with coenzyme Q_{10} during heart surgery. *Usa Clin. Invest. Suppl.* (Germany), 1993, 71/8 (S 155-S 161)

Effect of CoQ_{10} on myocardial ischemia/reperfusion injury in the isolated rat heart. *Journal of the Japanese Association for Thoracic Surgery* (Japan), 1995, 43/4 (466-472)

Free radical reaction products and antioxidant capacity in arterial plasma during coronary artery bypass grafting. *J. Thorac. Cardiovasc. Surg.* (USA) 1994, 108/1 (140-147)

Oxygen radicals in cerebral vascular injury. *Circ. R Res.*, 1985, 57/4 (508-516)

Postischemic tissue injury by iron-mediated free radical lipid peroxidation. *Ann. Emerg. Med.*, 1985, 14/8 (804-809)

Oxygen free radical-induced histamine release during intestinal ischemia and reperfusion. *Eur. Surg. Res.* (Switzerland), 1989, 21/6 (297-304)

Role of iron ions in the genesis of reperfusion injury following successful cardiopulmonary resuscitation: Preliminary data and a biochemical hypothesis. *Ann. Emerg. Med.*, 1985, 14/8 (777-783)

The biological significance of zinc. *Anaesthesist* (Berl.) (Germany, West), 1975, 24/8 (329-342)

Cortical pO_2 distribution during oligemic hypotension and its pharmacological modifications (Hydergine). *Switzerland Arzneim.-Forsch.* (Germany, West), 1978, 28/5 (768-770)

The use of piracetam (Nootrop) in post-anesthetic recovery of elderly patients. (A preliminary study). *Greece Acta Anaesthesiol. Hell.* (Greece), 1981, 15/1-2 (76-80)

Free radical reaction products and antioxidant capacity in arterial plasma during coronary artery bypass grafting. *J. Thorac. Cardiovasc. Surg.*, 1994, 108/1 (140-147)

Free radical trapping agents in myocardial protection in cardiac surgery. *France Ann. Cardiol. Angeiol.* (France), 1986, 35/7 BIS (447-452)

Biochemical studies of cerebral ischemia in the rat—Changes in cerebral free amino acids, catecholamines and uric acid. *Japan Brain Nerve* (Japan), 1986, 38/3 (253-258)

Glutathione status in human blood during surgery. *Clin. Chem. Enzymol. Commun.* (UK), 1988, 1/2 (71-76)

Effect of supplemental vitamin A on colon anastomotic healing in rats given preoperative irradiation. *Am. J. Surg.*, 1987, 153/2 (153-156)

Effect of reduced glutathione on endocrine and renal functions following halothane anesthesia and surgery in man. *Jpn. J. Anesthesiol.* (Japan), 1982, 31/8 (830-839)

Intraocular irrigating solutions and lens clarity. *Amer.J.Ophthal.*, 1976, 82/4 (594-597)

Intraocular irrigating solutions. Their effect on the corneal endothelium. *Arch.Ophthal.*, 1975, 93/8 (648-657)

Anticancer Activity of PC Spes

See references under Prostate Cancer.

Anxiety and Stress

The impact of a new emotional self-management program on stress, emotions, heart rate variability, DHEA and cortisol. *Integr Physiol Behav Sci* Apr-Jun 1998, 33 (2) p151-70

An open non-comparative study on the efficacy of an oral multivitamin combination containing calcium and magnesium on persons permanently exposed to occupational stress-predisposing factors. *Journal of Clinical Research* (UK), 1998, 1/303-315 (303-313)

Age-related neurodegeneration and oxidative stress: putative nutritional intervention. *Neurol Clin* Aug 1998, 16 (3) p747-55

Oxidative stress and advancing age: results in healthy centenarians. *J Am Geriatr Soc* Jul 1998, 46 (7) p833-8

How controlled stress affects healing tissues. *J Hand Ther* Apr-Jun 1998, 11 (2) p125-30

Second World Congress on Stress, Melbourne, Australia, October 1998: Adversity over the life course: Assessment and quantification issues. *Stress Medicine* (UK), 1998, 14/4 (205-211)

Oxidative stress in critical care: Is antioxidant supplementation beneficial? *Journal of the American Dietetic Association*, 1998, 98/9 (1001-1008)

Psychometric evidence that dental amalgam mercury may be an etiological factor in manic depression. *Journal of Orthomolecular Medicine* (Canada), 1998, 13/1 (31-40)

Over-the-counter psychotropics: A review of melatonin, St John's wort, valerian, and kava-kava. *Journal of American College Health*, 1998, 46/6 (271-276)

Stress, relaxation states, and creativity. *Percept Mot Skills* 1999 Apr;88(2):409-16 Exercise and the experience and appraisal of daily stressors: a naturalistic study. *J Behav Med* 1998 Aug;21(4):363-74

Effect of aerobic exercise on negative affect, positive affect, stress, and depression. *Percept Mot Skills* 1992 Oct;75(2): 355-61

The effects of physical activity and exercise training on psychological stress and well-being in an adolescent population. *J Psychosom Res* 1992 Jan;36(1):55-65

A biopsychosocial model of glycemic control in diabetes: stress, coping and regimen adherence. *J Health Soc Behav* 1999 Jun;40(2):141-58

Endocrine correlates of personality traits: A comparison between emotionally stable and emotionally labile healthy young men. *Neuropsychobiology* (Switzerland), 1997, 35/4 (205-210)

Tissue changes in glutathione metabolism and lipid peroxidation induced by swimming are partially prevented by melatonin. *Pharmacology and Toxicology* (Denmark), 1996, 78/5 (308-312)

The role of beta-adrenoceptor blockers in the treatment of psychiatric disorders. *CNS Drugs* (New Zealand), 1996, 5/2 (115-136)

At least three neurotransmitter systems mediate a stress-induced increase in c-fos mRNA in different rat brain areas. *Cellular and Molecular Neurobiology*, 1997, 17/2 (157-169)

Calcitonin gene-related peptide is an adipose-tissue neuropeptide with lipolytic actions. *Endocrinology and Metabolism* (UK), 1996, 3/4 (235-242)

Adverse CNS-effects of beta-adrenoceptor blockers. *Pharmacopsychiatry* (Germany), 1996, 29/6 (201-211)

Acute effects of beta blockade and exercise on mood and anxiety. *British Journal of Sports Medicine* (UK), 1996, 30/3 (238-242)

Stressor-induced alterations of the splenic plaque-forming cell response: Strain differences and modification by propranolol. *Pharmacology Biochemistry and Behavior*, 1996, 53/2 (235-241)

Propranolol reduces the anxiety associated with day case surgery. European Journal of Surgery, *Acta Chirurgica* (Norway), 1996, 162/1 (11-14)

Nutritional management of the metabolically stressed patient. *Crit. Care Nurs. Q.*, 1995, 17/4 (79-90)

Propranolol in psychiatry. Therapeutic uses and side effects. *Neuropsychobiology* (Switzerland) 1986, 15 (1) p20-7

Propranolol in experimentally induced stress. *Br J Psychiatry* (England) Dec 1981, 139 p545-9

Modulation of the immunologic response to acute stress in humans by beta-blockade or benzodiazepines. *Faseb J* Mar 1996, 10 (4) p517-24

Beta-adrenergic receptors are involved in stress-related behavioral changes. *Pharmacol Biochem Behav* May 1993, 45 (1) p1-7

The effect of beta blockade on stress-induced cognitive dysfunction in adolescents. *Clin Pediatr* (Phila) Jul 1991, 30 (7) p441-5

Modulation of baseline behavior in rats by putative serotonergic agents in three ethoexperimental paradigms. *Behav Neural Biol* Nov 1990, 54 (3) p234-53

Effects of propranolol, atenolol, and chlordesmethyldiazepam on response to mental stress in patients with recent myocardial infarction. *Clin Cardiol* Jun 1987, 10 (6) p293-302

Clinical Trials For Chronic Fatigue and Anxiety. Life Extension Update-February 1996

Nutritional management of the metabolically stressed patient. *Crit. Care Nurs. Q.*, 1995, 17/4 (79-90)

Propranolol in psychiatry. Therapeutic uses and side effects. *Neuropsychobiology* (Switzerland) 1986, 15 (1) p20-7

Propranolol in experimentally induced stress. *Br J Psychiatry* Dec 1981, 139 p545-9

Modulation of the immunologic response to acute stress in humans by beta-blockade or benzodiazepines. *Faseb J* Mar 1996, 10 (4) p517-24

Beta-adrenergic receptors are involved in stress-related behavioral changes. *Pharmacol Biochem Behav* May 1993, 45 (1) p1-7

The effect of beta blockade on stress-induced cognitive dysfunction in adolescents. *Clin Pediatr* (Phila) Jul 1991, 30 (7) p441-5

Modulation of baseline behavior in rats by putative serotonergic agents in three ethoexperimental paradigms. *Behav Neural Biol* Nov 1990, 54 (3) p234-53

Effects of propranolol, atenolol, and chlordesmethyldiazepam on response to mental stress in patients with recent myocardial infarction. *Clin Cardiol* Jun 1987, 10 (6) p293-302

Clinical Trials For Chronic Fatigue and Anxiety. *Life Extension Update-February* 1996

Dr. J. Bory, *Journees de Biochimie medicale de l'Ouest, Brest*, 1981

Ph. Darcet et al (*Ann. Nutr. Alim.*), 1980, 34 277.901

G. Durant, G. Pascal N. Vodovar, H. Gounelle De Pontanel (*Med. et Nutr.*), 1978, vol. XIV, 1 95-204)

Growford and Sinclair,1972 (*J. Nutrition*, 102-1315)

M. Henry, researcher, Personal contribution

Lamptey and Walter, 1976 l (*J. Nutrition*, 106-86)

Professor P Metais (*Cahiers de Nutrition et Dietetique)*, 1980, vol. XV, n 3, 227

Prostaglandines et physiologic de la reproduction, International Inserm Symposium (*Revue francaise des laboratoires-*January 1980, n 77 4-5-6)

Arrhythmia (Cardiac)

Prevention of cardiac arrhythmia by dietary (n-3) polyunsaturated fatty acids and their mechanism of action. *Journal of Nutrition*, 1997, 127/3 (383-393)

Fatty acids suppress voltage-gated Na+ currents in HEK293t cells transfected with the alpha-subunit of the human cardiac Na+ channel. *Proceedings of the National Academy of Sciences of the United States of America,* 1998, 95/5 (2680-2685)

n-3 Polyunsaturated fatty acids, heart rate variability and ventricular arrhythmias in patients with previous myocardial infarcts. *Ugeskrift for Laeger* (Denmark), 1997, 159/37 (5525-5529)

Randomized, double-blind, placebo-controlled trial of fish oil and mustard oil in patients with suspected acute myocardial infarction: The Indian experiment of infarct survival - 4. *Cardiovascular Drugs and Therapy,* 1997, 11/3 (485-491)

omega3 fatty acids in the prevention-management of cardiovascular disease. *Canadian Journal of Physiology and Pharmacology* (Canada), 1997, 75/3 (234-239)

Omega-3 fatty acids and prevention of cardiovascular disease. *Cahiers de Nutrition et de Dietetique* (France), 1997, 32/2 (107-114)

Vitamin E analogues reduce the incidence of ventricular fibrillations and scavenge free radicals. *Fundamental and Clinical Pharmacology* (France), 1998, 12/2 (164-172)

Antioxidant activity of U-83836E, a second generation lazaroid, during myocardial Ischemia/Reperfusion injury. *Free Radical Research* (UK), 1997, 27/6 (577-590)

Trace elements and cardioprotection: Increasing endogenous glutathione peroxidase activity by oral selenium supplementation in rats limits reperfusion-induced arrhythmias. *Journal of Trace Elements in Medicine and Biology* (Germany), 1998, 12/1 (28-38)

Randomized, double-blind placebo-controlled trial of coenzyme Q_{10} in patients with acute myocardial infarction. *Cardiovascular Drugs and Therapy,* 1998, 12/4 (347-353)

Effect of coenzyme Q_{10} therapy in patients with congestive heart failure: A long-term multicenter randomized study. *Clin. Invest. Suppl.* (Germany), 1993, 71/8 (S 134-S 136)

Serum concentration of lipoprotein(a) decreases on treatment with hydrosoluble coenzyme Q_{10} in patients with coronary artery disease: discovery of a new role. *Int J Cardiol* 1999 Jan;68(1):23-9

Coenzyme Q_{10} administration increases brain mitochondrial concentrations and exerts neuroprotective effects. *Proc Natl Acad Sci U S A* 1998 Jul 21;95(15):8892-7

Fish oil and other nutritional adjuvants for treatment of congestive heart failure. *Medical Hypotheses* (UK), 1996, 46/4 (400-406)

Evidence on the participation of the 3',5'-cyclic AMP pathway in the non-genomic action of 1,25-dihydroxy-vitamin D3 in cardiac muscle. *Mol Cell Endocrinol* (Netherlands) Dec 1991, 82 (2-3) p229-35

1,25(OH)2 vitamin D3, and retinoic acid antagonize endothelin-stimulated hypertrophy of neonatal rat cardiac myocytes. *J Clin Invest* Apr 1 1996, 97 (7) p1577-88

[Effect of vitamin E deficiency on the development of cardiac arrhythmias as affected by acute ischemia]. *Biull Eksp Biol Med* (USSR) Nov 1986, 102 (11) p530-2

Antioxidant protection against adrenaline-induced arrhythmias in rats with chronic heart hypertrophy. *Can J Cardiol* (Canada) Mar 1990, 6 (2) p71-4

The antiarrhythmic effects of taurine alone and in combination with magnesium sulfate on ischemia/reperfusion arrhythmia. *Chinese Pharmacological Bulletin* (China), 1994, 10/5 (358-362)

Prophylactic effects of taurine and diltiazem, alone or combined, on reperfusion arrhythmias in rats. *Acta Pharmacologica Sinica* (China), 1996, 17/2

The effects of antioxidants on reperfusion dysrhythmias. *Ceska a Slovenska Farmacie* (Czech Republic), 1995, 44/5 (257-260)

Protective effects of all-trans-retinoic acid against cardiac arrhythmias induced by isoproterenol, lysophosphatidylcholine or ischemia and reperfusion. *Journal of Cardiovascular Pharmacology,* 1995, 26/6

Effects of dietary supplementation with alpha-tocopherol on myocardial infarct size and ventricular arrhythmias in a dog model of ischemia-reperfusion. *J. Am. Coll. Cardiol.*, 1994, 24/6 (1580-1585)

Magnesium flux during and after open heart operations in children. *Ann Thorac Surg* Apr 1995, 59 (4) p921-7

Sino-atrial Wenckebach conduction in thyrotoxic periodic paralysis: a case report. *Int J Cardiol* (Ireland) Jan 6 1995, 47 (3) p285-9

A possible beneficial effect of selenium administration in antiarrhythmic therapy. *J Am Coll Nutr* Oct 1994, 13 (5) p496-8

Omega-3 fatty acids and prevention of ventricular fibrillation. *Prostaglandins Leukot Essent Fatty Acids* (Scotland) Feb-Mar 1995, 52

[Effect of anti-arrhythmia drugs on the beta2 receptor-dependent adenyl cyclase system of lymphocytes in patients with cardiac rhythm disorders]. *Kardiologiia* (USSR) Jul 1989, 29 (7) p25-9

An expanded concept of "insurance" supplementation—broad-spectrum protection from cardiovascular disease. *Med Hypotheses* (England) Oct 1981, 7 (10) p1287-1302

Italian multicenter study on the safety and efficacy of Coenzyme Q_{10} as adjunctive therapy in heart failure (interim analysis). *Clin Investig* (Germany) 1993, 71 (8 Suppl) pS145-9

Isolated diastolic dysfunction of the myocardium and its response to CoQ_{10} treatment. *Clin Investig* (Germany) 1993, 71 (8 Suppl) pS140-4

Protective effects of propionyl-L-carnitine during ischemia and reperfusion. *Cardiovasc Drugs Ther* Feb 1991, 5 Suppl 1 p77-83

Consequences of magnesium deficiency on the enhancement of stress reactions; preventive and therapeutic implications (a review). *J Am Coll Nutr* Oct 1994

Community-based prevention of stroke: nutritional improvement in Japan. *Health Rep* (Canada) 1994, 6 (1)

Effect of dietary magnesium supplementation on intralymphocytic free calcium and magnesium in stroke-prone spontaneously hypertensive rats. *Clin Exp Hypertens* May 1994

Clinical study of cardiac arrhythmias using a 24-hour continuous electrocardiographic recorder (5th report)—antiarrhythmic action of Coenzyme Q_{10} in diabetics. *Tohoku J Exp Med* (Japan) Dec 1983, 141 Suppl p453-63

Usefulness of Coenzyme Q_{10} in clinical cardiology: a long-term study. *Mol Aspects Med* (England) 1994, 15 Suppl

Isolated diastolic dysfunction of the myocardium and its response to CoQ_{10} treatment. *Clin Investig* (Germany) 1993, 71 (8 Suppl) pS140-4

Effect of coenzyme Q_{10} on structural alterations in the renal membrane of stroke-prone spontaneously hypertensive rats. *Biochem Med Metab Biol* Apr 1991

Coenzyme Q_{10}: a new drug for cardiovascular disease. *J Clin Pharmacol* Jul 1990

[Effects of 2,3-dimethoxy-5-methyl-6-(10'-hydroxydecyl)-1,4-benzoquinone (CV-2619) on adriamycin-induced ECG abnormalities and myocardial energy metabolism in spontaneously hypertensive rats] *Nippon Yakurigaku Zasshi* (Japan) Oct 1982

Bioenergetics in clinical medicine. III. Inhibition of coenzyme Q_{10}-enzymes by clinically used anti-hypertensive drugs. *Res Commun Chem Pathol Pharmacol* Nov 1975

Bioenergetics in clinical medicine. Studies on coenzyme Q_{10} and essential hypertension. *Res Commun Chem Pathol Pharmacol* Jun 1975

[Prevention of cerebrovascular insults]. *Schweiz Med Wochenschr* (Switzerland) Nov 12 1994

[Essential antioxidants in cardiovascular diseases—lessons for Europe] *Ther Umsch* (Switzerland) Jul 1994

Antioxidant vitamin intake and coronary mortality in a longitudinal population study. *Am J Epidemiol* Jun 15 1994

Decline in stroke mortality. An epidemiologic perspective. *Ann Epidemiol* Sep 1993

Can antioxidants prevent ischemic heart disease? *J Clin Pharm Ther* (England) Apr 1993

Antioxidant therapy in the aging process. *Exs* (Switzerland) 1992, 62

Effect of flosequinan on ischaemia-induced arrhythmias and on ventricular cyclic nucleotide content in the anaesthetized rat. *Br J Pharmacol* (England) Apr 1993, 108 (4) p1111-6

What do the newer inotropic drugs have to offer? *Cardiovasc. Drugs Ther.*, 1992, 6/1 (15-18)

Arrhythmogenic effect of forskolin in the isolated perfused rat heart: Influence of nifedipine reduction of external calcium. *Clin. Exp. Pharmacol. Physiol.* (Australia), 1989, 16/10 (751-757)

Hormone secretagogues increase cytosolic calcium by increasing cAMP in corticotropin-secreting cells. *Proc. Natl Acad. Sci. U. S. A.*, 1985, 82/23 (8034-8038)

The genesis of arrhythmias during myocardial ischemia. Dissociation between changes in cyclic adenosine monophosphate and electrical instability in the rat. *Circ. Res.*, 1985, 57/5 (668-675)

Effects of high K on relaxation produced by drugs in the guinea-pig tracheal muscle. *Respir. Physiol.* (Netherlands), 1985, 61/1 (43-55)

Forskolin inhibits ouabain-sensitive ATPase in the medulla of rat kidney. *Ircs Med. Sci.* (England), 1983, 11/11 (957-958)

Arthritis

Ginger (Zingiber officinale) and rheumatic disorders. *Med Hypotheses* 1989 May;29(1):25-8

Ginger (Zingiber officinale) in rheumatism and musculoskeletal disorders. *Med Hypotheses* 1992 Dec;39(4):342-8

Suppressive effects of eugenol and ginger oil on arthritic rats. *Pharmacology* 1994 Nov;49(5):314-8

Plant extracts from stinging nettle (Urtica dioica), an antirheumatic remedy, inhibit the proinflammatory transcription factor NF-kappaB. *FEBS Lett* 1999 Jan 8;442(1):89-94

[Anti-inflammatory effect of Urtica dioica folia extract in comparison to caffeic malic acid]. *Arzneimittelforschung* 1996 Jan;46(1):52-6

The effect of aurotherapy on the level of unsaturated fatty acids during the treatment of rheumatoid arthritis patients. *Lik Sprava* (Ukraine) Sep-Oct 1997, (5) p166-70

Putative analgesic activity of repeated oral doses of vitamin E in the treatment of rheumatoid arthritis. Results of a prospective placebo controlled double blind trial. *Ann Rheum Dis* (England) Nov 1997, 56 (11) p649-55

Inadequate calcium, folic acid, vitamin E, zinc, and selenium intake in rheumatoid arthritis patients: results of a dietary survey. *Semin Arthritis Rheum* Dec 1997, 27 (3) p180-5

Dietary n-3 fatty acids and therapy for rheumatoid arthritis. *Semin Arthritis Rheum* Oct 1997, 27 (2) p85-97

[Selenium concentration in erythrocytes of patients with rheumatoid arthritis . Clinical and laboratory chemistry infection markers during administration of selenium]. *Med Klin* (Germany) Sep 15 1997, 92 Suppl 3 p29-31

Abnormalities in skeletal growth in children with juvenile rheumatoid arthritis. *Rheum Dis Clin North Am* Aug 1997, 23 (3) p499-522

Availability of iron and degree of inflammation modifies the response to recombinant human erythropoietin when treating anemia of chronic disease in patients with rheumatoid arthritis. *Rheumatol Int* (Germany) 1997, 17 (2) p67-73

Serum concentrations of alpha tocopherol, beta carotene, and retinol preceding the diagnosis of rheumatoid arthritis and systemic lupus erythematosus. *Ann Rheum Dis* (England) May 1997, 56 (5) p323-5

Faecal microbial flora and disease activity in rheumatoid arthritis during a vegan diet. *Br J Rheumatol* (England) Jan 1997, 36 (1) p64-8

Dietary therapy with Lactobacillus GG, bovine colostrum or bovine immune colostrum in patients with juvenile chronic arthritis: Evaluation of effect on gut defence mechanisms. *Inflammopharmacology* (Netherlands), 1997, 5/3 (219-236)

Inflammation and bone metabolism in rheumatoid arthritis. Pathogenetic aspects and therapeutic options. *Medizinische Klinik* (Germany), 1997, 92/10 (607-614)

Serum-concentration of 25-hydroxy- vitamin D in elderly people with rheumatoid arthritis. *Geriatrie Forschung* (Germany), 1997, 7/3 (129-133)

Vitamin E in activated arthrosis and rheumatoid arthritis: What is the therapeutic value of alpha-tocopherol? *Fortschritte der Medizin* (Germany), 1997, 115/26 (39-42)

Concentration of selenium in erythrocytes of patients with rheumatoid arthritis in relation to clinical and laboratory signs of inflammation. *Medizinische Klinik* (Germany), 1997, 92/ Suppl. 3 (29-31)

Methyl-vitamin B12 blocks the CD28 co-stimulatory pathway in human T cells and its possible therapeutic application for T cell-mediated diseases, including rheumatoid arthritis. *Japanese Journal of Rheumatology* (Netherlands), 1997, 7/1 (35-45)

Effects of cyclosporin on joint damage in rheumatoid arthritis. The Italian Rheumatologists Study Group on Rheumatoid Arthritis. *Clin Exp Rheumatol* (Italy) May-Jun 1997, 15 Suppl 17 pS83-9

Management of rheumatoid arthritis: Rationale for the use of colloidal metallic gold. *Journal of Nutritional and Environmental Medicine* (UK), 1997, 7/4 (295-305)

Methotrexate in rheumatoid arthritis. Folate supplementation should always be given. *BioDrugs* (New Zealand), 1997, 8/3 (164-175)

The influence of topical application of Oeparol (R) (evening primrose oil) on skin neovascular response induced in mice by leucocytes of rheumatoid arthritis patients. *Reumatologia* (Poland), 1997, 35/2 (166-170)

Periarthritis humeroscapularis: Alternative pain treatment with magnet plasters. *Ther. Ggw.* (Germany, West), 1982, 121/8 (487-492)

Substances reactive with mannose-binding protein (MBP) in sera of patients with rheumatoid arthritis. *Fukushima J Med Sci* (Japan) Dec 1997, 43 (2) p99-111

Putative analgesic activity of repeated oral doses of vitamin E in the treatment of rheumatoid arthritis. Results of a prospective placebo controlled double blind trial. *Ann Rheum Dis* (England) Nov 1997, 56 (11) p649-55

Renal stones in patients with rheumatoid arthritis. *J Rheumatol* (Canada) Nov 1997, 24 (11) p2123-8

[Inflammation and bone metabolism in rheumatoid arthritis. Pathogenetic viewpoints and therapeutic possibilities]. *Med Klin* (Germany) Oct 15 1997, 92 (10) p607-14

Predictors of total body bone mineral density in non-corticosteroid-treated prepubertal children with juvenile rheumatoid arthritis. *Arthritis Rheum* Nov 1997, 40 (11) p1967-75

Nutrient intake patterns, body mass index, and vitamin levels in patients with rheumatoid arthritis. *Arthritis Care Res* Feb 1997, 10 (1) p9-17

Effects of low dose methotrexate on the bone mineral density of patients with rheumatoid arthritis. *J Rheumatol* (Canada) Aug 1997, 24 (8) p1489-94

Correlation between blood antioxidant levels and lipid peroxidation in rheumatoid arthritis. *Clin Biochem* Jun 1997, 30 (4) p351-5

Emerging treatments for rheumatoid arthritis. *Am J Med* Jan 27 1997, 102 (1A) p11S-15S

Zinc metabolism in rheumatoid arthritis: plasma and urinary zinc and relationship to disease activity [see comments]. *J Rheumatol* (Canada) Apr 1997, 24 (4) p643-6

Increased serum *NG*-hydroxy-*L*-arginine in patients with rheumatoid arthritis and systemic lupus erythematosus as an index of an increased nitric oxide synthase activity. *Ann Rheum Dis* (England) May 1997, 56 (5) p330-2

Management of oral complications of disease-modifying drugs in rheumatoid arthritis. *Br J Rheumatol* (England) Apr 1997, 36 (4) p473-8

Comparison between intravenous and subcutaneous recombinant human erythropoietin (Epoetin alfa) administration in presurgical autologous blood donation in anemic rheumatoid arthritis patients undergoing major orthopedic surgery. *Vox Sang* (Switzerland) 1997, 72 (2) p93-100

Abnormal homocysteine metabolism in rheumatoid arthritis. *Arthritis Rheum* Apr 1997, 40 (4) p718-22

Prediction of articular destruction in rheumatoid arthritis: disease activity markers revisited [see comments]. *J Rheumatol* (Canada) Jan 1997, 24 (1) p28-34

Intractable diarrhoea associated with secondary amyloidosis in rheumatoid arthritis. *Ann Rheum Dis* (England) Sep 1997, 56 (9) p535-41

An open study of the anti-TNF alpha agent pentoxifylline in the treatment of rheumatoid arthritis. *Rev Rhum Engl Ed* (France) Dec 1997, 64 (12) p789-93

Life-table analysis of cyclosporin A treatment in psoriatic arthritis: comparison with other disease-modifying antirheumatic drugs. *Clin Exp Rheumatol* (Italy) Nov-Dec 1997, 15 (6) p609-14

Methotrexate as the initial second-line disease modifying agent in the treatment of rheumatoid arthritis patients. *Clin Exp Rheumatol* (Italy) Nov-Dec 1997, 15 (6) p597-601

The relationship between variations in knee replacement utilization rates and the reported prevalence of arthritis in Ontario, Canada. *J Rheumatol* (Canada) Dec 1997, 24 (12) p2403-12

Differences in the use of second-line agents and prednisone for treatment of rheumatoid arthritis by rheumatologists and non-rheumatologists. *J Rheumatol* (Canada) Dec 1997, 24 (12) p2283-90

Destruction of the first carpometacarpal joint behaves differently from that of the entire carpus in rheumatoid arthritis. A 20-year follow-up study. *Scand J Rheumatol* (NORWAY) 1997, 26 (5) p361-3

Combination treatment of severe rheumatoid arthritis with cyclosporine and methotrexate for forty-eight weeks: an open-label extension study. The Methotrexate-Cyclosporine Combination Study Group. *Arthritis Rheum* Oct 1997, 40 (10) p1843-51

Patient education and disease activity: a study among rheumatoid arthritis patients. *Arthritis Care Res* Oct 1997, 10 (5) p320-4

Acetabular pressures during hip arthritis exercises. *Arthritis Care Res* Oct 1997, 10 (5) p308-19

Magnetic resonance imaging of the wrist in defining remission of rheumatoid arthritis. *J Rheumatol* (Canada) Jul 1997, 24 (7) p1303-8

Commercial wrist extensor orthoses: a descriptive study of use and preference in patients with rheumatoid arthritis. *Arthritis Care Res* Feb 1997, 10 (1) p27-35

Effect of treatment with methotrexate, hydroxychloroquine, and prednisone on lymphocyte polyamine levels in rheumatoid arthritis: correlation with the clinical response and rheumatoid factor synthesis. *Clin Exp Rheumatol* (Italy) Jul-Aug 1997, 15 (4) p343-7

Prognostic criteria in rheumatoid arthritis: can we predict which patients will require specific anti-rheumatoid treatment?. *Clin Exp Rheumatol* (Italy) May-Jun 1997, 15 Suppl 17 pS15-25

Financial and career losses due to rheumatoid arthritis: a pilot study. *J Rheumatol* (Canada) Aug 1997, 24 (8) p1527-30

Comparative usefulness of C-reactive protein and erythrocyte sedimentation rate in patients with rheumatoid arthritis. *J Rheumatol* (Canada) Aug 1997, 24 (8) p1477-85

Off-the-shelf orthopedic footwear for people with rheumatoid arthritis. *Arthritis Care Res* Aug 1997, 10 (4) p250-6

Radiographic results from the Minocycline in Rheumatoid Arthritis (MIRA) Trial. *J Rheumatol* (Canada) Jul 1997, 24 (7) p1295-302

Reference curves of radiographic damage in patients with rheumatoid arthritis: application of quantile regression and fractional polynomials. *J Rheumatol* (Canada) Jul 1997, 24 (7) p1288-94

Measurement of morning stiffness in rheumatoid arthritis clinical trials. *J Clin Epidemiol* (England) Jul 1997, 50 (7) p757-63

Oral contraceptives and rheumatoid arthritis: results from a primary care-based incident case-control study. *Semin Arthritis Rheum* Jun 1997, 26 (6) p817-23

Effect of disease modifying agents on the lipid profiles of patients with rheumatoid arthritis [see comments]. *Ann Rheum Dis* (England) Jun 1997, 56 (6) p374-7

[Favorable results of early 2nd-stage medication in rheumatoid arthritis]. *Ned Tijdschr Geneeskd* (Netherlands) Apr 12 1997, 141 (15) p732-6

Direct costs of medical attention to Mexican patients with rheumatoid arthritis in a tertiary care center. *Clin Exp Rheumatol* (Italy) Jan-Feb 1997, 15 (1) p75-8

Cardiovascular morbidity and mortality in patients with seropositive rheumatoid arthritis in Northern Sweden. *J Rheumatol* (Canada) Mar 1997, 24 (3) p445-51

The two-year follow-up of a randomized comparison of in-patient multidisciplinary team care and routine out-patient care for active rheumatoid arthritis. *Br J Rheumatol* (England) Jan 1997, 36 (1) p82-5

Rheumatology visit frequency and changes in functional disability and pain in patients with rheumatoid arthritis. *J Rheumatol* (Canada) Jan 1997, 24 (1) p35-42

Limited effect of sulphasalazine treatment in reactive arthritis. A randomised double blind placebo controlled trial. *Ann Rheum Dis* (England) Jan 1997, 56 (1) p32-6

Diagnostic value of antiperinuclear factor and anti-stratum corneum antibody in rheumatoid arthritis. Part 1. *Revista Brasileira de Reumatologia* (Brazil), 1997, 37/5 (251-259)

Appraisal and coping in immunologically distinct subgroups of women with rheumatoid arthritis. *British Journal of Health Psychology* (UK), 1997, 2/4 (327-331)

Disposition and clinical efficacy of methotrexate in patients with rheumatoid arthritis following weekly, low, intramuscular dosing: A pilot study. *Current Therapeutic Research—Clinical and Experimental*, 1997, 58/7 (434-445)

Pathogenesis of rheumatoid arthritis. *Medizinische Klinik* (Germany), 1997, 92/6 (347-353)

Effects of therapeutic ultrasound in a water bath on skin microcirculation and skin temperature in rheumatoid arthritis. *European Journal of Physical Medicine and Rehabilitation* (Austria), 1997, 7/2 (46-49)

Improving arthritis self-management among older adults: 'Just what the doctor didn't order'. *British Journal of Health Psychology* (UK), 1997, 2/2 (175-186)

Brucellar septic arthritis: Evolutive course of 27 cases. *Revista Espanola de Reumatologia* (Spain), 1997, 24/3 (82-86)

Favourable results of early second-phase antirheumatic drugs in rheumatoid arthritis. *Nederlands Tijdschrift voor Geneeskunde* (Netherlands), 1997, 141/15 (732-736)

Favourable effect of a short period of inpatient multidisciplinary team care in rheumatoid arthritis: A randomized trial. *Nederlands Tijdschrift voor Geneeskunde* (Netherlands), 1997, 141/15 (727-731)

Effects of unsaturated fatty acids on interleukin-1beta production by human monocytes. *Cytokine* (UK), 1997, 9/12 (1008-1012)

Oral administration of unsaturated fatty acids: Effects on human peripheral blood T lymphocyte proliferation. *Journal of Leukocyte Biology*, 1997, 62/4 (438-443)

Gammalinolenic acid and dihomogammalinolenic acid suppress the CD3-mediated signal transduction pathway in human T cells. *Clinical Immunology and Immunopathology*, 1997, 83/3 (237-244)

Omega-3 fatty acids in rheumatoid arthritis: An overview. *Seminars in Arthritis and Rheumatism*, 1998, 27/6 (366-370)

Over-the-counter complementary remedies used for arthritis. *Pharmaceutical Journal* (UK), 1998, 260/6997 (830-831)

Plasma omega-3 fatty acids before and after nutritional therapy. *Journal of Nutritional and Environmental Medicine* (UK), 1998, 8/1 (25-34)

Modulation of pro-inflammatory cytokine biology by unsaturated fatty acids. *Zeitschrift fur Ernahrungswissenschaft* (Germany), 1998, 37/Suppl. 1 (57-65)

Anti-inflammatory activity of a lipid fraction (Lyprinol) from the NZ green-lipped mussel. *Inflammopharmacology* (Netherlands), 1997, 5/3 (237-246)

n-3 polyunsaturated fatty acids and cytokine production in health and disease. *Annals of Nutrition and Metabolism* (Switzerland), 1997, 41/4 (203-234)

Nutritional management of osteoarthritis. *Veterinary Clinics of North America—Small Animal Practice*, 1997, 27/4 (883-911)

Lipid mediators in inflammatory disorders. *Drugs* (New Zealand), 1998, 55/4 (487-496)

Glucosamine sulfate for osteoarthritis. *Annals of Pharmacotherapy*, 1998, 32/5 (580-587)

Arthritis with nutritional rehabilitation: A case report. *Journal of Sports Chiropractic and Rehabilitation*, 1998, 12/1 (20-23)

Critical roles of glycosaminoglycan side chains of cartilage proteoglycan (aggrecan) in antigen recognition and presentation. *Journal of Immunology*, 1998, 160/8 (3812-3819)

Glycosaminoglycan components in temporomandibular joint synovial fluid as markers of joint pathology. *Journal of Oral and Maxillofacial Surgery*, 1998, 56/2 (209-213)

Synovial fluid chondroitin and keratan sulphate epitopes, glycosaminoglycans, and hyaluronan in arthritic and normal knees. *Annals of the Rheumatic Diseases* (UK), 1997, 56/5 (299-307)

Modulation of adjuvant-induced arthritis by dietary arachidonic acid in essential fatty acid-deficient rats. *Lipids*, 1997, 32/9 (979-988)

Clinical trials of herbs. *Primary Care—Clinics in Office Practice*, 1997, 24/4 (889-903)

hprt-Mutant T cells in the peripheral blood and synovial tissue of patients with rheumatoid arthritis. *Arthritis and Rheumatism*, 1998, 41/10 (1772-1782)

Therapeutic advances in systemic lupus erythematosus. *Current Opinion in Rheumatology*, 1998, 10/5 (435-441)

Physiological characterization of mBSA antigen induced arthritis in the rat. I. Vascular leakiness and pannus growth. *Journal of Rheumatology* (Canada), 1998, 25/9 (1772-1777)

Folic acid supplementation prevents deficient blood folate levels and hyperhomocysteinemia during longterm, low dose methotrexate therapy for rheumatoid arthritis: Implications for cardiovascular disease prevention. *Journal of Rheumatology* (Canada), 1998, 25/3 (441-446)

The efficacy of folic acid and folinic acid in reducing methotrexate gastrointestinal toxicity in rheumatoid arthritis. A metaanalysis of randomized controlled trials. *Journal of Rheumatology* (Canada), 1998, 25/1 (36-43)

The effects of daily intake of folic acid on the efficacy of methotrexate therapy in children with juvenile rheumatoid arthritis. A controlled study. *Journal of Rheumatology* (Canada), 1997, 24/11 (2230-2232)

Perioperative use of methotrexate—A survey of clinical practice in the UK. *British Journal of Rheumatology* (UK), 1997, 36/9 (1009-1011)

Methotrexate in rheumatoid arthritis: When are liver biopsies needed? *BioDrugs* (New Zealand), 1997, 7/2 (85-90)

Lymphoma in patients with rheumatoid arthritis: Association with the disease state or methotrexate treatment. *Seminars in Arthritis and Rheumatism*, 1997, 26/6 (794-804)

Rheumatoid arthritis and metal compounds—Perspectives on the role of oxygen radical detoxification. *Analyst* (UK), 1998, 123/1 (3-6)

Effect of Santolina oblongifola on ACII-immunized animals. *Inflammopharmacology* (Netherlands), 1997, 5/4 (351-361)

Matrix metalloproteinases in skin. *Experimental Dermatology* (Denmark), 1997, 6/5 (199-213)

Matrix metalloproteinases: Novel targets for directed cancer therapy. *Drugs and Aging* (New Zealand), 1997, 11/3 (229-244)

Matrix metalloproteinases. *Journal of UOEH* (Japan), 1997, 19/3 (229-232)

Mechanism of inhibition of the human matrix metalloproteinase stromelysin-1 by TIMP-1. *Nature* (UK), 1997, 389/6646 (77-81)

Antioxidant functions of micronutriments in the general population and critically ill patients. *Nutrition Clinique et Metabolisme* (France), 1997, 11/2 (125-132)

A novel series of matrix metalloproteinase inhibitors for the treatment of inflammatory disorders. *Bioorganic and Medicinal Chemistry Letters* (UK), 1997, 7/7 (897-902)

Anti-inflammatory activity of the aqueous extract from Rhizoma smilacis glabrae. *Pharmacological Research* (UK), 1997, 36/4 (309-314)

Salubrious effect of Semecarpus anacardium against lipid peroxidative changes in adjuvant arthritis studied in rats. *Molecular and Cellular Biochemistry* (Netherlands), 1997, 175/1-2 (65-69)

Antioxidant functions of micronutriments in the general population and critically ill patients. *Nutrition Clinique et Metabolisme* (France), 1997, 11/2 (125-132)

High-risk subjects for vitamin deficiency. *European Journal of Cancer Prevention* (UK), 1997, 6/Suppl. 1 (S37-S42)

Efficacy of vitamin E versus diclofenac-sodium in the treatment of patients with chronic rheumatoid arthritis. *Zeitschrift fur Rheumatologie* (Germany), 1998, 57/4 (215-221)

Vitamin E in the treatment of rheumatic diseases. *Zeitschrift fur Rheumatologie* (Germany), 1998, 57/4 (207-214)

Oxidant-antioxidant imbalance in blood of children with juvenile rheumatoid arthritis. *BioFactors* (Netherlands), 1998, 8/1-2 (155-159)

Effect of vitamin E on vascular responses of thoracic aorta in rat experimental arthritis. *General Pharmacology,* 1998, 31/1 (149-153)

Abnormal vitamin B6 status in rheumatoid cachexia. Association with spontaneous tumor necrosis factor alpha production and markers of inflammation. *Arthritis Rheum* 1995 Jan;38(1):105-9

Supplementation with folic acid during methotrexate therapy for rheumatoid arthritis. A double-blind, placebo-controlled trial. *Ann Intern Med* 1994 Dec 1;121(11):833-41

Calcium and vitamin D3 supplementation prevents bone loss in the spine secondary to low-dose corticosteroids in patients with rheumatoid arthritis. A randomized, double-blind, placebo-controlled trial. *Ann Intern Med* 1996 Dec 15;125(12):961-8

Matrix metalloproteinase inhibitors. *Expert Opinion on Therapeutic Patents* (UK), 1997, 7/10 (1213-1216)

Treatment of rheumatoid arthritis with blackcurrant seed oil. *Br. J. Rheumatol.* (UK), 1994, 33/9 (847-852)

Treatment of rheumatoid arthritis with gammalinolenic acid. *Ann. Intern. Med.*, 1993, 119/9 (867-873)

Validation of a meta-analysis: The effects of fish oil in rheumatoid arthritis. *Journal of Clinical Epidemiology,* 1995, 48/11 (1379-1390)

Botanical lipids: Effects on inflammation, immune responses, and rheumatoid arthritis. *Seminars in Arthritis and Rheumatism*, 1995, 25/2 (87-96)

n-3 Polyunsaturated fatty acids: Update 1995. *European Journal of Clinical Investigation* (UK), 1995, 25/9

Marine and botanical lipids as immunomodulatory and therapeutic agents in the treatment of rheumatoid arthritis. *Rheumatic Disease Clinics of North America*, 1995, 21/3 (759-777)

Attenuation of adjuvant arthritis in rats by treatment with oxygen radical scavengers. *Immunol. Cell Biol.* (Australia), 1994, 72/5

Alteration of the cellular fatty acid profile and the production of eicosanoids in human monocytes by gamma-linolenic acid. *Arthritis Rheum.* 1990, 33/10 (1526-1533)

Suppression of acute and chronic inflammation by dietary gamma linolenic acid. *J. Rheumatol.* (Canada), 1989, 16/6 (729-733)

Reactive oxygen species, lipid peroxides and essential fatty acids in patients with rheumatoid arthritis and systemic lupus erythematosus. *Prostaglandins Leukotrienes Essent. Fatty Acids* (UK), 1991, 43/4

Suppression of acute and chronic inflammation by dietary gamma linolenic acid. *J. Rheumatol.* (Canada), 1989, 16/6 (729-733)

Effects of fish oil supplementation on non-steroidal anti-inflammatory drug requirement in patients with mild rheumatoid arthritis—a double-blind placebo controlled study. *Br J Rheumatol* (England) Nov 1993, 32 (11) p982-9

Association of etretinate and fish oil in psoriasis therapy. Inhibition of hypertriglyceridemia resulting from retinoid therapy after fish oil supplementation. *Acta Derm Venereol Suppl* (Stockh) (Norway) 1994, 186 p151-3

Intravenous infusion of n-3 polyunsaturated fatty acids. *Proc Soc Exp Biol Med* Jun 1992, 200 (2) p171-3

Effects of dietary fish oil lipids on allergic and inflammatory diseases. *Allergy Proc* Sep-Oct 1991, 12 (5) p299-303

Omega-3 fatty acids in health and disease and in growth and development. *Am J Clin Nutr* Sep 1991, 54 (3) p438-63

The effect of dietary fish oil supplement upon the content of dihomo-gammalinolenic acid in human plasma phospholipids. *Prostaglandins Leukot Essent Fatty Acids* (Scotland) May 1990, 40 (1) p9-12

Summary of the NATO advanced research workshop on dietary omega 3 and omega 6 fatty acids: biological effects and nutritional essentiality. *J Nutr* Apr 1989, 119 (4) p521-8

Health effects and metabolism of dietary eicosapentaenoic acid. *Prog Food Nutr Sci* (England) 1988, 12 (2) p111-50

[Potential value of eicosapentaenoic acid]. *Allerg Immunol* (Paris) (France) Oct 1987, 19 (8 Suppl) p12-3

Collagen antibodies in Ross River virus disease (epidemic polyarthritis). *Rheumatol Int* (Germany, West) 1987, 7 (6) p267-9

Effects of dietary supplementation with marine fish oil on leukocyte lipid mediator generation and function in rheumatoid arthritis. *Arthritis Rheum* Sep 1987, 30 (9) p988-97

Low prevalences of coronary heart disease (CHD), psoriasis, asthma and rheumatoid arthritis in Eskimos: are they caused by high dietary intake of eicosapentaenoic acid (EPA), a genetic variation of essential fatty acid (EFA) metabolism or a combination of both? *Med Hypotheses* (England) Apr 1987, 22 (4) p421-8

Inhibition of elastase enzyme release from human polymorphonuclear leukocytes by *N*-acetyl-galactosamine and *N*-acetylglucosamine. *Clin Exp Rheumatol* (Italy) Jan-Feb 1991, 9 (1) p17-21

Severe rheumatoid arthritis: current options in drug therapy. *Geriatrics* Dec 1990, 45 (12) p43-8

Terminal *N*-acetylglucosamine in chronic synovitis. *Br J Rheumatol* (England) Feb 1990, 29 (1) p25-31

Membrane *N*-acetylglucosamine: expression by cells in rheumatoid synovial fluid, and by pre-cultured monocytes. *Br J Exp Pathol* (England) Oct 1989, 70 (5) p567-77

Serum levels of interleukin-2 receptor and activity of rheumatic diseases characterized by immune system activation. *Arthritis Rheum* Nov 1988, 31 (11) p1358-64

[Therapy of gonarthrosis using chondroprotective substances. Prospective comparative study of glucosamine sulphate and glycosaminoglycan polysulphate]. *Fortschr Med* (Germany, East) Jun 28 1984, 102 (24) p676-82

Oral glucosamine sulphate in the management of arthrosis: report on a multi-centre open investigation in Portugal. *Pharmatherapeutica* (England) 1982, 3 (3) p157-68

Double-blind clinical evaluation of intra-articular glucosamine in outpatients with gonarthrosis. *Clin Ther* 1981, 3 (5) p336-43

A double-blind placebo controlled trial of Efamol Marine on skin and joint symptoms of psoriatic arthritis. *Br J Rheumatol* (England) Oct 1994, 33 (10) p954-8

Evening primrose oil in patients with rheumatoid arthritis and side-effects of non-steroidal anti-inflammatory drugs. *Br J Rheumatol* (England) Oct 1991, 30 (5) p370-2

Essential fatty acid and prostaglandin metabolism in Sjogren's syndrome, systemic sclerosis and rheumatoid arthritis. *Scand J Rheumatol Suppl* (Sweden) 1986, 61 P242-5

Beneficial effect of eicosapentaenoic and docosahexaenoic acids in the management of systemic lupus erythematosus and its relationship to the cytokine network. *Prostaglandins Leukot Essent Fatty Acids* (SCOT) Sep 199451 (3) p207-13

Fish-oil fatty acid supplementation in active rheumatoid arthritis. A double-blinded, controlled, crossover study. *Ann Intern Med* Apr 1987, 106 (4) p497-503

Zonal distribution of chondroitin-4-sulphate/dermatan sulphate and chondroitin-6- sulphate in normal and diseased human synovium. *Ann Rheum Dis* (England) Jan 1994, 53 (1) p35-8

Asthma

Mortality associated with low plasma concentration of beta carotene and the effect of oral supplementation. *JAMA* 1996 Mar 6;275(9):699-703

Local and systemic effects of cigarette smoking on folate and vitamin B-12. *Am J Clin Nutr* 1994 Oct;60(4):559-66

Influence of smoking on folate intake and blood folate concentrations in a group of elderly Spanish men. *J Am Coll Nutr* 1994 Feb;13(1):68-72

Reduced plasma ascorbic acid concentrations in nonsmokers regularly exposed to environmental tobacco smoke. *Am J Clin Nutr* 1993 Dec;58(6):886-90

Vitamin C pharmacokinetics in healthy volunteers: evidence for a recommended dietary allowance. *Proc Natl Acad Sci U S A* 1996 Apr 16;93(8):3704-9

Vitamin C status and respiratory function. *Eur J Clin Nutr* 1996 Sep;50(9):573-9

Does dietary intake of vitamins C and E influence lung function in older people? *Am J Respir Crit Care Med* 1996 Nov;154(5):1401-4

Ascorbic acid and dehydroascorbic acid as biomarkers of oxidative stress caused by smoking. *Am J Clin Nutr* 1997 Apr;65(4):959-63

Blocking effect of vitamin C in exercise-induced asthma. *Arch Pediatr Adolesc Med* 1997 Apr;151(4):367-70

Assessment of vitamin A status in chronic obstructive pulmonary disease patients and healthy smokers. *Am J Clin Nutr* 1996 Dec;64(6):928-34

Ascorbic acid in bronchial asthma. *S Afr Med J* 1983 Apr 23;63(17):649-52

A diet free from additives in the management of allergic disease. *Clin Allergy* 1977 Sep;7(5):417-21

Co-oxidation of carotenes requires one soybean lipoxygenase isoenzyme. *Biochim Biophys Acta* 1979 Dec 18;575(3):439-45

Vegan regimen with reduced medication in the treatment of bronchial asthma. *J Asthma* 1985;22(1):45-55

Capsaicin-induced desensitization of airway mucosa to cigarette smoke, mechanical and chemical irritants. *Nature* 1983 Mar 17-23;302(5905):251-3

Can dietary selenium reduce leukotriene production? *Med Hypotheses* 1984 Jan;13(1):45-50

Children with allergic rhinitis and/or bronchial asthma treated with elimination diet: a five-year follow-up. *Ann Allergy* 1980 May;44(5):273

The effects of vitamin E on arachidonic acid metabolism. *Ann N Y Acad Sci* 1982;393:376-91

Sensitivity to ingested metabisulfites in asthmatic subjects. *J Allergy Clin Immunol* 1981 Jul;68(1):26-32

Aspirin-induced asthma in children. *Ann Allergy* 1982 Jan;48(1):1-5

Inhibition of fatty acid oxygenases by onion and garlic oils. Evidence for the mechanism by which these oils inhibit platelet aggregation. *Biochem Pharmacol* 1980 Dec 1;29(23):3169-73

Depressed plasma pyridoxal phosphate concentrations in adult asthmatics. *Am J Clin Nutr* 1985 Apr;41(4):684-8

Pyridoxine treatment of childhood bronchial asthma. *Ann Allergy* 1975 Aug;35(2):93-7

Histamine and ascorbic acid in human blood. *J Nutr* 1980 Apr;110(4):662-8

Plasma vitamin C (ascorbic acid) levels in asthmatic children. *Afr J Med Med Sci* 1985 Sep-Dec;14(3-4):115-20

Plasma and white blood cell ascorbic acid concentrations in patients with bronchial asthma. *Clin Chim Acta* 1979 Mar 1;92(2):161-6

Effect of ascorbic acid on response to methacholine challenge in asthmatic subjects. *Am Rev Respir Dis* 1983 Feb;127(2):143-7

High dose ascorbic acid in Nigerian asthmatics. *Trop Geogr Med* 1980 Jun;32(2):132-7

Inhibition of histamine-induced airway constriction by ascorbic acid. *J Allergy Clin Immunol* 1973 Apr;51(4):218-26

The attenuation of exercise-induced bronchospasm by ascorbic acid. *Ann Allergy* 1982 Sep;49(3):146-51

The effect of vitamin C on antigen-induced bronchospasm. *J Allergy Clin Immunol* 1979 Jan;63(1):61-4

Bronchodilating effect of intravenous magnesium sulfate in bronchial asthma. *JAMA* 1987 Feb 27;257(8):1076-8

Effect of parenteral magnesium on pulmonary function, plasma cAMP, and histamine in bronchial asthma. *J Asthma* 1985;22(1):3-11

Prospects for modifying the allergic response by fish oil diets. *Clin Allergy* 1986 Mar;16(2):89-100

Objective clinical and laboratory studies of immediate hypersensitivity reactions to foods in asthmatic children. *J Allergy Clin Immunol* 1976 Oct;58(4):500-15

Importance of food allergy in childhood asthma. *Allergol Immunopathol* (Madr) 1981;Suppl 9:71-3

Validation of a rhinitis symptom questionnaire (ISAAC core questions) in a population of Swiss school children visiting the school health services. SCARPOL-team. Swiss Study on Childhood Allergy and Respiratory Symptom with respect to Air Pollution and Climate. International Study of Asthma and Allergies in Childhood. *Pediatr Allergy Immunol* (Denmark) May 1997, 8 (2) p75-82

Worldwide variations in prevalence of symptoms of allergic rhinoconjunctivitis in children: the International Study of Asthma and Allergies in Childhood (ISAAC). *Pediatr Allergy Immunol* (Denmark) Nov 1997, 8 (4) p161-76

[Fatal asthma. Description and study of risk factors, in the heart of an asthmatic population followed by the College of Pneumonology of the Southwest]. *Rev Mal Respir* (France) Dec 1997, 14 (6) p473-80

Asthma among secondary schoolchildren in relation to the school environment. *Clin Exp Allergy* (England) Nov 1997, 27 (11) p1270-8

Use of herbal products, coffee or black tea, and over-the-counter medications as self-treatments among adults with asthma. *J Allergy Clin Immunol* Dec 1997, 100 (6 Pt 1) p789-91

Efficacy and safety of loratadine plus pseudoephedrine in patients with seasonal allergic rhinitis and mild asthma. *J Allergy Clin Immunol* Dec 1997, 100 (6 Pt 1) p781-8

Occupational asthma induced by garlic dust. *J Allergy Clin Immunol* Dec 1997, 100 (6 Pt 1) p734-8

Gastro-oesophageal reflux prevalence and relationship with bronchial reactivity in asthma. *Eur Respir J* (Denmark) Oct 1997, 10 (10) p2255-9

Do specialists order too many tests? The case of allergists and pediatric asthma. *Ann Allergy Asthma Immunol* Dec 1997, 79 (6) p496-502

Sensitization to indoor allergens and the risk for asthma hospitalization in children. *Ann Allergy Asthma Immunol* Nov 1997, 79 (5) p455-9

Airways obstruction in patients with long-term asthma consistent with 'irreversible asthma'. *Chest* Nov 5 1997, 112 (5) p1234-40

Intravenous magnesium sulfate in acute severe asthma not responding to conventional therapy. *Indian Pediatr* (India) May 1997, 34 (5) p389-97

The safety of asthma and allergy medications during pregnancy. *J Allergy Clin Immunol* Sep 1997, 100 (3) p301-6

Prevalence of childhood asthma in Istanbul, Turkey. *Allergy* (Denmark) May 1997, 52 (5) p570-5

Asthma and allergy avoidance knowledge and behavior in postpartum women. *Ann Allergy Asthma Immunol* Jul 1997, 79 (1) p35-42

The effect of polyunsaturated fatty acids of the omega-3 class on the late phase of the allergic reaction in bronchial asthma patients] *Ter Arkh* (Russia) 1997, 69 (3) p31-3

Occupational asthma caused by triglycidyl isocyanurate (TGIC). *Clin Exp Allergy* (England) May 1997, 27 (5) p510-4

Sensitization to inhaled allergens as a risk factor for asthma and allergic diseases in Chinese population. *J Allergy Clin Immunol* May 1997, 99 (5) p594-9

Effect of inhaled magnesium sulfate on sodium metabisulfite-induced bronchoconstriction in asthma. *Chest* Apr 1997, 111 (4) p858-61

Parental smoking behavior and passive smoke exposure in children with asthma. *Ann Allergy Asthma Immunol* Apr 1997, 78 (4) p419-23

Care of asthma: allergy clinic versus emergency room. *Ann Allergy Asthma Immunol* Apr 1997, 78 (4) p373-80

Incidence and outcomes of asthma in the elderly. A population-based study in Rochester, Minnesota. *Chest* Feb 1997, 111 (2) p303-10

Occupational allergic rhinoconjunctivitis and asthma due to fennel seed. *Ann Allergy Asthma Immunol* Jan 1997, 78 (1) p37-40

Differences in nonspecific bronchial responsiveness between patients with asthma and patients with rhinitis are not explained by type and degree of inhalant allergy. *Int Arch Allergy Immunol* (Switzerland) Jan 1997, 112 (1) p65-72

Fatal asthma. A clinical study in the south of France. *Revue des Maladies Respiratoires* (France), 1997, 14/6 (473-480)

Genes for asthma? An analysis of the European Community Respiratory Health Survey. *American Journal of Respiratory and Critical Care Medicine*, 1997, 156/6 (1773-1780)

Recruitment of circulating allergen-specific T lymphocytes to the lung on allergen challenge in asthma. *Journal of Allergy and Clinical Immunology*, 1997, 100/5 (669-678)

Reduced interferon-gamma but normal IL-4 and IL-5 release by peripheral blood mononuclear cells from Xhosa children with atopic asthma. *Journal of Allergy and Clinical Immunology*, 1997, 100/5 (662-668)

Potentiation of histamine release against inhalant allergens (Dermatophagoides pteronyssinus) with bacterial antigens in bronchial asthma. *Journal of Investigational Allergology and Clinical Immunology* (Spain), 1997, 7/4 (210-215)

House dust mite avoidance measures improve peak flow and symptoms in patients with allergy but without asthma: A possible delay in the manifestation of clinical asthma? *Journal of Allergy and Clinical Immunology*, 1997, 100/3 (313-319)

Exposure chamber for allergen challenge. A placebo-controlled, double-blind trial in house-dust-mite asthma. *Allergy: European Journal of Allergy and Clinical Immunology* (Denmark), 1997, 52/8 (821-828)

Asthma, bronchial hyperreactivity and mediator release in children with birch pollinosis. ECP and EPX levels are not related to bronchial hyperreactivity. *Clinical and Experimental Allergy* (UK), 1997, 27/5 (530-539)

Birthweight and preterm birth in relation to indicators of childhood asthma. *Canadian Respiratory Journal* (Canada), 1997, 4/2 (91-97)

The role of cockroach allergy and exposure to cockroach allergen in causing morbidity among inner-city children with asthma. *New England Journal of Medicine*, 1997, 336/19 (1356-1363)

Purification and characterization of a soybean hull allergen responsible for the Barcelona asthma outbreaks. II. Purification and sequencing of the Gly m 2 allergen. *Clinical and Experimental Allergy* (UK), 1997, 27/4 (424-430)

Comparative degree and type of sensitization to common indoor and outdoor allergens in subjects with allergic rhinitis and/or asthma. *Clinical and Experimental Allergy* (UK), 1997, 27/1 (52-59)

A controlled trial of immunotherapy for asthma in allergic children. *New England Journal of Medicine*, 1997, 336/5 (324-331)

Occupational asthma due to chrome and nickel electroplating. *Thorax* (UK), 1997, 52/1 (28-32)

[Treatment possibilities in bronchial asthma. Alternative methods, naturopathy methods, academic medicine. German Respiratory Tract Group e.V., German Allergy and Asthma Society e.V., Patient Group of Respiratory Tract Diseases e.V.] *Med Monatsschr Pharm* (Germany) Nov 1997, 20 (11) p310-4

Influence of inhaled corticosteroids and dietary intake on bone density and metabolism in patients with moderate to severe asthma. *J Am Diet Assoc* Dec 1997, 97 (12) p1401-6

Nebulized glutathione induces bronchoconstriction in patients with mild asthma. *American Journal of Respiratory and Critical Care Medicine*, 1997, 156/2 I (425-430)

Oxidant stress, anti-oxidants, nitric oxide and essential fatty acids in bronchial asthma. *Medical Science Research* (UK), 1997, 25/5 (307-309)

[Effects of laser therapy on lipids and antioxidants in blood of patients with bronchial asthma] *Ter Arkh* (Russia) 1997, 69 (12) p49-50

The role of magnesium in the pathogenesis and therapy of bronchial asthma. *Przegl Lek* (Poland) 1997, 54 (9) p630-3

Investigation of the effect of short-term change in dietary magnesium intake in asthma. *Eur Respir J* (Denmark) Oct 1997, 10 (10) p2225-9

Alternative therapies for asthma. *Curr Opin Pulm Med* Jan 1997, 3 (1) p61-71

Nutrition and asthma. *Arch Intern Med* Jan 13 1997, 157 (1) p23-34

Bronchial reactivity and intracellular magnesium: A possible mechanism for the bronchodilating effects of magnesium in asthma. *Clinical Science* (UK), 1998, 95/2 (137-142)

Use of intravenous magnesium sulfate in acute asthma. *Farmacia Hospitalaria* (Spain), 1998, 22/1 (39-42)

Contemporary issues in the emergency care of children with asthma. *Immunology and Allergy Clinics of North America*, 1998, 18/1 (211-240)

Effect of gammalinolenic acid, dihomogammalinolenic acid, ascorbyl-6-gammalinolenic acid and ascorbyl-6-dihomo gammalinolenic acid on histamine-and methacholine-induced contraction of the isolated guinea pig tracheal chain. *Prostaglandins Leukotrienes and Essential Fatty Acids* (UK), 1998, 58/4 (327-331)

New antiasthmatic drugs from traditional medicine? *Int Arch Allergy Appl Immunol* 1991;94(1-4):262-5

Antiasthmatic effects of onions. Prevention of platelet-activating factor induced bronchial hyperreactivity to histamine in guinea pigs by dyphenylthiosulfinate. *Int. Arch. Allergy Appl. Immunol* (Switzerland), 1989, 88/1-2 (228-230)

Antiasthmatic effects of onions. Alk(en)ylsulfinothioic acid alk(en)yl-esters inhibit histamine release, leukotriene and thromboxane biosynthesis in vitro and counteract PAF and allergen-induced bronchial obstruction in vivo. *Biochem. Pharmacol.* (UK), 1988, 37/23 (4479-4486)

Onion extracts as antiasthmatic drugs? *Allergologie* (Germany, West), 1987, 10/8 (316-324)

Antiasthmatic effects of onions. Inhibition of platelet-activating factor-induced bronchial obstruction by onion oils. *Int. Arch. Allergy Appl. Immunol.* (Switzerland), 1987, 82/3-4 (535-536)

Antiasthmatic effects of onion extracts—Detection of benzyl- and other isothiocyanates (mustard oils) as antiasthmatic compounds of plant origin. *Germany, West Eur. J. Pharmacol.* (Netherlands), 1985, 107/1 (17-24)

Vitamin E: Immunomodulating effect in patients with bronchial asthma. *Voprosy Meditsinskoj Khimii* (Russian Federation), 1995, 41/4 (33-36)

The role of free radicals in disease. *Australian and New Zealand Journal of Ophthalmology* (Australia), 1995, 23/1 (3-7)

Increased lipid peroxidation and decreased antioxidants in lungs of guinea pigs following an allergic pulmonary response. *Toxicology and Applied Pharmacology,* 1995, 132/1 (72-81)

A prospective study of diet and adult-onset asthma. *American Journal of Respiratory and Critical Care Medicine,* 1995, 151/5 (1401-1408)

Oxygen radicals in lung pathology. *Free Radic. Biol. Med.*, 1990, 9/5 (381-400)

Effects of the ozone on the respiratory tract. *Zentralbl. Arbeitsmed.Arbeitssch.Prophyl.Ergonomie* (Germany, Federal Republic of), 1988, 38/3 (62-73)

Genetics and respiratory diseases. *Jpn. J. Thorac. Dis.* (JA), 1985, 23/9 (991-997)

Vitamin therapy in the absence of obvious deficiency. What is the evidence? *Denmark Drugs* (Australia), 1984, 27/2 (148-170)

Nutritional influences on the toxicity of environmental pollutants. The effect of vitamin A on NO_2 induced lung injury. A review. *J. Appl. Nutr.*, 1978, 30/3-44 (88-113)

Phosphodiesterase IV inhibitors synergistically potentiate relaxation induced by forskolin in guinea pig trachea. *Clinical and Experimental Pharmacology and Physiology* (Australia), 1998, 25/2 (114-119)

The role of prostaglandin F(2alpha) in byssinosis. *Am. Ind. Hyg. Assoc. J.*, 1980, 41/5 (382-384)

The scientific rediscovery of an ancient Chinese herbal medicine. *J Altern Complement Med* Fall 1998, 4 (3) p289-303

The hypochlorhydria of asthma in childhood. *Quart. J. Med.* 24:181-197, 1931

Encyclopedia of Natural Medicine. Rocklin, CA: Prima Publishing, 1990

Sulfite-sensitive asthma. *Res. Instit. Of Scripps Clinic Scientific Report 39*:57-58, 1982-1983

Vitamin B12 therapy in allergy and chronic dermatoses. *J. Allergy* 2:183-5, 1951

Upon therapy for asthma using vitamin B12. *Riforma Medica* August 2, 1952, pp. 849-51

G B reported in Med. *World News*, July 14, 1986

Hypochlorhydria in asthma with special reference to the age incidence. *Quart. J. Med.* 4:397-405, 1935

Alterations in human leukocyte function induced by ingestion of eicosapentaenoic acid. *J Clin Immunol* Sep 1986, 6 (5) p402-10

The treatment of asthmatic patients using an alpha-adrenergic receptor blocking agent, co-dergocrine mesylate ('Hydergine'). *Pharmatherapeutica* (England) 1980, 2 (5) p330-6

Plasma vitamin C (ascorbic acid) levels in asthmatic children. *Afr J Med Med Sci* (England) Sep-Dec 1985, 14 (3-4)

Intravenous magnesium sulfate as an adjunct in the treatment of acute asthma. *Chest* Jun 1995, 107 (6) p1576-81

[Magnesium in lung diseases]. *Tidsskr Nor Laegeforen* (Norway) Mar 10 1995, 115 (7) p827-8

Asthma, inhaled oxidants, and dietary antioxidants. *Am J Clin Nutr* Mar 1995, 61 (3 Suppl) p625S-630S

Relaxant effects of forskolin on guinea pig tracheal smooth muscle. *Lung* (Germany, West), 1987, 165/4 (225-237)

Bronchial asthma: Factors which contribute to 'intractable asthma' and approach to new treatments, from the standpoint of the bronchial pathophysiology. *Jpn. J. Thorac. Dis.* (Japan), 1985, 23/9 (971-980)

Bronchodilator and antiallergy activity of forskolin. *Eur. J. Pharmacol.* (Netherlands), 1985, 111/1 (1-8)

Activation of cAMP-dependent pathways in human airway smooth muscle cells inhibits TNF-alpha-induced ICAM-1 and VCAM-1 expression and T lymphocyte adhesion. *J Immunol* Mar 1 1995, 154 (5) p2358-65

Consequences of magnesium deficiency on the enhancement of stress reactions; preventive and therapeutic implications (a review). *J Am Coll Nutr* Oct 1994, 13 (5) p429-46

Rapid infusion of magnesium sulfate obviates need for intubation in status asthmaticus. *Am J Emerg Med* Mar 1994, 12 (2)

Magnesium sulfate for the treatment of bronchospasm complicating acute bronchitis in a four-months'-pregnant woman. *Ann Emerg Med* Aug 1993, 22 (8) p1365-7

Acetylcysteine for life-threatening acute bronchial obstruction. *Ann. Intern. Med.*, 1978, 88/5 (656)

Effect of the combination of human thioredoxin and *L*-cysteine on ischemia- reperfusion injury in isolated rat lungs. *European Surgical Research* (Switzerland), 1995, 27/6 (363-370)

Effects of *N*-acetyl-*L*-cysteine on regional blood flow during endotoxic shock. *European Surgical Research* (Switzerland), 1995, 27/5 (292-300)

A combination of cefuroxime and *N*-acetyl-cysteine for the treatment of lower respiratory tract infections in children. *Int. J. Clin. Pharmacol. Ther. Toxicol.* (Germany, West), 1985, 23/5

Irish general practice study of acetylcysteine (Fabrol) in chronic bronchitis. *J. Int. Med. Res.* (England), 1984, 12/2 (96-101)

Regulation of Ca2+-dependent K+-channel activity in tracheal myocytes by phosphorylation. *Nature* (UK), 1989, 341/6238 (152-154)

Effects of *N*-acetyl-*L*-cysteine on regional blood flow during endotoxic shock. *European Surgical Research* (Switzerland), 1995, 27/5 (292-300)

Irish general practice study of acetylcysteine (Fabrol) in chronic bronchitis. *J. Int. Med. Res.* (England), 1984, 12/2 (96-101)

Atherosclerosis

The role of homocysteine, folate and other B-vitamins in the development of atherosclerosis. *Arch Latinoam Nutr* (Venezuela) Jun 1997, 47 (2 Suppl 1) p9-12

Effect of gemfibrozil on early carotid atherosclerosis in diabetic patients with hyperlipidaemia. *Int Angiol* (Italy) Dec 1997, 16 (4) p258-61

Erythrocyte selenium-glutathione peroxidase activity is lower in patients with coronary atherosclerosis. *Jpn Heart J* (Japan) Nov 1997, 38 (6) p793-8

[Prevention of atherosclerosis in diabetics]. *Cas Lek Cesk* (Czech Republic) Sep 10 1997, 136 (17) p523-6

Insulin sensitivity and intake of vitamins E and C in African American, Hispanic, and non-Hispanic white men and women: the Insulin Resistance and. *Am J Clin Nutr* Nov 1997, 66 (5) p1224-31

Moderate beer consumption and positive biochemical changes in patients with coronary atherosclerosis. *J Intern Med* (England) Sep 1997, 242 (3) p219-24

Prevention of the angiographic progression of coronary and vein-graft atherosclerosis by gemfibrozil after coronary bypass surgery in men with low levels of HDL cholesterol. Lopid Coronary Angiography Trial (LOCAT) Study Group [see comments]. *Circulation* Oct 7 1997, 96 (7) p2137-43

Effects of malnutrition and atherosclerosis on the fatty acid composition of plasma phospholipids in the elderly. *Ann Nutr Metab* (Switzerland) 1997, 41 (3) p166-72

Effects of fluvastatin on coronary atherosclerosis in patients with mild to moderate cholesterol elevations (Lipoprotein and Coronary. *Am J Cardiol* Aug 1 1997, 80 (3) p278-86

Association of serum vitamin levels, LDL susceptibility to oxidation, and autoantibodies against MDA-LDL with carotid atherosclerosis. A case-control study. The ARIC Study Investigators. Atherosclerosis Risk in Communities. *Arterioscler Thromb Vasc Biol* Jun 1997, 17 (6) p1171-7

Relation of plasma phospholipid and cholesterol ester fatty acid composition to carotid artery intima-media thickness: the Atherosclerosis. *Am J Clin Nutr* Feb 1997, 65 (2) p551-9

LDL-containing immune complexes and atherosclerosis in diabetes. *Diabetes Reviews*, 1997, 5/4 (410-424)

Small, dense LDL, risk factor for atherosclerosis disease. Therapeutical management. *Revue Francaise d'Endocrinologie Clinique—Nutrition et Metabolisme* (France), 1997, 38/4-5 (307-314)

Bezafibrate following acute myocardial infarction: Important findings from the Bezafibrate Coronary Atherosclerosis Intervention Trial. *Fibrinolysis and Proteolysis* (UK), 1997, 11/ Suppl. 1 (159-162)

Atherosclerosis: From a purely metabolic disease to chronic inflammation with aspects of a storage disease. *Prakticky Lekar* (Czech Republic), 1997, 77/6 (266-275)

The effect of dietary fat, antioxidants, and pro-oxidants on blood lipids, lipoproteins, and atherosclerosis. *Journal of the American Dietetic Association*, 1997, 97/7 Suppl. (S31-S41)

Coronary risk factors, endothelial function, and atherosclerosis: A review. *Clinical Cardiology*, 1997, 20/5 (426-432)

Role of the natural antioxidants in the prevention of atherosclerosis. *Farmacia Clinica* (Spain), 1997, 14/1 (43-48)

Antioxidant content in low density lipoprotein and lipoprotein oxidation in vivo and in vitro. *Free Radical Research* (UK), 1998, 29/2 (165-173)

Are there protective environmental factors? *Archives des Maladies du Coeur et des Vaisseaux* (France), 1998, 91/Spec. Iss. 5 (27-31)

Functional food science and the cardiovascular system. *British Journal of Nutrition* (UK), 1998, 80/Suppl. 1 (S113-S146)

Folate deficiencies and cardiovascular pathologies. *Clinical Chemistry and Laboratory Medicine* (Germany), 1998, 36/7 (419-429)

Homocysteine vs cholesterol: Competing views, or a unifying explanation of arteriosclerotic cardiovascular disease? *Laboratory Medicine*, 1998, 29/7 (410-417)

Hyperhomocysteinemia and atherosclerotic vascular disease: Pathophysiology, screening, and treatment. *Archives of Internal Medicine*, 1998, 158/12 (1301-1306)

Emerging approaches in the prevention of atherosclerotic cardiovascular diseases. *International Journal of Clinical Practice, Supplement* (UK), 1998, -/94 (7-19)

Homocyst(e)inemia and risk of atherosclerosis: A clinical approach to evaluation and management. *Endocrinologist*, 1998, 8/3 (170-177)

High homocysteine, low folate, and low vitamin B6 concentrations. *Transplantation*, 1998, 65/4 (544-550)

Recommended dietary allowance of folic acid sufficient for low homocysteine level. *Netherlands Nederlands Tijdschrift voor Geneeskunde* (Netherlands), 1998, 142/14 (782-786)

Homocysteine and cardiovascular disease. *Annual Review of Medicine*, 1998, 49/- (31-62)

Vitamin supplementation reduces blood homocysteine levels: A controlled trial in patients with venous thrombosis and healthy volunteers. *Arteriosclerosis, Thrombosis, and Vascular Biology*, 1998, 18/3 (356-361)

Hyperhomocysteinaemia—A new risk factor for atherosclerosis. *Klinikarzt* (Germany), 1998, 27/3 (64-71)

Homocysteine and vascular diseases. *Hematologie* (France), 1998, 4/1 (7-16)

Effects of folic acid supplementation on hyperhomocysteinemia in CAPD patients: Effects on unsaturated fatty acids. *Japanese Journal of Nephrology* (Japan), 1998, 40/1 (8-16)

Low circulating folate and vitamin B6 concentrations risk factors for stroke, peripheral vascular disease, and coronary artery disease. *Circulation*, 1998, 97/5 (437-443)

Vitamins B6, B12, and folate: Association with plasma total homocysteine and risk of coronary atherosclerosis. *Journal of the American College of Nutrition*, 1998, 17/5 (435-441)

Prospective study of coronary heart disease incidence in relation to fasting total homocysteine, related genetic polymorphisms, and B vitamins: The atherosclerosis risk in communities (ARIC) study. *Circulation*, 1998, 98/3 (204-210)

Decreased prevalence of symptomatic atherosclerosis in arthritis patients on long-term aspirin therapy. *Angiology*, 1998, 49/ 10 (827-832)

Hypothesis: Cis-unsaturated fatty acids as potential anti-peptic ulcer drugs. *Prostaglandins Leukotrienes and Essential Fatty Acids* (UK), 1998, 58/5 (377-380)

Influence of long-chain polyunsaturated fatty acids on oxidation of low density lipoprotein. *Prostaglandins Leukotrienes and Essential Fatty Acids* (UK), 1998, 59/2 (143-151)

Effects of eicosapentaenoic acids on remnant-like particles, cholesterol concentrations and plasma fatty acid composition in patients with diabetes mellitus. *In Vivo* (Greece), 1998, 12/3 (311-314)

Omega-3 ethyl ester concentrate decreases total apolipoprotein CIII and increases antithrombin III in postmyocardial infarction patients. *Clinical Drug Investigation* (New Zealand), 1998, 15/6 (473-482)

A central role for protein kinase c overactivity in diabetic glomerulosclerosis: Implications for prevention with antioxidants, fish oil, and ACE inhibitors. *Medical Hypotheses* (UK), 1998, 50/2 (155-165)

Taurine in management of diffuse cerebral arteriopathy. Clinical and electroencephalographic observations, and mental test results. *Clin.Ter.* (Italy), 1974, 71/5 (427-436)

Effect of taurine on incipient senile involution of the brain. *Clin.Ter.* (Italy), 1974, 70/5 (425-433)

Ginkgo—Myth and reality. *Schweiz. Rundsch. Med. Prax.* (Switzerland), 1995, 84/1 (1-6)

Phytotherapy in cardiovascular diseases. Supportive therapy in early stages. *Therapiewoche* (Germany), 1994, 44/29 (1650-1653)

Study of the antiischemic action of EGb 761 in the treatment of peripheral arterial occlusive disease by TcPO2 determination. *Angiology*, 1994, 45/6 (413-417)

Up-regulation of intracellular signalling pathways may play a central pathogenic role in hypertension, atherogenesis, insulin resistance, and cancer promotion—the 'PKC syndrome'. *Medical Hypotheses* (UK), 1996, 46/3 (191-221)

Evaluation of the evidence on the role of tomato products in disease prevention. *Proceedings of the Society for Experimental Biology and Medicine*, 1998, 218/2 (140-143)

Copper: An antioxidant nutrient for cardiovascular health. *Curr. Opin. Lipidology* (UK), 1994, 5/1 (22-28)

Trace elements and cardiovascular diseases. *Acta Pharmacol. Toxicol.* (Denmark), 1986, 59/Suppl. 7 (317-324)

Increased cholesterol in plasma in a young man during experimental copper depletion. *Metab. Clin. Exp.*, 1984, 33/12 (1112-1118)

Antioxidant vitamin levels in plasma and low density lipoprotein of obese girls. *Free Radical Research* (UK), 1998, 28/1 (81-86)

Dietary iron concentration alters LDL oxidatively the effect of antioxidants. *Research Communications in Molecular Pathology and Pharmacology*, 1998, 99/1 (69-80)

Plasma antioxidant and trace element status in familial hypercholesterolemic patients treated with LDL-apheresis. *Annales Pharmaceutiques Francaises* (France), 1998, 56/1 (18-25)

Ascorbic acid clearance in diabetic nephropathy. *Journal of Diabetes and its Complications*, 1998, 12/5 (259-263)

Vascular damage from smoking: Disease mechanisms at the arterial wall. *Vascular Medicine* (UK), 1998, 3/1 (21-28)

Dynamics of vitamin E action against LDL oxidation. *Free Radical Research* (UK), 1998, 28/6 (561-572)

Cost-effectiveness of vitamin E therapy in the treatment of patients with angiographically proven coronary narrowing (CHAOS trial). *American Journal of Cardiology*, 1998, 82/4 (414-417)

Alpha-Tocopherol induces oxidative damage to DNA in the presence of copper(II) ions. *Chemical Research in Toxicology*, 1998, 11/8 (855-862)

Induction by lysophosphatidylcholine, a major phospholipid component of atherogenic lipoproteins, of human coronary artery smooth muscle cell migration. *Circulation*, 1998, 98/4 (353-359)

Erythrocyte antioxidant status in asymptomatic hypercholesterolemic men. *Atherosclerosis* (Ireland), 1998, 138/2 (375-381)

Monocyte superoxide production is inversely related to normal content of alpha-tocopherol in low-density lipoprotein. *Atherosclerosis* (Ireland), 1998, 138/2 (263-269)

Dehydroepiandrosterone protects low density lipoproteins against peroxidation by free radicals produced by gamma-radiolysis of ethanol-water mixtures. *Atherosclerosis* (Ireland), 1998, 136/1 (99-107)

Oxidation of low density lipoproteins in the pathogenesis of atherosclerosis. *Atherosclerosis* (Ireland), 1998, 137/Suppl. (S33-S38)

Vitamin E in diabetes mellitus. *Medizinische Welt* (Germany), 1998, 49/5 (250-255)

Metabolic consequences of reduced plasma LDL-C during hypolipidaemic therapy: Assessment of lipoperoxidation activity and vitamin E in lipoprotein fractions. *Klinicka Biochemie a Metabolismus* (Czech Republic), 1998, 6/2 (77-81)

Where are we with vitamin E? *Journal of Thrombosis and Thrombolysis* (Netherlands), 1998, 5/3 (209-214)

The antioxidative effects of the isoflavan glabridin on endogenous constituents of LDL during its oxidation. *Atherosclerosis* (Ireland), 1998, 137/1 (49-61)

Effect of vitamin E and beta carotene on the incidence of primary nonfatal myocardial infarction and fatal coronary heart disease. *Archives of Internal Medicine*, 1998, 158/6 (668-675)

Low-density lipoprotein oxidation and vitamins E and C in sustained and white-coat hypertension. *Hypertension*, 1998, 31/2 (621-626)

Progress in cardiology. *Medecine et Hygiene* (Switzerland), 1998, 56/2191 (16-20)

Effect of supplementation with vitamin E on LDL oxidizability and prevention of atherosclerosis. *BioFactors* (Netherlands), 1998, 7/1-2 (51-54)

Action of vitamin E as antioxidant against oxidative modification of low density lipoprotein. *BioFactors* (Netherlands), 1998, 7/1-2 (41-50)

Atherogenic lipoproteins support assembly of the prothrombinase complex and thrombin generation: Modulation by oxidation and vitamin E. *Blood*, 1998, 91/2 (508-515)

A double-blind crossover study in moderately hypercholesterolemic men that compared the effect of aged garlic extract and placebo administration on blood lipids. *Am J Clin Nutr* 1996 Dec;64(6):866-70

Plasma homocysteine levels and mortality in patients with coronary artery disease. *N Engl J Med* 1997 Jul 24;337(4):230-6 Comment in: *N Engl J Med* 1997 Nov 27;337(22):1631-2; discussion 1632-3

The effect of folic acid fortification on plasma folate and total homocysteine concentrations. *N Engl J Med* 1999 May 13;340(19):1449-54

Dietary supplement with vitamin C prevents nitrate tolerance. *J Clin Invest* 1998 Jul 1;102(1):67-71

Randomized, double-blind, placebo-controlled study of the preventive effect of supplemental oral vitamin C on attenuation of development of nitrate tolerance. *J Am Coll Cardiol* 1998 May;31(6):1323-9

Coenzyme Q_{10}: a new drug for cardiovascular disease. *J Clin Pharmacol* 1990 Jul;30(7):596-608

Italian multicenter study on the safety and efficacy of Coenzyme Q_{10} as adjunctive therapy in heart failure. CoQ_{10} Drug Surveillance Investigators. *Mol Aspects Med* 1994;15 Suppl:s287-94

Italian multicenter study on the safety and efficacy of coenzyme Q_{10} as adjunctive therapy in heart failure (interim analysis). The CoQ_{10} Drug Surveillance Investigators. *Clin Investig* 1993;71(8 Suppl):S145-9

Clinical experience of Coenzyme Q_{10} to enhance intraoperative myocardial protection in coronary artery revascularization. *Cardiovasc Drugs Ther* 1991 Mar;5 Suppl 2:297-300

Association between plasma homocysteine concentrations and extracranial carotid-artery stenosis. *N Engl J Med* 1995 Feb 2;332(5):286-91 Comment in: *N Engl J Med* 1995 Feb 2;332(5):328-9 Comment in: *N Engl J Med* 1995 Aug 3;333(5):325

Vitamin B-12, vitamin B-6, and folate nutritional status in men with hyperhomocysteinemia. *Am J Clin Nutr* 1993 Jan;57(1):47-53

Carotid and femoral artery wall thickness and stiffness in patients at risk for cardiovascular disease, with special emphasis on hyperhomocysteinemia. *Arterioscler Thromb Vasc Biol* 1998 Dec;18(12):1958-63

Serum homocysteine and risk of coronary heart disease and cerebrovascular disease in elderly men: a 10-year follow-up. *Arterioscler Thromb Vasc Biol* 1998 Dec;18(12):1895-901

Vitamin supplementation reduces blood homocysteine levels: a controlled trial in patients with venous thrombosis and healthy volunteers. *Arterioscler Thromb Vasc Biol* 1998 Mar;18(3):356-61

Plasma homocysteine levels related to interactions between folate status and methylenetetrahydrofolate reductase: a study in 52 healthy subjects. *Metabolism* 1998 Nov;47(11):1413-8

Vitamins B6, B12, and folate: association with plasma total homocysteine and risk of coronary atherosclerosis. *J Am Coll Nutr* 1998 Oct;17(5):435-41

Vitamins B6, B12, and folate: association with plasma total homocysteine and risk of coronary atherosclerosis. *J Am Coll Nutr* 1998 Oct;17(5):435-41

Effectiveness of low-dose crystalline nicotinic acid in men with low high-density lipoprotein cholesterol levels. *Arch Intern Med* 1996 May 27;156(10):1081-8

Clinical trial experience with extended-release niacin (Niaspan): dose-escalation study. *Am J Cardiol* 1998 Dec 17;82(12A):35U-38U; discussion 39U-41U

Vitamin E and atherosclerosis. *J Nutr* 1998 Oct;128(10):1593-6

Dynamics of vitamin E action against LDL oxidation. *Free Radic Res* 1998 Jun;28(6):561-72

Cost-effectiveness of vitamin E therapy in the treatment of patients with angiographically proven coronary narrowing (CHAOS trial). Cambridge Heart Antioxidant Study. *Am J Cardiol* 1998 Aug 15;82(4):414-7

Antioxidant vitamin intake and coronary mortality in a longitudinal population study. *Am J Epidemiol* 1994 Jun 15;139(12):1180-9

Will the 'good fairies' please prove to us that vitamin E lessens human degenerative disease? *Free Radic Res* 1997 Nov;27(5):511-32 Corrected and republished article originally printed in *Free Radic Res* 1997 Jun;26(6):565-83

Probucol and multivitamins in the prevention of restenosis after coronary angioplasty. Multivitamins and Probucol Study Group. *N Engl J Med* 1997 Aug 7;337(6):365-72 Comment in: *N Engl J Med* 1997 Dec 25;337(26):1918; discussion 1919

Effects of intravenous perilla oil emulsion on nutritional status, polyunsaturated fatty acid composition of tissue phospholipids, and thromboxane A2 production in streptozotocin-induced diabetic rats. *Nutrition* 1995 Sep-Oct;11(5):450-5

Homocysteine metabolism and risk of myocardial infarction: relation with vitamins B6, B12, and folate. *Am J Epidemiol* 1996 May 1;143(9):845-59

Homocysteine and atherothrombosis. *N Engl J Med* 1998 Apr 9;338(15):1042-50 Comment in: *N Engl J Med* 1998 Aug 13;339(7):477-8; discussion 479

Homocysteine and cardiovascular disease. *Annu Rev Med* 1998;49:31-62

The antiatherosclerotic effect of Allium sativum. *Atherosclerosis* 1999 May;144(1):237-49

Hyperhomocysteinaemia and end stage renal disease. *Journal of Nephrology* (Italy), 1997, 10/2 (77-84)

Dietary pectin influences fibrin network structure in hypercholesterolaemic subjects. *Thrombosis Research* (UK), 1997, 86/3 (183-196)

Possible participation of Fas-mediated apoptosis in the mechanism of atherosclerosis. *Gerontology* (Switzerland), 1997, 43/ Suppl. 1 (35-42)

Omega3 fatty acids in the prevention-management of cardiovascular disease Simopoulos *A.P. Canadian Journal of Physiology and Pharmacology* (Canada), 1997, 75/3 (234-239)

Vitamin intake: A possible determinant of plasma homocyst(e)ine among middle-aged adults. *Annals of Epidemiology*, 1997, 7/4 (285-293)

Dietary soy protein and estrogen replacement therapy improve cardiovascular risk factors and decrease aortic cholesteryl ester content in ovariectomized cynomolgus monkeys. *Metabolism: Clinical and Experimental*, 1997, 46/6 (698-705)

Augmented Ca2+ in-flux is involved in the mechanism of enhanced proliferation of cultured vascular smooth muscle cells from spontaneously diabetic Goto-Kakizaki rats. *Atherosclerosis* (Ireland), 1997, 131/2 (167-175)

Atherogenesis and the homocysteine-folate-cobalamin triad: Do we need standardized analyses? *Journal of the American College of Nutrition*, 1997, 16/3 (258-267)

Regulation of leucocyte-endothelial interactions of special relevance to atherogenesis. *Clinical and Experimental Pharmacology and Physiology* (Australia), 1997, 24/5 (A33-A35)

Fasting total plasma homocysteine and atherosclerotic peripheral vascular disease. *Annals of Vascular Surgery*, 1997, 11/3 (217-223)

Estrogen inhibin and proliferation of vascular smooth muscle cells. *Atherosclerosis* (Ireland), 1997, 130/1 (1-10)

Plasma total homocysteine, B vitamins, and risk of coronary atherosclerosis. *Arteriosclerosis, Thrombosis, and Vascular Biology*, 1997, 17/5 (989-995)

Correlation between plasma homocyst(e)ine and aortic atherosclerosis. *American Heart Journal*, 1997, 133/5 (534-540)

Estrogen reduces proliferation and agonist-induced calcium increase in coronary artery smooth muscle cells. *American Journal of Physiology—Heart and Circulatory Physiology*, 1997, 272/4 41-4 (H1996-H2003)

Cell cycle effects of nitric oxide on vascular smooth muscle cells. *American Journal of Physiology—Heart and Circulatory Physiology*, 1997, 272/4 41-4 (H1810-H1818)

Transcriptional and post-transcriptional control of lysyl oxidase expression in vascular smooth muscle cells: Effects of TGF-beta1 and serum deprivation. *Journal of Cellular Biochemistry*, 1997, 65/3 (395-407)

Effects of dehydroepiandrosterone on proliferation of human aortic smooth muscle cells. *Life Sciences*, 1997, 60/11 (833-838)

Dietary fish oil: Influence on lesion regression in the porcine model of atherosclerosis. *Arteriosclerosis, Thrombosis, and Vascular Biology*, 1997, 17/4 (688-694)

Additive hypocholesterolemic effect of psyllium and cholestyramine in the hamster: Influence on fecal sterol and bile acid profiles. *Journal of Lipid Research*, 1997, 38/3 (491-502)

Calcifying subpopulation of bovine aortic smooth muscle cells is responsive to 17beta-estradiol. *Circulation*, 1997, 95/7 (1954-1960)

Influence of lifestyle modification on atherosclerotic progression determined by ultrasonographic change in the common carotid intima-media thickness. *American Journal of Clinical Nutrition*, 1997, 65/4 (1000-1004)

Angiotensin-converting enzyme inhibition prevents arterial nuclear factor-kappaB activation, monocyte chemoattractant protein-1 expression, and macrophage infiltration in a rabbit model of early accelerated atherosclerosis. *Circulation*, 1997, 95/6 (1532-1541)

Tumor necrosis factor-alpha activates smooth muscle cell migration in culture and is expressed in the balloon-injured rat aorta. *Arteriosclerosis, Thrombosis, and Vascular Biology*, 1997, 17/3 (490-497)

Vitamin E inhibits low-density lipoprotein-induced adhesion of monocytes to human aortic endothelial cells in vitro. *Arteriosclerosis, Thrombosis, and Vascular Biology*, 1997, 17/3 (429-436)

Vascular myofibroblasts: Lessons from coronary repair and remodeling. *Arteriosclerosis, Thrombosis, and Vascular Biology*, 1997, 17/3 (417-422)

Functional CD40 ligand is expressed on human vascular endothelial cells, smooth muscle cells, and macrophages: Implications for CD40-CD40 ligand signaling in atherosclerosis. *Proceedings of the National Academy of Sciences of the United States of America*, 1997, 94/5 (1931-1936)

Nitric oxide synthase: Role in the genesis of vascular disease. *Annual Review of Medicine*, 1997, 48/- (489-509)

Endothelial function. General considerations. *Drugs* (New Zealand), 1997, 53/Suppl. 1 (1-10)

Hyperhomocyst(e)inemia is associated with impaired endothelium- dependent vasodilation in humans. *Circulation*, 1997, 95/5 (1119-1121)

The role of folic acid in deficiency states and prevention of disease. *Journal of Family Practice*, 1997, 44/2 (138-144)

Lipid-lowering trials in the primary and secondary prevention of coronary heart disease: New evidence, implications and outstanding issues. *Current Opinion in Lipidology* (UK), 1996, 7/6 (341-355)

Effects of vitamin D on aortic smooth muscle cells in culture. *Toxicology in Vitro* (UK), 1996, 10/6 (701-711)

Antagonistic effects of tetrahydropyrans on platelet activating factor-induced DNA synthesis and proliferation of cerebromicrovascular smooth muscle cells. *Chinese Journal of Pharmacology and Toxicology* (China), 1996, 10/4 (251-254)

Soy isoflavones enhance coronary vascular reactivity in atherosclerotic female macaques. *Fertility and Sterility*, 1997, 67/1 (148-154)

Common mutation in methylenetetrahydrofolate reductase: Correlation with homocysteine metabolism and late-onset vascular disease. *Circulation*, 1996, 94/12 (3074-3078)

Hyperhomocysteinemia confers an independent increased risk of atherosclerosis in end-stage renal disease and is closely linked to plasma folate and pyridoxine concentrations. *Circulation*, 1996, 94/11 (2743-2748)

Endothelin receptors and atherosclerosis: A potential target for therapeutic intervention. *Expert Opinion on Investigational Drugs* (UK), 1996, 5/11 (1495-1508)

Endothelium and atherosclerosis: Monocyte accumulation as a target for therapeutic intervention. *Expert Opinion on Investigational Drugs* (UK), 1996, 5/11 (1487-1494)

Upregulation of IGF-I and collagen I mRNA in human atherosclerotic tissue is not accompanied by changes in type 1 IGF receptor or collagen III mRNA: An in situ hybridization study. *Coronary Artery Disease* (UK), 1996, 7/8 (569-572)

150-kD oxygen-regulated protein is expressed in human atherosclerotic plaques and allows mononuclear phagocytes to withstand cellular stress on exposure to hypoxia and modified low density lipoprotein. *Journal of Clinical Investigation*, 1996, 98/8 (1930-1941)

Dietary fats and coronary heart disease. *Biomedicine and Pharmacotherapy* (France), 1996, 50/6-7 (261-268)

Interferon-inducible protein-10 involves vascular smooth muscle cell migration, proliferation, and inflammatory response. *Journal of Biological Chemistry*, 1996, 271/39 (24286-24293)

Basic science of abdominal aortic aneurysms: Emerging therapeutic strategies for an unresolved clinical problem. *Current Opinion in Cardiology* (UK), 1996, 11/5 (504-518)

Homocystinuria: What about mild hyperhomocysteinaemia? *Postgraduate Medical Journal* (UK), 1996, 72/851 (513-518)

Pathogenesis of atherosclerosis. *Maturitas* (Ireland), 1996, 23/ Suppl. (S47-S49)

Effect of low dose omega-3 fatty acid supplementations on plasmalipids and lipoproteins in patients with coronary sclerosis and dyslipoproteinaemia. *Zeitschrift fur Ernahrungswissenschaft* (Germany), 1996, 35/2 (191-198)

Antioxidant of the coronary diet and disease. *Clinica Cardiovascular* (Spain), 1996, 14/2 (29-38)

Gamma imaging of atherosclerotic lesions: The role of antibody affinity in in vivo target localization. *Journal of Nuclear Cardiology,* 1996, 3/3 (231-241)

Enhanced capacity of n-3 fatty acid-enriched macrophages to oxidize low density lipoprotein mechanisms and effects of antioxidant vitamins. *Atherosclerosis* (Ireland), 1996, 124/2 (157-169)

Prevention of preatheromatous lesions in sand rats by treatment with a nutritional supplement. *Arzneimittel-Forschung / Drug Research* (Germany), 1996, 46/6 (610-614)

Dietary methionine imbalance, endothelial cell dysfunction and atherosclerosis. *Nutrition Research*, 1996, 16/7 (1251-1266)

Evidence for cultured human vascular smooth muscle cell heterogeneity: Isolation of clonal cells and study of their growth characteristics. *Thrombosis and Haemostasis* (Germany), 1996, 75/5 (854-858)

Adenosine inhibitory effect on enhanced growth of aortic smooth muscle cells from streptozotocin-induced diabetic rats. *British Journal of Pharmacology* (UK), 1996, 118/3 (783-789)

Fish oil supplementation in patients with heterozygous familial hypercholesterolemia. *Recenti Progressi in Medicina* (Italy), 1996, 87/3 (102-105)

Pathology induced by high vitamin doses. *Cahiers de Nutrition et de Dietetique* (France), 1996, 31/2 (76-80)

Smooth muscle cell migration and proliferatlon is enhanced in abdominal aortic aneurysms. *Australian and New Zealand Journal of Surgery* (Australia), 1996, 66/5 (305-308)

Eicosanoid precursors: Potential factors for atherogenesis in diabetic CAPD patients? *Peritoneal Dialysis International* (Canada), 1996, 16/Suppl. 1 (S250-S253)

Increased serum level of total homocysteine in CAPD patients: Despite fish oil therapy. *Peritoneal Dialysis International* (Canada), 1996, 16/Suppl. 1(S246-S249)

The central role of calcium in the pathogenesis of cardiovascular disease. *Journal of Human Hypertension* (UK), 1996, 10/3 (143-155)

Shosaikoto (Kampo medicine) protects macrophage function from suppression by hypercholesterolemia. *Biological and Pharmaceutical Bulletin* (Japan), 1996, 19/4 (652-654)

Metabolism of linoleic and alpha-linolenic acids in cultured cardiomyocytes: Effect of different n-6 and n-3 fatty acid supplementation. *Molecular and Cellular Biochemistry,* 1996, 157/1-2 (217-222)

17beta-estradiol and smooth muscle cell proliferation in aortic cells of male and female rats. *Biochemical and Biophysical Research Communications*, 1996, 221/1 (8-14)

Homocysteine, folate, and vascular disease. *Journal of Myocardial Ischemia*, 1996, 8/2 (60-63)

Effect of etofibrate and nicanartine on plasminogen activator inhibitor type-1 production in vitro by cultured vascular cells and on plasma plasminogen activator inhibitor type-1 activity in vivo in rabbits. *Current Therapeutic Research—Clinical and Experimental*, 1996, 57/3 (192-202)

Phorbol ester inhibits the phosphorylation of the retinoblastoma protein without suppressing cyclin D-associated kinase in vascular smooth muscle cells. *Journal of Biological Chemistry,* 1996, 271/14 (8345-8351)

Inhibitory effects of NB-818 on migration and proliferation of smooth muscle cells. *Japanese Pharmacology and Therapeutics* (Japan), 1996, 24/2 (213-217)

A novel cis-acting element is essential for cytokine-mediated transcriptional induction of the serum amyloid A gene in nonhepatic cells. Veterinary Pathobiology Department, University of Missouri US6/4 (1584-1594)

Nutritional interest of flavonoids. *Medecine et Nutrition* (France), 1996, 32/1 (17-27)

Study of causes underlying the low atherosclerotic response to dietary hypercholesterolemia in a selected strain of rabbits. *Atherosclerosis* (Ireland), 1996, 121/1 (63-73)

Simvastatin releases Ca2+ from a thapsigargin-sensitive pool and inhibits InsP3-dependent Ca2+ mobilization in vascular smooth muscle cells. *Journal of Cardiovascular Pharmacology,* 1996, 27/3 (383-391)

The effect of reduced glomerular filtration rate on plasma total homocysteine concentration. *Scandinavian Journal of Clinical and Laboratory Investigation* (Norway), 1996, 56/1 (41-46)

Effects of diet and exercise on qualitative and quantitative measures of LDL and its susceptibility to oxidation. *Arteriosclerosis, Thrombosis, and Vascular Biology,* 1996, 16/2 (201-207)

Homocysteine: Relation with ischemic vascular diseases. *Revue de Medecine Interne* (France), 1996, 17/1 (34-45)

Evaluation of hydroxyl radical-scavenging property of garlic. *Molecular and Cellular Biochemistry,* 1996, 154/1 (55-63)

Effects of interaction of RRR-alpha-tocopheryl acetate and fish oil on low-density-lipoprotein oxidation in postmenopausal women with and without hormone-replacement therapy. *American Journal of Clinical Nutrition,* 1996, 63/2 (184-193)

Therapeutic actions of garlic constituents. *Medicinal Research Reviews*, 1996, 16/1 (111-124)

Soybean isoflavones improve cardiovascular risk factors without affecting the reproductive system of peripubertal rhesus monkeys. *Journal of Nutrition*, 1996, 126/1 (43-50)

Endothelin-1 and angiotensin II act as progression but not competence growth factors in vascular smooth muscle cells. *European Journal of Pharmacology* (Netherlands), 1996, 295/2-3 (261-269)

Apoptosis of vascular smooth muscle cells induced by in vitro stimulation with interferon-gamma, tumor necrosis factor-alpha, and interleukin-1beta. *Arteriosclerosis, Thrombosis, and Vascular Biology*, 1996, 16/1 (19-27)

High dose B-vitamin treatment of hyperhomocysteinemia in dialysis patients. *Kidney International,* 1996, 49/1 (147-152)

Long-term folic acid (but not pyridoxine) supplementation lowers elevated plasma homocysteine level in chronic renal failure. *Mineral and Electrolyte Metabolism* (Switzerland), 1996, 22/1-3 (106-109)

The mechanism of apolipoprotein B-100 thiol depletion during oxidative modification of low-density lipoprotein. *Archives of Biochemistry and Biophysics*, 1997, 341/2 (287-294)

Ascorbate and urate are the strongest determinants of plasma antioxidative capacity and serum lipid resistance to oxidation in Finnish men. *Atherosclerosis* (Ireland), 1997, 130/1 (223-233)

Antioxidants in the prevention of atherosclerosis. *Current Opinion in Lipidology* (UK), 1996, 7/6 (374-380)

The carotenoids beta-carotene, canthaxanthin and zeaxanthin inhibit macrophage-mediated LDL oxidation. *FEBS Letters* (Netherlands), 1997, 401/2-3 (262-266)

Polyunsaturated fatty acids, antioxidants, and cognitive function in very old men. *American Journal of Epidemiology*, 1997, 145/1 (33-41)

Animal studies on antioxidants. *Journal of Cardiovascular Risk* (UK), 1996, 3/4 (358-362)

Alpha-Tocopherol and beta-carotene serum levels in post-menopausal women treated with transdermal estradiol and oral medroxyprogesterone acetate. *Hormone and Metabolic Research* (Germany), 1996, 28/10 (558-561)

Time-course studies by synchrotron X-ray solution scattering of the structure of human low-density lipoprotein during Cu2+-induced oxidation in relation to changes in lipid composition. *Biochemical Journal* (UK), 1996, 319/1 (217-227)

Antioxidant status of hypercholesterolemic patients treated with LDL apheresis. *Cardiovascular Drugs and Therapy*, 1996, 10/5 (567-571)

Abnormal antioxidant vitamin and carotenoid status in chronic renal failure. QJM—*Monthly Journal of the Association of Physicians* (UK), 1996, 89/10 (765-769)

Antioxidants in cardiovascular disease: Randomized trials. *Nutrition*, 1996, 12/9 (583-588)

Dietary antioxidants and cognitive function in a population-based sample of older persons: The Rotterdam study. *American Journal of Epidemiology*, 1996, 144/3 (275-280)

Lack of correlation between the alpha-tocopherol content of plasma and LDL, but high correlations for gamma-tocopherol and carotenoids. *Journal of Lipid Research*, 1996, 37/9 (1936-1946)

Oxidized low density lipoproteins in atherogenesis: Role of dietary modification. *Annual Review of Nutrition*, 1996, 16/-(51-71)

Effect of dietary supplementation of beta-carotene on human monocyte-macrophage-mediated oxidation of low density lipoprotein. *Israel Journal of Medical Sciences* (Israel), 1996, 32/6 (473-478)

Increased oxidation resistance of atherogenic plasma lipoproteins at high vitamin E levels in non-vitamin E supplemented men. *Atherosclerosis* (Ireland), 1996, 124/1 (83-94)

Increased levels of autoantibodies to cardiolipin and oxidised low density lipoprotein are inversely associated with plasma vitamin C status in cigarette smokers. *Atherosclerosis* (Ireland), 1996, 124/1 (75-81)

Antioxydant vitamins and risk of cardiovascular diseases. The significance of oxidised low-density lipoprotein in atherosclerosis. *Ugeskrift for Laeger* (Denmark), 1996, 158/19 (2706-2710)

Prevention of atherosclerosis with dietary antioxidants: Fact or fiction? *Journal of Nutrition*, 1996, 126/4 Suppl. (1067S-1071S)

Nutritional supplement program halts progression of early coronary atherosclerosis documented by ultrafast computed tomography. *Journal of Applied Nutrition*, 1996, 48/3 (68-78)

Metal excretion and magnesium retention in patients with intermittent claudication treated with intravenous disodium EDTA. *Clinical Chemistry*, 1996, 42/12 (1938-1942)

Therapy for acute myocardial infarction. *Clinics in Geriatric Medicine*, 1996, 12/1 (141-168)

Vitamin E consumption and the risk of coronary disease in women. *New Engl. J. Med.*, 1993, 328/20 (1444-1449)

The role of free radicals in disease. *Australian and New Zealand Journal of Ophthalmology* (Australia), 1995, 23/1

Coenzyme Q_{10} and coronary artery disease. *Clin. Invest. Suppl.* (Germany), 1993, 71/8

Dietary antioxidant vitamins and death from coronary heart disease in postmenopausal women. *New England Journal of Medicine*, 1996, 334/18

Vitamin E and atherosclerosis: Potential role of vitamin E in the prevention of cardiovascular diseases. *Nutrition Clinique et Metabolisme* (France), 1996, 10/1 (43-44)

Randomized, controlled trial of antioxidant vitamins and cardioprotective diet on hyperlipidemia, oxidative stress, and development of experimental atherosclerosis: The diet and antioxidant trial on atherosclerosis (DATA). *Cardiovascular Drugs and Therapy*, 1995, 9/6

Serum levels of vitamin E in relation to cardiovascular diseases. *Journal of Clinical Pharmacy and Therapeutics* (UK), 1995, 20/6

Oxidative susceptibility of low density lipoprotein from rabbits fed atherogenic diets containing coconut, palm, or soybean oils. *Lipids,* 1995, 30/12 (1145-1150)

Coantioxidants make alpha-tocopherol an efficient antioxidant for low-density lipoprotein. *American Journal of Clinical Nutrition*, 1995, 62/6 Suppl

Optimal diet for reducing the risk of arteriosclerosis. *Canadian Journal of Cardiology* (Canada), 1995, 11/Suppl. G

Effect of vitamin E, vitamin C and beta-carotene on LDL oxidation and atherosclerosis. *Canadian Journal of Cardiology* (Canada), 1995, 11/Suppl. G (97G-103G)

Atherosclerosis: Vitamin E protects coronary arteries. *Deutsche Apotheker Zeitung* (Germany), 1995, 135/41 (42+44)

Effects on health of dietary supplementation with 100 mg d-alpha-tocopheryl acetate, daily for 6 years. *Journal of International Medical Research* (UK), 1995, 23/5

Mechanisms of the cardioprotective effect of a diet enriched with omega-3 polyunsaturated fatty acids. *Pathophysiology* (Netherlands), 1995, 2/3 (131-140)

Prevention of atherosclerosis: The potential role of antioxidants. *Postgraduate Medicine*, 1995, 98/1

Vitamin E: Metabolism and role in atherosclerosis. *Ann. Biol. Clin.* (France), 1994, 52/7-8

Vitamin C prevents cigarette smoke-induced leukocyte aggregation and adhesion to endothelium in vivo. *Proc. Natl. Acad. Sci. U. S. A.*, 1994, 91/16 (7688-7692)

Homocysteine and coronary atherosclerosis. *J Am Coll Cardiol* Mar 1 1996, 27 (3) p517-27

Hyperhomocysteinaemia: a role in the accelerated atherogenesis of chronic renal failure? *Neth J Med* (Netherlands) May 1995, 46 (5) p244-51

Hyperhomocysteinaemia and endothelial dysfunction in young patients with peripheral arterial occlusive disease. *Eur J Clin Invest* (England) Mar 1995, 25 (3) p176-81

Homocysteine and coronary atherosclerosis. *J Am Coll Cardiol* Mar 1 1996, 27 (3) p517-27

Vitamin nutrition status and homocysteine: an atherogenic risk factor. *Nutr Rev* Nov 1994, 52 (11) p383-7

Homocysteine and coronary artery disease. *Cleve Clin J Med* Nov-Dec 1994, 61 (6) p438-50

Treatment of atherosclerosis and thrombosis with aspirin. *Lancet* (England) Sep 9 1972, 2 (776) p532-4

[Progress in the prevention and treatment of ischemic cerebrovascular diseases with garlic extract]. *Chung Kuo Chung Hsi I Chieh Ho Tsa Chih* (China) Feb 1995, 15 (2) p124-6 (24 Refs.)

Platelets, carotids, and coronaries. Critique on antithrombotic role of antiplatelet agents, exercise, and certain diets. *Am J Med* Sep 1984, 77 (3) p513-23

Effects of 11-week increases in dietry eicosapentaenoic acid on bleeding time, lipids, and platelet aggregation. *Lancet* (England) Nov 28 1981, 2 (8257) p1190-3

N-3 but not N-6 fatty acids reduce the expression of the combined adhesion and scavenger receptor CD36 in human monocytic cells. *Cell Biochem Funct* (England) Sep 1995, 13 (3) p211-6

Essential fatty acid metabolism in patients with essential hypertension, diabetes mellitus and coronary heart disease. *Prostaglandins Leukot Essent Fatty Acids* (Scotland) Jun 1995, 52 (6) p387-91

[Changes in fatty acid composition, platelet aggregability and RBC function in elderly subjects with administration of low-dose fish oil concentrate and comparison with younger subjects]. *Ronen Igakkai Zasshi* (Japan) Aug 1994, 31 (8) p596-603

Do fish oils prevent restenosis after coronary angioplasty? *Circulation* Nov 1994, 90 (5) p2248-57

N-3 fatty acid incorporation into LDL particles renders them more susceptible to oxidation in vitro but not necessarily more atherogenic in vivo. *Arterioscler Thromb* Jul 1994, 14 (7) p1170-6

Human atherosclerotic plaque contains both oxidized lipids and relatively large amounts of alpha-tocopherol and ascorbate. *Arterioscler Thromb Vasc Biol* Oct 1995, 15 (10) p1616-24

Attention Deficit Disorder (ADD)

Subclinical hyperthyroidism and hyperkinetic behavior in children. *Pediatr Neurol* 1999 Mar;20(3):192-4

Dietary replacement in preschool-aged hyperactive boys. *Pediatrics* 1989 Jan;83(1):7-17

Social skills training with parent generalization: treatment effects for children with attention deficit disorder. *J Consult Clin Psychol* 1997 Oct;65(5):749-57

Coincidence of attention deficit disorder and atopic disorders in children: empirical findings and hypothetical background. *J Abnorm Child Psychol* 1991 Feb;19(1):1-13

Stimulants and antidepressant pharmacokinetics in hyperactive children. *Psychopharmacol Bull* 1991;27(4):411-5

Clinical trial of piracetam in patients with myoclonus: nationwide multiinstitution study in Japan. The Myoclonus/Piracetam Study Group. *Mov Disord* 1996 Nov;11(6):691-700

Psychopharmacology of the psychiatric disorders of childhood and adolescence. *Med J Aust* 1990 Jan 1;152(1):32-9

Dietary correlates of hyperactive behavior in children. *J Consult Clin Psychol* 1980 Dec;48(6):760-9

Foods and additives are common causes of the attention deficit hyperactive disorder in children. *Ann Allergy* 1994 May;72(5):462-8

Megavitamins and learning disorders: a controlled double-blind experiment. *J Nutr* 1979 May;109(5):819-26

Behavioral effects of dietary neurotransmitter precursors: basic and clinical aspects. *Neurosci Biobehav Rev* 1996 Summer;20(2):313-23

Plasma amino acids in attention deficit disorder. *Psychiatry Res* 1990 Sep;33(3):301-6

Amino acid supplementation as therapy for attention deficit disorder. *J Am Acad Child Psychiatry* 1986 Jul;25(4):509-13

Plasma free tryptophan concentration in children with attention deficit disorder. *Folia Psychiatr Neurol Jpn* 1985;39(4):531-5

The effect of pyridoxine hydrochloride on blood serotonin and pyridoxal phosphate contents in hyperactive children. *Pediatrics* 1975 Mar;55(3):437-41

Trace mineral levels in hyperactive children responding to the Feingold diet. *J Pediatr* 1979 Jun;94(6):944-5

Assessment of chemical factors in relation to child hyperactivity. *Journal of Nutritional and Environmental Medicine*, 1997, 7/4 (333-342)

Aspartame, behavior, and cognitive function in children with attention deficit disorder. *Pediatrics* 1994 Jan;93(1):70-5

Phenylethylaminergic mechanisms in attention-deficit disorder. *Biol Psychiatry* 1991 Jan 1;29(1):15-22

Attention deficit disorder and hyperactivity—changes in hypothalamic function in hyperactive children: a new model. *Med Hypotheses* 1997 Mar;48(3):267-75

Right hemisphere dysfunction in subjects with attention-deficit disorder with and without hyperactivity. *J Child Neurol* 1997 Feb;12(2):107-15

The role of intelligence and hyperactivity in diagnosis of attention deficit disorder in children and adolescents. *International Journal of Adolescent Medicine and Health* 1997, 9/3 (165-171)

Omega-3 fatty acids in boys with behavior, learning, and health problems. *Physiology and Behavior,* 1996, 59/4-5 (915-920)

Behavioral effects of dietary neurotransmitter precursors: Basic and clinical aspects. *Neuroscience and Biobehavioral Reviews*, 1996, 20/2 (313-323)

Coloboma hyperactive mutant mice exhibit regional and transmitter-specific deficits in neurotransmission. *Journal of Neurochemistry,* 1997, 68/1 (176-186)

Clinical trial of piracetam in patients with myoclonus: Nationwide multiinstitution study in Japan. *Movement Disorders*, 1996, 11/6 (691-700)

Neurobehavioral aspects of lead neurotoxicity in children. *Central European Journal of Public Health* (Czech Republic), 1997, 5/2 (65-69)

Hair lead levels related to children's classroom attention-deficit behavior. *Archives of Environmental Health*, 1996, 51/3 (214-220)

Bone lead levels and delinquent behavior. *Journal of the American Medical Association*, 1996, 275/5 (363-369)

Zinc deficiency in attention-deficit hyperactivity disorder. *Biological Psychiatry,* 1996, 40/12 (1308-1310)

Iron treatment in children with attention deficit hyperactivity disorder: A preliminary report. *Neuropsychobiology* (Switzerland), 1997, 35/4 (178-180)

Attention-deficit hyperactivity disorder: Pharmacotherapy and beyond. *Postgraduate Medicine*, 1997, 101/5 (201+213+222)

Do nutrient supplements and dietary changes affect learning and emotional reactions of children with learning difficulties? A controlled series of 16 cases. *Nutr Health* (England) 1984, 3 (1-2) p69-77

[Effect of supplementary intake of vitamins for 6 months on physical and mental work capacity of children beginning school education at the age of 6 years]. *Vopr Pitan* (USSR) Jul-Aug 1988

Nutritional therapy for selected inborn errors of metabolism. *J Am Coll Nutr* 1989, 8 Suppl

Vitamin supplements and purported learning enhancement in mentally retarded children. *J Nutr Sci Vitaminol* (Tokyo) (Japan) Jun 1989

Vitamin B6 in clinical neurology. *Ann N Y Acad Sci* 1990, 585 p250-60

[Vitamin B12 deficiency due to abnormal eating habits]. *Ned Tijdschr Geneeskd* (Netherlands) Feb 26 1994

Use and safety of elevated dosages of vitamin E in infants and children. *Int J Vitam Nutr Res Suppl* (Canada) 1989, 30 p69-80

Experience over 17 years with antioxidant treatment in Spielmeyer-Sjogren disease. *Am J Med Genet Suppl* 1988, 5 p265-74

Vitamin E and the nervous system. *Crit Rev Neurobiol* 1987, 3 (1)

Clinical uses of vitamin E. *Acta Vitaminol Enzymol* (Italy) 1985, 7 Suppl p33-43

Neurologic complications of vitamin E deficiency: case report and review of the literature. *Bull Clin Neurosci* 1985, 50 p53-60

A progressive neurological syndrome associated with an isolated vitamin E deficiency *Can J Neurol Sci* (Canada) Nov 1984, 11 (4 Suppl) p561-4

[Evaluation of the effectiveness of prophylactic vitamin administration to school children in Moscow]. *Vopr Pitan* (USSR) May-Jun 1992

The assessment of the vitamin B6 status among Egyptian school children by measuring the urinary cystathionine excretion. *Int J Vitam Nutr Res* (Switzerland) 1984, 54 (4) p321-7

Dramatic favorable responses of children with learning disabilities or dyslexia and attention deficit disorder to antimotion sickness medications: four case reports. *Percept Mot Skills* Dec 1991, 73 (3 Pt 1) p723-38

New developments in pediatric psychopharmacology. *J Dev Behav Pediatr* Sep 1983, 4 (3) p202-9

Piracetam in the management of minimal brain dysfunction [letter]. *S Afr Med J* (South Africa) Aug 7 1976, 50 (34) p1312

Altered dopaminergic function in the prefrontal cortex, nucleus accumbens and caudate-putamen of an animal model of attention-deficit hyperactivity disorder? The spontaneously hypertensive rat. *Brain Res* (Netherlands) Apr 10 1995, 676 (2) p343-51

Deanol and methylphenidate in minimal brain dysfunction. *Clin Pharmacol Ther* May 1975, 17 (5) p534-40

Effect of dextroamphetamine and methylphenidate on calcium and magnesium concentration in hyperactive boys. *Psychiatry Res* (Ireland) Nov 1994, 54 (2) p199-210

[Deficiency of certain trace elements in children with hyperactivity]. *Psychiatr Pol* (Poland) May-Jun 1994, 28 (3) p345-53

[Level of magnesium in blood serum in children from the province of Rzesz?ow]. *Wiad Lek* (Poland) Feb 1993, 46 (3-4) p120-2

Gamma-linolenic acid for attention-deficit hyperactivity disorder: placebo-controlled comparison to D-amphetamine. *Biol Psychiatry* Jan 15 1989, 25 (2) p222-8

Megavitamins and hyperactivity [letter]. *Pediatrics* Aug 1986, 78 (2) p374-5

Vitamin E and Alzheimer's disease in subjects with Down syndrome. *Journal of Mental Deficiency Research,* 1988 Dec Vol 32(6) 479-484

Behavioral disorders, learning disabilities and megavitamin therapy. *Adolescence* 1987 Fal Vol 22(87) 729-738

Macrocytosis and cognitive decline in Down syndrome. *British Journal of Psychiatry* 1986 Dec Vol 149 797-798

Treatment approaches in Down syndrome: A review. *Australia & New Zealand Journal of Developmental Disabilities*

A double blind study of vitamin B_6 in Down syndrome infants: I. Clinical and biochemical results. *Journal of Mental Deficiency Research* 1985 Sep Vol 29(3) 233-240

A double blind study of vitamin B-sub-6 in Down syndrome infants: II. Cortical auditory evoked potentials. *Journal of Mental Deficiency Research* 1985 Sep Vol 29(3) 241-246

Xylose absorption in Down syndrome. *Journal of Mental Deficiency Research* 1985 Jun Vol 29(2) 173-177

Nutritional aspects of Down syndrome with special reference to the nervous system. *British Journal of Psychiatry* 1984 Aug Vol 145 115-120

Children's mental retardation study is attacked: A closer look. *International Journal of Biosocial Research* 1982 Vol 3(2) 75-86

Effects of nutritional supplementation on IQ and certain other variables associated with Down syndrome. *American Journal of Mental Deficiency* 1983 Sep Vol 88(2) 214-217

Vitamin A and carotene values of institutionalized mentally retarded subjects with and without Down syndrome. *Journal of Mental Deficiency Research* 1977 Mar Vol 21(1) 63-74

Sodium-dependent glutamate binding in senile dementia. *Neurobiology of Aging* 1987 May-Jun Vol 8(3) 219-223

Alzheimer-like neurotransmitter deficits in adult Down syndrome brain tissue. *Journal of Neurology, Neurosurgery & Psychiatry* 1987 Jun Vol 50(6) 775-778

A report on phosphatidylcholine therapy in a Down Syndrome child. *Psychological Reports* 1986 Feb Vol 58(1) 207-217

Autism

The biochemistry of unsaturated fatty acids and development of preterm infants. *British Journal of Clinical Practice* 1995, 49/Suppl. 80 (3-6)

Dietary intervention in autistic syndromes. *Brain Dysfunction* 1990, 3/5-6 (315-327)

Effects of pyridoxine and magnesium on autistic symptoms: Initial observations. *Journal of Autism and Developmental Disorders* 1981, 11/2 (219-230)

Efficacy in endogenous depression and Parkinson's disease. *J. Neural Trans* 55:301-8, 1982

Behavioral and biochemical effects of oral magnesium, vitamin B6 and magnesium. Vitamin B6 administration in autistic children. *Magnesium Bulletin* 3:23-4, 1981

Goth A: *Medical Pharmacology,* 11th ed. CV Mosby, St Louis, Mo, 1984. Pp226-33

Coulter, H. L. *Vaccination, Social Violence and Criminality: The Medical Assault on the American Brain*. Berkely, CA : North Atlantic Books, 1990

Werbach, M. R., M.D. *Nutritional Influences on Mental Illness.* Tarzana, CA: Third Line Press, 1991, 75

Petersdorg R; Harrison S, *Principles of Internal Medicine.* P2141, New York, NY: McGraw-Hill 1983

Berkow R: *Merck Manual*, Rahway, NJ: Merck and Co., 1982. P 1900-1

Lipton M, Mailman R, and Numeroff C: Vitamins, megavitamin therapy, and the nervous system. In: *Nutrition and the Brain*, vol 3, Wurtman R and Wurtman J, eds, New York, NY: Raven Press, 1979. Pp183-264

[Rett's syndrome—differential diagnosis of autism in a case report]. *Divcic B Lijec Vjesn* Dec 1989, 111 (12) p458-60

Pica and Elevated Blood Lead Level in Autistic and Atypical. *American Journal of Diseases of Children 130 no. 1 (Jan, 1976): 47-8*

Autism in a Child with Congenital Cytomegalovirus Infection. *Journal of Autism and Developmental Disorders* 13 no. 3 Sep, (1983): 249-53

Autism in Fetal Alcohol Syndrome: A Report of Six Cases. *Alcoholism, Clinical and Experimental Research.* 16 no. 3 (1992): 558-565

Reduced Brain Stem Size in Chilren with Autism. *Brain and Development* 14 no. 2 (1992); 94-97

Central Conduction Time in Childhood Autism. *British Journal of Psychiatry* 160 (May, 1992): 659-63

Cerebral Blood Flow Abnormalities in Adults with Infantile Autism. *Journal of Nervous and Mental Disease* 180 no. 7 (Jul, 1992); 413-17

Dietary influences on neurotransmission. *Adv Pediatr* 1986, 33 p23-47

Brief report: circadian melatonin, thyroid-stimulating hormone, prolactin, and cortisol levels in serum of young adults with autism. *Autism Dev Disord* Dec 1995, 25 (6) p641-54

Blood serotinin and free tryptophan concentration in autistic children. *Neuropsychobiol* 11:22-7, 1984

McGraw-Hill, New York, NY 1983 *Harrison's Principles of Internal Medicine* P2141

Tetrahydrofolate and hydroxycobalamin in the management of Dihydropteridine reductase deficiency. *J Ment Def Res* 26:21-5, 1982

The effects of high doses of vitamin B6 on autistic children: A double-blind crossover study. *Am J Psychiatry* 135:472-5, 1979

Clinical and biological effects of high doses of vitamin B6 and magnesium on autistic children. *Acta Vitaminol Enzymol* 4:27-44, 1982

Vitamin B6, magnesium, and combined B6-magnesium: Therapeutic effects in childhood autism. *Biol Psychiatry* 20:467-8, 1985

Improved social and language skills after secretin administration in patients with autistic spectrum disorders. *Journal of the Association for Academic Minority Physicians* 1998;9(1):9-15

High-dose pyridoxine and magnesium administration in children with autistic disorder: an absence of salutary effects in a double-blind, placebo-controlled study. *J Autism Dev Disord* Aug 1997, 27 (4) p467-78

Shott S: Efficacy of vitamin B6 and magnesium in the treatment of autism: a methodology review and summary of outcomes. *J Autism Dev Disord* Oct 1995, 25 (5) p481-93

[Clinical heterogeneity of the autistic syndrome: a study of 60 families]. *Invest Clin* 1992, 33 (1) p13-31

Niacin and vitamin B6 in mental functioning: A review of controlled trials in humans. *Biological Psychiatry* 1991, 29/9 (931-941)

Abnormal intestinal permeability in children with autism. *Acta Paediatrica, International Journal of Paediatrics* 1996, 85/9 (1076-1079)

Plasma excitatory amino acids in autism. *Invest Clin* Jun 1996, 37 (2) p113-28

Efficacy of vitamin B6 and magnesium in the treatment of autism: a methodology review and summary of outcomes

Lead intoxication in children with pervasive developmental disorders. *J Toxicol Clin Toxicol* 1996, 34 (2) p177-81

A review of adverse events. *Drug Safety* 1998, 19/6 (435-454)

Autism and genetic disorders. *Schizophr Bull* 1986, 12 (4) p724-38

Behavioral disorders, learning disabilities and megavitamin therapy. *Adolescence Fall* 1987, 22 (87) p729-38

Low serum tryptophan to large neutral amino acids: Ratio in idiopathic infantile autism. *Biomedicine and Pharmacotherapy* 1995, 49/6 (288-292)

Brief report: circadian melatonin, thyroid-stimulating hormone, prolactin, and cortisol levels in serum of young adults with autism. *J Autism Dev Disord* Dec 1995, 25 (6) p641-54

Thyroid hormone in autistic children.*J Autism Dev Disord* Dec 1980, 10 (4) p445-50

Hypothyroidism and autism spectrum disorders. *Journal of Child Psychology and Psychiatry and Allied Disciplines* 1992, 33/3 (531-542)

Autoimmune Diseases

Cyclosporine and therapeutic plasma exchange in treatment of progressive autoimmune diseases. *Artif Organs* Sep 1997, 21 (9) p983-8

Plasmapheresis in autoimmune inner ear disease: long-term follow-up. *Am J Otol* Sep 1997, 18 (5) p572-6

Autoimmune pancreatitis as a new clinical entity. Three cases of autoimmune pancreatitis with effective steroid therapy. *Dig Dis Sci* Jul 1997, 42 (7) p1458-68

Clonal accumulation of V beta 5.1-positive cells in the liver of a patient with autoimmune cholangiopathy. *Liver* (Denmark) Feb 1997, 17 (1) p7-12

[Autoimmune hepatitis treated with cyclosporin revealed by acute hepatocellular failure] *Arch Pediatr* (France) Jan 1997, 4 (1) p40-3

A case of acute inflammatory demyelinating neuropathy associated with autoimmune-type chronic active hepatitis. *Clinical Neurology* (Japan), 1997, 37/11 (976-981)

Antiphospholipid antibodies in autoimmune and infectious diseases: Participation of beta-2-glycoprotein I. *Revista Brasileira de Reumatologia* (Brazil), 1997, 37/5 (282-286)

Hemopoietic blood and marrow transplants in the treatment of severe autoimmune disease. *Current Opinion in Hematology*, 1997, 4/6 (390-394)

Clonal accumulation of Vbetleft arrow over right arrow.1-positive cells in the liver of a patient with autoimmune cholangiopathy. *Liver* (Denmark), 1997, 17/1 (7-12)

Cyclosporin treatment of an acute hepatic failure revealing an autoimmune hepatitis. *Archives de Pediatrie* (France), 1997, 4/1 (40-43)

Whole thymus extract (Thymex-L) in the treatment of autoimmune hepatitis. *International Journal of Thymology* (Germany), 1997, 4/1 (386-389)

Hematopoietic stem cell transplants for autoimmune disease: Role of EULAR. *Journal of Rheumatology* (Canada), 1997, 24/ Suppl. 48 (98-99)

Autoimmune diseases: Tracing the shared threads. *Hospital Practice*, 1997, 32/4 (147-154)

Age-related changes in cobalamin (vitamin B12) handling: Implications for therapy. *Drugs and Aging* (New Zealand), 1998, 12/4 (277-292)

Adrenal insufficiency after recurrent post-partum thyroiditis (post-partum Schmidt syndrome): A case report. *Thyroid*, 1998, 8/3 (269-272)

Osteomalacia secondary to celiac disease, primary hyperparathyroidism, and graves' disease. *American Journal of the Medical Sciences*, 1998, 315/2 (136-139)

Selenoproteins in human bone, intestine and thyroid. *Medizinische Klinik* (Germany), 1997, 92/Suppl. 3 (24-26)

Modulation of antioxidant enzymes and programmed cell death by n-3 fatty acids. *Lipids*, 1996, 31/3 Suppl. (S91-S96)

Endotoxin induced production of interleukin-6 is enhanced by vitamin E deficiency and reduced by black tea extract. *Inflammation Research* (Switzerland), 1995, 44/7 (301-305)

Lipid peroxidase and erythrocyte redox system in systemic vasculitides treated with corticoids. Effect of vitamin E administration. *Romanian Journal of Internal Medicine* (Romania), 1994, 32/4 (283-289)

The pathogenesis of inflammatory disease: Surgical shock and multiple system organ failure. *Inflammopharmacology* (Netherlands), 1995, 3/2 (149-168)

Effects of n-3 and n-6 fatty acids on the activities and expression of hepatic antioxidant enzymes in autoimmune-prone NZBxNZW F1 mice. *Lipids*, 1994, 29/8 (561-568)

Decreased pro-inflammatory cytokines and increased antioxidant enzyme gene expression by omega-3 lipids in murine lupus nephritis. *Biochem. Biophys. Res. Commun.*, 1994, 200/2 (893-898)

Glutathione and lymphocyte activation: A function of ageing and auto-immune disease. *Immunology* (UK), 1987, 61/4 (503-508)

D-penicillamine-induced increase in intracellular glutathione correlating to clinical response in rheumatoid arthritis. *J. Rheumatol.* (Canada), 1981, 8/Suppl. 7 (14-19)

Suppression of interleukin-1 and tumor necrosis factor-alpha production by acanthoic acid, (-)-pimara-9(11), 15-dien-19-oic acid, and its antifibrotic effects in vivo. *Cellular Immunology*, 1996, 170/2 (212-221)

Low incidence of autoimmune type I diabetes in BB rats fed a hydrolysed casein-based diet associated with early inhibition of non-macrophage-dependent hyperexpression of MHC class I molecules on beta cells. *Diabetologia* (Germany), 1995, 38/10 (1138-1147)

A modified determination of coenzyme Q_{10} in human blood and CoQ_{10} blood levels in diverse patients with allergies. *Biofactors* (UK), 1988, 1/4 (303-306)

Should dehydroepiandrosterone replacement therapy be provided with glucocorticoids? *Rheumatology* (Oxford) 1999 Jun;38(6):488-95

Dehydroepiandrosterone (DHEA) inhibits IL-6 secretion from monocytes and peripheral blood mononuclear cells (PBL) in man. *Journal of Neuroimmunology* 90 (1): p 44 Sept. 1, 1998

Regulation of interleukin-6 expression in human osteoblastic cells in vitro. *Exp Clin Endocrinol Diabetes* 1998;106(4):324-33

Modulation of cytokine production by dehydroepiandrosterone (DHEA) plus melatonin (MLT) supplementation of old mice. *Proc Soc Exp Biol Med* 1998 May;218(1):76-82

Modulation of immune dysfunction during murine leukaemia retrovirus infection of old mice by dehydroepiandrosterone sulphate (DHEAS). *Proc Soc Exp Biol Med* 1998 May;218(1):76-82

IL-6, DHEA and the ageing process. *Mech Ageing Dev* 1997 Feb;93(1-3):15-24

Serum dehydroepiandrosterone (DHEA) and DHEA sulfate are negatively correlated with serum interleukin-6 (IL-6), and DHEA inhibits IL-6 secretion from mononuclear cells in man in vitro: possible link between endocrinosenescence and immunosenescence. *J Clin Endocrinol Metab* 1998 Jun;83(6):2012-7

Serum levels of IL-6 and development of disability in older persons. *J Am Geriatr Soc* 1999 Jun;47(6):755-6

[Selenoproteins in bone, gastrointestinal tract and thyroid gland of the human]. *Med Klin* 1997 Sep 15;92 Suppl 3:24-6

Role of sugars in human neutrophilic phagocytosis. *Am J Clin Nutr* 1973 Nov;26(11):1180-4

Sucrose, neutrophilic phagocytosis and resistance to disease. *Dent Surv* 1976 Dec;52(12):46-8

Obesity, plasma lipids and polymorphonuclear (PMN) granulocyte functions. *Scand J Haematol* 1977 Sep;19(3):293-303

Inhibition of lymphoproliferation by hyperlipoproteinemic plasma. *J Clin Invest* 1976 Oct;58(4):950-4

Vitamins and immunity: II. Influence of *L*-carnitine on the immune system. *Acta Vitaminol Enzymol* 1982;4(1-2):135-40

Reversibility by *L*-carnitine of immunosuppression induced by an emulsion of soya bean oil, glycerol and egg lecithin. *Arzneimittelforschung* 1982;32(11):1485-8

On the biochemical similarities of ascorbic acid and interferon. *J Theor Biol* 1982 Sep 21;98(2):235-8

The Third Face of Vitamin C. *J Orthomol Med* 7 (1992): 197-200

Treatment of Hepatitis with Infusions of Ascorbic Acid: Comparison with Other Therapies. *JAMA* 156 (1954): 565

Depression of Lymphocyte Transformation Following Oral Glucose Ingestion. *Am J Clin Nutr* 30 (1977): 613

Vitamin C and Immune Responses. *Food Technol* 41 (1987): 112-4

Androgen and progesterone levels in females with rheumatoid arthritis. *Reumatismo* (Italy), 1994, 46/2 (65-69)

Docosahexaenoic and eicosapentaenoic acids inhibit human lymphoproliferative responses in vitro but not the expression of T cell surface activation markers. *Scandinavian Journal of Immunology* (UK), 1996, 43/3

Modulation of antioxidant enzymes and programmed cell death by n-3 fatty acids. *Lipids*, 1996, 31/3 Suppl. (S91-S96)

Dietary marine lipids suppress continuous expression of interleukin-1beta gene transcription. *Lipids*, 1996, 31/3 Suppl. (S23-S31)

Tissue specific regulation of transforming growth factor beta by omega-3 lipid-rich krill oil in autoimmune murine lupus. *Nutrition Research*, 1996, 16/3 (489-503)

The effects of dietary lipid manipulation on the production of murine T cell-derived cytokines. *Cytokine* (UK), 1995, 7/6 (548-553)

Dietary omega-3 lipids delay the onset and progression of autoimmune lupus nephritis by inhibiting transforming growth factor beta mRNA and protein expression. *Journal of Autoimmunity* (UK), 1995, 8/3 (381-393)

Fish oil feeding modulates leukotriene production in murine lupus nephritis. *Prostaglandins,* 1994, 48/5 (331-348)

Effects of n-3 and n-6 fatty acids on the activities and expression of hepatic antioxidant enzymes in autoimmune-prone NZBxNZW F1 mice. *Lipids*, 1994, 29/8 (561-568)

Increased TGF-beta and decreased oncogene expression by omega-3 fatty acids in the spleen delays onset of autoimmune disease in B/W mice. *J. Immunol.*, 1994, 152/12 (5979-5987)

Decreased pro-inflammatory cytokines and increased antioxidant enzyme gene expression by omega-3 lipids in murine lupus nephritis. *Biochem. Biophys. Res. Commun.,* 1994, 200/2 (893-898)

Suppression of autoimmune disease by dietary n-3 fatty acids. *J. Lipid Res.*, 1993, 34/8 (1435-1444)

Role of omega-3 fatty acids in health and disease. *Nutr. Res.*, 1993, 13/Suppl. 1 (S19-S45)

Omega-3 polyunsaturated fatty acids: A potential new treatment of immune renal disease. *Mayo Clin. Proc.*, 1991, 66/10 (1018-1028)

Practicalities of lipids: ICU patient, autoimmune disease, and vascular disease. *J. Parenter. Enter. Nutr.*, 1990, 14/5 Suppl

Dietary marine lipids suppress murine autoimmune disease. *J. Intern. Med. Suppl.* (UK), 1989, 225/731

Depression of humoral responses and phagocytic functions in vivo and in vitro by fish oil and eicosapentanoic acid. *Clin. Immunol. Immunopathol.*, 1989, 52/2 (257-270)

The type of dietary fat affects the severity of autoimmune disease in NZB/NZW mice. *Am. J. Pathol.*, 1987, 127/1 (106-121)

Effects of dietary supplementation on autoimmunity in the MRL/lpr mouse: A preliminary investigation. *Ann. Rheum. Dis.* (UK), 1986, 45/12 (1019-1024)

A fish oil diet rich in eicosapentaenoic acid reduces cyclooxygenase metabolites, and suppresses lupus in MRL-lpr mice. *J. Immunol.*, 1985, 134/3 (1914-1919)

The protective effect of dietary fish oil on murine lupus. *Prostaglandins*, 1985, 30/1 (51-75)

Modulation of antioxidant enzymes and programmed cell death by n-3 fatty acids. *Lipids*, 1996, 31/3 Suppl. (S91-S96)

Effect of (n-3) polyunsaturated fatty acids on cytokine production and their biologic function. *Nutrition*, 1996, 12/1 Suppl. (S8-S14)

Lipid peroxidase and erythrocyte redox system in systemic vasculitides treated with corticoids. Effect of vitamin E administration. *Romanian Journal Of Internal Medicine* (Romania), 1994, 32/4 (283-289)

Free radical tissue damages in the anterior segment of the eye in experimental autoimmune uveitis. *Investigative Ophthalmology and Visual Science*, 1996, 37/4

Intervention at diagnosis of type I diabetes using either antioxidants or photopheresis. *Diabetes Metab. Rev.* (UK), 1993, 9/4 (329-336)

Free radical theory of aging: Beneficial effect of antioxidants on the life span of male NZB mice: Role of free radical reactions in the deterioration of the immune system with age and in the pathogenesis of systemic lupus erythematosus. *Age,* 1980, 3/3 (64-73)

The connective tissue diseases and the overall influence of gender. *Int J of Fertility and Menopausal Studies,* 1996, 41/2

Blood dehydroepiandrosterone sulphate (DHEAS) levels in pemphigoid/pemphigus and psoriasis. *Clinical And Experimental Rheumatology* (Italy), 1995, 13/3

Neuroendocrine-immune system interactions and autoimmunity. *Annual Review of Immunology,* 1995, 13/- (307-338)

Low serum levels of dehydroepiandrosterone may cause deficient IL-2 production by lymphocytes in patients with systemic lupus erythematosus (SLE). *Clinical and Experimental Immunology* (UK), 1995, 99/2

Bacterial Infections

Bromelain prevents secretion caused by Vibrio cholerae and Escherichia coli enterotoxins in rabbit ileum in vitro. *Gastroenterology* 1997, 113/1 (175-184)

Bromelain protects piglets from diarrhoea caused by oral challenge with K88 positive enterotoxigenic Escherichia coli. *Gut* (UK) 1998, 43/2 (196-202)

Oral administration of protease inhibits enterotoxigenic Escherichia coli receptor activity in piglet small intestine. *Gut* (UK) 1996, 38/1 (28-32)

Mycobacteria-induced autoantibody production is associated with susceptibility to infection but not with host propensity to develop autoimmune disease. *Clinical and Experimental Immunology* (UK) 1995, 100/1 (75-80)

Therapy of chlamydia infections with tetracyclines. *International Journal of Experimental and Clinical Chemotherapy* (Germany) 1990, 3/2 (101-106)

Activation of normal murine B cells by Echinococcus granulosus. *Immunology* (UK) 1989, 67/1 (16-20)

Evidence for autoantibody production associated with polyclonal B-cell activation by Pseudomonas aeruginosa. *Infection and Immunity* 1982, 35/1 (13-19)

Treatment of chronic obstructive respiratory disease. *Ars Medici* (Switzerland) 1977, 67/9 (389-390)

Clinical experience with an anti inflammatory enzyme for treating urethral infection. *Yokohama Medical Bulletin* 1972, 23/3-4 (53-65)

Protective effect of bromelain in combination with antibiotics on experimental infection in mice induced by Streptococcus hemolyticus,. *Japanese Journal of Antibiotics* 1974, 27/2 (118-121)

A study of an antibiotic and enzyme combination in 51 patients with otorrhinolaryngologic infections. *Revista Brasileira de Clinica e Terapeutica* 1973, 2/8 (349-354)

[Simultaneous therapy of inflammation and bacterial infection. Proteolytic activity of the saliva after administration of bromelain]. *G Stomatol Ortognatodonzia* (Italy) Oct-Dec 1984, 3 (4) p653-4

[Simultaneous therapy of inflammation and bacterial infection. Proteolytic activity of the saliva after administration of bromelain]. *G Stomatol Ortognatodonzia* (Italy) Jul-Sep 1984, 3 (3) p382-3

One-step synthesis of novel 2,4-diaminopyrimidine antifolates from bridged alicyclic ketones and cyanoguanidine. *Journal of Heterocyclic Chemistry* 1999, 36/3 (723-728)

Occurrence of an incomplete C8 molecule in homozygous C8 deficiency in man. *Journal of Experimental Medicine* 1981, 154/5 (1599-1607)

Bleomycin: Discovery, chemistry, and action. *Gann Monographs on Cancer Research* 1976, vol.19/- (3-36)

Probiotics. Antistaphylococcal and antifibrinolytic activities of omega amino and omega guanidinoalkanesulfonic acids. *Journal of Medicinal Chemistry* 1975, 18/5 (502-505)

[Leukocyte cytoskeleton under normal and pathological conditions]. *Arkh Patol* (USSR) 1983, 45 (6) p81-7

[In vitro activity of Mercurius cyanatus complex against relevant pathogenic bacterial isolates]. *Arzneimittelforschung* (Germany) Sep 1995, 45 (9) p1018-20

New support for a folk remedy: Cranberry juice reduces bacteriuria and pyuria in elderly women. *Nutrition Reviews* 1994, 52/5 (168-170)

Leishmania donovani possess a NADPH-dependent alkylglycerol cleavage enzyme. *Biochemical and Biophysical Research Communications* 1996, 227/3 (885-889)

Structure and antigenicity of the lipophosphoglycan from Leishmania major amastigotes. *Glycobiology* (UK) 1991, 1/4 (419-424)

Recommendations for preventing the spread of vancomycin resistance. *Infect Control Hosp Epidemiol* Feb 1995, 16 (2) p105-13

Vancomycin added to empirical combination antibiotic therapy for fever in granulocytopenic cancer patients. European

Organization for Research and Treatment of Cancer (EORTC) International Antimicrobial Therapy Cooperative Group and the National Cancer Institute of Canada-Clinical Trials Group [published erratum appears in *J Infect Dis* 1991 Oct;164(4):832] [see comments]. *J Infect Dis* May 1991, 163 (5) p951-8

Anti tubercular activity of garlic oil. *Indian Journal of Pathology and Microbiology* (India), 1998, 41/1 (131)

Sensitivity of food pathogens to garlic (Allium sativum). *Journal of Applied Microbiology* (UK), 1998, 84/2 (213-215)

Outer membrane permeability and effect of basic amino acids on antipseudomonal activity of carbapenems. *Japanese Journal of Chemotherapy* (Japan), 1998, 46/2 (73-80)

Antigen-specific lymphocytes enhance nitric oxide production in Mycobacterium bovis BCG-infected bovine macrophages. *Immunology and Cell Biology* (Australia), 1998, 76/4 (363-368)

Effects of copper and zinc ions on the germicidal properties of two popular pharmaceutical antiseptic agents—cetylpyridinium chloride and povidone-iodine. *Analyst* (UK), 1998, 123/3 (503-507)

Relationship between residual metal ions in a solution and the inhibitory capability of the metal ions for pathogenic bacterial growth. *Bulletin of the Chemical Society of Japan* (Japan), 1998, 71/4 (939-945)

Effects of zinc oxide on the attachment of Staphylococcus aureus strains. *Journal of Dermatological Science* (Ireland), 1998, 17/1 (67-74)

Toxicity of hydrogen peroxide produced by electroplated coatings to pathogenic bacteria. *Canadian Journal of Microbiology* (Canada), 1998, 44/5 (441-447)

Comparison of a topical benzoyl peroxide gel, oral minocycline, oral doxycycline and a combination for suppression of P. acnes in acne patients. *Journal of Dermatological Treatment* (UK), 1998, 9/3 (187-191)

Clinical evaluation of ceftazidime in the treatment of pediatric infections. *Jpn. J. Antibiot.* (Japan), 1984, 37/3 (363-376)

Small bowel bacterial overgrowth syndrome. *Scand. J. Gastroenterol. Suppl.* (Norway), 1983, 18/85 (83-93)

Effect of compounds with antibacterial activities in human milk on respiratory syncytial virus and cytomegalovirus in vitro. *Journal of Medical Microbiology* (UK), 1998, 47/11 (1015-1018)

Anti-inflammatory activity in rats and mice of phenolic acids isolated from Scrophularia frutescens. *Journal of Pharmacy and Pharmacology* (UK), 1998, 50/10 (1183-1186)

Effects of bacterial DNA on cytokine production by (NZB/NZW)F1 mice. *Journal of Immunology*, 1998, 161/8 (3890-3895)

The utility of aminoglycosides in an era of emerging drug resistance. *International Journal of Antimicrobial Agents* (Netherlands), 1998, 10/2 (95-105)

Screening of oriental herbal medicines for antibacterial activities. *Natural Product Sciences* (South Korea), 1998, 4/1 (32-37)

Antimicrobial activity of honey on selected microorganisms: A preliminary study. *Biomedical Research* (India), 1998, 9/1 (51-54)

Malnutrition and bacterial infections in hepatic cirrhosis *GED - Gastrenterologia Endoscopia Digestiva* (Brazil), 1997, 16/6 226-230)

Momordica charantia and Allium sativum: Broad spectrum antibacterial activity. *Korean Journal of Pharmacognosy* (South Korea), 1998, 29/3 (155-158)

Surveillance of susceptibility of clinical isolates of various bacterial species to antibacterial agents. *Japanese Journal of Chemotherapy* (Japan), 1998, 46/9 (343-363)

The antimicrobial susceptibilities and serotypes of Pseudomonas aeruginosa isolated from sputum. *Japanese Journal of Antibiotics* (Japan), 1998, 51/1 (26-36)

Probing the specificity of aminoglycoside-ribosomal RNA interactions with designed synthetic analogs. *Journal of the American Chemical Society*, 1998, 120/9 (1965-1978)

A single 16S ribosomal RNA substitution is responsible for resistance to amikacin and other 2-deoxystreptamine aminoglycosides in Mycobacterium abscessus and Mycobacterium chelonae. *Journal of Infectious Diseases*, 1998, 177/6 (1573-1581)

Influence of subinhibitory concentrations of antibiotics on surface hydrophobicity of Salmonella enteritidis. *Arzneimittel-Forschung / Drug Research* (Germany), 1998, 48/6 (697-700)

Protein synthesis as a target for antibacterial drugs: Current status and future opportunities. *Expert Opinion on Investigational Drugs* (UK), 1998, 7/8 (1237-1244)

In vitro activity of piperacillin/tazobactam versus other broad-spectrum antibiotics against nosocomial gram-negative pathogens isolated from burn patients. *Journal of Chemotherapy* (Italy), 1998, 10/3 (208-214)

The fourth-generation cephalosporins: What's the true progress. *Arquivos Brasileiros de Medicina* (Brazil), 1998, 72/3 (111-116)

Loss of fimbrial adhesion with the addition of Vaccinum macrocarpon to the growth medium of P-fimbriated Escherichia coli. *Journal of Urology*, 1998, 159/2 (559-562)

Evaluation of the effect of arginine-enriched amino acid solution on tumor growth. *J. Parenter. Enter. Nutr.*, 1985, 9/4 (428-434)

Activation of mouse macrophages by alkylglycerols, inflammation products of cancerous tissues. *Cancer Research*, 1988 Nov 1, 48(21):6044-9

Activation of mouse peritoneal macrophages by lysophospholipids and ether derivatives of neutral lipids and phospholipids. *Cancer Research*, 1987 Apr 15, 47(8):2008-13

Activation of macrophages by ether analogueues of lysophospholipids. *Cancer Immunology, Immunotherapy*, 1987, 25(3):185-92

Interactions between alkylglycerols and human neutrophil granulocytes. *Scandinavian Journal of Clinical and Laboratory Investigation*, 1990 Jun, 50(4):363-70

The effect of antioxidants on bleomycin treatment in in vitro and in vivo genotoxicity assays. *Mutation Research—Fundamental and Molecular Mechanisms of Mutagenesis* (Netherlands), 1995, 329/1 (37-47)

Inhibitory effect of vitamin C on the mutagenicity and covalent DNA binding of the electrophilic and carcinogenic metabolite, 6-sulfooxymethylbenzo(a)pyrene. *Carcinogenesis* (UK), 1994, 15/5 (917-920)

Few aspects of bacterial colonies in the stomach during the treatment with acidoinhibitors. *Boll. Chim. Farm.* (Italy), 1992, 131/8 (302-303)

The prevention and management of pressure ulcers. *Med. Clin. North Am.*, 1989, 73/6 (1511-1524)

The inhibition of bacterially mediated *N*-nitrosation by vitamin C: Relevance to the inhibition of endogenous *N*-nitrosation in the achlorhydric stomach. *Carcinogenesis* (UK), 1989, 10/2 (397-399)

Partial purification and some properties of an antibacterial compound from Aloe vera. *Phytother. Res.* (UK), 1988, 2/2 (67-69)

Activation of serum complement leads to inhibition of ascorbic acid transport (42530). *Proc. Soc. Exp. Biol. Med.*, 1987, 185/2 (153-157)

Effects of vitamins A, C, and E on aflatoxin B_1-induced mutagenesis in Salmonella typhimurium TA-98 and TA-100. *Teratog. Carcinog. Mutag.*, 1985, 5/1 (29-40)

Effect of vitamin A supplementation on lectin-induced diarrhoea and bacterial translocation in rats. *Nutrition Research*, 1996, 16/3 (459-465)

Increased translocation of Escherichia coli and development of arthritis in vitamin A-deficient rats. *Infection and Immunity*, 1995, 63/8 (3062-3068)

Gastrointestinal infections in children. *Curr. Opin. Gastroenterol.* (UK), 1994, 10/1 (88-97)

Intestinal malabsorption presenting with night blindness. *Br. J. Clin. Pract.* (UK), 1993, 47/5 (275-276)

Etiology of acute lower respiratory tract infection in children from Alabang, Metro Manila. *Rev. Infect. Dis.*, 1990, 12/Suppl. 8 (S929-S939)

Effect of vitamin A in enteral formulae for burned guinea-pigs. *Burns* (UK), 1990, 16/4 (265-272)

Vitamin A supplementation improves macrophage function and bacterial clearance during experimental salmonella infection. *Proc. Soc. Exp. Biol. Med.*, 1989, 191/1 (47-54)

Inhibition by retinoic acid of multiplication of virulent tubercle bacilli in cultured human macrophages. *Infect. Immun.*, 1989, 57/3 (840-844)

Corneal ulceration, measles, and childhood blindness in Tanzania. *Br. J. Ophthalmol.* (UK), 1987, 71/5 (331-343)

Impact of vitamin A supplementation on childhood mortality. A randomised controlled community trial. *Lancet* (UK), 1986, 1/8491 (1169-1173)

Impaired blood clearance of bacteria and phagocytic activity in vitamin A-deficient rats (41999). *Proc. Soc. Exp. Biol. Med.*, 1985, 178/2 (204-208)

Chronic salmonella septicemia and malabsorption of vitamin A. *Am. J. Clin. Nutr.*, 1979, 32/2 (319-324)

Retinol level in patients with psoriasis during treatment with B group vitamins, a bacterial polysaccharide (pyrogenal) and methotrexate (Russian). *Vestn.Derm.Vener.* (USSR), 1975, 51/1 (55-58)

Essential fatty acids: Biology and their clinical implications. *Asia Pac. J. Pharmacol.* (Singapore), 1991, 6/4 (317-330)

Essential fatty acid deficiency in children. *tijdschr. kindergeneeskd.* (Netherlands), 1981, 49/1 (10-15)

Nitric oxide-dependent killing of Candida albicans by murine peritoneal cells during an experimental infection. *FEMS Immunology and Medical Microbiology* (Netherlands), 1995, 11/3 (157-162)

Biosynthesis and interaction of endothelium-derived vasoactive mediators. *Eicosanoids* (Germany), 1991, 4/4 (187-202)

Regulation of macrophage physiology by *L*-arginine: Role of the oxidative *L*-arginine deiminase pathway. *J. Immunol.*, 1989, 143/11 (3641-3646)

Comparative evaluation of aloe vera in the management of burn wounds in guinea pigs. *Plast. Reconstr. Surg.*, 1988, 81/3 (386-389)

Effect of topical zinc oxide on bacterial growth and inflammation in full-thickness skin wounds in normal and diabetic rats. Agren MS; Soderberg TA; Reuterving CO; Hallmans G; Tengrup I, Department of Pathology, University of Linkoping, Sweden. *Eur J Surg* (Sweden) Feb 1991, 157 (2) p97-101

Antimicrobial activity of some commercial extracts of propolis prepared with different solvents. *Phytotherapy Research* (UK), 1996, 10/4 (335-336)

Antibacterial action of a formulation containing propolis of Apis mellifera. *L. Rev. Farm. Bioquim. Univ. Sao Paulo* (Brazil), 1994, 30/1 (19-21)

Electron microscopic and microcalorimetric investigations of the possible mechanism of the antibacterial action of a defined propolis provenance. *Planta Med.* (Germany), 1994, 60/3 (222-227)

Synergistic effect of ethanolic extract of propolis and antibiotics on the growth of Staphylococcus aureus. *Arzneim.-Forsch. Drug Res.* (Germany), 1993, 43/5 (607-609)

Antibacterial, antifungal, antiamoebic, antiinflammatory and antipyretic studies on propolis bee products. *J. Ethnopharmacol.* (Ireland), 1991, 35/1 (77-82)

Antibacterial properties of propolis (bee glue). *J. R. Soc. Med.* (UK), 1990, 83/3 (159-160)

Biological properties and clinical application of propolis. III. Investigation of the sensitivity of staphylococci isolated from pathological cases to ethanol extract of propolis (EEP). *Arzneim.-Forsch.* (Germany, West), 1977, 27/7 (1395)

Biological properties and clinical application of propolis. I. Some physico chemical properties of propolis. *Arzneimittel-Forsch.* (Germany, West), 1977, 27/4 (889-890)

Balding

Balding hair follicle dermal papilla cells contain higher levels of androgen receptors than those from non-balding scalp. *J Endocrinol* (England) Jan 1998, 156 (1) p59-65

United States Patent: [19][11]

Patent Number: 5,352,442

Proctor: [45]

Date of Patent: Oct. 4,1994

Various other U.S. and foreign patents

Further references:

Anderson, *Chemical Abstracts*, vol. 90, p. 311K (1979)

Ando et al., *Chemical Abstracts* 93:79872n (1980)

Bazzano et al., *Journal of American Academy of Dermatology*, vol. 15, pp. 880-883 (1986)

Barry, *Pharmacology of the Skin*, vol. 1, pp. 121-137 (1987)

Cheng et al., *Archives of Dermatological Research*, vol. 278, pp. 470-473 (1986)

Cumming. et al., *Journal of American Medical Association*, vol. 247, pp. 1295-1298 (1982)

Dawber, *Dermatologica*, vol. 175 suppl. 2, pp. 23-28 (1987)

DeVillez, *Archives of Dermatology*, vol 121, pp. 197-202, (1985)

Dostert a d., *Xenobiotica*, vol. 15, No. 10, pp. 799-803 (1985)

Ehman et d., *Investigative Radiology*, vol. 21, pp. 125-131 (1986)

Feelisch et al., *Evr. Journal of Pharmacology*, vol. 139, pp. 19-30 (1987)

Feelisch et al., *Evr. Journal of Pharmacology*, vol. 142, pp. 405-409 (1987)

Fox et al., *Annals of the New York Academy of Sciences*, vol. 411, pp. 14-19 (1983)

Goffman et al., *International Journal of Radiation, Oncology, Biology and Physics*, vol. 22, pp. 803-806 (Nov. 4, 1992)

Headington, *Current Therapeutic Research,* vol. 36, pp. 1098-1105 (1984)

Hearse et al., *Circulation Research*, vol. 60, pp. 375-383 (1987)

Heschler, *Chemical Abstracts*, vol. 78, pp. 115-239 (1973)

Ignarro et al., *Biochemica ct. Biophysica Acta*, vol. 631, pp. 221-231 (1980)

J., Soc. Cosmetology Chem., (Italy) vol. 33, pp. 95-96 (Mar./Apr. 1982)

Journal of American Medical Association, vol. 260, No. 20 (1988)

Karlsson et al., *Journal of Cyclic Nucleotide and Protein Res.*, vol. 10, No. 4, pp. 309-315 (1985)

Kvedar, *Journal of American Academic Dermatology*, vol. 12, pp. 215-225 (1985)

Longevity, vol. 2, No. 3, p. 26 (Jan. 1988)

Lucky, *Archives of Dermatology*, vol. 121, pp.57-62 (1985). Messina, *Current Therapeutic Research* vol. 34, pp. 319-324 (1983)

Messina, *Current Therapeutic Research*, vol. 38, pp. 269-282 (1985)

Mitchell et al., *IBC USA Conference*, South Natick, Mass: (Jun. 27, 1991)

Mittal et al., *Proc. of National Academy of Science USA,* vol. 74, No. 10 pp. 4360-4364 (1977)

Bell's Palsy

F-waves of the facial muscles in healthy control subjects and in patients with peripheral facial nerve disturbance. *Electromyogr Clin Neurophysiol* (Belgium) Apr-May 1999, 39 (3) p167-74,

An unusual manifestation of diabetes mellitus. *Hosp Pract* (Off Ed) May 15 1999, 34 (5) p39-40

The illness known as "twisted mouth" among the Nehinaw (Cree). *Int J Circumpolar Health* (Finland) 1998, 57 Suppl 1 p67-71

Blink reflex recovery in facial weakness: an electrophysiologic study of adaptive changes. *Neurology* Mar 10 1999, 52 (4) p834-8

A clinical study on the magnetic stimulation of the facial nerve. *Laryngoscope* Mar 1999, 109 (3) p492-7

Peripheral facial palsy: etiology, diagnosis and treatment. *Eur Neurol* (Switzerland) Jan 1999, 41 (1) p3-9

Seasonal patterns of idiopathic facial paralysis: a 16-year study. *Otolaryngol Head Neck Surg* Feb 1999, 120 (2) p269-71

Methylcobalamin. *Altern Med Rev* Dec 1998, 3 (6) p461-3

[Bell's palsy: diagnostic and therapeutical trial in childhood] *Minerva Pediatr* (Italy) Jun 1996, 48 (6) p245-50

Methylcobalamin treatment of Bell's palsy. *Methods Find Exp Clin Pharmacol* (Spain) Oct 1995, 17 (8) p539-44

Treatment for facial neuronitis: a new approach to Bell's palsy. *An Otorrinolaringol Ibero Am* (Spain) 1991, 18 (4) p361-74

[Conservative treatment of Bell's palsy—high dose steroid infusion with low-molecular dextran] *Nippon Jibiinkoka Gakkai Kaiho* (Japan) May 1989, 92 (5) p694-702

Medical treatment of Bell's palsy. Oral vs. intravenous administration. *Acta Otolaryngol Suppl* (Stockh) (Sweden) 1988, 446 p114-8

An animal model of type-1 herpes simplex virus infection of facial nerve. *Acta Otolaryngol Suppl* (Stockh) (Sweden) 1988, 446 p157-64

Susceptibility of isolated rat facial nerve to anaerobic stress. *Eur Arch Otorhinolaryngol Suppl* (Germany) 1997, 1 pS64-7

An accidental tarsorrhaphy caused by acrylic adhesive. *Am J Ophthalmol* Sep 1976, 82 (3) p501

Administration of mecobalamin after surgical repair of the facial nerve. *Practica Otologica* (Japan) 1981, 74/10 (2301-2307)

Management on Bell's palsy. *Revue de Medecine* (France) 1981, 22/23 (1417-1419)

Prognosis in Bell's palsy. Influence of early treatment *Journal of the Indian Medical Association* 1974, 62/8 (281-282)

[Idiopathic facial paralysis]. *HNO* (Germany) Sep 1998, 46 (9) p786-98

Bell's palsy: an update on idiopathic facial paralysis. *Nurse Pract* Aug 1997, 22 (8) p88, 97-100, 102-5; quiz 106-7

[Diagnosis and treatment of facial palsy]. *Neurologia* (Spain) Jan 1997, 12 (1) p23-30

Hemifacial spasm: clinical findings and treatment. *Muscle Nerve Dec* 1998, 21 (12) p1740-7

[6 years experience with reversible and surgical upper eyelid weighting in lagophthamos]. *Ophthalmologe* (Germany) Apr 1997, 94 (4) p295-9

[Early corticoid treatment of idiopathic facial palsy (Bell)]. *Acta Otorrinolaringol Esp* (SPAIN) Apr 1997, 48 (3) p177-81

The use of low-dose histamine therapy in otolaryngology. *Ear, Nose and Throat Journal* 1999, 78/5 (366-370)

Bladder Conditions

See references under Urinary Tract Infections.

Breast Cancer

Progress on therapy of breast cancer with vitamin Q_{10} and the regression of metastases. *Biochem Biophys Res Commun* Jul 6 1995

Apparent partial remission of breast cancer in 'high risk' patients supplemented with nutritional antioxidants, essential fatty acids and coenzyme Q_{10}. *Mol Aspects Med* (England) 1994, 15 Suppl

Effects of isoprenoids (CoQ_{10}) on growth of normal human mammary epithelial cells and breast cancer cells in vitro. *Anticancer Res* (Greece) Jan-Feb 1994

Partial and complete regression of breast cancer in patients in relation to dosage of Coenzyme Q_{10}. *Biochem Biophys Res Commun* Mar 30 1994

Modulation of the length of the cell cycle time of MCF-7 human breast cancer cells by melatonin. *Life Sci* (England) 1996, 58 (9)

Melatonin blocks the stimulatory effects of prolactin on human breast cancer cell growth in culture. *Br J Cancer* (England) Dec 1995

Melatonin modulation of estrogen-regulated proteins, growth factors, and proto-oncogenes in human breast cancer. *J Pineal Res* (Denmark) Mar 1995

Melatonin inhibition of MCF-7 human breast-cancer cells growth: influence of cell proliferation rate. *Cancer Lett* (Ireland) Jul 13 1995

Serial transplants of DMBA-induced mammary tumors in Fischer rats as model system for human breast cancer. IV. Parallel changes of biopterin and melatonin indicate interactions between the pineal gland and cellular immunity in malignancy. *Oncology* (Switzerland) Jul-Aug 1995

Modulation of cancer endocrine therapy by melatonin: a phase II study of tamoxifen plus melatonin in metastatic breast cancer patients progressing under tamoxifen alone. *Br J Cancer* (England) Apr 1995

Modulation of estrogen receptor mRNA expression by melatonin in MCF-7 human breast cancer cells. *Mol Endocrinol* Dec 1994

Melatonin modulates growth factor activity in MCF-7 human breast cancer cells. *J Pineal Res* (Denmark) Aug 1994

Differences between pulsatile or continuous exposure to melatonin on MCF-7 human breast cancer cell proliferation. *Cancer Lett* (Ireland) Sep 30 1994

Effects of melatonin on cancer: studies on MCF-7 human breast cancer cells in culture. *J Neural Transm Suppl* (Austria) 1986, 21 p433-49

Role of pineal gland in aetiology and treatment of breast cancer. *Lancet* (England) Oct 14 1978

Beta-interferon, retinoids and tamoxifen as maintenance therapy in metastatic breast cancer. A pilot study. *Clin Ter* (Italy) Oct 1995

The effects of retinoids on proliferative capacities and macromolecular synthesis in human breast cancer MCF-7 cells. *Cancer* Nov 15 1980

The anti-proliferative effect of vitamin D3 analogueues is not mediated by inhibition of the AP-1 pathway, but may be related to promoter selectivity. *Oncogene* (England) Nov 2 1995

Epidemiology of soy and cancer: perspectives and directions. *J Nutr* Mar 1995, 125 (3 Suppl)

Effects of tyrosine kinase inhibitors on the proliferation of human breast cancer cell lines and proteins important in the ras signaling pathway. *Int J Cancer* Jan 17 1996

Selective responsiveness of human breast cancer cells to indole-3-carbinol, a chemopreventive agent. *J Natl Cancer Inst* Jan 19 1994

Differential stimulatory and inhibitory responses of human MCF-7 breast cancer cells to linoleic acid and conjugated linoleic acid in culture. *Anticancer Res.* (Greece), 1992, 12/6 B

Inhibitory effect of conjugated dienoic derivatives of linoleic acid and beta-carotene on the in vitro growth of human cancer cells. *Cancer Lett.* (Ireland), 1992, 63/2 (125-133)

Preferential cytotoxicity on tumor cells by caffeic acid phenethyl ester isolated from propolis. *Experientia* (Switzerland), 1988, 44/3 (230-232)

Effect of caffeic acid esters on carcinogen-induced mutagenicity and human colon adenocarcinoma cell growth. *Chem.-Biol. Interact.* (Ireland), 1992, 84/3 (277-290)

Bursitis

See references under Arthritis.

Cancer Chemotherapy

Treatment of cancer chemotherapy-induced toxicity with the pineal hormone melatonin. *Support Care Cancer* Mar 1997, 5 (2) p126-9

The protective role of selenium on the toxicity of cisplatin-contained chemotherapy regimen in cancer patients. *Biol Trace Elem Res* Mar 1997, 56 (3) p331-41

Supplementation with antioxidants prior to bone marrow transplantation. *Wiener Klinische Wochenschrift* 1997, 109/19 (771-776)

The role of natrium selenite as adjuvants in radiotherapy of rectal cancer. *Medizinische Klinik*, 1997, 92/Suppl. 3 (48-49)

Ascorbic acid in the prevention and treatment of cancer. *Altern Med Rev* Jun 1998, 3 (3) p174-86

Characteristics of green tea—A review. *Zeitschrift fur Onkologie*, 1998, 30/3 (57-63)

Antioxidants enhance the cytotoxicity of chemotherapeutic agents in colorectal cancer : a p53-independent induction of p21WAF1/CIP1 via C/EBPbeta [see comments]. *Nat Med* Nov 1997, 3 (11) p1233-41

Selenium (Se) deficiency in women with ovarian cancer undergoing chemotherapy and the influence of supplementation with this micro-element on biochemical parameters. *Pharmazie* Jul 1998, 53 (7) p473-6

Melatonin as biological response modifier in cancer patients. *Anticancer Res* Mar-Apr 1998, 18 (2B) p1329-32

A randomized study of chemotherapy with cisplatin plus etoposide versus chemoendocrine therapy with cisplatin, etoposide and the pineal hormone melatonin as a first-line treatment of advanced non-small cell lung cancer patients in a poor clinical state. *J Pineal Res* Aug 1997, 23 (1) p15-9

Melatonin in osteosarcoma: an effective drug? *Med Hypotheses* Jun 1997, 48 (6) p523-5

The validity of melatonin as an oncostatic agent. *J Pineal Res* May 1997, 22 (4) p184-202

Retinoids: use in combating cancer. *Ned Tijdschr Geneeskd* Jun 14 1997, 141 (24) p1183-8

Treatment of hepatocellular carcinoma: Medical options. *Liver Transplantation and Surgery*, 1998, 4/5 Suppl. 1 (S92-S97)

Effects of glutamine supplements and radiochemotherapy on systemic immune and gut barrier function in patients with advanced esophageal cancer. *Annals of Surgery* 1998, 227/4 (485-491

[Effect of biological membrane stabilizing drugs (Coenzyme Q_{10}, dextran sulfate and reduced glutathione) on adriamycin (doxorubicin)-induced toxicity and microsomal lipid peroxidation in mice] *Gan To Kagaku Ryoho*. 1996 Jan. 23(1). P 93-8

Coenzyme Q_{10}, plasma membrane oxidase and growth control. *Mol Aspects Med*. 1994. 15 SupplP s1-11

Protective effects of various drugs on adriamycin (doxorubicin)-induced toxicity and microsomal lipid peroxidation in mice and rats. *Biol Pharm Bull*. 1993 Nov. 16(11). P 1114-7

Tissue concentration of doxorubicin (adriamycin) in mouse pretreated with alpha- tocopherol or coenzyme Q_{10}. *Acta Med Okayama*. 1991 Jun. 45 (3). P 195-9

[Electrocardiogram analysis of adriamycin cardiotoxicity in 160 cases] *Chung Hua Chung Liu Tsa Chih*. 1991 Jan. 13 (1). p71-3

Adriamycin-Fe3+-induced mitochondrial protein damage with lipid peroxidation. *Biol Pharm Bull*. 1995 Apr. 18(4). P 514-7

Effect of antioxidants on adriamycin-induced microsomal lipid peroxidation. *Biol Trace Elem Res*. 1995 Jan-Mar. 47(1-3). P 111-6

Alpha tocopherol improves focal glomerulosclerosis in rats with adriamycin-induced progressive renal failure. *Nephron*. 1994. 68(3). P 347-52

Adriamycin-induced oxidative stress in rat central nervous system. *Biochem Mol Biol Int*. 1993 Apr. 29(5). P 807-20

[Cardioprotection in chemo- and radiotherapy for malignant diseases—an echocardiographic pilot study] *Schweiz Rundsch Med Prax*. 1995 Oct 24. 84(43). P 1220-3

Randomised comparison of fluorouracil, epidoxorubicin and methotrexate (FEMTX) plus supportive care with supportive care alone in patients with non-resectable gastric cancer. *Br J Cancer*. 1995 Mar. 71(3). P 587-91

Enhancement of the antineoplastic effect of anticarcinogens on benzo[a]pyrene-treated Wistar rats, in relation to their number and biological activity. *Cancer Lett*. 1994 Jul 29. 82(2). P 153-65

Critical reappraisal of vitamins and trace minerals in nutritional support of cancer patients. *Support Care Cancer*. 1993 Nov. 1(6). P 295-7

The effects of chemotherapy including cisplatin on vitamin D metabolism. *Endocr J*. 1993 Dec. 40(6). P 737-42

Vitamin A, a useful biochemical modulator capable of preventing intestinal damage during methotrexate treatment. *Pharmacol Toxicol*. 1993 Aug. 73(2). P 69-74

Chemotherapy-induced alopecia: new developments *South Med J*. 1993 May. 86(5). P 489-96

Vitamin E enhances the chemotherapeutic effects of adriamycin on human prostatic carcinoma cells in vitro. *J. Urol*. (Baltimore), 1986, 136/2 (529-531)

Hematological aspects of vitamin E, continued. Adriamycin cardiotoxicity amelioration by alpha-tocopherol. *Am. J. Pediatr. Hematol. Oncol*., 1979, 1/2 (151-153)

Treatment of cancer-related thrombocytopenia by low-dose subcutaneous Interleukin-2 plus the pineal hormone melatonin: A biological phase II study. *Journal of Biological Regulators and Homeostatic Agents* (Italy), 1995, 9/2 (52-54)

Type 2 Th cells as target of the circadian melatonin signal: Relevance in local immunity. *Regional Immunology*, 1995, 6/5-6 (350-354)

Hematopoietic rescue via T-cell-dependent, endogenous granulocyte-macrophage colony-stimulating factor induced by the pineal neurohormone melatonin in tumor-bearing mice. *Cancer Res*., 1994, 54/9 (2429-2432)

Randomized study with the pineal hormone melatonin versus supportive care alone in advanced nonsmall cell lung cancer resistant to a first-line chemotherapy containing cisplatin. *Oncology* (Switzerland), 1992, 49/5 (336-339)

Preliminary studies on melatonin in the treatment of myelodysplastic syndromes following cancer chemotherapy. *J. Pineal Res*. (Denmark), 1990, 8/4 (347-354)

Melatonin increase as predictor for tumor objective response to chemotherapy in advanced cancer patients. *Tumori* (Italy), 1988, 74/3 (339-345)

Induction of cyclo-oxygenase-2 mRNA by prostaglandin E-2 in human prostatic carcinoma cells. *British Journal of Cancer* 75(8): p1111-1118 1997

Tjandrawinata R R; Dahiya R; Hughes-Fulford M, Abstract: Prostaglandins are synthesized from arachidonic acid by the enzyme cyclo-oxygenase. Lab. Cell Growth, Veterans Affairs Med. Cent., 4150 Clement St., San Francisco, CA 94121

Inhibition of the 3-hydroxy-3-methylglutaryl-coenzyme A reductase pathway induces p53-independent transcriptional regulation of p21(WAF1/CIP1) in human prostate carcinoma cells, *Journal of Biological Chemistry* (United States) 24 Apr;1998, 273/17

Cyclooxygenase-2 expression is up-regulated in human pancreatic cancer. *Cancer Res* 1999 Mar 1;59(5):987-90

COX-2 and colon cancer. *Inflammation Research* 1998 Oct;47 Suppl 2:S112-6

Chemopreventive effect of N-(2-cyclohexyloxy-4-nitrophenyl)methane

sulfonamide (NS-398), a selective cyclooxygenase-2 inhibitor, in rat colon carcinogenesis induced by azoxymethane. *Japanese J Cancer Res* 1999 Apr;90(4):

406-12

Lovastatin Augments Sulindac-Induced Apoptosis in Colon Cancer Cells and Potentiates Chemopreventive Effects of Sulindac. *Gastroenterology* 1999 Oct;117(4):838-847

ras Oncogenes in human cancer: a review. Published erratum appears in *Cancer Res* 1990 Feb 15;50(4):1352

Lovastatin-induced proliferation inhibition and apoptosis in C6 glial cells. *J Pharmacol Exp Ther* 1999 Apr;289(1):572-9

Etodolac (Lodine) in the treatment of osteoarthritis: recent studies. *J Rheumatol* (Suppl) 1997 Feb;47:23-31

Double blind evaluation of the long-term effects of etodolac versus ibuprofen in patients with rheumatoid arthritis. *J Rheumatol* (Suppl) 1997 Feb;47:17-22

The relationship between cyclooxygenase-2 expression and colorectal cancer. *JAMA* 1999 Oct 6;282(13):1254-7

Cancer Radiation Therapy

Oxygenation of cervical cancers during radiotherapy and radiotherapy + cis-retinoic acid/interferon. *Int J Radiat Oncol Biol Phys* 1999 Jan 15;43(2):367-73

A 2-week pretreatment with 13-cis-retinoic acid + interferon-alpha-2a prior to definitive radiation improves tumor tissue oxygenation in cervical cancers. *Strahlenther Onkol* 1998 Nov;174(11):571-4

Melatonin and protection from whole-body irradiation: survival studies in mice. *Mutat Res* 1999 Mar 10;425(1):21-7

Increased survival time in brain glioblastomas by a radioneuroendocrine strategy with radiotherapy plus melatonin compared to radiotherapy alone. *Oncology* 1996 Jan-Feb;53(1):43-6

Vitamin A inhibits radiation-induced pneumonitis in rats. *J Nutr* 1998 Oct;128(10):1661-4

Sexual dysfunction after radical radiation therapy for prostate cancer: a prospective evaluation. *Urology* 1999 Jul;54(1):124-9

Striking regression of radiation-induced fibrosis by a combination of pentoxifylline and tocopherol. *Br J Radiol* 1998 Aug;71(848):892-4

Taurine deficiency after intensive chemotherapy and/or radiation. *Am J Clin Nutr*; 55(3):708-11 1992

Effect of glutaurine and its derivatives and their combinations with radiation protective substances upon irradiated mice. *Acta Radiol Oncol Radiat Phys Biol*; 20(5):319-324 1981

[Effect of mixed gamma-neutron irradiation on taurine penetration through cellular membranes of rat peripheral blood leukocytes]. Res. Inst. Biology and Biophysics, V. V. Kuibyshev Tomsk State Univ., Tomsk, USSR

[Sources of taurine hyperexcretion in irradiated rats] *Radiobiologiia*; 20(3):455-459 1980

[Taurine and sh-group content in the platelets of irradiated rats] *Radiobiologiia;* 18(2):271-274

Biological Effects of Alkylglycerols I. Prog Biochem Pharmacol; 22:48-57 1988, (37 Refs)

Effect of alkoxyglycerols on the frequency of injuries following radiation therapy for carcinoma of the uterine cervix. *Acta Obstet Gynecol Scand*; 56(4):441-448 1977

In vivo radioprotective activity of Panax ginseng and diethyldithiocarbamate. *In Vivo*; 7(5):467-70 1993

Inhibition of mutagenesis and transformation by root extracts of panax ginseng in vitro. *Planta Med*; 57(2):125-8 1991

Restoration of radiation injury by ginseng. Ii. Some properties of the radioprotective substances. *J Radiat Res* (Tokyo); 22(3):336-343

Restoration of radiation injury by ginseng. I. Responses of x-irradiated mice to ginseng extract. *J Radiat Res* (Tokyo); 22(3):323-335

[Substances stimulating recovery from radiation injury]. *Radioisotopes*; 27(11):666-675 1978

Acemannan Immunostimulant in combination with surgery and radiation therapy on spontaneous canine and feline fibrosarcomas. *J Am Anim Hosp Assoc*; 31(5):439-47 1995

Acemannan-containing wound dressing gel reduces radiation-induced skin reactions in C3H mice. *Int J Radiat Oncol Biol Phys*; 32(4):1047-52 1995

Cancer Surgery

Preoperative oral supplement with immunonutrients in cancer patients. *JPEN J Parenter Enteral Nutr Jul*-Aug 1998, 22 (4) p206-11

Ascorbic acid in the prevention and treatment of cancer. *Altern Med Rev* Jun 1998, 3 (3) p174-86

Effect of a fish oil structured lipid-based diet on prostaglandin release from mononuclear cells in cancer patients after surgery. *JPEN J Parenter Enteral Nutr* Sep-Oct 1997, 21 (5) p266-74

Eating to beat breast cancer: potential role for soy supplements. *Ann Oncol* Mar 1997, 8 (3) p223-5

Dietary supplement use by women at risk for breast cancer recurrence. *Journal of the American Dietetic Association*, 1998, 98/3 (285-292)

Fiber and its effect on colonic function in health and disease. *Current Opinion in Gastroenterology*, 1998, 14/1 (1-5)

Potentiation of the response to chemotherapy in patients with breast cancer by dietary supplementation with *L*-arginine: Results of a randomised controlled trial. *International Journal of Oncology*, 1998, 12/1 (221-225)

Vitamin B12 and folic acid plasma levels after ileocecal and ileal neobladder reconstruction. *Urology*, 1997, 50/6 (888-892)

Dietary iron and recurrence of colorectal adenomas. *Cancer Epidemiology Biomarkers and Prevention*, 1997, 6/12 (1029-1032)

Immuno-nutrition: Designer diets in cancer. *Supportive Care in Cancer*, 1997, 5/5 (381-386)

Dietary supplementation with *L*-arginine: Modulation of tumour-infiltrating lymphocytes in patients with colorectal cancer. *British Journal of Surgery*, 1997, 84/2 (238-241)

Subcutaneous, omentum and tumor fatty acid composition, and serum insulin status in patients with benign or cancerous ovarian or endometrial tumors. Do tumors preferentially utilize polyunsaturated fatty acids? *Cancer Letters*, 1997, 111/1-2 (179-185)

Glutathione metabolism in patients with non-small cell lung cancers. *Cancer Research*, 1997, 57/1 (152-155)

The effect of folic acid supplementation on the risk for cancer or dysplasia in ulcerative colitis. *Gastroenterology*, 1997, 112/1 (29-32)

Interleukin 2 treatment in colorectal cancer: current results and future prospects. *Eur J Surg Oncol*; 20(6):622-9 1994

Perioperative immunomodulation in cancer surgery. *Am J Surg*; 167(1):174-9 1994

Immune defects in patients with head and neck cancer. *Anticancer Res*; 13(6B):2507-19 1993

Effects of alprazolam on cellular immune response to surgical stress in mice. *Cancer Lett*; 73(2-3):155-60 1993

Morphine attenuates surgery-induced enhancement of metastatic colonization in rats. *Pain*; 54(1):21-8 1993

Narcotic-induced suppression of natural killer cell activity in ventilated and nonventilated rats. *Clin Immunol Immunopathol*; 64(2):173-6 1992

The impact of surgery on natural killer cell cytotoxicity and tumor metastasis in rats. *Diss Abstr Int [B]*; 53(4):1776 1992

Altered lymphocyte subsets and natural killer cells of patients with obstructive jaundice in perioperative period. *J Tongji Med Univ*; 11(3):145-9 1991

Hierarchical immunosuppression of regional lymph nodes in patients with head and neck squamous cell carcinoma. *Otolaryngol Head Neck Surg*; 105(4):517-27 1991

Effects of alprazolam on t-cell immunosuppressive response to surgical stress in mice. *Cancer Lett*; 58(3):183-7 1991

Blood transfusion and survival after laryngectomy for laryngeal carcinoma. *J Laryngol Otol*; 105(4):293-4 1991

[The effect of surgical intervention on the state of the immune system in brain tumors]. *Klin Khir*; (12):4-6 1990

[Dynamics of various indicators of immunity in relation to the type of anesthesia during surgical treatment of patients with lung cancer after irradiation]. *Vestn Khir Im I I Grek*; 145(8):99-102 1990

Mechanism of surgical stress impairment of murine natural killer cell cytotoxicity. *Diss Abstr Int [B]*; 51(6):2809 1990

Highly immunogenic regressor tumor cells can prevent development of postsurgical tumor immunity. *Cell Immunol*; 119(1):101-13 1989

General concepts in cancer treatment. *Surgical Oncology: A European Handbook*, p. 121-305, 1989

Effects of low dose perioperative interferon on the surgically induced suppression of antitumour immune responses. *Br J Surg*; 75(10):976-81 1988

Lymphocyte subsets, natural killer cytotoxicity, and perioperative blood transfusion for elective colorectal cancer surgery. *Cancer Detect Prev Suppl*; 1:571-6 1987

Effect of surgical stress on murine natural killer cell cytotoxicity. *J Immunol*; 138(1):171-8 1987

Immune suppression: *therapeutic alterations. Principles of Cancer Biotherapy*, p. 93-162, 1987

Suppression of natural killer cell activity by surgical stress in cancer patients and the underlying mechanisms. *Acta Med Okayama*; 40(2):113-9 1986

Surgical stress-mediated suppression of murine natural killer cell cytotoxicity. *Cancer Res*; 44(9):3888-91 1984

Surgery, trauma and immune suppression. Evolving the mechanism. *Ann Surg*; 197(4):434-8 1983

Surgical essentials in the care of the elderly cancer patient. *Aging;* 24:57-61 1983

[Postoperative treatment of malignant brain tumors with acnu and psk-particularly immunological follow-up research]. *Gan To Kagaku Ryoho*; 9(6):1081-90 1982

Principles of pathology in surgery. *Principles of Pathology in Surgery*, 453 pp., 1980

Small cell carcinoma of the lung. *Ann Thorac Surg*; 30(6):602-610 1980

Cancer and immunocompetence. *Acta Chir Scand Suppl*; (498):146-150 1980

Alteration of lymphocyte function due to anesthesia: in vivo and in vitro suppression of mitogen-induced blastogenesis by sodium pentobarbital. *Surgery*; 87(5):573-580 1980

A mechanism of suppression of antitumor immunity (lai reactivity) by surgery. *Cancer Immunol Immunother*; 7(4):263-269 1980

[The state of immune responsiveness in various course of stomach cancer]. *Vopr Onkol*; 23(4):72-76 1977

Effects of operation on immune response in cancer patients: sequential evaluation of in vitro lymphocyte function. *Surgery*; 79(1):46-51 1976

[Surgery, hormone therapy, and irradiation in a patient with metastasizing mammary carcinoma]. *Fortschr Med*; 92(14):615-616 1974

Renal impairment associated with the pre-operative administration of recombinant interleukin-2. *Clin Sci* (Colch); 87(5):513-8 1994

Cancer (Adjuvant) Treatment

Gut bacteria and aetiology of cancer of the breast. *Lancet* 1971 Aug 28;2(7722):472-3

Soybean phytochemicals inhibit the growth of transplantable human prostate carcinoma and tumor angiogenesis in mice. *J Nutr* 1999 Sep;129(9):1628-35

The two phyto-oestrogens genistein and quercetin exert different effects on oestrogen receptor function. *Br J Cancer* 1999 Jun;80(8):1150-5

p53-independent apoptosis induced by genistein in lung cancer cells. *Nutr Cancer* 1999;33(2):125-31

Effects of a soybean isoflavone mixture on carcinogenesis in prostate and seminal vesicles of F344 rats. *Jpn J Cancer Res* 1999 Apr;90(4):393-8

Differentiating agents and nontoxic therapies. Myers CE *Urol Clin North Am* 1999 May;26(2):341-51

Tocotrienol: a review of its therapeutic potential. *Clin Biochem* 1999 Jul;32(5):309-19

Vitamins and lung cancer. *Proc Nutr Soc* 1999 May;58(2): 329-33

Vitamins A, C and E and the risk of breast cancer: results from a case-control study in Greece. *Br J Cancer* 1999 Jan;79(1):23-9

Health-promoting properties of common herbs. *Am J Clin Nutr* 1999 Sep;70(3 Suppl):491S-9S

Mechanistic aspects of green tea as a cancer preventive: effect of components on human stomach cancer cell lines. *Jpn J Cancer Res* 1999 Jul;90(7):733-9

Prostate cancer chemoprevention by green tea. *Semin Urol Oncol* 1999 May;17(2): 70-6

[Protective effect of tea on immune function in mice]. *Chung Hua Yu Fang I Hsueh Tsa Chih* 1998 Sep;32(5):270-4

[Chemoprotection by green tea against the formation of food-borne carcinogen 2-amino-1-methyl-6-phenylimidazo [4,5-b] pyridine (PhIP)-DNA adducts in rats]. *Chung Hua Yu Fang I Hsueh Tsa Chih* 1998 Sep;32(5):261-4

Tea and health: the underlying mechanisms. *Proc Soc Exp Biol Med* 1999 Apr;220(4):271-5

Cancer chemopreventive mechanisms of tea against heterocyclic amine mutagens from cooked meat. *Proc Soc Exp Biol Med* 1999 Apr;220(4):239-43

Protective effect of allium vegetables against both esophageal and stomach cancer: a simultaneous case-referent study of a high-epidemic area in Jiangsu Province, China. *Jpn J Cancer Res* 1999 Jun;90(6):614-21

Selenium. *J Toxicol Clin Toxicol* 1999;37(2):145-72

The effects of garlic preparations against human tumor cell proliferation. *Phytomedicine* 1999 Mar;6(1):7-11

[The preventing function of garlic on experimental oral precancer and its effect on natural killer cells, T-lymphocytes and interleukin-2]. *Hunan I Ko Ta Hsueh Hsueh Pao* 1997;22(3):246-8

Effects of the garlic components diallyl sulfide and diallyl disulfide on arylamine *N*-acetyltransferase activity in human colon tumour cells. *Food Chem Toxicol* 1998 Sep-Oct;36(9-10):761-70

Conjugated linoleic acid inhibits proliferation and induces apoptosis of normal rat mammary epithelial cells in primary culture. *Exp Cell Res* 1999 Jul 10;250(1):22-34

Inhibitory action of melatonin on H2O2- and cyclophosphamide-induced DNA damage. *Mutagenesis* 1999 Jan;14(1): 107-12

Melatonin increases p53 and p21WAF1 expression in MCF-7 human breast cancer cells in vitro. *Life Sci* 1999;65(4):415-20

Melatonin administration in tumor-bearing mice (intact and pinealectomized) in relation to stress, zinc, Thymulin and IL-2. *Int J Immunopharmacol* 1999 Jan;21(1):27-46

[Melatonin and its wide-spectrum effects: use of melatonin in the treatment of tumors]. *Cesk Fysiol* 1999 Feb;48(1):27-40

Meditation and prostate cancer: integrating a mind/body intervention with traditional therapies. *Semin Urol Oncol* 1999 May;17(2):111-8

Meloxicam inhibits the growth of colorectal cancer cells. *Carcinogenesis* 1998 Dec;19(12):2195-9

COX-2 and colon cancer. *Inflamm Res* 1998 Oct;47 Suppl 2:S112-6

Etodolac (Lodine) in the treatment of osteoarthritis: recent studies. *J Rheumatol Suppl* 1997 Feb;47:23-31

Laboratory of Angiogenesis Research, Microbiology and Tumor Biology Center, Karolinska Institute, S-171 77, *Haematologica* 1999 Jul;84(7):643-50

Angiogenesis and Tumor matastasis. *Annu Rev Med,* 1998, 49: 407-24

Angiostatin induces and sustains dormancy of human primary tumors in mice. *Nat Med,* 1996 Jun, 2:6, 689-92

Systemic inhibition of tumor growth and tumor metastases by intramuscular administration of the endostatin gene. *Nat Biotechnol* 1999 Apr;17(4):343-8

Endostatin: an endogenous inhibitor of angiogenesis and tumor growth. *Cell*, 1997 Jan, 88:2, 277-85

Expression of angiostatin cDNA in a murine fibrosarcoma suppresses primary tumor growth and produces long-term dormancy of metastases. *J Clin Invest*, 1998 Mar, 101:5, 1055-63

Liposomes complexed to plasmids encoding angiostatin and endostatin inhibit breast cancer in nude mice. *Cancer Res* 1999 Jul 15;59(14):3308-12

Human angiostatin inhibits murine hemangioendothelioma tumor growth in vivo *Cancer Res*, 1997 Dec, 57:23, 5277-80

Effects of angiogenesis inhibitors on multistage carcinogenesis in mice. *Science* 1999 Apr 30;284(5415):808-12.

Anti-angiogenesis therapy and strategies for integrating it with adjuvant therapy. *Recent Results Cancer Res* 1998;152:341-52

Regulation of angiogenesis by SPARC and angiostatin: implications for tumor cell biology. *Semin Cancer Biol,* 1996 Jun, 7:3, 139-46

[Tumoral angiogenesis: physiopathology, prognostic value and therapeutic perspectives]. *Rev Med Interne* 1998 Dec;19(12):904-13

The mechanism of cancer-mediated conversion of plasminogen to the angiogenesis inhibitor angiostatin. *Proc Natl Acad Sci U S A*, 1997 Sep, 94:20, 10868-72

Suppression of tumor growth with recombinant murine angiostatin. *Biochem Biophys Res Commun*, 1997 Jul, 236:3, 651-4

Angiostatin: an endogenous inhibitor of angiogenesis and of tumor growth. *EXS*, 1997, 79:, 273-94

Human prostate carcinoma cells express enzymatic activity that converts human plasminogen to the angiogenesis inhibitor, angiostatin. *Cancer Res*, 1996 Nov, 56:21, 4887-90

Kringle domains of human angiostatin. Characterization of the anti-proliferative activity on endothelial cells. *J Biol Chem,* 1996 Nov, 271:46, 29461-7

Angiostatin-converting enzyme activities of human matrilysin (MMP-7) and gelatinase B/type IV collagenase (MMP-9). *J Biol Chem*, 1997 Nov, 272:46, 28823-5

Generation of angiostatin by reduction and proteolysis of plasmin. Catalysis by a plasmin reductase secreted by cultured cells. *J Biol Chem*, 1997 Aug, 272:33, 20641-5

A recombinant human angiostatin protein inhibits experimental primary and metastatic cancer. *Cancer Res*, 1997 Apr, 57:7, 1329-34

Macrophage-derived metalloelastase is responsible for the generation of angiostatin in Lewis lung carcinoma. *Cell*, 1997 Mar, 88:6, 801-10

Angiostatin induces and sustains dormancy of human primary tumors in mice. *Nat Med,* 1996 Jun, 2:6, 689-92

Limited plasmin proteolysis of vitronectin. Characterization of the adhesion protein as morpho-regulatory and angiostatin-binding factor. *Eur J Biochem*, 1996 Mar, 236:2, 682-8

Kringle 5 of plasminogen is a novel inhibitor of endothelial cell growth. *J Biol Chem*, 1997 Sep, 272:36, 22924-8

Limited proteolysis of angiogenin by elastase is regulated by plasminogen. *J Protein Chem*, 1997 Oct, 16:7, 669-79

Apolipoprotein(a) kringle 4-containing fragments in human urine. Relationship to plasma levels of lipoprotein(a). *J Clin Invest*, 1996 Feb, 97:3, 858-64

Mechanisms and therapeutic implications of angiogenesis. *Curr Opin Oncol*, 1996 Jan, 8:1, 60-5

The rationale and future potential of angiogenesis inhibitors in neoplasia. *Drugs* 1999 Jul;58(1):17-38

Liposomes complexed to plasmids encoding angiostatin and endostatin inhibit breast cancer in nude mice. *Cancer Res* 1999 Jul 15:59(14):3308-12

Therapeutic potentials of angiostatin in the treatment of cancer. *Haematologica* 1999 Jul;84(7):643-50

Tumor Growth: A Putative Role for Platelets? *Oncologist* 1998;3(2):II

Investment in Research as a National Priority. *Oncologist* 1998;3(1):I

Enhanced activity of estramustine, vinblastine, etoposide, and suramin in prostate carcinoma. *Neoplasma* 1999;46(2):117-23

Suramin in combination with weekly epirubicin for patients with advanced hormone-refractory prostate carcinoma. *Cancer* 1999 Aug 1;86(3):470-6

Distinct mechanisms underlay DNA disintegration during apoptosis induced by genotoxic and nongenotoxic agents in neuroblastoma cells. *Neurochem Int* 1999 Jun;34(6):465-72

Differentiation-inducing effect of retinoic acid, difluoromethyl ornithine, sodium butyrate and sodium suramin in human colon cancer cells. *Cancer Lett* 1998 Dec 11;134(1):53-60

Serologic tumor markers, clinical biology, and therapy of prostatic carcinoma. *Urol Clin North Am* 1999 May;26(2):281-90

Suramin treatment in hormone- and chemotherapy-refractory prostate cancer. *Urology* 1999 Mar;53(3):535-41

Mechanisms of growth stimulation by suramin in non-small-cell lung cancer cell lines. *Cancer Chemother Pharmacol* 1999;43(4):341-7

Treatment options in androgen-independent prostate cancer. *Cancer Invest* 1999;17(2):137-44

Suramin blocks hepatitis C binding to human hepatoma cells in vitro. *J Med Virol* 1999 Mar;57(3):238-42

Impact of Westernization on the Nutrition of Japanese: Changes in Physique. *Cancer, Longevity, and Centenarians, Prev Med* 7 (1978): 205

Nutrition and cancer—on the mechanisms bearing on causes of cancer of the colon, breast, prostate, and stomach. *Bull N Y Acad Med* 1980 Oct;56(8):673-96

The national economic burden of cancer: an update. *J Natl Cancer Inst* 1990 Dec 5;82(23):1811-4

Natural history of breast cancer. Progression from hyperplasia to neoplasia as predicted by angiogenesis. *Cancer* 1977 Jun;39(6 Suppl):2697-703

The natural history of mammary carcinoma. *Am J Surg* 1966 Mar;111(3):435-42

Breast cancer in 3,558 women: age as a significant determinant in the rate of dying and causes of death. *Surgery* 1978 Feb;83(2):123-32

Present Trends in Cancer Epidemiology, *Proc Can Cancer Conf* 8 (1969): 40

Contribution of the Environment to Cancer Incidence: An Epidemiologic Exercise, *J Nat Ca Inst* 58 (1977): 825

W. J. Diamond M.D., W. Lee Cowden M.D., Burton Goldberg, M.D., *"An Alternative Medicine—Definitive Guide to Cancer,"* Ch 24, p 518

Cross Currents: The Promise of Electromedicine, The Perils of Electropollution (Los Angeles: Jeremy P. Tarcher, 1990), 206

Morra, M., and E. Potts, *Diagnostic Test, Choices: Realistic Alternatives in Cancer Treatment* (New York): Avon, 1987), 97

Cancer Tumor Risk Development Increases with Surgical Stress, Reuters April 19, 1999, *International Journal of Cancer* (1999); 80; 880-888

Blood Group MN Antigens and Precursors in Normal and Malignant Human Breast. *Journal of the National Cancer Institute* 40 (1975), 183-192

Return of Elevated Antimalignin Antiboby to Normal Indicates Remission of Breast Cancer, Bogoch, S., et al, (Boston: *Foundation for Research on the Nervous System and Oncolab*, 1996). Unpublished manuscript

"Computer-assisted Rescreening of Clinically Important False Negative Cervical Smears Using the PAPNET Testing System," Rosenthal, Dorothy, M.D. et al, *Acta Cytologica* 40:1 (January-February 1996) *See also Reducing the Error Rate in Papanicolaou Smears, The Female Patient, Koss, Leopold G., M.D.,19:6 (June 1994)

Screening for Prostate Cancer, *Technology Review* 8-9 (1994), 16-17

Editorial, The PSA Debate Continues, *Johns Hopkins Medical Letter* (February 1995), 3

[No Title]. *Cancer Letters* (Ireland) 1997, 114/1-2 (11-17)

Low Serum — Vitamin A and Subsequent Risk of Cancer, Preliminary results of a prospective study., *Lancet* 2 (1980): 813

The Interaction of Vitamins with Cancer Chemotherapy. *Cancer J for Clinicians* 29 (1979): 280

Prevention of Chemical Carcinogenesis by Vitamin A and Its Synthetic Analogs, (Retinoids). *Fed Proc* 35 (1976): 1332

Vitamin E Increases the Growth Inhibitory and Differentiating Effects of Tumor Therapeutic Agents on Neuroblastoma and Glioma Cells in Culture, *Proceedings for the Society for Experimental Biology and Medicine* 164:2 (1980), 158 B163

Vitamin E Deficiency Accentuates Adriamycin Cardiotoxicity. *Cancer Research* 41 (1981), 3395

Effect on Vitamin E and Selenium on Defenses Against Reactive Oxygen Species and heir Effect on Radiontion Sensitivity, *Annals of the New York Academy of Science* 393 (1982), 419-425

[No Title]. *Endocrinology* Apr 1998, 129 (4) p2102-10

Community-based Study of Vitamin C (ascorbic acid)—Therapy in Patients with Advanced Cancer. *Proceedings of the American Society of Clinical Oncology* 2 (1983), 92. See also: Vitamin C and Cancer. *International Journal of Environmental Studies* 75 (1977), 4538-4542

L-ascorbic acid (vitamin C) Augmentation of Anticancer Activity of Methoxy-substituted Benzoquinones, Adriamycin, and a Dihydroxyulated Amino Substituted Quinone(DHAQ), Unpublished, Cited in: Pelton, R., and L. Overholser, *Alternatives in Cancer Therapy* (New York: Fireside/Simon & Shuster, 1994)

Selenium in Nutritional Cancer Prophylaxis: An Update. *Vitamins, Nutrition and Cancer*, Basel, Swtrizerland: Karger, 1984

Cell injury by antineoplastic agents and influence of Coenzyme Q_{10} on cellular potassium activity and potential difference across the membrane in rat liver cells. *Cancer Res* 1980 May;40(5):1663-7

Anti-tumor Action of Alkyl-lysophospholipids, *Anticancer Research* 1:6 (1981), 345-352

Regression of Tumor Growth after Administration of Alkoxy glycerols, *Acta Obstetrica et Gynecologica* Scandinavica 57 (1978), 79-83

Alkoxyglycerols and Their Use in Radiation Treatment, *Acta Radiologica* 223 (1963) 7-99

Adriamycin cardiotoxicity: early detection by systolic time interval and possible prevention by Coenzyme Q_{10}. *Cancer Treat Rep*. 1978; 62:887-91

[No Title]. *Am J Cli Nutr* Jul 1997, 66 (1) p46 51

Lignans and isflavonoids in the plasma and prostatic fluid of men: Samples from Protugal, Hong Kong, and the United Kingdom. *Prostate* 1997 Jul 1;32(2):122-8

Long Term Follow-up of Cancer patients Using Contreras, Hoxsey, and Gerson Therapies, *Journal of Naturopathic Medicine* 5:1 (1994), 74-76

Office of Technology Assessment, Unconventional Cancer Treatments, Washington, DC: US Government Printing Office, 1990, 83

Walters, R. *Essiac Options: The Alternative Cancer Therapy Book* (Garden City, NY: Avery Publishing, 1993, 112

Biochemical Study of Chinese Rhubarb XXIX, Inhibitory Effects of Anthraquinone Derivatives on P338 Leukemia in Mice, *Journal of Chinese Pharmacology University* 20 (1989), 155-157

Macrophage Activation by the Polysaccharide Arabinogalactan Isolated from Plant Cell Cultures of Echinacea purpurea, *Journal of the National Cancer Institute* 81:9 (1989), 669-675

Greater Health and Longevity: Chlorella, the Green Algae Superfood, May be the Answer, *Alternative Medicine Digest* 12 (1996), 56

Wilner, J. Suggested Nutritional Supplements: Algae, *The Cancer Solution* (Boca Raton), FL: Peltec Publishing, 1994

[No title], *Japan Pre Med* Nov-Dec 1997, 26 (6) p769-75

Chisaka, T. et al, Chemical and Pharmaceutical Bulletin (1998), Cited in: Wilner, J. A Green Tea, *The Cancer Solution* (Boca Raton, FL: Peltec Publishing, 1994), 75

Marked Antimutagenic Potential of Aqueous Green Tea Extracts: Mechanism of Action, *Mutagenesis* 9 (1994), 325-331

Green Tea and Skin Anticarcinogenic Effects. *Journal of Investigative Dermatology* 102 (1994), 3-7

Green tea and skin—anticarcinogenic effects. *Invest Dermatol* 1994 Jan;102(1):3-7

Green tea polyphenols inhibit oxidant-induced DNA strand breakage in cultured lung cells. *Free Radic Biol Med* 1997;23(2):235-42

Mechanisms of growth inhibition of human lung cancer cell line, PC-9, by tea polyphenols. *Jpn J Cancer Res* 1997 Jul;88(7):639-43

Mechanistic aspects of green tea as a cancer preventive: effect of components on human stomach cancer cell lines. *Jpn J Cancer Res* 1999 Jul;90(7):733-9

Aryl hydrocarbon receptor-mediated antiestrogenic and antitumorigenic activity of diindolylmethane. *Carcinogenesis* 1998 Sep;19(9):1631-9

Induction of apoptosis in prostate cancer cell lines by the green tea component, (-)-epigallocatechin-3-gallate. *Cancer Lett* 1998 Aug 14;130(1-2):1-7

Green tea epigallocatechin gallate shows a pronouced growth inhibitory effect on cancerous cells but not on their normal counterparts. *Cancer Lett* Jul 17, 1998, 129 (2) p223-8

A randomized study of chemotherapy with cisplatin plus etoposide versus chemoendocrine therapy with cisplatin, etoposide and the pineal hormone melatonin as a first-line treatment of advanced non-small cell lung cancer patients in a poor clinical state. *J Pineal Res* 1997 Aug;23(1):15-9

Treatment of cancer chemotherapy-induced toxicity with the pineal hormone melatonin. *Support Care Cancer* 1997 Mar;5(2):126-9

[No Title]. *Journal of Nutraceuticals, Functional and Medical Foods* 1997, 1/3 (73-99)

[No Title]. *Drugs of Today* (Spain) 1997, 33/1 (25-39)

Potent antitumor activity of 2-methoxyestradiol in human pancreatic cancer cell lines. *Clin Cancer Res* 1999 Mar;5(3):493-9

[No Title]. *Arzneimittelforschung* 1999 Aug;49(8):649-62

Inhibition of tumor necrosis factor alpha-stimulated aromatase activity by microtubule-stabilizing agents, paclitaxel and 2-methoxyestradiol. *Biochem Biophys Res Commun* 1999 Jul 22;261(1):214-7

Cyclooxygenase-2 expression is up-regulated in human pancreatic cancer. *Cancer Research* (1999; Mar 1;59(5):987-90)

A comparative study of the effects of genistein and 2-methoxy estradiol on the proteolytic balance and tumour cell proliferation. *Br J Cancer* 1999 Apr;80(1-2):17-24

Potent antitumor activity of 2-methoxyestradiol in human pancreatic cancer cell lines. *Clin Cancer Res* 1999 Mar;5(3):493-9

Fish oil-enriched nutritional supplement attenuates progression of the acute-phase response in weight-losing patients with advanced pancreatic cancer. *J Nutr* 1999 Jun;129(6):1120-5

Practices influencing iron status in university women. *Nutrition Research*, 1997, 17/1 (9-22)

Protease inhibitors and carcinogenesis. *Cancer Investigation*, 1996, 14/6 (597-608)

Inhibition of epidermal growth factor receptor-associated tyrosine kinase blocks glioblastoma invasion of the brain. *Neurosurgery*, 1997, 40/1 (141-151)

The fatty acid composition of human gliomas differs from that found in nonmalignant brain tissue. *Lipids*, 1996, 31/12 (1283-1288)

Microdosimetric evaluation of relative biological effectiveness. *International Journal of Radiation Oncology Biology Physics*, 1996, 36/3 (689-697)

Whole-grain consumption and chronic disease: Protective mechanisms. *Nutrition and Cancer*, 1997, 27/1 (14-21)

Effect of oestradiol and insulin on the proliferative pattern and on oestrogen and progesterone receptor contents in MCF-7 cells. *Journal of Cancer Research and Clinical Oncology* (Germany), 1996, 122/12 (745-749)

Vegetable, fruit, and grain consumption to colorectal adenomatous polyps. *American Journal of Epidemiology*, 1996, 144/11 (1015-1025)

Improvement by eicosanoids in cancer cachexia induced by LLC-IL6 transplantation. *Journal of Cancer Research and Clinical Oncology* (Germany), 1996, 122/12 (711-715)

Diet and risk of esophageal cancer by histologic type in a low-risk Group. *International Journal of Cancer*, 1996, 68/3 (300-304)

The effect of unsaturated fatty acids on membrane composition and signal transduction in HT-29 human colon cancer cells. *Cancer Letters* (Ireland), 1996, 108/1 (25-33)

Genistein-stimulated adherence of prostate cancer cells is associated with the binding of focal adhesion kinase to beta-1-integrin. *Clinical and Experimental Metastasis* (UK), 1996, 14/4 (389-398)

Chemoprevention of mammary cancer by diallyl selenide, a novel organoselenium compound. *Anticancer Research* (Greece), 1996, 16/5 A (2911-2915)

Tofu and risk of breast cancer in Asian-Americans. *Cancer Epidemiology Biomarkers and Prevention*, 1996, 5/11(901-906)

Dietary calcium, vitamin D, and the risk of colorectal cancer in Stockholm, Sweden. *Cancer Epidemiology Biomarkers and Prevention*, 1996, 5/11(897-900)

Effect of omega-3 fatty acids on the progression of metastases after the surgical excision of human breast cancer cell solid tumors growing in nude mice. *Clinical Cancer Research*, 1996, 2/10 (1751-1756)

Regulation of human colonic cell line proliferation and phenotype by sodium butyrate. *Digestive Diseases and Sciences*, 1996, 41/10 (1986-1993)

Curcumin inhibits the proliferation and cell cycle progression of human umbilical vein endothelial cell. *Cancer Letters* (Ireland), 1996, 107/1 (109-115)

Cell cycle arrest and induction of apoptosis in pancreatic cancer cells exposed to eicosapentaenoic acid in vivo. *British Journal of Cancer* (UK), 1996, 74/9 (1375-1383)

Effects of dietary conjugated linoleic acid on lymphocyte function and growth of mammary tumors in mice. *Anticancer Research* (Greece), 1997, 17/2 A (987-993)

Conjugated linoleic acid suppresses the growth of human breast adenocarcinoma cells in SCID mice. *Anticancer Research* (Greece), 1997, 17/2 A (969-973)

Lymphatic recovery, tissue distribution, and metabolic effects of conjugated lioleic acid in rats. *Journal of Nutritional Biochemistry*, 1997, 8/1 (38-43)

Proliferative responses of normal human mammary and MCF-7 breast cancer cells to linoleic acid, conjugated linoleic acid and eicosanoid synthesis inhibitors in culture. *Anticancer Research* (Greece), 1997, 17/1 A (197-203)

Conjugated linoleic acid modulates hepatic lipid composition in mice. *Lipids*, 1997, 32/2 (199-204)

Dietary conjugated linoleic acid modulation of phorbol ester skin tumor promotion. *Nutrition and Cancer*, 1996, 26/2 (149-157)

The efficacy of conjugated linoleic acid in mammary cancer prevention is independent of the level or type of fat in the diet. *Carcinogenesis* (UK), 1996, 17/5 (1045-1050)

Dietary modifiers of carcinogenesis. *Environmental Health Perspectives*, 1995, 103/Suppl. 8 (177-184)

Effects of C18 fatty acid isomers on DNA synthesis in hepatoma and breast cancer cells. *Anticancer Research* (Greece), 1995, 15/5 B (2017-2021)

Effect of timing and duration of dietary conjugated linoleic acid on mammary cancer prevention. *Nutrition and Cancer*, 1995, 24/3 (241-247)

Reinvestigation of the antioxidant properties of conjugated linoleic acid. *Lipids*, 1995, 30/7 (599-605)

Furan fatty acids determined as oxidation products of conjugated octadecadienoic acid. *Lipids*, 1995, 30/7 (595-598)

The role of phenolics, conjugated linoleic acid, carnosine, and pyrroloquinoline quinone as nonessential dietary antioxidants. *Nutrition Reviews*, 1995, 53/3 (49-58)

Conjugated linoleic acid is a growth factor for rats as shown by enhanced weight gain and improved feed efficiency. *J. Nutr.*, 1994, 124/12 (2344-2349)

Conjugated linoleic acid: A powerful anticarcinogen from animal fat sources. *Cancer*, 1994, 74/3 (1050-1054)

Effect of cheddar cheese consumption on plasma conjugated linoleic acid concentrations in men. *Nutr. Res.*, 1994, 14/3 (373-386)

Intake of selected micronutrients and the risk of endometrial carcinoma. *Cancer*, 1996, 77/5 (917-923)

Tea in chemoprevention of cancer: Epidemiologic and experimental studies. *International Journal of Oncology* (Greece), 1996, 8/2 (221-238)

Genistein suppresses growth stimulatory effect of growth factors in HCE 16/3 cells. *Chinese Journal of Oncology* (China), 1997, 19/2 (118-122)

Intestinal immunocompetency and/or cancer control. *Biotherapy* (Japan), 1997, 11/4 (524-525)

Chemoprotection against the formation colon DNA adducts from the food-borne carcinogen 2-amino-1-methyl-6-phenylimidazo(4,5-b)pyridine (PhIP) in the rat. *Mutation Research—Fundamental and Molecular Mechanisms of Mutagenesis* (Netherlands), 1997, 376/1-2 (115-122)

Effects of protein kinase and phosphatase inhibitors on the growth of human prostatic cancer cells. *Medical Science Research* (UK), 1997, 25/5 (353-354)

Estrogenic activity of natural and synthetic estrogens in human breast cancer cells in culture. *Environmental Health Perspectives*, 1997, 105/Suppl. 3 (637-645)

Dietary estrogens stimulate human breast cells to enter the cell cycle. *Environmental Health Perspectives*, 1997, 105/Suppl. 3 (633-636)

Medical hypothesis: Bifunctional genetic-hormonal pathways to breast cancer. *Environmental Health Perspectives*, 1997, 105/Suppl. 3 (571-576)

Natural products and their derivatives as cancer chemopreventive agents. *Progress in Drug Research* (Switzerland), 1997, 48/-(147-171)

Isolation of isoflavones from soy-based fermentations of the erythromycin-producing bacterium Saccharopolyspora erythraea. *Applied Microbiology and Biotechnology* (Germany), 1997, 47/4 (398-404)

Migration of highly aggressive MV3 melanoma cells in 3-dimensional collagen lattices results in local matrix reorganization and shedding of alpha2 and beta1 integrins and CD44. *Cancer Research*, 1997, 57/10 (2061-2070)

Inhibition of growth and induction of differentiation of metastatic melanoma cells in vitro by genistein: Chemosensitivity is regulated by cellular p53. *British Journal of Cancer* (UK), 1997, 75/11 (1559-1566)

Phyto-oestrogens and Western diseases. *Annals of Medicine* (UK), 1997, 29/2 (95-120)

Preclinical studies of the combination of angiogenic inhibitors with cytotoxic agents. *Investigational New Drugs*, 1997, 15/1 (39-48)

Curcumin and genistein, plant natural produbreast cancer MCF-7 cells induced by estrogenic pesticides. *Biochemical and Biophysical Research Communications*, 1997, 233/3 (692-696)

New agents for cancer chemoprevention. *Nation* 996, 63/Suppl. 26 (1-28)

Glutathione *S*-transferases of female A/J mouse lung and their induction by anticarcinogenic organosulfides from garlic. *Archives of Biochemistry and Biophysics*, 1997, 340/2 (279-286)

Metabolic support of the gastrointestinal tract: Potential gut protection during intensive cytotoxic therapy. *Cancer*, 1997, 79/9 (1794-1803)

Inhibition of malignant cell proliferation by culture media conditioned by cardiac or skeletal muscle. *Cell Biology International* (UK), 1997, 21/3 (133-144)

A diet rich in fat and poor in dietary fiber increases the in vitro formation of reactive oxygen species in human feces. *Journal of Nutrition*, 1997, 127/5 (706-709)

Inhibition of 12-O-tetradecanoylphorbol-13-acetate induced Epstein-Barr virus early antigen activation by natural colorants. *Cancer Letters* (Ireland), 1997, 115/2 (173-178)

The bovine papillomavirus E6 oncoprotein interacts with paxillin and disrupts the actin cytoskeleton. *Proceedings of the National Academy of Sciences of the United States of America*, 1997, 94/9 (4412-4417)

Genistein inhibits proliferation and in vitro invasive potential of human prostatic cancer cell lines. *Anticancer Research* (Greece), 1997, 17/2 A (1199-1204)

Assessment of cyclooxygenase inhibitors using in vitro assay systems. *Methods in Cell Science* (Netherlands), 1997, 19/1 (25-31)

Activation of gelatinase A (72-kDa type IV collagenase) induced by monensin in normal human fibroblasts. *Experimental Cell Research*, 1997, 232/2 (322-330)

Selective modulation of cell adhesion molecules on lymphocytes by bromelain protease 5. *Pathobiology* (Switzerland), 1996, 64/6 (339-346)

Overview of the epidemiology of colorectal cancer. *Diseases of the Colon and Rectum*, 1997, 40/4 (483-493)

Suppression of nitric oxide production in lipopolysaccharide-stimulated macrophage cells by omega3 polyunsaturated fatty acids. *Japanese Journal of Cancer Research* (Japan), 1997, 88/3 (234-237)

The effect of nutritional intervention on immune functions and other biomarkers in high cancer risk individuals

Adenocarcinomas of the esophagus and gastric cardia: The role of diet. *Nutrition and Cancer,* 1997, 27/3 (298-309)

Effects of high- and low-risk diets on gut microflora-associated biomarkers of colon cancer in human flora-associated rats. *Nutrition and Cancer,* 1997, 27/3 (250-255)

Eating to beat breast cancer: Potential role for soy supplements. *Annals of Oncology* (Netherlands), 1997, 8/3 (223-225)

Position of the American Dietetic Association: Phytochemicals and functional foods. *Journal of Nutraceuticals, Functional and Medical Foods,* 1997, 1/1 (33-45)

Angiogenesis as a target for tumor treatment. *Oncology* (Switzerland), 1997, 54/3 (177-184)

Identification of compounds with preferential inhibitory activity against low-Nm23-expressing human breast carcinoma and melanoma cell lines. *Nature Medicine,* 1997, 3/4 (395-401)

Activation of mitogenic signaling by endothelin 1 in ovarian carcinoma cells. *Cancer Research,* 1997, 57/7 (1306-1311)

Modulation of apoptosis by sulindac, curcumin, phenylethyl-3-methylcaffeate, and 6-phenylhexyl isothiocyanate: Apoptotic index as a biomarker in colon cancer chemoprevention and promotion. *Cancer Research,* 1997, 57/7 (1301-1305)

Reduction of urinary mutagen excretion in rats fed garlic. *Cancer Letters* (Ireland), 1997, 114/1-2 (185-186)

Meat, starch and non-starch polysaccharides, are epidemiological and experimental findings consistent with acquired genetic alterations in sporadic colorectal cancer? *Cancer Letters* (Ireland), 1997, 114/1-2 (25-34)

Induction of human adenocarcinoma cell differentiation by the phytoestrogen genistein is independent of its antiestrogenic function. *International Journal of Oncology* (Greece), 1997, 10/4 (753-757)

Metabolism of the chemoprotective agent diallyl sulfide to glutathione conjugates in rats. *Chemical Research in Toxicology,* 1997, 10/3 (318-327)

Incorporation of long-chain n-3 fatty acids in tissues and enhanced bone marrow cellularity with docosahexaenoic acid feeding in post-weanling Fischer 344 rats. *Lipids,* 1997, 32/3 (293-302)

Differential effects of polyunsaturated fatty acids on chemosensitivity of NIH3T3 cells and its transformants. *International Journal of Cancer,* 1997, 70/3 (357-361)

The new dietary fats in health and disease. *Journal of the American Dietetic Association,* 1997, 97/3 (280-286)

Inhibition of proliferation of estrogen receptor-positive MCF-7 human breast cancer cells by flavonoids in the presence and absence of excess estrogen. *Cancer Letters* (Ireland), 1997, 112/2 (127-133)

S-allylmercaptocysteine inhibits cell proliferation and reduces the viability of erythroleukemia, breast, and prostate cancer cell lines. *Nutrition and Cancer,* 1997, 27/2 (186-191)

Inhibition of *N*-methyl-*N*-nitrosourea-induced mammary tumors in rats by the soybean isoflavones. *Anticancer Research* (Greece), 1996, 16/6 A (3293-3298)

Experimental approaches to therapy and prophylaxis for heat stress and heatstroke. *Wilderness and Environmental Medicine,* 1996, 7/4 (312-334)

Genistein-induced apoptosis of prostate cancer cells is preceded by a specific decrease in focal adhesion kinase activity. *Molecular Pharmacology,* 1997, 51/2 (193-200)

Male rats fed methyl- and folate-deficient diets with or without niacin develop hepatic carcinomas associated with decreased tissue NAD concentrations and altered poly(ADP-ribose) polymerase activity. *Journal of Nutrition,* 1997, 127/1 (30-36)

Nutritional and lifestyle habits and water-fiber interaction in colorectal adenoma etiology. *Cancer Epidemiology Biomarkers and Prevention,* 1997, 6/2 (79-85)

Prevention of mammary preneoplastic transformation by naturally-occurring tumor inhibitors. *Cancer Letters* (Ireland), 1997, 111/1-2 (141-147)

Nitric oxide scavenging by curcuminoids. *Journal of Pharmacy and Pharmacology* (UK), 1997, 49/1 (105-107)

Antiproliferative potency of structurally distinct dietary flavonoids on human colon cancer cells. *Cancer Letters* (Ireland), 1996, 110/1-2 (41-48)

Dietary fat and colon cancer: Modulating effect of types and amount of dietary fat on ras-p21 function during promotion and progression stages

Short-chain fructo-oligosaccharides reduce the occurrence of colon tumors and develop gut-associated lymphoid tissue in Min mice. *Cancer Research,* 1997, 57/2 (225-228)

Usage and users of natural remedies in a middle-aged population: Demographic and psychosocial characteristics. Results from the Malmo Diet and Cancer Study. *Pharmacoepidemiology and Drug Safety* (UK), 1996, 5/5 (303-314)

T-cell adjuvants. *Int J Immunopharmacol*; 16(9):703-10 1994

Therapy of secondary t-cell immunodeficiencies with biological substances and drugs. *Med Oncol Tumor Pharmacother*; 6(1):11-7 1989

Immunological effects of isoprinosine as a pulse immunotherapy in melanoma and arc patients. *Cancer Detect Prev Suppl*; 1:457-62 1987

Isoprinosine as an immunopotentiator in an animal model of human osteosarcoma. *Int J Immunopharmacol*; 3(4):383-389 1981

Immune effects of preoperative immunotherapy with high-dose subcutaneous interleukin-2 versus neuroimmunotherapy with low-dose interleukin-2 plus the neurohormone melatonin in gastrointestinal tract tumor patients. *J Biol Regul Homeost Agents*; 9(1):31-3 1995

The immunoneuroendocrine role of melatonin. *J Pineal Res*; 14(1):1-10 1993

Endocrine and immune effects of melatonin therapy in metastatic cancer patients. *Eur J Cancer Clin Oncol;* 25(5):789-95 1989

Potential of tyrosine kinase receptors as therapeutic targets in cancer. *Cancer Therapy in the Twenty-First Century,* Vol 1, p.49-81, 1994

In vitro inhibition of proliferation of MDA-MB-435 human breast cancer cells by combinations of tocotrienols and flavonoids (Meeting abstract). *Faseb J*; 9(4):A868 1995

Effects of tyrosine kinase inhibitors on the proliferation of human breast cancer cell lines and proteins important in the ras signaling pathway. *Int J Cancer*; 65(2):186-91 1996

Reversal of multidrug resistance in vivo by dietary administration of the phytochemical indole-3-carbinol. *Cancer Res*; 56(3):574-81 1996

Differential sensitivity of human prostatic cancer cell lines to the effects of protein kinase and phosphatase inhibitors. *Cancer Lett*; 98(1):103-10 1995

Growth regulation of the human papillary thyroid cancer cell line by protein tyrosine kinase and cAMP-dependent protein kinase. *Endocr J*; 41(4):399-407 1994

The effects of different combinations of flavonoids on the proliferation of MDA-MB-435 human breast cancer cells (Meeting abstract). *Proc Annu Meet Am Assoc Cancer Res*; 36:A3538 1995

Preferential requirement for protein tyrosine phosphatase activity in the 12-O- tetradecanoylphorbol-13-acetate-induced differentiation of human colon cancer cells. *Biochem Pharmacol*; 50(8):1217-22 1995

Bioactive organosulfur phytochemicals in Brassica oleracea vegetables—a review. *Food Chem Toxicol*; 33(6):537-43 1995

[Growth and invasion of differentiated thyroid gland carcinoma: importance of signal transduction]. *Langenbecks Arch Chir*; 380(2):96-101 1995

Nerve growth factor stimulates clonal growth of human lung cancer cell lines and a human glioblastoma cell line expressing high-affinity nerve growth factor binding sites involving tyrosine kinase signaling. *Cancer Res*; 55(10):2212-9 1995

Evaluation of the biochemical targets of genistein in tumor cells. *J Nutr*; 125(3 Suppl):784S-789S 1995

In vitro hormonal effects of soybean isoflavones. *J Nutr*; 125(3 Suppl):751S-756S 1995

Resistance of melanoma cell lines to interferons correlates with reduction of IFN-induced tyrosine phosphorylation. Induction of the anti-viral state by IFN is prevented by tyrosine kinase inhibitors. *J Immunol*; 154(5):2248-56 1995

Biotherapy of B-cell precursor leukemia by targeting genistein to CD19-associated tyrosine kinases. *Science*; 267(5199):886-91 1995

Genistein inhibits the growth of prostate cancer cells. What is the mechanism? *Proc Annu Meet Am Assoc Cancer Res*; 36:A2310 1995

Growth-inhibitory effects of the natural phyto-oestrogen genistein in MCF-7 human breast cancer cells. *Eur J Cancer*; 30A(11):1675-82 1994

Natural flavonoids and lignans are potent cytostatic agents against human leukemic HL-60 cells. *Life Sci*; 55(13):1061-9 1994

The natural tyrosine kinase inhibitor genistein produces cell cycle arrest and apoptosis in Jurkat T-leukemia cells. *Leuk Res*; 18(6):431-9 1994

Selective responsiveness of human breast cancer cells to indole-3-carbinol, a chemopreventive agent. *J Natl Cancer Inst;* 86(2):126-31 1994

Genistein is an effective stimulator of sex hormone-binding globulin production in hepatocarcinoma human liver cancer cells and suppresses proliferation of these cells in culture. *Steroids*; 58(7):301-4 1993

Lycopene is a more potent inhibitor of human cancer cell proliferation than either alpha-carotene or beta-carotene. *Nutr Cancer*; 24(3):257-66 1995

Inhibitory effect of 220-oxa-1,25-dihydroxyvitamin D3 on the proliferation of pancreatic cancer cell lines. *Gastroenterology*; 110(5):1605-13 1996

Antiproliferative responses to two human colon cancer cell lines to vitamin D3 are differently modified by 9-cis-retinoic acid. *Cancer Res*; 56(3):623-32 1996

Vitamin D: a modulator of cell proliferation and differentiation. *J Steroid Biochem Mol Biol*; 37(6):873-6 1990

Preferential cytotoxicity on tumor cells by caffeic acid phenethyl ester isolated from propolis. *Experientia* (Switzerland), 1988, 44/3 (230-232)

Effect of caffeic acid esters on carcinogen-induced mutagenicity and human colon adenocarcinoma cell growth. *Chem.-Biol. Interact*. (Ireland), 1992, 84/3 (277-290)

Candida (Fungal, Yeast) Infections

Vitamin C inhibits arylamine *N*-acetyltransferase activity in the fungus Candida albicans. *Research Communications in Pharmacology and Toxicology*, 1998, 3/1-2 (45-54)

Vitamin C and cervico-vaginal infections in pregnant women. *Nutrition Research*, 1998, 18/6 (939-944)

Tea tree oil causes K+ leakage and inhibits respiration in Escherichia coli. *Lett Appl Microbiol* (England) May 1998, 26 (5) p355-8

Effects of tea tree oil on Escherichia coli. *Lett Appl Microbiol* (England) Mar 1998, 26 (3) p194-8

In vitro susceptibility of Malassezia furfur to the essential oil of Melaleuca alternifolia. *J Med Vet Mycol* (England) Sep-Oct 1997, 35 (5) p375-7

In-vitro activity of essential oils, in particular Melaleuca alternifolia (tea tree) oil and tea tree oil products, against Candida spp. *Journal of Antimicrobial Chemotherapy* (UK), 1998, 42/5 (591-595)

Australian tea tree oil. *Canadian Pharmaceutical Journal* (Canada), 1998, 131/2 (42-46)

The future of medicine: The effect of tea tree oil extract on the growth of fungi. *Lower Extremity*, 1997, 4/2 (113-116)

A new protocol for antimicrobial testing of oils. *Journal of Microbiological Methods* (Netherlands), 1997, 28/1 (21-24)

[Fecal microflora in healthy young people]. *Zh Mikrobiol Epidemiol Immunobiol* (USSR) Feb 1983, (2) p36-40

Biotherapeutic agents. A neglected modality for the treatment and prevention of selected intestinal and vaginal infections. *Jama* Mar 20 1996, 275 (11) p870-6

Influence of lactobacilli on the adhesion of Staphylococcus aureus and Candida albicans to fibers and epithelial cells. *J Ind Microbiol* (England) Sep 1995, 15 (3) p248-53

Effect of Lactobacillus acidophilus on antibiotic-associated gastrointestinal morbidity: a prospective randomized trial. *J Otolaryngol* (Canada) Aug 1995, 24 (4) p230-3

Inhibition of Candida albicans by Lactobacillus acidophilus: evidence for the involvement of a peroxidase system. *Microbios* (England) 1994, 80 (323) p125-33

Ingestion of yogurt containing Lactobacillus acidophilus as prophylaxis for candidal vaginitis [see comments]. *Ann Intern Med* Mar 1 1992, 116 (5) p353-7

Evidence for the involvement of thiocyanate in the inhibition of Candida albicans by Lactobacillus acidophilus. *Microbios* (England) 1990, 62 (250) p37-46

Viricidal effects of Lactobacillus and yeast fermentation. *Appl Environ Microbiol* Aug 1983, 46 (2) p452-8

Inhibition of Candida albicans by Lactobacillus acidophilus. *J Dairy Sci* May 1980, 63 (5) p830-2

Thrush bowel infection: existence, incidence, prevention and treatment, particularly by a Lactobacillus acidophilus preparation. *Curr Med Drugs* (England) Dec 1967, 8 (4) p3-11

[Candida infection of the female genitalia. Complaints and clinical findings] Candidainfektion des weiblichen Genitales. *Beschwerden und Befund. Med Klin* (Germany, West) Jan 31 1969, 64 (5) p203-6

Dietary supplement of neosugar alters the fecal flora and decreases activities of some reductive enzymes in human subjects. *Am J Clin Nutr* May 1996, 63 (5) p709-16

In vitro fructooligosaccharide utilization and inhibition of Salmonella spp. by selected bacteria. *Poult Sci* Sep 1995, 74 (9) p1418-25

Dietary fructooligosaccharide, xylooligosaccharide and gum arabic have variable effects on cecal and colonic microbiota and epithelial cell proliferation in mice and rats. *J Nutr* Oct 1995, 125 (10) p2604-9

A comparison of susceptibility to five antifungal agents of yeast cultures from burn patients. *Burns* (England) May 1995, 21 (3) p167-70

[A trial of the use of diflucan (fluconazole) in patients with vaginal candidiasis]. *Antibiot Khimioter.* 1993 Dec. 38(12). P 39-41

[Fluconazole—a new antifungal agent]. *Tidsskr Nor Laegeforen*. 1992 Jun 10. 112(15). P 1961-3

[Endogenous candida endophthalmitis: a new therapy]. *Klin Monatsbl Augenheilkd*. 1991 Dec. 199(6). P 446-9

Perspective Evaluation of Candida Antigen Detection Test For Invasive Candidiasis and Immunocompromised Adult Patients With Cancer. *The American Journal of Medicine*, December 1989;87(621-627)

Pathogenesis of Candidiasis: Immunosuppression By Cell Wall Mannan Catabolites, *Archives of Surgery, November* 1989; 124:1290-1294

Ingestion of Yogurt Containing Lactobacillus Acidophilus as Prophylaxis for Candidal Vaginitis. *Annals Of Internal Medicine*, March 1, 1992;116(5):353-357

Garlic: A Review of Its Relationship to Malignant Disease. *Preventive Medicine*, May 1990;19(3):346-361

Anticandidal and Anticarcinogenic Potentials For Garlic. *International Clinical Nutrition Review,* October 1990;10(4):423-429

Vaginal Flora and Urinary Tract Infections. *Current Opinion in Infectious Disease*, 1991;4:37-41

Regulation of The Immune Response to Candida Albicans by Monocyte and Progesterone. *American Journal of Obstetrics and Gynecology,* 1991;164:1351-4

Hydrogen Peroxide-Producing Organisms Toxic To Vaginal Bacteria. *Infectious Disease News*, August 8, 1991;5

The Vaginal Ecosystem. Mardh, Per-Anders, M.D., *American Journal of Obstetrics and Gynecology,* October 1991;165(4): Part II:1163-1168

Ingestion of Yogurt Containing Lactobacillus Acidophilus as Prophylaxis for Candidal Vaginitis. *Annals of Internal Medicine*, March 1, 1992;116(5);353-357

Catabolic Wasting

Muscle glutamine concentration and protein turnover in vivo in malnutrition and endotoxemia. *Metabolism* 1989 Aug;38(8 Suppl 1):6-13

Catabolic aspects of cranial trauma. *Ann Fr Anesth Reanim* (France) 1998, 17 (2) p180-5

Potential benefits of resistance exercise training on nutritional status in renal failure. *J Ren Nutr Jan* 1998, 8 (1) p2-10

Serum creatine kinase activity is not a reliable marker for muscle damage in conditions associated with low extracellular glutathione concentration [see comments] *Clin* Chem May 1998, 44(5) p939-43, Comment in *Clin Chem* 1998 May;44(5):905

Growth hormone therapy may benefit protein metabolism in mitochondrial encephalomyopathy. *Clin Endocrinol* (Oxf) (England) Jul 1997, 47 (1) p113-7

Inducible nitric oxide synthase in skeletal muscle of patients with chronic heart failure. *Journal of the American College of Cardiology,* 1998, 32/4 (964-969)

Plasma and muscle amino acid levels in relation to resting energy expenditure and inflammation in stable chronic obstructive pulmonary disease. *American Journal of Respiratory and Critical Care Medicine,* 1998, 158/3 (797-801)

Role of cysteine and glutathione in signal transduction, immunopathology and cachexia. *BioFactors* (Netherlands), 1998, 8/ 1-2 (97-102)

The role of IGFs in catabolism. *Bailliere's Clinical Endocrinology and Metabolism* (UK), 1997, 11/4 (679-697)

Age-related sarcopenia in humans is associated with reduced synthetic rates of specific muscle proteins. *Journal of Nutrition*, 1998, 128/2 Suppl. (351S-355S)

Metabolic acidosis and protein catabolism: Mechanisms and clinical implications. *Mineral and Electrolyte Metabolism* (Switzerland), 1998, 24/1 (13-19)

Outcome of critically ill patients after supplementation with glutamine. *Nutrition*, 1997, 13/7-8 (752-754)

The search for the uremic toxin: The case for metabolic acidosis. *Wiener Klinische Wochenschrift* (Austria), 1997, 109/1 (7-12)

Biology of cachexia. *J Natl Cancer Inst* Dec 3 1997, 89 (23) p1763-73

Human growth hormone prevents the protein catabolic side effects of prednisone in humans. *J Clin Invest* Jul 1990, 86 (1) p265-72

Feeding conjugated linoleic acid to animals partially overcomes catabolic responses due to endotoxin injection. *Biochem Biophys Res Commun* Feb 15 1994, 198 (3) p1107-12

Evidence for a nutritional need for glutamine in catabolic patients. *Kidney Int Suppl* Nov 1989, 27 pS287-92

The role of glutamine in the immune system and in intestinal function in catabolic states. *Amino Acids* (Austria), 1994, 7/3 (231-243)

Feeding conjugated linoleic acid to animals partially overcomes catabolic responses due to endotoxin injection. *Biochem Biophys Res Commun* Feb 15 1994, 198

Inhibition of lipolysis and muscle protein degradation by EPA in cancer cachexia. *Nutrition,* 1996, 12/1 Suppl. (S31-S33)

The effect of polyunsaturated fatty acids on the progress of cachexia in patients with pancreatic cancer. *Nutrition*, 1996, 12/1 Suppl. (S27-S30)

Comparison of the effectiveness of eicosapentaenoic acid administered as either the free acid or ethyl ester as an anticachectic and antitumour agent. *Prostaglandins Leukotrienes Essent Fatty Acids* (UK), 1994, 51/2 (141-145)

Kinetics of the inhibition of tumour growth in mice by eicosapentaenoic acid-reversal by linoleic acid. *Biochem. Pharmacol.* (UK), 1993, 45/11 (2189-2194)

Anticachectic and antitumor effect of eicosapentaenoic acid and its effect on protein turnover. *Cancer Res.*, 1991, 51/22 (6089-6093)

Muscle wasting and dedifferentiation induced by oxidative stress in a murine model of cachexia is prevented by inhibitors of nitric oxide synthesis and antioxidants. *EMBO Journal* (UK), 1996, 15/8 (1753-1765)

Modulation of immune function and weight loss by *L*-arginine in obstructive jaundice in the rat. *Br. J. Surg.* (UK), 1994, 81/8 (1199-1201)

Effects of *L*-carnitine on serum triglyceride and cytokine levels in rat models of cachexia and septic shock. *British Journal of Cancer* (UK), 1995, 72/5

L-carnitine deficiency in AIDS patients. *AIDS* (UK), 1992, 6/2 (203-205)

The enzymatic activities of branched-chain amino acid catabolism in tumour-bearing rats. *Cancer Lett.* (Ireland), 1992, 61/3 (239-242)

Branched chain amino acids as the protein component of parenteral nutrition in cancer cachexia. *Br. J. Surg.* (UK), 1989, 76/2 (149-153)

Zinc in different tissues: Relation to age and local concentrations in cachexia, liver cirrhosis and long-term intensive care. *Infusionsther. Klin. Ernahr.* (Switzerland), 1979, 6/4 (225-229)

The role of serum protein in congestive heart failure. Nutritional support in organ failure: proceedings of the International Symposium, 1990, -/- (45- 52)

Clinical rise of a combination containing phosphocreatinine as adjuvant to physiokinesiotherapy. *Riabilitazione* (Italy), 1976, 9/2 (51-62)

Myopathy and HIV infection. *Current Opinion in Rheumatology,* 1995, 7/6 (497-502)

Effects of *L*-carnitine on serum triglyceride and cytokine levels in rat models of cachexia and septic shock. *British Journal of Cancer* (UK), 1995, 72/5

Cataract

Alex Duarte, OD, Ph.D., *Cataract Breakthrough*, 1994

The Hadley School for the Blind, Inc., *The Truth About Your Eyes*, First Collier Books Edition, C. 1962

Karen Timberlake, *Chemistry, Third Edition,* Los Angeles Valley College: Harper & Row, Publishers Inc, C. 1983

Dorland's Illustrated Medical Dictionary, 25th Edition, W. B. Saunders Company, C. 1974

Gary A. Thibodeau, Ph.D., and Catherine Parker Anthony, RN, BA, MS, *Structure & Function of the Body, Eighth Edition,* Times Mirror/Mosby College Publishing, C. 1988

Contemporary views on the pathogenesis and possible prophylaxis of age related cataracts. *Pol Merkuriusz Lek* (Poland) Jan 1997, 2 (7) p76-8

Antioxidant functions of micronutriments in the general population and critically ill patients. *Nutrition Clinique et Metabolisme* (Nutr. Clin. Metab.) (France) 1997, 11/2 (125-132)

Aqueous humour and serum zinc and copper concentrations of patients with glaucoma and cataract. *British Journal of Ophthalmology* (UK) 1990, 74/11 (661-662)

Antioxidants and cataract: cataract induction in space environment and application to terrestrial aging cataract. *Biochem Mol Biol Int* (Australia) Sep 1997, 42 (6) p1189-97

A glutathione deficiency in open-angle glaucoma and the approaches to its correction. *Vestn Oftalmol* (Russia) Jul-Dec 1992, 108 (4-6) p13-5

Alpha-lipoic acid as a biological antioxidant. *Free Radical Biology and Medicine* 1995, 19/2 (227-250)

Relations among aging, antioxidant status, and cataract. *Am J Clin Nutr* Dec 1995, 62 (6 Suppl) p1439S-1447S

Food and nutrient intake and risk of cataract. *Ann Epidemiol* Jan 1996, 6 (1) p41-6

Epidemiologic evidence of a role for the antioxidant vitamins and carotenoids in cataract prevention. *Am J Clin Nutr* Jan 1991, 53 (1 Suppl) p352S-355S

Health implications of Mediterranean diets in light of contemporary knowledge. 1. Plant foods and dairy products. *American Journal of Clinical Nutrition* 1995, 61/6 Suppl. (1407S-1415S)

Cataract eye camp in India and xerophthalmia projects. Experience of a visiting ophthalmologist in January 91 in Sitapur, Uttar Pradesh, India. *Klinische Monatsblatter fur Augenheilkunde* (Germany) 1992, 200/5 (585-587)

Antioxidant functions of vitamins. Vitamins E and C, beta-carotene, and other carotenoids. *Ann N Y Acad Sci* Sep 30 1992, 669 p7-20

Successful treatment of severe atopic dermatitis-complicated cataract and male infertility with a natural product antioxidant. *Int J Tissue React* (Switzerland) 1998, 20 (2) p63-9

Antioxidant vitamins and nuclear opacities: the longitudinal study of cataract. *Ophthalmology* May 1998, 105 (5) p831-6

Dietary carotenoids, vitamins A, C, and E, and advanced age-related macular degeneration. Eye Disease Case-Control Study Group. *JAMA* 1994 Nov 9;272(18):1413-20

The use of vitamin supplements and the risk of cataract among US male physicians. *Am J Public Health* 1994 May;84(5):788-92

Association between low plasma vitamin E concentration and progression of early cortical lens opacities. *Am J Epidemiol* 1996 Sep 1;144(5):496-500

Stereospecific effects of R-lipoic acid on buthionine sulfoximine-induced cataract formation in newborn rats. *Biochem Biophys Res Commun* Apr 16 1996, 221 (2) p422-9

Alpha-Lipoic acid as a biological antioxidant. *Free Radic Biol Med* Aug 1995, 19 (2) p 227-50

Alpha-lipoic acid supplementation prevents symptoms of vitamin E deficiency. *Biochem Biophys Res Commun* Oct 14 1994

A review of the evidence supporting melatonin's role as an antioxidant. *J Pineal Res* (Denmark) Jan 1995, 18 (1) p1-11

Glutathione deficiency decreases tissue ascorbate levels in newborn rats: ascorbate spares glutathione and protects against oxidative damage. *Proc Natl Acad Sci U S A* Jun 1 1991, 88 (11) p4656-60

51Cr release and oxidative stress in the lens. *Lens Eye Toxic Res* 1989, 6 (1-2) p183-202

Free radical tissue damage: protective role of antioxidant nutrients. *FASEB J* Dec 1987, 1 (6) p441-5

Oxidative damage and defense. *Am J Clin Nutr* (US) Jun 1996, 63 (6) p985S-990S

[Antioxidative vitamins and cataracts in the elderly]. *Z Ernahrungswiss* (Germany) Sep 1995, 34 (3) p167-76

Alpha-lipoic acid prevents buthionine sulfoximine-induced cataract formation in newborn rats. *Free Radic Biol Med* Apr 1995, 18 (4) p823-9

Prevention of cataracts by nutritional and metabolic antioxidants. *Crit Rev Food Sci Nutr* 1995, 35 (1-2) p111-29

Free radicals, exercise, and antioxidant supplementation. *Int J Sport Nutr* Sep 1994, 4 (3) p205-20, *Comment in Int J Sport Nutr* 1994 Sep;4(3):203-4

The use of vitamin supplements and the risk of cataract among US male physicians. *Am J Public Health* May 1994, 84 (5) p788-92

Modelling cortical cataractogenesis VII: Effects of vitamin E treatment on galactose-induced cataracts. *Exp Eye Res* (England) Feb 1985, 40 (2) p213-22

Modeling cortical cataractogenesis. V. Steroid cataracts induced by solumedrol partially prevented by vitamin E in vitro. *Exp Eye Res* (England) Jul 1983, 37 (1) p65-76

Antioxidant vitamins in cataract prevention. *Z Ernahrungswiss* (Germany, West) Mar 1989, 28 (1) p56-75

Biochemical and morphological changes in the lenses of selenium and/or vitamin E deficient rats. *Biomed Environ Sci* Jun 1994, 7 (2) p109-15

Biochemical changes and cataract formation in lenses from rats receiving multiple, low doses of sodium selenite. *Exp Eye Res* (England) Nov 1992, 55 (5) p671-8

Defense system of the lens against oxidative damage: effect of oxidative challenge on cataract formation in glutathione peroxidase deficient-acatalasemic mice. *Exp Eye Res* (England) Oct 1980, 31 (4) p425-33 (no abstract)

Intraocular irrigating solutions and lens clarity. *Amer. J. Ophthal.*, 1976, 82/4 (594-597)

Intraocular irrigating solutions. Their effect on the corneal endothelium. *Arch. Ophthal.*, 1975, 93/8 (648-657)

Cerebral Vascular Disease

Ginkgo biloba L. *Fitoterapia* (Italy), 1998, 69/3 (195-244)

Antioxidant status and alpha1-antiproteinase activity in subarachnoid hemorrhage patients. *Life Sci* 1998;63(10):821-6

The effect of hypertension on cerebral atherosclerosis in the cynomolgus monkey. *Stroke*, 1993, 24/8 (1218-1227)

The case for intravenous magnesium treatment of arterial disease in general practice: Review of 34 years of experience. *J. Nutr. Med.* (UK), 1994, 4/2 (169-177)

Neuropsychiatric complications of cardiac surgery. *J. Cardiothorac. Vasc. Anesth.*, 1994, 8/1 Suppl. 1 (13-18)

Effects of the dipyridamol-dihydroergotoxine (Hydergine) methane sulphonate associations on pO_2 and its incidence in brain tissue. *Gen. Pharmacol.* (England), 1983, 14/6 (579-583)

The protective effects of dietary fish oil on focal cerebral infarction. *Prostaglandins Med.*, 1979, 3/5 (257-268)

What causes infarction in ischemic brain? *Neurology*, 1983, 33/2 (222-233)

Effects of antihypertensive drugs on blood velocity: implications for prevention of cerebral vascular disease. *Canad. J. Neurol.Sci.* (Canada), 1977, 4/2 (93-97)

Oxygen radicals in cerebral vascular injury. *Circ. Res.*, 1985, 57/4 (508-516)

Postischemic tissue injury by iron-mediated free radical lipid peroxidation. *Usa Ann. Emerg. Med.*, 1985, 14/8 (804-809)

Role of iron ions in the genesis of reperfusion injury following successful cardiopulmonary resuscitation: Preliminary data and a biochemical hypothesis. *Ann. Emerg. Med.*, 1985, 14/8 (777-783)

Cortical pO_2 distribution during oligemic hypotension and its pharmacological modifications (Hydergine). *Switzerland Arzneim.-Forsch.* (Germany, West), 1978, 28/5 (768-770)

The use of piracetam (Nootropil) in post-anesthetic recovery of elderly patients. (A preliminary study). *Greece Acta Anaesthesiol. Hell.* (Greece), 1981, 15/1-2 (76-80)

Free radical reaction products and antioxidant capacity in arterial plasma during coronary artery bypass grafting. *J. Thorac. Cardiovasc. Surg.*, 1994, 108/1 (140-147)

Biochemical studies of cerebral ischemia in the rat—Changes in cerebral free amino acids, catecholamines and uric acid. *Japan Brain Nerve* (Japan), 1986, 38/3 (253-258)

Free radicals scavenging action and anti-enzyme activities of procyanidines from Vitis vinifera. A mechanism for their capillary protective action. *Arzneimittelforschung* (Germany) May 1994, 44 (5) p592-601

Prevention of postischemic cardiac injury by the orally active iron chelator 1,2- dimethyl-3-hydroxy-4-pyridone (L1) and the antioxidant (+)-cyanidanol-3. *Circulation*, 1989, 80/1 (158-164)

Iron-load increases the susceptibility of rat hearts to oxygen reperfusion damage. Protection by the antioxidant (+)-cyanidanol-3 and deferoxamine. *Circulation*, 1988, 78/2 (442-449)

Cervical Dysplasia

Cigarette smoking and dysplasia and carcinoma in situ of the uterine cervix. *JAMA* Jul 22-29 1983, 250 (4) p499-502

Smoking and carcinoma in situ of the uterine cervix. *Am J Public Health* May 1983, 73 (5) p558-62

Genetic damage in exfoliated cells of the uterine cervix. Association and interaction between cigarette smoking and progression to malignant transformation? *Acta Cytologica* 1998, 42/3 (639-649)

Smoking and the antioxidant ascorbic acid: plasma, leukocyte, and cervicovaginal cell concentrations in normal healthy women. *Am J Obstet Gynecol* Dec 1990, 163 (6 Pt 1) p1948-52

Annual variation of serum selenium in patients with gynaecological cancer during 1978-1983 in Finland, a low selenium area. *Int J Vitam Nutr Res* 1985, 55 (4) p433-8,

A case-control study of nutrient status and invasive cervical cancer. I. Dietary indicators. *American Journal of Epidemiology* 1991, 134/11 (1335-1346)

The association of plasma micronutrients with the risk of cervical dysplasia in Hawaii. *Cancer Epidemiol Biomarkers Prev* Jun 1998, 7 (6) p537-44

Can cervical dysplasia and cancer be prevented with nutrients? *Nutr Rev* Jan 1998, 56 (1 Pt 1) p9-16

Can cervical dysplasia and cancer be prevented with nutrients? *Nutr Rev* Jan 1998, 56 (1 Pt 1) p9-16

Dietary factors in women with dysplasia colli uteri associated with human papillomavirus infection. *Nutr Cancer* 1998, 30 (1) p39-45

Cervical intraepithelial neoplasia, cervical cancer, and HPV. *Annual Review of Public Health* 1996, 17/- (69-84)

Human papillomavirus and invasive cervical cancer in Brazil. *Br J Cancer* (Scotland) Jan 1994, 69 (1) p114-9

Herpes simplex virus type 2: a possible interaction with human papillomavirus types 16/18 in the development of invasive cervical cancer. *Int J Cancer* Sep 30 1991, 49 (3) p335-40

Epidemiologic evidence showing that human papillomavirus infection causes most cervical intraepithelial neoplasia [see comments]. *J Natl Cancer Inst* Jun 16 1993, 85 (12) p958-64

Viral characteristics of human papillomavirus infection and antioxidant levels as risk factors for cervical dysplasia. *Int J Cancer* Nov 23 1998, 78 (5) p594-9

A case-control study of nutrient status and invasive cervical cancer. II. Serologic indicators. *American Journal of Epidemiology* 1991, 134/11 (1347-1355)

The role of sexual factors in the aetiology of cervical dysplasia [see comments]. *Int J Epidemiol* (England) Oct 1993, 22 (5) p798-803

Risk factors for cervical dysplasia: implications for prevention. *Public Health* (England) Jul 1994, 108 (4) p241-9

Risk factors in the development of cervical intraepithelial neoplasia in women with vulval warts. *Genitourin Med* (England) Oct 1988, 64 (5) p316-20

Quantification of HPV-16 E6-E7 transcription in cervical intraepithelial neoplasia by reverse transcriptase polymerase chain reaction. *Int J Cancer* Sep 30 1993, 55 (3) p397-401

[A cohort study on cancer of uterine cervix in Jingan county, Jiangxi province]. *Chung Hua Chung Liu Tsa Chih* (China) Nov 1992, 13 (6) p409-12

A nuclear DNA study of uterine cervical dysplasia with reference to its prognostic significance. *Nippon Sanka Fujinka Gakkai Zasshi* (Japan) Nov 1988 , 40 (11) p1760-6

Risk factors for cervical intraepithelial neoplasia. *Cancer* May 1 1992, 69 (9) p2276-82

Risk factors for cervical neoplasia in Denmark. *APMIS* Suppl (Denmark) 1998, 80 p1-41

Correlation of cervical cancer mortality with reproductive and dietary factors, and serum markers in China. *International Journal of Epidemiology* (United Kingdom) 1994, 23/6 (1127-1132)

Spontaneous evolution of intraepithelial lesions according to the grade and type of the implicated human papillomavirus (HPV) *European Journal of Obstetrics Gynecology and Reproductive Biology* (Ireland) 1996, 65/1 (45-53)

A case-control study of nutrient status and invasive cervical cancer. II. Serologic indicators. *American Journal of Epidemiology* 1991, 134/11 (1347-1355)

Plasma ascorbic acid and beta- carotene levels in women evaluated for HPV infection, smoking, and cervix dysplasia. *Cancer Detect Prev* 1991, 15 (3) p165-70

Nutrients in diet and plasma and risk of in situ cervical cancer. *Journal of the National Cancer Institute* 1988, 80/8 (580-585)

The role of vitamins in the etiology of cervical neoplasia: An epidemiological review. *Archives of Gynecology and Obstetrics* (Germany) 1989, 246/1 (1-13)

Beta-carotene levels in exfoliated cervicovaginal epithelial cells in cervical intraepithelial neoplasia and cervical cancer. *Am J Obstet Gynecol* Dec 1992, 167 (6) p1899-903

Dietary vitamin C and uterine cervical dysplasia. *American Journal of Epidemiology* 1981, 114/5 (714-724)

Cervical Dysplasia

Dietary and serum carotenoids and cervical intraepithelial neoplasia. *Int J Cancer* Apr 22 1991, 48 (1) p34-8

Plasma vitamin C and uterine cervical dysplasia. *Am J Obstet Gynecol* Apr 1 1985, 151 (7) p976-80

Viral characteristics of human papillomavirus infection and antioxidant levels as risk factors for cervical dysplasia. *Int J Cancer* Nov 23 1998, 78 (5) p594-9

Dietary intake and blood levels of lycopene: association with cervical dysplasia among non-Hispanic, black women. *Nutr Cancer* 1998, 31 (1) p31-40

Dietary intake and blood levels of lycopene: association with cervical dysplasia among non-Hispanic, black women. *Nutr Cancer* 1998, 31 (1) p31-40

Serum micronutrients and the subsequent risk of cervical cancer in apopulation-based nested case-control study. *Cancer Epidemiol Biomarkers Prev* Jul-Aug 1993, 2 (4) p335-9

Change of vitamin a status and its influence on cervical dysplasia. *Zentralblatt fur Gynakologie* (Germany) 1995, 117/9 (472-475)

Folates: supplemental forms and therapeutic applications. *Altern Med Rev* Jun 1998, 3 (3) p208-20

Folic acid and ceervical dysplasia. *Minerva Ginecologica* (Italy) 1996, 48/10 (397-400)

Folate status, women's health, pregnancy outcome, and cancer. *Journal of the American College of Nutrition* 1993, 12/4 (438-441)

Epidemiologic studies of vitamins and cancer of the lung, esophagus, and cervix.

Adv Exp Med Biol 1986, 206 p11-26

Folate deficiency and cervical dysplasia. *Journal of the American Medical Association* 1992, 267/4 (528-533)

Antineoblastic activity of antioxidant vitamins: the role of folic acid in the prevention of cervical dysplasia. *Panminerva Med* (Italy) Dec 1993, 35 (4) p193-6

Folate status, women's health, pregnancy outcome, and cancer. *J Am Coll Nutr* Aug 1993, 12 (4) p438-41

Folate deficiency, cancer and congenital abnormalities. Is there a connection? (see comments)]. *Tidsskr Nor Laegeforen* (Norway) Jan 20 1996, 116 (2) p250-4

Oral folic acid supplementation for cervical dysplasia: A clinical intervention trial

American Journal of Obstetrics and Gynecology 1992, 166/3 (803-809)

Hypomethylation in cervical tissue: is there a correlation with folate status? *Cancer Epidemiol Biomarkers Prev* Oct 1998, 7 (10) p901-6

Improvement in cervical dysplasia associated with folic acid therapy in users of oral contraceptives. *Am J Clin Nutr* Jan 1982, 35 (1) p73-82

Megaloblastic changes in the cervical epithelium: association with oral contraceptive therapy and reversal with folic acid. *J. Am. Med. Assoc.*; VOL 226 ISS Dec 17 1973, P1421-1424, (REF 20)

Improvement in cervical dysplasia associated with folic acid therapy in users of oral contraceptives. *Am J Clin Nutr* Jan 1982, 35 (1) p73-82

Megaloblastic changes in the cervical epithelium: association with oral contraceptive therapy and reversal with folic acid. *J. Am. Med. Assoc.;* VOL 226 ISS Dec 17 1973, P1421-1424

Folic Acid Deficiency Megaloblastic Anemia And Peripheral Polyneuropathy Due To Oral Contraceptives. *ISR J MED SCI* 25 (3). 1989. 142-145.

Megaloblastic anemia in a vegetarian taking oral contraceptives. *South Med J*; VOL 68, ISS 2, 1975, P249-50

Folate deficiency and oral contraceptives. *J. Am. Med. Assoc.*; VOL 214 ISS Oct 5 1970, P105-108, (REF 38)

Improvement in cervical dysplasia associated with folic acid therapy in users of oral contraceptives. *American Journal of Clinical Nutrition* 1982, 35/1 (73-82)

Influence of vitamin A on cervical dysplasia and carcinoma in situ. *Nutrition and Cancer* 1984, 6/1 (49-57)

Enhancement of regression of cervical intraepithelial neoplasia II (moderate dysplasia) with topically applied all-trans-retinoic acid: a randomized trial [see comments]. *J Natl Cancer Inst* Apr 6 1994, 86 (7) p539-43

Phase II trial of beta- all- trans- retinoic acid for cervical intraepithelial neoplasia delivered via a collagen sponge and cervical cap. *Western Journal of Medicine* 1986, 145/2 (192-195)

A phase I trial of topically applied trans-retinoic acid in cervical dysplasia-clinical efficacy. *Invest New Drugs* 1986, 4 (3) p241-4

Retinoids and the prevention of cervical dysplasias. *Am J Obstet Gynecol* Dec 15 1981, 141 (8) p890-4

Influence of vitamin A on cervical dysplasia and carcinoma in situ. *Nutr Cancer* 1984, 6 (1) p49-57

Use of vitamins A and D in chemoprevention and therapy of cancer: control of nuclear receptor expression and function. Vitamins, cancer and receptors. *Adv Exp Med Biol* 1995, 375 p1-15

Specificity of retinoid receptor gene expression in mouse cervical epithelia. *Endocrinology* May 1994, 134 (5) p2018-25

Studies of retinoids in the prevention and treatment of cancer. *J Am Acad Dermatol* Apr 1982, 6 (4 Pt 2 Suppl) p824-7

Antioxidant nutrients: associations with persistent human papillomavirus infection. *Cancer Epidemiol Biomarkers Prev* Nov 1997, 6 (11) p917-23

Content of beta-carotene in blood serum of human papillomavirus infected women with cervical dysplasias. *Arch Immunol Ther Exp* (Warsz) (Poland) 1996, 44 (5-6) p309-13

Premalignant lesions: role of antioxidant vitamins and beta-carotene in risk reduction and prevention of malignant transformation. *Am J Clin Nutr* Jan 1991, 53 (1 Suppl) p386S-390S

Growth retardation in human cervical dysplasia-derived cell lines by beta-carotene through down-regulation of epidermal growth factor receptor. *Am J Clin Nutr* Dec 1995, 62 (6 Suppl) p1535S-1540S

Growth suppression and induction of heat-shock protein-70 by 9-cis beta-carotene in cervical dysplasia-derived cells. *Life Sci* (England) 1997, 61 (8) p839-45

Oral contraceptive use and adenocarcinoma of cervix [see comments]. *Lancet* (England) Nov 19 1994, 344 (8934) p1390-4

Comparison of oral contraceptive use in women with adenocarcinoma and squamous cell carcinoma of the uterine cervix. *Gynecol Obstet Invest* (Switzerland) 1991, 32 (2) p98-101

Comparison of oral contraceptive use in women with adenocarcinoma and squamous cell carcinoma of the uterine cervix. *Gynecol Obstet Invest* (Switzerland) 1991, 32 (2) p98-101

Oral contraceptive use and invasive cervical cancer. *Int J Epidemiol* (England) Jun 1990, 19 (2) p259-63

Oral contraceptive use and risk of invasive cervical cancer. *Int J Epidemiol* (England) Mar 1990, 19 (1) p4-11

Use of oral contraceptives and risk of invasive cervical cancer in previously screened women. *Int J Cancer* Apr 15 1987, 39 (4) p427-30

Risk factors for cervical neoplasia in Denmark. *APMIS* Suppl (Denmark) 1998, 80 p1-41

Long-term use of oral contraceptives and cervical neoplasia: an association confounded by other risk factors? *Contraception* Oct 1985, 32 (4) p337-46

Oral contraceptives and cervical neoplasia. *Contraception* 1991, 43/6 (581-595)

Case-control study of risk factors for cervical squamous- cell neoplasia in Denmark. III. Role of oral contraceptive use. *Cancer Causes Control* (England) Nov 1993, 4 (6) p513-9

Oral contraceptive use and cervical intraepithelial neoplasia. *J Clin Epidemiol* (England) Oct 1992, 45 (10) p1111-8

Oral contraceptive use and the incidence of cervical intraepithelial neoplasia [see comments]. *Am J Obstet Gynecol* Jul 1992, 167 (1) p40-4

A case-control study of oral contraceptive use in women with adenocarcinoma of the uterine cervix. *Eur J Obstet Gynecol Reprod Biol* (Netherlands) Sep 1987, 26 (1) p85-90

A longitudinal analysis of human papillomavirus 16 infection, nutritional status, and cervical dysplasia progression. *Cancer Epidemiol Biomarkers Prev* Jun 1995, 4 (4) p373-80

Zinc concentration in plasma and erythrocytes of subjects receiving folic acid supplementation. *American Journal of Clinical Nutrition* 1988, 47/3 (484-486)

Stress and hopelessness in the promotion of cervical intraepithelial neoplasia to invasive squamous cell carcinoma of the cervix [published erratum appears in *J Psychosom Res* 1987;31(5):659]. *J Psychosom Res* (England) 1986, 30 (1) p67-76

[Relation between selenium and cancer of uterine cervix]. *Chung Hua Chung Liu Tsa Chih* (China) Mar 1995, 17 (2) p112-4

Serum selenium and the risk of cancer, by specific sites: case-controlanalysis of prospective data. *J Natl Cancer Inst* Jul 1987, 79 (1) p103-8

Chemopreventive action of selenium on methylcholanthrene-induced carcinogenesis in the uterine cervix of mouse. *Oncology* (Switzerland) 1992, 49 (3) p237-40,

Dietary vitamins A, C, and E and selenium as risk factors for cervical cancer.*Epidemiology* Jan 1990, 1 (1) p8-15

[Concentration of selenium and vitamin E in the serum of women with malignant genital neoplasms and their family members]. *Ginekol Pol* (Poland) Jun 1989, 60 (6) p301-5

Relationship between the cervical uterine cancer evolution and seleniumconcentration in urine determined by NAA. *Journal of Radioanalytical and Nuclear Chemistry* (Hungary) 1997, 217/2 (167-169)

Activation analysis of selenium in cancer research. *Journal of Radioanalytical and Nuclear Chemistry* (Hungary) 1995, 195/1 (91-95)

Low serum selenium concentration in patients with cervical or endometrialcancer. *Int J Gynaecol Obstet* (Ireland) Feb 1984, 22 (1) p35-40

Pyridoxine, the pill and depression. *Journal of Pharmacotherapy* 1980, 3/1 (20-29)

Physiological And Psychological Effects Of Vitamins E And B-6 On Women Taking Oral Contraceptives. *Int J Vitam Nutr Res* 49 (1). 1979. 43-50

Influence of oral contraceptives, pyridoxine (vitamin B6), and tryptophanon carbohydrate metabolism. *Lancet* (England) Apr 10 1976, 1 (7963) p759-64,

Does use of oral contraceptives enhance the toxicity of carbon disulfidethrough interactions with pyridoxine and tryptophan metabolism? *Med Hypotheses* (England) Jan 1980, 6 (1) p21-33

Drug–vitamin B6 interaction. *Curr Concepts Nutr* 1983, 12 p1-12, The effect of oral contraceptives on the apparent vitamin B6 status insome Sudanese women. *Br J Nutr* (England) Sep 1986, 56 (2) p363-7

Cholesterol Reduction

Dietary isoflavones reduce plasma cholesterol and atherosclerosis in C57BL/6 mice but not LDL receptor-deficient mice. *J Nutr* Jun 1998, 128 (6) p954-9

Evolution of the health benefits of soy isoflavones. *Proceedings of the Society for Experimental Biology and Medicine*, 1998, 217/3 (386-392)

Polyphenols produced during red wine ageing. *Biofactors* (Netherlands) 1997, 6 (4) p403-10

Lipemic and lipoproteinemic effects of natural and synthetic androgens in humans. *Clin Exp Pharmacol Physiol* (England) Jul 1986, 13 (7) p513-8

Fats in indian diets and their nutritional and health implications. *Lipids*, 1996, 31/3 Suppl. (S287-S291)

The effects of natural dietary fiber from fruit and vegetables with oxalate from spinach on plasma minerals, lipids and other metabolites in men. *Nutr. Res.*, 1990, 10/4 (367-378)

Medical nutrition therapy lowers serum cholesterol and saves medication costs in men with hypercholesterolemia. *J Am Diet Assoc* Aug 1998, 98 (8) p889-94; quiz 895-6

Perspectives in the treatment of dyslipidemias in the prevention of coronary heart disease. *Angiology* May 1998, 49 (5) p339-48

Effects of crystalline nicotinic acid-induced hepatic dysfunction on serum low-density lipoprotein cholesterol and lecithin cholesteryl acyl transferase. *Am J Cardiol* Mar 15 1998, 81 (6) p805-7

A randomized trial of the effects of atorvastatin and niacin in patients with combined hyperlipidemia or isolated hypertriglyceridemia. Collaborative Atorvastatin Study Group. *Am J Med* Feb 1998, 104 (2) p137-43

Use of niacin, statins, and resins in patients with combined hyperlipidemia. *Am J Cardiol* Feb 26 1998, 81 (4A) p52B-59B

Triglyceride as a risk factor for coronary artery disease. *American Journal of Cardiology*, 1998, 82/9 A (22Q-25Q)

The antiatherogenic role of high-density lipoprotein cholesterol. *American Journal of Cardiology*, 1998, 82/9 A (13Q-21Q)

Atorvastatin in the treatment of primary hypercholesterolemia and mixed dyslipidemias. *Annals of Pharmacotherapy*, 1998, 32/10 (1030-1043)

Atorvastatin: A potent new HMG-CoA reductase inhibitor. *Cardiovascular Reviews and Reports*, 1998, 19/5 (32-48)

Hypocoagulant and lipid-lowering effects of dietary n-3 polyunsaturated fatty acids with unchanged platelet activation in rats. *Arterioscler Thromb Vasc Biol* Sep 1998, 18 (9) p1480-9

Effects of dietary fish oil on serum lipids and VLDL kinetics in hyperlipidemic apolipoprotein E*3-Leiden transgenic mice. *J Lipid Res* Jun 1998, 39 (6) p1181-8

Effect of fish-oil-enriched margarine on plasma lipids, low-density-lipoprotein particle composition, size, and susceptibility to oxidation. *Am J Clin Nutr* Aug 1998, 68 (2) p235-41

Abnormal content of n-6 and n-3 long-chain unsaturated fatty acids in the phosphoglycerides and cholesterol esters of parahippocampal cortex from Alzheimer's disease patients and its relationship to acetyl CoA content. *Int J Biochem Cell Biol* (England) Feb 1998, 30 (2) p197-207

Mediterranean dietary pattern in a randomized trial: prolonged survival and possible reduced cancer rate [see comments]. *Arch Intern Med* Jun 8 1998, 158 (11) p1181-7

Dietary (n-3) and (n-6) polyunsaturated fatty acids rapidly modify fatty acid composition and insulin effects in rat adipocytes. *J Nutr* Mar 1998, 128 (3) p512-9

The triphasic effects of exercise on blood rheology: Which relevance to physiology and pathophysiology? *Clinical Hemorheology and Microcirculation*, 1998, 19/2 (89-104)

Hyperlipidemia and diabetes mellitus. *Mayo Clinic Proceedings*, 1998, 73/10 (969-976)

Insulin therapy for a non-diabetic patient with severe hypertriglyceridemia. *Journal of the American College of Nutrition*, 1998, 17/5 (458-461)

Effects of omega-3 fatty acids and/or antioxidants on endothelial cell markers. *European Journal of Clinical Investigation* (UK), 1998, 28/8 (629-635)

Omega-3 ethyl ester concentrate decreases total apolipoprotein CIII and increases antithrombin III in postmyocardial infarction patients. *Clinical Drug Investigation* (New Zealand), 1998, 15/6 (473-482)

One-year treatment with ethyl esters of n-3 fatty acids in patients with hypertriglyceridemia and glucose intolerance reduced triglyceridemia, total cholesterol and increased HDL-C without glycemic alterations. *Atherosclerosis* (Ireland), 1998, 137/2 (419-427)

Soluble cell adhesion molecules in hypertriglyceridemia and potential significance on monocyte adhesion. *Arteriosclerosis, Thrombosis, and Vascular Biology*, 1998, 18/5 (723-731)

The effects of an omega-3 ethyl ester concentrate on blood lipid concentrations in patients with hyperlipidaemia. *Clinical Drug Investigation* (New Zealand), 1998, 15/5 (397-404)

On the effect of 2-deuterium- and 2-methyl-eicosapentaenoic acid derivatives on triglycerides, peroxisomal beta-oxidation and platelet aggregation in rats. *Biochimica et Biophysica Acta —Biomembranes* (Netherlands), 1998, 1369/2 (193-203)

Effect of garlic (Allium sativum) on blood lipids, blood sugar, fibrinogen and fibrinolytic activity in patients with coronary artery disease. *Prostaglandins Leukot Essent Fatty Acids* (Scotland) Apr 1998, 58 (4) p257-63

Garlic powder and plasma lipids and lipoproteins: a multicenter, randomized, placebo-controlled trial. *Arch Intern Med* Jun 8 1998, 158 (11) p1189-94

Effect of a garlic oil preparation on serum lipoproteins and cholesterol metabolism: a randomized controlled trial. *JAMA* Jun 17 1998, 279 (23) p1900-2

[Influence of lifestyle on the use of supplements in the Brandenburg nutrition and cancer study]. *Z Ernahrungswiss* (Germany) Mar 1998, 37 (1) p38-46

In vitro effect of garlic powder extract on lipid content in normal and atherosclerotic human aortic cells. *Lipids* Oct 1997, 32 (10) p1055-60

Modulation of lipid profile by fish oil and garlic combination. *J Natl Med Assoc* Oct 1997, 89 (10) p673-8

Effect of garlic and fish-oil supplementation on serum lipid and lipoprotein concentrations in hypercholesterolemic men [see comments]. *Am J Clin Nutr* Feb 1997, 65 (2) p445-50

Garlic powder in the treatment of moderate hyperlipidaemia: a controlled trial and meta-analysis. *J R Coll Physicians Lond* (England) Jul-Aug 1996, 30 (4) p329-34

Isolation of cholesteryl ester transfer protein inhibitors from Panax ginseng roots. *Chem Pharm Bull* (Tokyo) (Japan) Feb 1996, 44 (2) p444-5

A double-blind crossover study in moderately hypercholesterolemic men that compared the effect of aged garlic extract and placebo administration on blood lipids. *Am J Clin Nutr* Dec 1996, 64 (6) p866-70

Perspectives on soy protein as a nonpharmacological approach for lowering cholesterol. *J Nutr* Mar 1995, 125 (3 Suppl) p675S-678S

Consumption of a garlic clove a day could be beneficial in preventing thrombosis. *Prostaglandins Leukot Essent Fatty Acids* (Scotland) Sep 1995, 53 (3) p211-2

On the effect of garlic on plasma lipids and lipoproteins in mild hypercholesterolaemia. *Atherosclerosis* (Ireland) Mar 1995, 113 (2) p219-25

Direct anti-atherosclerosis-related effects of garlic. *Ann Med* (England) Feb 1995, 27 (1) p63-5

Cardiovascular disease. *JAMA* Jun 1 1994, 271 (21) p1660-1

Garlic as a lipid lowering agent—a meta-analysis. *J R Coll Physicians Lond* (England) Jan-Feb 1994, 28 (1) p39-45

Limitation of the deterioration of lipid parameters by a standardized garlic-ginkgo combination product. A multicenter placebo-controlled double-blind study. *Arzneimittelforschung* (Germany) Sep 1993, 43 (9) p978-81

Inter-relationships between haemostatic tests and the effects of some dietary determinants in the Caerphilly cohort of older men. *Blood Coagul Fibrinolysis* (England) Aug 1993, 4 (4) p529-36

Effect of garlic on total serum cholesterol. A meta-analysis [see comments]. *Ann Intern Med* Oct 1 1993, 119 (7 Pt 1) p599-605

Effects of garlic coated tablets in peripheral arterial occlusive disease. *Clin Investig* (Germany) May 1993, 71 (5) p383-6

Can garlic reduce levels of serum lipids? A controlled clinical study. *Am J Med* Jun 1993, 94 (6) p632-5

Hypertension and hyperlipidaemia: garlic helps in mild cases. *Br J Clin Pract Suppl* (England) Aug 1990, 69 p3-6

Therapy with garlic: results of a placebo-controlled, double-blind study. *Br J Clin Pract Suppl* (England) Aug 1990, 69 p7-11

The effect of a garlic preparation on the composition of plasma lipoproteins and erythrocyte membranes in geriatric subjects. *Br J Clin Pract Suppl* (England) Aug 1990, 69 p12-9

Comparison of the efficacy and tolerance of a garlic preparation vs. bezafibrate. *Arzneimittelforschung* (Germany) Dec 1992, 42 (12) p1473-7

[Postprandial lipemia under treatment with Allium sativum. Controlled double-blind study of subjects with reduced HDL2-cholesterol]. *Arzneimittelforschung* (Germany) Oct 1992, 42 (10) p1223-7

Effect of ingestion of raw garlic on serum cholesterol level, clotting time and fibrinolytic activity in normal subjects. *J Postgrad Med* (India) Jul 1991, 37 (3) p128-31

Effect of garlic on thrombocyte aggregation, microcirculation, and other risk factors. *Int J Clin Pharmacol Ther Toxicol* (Germany) Apr 1991, 29 (4) p151-5

[Garlic as phytogenic antilipemic agent. Recent studies with a standardized dry garlic powder substance]. *Fortschr Med* (Germany) Dec 20 1990, 108 (36) p703-6

Treatment of hyperlipidaemia with garlic-powder tablets. Evidence from the German Association of General Practitioners' multicentric placebo-controlled double-blind study. *Arzneimittelforschung* (Germany) Oct 1990, 40 (10) p1111-6

Garlic, onions and cardiovascular risk factors. A review of the evidence from human experiments with emphasis on commercially available preparations [see comments]. *Br J Clin Pharmacol* (England) Nov 1989, 28 (5) p535-44

Effect of dried garlic on blood coagulation, fibrinolysis, platelet aggregation and serum cholesterol levels in patients with hyperlipoproteinemia. *Atherosclerosis* (Netherlands) Dec 1988, 74 (3) p247-9

Lack of efficacy of dried garlic in patients with hyperlipoproteinemia. *Arzneimittelforschung* (Germany, West) Apr 1986, 36 (4) p766-8

Bulgarian traditional medicine: a source of ideas for phytopharmacological investigations. *J Ethnopharmacol* (Switzerland) Feb 1986, 15 (2) p121-32

Influence of garlic on serum cholesterol, serum triglycerides, serum total lipids and serum glucose in human subjects. *Nahrung* (Germany, East) 1984, 28 (2) p159-63

[Garlic therapy? Theories of a folk remedy (author's transl)]. *MMW Munch Med Wochenschr* (Germany, West) Oct 9 1981, 123 (41) p1537-8

The structure-hemolysis relationship of oleanolic acid derivatives and inhibition of the saponin-induced hemolysis with sapogenins. *J Pharmacobiodyn* (Japan) Nov 1981, 4 (11) p833-7

The long-term use of garlic in ischemic heart disease—an appraisal. *Atherosclerosis* (Netherlands) Oct 1981, 40 (2) p175-9

Comparative effect of clofibrate, garlic and onion on alimentary hyperlipemia. *Atherosclerosis* (Netherlands) Jul 1981, 39 (4) p447-52

Effect of garlic on normal blood cholesterol level. *Indian J Physiol Pharmacol* (India) Jul-Sep 1979, 23 (3) p211-4

Effect of the essential oils of garlic and onion on alimentary hyperlipemia. *Atherosclerosis* (Netherlands) Jan-Feb 1975, 21 (1) p15-9

Garlic extract therapy in children with hypercholesterolemia. *Archives of Pediatrics and Adolescent Medicine*, 1998, 152/11 (1089-1094)

Herbal 'health' products: What family physicians need to know. *American Family Physician*, 1998, 58/5 (1133-1140)

Changes in platelet function and susceptibility of lipoproteins to oxidation associated with administration of aged garlic extract. *Journal of Cardiovascular Pharmacology*, 1998, 31/6 (904-908)

The consumer market for functional foods. *Journal of Nutraceuticals, Functional and Medical Foods*, 1997, 1/3 (5-21)

Dietary therapy for preventing and treating coronary artery disease. *American Family Physician*, 1998, 57/6 (1299-1306)

Effect of garlic on some blood lipids and hmgcoa reductase activity. *Iranian Journal of Medical Sciences* (Iran), 1996, 21/3-4 (141-146)

Physical performance support with combined phytotherapy. Ginseng, whitethorn and mixed pollen combination against stress. *Therapiewoche* (Germany), 1996, 46/25 (1421-1425)

Antioxidant of the coronary diet and disease. *Clinica Cardiovascular* (Spain), 1996, 14/2 (29-38)

Satellite symposium 'International Garlic Research'. *Zeitschrift fur Phytotherapie* (Germany), 1996, 17/1 (13-25)

Garlic in hyperlipidemia. Influence of a garlic preparation on the lipid serum levels of patients with primary hyperlipidaemia. *Zeitschrift fur Phytotherapie* (Germany), 1995, 16/6 (343-348)

Therapeutic actions of garlic constituents. *Medicinal Research Reviews*, 1996, 16/1 (111-124)

Towards the control of the hypertension epidemic. The Philippine experience. *Philippine Journal of Internal Medicine* (Philippines), 1995, 33/2 (33-35)

How does garlic exert its hypocholesterolaemic action? The tellurium hypothesis. *Medical Hypotheses* (UK), 1995, 44/4 (295-297)

Efficacy of dietary recommendations and phytotherapy with Allium sativum in mild and moderate hypercholesterinemia. *Med. Welt* (Germany), 1994, 45/7-8 (327-323)

Dyslipidemias and the secondary prevention of coronary heart disease. *Dis. Mon.*, 1994, 40/8 (373-462)

Effect of garlic powder tablets on blood lipids and blood pressure—A six month placebo controlled, double blind study. *Br. J. Clin. Res.* (UK), 1993, 4/- (37-44)

Garlic supplementation and lipoprotein oxidation susceptibility. *Lipids*, 1993, 28/5 (475-477)

Postprandial lipaemia under treatment with allium sativum/ Controlled double-blind study in healthy volunteers with reduced HDL2- cholesterol levels. *Arzneim.-Forsch. Drug Res.* (Germany), 1992, 42/10 (1223-1227)

Garlic as a phytogenic lipid-lowering drug—A review of clinical trials with standardized garlic powder preparations. *Fortschr. Med.* (Germany, Federal Republic of), 1990, 108/36 (49-54)

Effect of an odor-modified garlic preparation on blood lipids. *Nutr. Res.*, 1987, 7/2 (139-149)

Oral guar gum treatment of intrahepatic cholestasis and pruritus in pregnant women: effects on serum cholestanol and other non-cholesterol sterols. *Eur J Clin Invest* (England) May 1998, 28 (5) p359-63

Increasing amounts of dietary fiber provided by foods normalizes physiologic response of the large bowel without altering calcium balance or fecal steroid excretion. *Am J Clin Nutr* Sep 1998, 68 (3) p615-22

[The use of dietary fiber as natural enterosorbents in diseases of the hepatobiliary system]. *Lik Sprava* (Ukraine) Mar-Apr 1998, (2) p80-2

Validity and reproducibility of a food frequency questionnaire to assess dietary intake of women living in Mexico City. *Salud Publica Mex* (Mexico) Mar-Apr 1998, 40 (2) p133-40

Oxidized LDL promotes vascular endothelial cell pinocytosis via a prooxidation mechanism. *FASEB J* Jul 1998, 12 (10) p823-30

[Dietary fibers in diet therapy]. *Vopr Pitan* (Russia) 1998, (1) p39-42

Definition of healthy eating in the Spanish adult population: a national sample in a pan-European survey. *Public Health* (England) Mar 1998, 112 (2) p95-101

Dietary sources of nutrients among US adults, 1989 to 1991. *J Am Diet Assoc* May 1998, 98 (5) p537-47

Fruit consumption, fitness, and cardiovascular health in female adolescents: the Penn State Young Women's Health Study. *Am J Clin Nutr* Apr 1998, 67 (4) p624-30

Zinc absorption, mineral balance, and blood lipids in women consuming controlled lactoovovegetarian and omnivorous diets for 8 wk. *Am J Clin Nutr* Mar 1998, 67 (3) p421-30

Long-term effects of consuming foods containing psyllium seed husk on serum lipids in subjects with hypercholesterolemia. *Am J Clin Nutr* Mar 1998, 67 (3) p367-76

Decreased serum total cholesterol concentration is associated with high intake of soy products in Japanese men and women. *J Nutr* Feb 1998, 128 (2) p209-13

Cholesterol, phospholipid, and protein changes in focal opacities in the human eye lens. *Invest Ophthalmol Vis Sci* Jan 1998, 39 (1) p94-103

A low-viscosity soluble-fiber fruit juice supplement fails to lower cholesterol in hypercholesterolemic men and women. *Journal of Nutrition,* 1998, 128/11 (1927-1932)

Food and nutrient intake of premenopausal female vegetarians and omnivores in Finland. *Scandinavian Journal of Nutrition / Naringsforskning* (Sweden), 1998, 42/3 (98-103)

Functional food science and the cardiovascular system. *British Journal of Nutrition* (UK), 1998, 80/Suppl. 1 (S113-S146)

Lipid- and glucose-lowering efficacy of Plantago Psyllium in type II diabetes. *Journal of Diabetes and its Complications,* 1998, 12/5 (273-278)

Impact of neuroendocrine activation on coronary artery disease. *American Journal of Cardiology,* 1998, 82/6 A (8H-14H)

Fruit and vegetable intake in young children. *Journal of the American College of Nutrition*, 1998, 17/4 (371-378)

Whole flaxseed consumption lowers serum LDL-cholesterol and lipoprotein(a) concentrations in postmenopausal women. *Nutrition Research*, 1998, 18/7 (1203-1214)

The potential role of soluble fibre in the treatment of hypercholesterolaemia. *Postgraduate Medical Journal* (UK), 1998, 74/ 873 (391-394)

Nutrition and coronary heart disease. *Comprehensive Therapy,* 1998, 24/4 (198-204)

Distribution and synthesis of apolipoprotein J in the atherosclerotic aorta. *Arteriosclerosis, Thrombosis, and Vascular Biology,* 1998, 18/4 (665-672)

Dietary fiber, the evolution of the human diet and coronary heart disease. *Nutrition Research,* 1998, 18/4 (633-652)

Managing hypercholesterolaemia: What role for dietary fibre? *British Journal of Cardiology* (UK), 1998, 5/3 (156-163)

Human fatty acid synthesis is reduced after the substitution of dietary starch for sugar. *American Journal of Clinical Nutrition*, 1998, 67/4 (631-639)

LDL oxidation: therapeutic perspectives. *Atherosclerosis* (Ireland) Apr 1998, 137 Suppl pS25-31

Influence of vitamin C status on ethanol metabolism in guinea-pigs. *Physiol Res* (Czech Republic) 1998, 47 (2) p137-41

Dietary antioxidants inhibit development of fatty streak lesions in the LDL receptor-deficient mouse. *Arterioscler Thromb Vasc Biol* Sep 1998, 18 (9) p1506-13

Vitamin E combined with selenium inhibits atherosclerosis in hypercholesterolemic rabbits independently of effects on plasma cholesterol concentrations. *Circ Res* Aug 24 1998, 83 (4) p366-77

Regulation of apolipoprotein B-containing lipoproteins by vitamin C level and dietary fat saturation in guinea pigs. *Metabolism* Jul 1998, 47 (7) p883-91

The nutritional health of New Zealand vegetarian and non-vegetarian Seventh-day Adventists: selected vitamin, mineral and lipid levels. *N Z Med J* (New Zealand) Mar 27 1998, 111 (1062) p91-4

Characteristics of survey participants with and without a telephone: findings from the third National Health and Nutrition Examination Survey. *J Clin Epidemiol* (England) Jan 1998, 51 (1) p55-60

Low-density lipoprotein oxidation and vitamins E and C in sustained and white-coat hypertension. *Hypertension* Feb 1998, 31 (2) p621-6

Citrus fruit supplementation reduces lipoprotein oxidation in young men ingesting a diet high in saturated fat: presumptive evidence for an interaction between vitamins C and E in vivo. *Am J Clin Nutr* Feb 1998, 67 (2) p240-5

Diet, antioxidant status, and smoking habits in French men [see comments]. *Am J Clin Nutr* Feb 1998, 67 (2) p231-9

Vitamin C supplementation restores the impaired vitamin E status of guinea pigs fed oxidized frying oil. *J Nutr* Jan 1998, 128 (1) p116-22

Antioxidant vitamins and coronary artery disease risk in South African males. *Clinica Chimica Acta* (Netherlands), 1998, 278/1 (55-60)

Nutrient losses and gains during frying: A review. *International Journal of Food Sciences and Nutrition* (UK), 1998, 49/2 (157-168)

Vitamins E plus C and interacting conutrients required for optimal health. *BioFactors* (Netherlands), 1998, 7/1-2 (113-174)

Hypolipidemic effects of synthetic gugulsterones in normal rats and assessment of its long-term toxicity at cellular levels in various organs. *Indian J Med Sci* (India) Mar 1996, 50 (3) p63-7

Effects of *S*-allyl cysteine sulfoxide isolated from Allium sativum Linn and gugulipid on some enzymes and fecal excretions of bile acids and sterols in cholesterol fed rats. *Indian J Exp Biol* (India) Oct 1995, 33 (10) p749-51

Antiperoxide effects of *S*-allyl cysteine sulphoxide isolated from Allium sativum Linn and gugulipid in cholesterol diet fed rats. *Indian J Exp Biol* (India) May 1995, 33 (5) p337-41

Clinical trials with gugulipid . A new hypolipidaemic agent [see comments]. *J Assoc Physicians India* (India) May 1989, 37 (5) p323-8

Reduction of cholesterol and Lp(a) and regression of coronary artery disease: A case study. *Journal of Orthomolecular Medicine* (Canada) 1996, 11/3 (173-179)

Recent trends in hyperlipoproteinemias and its pharmacotherapy. *Indian Journal of Pharmacology* (India) 1995, 27/1 (14-29)

Nicotinic acid treatment shifts the fibrinolytic balance favourably and decreases plasma fibrinogen in hypertriglyceridaemic men [see comments]. *J Cardiovasc Risk*, 1997 Jun, 4:3, 165-71

Clinical trial experience with extended-release niacin (Niaspan): dose-escalation study. *Am J Cardiol*, 1998 Dec 17, 82:12A, 35U-38U; discussion 39U-41U

Clinical trials with gugulipid. A new hypolipidaemic agent. *J Assoc Physicians India* (India) May 1989, 37 (5) p323-8

Hypolipidemic and antioxidant effects of Commiphora mukul as an adjunct to dietary therapy in patients with hypercholesterolemia. *Cardiovasc Drugs Ther* Aug 1994, 8 (4) p659-64

Beneficial effects of Allium sativum (garlic), Allium cepa and Commiphora mukul on experimental hyperlipidemia and atherosclerosis—a comparative evaluation. *J Postgrad Med* (India) Jul 1991, 37 (3) p132-5

Curcumin, a major component of food spice turmeric (Curcuma longa) inhibits aggregation and alters eicosanoid metabolism in human blood platelets. *Prostaglandins Leukotrienes and Essential Fatty Acids* (UK), 1995, 52/4 (223- 227)

Influence of capsaicin, eugenol, curcumin and ferulic acid on sucrose-induced hypertriglyceridemia in rats. *Nutr. Rep. Int.*, 1988, 38/3 (571-581)

Inhibitory effect of curcumin, an anti-inflammatory agent, on vascular smooth muscle cell proliferation. *Eur. J. Pharmacol.* (Netherlands), 1992, 221/2-3 (381-384)

Polyphenols as cancer chemopreventive agents. *J Cell Biochem Suppl* 1995, 22 p169-80

Anti-tumour and antioxidant activity of natural curcuminoids. *Cancer Lett* (Ireland) Jul 20 1995, 94 (1) p79-83

Phospholipid epitopes for mouse antibodies against bromelain-treated mouse erythrocytes. *Immunology* (England) Sep 1987, 62 (1) p11-6

The effect of spices on cholesterol 7 alpha-hydroxylase activity and on serum and hepatic cholesterol levels in the rat. *Int J Vitam Nutr Res* (Switzerland) 1991, 61 (4) p364-9

Effect of gugulipid on bioavailability of diltiazem and propranolol. *J Assoc Physicians India* (India) Jun 1994, 42 (6) p454-5

Clinical trials with gugulipid. A new hypolipidaemic agent. *J Assoc Physicians India* (India) May 1989, 37 (5) p323-8

Biological effects of isoflavones in young women: Importance of the chemical composition of soyabean products. *British Journal of Nutrition* (UK), 1995, 74/4 (587-601)

Overview of proposed mechanisms for the hypocholesterolemic effect of soy. *Journal of Nutrition*, 1995, 125/3 Suppl. (606S-611S)

Biological effects of a diet of soy protein rich in isoflavones on the menstrual cycle of premenopausal women. *Am. J. Clin. Nutr.*, 1994, 60/3 (333-340)

A review of the clinical effects of phytoestrogens. *Obstetrics and Gynecology*, 1996, 87/5 II Suppl. (897-904)

Nutritional interest of flavonoids. *Medecine et Nutrition* (France), 1996, 32/1 (17-27)

Inhibition of protein tyrosine kinase alters the effect of serum basic protein I on triacylglycerols and cholesterol differently in normal and hyperapoB fibroblasts. *Arteriosclerosis, Thrombosis, and Vascular Biology*, 1995, 15/8 (1195-1203)

Influence of dietary curcumin and cholesterol on the progression of experimentally induced diabetes in albino rat. *Molecular and Cellular Biochemistry*, 1995, 152/1 (13-21)

Effect of retinol deficiency and curcumin or turmeric feeding on brain Na+-K+ adenosine triphosphatase activity. *Mol. Cell. Biochem.*, 1994, 137/2 (101-107)

Bioactive substances in food: Identification and potential uses. *Can. J. Physiol. Pharmacol.* (Canada), 1994, 72/4 (423-434)

Mechanism of antiinflammatory actions of curcumine and boswellic acids. J. *Ethnopharmacol.* (Ireland), 1993, 38/2-3 (113-119)

Influence of dietary spices on adrenal steroidogenesis in rats. *Nutr. Res.*, 1993, 13/4 (435-444)

Differential effects of dietary lipids and curcumin on kidney microsomal fatty acids and Na+, K+ - ATPase activity in rat. *Nutr. Res.*, 1992, 12/7 (893-904)

Chronic Fatigue Syndrome

Fibromyalgia and chronic fatigue: the holistic perspective. *Holist Nurs Pract* Apr 1998, 12 (3)p55-63

Chronic fatigue syndrome: an update. *Annu Rev Med* 1998, 49 p1-13

Chronic fatigue syndrome. Helping patients cope with this enigmatic illness. *Postgrad Med* Jan 1998, 103 (1)p175-6, 179-84

Decreased immunoreactive beta-endorphin in mononuclear leucocytes from patients with chronic fatigue syndrome. *Clinical and Experimental Rheumatology* (Italy), 1998, 16/6 (729-732)

Chronic fatigue syndrome: An atopic state. *Journal of Chronic Fatigue Syndrome*, 1998, 4/3 (39-57)

Isolated diastolic dysfunction of the myocardium and its response to CoQ_{10} treatment. *Clin Investig* (Germany) 1993, 71 (8 Suppl) pS140-4

Analysis of dietary intake and selected nutrient concentrations in patients with chronic fatigue syndrome. *J Am Diet Assoc* Apr 1996, 96 (4) p383-6

[Chronic fatigue syndrome]. *Nippon Naika Gakkai Zasshi* (Japan) Sep 10 1993, 82 (9) p1571-6

Electron-microscopic investigation of muscle mitochondria in chronic fatigue syndrome. *Neuropsychobiology* (Switzerland) 1995, 32 (4) p175-81

Serum levels of carnitine in chronic fatigue syndrome: clinical correlates. *Neuropsychobiology* (Switzerland) 1995, 32 (3) p132-8

Acylcarnitine deficiency in chronic fatigue syndrome. *Clin Infect Dis* Jan 1994, 18 Suppl 1 pS62-7

Cirrhosis

See references under Liver (Cirrhosis).

Cognitive Enhancement

See references under Age-Associated Mental Impairment.

Common Cold

[Clinical evaluation of Olbas oil effect on nasal mucosa in acute rhinitis patients during common cold] *Otolaryngol Pol* (Poland) 1997, 51 Suppl 25 p312-4

Caffeine and the common cold. *J Psychopharmacol* (Oxf) 1997, 11 (4) p319-24

Vitamin C supplementation and the common cold—was Linus Pauling right or wrong? *Int J Vitam Nutr Res* (Switzerland) 1997, 67 (5) p329-35

Zinc lozenges reduce the duration of common cold symptoms. *Nutr Rev* Mar 1997, 55 (3) p82-5

Vitamin C intake and susceptibility to the common cold. *Br J Nutr* (England) Jan 1997, 77 (1) p59-72

Primary infection by human parvovirus B19 and cold agglutinins. *Annales de Dermatologie et de Venereologie (Ann. Dermatol. Venereol.)* (France) 1997, 124/3 (257-259)

Vitamin C and common cold in general practice. An update. *Huisarts en Wetenschap* (Netherlands), 1998, 41/11 (524-527)

Zinc gluconate and the common cold. Review of randomized controlled trials. *Can Fam Physician* (Canada) May 1998, 44 p1037-42

The role of zinc lozenges in treatment of the common cold. *Ann Pharmacother* Jan 1998, 32 (1) p63-9

Zinc gluconate lozenges for treating the common cold in children: a randomized controlled trial . *JAMA* Jun 24 1998, 279 (24) p1962-7

A meta-analysis of zinc salts lozenges and the common cold. *Arch Intern Med* Nov 10 1997, 157 (20) p2373-6

Serum dehydroepiandrosterone (DHEA) and DHEA sulfate are negatively correlated with serum interleukin- 6 (IL-6), and DHEA inhibits IL-6 secretion from mononuclear cells in man in vitro: possible link between endocrinosenescence and immunosenescence. *J Clin Endocrinol Metab* Jun 1998, 83 (6) p2012-7

Low serum levels of dehydroepiandrosterone may cause deficient IL-2 production by lymphocytes in patients with systemic lupus erythematosus (SLE). *Clin Exp Immunol* (England) Feb 1995, 99 (2) p251-5

Dehydroepiandrosterone modulates the spontaneous and IL-6 stimulated fibrinogen production of human hepatoma cells. *Acta Microbiol Immunol Hung* (Hungary) 1995, 42 (2) p229-33

Administration of dehydroepiandrosterone reverses the immune suppression induced by high dose antigen in mice. *Immunol Invest* May 1995, 24 (4) p583-93

Dehydroepiandrosterone synergizes with antioxidant supplements for immune restoration in old as well as retrovirus-infected mice. *Journal of Nutritional Biochemistry (J. Nutr. Biochem.)* 1998, 9/7 (362-369)

Autoimmunity: The Female Connection. *Medscape Womens Health* 1996 Nov;1(11):5

Exogenous dehydroepiandrosterone modified the expression of T helper-related cytokines in NZB/NZW F1 mice. *Immunol Invest* 1998 Jul-Sep;27(4-5):291-302

Psychological stress, cytokine production, and severity of upper respiratory illness. *Psychosom Med* 1999 Mar-Apr;61(2):175-80

Sambucol™ inhibited several strains of influenza virus and reduced symptoms during an outbreak of Influenza B Panama, *Weizmann Institute of Science* 2-15-94

The effect of Sambucol™ on HIV infection in vitro, *Congress of Microbiology* 2-6-95

Problems and prospects of developing effective therapy for common cold viruses. *Trends in Microbiology* (UK), 1997, 5/2 (58-63)

Vitamin C intake and susceptibility to the common cold. *British Journal of Nutrition* (UK), 1997, 77/1 (59-72)

Vitamin C supplementation and common cold symptoms: Problems with inaccurate reviews. *Nutrition*, 1996, 12/11-12 (804-809):

Vitamin C, the placebo effect, and the common cold: A case study of how preconceptions influence the analysis of results. *Journal of Clinical Epidemiology*, 1996, 49/10 (1079-1085,1087)

Vitamin C and common cold incidence: A review of studies with subjects under heavy physical stress. *International Journal of Sports Medicine* (Germany), 1996, 17/5 (379-383)

Herbal immuno-stimulants. *Zeitschrift fur Phytotherapie* (Germany), 1996, 17/2 (79-95)

Epidemiology, pathogenesis, and treatment of the common cold. *Annals of Allergy, Asthma and Immunology*, 1997, 78/6 (531-540)

Zinc lozenges for the common cold (4). *Journal of Family Practice*, 1997, 44/6 (526)

Zinc lozenges reduce the duration of common cold symptoms. *Nutrition Reviews*, 1997, 55/3 (82-85):

The age-associated decline in immune function of healthy individuals is not related to changes in plasma concentrations of beta-carotene, retinol, alpha-tocopherol or zinc. *Mechanisms of Ageing and Development* (Ireland), 1997, 94/1-3 (55-69)

Zinc gluconate lozenges for treating the common cold (1) (multiple letters). *Annals of Internal Medicine*, 1997, 126/9 (738-739)

Zinc for the common cold. *Medical Letter on Drugs and Therapeutics*, 1997, 39/993 (9-10)

The common cold. *Primary Care—Clinics in Office Practice*, 1996, 23/4 (657-675)

How does zinc modify the common cold? Clinical observations and implications regarding mechanisms of action. *Medical Hypotheses* (UK), 1996, 46/3 (295-302)

Zinc for treating the common cold: review of all clinical trials since 1984. *Altern Ther Health Med* Nov 1996, 2 (6) p63-72

Zinc gluconate lozenges for treating the common cold. A randomized, double-blind, placebo-controlled study [see comments]. *Ann Intern Med* Jul 15 1996, 125 (2) p81-8, Comment in *Ann Intern Med* 1996 Jul 15;125(2):142-4

Social ties and susceptibility to the common cold. *JAMA* Jun 25 1997, 277 (24) p1940-4

In vivo anti-influenza virus activity of a zinc finger peptide. *Antimicrob Agents Chemother* Mar 1997, 41 (3) p687-92

Common (but not always considered) viral infections of the lower respiratory tract. *Pediatr Ann* Oct 1996, 25 (10) p577-84

Vitamin C and the common cold: a retrospective analysis of Chalmers' review. *J Am Coll Nutr* Apr 1995

Interrelation of vitamin C, infection, haemostatic factors, and cardiovascular disease. *Bmj* (England) Jun 17 1995, 310 (6994) p1559-63

Does vitamin C alleviate the symptoms of the common cold?—a review of current evidence. *Scand J Infect Dis* (Sweden) 1994, 26 (1) p1-6

Recommended dietary allowance: support from recent research. *J Nutr Sci Vitaminol* (Tokyo) (Japan) 1992, Spec No p173-6

Vitamin C and the common cold. *Br J Nutr* (England) Jan 1992, 67 (1) p3-16

Vitamin C and the common cold: using identical twins as controls. *Med J Aust* (Australia) Oct 17 1981, 2 (8) p411-2

The effects of ascorbic acid and flavonoids on the occurrence of symptoms normally associated with the common cold. *Am J Clin Nutr* Aug 1979, 32 (8) p1686-90

Winter illness and vitamin C: the effect of relatively low doses. *Can Med Assoc J* (Canada) Apr 5 1975, 112 (7) p823-6

Acetylcysteine: a drug with an interesting past and a fascinating future. *Respiration* (Switzerland) 1986, 50 Suppl 1 p26-30

[Effect of Astragalus membranaceus on Ca2+ influx and coxsackie virus B3 RNA replication in cultured neonatal rat heart cells]. *Chung Kuo Chung Hsi I Chieh Ho Tsa Chih* (China) Aug 1995

The inhibitory effect of astragalus membranaceus on coxsackie B-3 virus RNA replication. *Chin Med Sci J* (China) Sep 1995, 10 (3) p146-50

[The effect of astragalus polysaccharides (APS) on cell mediated immunity (CMI) in burned mice]. *Chung Hua Cheng Hsing Shao Shang Wai Ko Tsa Chih* (China) Mar 1994

Immunomodulating Chinese herbal medicines. *Mem Inst Oswaldo Cruz* (Brazil) 1991, 86 Suppl 2 p159-64

[The effect of vitamin A and Astragalus on the splenic T lymphocyte-CFU of burned mice]. *Chung Hua Cheng Hsing Shao Shang Wai Ko Tsa Chih* (China) Jun 1989

Nutritional antioxidants and the modulation of inflammation: theory and practice. *New Horiz* May 1994

Evaluation of zinc complexes on the replication of rhinovirus 2 in vitro. *Res Commun Chem Pathol Pharmacol* Dec 1989

Zinc gluconate and the common cold: a controlled clinical study. *J Int Med Res* (England) Jun 1992, 20 (3) p234-46

Prophylaxis and treatment of rhinovirus colds with zinc gluconate lozenges. *J Antimicrob Chemother* (England) Dec 1987

Reduction in duration of common colds by zinc gluconate lozenges in a double-blind study. *Antimicrob Agents Chemother* Jan 1984, 25 (1) p20-4

Antivirals for the chemoprophylaxis and treatment of influenza. *Semin Respir Infect* (United States) Mar 1992

Utilization of pulse oximetry for the study of the inhibitory effects of antiviral agents on influenza virus in mice. *Antimicrob Agents Chemother* Feb 1992

Further studies with short duration ribavirin aerosol for the treatment of influenza virus infection in mice and respiratory syncytial virus infection in cotton rats. *Antiviral Res* (Netherlands) Jan 1992

High dose-short duration ribavirin aerosol treatment--a review. *Bull Int Union Tuberc Lung Dis* (France) Jun-Sep 1991

Viral pneumonia. *Infect Dis Clin North Am* Sep 1991

Aerosol and intraperitoneal administration of ribavirin and ribavirin triacetate: pharmacokinetics and protection of mice against intracerebral infection with influenza A/WSN virus. *Antimicrob Agents Chemother* Jul 1991

Antiviral drug therapy. *Am Fam Physician* Jan 1991

Molecular mechanisms of action of ribavirin. *Rev Infect Dis* Nov-Dec 1990

New acquisitions in the chemotherapy of viral infections. *Verh K Acad Geneeskd Belg* (Belgium) 1990

Comparison of oral and aerosol ribavirin regimens in the high risk elderly. *J Clin Pharmacol* Dec 1989

Comparative activities of several nucleoside analogues against influenza A, B, and C viruses in vitro. *Antimicrob Agents Chemother* Jun 1988

Antiviral drugs for common respiratory diseases. What's here, what's to come. *Postgrad Med* Feb 1 1988, 83 (2) p136-9, 142-3, 146-8

Oral ribavirin treatment of influenza A and B. *Antimicrob Agents Chemother* Aug 1987

Clinical review of ribavirin. *Infect Control* May 1987, 8 (5) p215-8

Clinical use of antiviral drugs. *Drug Intell Clin Pharm* May 1987

Protection of mice from lethal influenza virus infection with high dose-short duration ribavirin aerosol. *Antimicrob Agents Chemother* Dec 1986, 30 (6) p942-4

Ribavirin: a clinical overview. *Eur J Epidemiol* (Italy) Mar 1986

Effect of ribavirin triphosphate on primer generation and elongation during influenza virus transcription in vitro. *Antiviral Res* (Netherlands) Feb 1985, 5 (1) p39-48

Ribavirin. *Drug Intell Clin Pharm* Feb 1984

[Immunomodulating activity of ethanol-water extracts of the roots of Echinacea gloriosa L., Echinacea angustifolia DC. and Rudbeckia speciosa Wenderoth tested on the immune system in C57BL6 inbred mice]. *Cesk Farm* (Czech Republic) Aug 1993

Application of purified polysaccharides from cell cultures of the plant Echinacea purpurea to mice mediates protection against systemic infections with Listeria monocytogenes and Candida albicans. *Int J Immunopharmacol* (England) 1991, 13 (1)

Macrophage activation by the polysaccharide arabinogalactan isolated from plant cell cultures of Echinacea purpurea. *J Natl Cancer Inst* May 3 1989

Macrophage activation and induction of macrophage cytotoxicity by purified polysaccharide fractions from the plant Echinacea purpurea. *Infect Immun* Dec 1984

Combined antiviral and antimediator treatment of rhinovirus colds. *J Infect Dis* Oct 1992, 166 (4)

[Common cold: diagnostic steps? Antibiotics?]. *Ther Umsch* (Switzerland) Apr 1992, 49 (4)

Alpha 2-interferon for the common cold. *Ann Pharmacother* Mar 1992, 26 (3) (no abstract)

Managing viral upper respiratory infections. *Aust Fam Physician* (Australia) May 1991, 20 (5)

Immunological barriers in the nose and paranasal sinuses. *Acta Otolaryngol* (Stockh) (Sweden) May-Jun 1987, 103

Interferon for the treatment of infections. *Annu Rev Med* 1987, 38 p51-9

Effect of Astragalus membranaceus on electrophysiological activities of acute experimental coxsackie B-3 viral myocarditis in mice *Chin. Med. Sci. J.* (China), 1993, 8/4 (203-206)

Efficacy and safety of the standardized ginseng extract G 115 for potentiating vaccination against common cold and/or influenza syndrome. *Drugs under Experimental and Clinical Research* (Switzerland), 1996, 22/2 65-72)

An emerging green pharmacy: Modern plant medicines and health. *Laboratory Medicine*, 1996, 27/3 (170-176)

Immunity in myocardiac hypertrophy rat and effect of total saponins of panax ginseng in vivo and in vitro. *Chinese Pharmacological Bulletin* (China), 1996, 12/1 (84-86)

Treatment of experimental coxsackie B-3 viral myocarditis with astragalus membranaceus in mice. *Chin. Med. J.* (China), 1990, 103/1 (14-18)

Effect of Astragalus membranaceus injecta on coxsackie b-2 virus infected rat beating heart cell culture. *Chin. Med. J.* (Peking) (China), 1987, 100/7 (595-602)

Sambucol(tm) inhibited several strains of influenza virus and reduced symptoms during an outbreak of influenza b panama. *Weizmann Institute of Science* 2-15-94

The effect of sambucol(tm) on hiv infection in vitro. *Congress of Microbiology* 2-6-95

Interrelation of vitamin C, infection, haemostatic factors, and cardiovascular disease. *BMJ* (England) Jun 17 1995, 310 (6994) p1559-63

Does vitamin C alleviate the symptoms of the common cold?—a review of current evidence. *Scand J Infect Dis* (Sweden) 1994, 26 (1) p1-6

Recommended dietary allowance: support from recent research. *J Nutr Sci Vitaminol* (Tokyo) (Japan) 1992, Spec No p173-6

Interrelation of vitamin C, infection, haemostatic factors, and cardiovascular disease. *BMJ* (England) Jun 17 1995, 310 (6994) p1559-63

Does vitamin C alleviate the symptoms of the common cold?—a review of current evidence. *Scand J Infect Dis* (Sweden) 1994, 26 (1) p1-6

Recommended dietary allowance: support from recent research. *J Nutr Sci Vitaminol* (Tokyo) (Japan) 1992, Spec No p173-6

Congestive Heart Failure/Cardiomyopathy

Coenzyme Q_{10}: a vital therapeutic nutrient for the heart with special application in congestive heart failure. *Conn Med* Nov 1997, 61 (11) p707-11

Refractory congestive heart failure successfully managed with high-dose Coenzyme Q_{10} administration. *Mol Aspects Med* (England) 1997, 18 Suppl pS299-305

Treatment of congestive heart failure with Coenzyme Q_{10} illuminated by meta-analyses of clinical trials. *Mol Aspects Med* (England) 1997, 18 Suppl pS159-68

Magnesium supplementation in patients with congestive heart failure [see comments] *J Am Coll Nutr* Feb 1997, 16 (1) p22-31

Carvedilol update iv: Prevention of oxidative stress, cardiac remodeling and progression of congestive heart failure. *Drugs of Today (Drugs Today)* (Spain) 1997, 33/7 (453-473)

Focus on carvedilol: A novel beta-adrenergic blocking agent for the treatment of congestive heart failure. *Formulary (Formulary)* 1997, 32/8 (795-805)

The use of oral magnesium in mild-to-moderate congestive heart failure. *Congestive Heart Failure (Congestive Heart Fail.)* 1997, 3/2 (21-24)

Sympathetic deactivation by growth hormone treatment in patients with dilated cardiomyopathy. *Eur Heart J* (England) Apr 1998, 19 (4) p623-7

L-carnitine in children with idiopathic dilated cardiomyopathy. *Indian Heart J* (India) Jan-Feb 1998, 50 (1) p59-61

The prevention and management of iodine-induced hyperthyroidism and its cardiac features. *Thyroid* Jan 1998, 8 (1) p101-6

Thyroid hormone and cardiovascular disease. *Am Heart J* Feb 1998, 135 (2 Pt 1) p187-96

Comparison of effects of ascorbic acid on endothelium-dependent vasodilation in patients with chronic congestive heart failure secondary to idiopathic dilated cardiomyopathy versus patients with effort angina pectoris secondary to coronary artery disease. *Am J Cardiol* Sep 15 1998, 82 (6) p762-7

A study of fatty acid content in the myocardium of dilated cardiomyopathy. *Chinese Journal of Cardiology* (China), 1998, 26/1 (12-14)

Serum concentration of lipoprotein(a) decreases on treatment with hydrosoluble coenzyme Q_{10} in patients with coronary artery disease: discovery of a new role. *Int J Cardiol* 1999 Jan;68(1):23-9

Coenzyme Q_{10} administration increases brain mitochondrial concentrations and exerts neuroprotective effects. *Proc Natl Acad Sci U S A* 1998 Jul 21;95 (15):8892-7

The clinical and hemodynamic effects of Coenzyme Q_{10} in congestive cardiomyopathy. *American Journal of Therapeutics*, 1997, 4/2-3 (66-72)

Fish oil and other nutritional adjuvants for treatment of congestive heart failure. *Medical Hypotheses* (UK), 1996, 46/4 (400-406)

The use of oral magnesium in mild-to-moderate congestive heart failure. *Congestive Heart Failure*, 1997, 3/2 (21-24)

Guidelines on treatment of hypertension in the elderly, 1995—A tentative plan for comprehensive research projects on aging and health. *Japanese Journal of Geriatrics* (Japan), 1996, 33/12 (945-974)

Predictors of sudden death and death from pump failure in congestive heart failure are different. Analysis of 24 h Holter monitoring, clinical variables, blood chemistry, exericise test and radionuclide angiography. *International Journal of Cardiology* (Ireland), 1997, 58/2 (151-162)

Magnesium supplementation in patients with congestive heart failure. *Journal of the American College of Nutrition*, 1997, 16/1 (22-31)

How best to determine magnesium requirement: Need to consider cardiotherapeutic drugs that affect its retention. *Journal of the American College of Nutrition*, 1997, 16/1 (4-6)

Magnesium: A critical appreciation. *Zeitschrift fur Kardiologie* (Germany), 1996, 85/Suppl. 6 (147-151)

Sarcoplasmic reticular Ca2+ pump ATPase activity in congestive myocardial infarction. *Canadian Journal of Cardiology* (Canada), 1996, 12/10 (1065-1073)

Significance of magnesium in congestive heart failure. *American Heart Journal*, 1996, 132/3 (664-671)

The rationale of magnesium as alternative therapy for patients with acute myocardial infarction without thrombolytic therapy. *American Heart Journal*, 1996, 132/2 II (483-486)

Mortality risk and patterns of practice in 4606 acute care patients with congestive heart failure: The relative importance of age, sex, and medical therapy. *Archives of Internal Medicine*, 1996, 156/15 (1669-1673)

The study of renal magnesium handling in chronic congestive heart failure. *Sapporo Medical Journal* (Japan), 1996, 65/1 (23-32)

Management of acute myocardial infarction in the elderly. *Drugs and Aging* (New Zealand), 1996, 8/5 (358-377)

Supraventricular tachycardia after coronary artery bypass grafting surgery and fluid and electrolyte variables. *Heart and Lung: Journal of Acute and Critical Care*, 1996, 25/1 (31-36)

Growth hormone in end-stage heart failure (multiple letters) (6). *Lancet* (UK), 1997, 349/9068 (1841-1843)

Haemodynamic effects of intravenous growth hormone in congestive heart failure (1). *Lancet (UK)*, 1997, 349/9058 (1067-1068)

Skeletal muscle metabolism in experimental heart failure. *Journal of Molecular and Cellular Cardiology* (UK), 1996, 28/11 (2263-2273)

Hydralazine prevents nitroglycerin tolerance by inhibiting activation of a membrane-bound NADH oxidase: A new action for an old drug. *Journal of Clinical Investigation*, 1996, 98/6 (1465-1470)

Edema and principles of diuretic use. *Medical Clinics of North America*, 1997, 81/3 (689-704)

Alterations in ATP-sensitive potassium channel sensitivity to ATP in failing human hearts. *American Journal of Physiology—Heart and Circulatory Physiology*, 1997, 272/4 41-4 (H1656-H1665)

Effective water clearance and tonicity balance: The excretion of water revisited. *Clinical and Investigative Medicine* (Canada), 1997, 20/1 (16-24)

Hypertension update. *Survey of Ophthalmology*, 1996, 41/1 (79-89)

Does aspirin cause acute or chronic renal failure in experimental animals and in humans? *American Journal of Kidney Diseases*, 1996, 28/1 Suppl. (S24-S29)

Elevated myocardial interstitial norepinephrine concentration contributes to the regulation of Na+,K+-ATPase in heart failure. *European Journal of Pharmacology* (Netherlands), 1996, 309/3 (235-241)

[Magnesium: current studies—critical evaluation—consequences]. *Z Kardiol* (Germany) 1996, 85 Suppl 6 p147-51

Nonsustained polymorphous ventricular tachycardia during amiodarone therapy for atrial fibrillation complicating cardiomyopathy. Management with intravenous magnesium sulfate. *Chest* May 1997, 111 (5) p1454-7

Magnesium deficiency-related changes in lipid peroxidation and collagen metabolism in vivo in rat heart. *Int J Biochem Cell Biol* (England) Jan 1997, 29 (1) p129-34

[Value of magnesium in acute myocardial infarct]. *Z Kardiol* (Germany) 1996, 85 Suppl 6 p129-34

NADH-coenzyme Q reductase (complex I) deficiency: heterogeneity in phenotype and biochemical findings. *J Inherit Metab Dis* (Netherlands) 1996, 19 (5) p675-86

Familial cardiomyopathy with cataracts and lactic acidosis: a defect in complex I (NADH-dehydrogenase) of the mitochondria respiratory chain. *Pediatr Res* Mar 1996, 39 (3) p513-21

Comparison of calcium-current in isolated atrial myocytes from failing and nonfailing human hearts. *Mol Cell Biochem* (Netherlands) Apr 12-26 1996, 157 (1-2) p157-62

Mitochondrial complex I deficiency leads to increased production of superoxide radicals and induction of superoxide dismutase. *J Clin Invest* Jul 15 1996, 98 (2) p345-51

A preliminary study of growth hormone in the treatment of dilated cardiomyopathy. *N Engl J Med* Mar 28 1996, 334 (13) p809-14 Comment in: *N Engl J Med* 1996 Mar 28;334(13):856-7; Comment in: *N Engl J Med* 1996 Aug 29;335(9):672; discussion 673-4; Comment in: *N Engl J Med* 1996 Aug 29;335(9):672-3; discussion 673-4

Effect of protection and repair of injury of mitochondrial membrane-phospholipid on prognosis in patients with dilated cardiomyopathy. *Blood Press Suppl* (Norway) 1996, 3 p53-5

[Therapeutic effects of Coenzyme Q_{10} on dilated cardiomyopathy: assessment by 123I-BMIPP myocardial single photon emission computed tomography (SPECT): a multicenter trial in Osaka University Medical School Group]. *Kaku Igaku* (Japan) Jan 1996, 33 (1) p27-32

The effects of calcium channel blockers on blood fluidity. *J Cardiovasc Pharmacol* 1990, 16 Suppl 6 pS40-4

Increased whole blood and plasma viscosity in patients with angina pectoris and 'normal' coronary arteries. *Acta Med. Scand.* (Sweden), 1988, 224/2 (109-114)

Can lifestyle changes reverse coronary heart disease? *Lancet* (UK), 1990, 336/8708 (129-133)

The natural history of atherosclerosis: An ecologic perspective. *Atherosclerosis* (Ireland), 1990, 82/1-2 (157-164)

Concordant dyslipidemia, hypertension and early coronary disease in Utah families. *Klin. Wochenschr.* (Germany, Federal Republic of), 1990, 68/Suppl. 20 (53-59)

Correction: Mediterranean alpha-linolenic acid rich diet in secondary prevention of coronary heart disease (Lancet (1994) June 11 (1454). *Lancet* (UK), 1995, 345/8951 (738)

Mediterranean alpha-linolenic acid-rich diet in secondary prevention of coronary heart disease. *Lancet* (UK), 1994, 343/8911 (1454-1459)

Effect of antioxidant-rich foods on plasma ascorbic acid, cardiac enzyme, and lipid peroxide levels in patients hospitalized with acute myocardial infarction. *Journal of the American Dietetic Association*, 1995, 95/7 (775-780)

Dietary supplementation with orange and carrot juice in cigarette smokers lowers oxidation products in copper-oxidized low-density lipoproteins. *Journal of the American Dietetic Association*, 1995, 95/6 (671-675)

Women, hormones and blood pressure. *Canadian Journal of Cardiology* (Canada), 1996, 12/6 Suppl. D (9D-12D)

Protective effect of fruits and vegetables on development of stroke in men. *Journal of the American Medical Association*, 1995, 273/14 (1113-1117)

The effect of caffeine on ventricular ectopic activity in patients with malignant ventricular arrhythmia. *Arch. Intern. Med.*, 1989, 149/3 (637-639)

Coffee, cocktails and coronary candidates. *N. Engl. J. Med.*, 1977, 297/8 (443-444)

Concentrations of magnesium, calcium, potassium, and sodium in human heart muscle after acute myocardial infarction. *Clin Chem* Nov 1980, 26 (12) p1662-5

[Therapeutic efficacy of pantothenic acid preparations in ischemic heart disease patients]. *Vopr Pitan* (USSR) Mar-Apr 1987, (2) p15-7

Antifibrillatory effect of tetrahydroberberine. *Chung Kuo Yao Li Hsueh Pao* (China) Jul 1993, 14 (4) p301-5

Effects of tetrahydroberberine on ischemic and reperfused myocardium in rats. *Chung Kuo Yao Li Hsueh Pao* (China) Mar 1993, 14 (2) p130-3

[Ventricular tachyarrhythmias treated with berberine]. *Chung Hua Hsin Hsueh Kuan Ping Tsa Chih* (China) Jun 1990, 18 (3) p155-6, 190

[Effects of berberine on ischemic ventricular arrhythmia]. *Chung Hua Hsin Hsueh Kuan Ping Tsa Chih* (China) Oct 1989, 17 (5) p300-1, 319

[Protective effects of berberine on spontaneous ventricular fibrillation in dogs after myocardial infarction]. *Chung Kuo Yao Li Hsueh Pao* (China) Jul 1989, 10 (4) p320-4

Protective effects of berberine and phentolamine on myocardial reoxygenation damage. *Chin Med Sci J* (England) Dec 1992, 7 (4) p221-5

Beneficial effects of berberine on hemodynamics during acute ischemic left ventricular failure in dogs. *Chin Med J* (Engl) (China) Dec 1992, 105 (12) p1014-9

[The role and mechanism of berberine on coronary arteries]. *Chung Hua Hsin Hsueh Kuan Ping Tsa Chih* (China) Aug 1990, 18 (4) p231-4, 254-5

Effect of tincture of Crataegus on the LDL-receptor activity of hepatic plasma membrane of rats fed an atherogenic diet. *Atherosclerosis* (Ireland) Jun 1996, 123 (1-2) p235-41

Effect of a hawthorn extract on contraction and energy turnover of isolated rat cardiomyocytes. *Arzneimittelforschung* (Germany) Nov 1995, 45 (11) p1157-61

[Crataegus Special Extract WS 1442. Assessment of objective effectiveness in patients with heart failure (NYHA II)]. *Fortschr Med* (Germany) Aug 30 1996, 114 (24) p291-6

[Crataegus Special Extract WS 1442 in NYHA II heart failure. A placebo controlled randomized double-blind study]. *Fortschr Med* (Germany) Jul 20 1993, 111 (20-21) p352-4

Abnormal membrane concentrations of 20 and 22-carbon essential fatty acids: a common link between risk factors and coronary and peripheral vascular disease? *Prostaglandins Leukot Essent Fatty Acids* (Scotland) Dec 1995, 53 (6) p385-96

Differential changes in left and right ventricular adenylyl cyclase activities in congestive heart failure. *American Journal of Physiology—Heart and Circulatory Physiology*, 1997, 272/2 41-2 (H884-H893)

Chronic opiate-receptor inhibition in experimental congestive heart failure in dogs. *American Journal of Physiology—Heart and Circulatory Physiology*, 1997, 272/1 41-1 (H478-H484)

beta-adrenoceptor mediated signal transduction in congestive heart failure in cardiomyopathic (UM-X7.1) hamsters. *Molecular and Cellular Biochemistry*, 1996, 157/1-2 (191-196)

Pharmacology and inotropic potential of Forskolin in the human heart. *J Clin Invest* Jul 1984, 74 (1) p212-23

[Effects of Forskolin on canine congestive heart failure]. *Nippon Yakurigaku Zasshi* (Japan) Nov 1986, 88 (5) p389-94

Italian multicenter study on the safety and efficacy of Coenzyme Q_{10} as adjunctive therapy in heart failure. *Mol Aspects Med* (England) 1994, 15 Suppl ps287-94

[Coenzyme Q_{10} (ubiquinone) in the treatment of heart failure. Are any positive effects documented?]. *Tidsskr Nor Laegeforen* (Norway) Mar 20 1994, 114 (8) p939-42

Italian multicenter study on the safety and efficacy of Coenzyme Q_{10} as adjunctive therapy in heart failure (interim analysis). The CoQ_{10} Drug Surveillance Investigators. *Clin Investig* (Germany) 1993, 71 (8 Suppl) pS145-9

Isolated diastolic dysfunction of the myocardium and its response to CoQ_{10} treatment. *Clin Investig* (Germany) 1993, 71 (8 Suppl) pS140-4

Effect of Coenzyme Q_{10} therapy in patients with congestive heart failure: a long-term multicenter randomized study. *Clin Investig* (Germany) 1993, 71 (8 Suppl) pS134-6

Role of metabolic therapy in cardiovascular disease. *Clin Investig* (Germany) 1993, 71 (8 Suppl) pS124-8

Usefulness of Taurine in chronic congestive heart failure and its prospective application. *Jpn Circ J* (Japan) Jan 1992, 56 (1) p95-9

Coenzyme Q_{10}: a new drug for cardiovascular disease. *J Clin Pharmacol* Jul 1990, 30 (7) p596-608

Coenzyme Q_{10}: a new drug for myocardial ischemia? *Med Clin North Am* Jan 1988, 72 (1) p243-58

Cardiac performance and Coenzyme Q_{10} in thyroid disorders. *Endocrinol Jpn* (Japan) Dec 1984, 31 (6) p755-61

A clinical study of the effect of Coenzyme Q on congestive heart failure. *Jpn Heart J* (Japan) Jan 1976, 17 (1) p32-42

[Magnesium in cardiology]. *Schweiz Rundsch Med Prax* (Switzerland) May 2 1995, 84 (18) p526-32

Magnesium therapy in acute myocardial infarction when patients are not candidates for thrombolytic therapy. *J Cardiol* Feb 15 1995, 75 (5) p321-3

[Oral Magnesium supplementation to patients receiving diuretics—normalization of Magnesium, Potassium and sodium, and Potassium pumps in the skeletal muscles]. *Ugeskr Laeger* (Denmark) Jul 4 1994, 156 (27) p4007-10, 4013

Effects of intravenous Magnesium sulfate on arrhythmias in patients with congestive heart failure. *Am Heart J* Jun 1993, 125 (6) p1645-50

Magnesium-Potassium interactions in cardiac arrhythmia. Examples of ionic medicine. *Magnes Trace Elem* (Switzerland) 92 1991, 10 (2-4) p193-204

Clinical clues to Magnesium deficiency. *Isr J Med Sci* (Israel) Dec 1987, 23 (12) p1238-41

Platelet Taurine in patients with arterial hypertension, myocardial failure or infarction. *Acta Med Scand Suppl* (Sweden) 1980, 642 p79-84

Physiological and experimental regulation of Taurine content in the heart. *Fed Proc* Jul 1980, 39 (9) p2685-90

A relation between myocardial Taurine contest and pulmonary wedge pressure in dogs with heart failure. *Physiol Chem Phys* 1977, 9 (3) p259-63

Adrenergic stimulation of Taurine transport by the heart. *Science* Oct 28 1977, 198 (4315) p409-11

Effects of *L*-Carnitine administration on left ventricular remodeling after acute anterior myocardial infarction. *J Am Coll Cardiol* Aug 1995, 26 (2) p380-7

The myocardial distribution and plasma concentration of Carnitine in patients with mitral valve disease. *Surg Today* (Japan) 1994, 24 (4) p313-7

Myocardial Carnitine metabolism in congestive heart failure induced by incessant tachycardia. *Basic Res Cardiol* (Germany) Jul-Aug 1993, 88 (4) 362-70

[The clinical and hemodynamic effects of propionyl-L-Carnitine in the treatment of congestive heart failure]. *Clin Ter* (Italy) Nov 1992, 141 (11) p379-84

L-Carnitine treatment for congestive heart failure--experimental and clinical study. *Jpn Circ J* (Japan) Jan 1992, 56 (1) p86-94

The therapeutic potential of Carnitine in cardiovascular disorders. *Clin Ther* Jan-Feb 1991, 13 (1) p2-21; discussion 1

[Dilated cardiomyopathy due to primary Carnitine deficiency] Cardiomiopatia dilatativa da deficit primitivo di carnitina. *Squarcia Pediatr Med Chir* (Italy) Mar-Apr 1986, 8 (2) p157-61

Characterization of inwardly rectifying K+ channel in human cardiac myocytes. Alterations in channel behavior in myocytes isolated from patients with idiopathic dilated cardiomyopathy. *Circulation* Jul 15 1995, 92 (2) p164-74

Impaired forearm vasodilation to hyperosmolal stimuli in patients with congestive heart failure secondary to idiopathic dilated cardiomyopathy or to ischemic cardiomyopathy. *Am J Cardiol* Nov 15 1992, 70 (15) p1315-9

Usefulness of coenzyme Q_{10} in clinical cardiology: a long-term study. *Mol Aspects Med* (England) 1994, 15 Suppl

Bioenergetics in clinical medicine. Studies on coenzyme Q_{10} and essential hypertension. *Res Commun Chem Pathol Pharmacol* Jun 1975

Can antioxidants prevent ischemic heart disease? *J Clin Pharm Ther* (England) Apr 1993

Antioxidant therapy in the aging process. *EXS* (Switzerland) 1992, 62

Pharmacology and inotropic potential of Forskolin in the human heart. *J Clin Invest* Jul 1984, 74 (1) p212-23

[Effects of Forskolin on canine congestive heart failure]. *Nippon Yakurigaku Zasshi* (Japan) Nov 1986, 88 (5) p389-94

Italian multicenter study on the safety and efficacy of Coenzyme Q10 as adjunctive therapy in heart failure. CoQ10 Drug Surveillance Investigators. *Mol Aspects Med* (England) 1994, 15 Suppl ps287-94

[Coenzyme Q10 (ubiquinone) in the treatment of heart failure. Are any positive effects documented?]. *Tidsskr Nor Laegeforen* (Norway) Mar 20 1994, 114 (8) p939-42

Italian multicenter study on the safety and efficacy of Coenzyme Q10 as adjunctive therapy in heart failure (interim analysis). The CoQ10 Drug Surveillance Investigators. *Clin Investig* (Germany) 1993, 71 (8 Suppl) pS145-9

Isolated diastolic dysfunction of the myocardium and its response to CoQ10 treatment. *Clin Investig* (Germany) 1993, 71 (8 Suppl) pS140-4

Effect of coenzyme Q10 therapy in patients with congestive heart failure: a long-term multicenter randomized study. *Clin Investig* (Germany) 1993, 71 (8 Suppl) pS134-6

Role of metabolic therapy in cardiovascular disease. *Clin Investig* (Germany) 1993, 71 (8 Suppl) pS124-8

Usefulness of Taurine in chronic congestive heart failure and its prospective application. *Jpn Circ J* (Japan) Jan 1992, 56 (1) p95-9

Coenzyme Q10: a new drug for cardiovascular disease. *J Clin Pharmacol* Jul 1990, 30 (7) p596-608

Coenzyme Q10: a new drug for myocardial ischemia? *Med Clin North Am* Jan 1988, 72 (1) p243-58

Cardiac performance and coenzyme Q10 in thyroid disorders. *Endocrinol Jpn* (Japan) Dec 1984, 31 (6) p755-61

A clinical study of the effect of Coenzyme Q on congestive heart failure. *Jpn Heart J* (Japan) Jan 1976, 17 (1) p32-42

[Magnesium in cardiology]. *Schweiz Rundsch Med Prax* (Switzerland) May 2 1995, 84 (18) p526-32

Constipation

East-West mortality divide and its potential explanations: proposed research agenda. *BMJ* 1996 Feb 17;312(7028):421-5

Trends in mortality from major diseases in Europe, 1980-1993. *Eur J Epidemiol* 1998 Jan;14(1):1-8

Randomized controlled trial of silymarin treatment in patients with cirrhosis of the liver. *J Hepatol* 1989 Jul;9(1):105-13

Artichoke leaf extract: recent findings reflecting effect on lipid metabolism, liver, and gastrointestinal tracts. *Phytomedicine* 1997; 4(4):369-78

Two thousand years of artichoke (Zwei Jahrtausend Artischocke). *Austrian Pharmaceutical Magazine* 1965; 19:4

Nutritive and Therapeutic Value of Fruit and Vegetables, 144,. *Chem Abstr.* 1962; 57: 964

Immunomodulation par des produits natural, Note I: effect d'un extrait aqueux de Raphanus sativus niger sur l'infection grippale experimentale chez la souris. *Virologie* 1987; (Apr-Jun):38(2):115-20

Isolation and properties of raphanin, an antibacterial substance from radish seed. *Proc Soc Exp Biol Med* 1947; 66:625-31

Heartburn requiring frequent antacid use may indicate significant illness. *Arch Intern Med* 1998 Nov 23;158(21):2373-6

[No title]. *Deutshe Apotheker Zeitung* 1984; 124:1433-43

Constipation. Diagnosis and treatment. *Home Care Provid* Oct 1997, 2 (5) p250-5

Castleman M. *The Healing Herbs: The Ultimate Guide to the Curative Power of Mature's Medicines*. Sheldon Sault Hendler

Weiss R.F. *Herbal Medicine*. Gothenburg: AB Arcanum, 1988; Beaconsfield England: Beaconsfield Publishers, 1988

Stary, Frantisek. *The Natural Guide to Medicinal Herbs and Plants.* New York: Dorset Press, 1992

The Lawrence Review of Natural Products. St Louis MO: Lippincott Company, November 1992

Lemonick, M. "Fire in the belly." *Time* 1999 (April 26):108

Mowrey D. *Scientific Validation of Herbal Remedies.* USA: Keats Publishing, 1990

Mowrey D. *Herbal Tonic Therapies.* USA: Keats Publishing, 1993

Hobbs C. *Herbs for Health*, November/December 1998, p 22

[Intake of dietary fiber and other nutrients by children with and without functional chronic constipation]. *Arq Gastroenterol* (Brazil) Apr-Jun 1996, 33 (2) p93-101

The treatment of chronic constipation in adults. A systematic review. *J Gen Intern Med* Jan 1997, 12 (1) p15-24

Health help. Fluid + fiber = frequency. *Home Care Provid* Jan-Feb 1996, 1 (1) p30

Fecal incontinence in children. *Am Fam Physician* (United States) May 1 1997, 55 (6) p2229-38

Chronic constipation—is the work-up worth the cost? *Dis Colon Rectum* Mar 1997, 40 (3) p280-6

Changing bowel hygiene practice successfully: a program to reduce laxative use in a chronic care hospital. *Geriatr Nurs* Jan-Feb 1997, 18 (1) p12-7

[A clinical study of the use of a combination of glucomannan with lactulose in the constipation of pregnancy]. *Minerva Ginecol* (Italy) Dec 1996, 48 (12) p577-82

Clinical response to dietary fiber treatment of chronic constipation. *Am J Gastroenterol* Jan 1997, 92 (1) p95-8

Lack of influence of intestinal transit on oxidative status in premenopausal women. *Eur J Clin Nutr* (England) Aug 1996, 50 (8) p565-8

Dietary fiber and laxation in postop orthopedic patients. *Clin Nurs Res* Nov 1996, 5 (4) p428-40

[The relationship between intake of dietary fiber and chronic constipation in children]. *Ned Tijdschr Geneeskd* (Netherlands) Oct 12 1996, 140 (41) p2036-9

Assessment of the effect of increased dietary fibre intake on bowel function in patients with spinal cord injury. *Spinal Cord* (England) May 1996, 34 (5) p277-83

Chronic idiopathic constipation: pathophysiology and treatment. *J Clin Gastroenterol* Apr 1996, 22 (3) p190-6

Pediatric constipation. *Gastroenterol Nurs* May-Jun 1996, 19 (3) p88-95

Constipation and fecal incontinence in the elderly population. *Mayo Clin Proc* Jan 1996, 71 (1) p81-92

Therapeutic availability of iron administered orally as the ferrous gluconate together with magnesium-L-aspartate hydrochloride. *Arzneimittelforschung* (Germany) Mar 1996, 46 (3) p302-6

The osmotic and intrinsic mechanisms of the pharmacological laxative action of oral high doses of magnesium sulphate. Importance of the release of digestive polypeptides and nitric oxide. *Magnes Res* (England) Jun 1996, 9 (2) p133-8

Small bowel obstruction caused by a medication bezoar: report of a case. *Surg Today* (Japan) 1996, 26 (1) p68-70

Challenges in the treatment of colonic motility disorders. *American Journal of Health-System Pharmacy,* 1996, 53/22 Suppl. (S17-S26)

Acute hypermagnesemia after laxative use. *Annals of Emergency Medicine,* 1996, 28/5 (552-555)

The connection between dietary fibre intake and chronic constipation in children. *Nederlands Tijdschrift voor Geneeskunde* (Netherlands), 1996, 140/41 (2036-2039)

Constipation in children. *American Family Physician,* 1996, 54/2 (611-630)

Products for indigestion. *Pharmaceutical Journal* (UK), 1996, 256/6892 (678-682)

Antacids drugs: Multiple but too often unknown pharmacological properties. *Journal de Pharmacie Clinique* (France), 1996, 15/1 (41-51)

Treatment of retentive encopresis with diet modification and scheduled toileting vs. mineral oil and rewards for toileting: A clinical decision. *Ambulatory Child Health* (UK), 1996, 1/3 (214-222)

Comparison of the effects of magnesium hydroxide and a bulk laxative on lipids, carbohydrates, vitamins A and E, and minerals in geriatric hospital patients in the treatment of constipation. *J Int Med Res* (England) Sep-Oct 1989, 17 (5) p442-54

[Magnesium: current concepts of its physiopathology, clinical aspects and therapy]. *Acta Vitaminol Enzymol* (Italy) 1982, 4 (1-2) p87-97

[Treatment of constipation with vitamin B5 or dexpanthenol]. *Med Chir Dig* (France) 1979, 8 (7) p671-4

Endogenous nitric oxide modulates morphine-induced constipation. *Biochem Biophys Res Commun* Dec 16 1991, 181 (2) p889-93

Effectiveness of bran supplement on the bowel management of elderly rehabilitation patients. *J Gerontol Nurs* Oct 1995, 21 (10) p21-30

Mechanisms of constipation in older persons and effects of fiber compared with placebo. *J Am Geriatr Soc* Jun 1995, 43 (6)

Crohn's Disease

Dietary supplementation of nucleotides and arginine promotes healing of small bowel ulcers in experimental ulcerative ileitis. *Digestive Diseases and Sciences,* 1997, 42/7 (1530-1536)

Nutrition in inflammatory bowel disease. *Current Opinion in Gastroenterology,* 1997, 13/2 (140-145)

Metabolic adaptation of terminal ileal mucosa after construction of an ileoanal pouch. *British Journal of Surgery* (UK), 1997, 84/1 (71-73)

Enhanced apoptosis in transformed human lung fibroblasts after exposure to sodium butyrate. *In Vitro Cellular and Developmental Biology*—Animal, 1996, 32/8 (505-513)

Nutrition and gastrointestinal disease. *Scandinavian Journal of Gastroenterology, Supplement* (Norway), 1996, 31/220 (52-59)

Excretion of amino acid residues from diets based on wheat flour or oat bran in human subjects with ileostomies. *European Journal of Clinical Nutrition* (UK), 1995, 49/8 (596-604)

Efficacy of glutamine-enriched enteral nutrition in an experimental model of mucosal ulcerative colitis. *British Journal of Surgery* (UK), 1995, 82/6 (749-751)

Butyrate metabolism in the terminal ileal mucosa of patients with ulcerative colitis. *British Journal of Surgery* (UK), 1995, 82/1 (36-38)

Colonic mucin synthesis is increased by sodium butyrate. *Gut* (UK), 1995, 36/1 (93-99)

Pouchitis—A poorly understood entity. *Dis. Colon Rectum,* 1995, 38/1 (100-103)

Novel drug therapies in inflammatory bowel disease. *Eur. J. Gastroenterol. Hepatol.* (UK), 1995, 7/2 (169-182)

Butyrate oxidation is impaired in the colonic mucosa of sufferers of quiescent ulcerative colitis. *Gut* (UK), 1994, 35/1 (73-76)

Butyrate, mesalamine, and factor XIII in experimental colitis in the rat: Effects on transglutaminase activity. *Gastroenterology,* 1994, 106/2 (399-404)

Ileal and colonic epithelial metabolism in quiescent ulcerative colitis: Increased glutamine metabolism in distal colon but no defect in butyrate Metabolism. *Gut* (UK), 1993, 34/11 (1552-1558)

Dietary fiber and gastrointestinal disease. *Surg. Gynecol. Obstet.,* 1993, 177/2 (209-214)

The role of short-chain fatty acid metabolism in colonic disorders. *Am. J. Gastroenterol.,* 1992, 87/4 (419-423)

Serum and tissue transglutaminase correlates with the severity of inflammation in induced colitis in the rat. *Scand. J. Gastroenterol.* (Norway), 1992, 27/2 (111-114)

Operative and perioperative treatment of patients with inflammatory bowel Disease. *Curr. Opin. Gastroenterol.* (UK), 1991, 7/4 (635-641)

Nutritional issues in pediatric inflammatory bowel disease. *J. Pediatr. Gastroenterol. Nutr.,* 1991, 12/4 (424-438)

The starved colon—Diminished mucosal nutrition, diminished absorption, and colitis. *Dis. Colon Rectum*, 1990, 33/10 (858-862)

Serum transglutaminase inflammatory bowel diseases. *J. Clin. Gastroenterol.*, 1990, 12/4 (400-404)

The colonic epithelium in ulcerative colitis: An energy-deficiency disease? *Lancet* (England), 1980, 2/8197 (712-715)

Effect of arginine on toxin production by clostridium difficile in defined medium. *Microbiology and Immunology* (Japan), 1997, 41/8 (581-585)

Stress-induced enhancement of colitis in rats: CRF and arginine vasopressin are not involved. *American Journal of Physiology—Gastrointestinal and Liver Physiology* 1997, 272/1 35-1 (G84-G91)

Induction of nitric oxide synthase in colonic smooth muscle from patients with toxic megacolon. *Gastroenterology,* 1995, 109/5 (1497-1502)

Manipulation of the *L*-arginine-nitric oxide pathway in experimental Colitis. *British Journal of Surgery* (UK), 1995, 82/9 (1188-1191)

Experimental colitis is ameliorated by inhibition of nitric oxide synthase activity. *Gut* (UK), 1995, 37/2 (247-255)

Sulfhydryl blocker-induced rat colonic inflammation is ameliorated by inhibition of nitric oxide synthase. *Gastroenterology,* 1995, 109/1 (98-106)

Amino acid composition of the blood serum in patients with chronic colitis (Russian). *Ter.Arkh.* (USSR), 1974, 46/4 (141-147)

Probiotics. *Pediatria Polska* (Poland), 1997, 72/6 (535-539)

Intestinal microflora and antibiotic therapy. *Pediatria Polska* (Poland), 1995, 70/7 (547-552)

Use of lactobacilli in gastroenterology. *Gastroenterol.* (Germany), 1994, 48/4 (173-178)

Relapsing clostridium difficile enterocolitis cured by rectal infusion. *Scand. J. Infect. Dis.* (Sweden), 1984, 16/2 (211-215

Antibiotics and intestinal flora *Ther. Umsch.* (Switzerland), 1980, 37/3 (194-197)

Altered bone metabolism in inflammatory bowel disease. *American Journal of Gastroenterology,* 1997, 92/7 (1157-1163)

The major complications of coeliac disease. *Bailliere's Clinical Gastroenterology* (UK), 1995, 9/2 (351-369)

Osteoporosis, corticosteroids and inflammatory bowel disease. *Alimentary Pharmacology and Therapeutics* (UK), 1995, 9/3 (237-250)

Bone mineral density and calcium regulating hormones in patients with inflammatory bowel disease (Crohn's disease and ulcerative colitis.) *Exp. Clin. Endocrinol.* (Germany), 1994, 102/1 (44-49)

Gastrointestinal infections in children. *Curr. Opin. Gastroenterol.* (UK), 1994, 10/1 (88-97)

Medical management of severe inflammatory disease of the rectum: Nutritional aspects. *Bailliere's Clin. Gastroenterol.* (UK), 1992, 6/1 (27-41)

Metabolism of vitamin A in inflammatory bowel disease. *Hepato-Gastroenterology* (Germany), 1991, 38/5 (391-395)

Neurologic manifestations of gastrointestinal disease. *Neurol. Clin.,* 1989, 7/3 (525-548)

Vitamin status in patients with inflammatory bowel disease. *Am. J. Gastroenterol.,* 1989, 84/7 (744-748)

Wernicke's encehalopathy during total parenteral nutrition: Observation in one case. *J. Parenter. Enter. Nutr.,* 1988, 12/6 (626-627)

Optic neuropathy from thiamine deficiency in a patient with ulcerative colitis. *Doc. Ophthalmol.* (Netherlands), 1987, 67/1-2 (45-51)

Vitamin D status in Crohn's disease: Association with nutrition and disease activity. *Gut* (England), 1985, 26/11 (1197-1203)

Zinc and vitamin A deficiency in patients with Crohn's disease is correlated with activity but not with localization or extent of the disease. *Hepato-Gastroenterol.* (Germany, West), 1985, 32/1 (34-38)

The prevalence of vitamin K deficiency in chronic gastrointestinal disorders. *American Journal of Clinical Nutrition,* 1985, 41/3 (639-643)

Vitamin serum levels (B_{12} folic acid, 25-OH-D_3) in Crohn's disease and ulcerative colitis. *Arztl. Lab.* (Germany, West), 1985, 31/3 (100-102)

Sulfasalazine inhibits the absorption of folates in ulcerative colitis. *N. Engl. J. Med.,* 1981, 305/25 (1513-1517)

Clinical-pharmacological aspects, application and effectiveness of total parenteral nutrition in surgical patients. *Int. J. Clin. Pharmacol. Biopharm.* (Germany, West), 1979, 17/3 (107-118)

Iron deficiency in inflammatory bowel disease. Diagnostic efficacy of serum ferritin. *Am. J. Dig. Dis.,* 1978, 23/8 (705-709)

Ascorbic acid metabolism in ulcerative colitis of bacterial origin. *Zdravookhr.Tadzh.* (USSR), 1973, 20/4 (10-12)

Selenium supplementation in the diets of patients suffering from ulcerative colitis. *Journal of Radioanalytical and Nuclear Chemistry* (Hungary), 1997, 217/2 (189-191)

Nutrition and ulcerative colitis. *Bailliere's Clinical Gastroenterology* (UK), 1997, 11/1 (153-174)

An enteral formula containing fish oil, indigestible oligosaccharides, gum arabic and antioxidants affects plasma and colonic phospholipid fatty acid and prostaglandin profiles in pigs. *Journal of Nutrition,* 1997, 127/1 (137-145)

The effect of folic acid supplementation on the risk for cancer or dysplasia in ulcerative colitis. *Gastroenterology,* 1997, 112/1 (29-32)

The value of an elimination diet in the management of patients with ulcerative colitis. *South African Medical Journal* (South Africa), 1995, 85/11 (1176-1179)

Influence of nutrition in ulcerative colitis—The significance of nutritional care in inflammatory bowel disease. *Langenbecks Archiv fur Chirurgie* (Germany), 1995, 380/1 (4-11)

Soy fiber delays disease onset and prolongs survival in experimental Clostridium difficile ileocecitis. *J. Parenter. Enter. Nutr.,* 1994, 18/1 (55-61)

Influence of intravenous n-3 lipid supplementation on fatty acid profiles and lipid mediator generation in a patient with severe ulcerative colitis. *Eur. J. Clin. Invest.* (UK), 1993, 23/11 (706-715)

The role of marine fish oils in the treatment of ulcerative colitis. *Nutr. Rev.,* 1993, 51/2 (47-49)

Localized deficiencies of folic acid in aerodigestive tissues. *Ann. New York Acad. Sci.,* 1992, 669/- (87-96)

Fish oil fatty acid supplementation in active ulcerative colitis: A double-blind, placebo-controlled, crossover study. *Am. J. Gastroenterol.,* 1992, 87/4 (432-437)

Omega-3 fatty acids in health and disease and in growth and development. *American Journal of Clinical Nutrition,* 1991, 54/3 (438-463)

Does nutritional therapy in inflammatory bowel disease have a primary or an adjunctive role? *Scand. J. Gastroenterol. Suppl.* (Norway), 1990, 25/172 (29-34)

Food allergy: The major cause of infantile colitis. *Arch. Dis. Child.* (England), 1984, 59/4 (326-329)

Is continuous enteral alimentation effective in gastrointestinal patients? Results in a series of 92 consecutive patients treated for 3 to 7 weeks. *Gastroenterol. Clin. Biol.* (France), 1983, 7/12 (1003-1009)

The faecal flora of patients with Crohn's disease. *J. Hyg.* (England), 1981, 87/1 (1-12)

Elemental diet in gastrointestinal diseases: experience from a case material of 59 patients. *Infusionsther. Klin. Ernahr.* (Switzerland), 1977, 4/6 (313-318)

Elemental diet as an alternative to intravenous nutrition in severe gastrointestinal disease. *Schweiz. Med. Wschr.* (Switzerland), 1977, 107/2 (43-49)

Selective immunoglobulin A deficiency, ulcerative colitis, and gluten sensitive enteropathy. A unique association. *Gastroenterology,* 1975, 69/2 (503-506)

Absorption of medium chain triglyceride and its clinical appraisal. *Hirosaki Med.J.* (Japan), 1974, 26/2 (167-186)

Crohn's disease. *Ugeskr.Laeg.* (Denmark), 1974, 136/17 (912-920)

Disaccharidase deficiency in adults with gastrointestinal disease (Bulgarian). *Vatr.Bolesti* (Sofia) (Bulgaria), 1973, 12/2 (24-31)

Short chain fatty acid rectal irrigation for left-sided ulcerative colitis: A randomised, placebo controlled trial. *Gut* (UK), 1997, 40/4 (485-491)

Special issues in nutritional therapy of inflammatory bowel disease. *Can. J. Gastroenterol.* (Canada), 1993, 7/2 (196-199)

A randomized controlled study of evening primrose oil and fish oil in ulcerative colitis. *Aliment. Pharmacol. Ther.* (UK), 1993, 7/2 (159-166)

Treatment of ulcerative colitis with fish oil supplementation: A prospective 12 month randomised controlled trial. *Gut* (UK), 1992, 33/7 (922-928)

Incorporation of fatty acids from fish oil and olive oil into colonic mucosal lipids and effects upon eicosanoid synthesis in inflammatory bowel disease. *Gut* (UK), 1991, 32/10 (1151-1155)

Carlsbad mineral water drinking cure. *Fysiatr. Revmatol. Vestn.* (Czech Republic), 1993, 71/4 (195-212)

Intestinal epithelial cells contribute to the enhanced generation of platelet activating factor in ulcerative colitis. *Gut* (UK), 1993, 34/5 (665-668)

Inflammatory bowel disease, Part II; Clinical and therapeutic aspects. *Dis. Mon.,* 1991, 37/11 (673-675)

Contribution of sigmoidoscopy with bioptic microbiology to the etiologic diagnosis of acute diarrhea in adults. A prospective study in sixty-five patients. *Annales de Gastroenterologie et d'Hepatologie* (France), 1996, 32/1 (11-17)

Serologic testing for amoebiasis. *Gastroenterology,* 1980, 78/1 (136-141)

Autoimmune factors in inflammatory bowel disease. *Mt. Sinai J. Med.,* 1976, 43/5 (602-624)

The effect of exogenous administration of Lactobacillus reuteri R2LC and oat fiber on acetic acid-induced colitis in the rat. *Scand. J. Gastroenterol .* (Norway), 1993, 28/2 (155-162)

Gut hormones in inflammatory bowel disease. *Scand. J. Gastroenterol.* (Norway),1983, 18/7 (845-852)

Kinetics of primary bile acids in patients with non-operated Crohn's disease. *Eur. J. Clin. Invest.* (England), 1982, 12/2 (135-143

Bile acid studies in uncomplicated Crohn's disease. *Gut (England),* 1977, 18/9 (730-735)

Bile acid metabolism and vitamin B_{12} absorption in ulcerative colitis. *Scand. J. Gastroent.* (Norway), 1976, 11/8 (769-775)

Refined carbohydrate, smooth muscle spasm and disease of the colon. *Lancet* (England), 1976, 1/7956 (395-397)

Pantothenic acid, coenzyme A, and human chronic ulcerative and granulomatous colitis. *Amer. J. Clin. Nutr.,* 1976, 29/12 (1333-1338)

Disruption of sulphated glycosaminoglycans in intestinal inflammation. *Lancet* (UK), 1993, 341/8847 (711-714)

Sulfapyride and sulfones decrease glycosaminoglycans viscosity in dermatitis herpetiformis, ulcerative colitis, and pyoderma gangrenosum. *Med. Hypotheses* (UK), 1990, 31/2 (99-103)

The glycosaminoglycans of the human colon in inflammatory and neoplastic conditions. *Arch. Pathol. Lab. Med.,* 1978, 102/3 (146-149)

Inflammatory bowel disease: Another possible facet of the allergic diathesis. *Ann. Allergy,* 1981, 47/2 (92-94)

The effect of proctocolectomy on serum antibody levels against cow's milk proteins in patients with chronic ulcerative colitis, with special reference to liver changes. *Scand. J. Gastroenterol.* (Norway), 1994, 29/7 (646-650)

Isotypic analysis of antibody response to a food antigen in inflammatorybowel disease. *Int. Arch. Allergy Appl. Immunol.* (Switzerland), 1985, 78/1 (81-85)

The biological activity of bovine cartilage preparations. *Semin. Arthritis Rheum.,* 1974, 3/4 (287-321)

HLA-B27 related arthritis and bowel inflammation. Part 2. Ileocolonoscopy and bowel histology in patients with HLA-B27 related arthritis. *J. Rheumatol.* (Canada), 1985, 12/2 (294-298)

HLA-B27 related arthritis and bowel inflammation. Part 1. Sulfasalazine (salazopyrin) in HLA-B27 related reactive arthritis. *J. Rheumatol.* (Canada), 1985, 12/2 (287-293)

Circulating antioxidants in ulcerative colitis and their relationship to disease severity and activity. *Journal of Gastroenterology and Hepatology* (Australia),1997, 12/7 (490-494)

Nutritional assessment and disease activity for patients with inflammatory bowel disease. *Canadian Journal of Gastroenterology* (Canada), 1995, 9/3 (131-136)

The role of antioxidant agents on experimental ulcerative colitis. *Bulletin of Gulhane Military Medical Academy* (Turkey), 1994, 36/4 (452-457)

Does vitamin E supplementation modulate in vivo arachidonate metabolism in human inflammation? *Pharmacol. Toxicol.* (Denmark), 1987, 61/4 (246-249)

Rutoside as mucosal protective in acetic acid-induced rat colitis. *Planta Medica* (Germany), 1997, 63/5 (409-414)

Effect of Quercitrin on acute and chronic experimental colitis in the rat. *Journal of Pharmacology and Experimental Therapeutics,* 1996, 278/2 (771-779)

The friendly anaerobes. *Clin. Infect. Dis.* 1993, 16/SUPPL. 4 (S427-S434)

Circulating antioxidants in ulcerative colitis and their relationship to disease severity and activity. *Journal of Gastroenterology and Hepatology* (Australia), 1997, 12/7 (490-494)

Serum zinc, copper, and selenium levels in inflammatory bowel disease: Effect of total enteral nutrition on trace element status *Am. J. Gastroenterol.* 1990, 85/12 (1584-1589)

Nutritional status of gastroenterology outpatients: Comparison of inflammatory bowel disease with functional disorders. *J. Am. Diet. Assoc.,* 1985, 85/12 (1591-1599)

Reactivity of infiltrating T lymphocytes with microbial antigens in Crohn's disease. *Lancet* 1991 Nov 16;338(8777):1238-9

Association of humoral markers of inflammation and dehydroepiandrosterone sulfate or cortisol serum levels in patients with chronic inflammatory bowel disease. *Am J Gastroenterol* 1998 Nov;93(11):2197-202

Antagonistic effects of sulfide and butyrate on proliferation of colonic mucosa: a potential role for these agents in the pathogenesis of ulcerative colitis. *Dig Dis Sci* (1996 Dec) 41(12):2477-81I

Increased rate of spinal trabecular bone loss in patients with inflammatory bowel disease. *Gut* (1988 Oct) 29 (10):1332-6

Distal procto-colitis, natural cytotoxicity, and essential fatty acids. *Am J Gastroenterol* 1998 May;93(5):804-9

Acetic acid-induced colitis in normal and essential fatty acid deficient rats. *J Pharmacol Exp Ther* 1995 Jan;272(1):469-75

Essential fatty acids in health and chronic disease. *Am J Clin Nutr* 1999 Sep;70(3 Suppl):560S-9S

Nutrition and inflammatory bowel disease. *Gastroenterol Clin North Am* 1999 Jun;28(2):423-43

Dietary monounsaturated n-3 and n-6 long-chain polyunsaturated fatty acids affect cellular antioxidant defense system in rats with experimental ulcerative colitis induced by trinitrobenzene sulfonic acid. *Dig Dis Sci* 1998 Dec;43 (12):2676-87

Effect of dietary n-3 fatty acids on hypoxia-induced necrotizing enterocolitis in young mice. n-3 fatty acids alter platelet-activating factor and leukotriene B4 production in the intestine. *Biol Neonate* 1998;74(1):31-8

Nutritional factors in inflammatory bowel disease. *Eur J Gastroenterol Hepatol* 1998 Mar;10(3):235-7

[Inflammatory bowel disease: importance of nutrition today]. *Nutr Hosp* 1997 Nov-Dec;12(6):289-98

Deafness

See references under Hearing Loss.

Depression

A population-based twin study of lifetime major depression in men and women. *Arch Gen Psychiatry* Jan 1999, 56 (1) p39-44

Narcolepsy and depression. *Arq Neuropsiquiatr* Sep 1997, 55 (3A) p423-6

Depression and openness to experience. *J Pers Assess* Dec 1997, 69 (3) p614-32

Winter depression and phototherapy. The state of the art. *Acta Med Port* Dec 1997, 10 (12) p887-93

Experiencing depression: women's perspectives in recovery. *J Psychiatr Ment Health Nurs* Dec 1997, 4 (6) p393-400

The role of noradrenaline in depression: a review. *J Psychopharmacol* 1997, 11 (4 Suppl) pS39-47

An experimental study of the effects of distant, intercessory prayer on self-esteem, anxiety, and depression. *Altern Ther Health Med* Nov 1997, 3 (6) p38-53

Religiosity and depression: ten-year follow-up of depressed mothers and offspring. *J Am Acad Child Adolesc Psychiatry* Oct 1997, 36 (10) p1416-25

In vivo evidence for the involvement of dopamine-D2 receptors in striatum and anterior cingulate gyrus in major depression. *Neuroimage* May 1997, 5 (4 Pt 1) p251-60

Specificity of the pyridostigmine/growth hormone challenge in the diagnosis of depression. *Biol Psychiatry* Nov 1 1997, 42 (9) p827-33

Subjective sleep quality and suicidality in patients with major depression. *J Psychiatr Res* May-Jun 1997, 31 (3) p377-81

Forskolin-stimulated platelet adenylyl cyclase activity is lower in persons with major depression. *Biol Psychiatry* Jul 1 1997, 42 (1) p30-8

Religiosity as a protective or prognostic factor of depression in later life; results from a community survey in The Netherlands. *Acta Psychiatr Scand* Sep 1997, 96 (3) p199-205

Anxiety and depression. Diagnosis and treatment during pregnancy. *Obstet Gynecol Clin North Am* Sep 1997, 24 (3) p535-58

Religious involvement and depression in older Dutch citizens. *Soc Psychiatry Psychiatr Epidemiol* Jul 1997, 32 (5)p284-91

Do plasma polyunsaturates predict hostility and depression? *World Rev Nutr Diet* 1997, 82 p175-86

Parasuicide, depression and the anticipation of positive and negative future experiences. *Psychol Med* Jul 1997, 27 (4) p973-7

Sleep disturbances and suicidal behavior in patients with major depression. *J Clin Psychiatry* Jun 1997, 58 (6) p249-51

Spiritual well-being, religiosity, hope, depression, and other mood states in elderly people coping with cancer. *Oncol Nurs Forum* May 1997, 24 (4) p663-71

Corticotropin-releasing hormone inhibits melatonin secretion in healthy volunteers—a potential link to low-melatonin syndrome in depression? *Neuroendocrinology* Apr 1997, 65 (4) p284-90

[St John's wort against depression in favour again] Johannesort till heders igen mot depression. *Lakartidningen* Jun 18 1997, 94 (25) p2365-7

Dehydroepiandrosterone (DHEA) treatment of depression. *Biol Psychiatry* Feb 1 1997, 41 (3) p311-8

Single mothers, poverty and depression. *Psychol Med* Jan 1997, 27 (1) p21-33

Self-esteem, optimism, and postpartum depression. *J Clin Psychol* Jan 1997, 53 (1) p59-63

Melatonin as a therapeutic agent in the treatment of sleep disturbance in depression. *J Nerv Ment Dis Mar* 1997, 185 (3) p201-2

Hypericum extract in the therapy of depression. *Nervenheilkunde* 1997, 16/9 (98-101)

Lipids, depression and physical diseases. *Current Opinion in Psychiatry* 1997, 10/6 (477-480)

St John's wort against depression. *Zeitschrift fur Allgemeinmedizin* 1997, 73/13 (766-767)

Psychology; suicidal behavior relapse of depression after vapid depletion of tryptophan. *Lancet* 1997, 349/9056 (915-919)

Randomized trial of physical exercise alone or combined with bright light on mood and health-related quality of life. *Psychological Medicine*, 1998, 28/6 (1359-1364)

Physical fitness: Benefits of exercise for the older patient. Part 2 of a roundtable discussion., *Geriatrics*, 1998, 53/10 (46-62)

Age-associated testosterone decline in men: Clinical issues for psychiatry. *American Journal of Psychiatry*, 1998, 155/10(1310-1318)

Serum thyroid hormones in patients with affective disorder before and after treatment. *Chinese Journal of Psychiatry*, 1998, 31/1 (19-22)

Bright light treatment of winter depression: A placebo-controlled trial. *Archives of General Psychiatry*, 1998, 55/10 (883-889)

A controlled trial of timed bright light and negative air ionization for treatment of winter depression. *Archives of General Psychiatry*, 1998, 55/10 (875-882)

The measurement of retardation in depression. *Journal of Clinical Psychiatry*, 1998, 59/Suppl. 14(19-25)

Late-life depression in primary care: Where do we go from here? *Journal of the American Osteopathic Association*, 1998, 98/9 (489-497)

The role of exercise training in aged subjects with anxiety-depression syndrome. *Archives of Gerontology and Geriatrics*, 1998, 27/Suppl. 6(381-384)

Workplace performance effects from chronic depression and its treatment. *Journal of Health Economics*, 1998, 17/5 (511-535)

Implementation and evaluation of an exercise rehabilitation training for breast cancer patients. *PPmP Psychotherapie Psychosomatik Medizinische Psychologie*, 1998, 48/9-10 (398-407)

Critical review of psycho-oncological interventions. *PPmP Psychotherapie Psychosomatik Medizinische Psychologie*, 1998, 48/9-10 (381-389)

Emotion and immunity. *Journal of Psychosomatic Research* 1998, 45/2(107-115)

From cognitive information to shared meaning: Healing principles in prevention intervention. *Psychiatry*, 1998, 61/2 (112-129)

Dawn simulation vs. lightbox treatment in winter depression: A comparative study. *Acta Psychiatrica Scandinavica* 1998, 98/1 (73-80)

Risk indicators for malnutrition are associated inversely with quality of life for participants in meal programs for older adults. *J Am Diet Assoc*May 1998, 98 (5) p548-53

Religious commitment and health status: a review of the research and implications for family medicine. *Arch Fam Med* Mar-Apr 1998, 7 (2) p118-24

The role of exercise training in aged subjects with anxiety-depression syndrome. *Archives of Gerontology and Geriatrics* 1998, 27/Suppl. 6(381-384)

Bright light treatment of winter depression: A placebo-controlled trial *Archives of General Psychiatry* 1998, 55/10 (883-889)

Effects of cardiac rehabilitation and exercise training programs in women with depression. *Am J Cardiol* 1999 May 15;83(10):1480-3, A7

Natural product formulations available in Europe for psychotropic indications. *Psychopharmacology Bulletin*, 1995, 31/4 (745-751)

Antidepressive effectiveness of a highly dosed hypericum extract. *Munchener Medizinische Wochenschrift* (Germany), 1996, 138/3 (35-39)

St. John's Wort in the treatment of depression. *Johanniskraut zur antidepressiven therapie. Fortschritte der Medizin* (Germany), 1995, 113/25 (32-33)

Hypericum perforatum. *Fitoterapia* (Italy), 1995, 66/1 (43-68)

Psychomotoric performance improvement: Antidepressant therapy with St John's wort. *Therapiewoche* (Germany), 1995, 45/2 (106+108+110+112)

Hypericum in the treatment of seasonal affective disorders. *J. Geriatr. Psychiatry Neurol*. (Canada), 1994, 7/Suppl. 1 (S29-S33)

Effectiveness and tolerance of the hypericum extract LI 160 compared to maprotiline: A multicenter double-blind study. *J. Geriatr. Psychiatry Neurol*. (Canada), 1994, 7/Suppl. 1 (S24-S28)

Effectiveness and tolerance of the hypericum extract LI 160 in comparison with imipramine: Randomized double-blind study with 135 outpatients. *J. Geriatr. Psychiatry Neurol*. (Canada), 1994, 7/Suppl. 1 (S19-S23)

Multicenter double-blind study examining the antidepressant effectiveness of the hypericum extract LI 160. *J. Geriatr. Psychiatry Neurol.* (Canada), 1994, 7/Suppl. 1 (S15-S18)

Hypericum treatment of mild depressions with somatic symptoms. *J. Geriatr. Psychiatry Neurol.* (Canada), 1994, 7/Suppl. 1 (S12-S14)

St. John's wort: A prescription from nature against depressions. Johanniskraut: ein rezept der natur gegen depressionen. *Therapiewoche* (Germany), 1994, 44/14 (808+811-815)

Psychopharmacological therapy after acquired brain damage. *Munch. Med. Wochenschr.* (Germany), 1994, 136/4 (51-55)

Extract of St. John's wort in the treatment of depression—Attention and reaction remain unimpaired. *Fortschr. Med.* (Germany), 1993, 111/19 (37-40)

Investigations of the antidepressive effects of St. Johns Wort. *Pz Wiss.* (Germany), 1993, 138/2 (50-54)

Experimental animal studies of the psychotropic activity of a Hypericum extract. *Arzneim.-Forsch. / Drug Res.* (Germany, West), 1987, 37/1 (10-13)

Plasma tryptophan and five other amino acids in depressed and normal subjects. *Archives of General Psychiatry* 38(6):642-646, 1981

Trace amine deficit in depressive illness: the phenylalanine connexion. *Acta Psychiatrica Scandinavica 61*(Suppl. 280):29-39, 1980

Phenylalanine levels in endogenous psychoses. *Psychiatrie, Neurologie und Medizinische Psychologie* 32(10):631-633, 1980

Evaluation of the relative potency of individual competing amino acids to tryptophan transport in endogenously depressed patients. *Psychiatry Research* 3(2):141-150, 1980

Amino acids in mental illness. *Biological Psychiatry Today.* Vol. B Amsterdam, Elsevier/North Holland, 1979, p1581-4

Lithium prevention of amphetamine-induced 'manic' excitement and of reserpine-induced 'depression' in mice: possible role of 2-phenylethylamine. *Psychopharmacology* (Berlin) 59(3):259-262, 1978

Depression, pregnancy and phenylalanine. *Neuropisiquiatria* (Buenos Aires) 8(1):60-64, 1977

Theoretical and therapeutic potential of indoleamine precursors in affective disorders. *Neuropsychobiology* (Basel) 3(4):199-233, 1977

Phenylethylamine and glucose in true depression. *Journal of Orthomolecular Psychiatry* (Regina) 5(3):199-202, 1976

Therapeutic action of D-phenylalanine in Parkinson's disease. *Arzneimittel-Forschung* (Aulendorf) 26(4):577-579, 1976

Effects of D-phenylalanine on clinical picture and phenethylaminuria in depression. *Biological Psychiatry* 10(2):235-239, 1975

Phenylalanine for endogenous depression. *Journal of Orthomolecular Psychiatry* (Regina) 3(2):80-81, 1974

Rapidity of onset of the antidepressant effect of parenteral S-adenosyl-L-methionine. *Psychiatry Research* (Ireland), 1995, 56/3

The clinical potential of ademetionine (S-adenosylmethionine) in neurological disorders. *Drugs* (New Zealand), 1994, 48/2 (137-152)

Primary fibromyalgia is responsive to S-adenosyl-L-methionine. *Curr. Ther. Res. Clin. Exp.*, 1994, 55/7

S-adenosyl-L-methionine in Sjogren's syndrome and fibromyalgia. *Curr. Ther. Res. Clin. Exp.*, 1994, 55/6

Effects of *S*-adenosyl-*L*-methionine on cognitive and vigilance functions in the elderly. *Curr. Ther. Res. Clin. Exp.*, 1994, 55/6

Results of treatment with *S*-adenosyl-*L*-methionine in patients with major depression and internal illnesses. *Curr. Ther. Res. Clin. Exp.*, 1994, 55/6

S-adenosyl-l-methionine (SAM) as antidepressant: Meta-analysis of clinical studies. *Acta Neurol. Scand. Suppl.* (Denmark), 1994, 89/154

S-adenosyl-L-methionine in the treatment of major depression complicating chronic alcoholism. *Curr. Ther. Res. Clin. Exp.*, 1994, 55/1

Clinical evaluation of *S*-adenosyl-*L*-methionine versus transcutaneous electrical nerve stimulation in primary fibromyalgia. *Curr. Ther. Res. Clin. Exp.*, 1993, 53/2

Double blind, placebo-controlled study of *S*-adenosyl-*L*-methionine in depressed postmenopausal women. *Psychother. Psychosom.* (Switzerland), 1993, 59/1

S-Adenosyl-methionine (SAMe) as antidepressant. *New Trends Clin. Neuropharmacol.* (Italy), 1992, 6/1-4

Efficacy of *S*-adenosyl-*L*-methionine in speeding the onset of action of imipramine. *Psychiatry Res.* (Ireland), 1992, 44/3

Oral S-adenosyl-L-methionine in depression. *Curr. Ther. Res. Clin. Exp.*, 1992, 52/3

Neuroendocrine effects of *S*-adenosyl-*L*-methionine, a novel putative antidepressant. *J. Psychiatr. Res.* (UK), 1990, 24/2

The antidepressant potential of oral *S*-adenosyl-l-methionine. *Acta Psychiatr. Scand.* (Denmark), 1990, 81/5

S-Adenosyl-*L*-methionine. A review of its pharmacological properties and therapeutic potential in liver dysfunction and affective disorders in relation to its physiological role in cell metabolism. *Drugs* (New Zealand), 1989, 38/3

Antidepressants: A Comparative review of the clinical pharmacology and therapeutic use of the 'newer' versus the 'older' drugs. *Drugs* (New Zealand), 1989, 37/5 (713-738)

Neuropharmacology of *S*-adenosyl-*L*-methionine. *Am. J. Med.*, 1987, 83/5 A (95-103)

Vitamins in psychiatry. Do they have a role? *Drugs* (Australia), 1985, 30/1

S-adenosyl-*L*-methionine (SAM) in clinical practice: Preliminary report on 75 minor depressives. *Curr. Ther. Res., Clin. Exp.*, 1985, 37/4

S-Adenosyl-*L*-Methionine (SAMe) treatment in psychogeriatry: a controlled clinical trial in depressed patients. *G.Gerontol.* (Italy), 1977, 25/3

A methyl donor, adenosylmethionine, in depression. *Folia Neuropsychiat.*(Lecce) (Italy), 1973, 16/4

Therapeutic effects and mechanism of action of S adenosyl l methionine in depressive syndromes. *Minerva Med.* (Italy), 1973, 64/29 (1515-1529)

S-Adenosyl-methionine (SAM) as antidepressant. *New Trends Clin. Neuropharmacol.* (Italy), 1992, 6/1-4

Monitoring *S*-adenosyl-methionine blood levels and antidepressant effect. *Acta Neurol.* (Italy), 1980, 35/6 (488-495)

Long-term high dose treatment of depression with St John's wort extract. *TW Neurologie Psychiatrie* (Germany), 1995, 9/4 (220-221)

Effective phytotherapy for depressive patients. Effiziente phytotherapie fur depressive. *Munchener Medizinische Wochenschrift* (Germany), 1996, 138/7 (58)

St John's wort—An effective alternative with almost no side-effects for the treatment of depression. Depressionen: johanniskraut—die effektive und nebenwirkungsarme alternative. *Zeitschrift fur Allgemeinmedizin* (Germany), 1996, 72/1 (63)

Hypericum perforatum (Saint Johns wort) in the treatment of depression. *Therapiewoche* (Germany), 1993, 43/17 (962)

Good results with Hypericum perforatum in the treatment of depressions. *Fortschr. Med.* (Germany), 1993, 111/8 (57-58)

The efficacy of hypericum extract is double-blind verified. *Prax. Mag. Med.* (Germany), 1993, -/4 (46)

Medicinal plants improve the results of brain performance test. *Fortschr. Med.* (Germany), 1993, 111/6 (50)

The efficacy of Hypericum extract in the treatment of depression. *Munch. Med. Wochenschr.* (Germany), 1993, 135/8 (65)

Phytotherapeutic antidepressive agent with few side-effects. *Fortschr. Med.* (Germany), 1993, 111/3 (54+56)

Depression—To brighten up the mind with Saint-John's-Wort. *Tw Neurol. Psychiatr.* (Germany), 1992, 6/12 (793-794)

Saint Johns wort in the treatment of depressions. *Therapiewoche* (Germany), 1992, 42/51-52 (3074-3075)

Saint Johns wort (Hypericum perforatum extract) in the treatment of depressions. *Fortschr. Med.* (Germany), 1992, 110/31 (68-69)

Herbal medicine in depressions? *Pharm. Ztg.* (Germany), 1992, 137/41 (78-79)

Identification of selective MAO-type-A inhibitors in Hypericum perforatum. *Pharmacopsychiatry* (Germany, Federal Republic of), 1989, 22/5 (194)

DHEA and Pregnenolone Precautions

Neuropsychiatric function and dehydroepiandrosterone sulfate in elderly women: a prospective study. *Biol Psychiatry* 1998 May 1;43(9):694-700

Effect of acute and chronic administration of dehydeoepiandrosterone on (+/-)-1-(2,5-dimethosy-4-iodophenyl)-2-aminopropane-induced wet dog shaking behavior in rats. *J Neural Transm* 1999;106(1):23-33

Adrenal secretion during major depression in 8-to16-year olds. Altered diurnal rhythms in salivary cortisol and dehydroepi androsterone (DHEA) at presentation. *Psychol Med* 1996 Mar;26(2):245-56

Use of dehydroepiandrosterone in psychiatric practice. *J Neurol Neurosurg Psychiatry* 1955 18:137-44

Effects of replacement dose of dehydroepiandrosterone in men and women of advancing age. Published erratum appears in *J Clin Endocrinol Metab* 1995 Sep;80(9):2799

1952. Treatment of inadequate personality in juveniles by dehydroisoandrosterone: preliminary report. *BMJ* 2:66-68

Endogenous levels of dehydroepiandrosterone sulfate, but not other sex hormones, are associated with with depressed mood in older women: the Rancho Bernardo Study. *Am Geriatr Soc* 1999 Jun;47(6):685-91

1995. Antidepressant and cognition-enhancing effects of DHEA in major depression. *Ann NY Acad Sci* 477:337-39

Double-blind treatment of major depression with dehydroepiandrosterone. *Am J Psychiatry* 1999 Apr;156(4):646-9

Elevated serum dehydroepiandrosterone sulfate levels in practitioners of the Transcendental Meditation (TM) and TM-Sidhi programs. *J Behav Med* 1992 Aug;15(4):327-41

The impact of a new emotional self-management program on stress, emotions, heart rate variability, DHEA and cortisol. *Integr Physiol Behav Sci* 1998 Apr-Jun;33(2):151-70

Effects of estrogen replacement therapy on dehydroepiandrosterone, dehydroepiandrosterone sulfate, and cortisol responses to exercise in postmenopausal women [published erratum appears in Fertil Steril 1998 Mar;69:606]. *Fertil Steril* 68: 836-43

Inhibition of migration and proliferation of vascular smooth muscle cells by dehydroepiandrosterone sulfate. *Biochim Biophys Acta* 1998 Feb 27;1406(1):107-14

Endogenous androgens and carotid intimal-medial thickness in women. *J Clin Endocrinol Metab* 1999 Jun;84(6):2008-12

Dehydroepiandrosterone treatment of midlife dysthymia. *Biol Psychiatry* 1999 Jun 15;45(12):1533-41

Diabetes Type I (Juvenile Diabetes)

Effect of ginger (Zingiber officinale Rosc.) and fenugreek (Trigonella foenumgraecum L.) on blood lipids, blood sugar and platelet aggregation in patients with coronary artery disease. *Prostaglandins Leukot Essent Fatty Acids* 1997 May;56(5):379-84

Effects of non-steroidal anti-inflammatory drugs on the in vivo synthesis of thromboxane and prostacyclin in humans. *Adv Prostaglandin Thromboxane Leukot Res* 1991;21A:153-6

alpha-Lipoic acid corrects neuropeptide deficits in diabetic rats via induction of trophic support. *Neurosci Lett* 1997 Feb 7;222(3):191-4

Biotin for diabetic peripheral neuropathy. *Biomed Pharmacother* 1990;44(10):511-4

The inhibition of sugar-induced structural alterations in collagen by aspirin and other compounds. *Biochem Biophys Res Commun* 1994 Mar 15;199(2):683-6

Combined high blood pressure and glucose in type 2 diabetes: double jeopardy. British trial shows clear effects of treatment, especially blood pressure reduction. *BMJ* 1998 Sep 12;317(7160):693-4

Meta-analysis of nicotinamide treatment in patients with recent-onset IDDM. The Nicotinamide Trialists. *Diabetes Care* 1996 Dec;19(12):1357-63

Acetyl-L-carnitine for symptomatic diabetic neuropathy. *Diabetologia* 1995 Jan;38(1):123

Inhibition of development of peripheral neuropathy in streptozotocin-induced diabetic rats with *N*-acetylcysteine. *Diabetologia* 1996 Mar;39 (3):263-9

Carbohydrate feeding before exercise: effect of glycemic index. *Int J Sports Med* 1991 Apr;12(2):180-6

Effect of intensive blood-glucose control with metformin on complications in overweight patients with type 2 diabetes (UKPDS 34). *Lancet* 1998 Sep 12;352(9131):854-65. Published erratum appears in *Lancet* 1998 Nov 7;352(9139):1557

Recent progress on the biologic and clinical significance of advanced glycosylation end products. *J Lab Clin Med* 1994 Jul;124(1):19-30

The Deutsche Nicotinamide Intervention Study: an attempt to prevent type 1 diabetes. DENIS Group. *Diabetes* Jun 1998, 47 (6) p980-4

Prevention of type 2 diabetes in childhood. *Clinical Pediatrics*, 1998, 37/2 (123-130)

[Prevention of juvenile diabetes (type 1): reality or fiction?] *Bull Mem Acad R Med Belg* (Belgium) 1994, 149 (12) p435-43; discussion 443-4

Insulin-like effect of vanadyl ion on streptozotocin-induced diabetic rats. *J Endocrinol* (England) Sep 1990, 126 (3) p451-9

Pathogenesis of type 1 and type 2 diabetes mellitus. *Ann Acad Med Singapore* (Singapore) Jul 1990, 19 (4) p506-11

Taurine and kynureninase. *Advances in Experimental Medicine and Biology* 1996, 403/- (55-58)

Sulfur amino acid metabolism in juvenile-onset nonketotic and ketotic diabetic patients. *Metabolism: Clinical and Experimental* 1984, 33/5 (425-428)

The correlation between EDTA chelation therapy and improvement in cardiovascular function: a meta-analysis. *J Adv Med* 1993, 6, 139

Benefits of EDTA chelation therapy in arteriosclerosis: a retrospective study of 470 patients. *J Advancement in Medicine*, 1993 Fall, 6:3

Oral alpha lipoic acid preparation proves good bioavailability in diabetic polyneuropathy. *Therapiewoche* (Germany), 1995, 45/23 (1367-1370)

Lipoic acid improves nerve blood flow, reduces oxidative stress, and improves distal nerve conduction in experimental diabetic neuropathy. *Diabetes Care*, 1995, 18/8 (1160-1167)

Thioctic (lipoic) acid: A therapeutic metal-chelating antioxidant? *Biochemical Pharmacology* (UK), 1995, 50/1 (123-126)

Diabetic polyneuropathy. Most effective measure: Keep blood sugar close to normal from the start. *Munchener Medizinische Wochenschrift* (Germany), 1995, 137/6

Primary preventive and secondary interventionary effects of acetyl-L-carnitine on diabetic neuropathy in the bio-breeding Worcester rat. *Journal of Clinical Investigation*, 1996, 97/8 (1900-1907)

Effects of acetyl- and proprionyl-L-carnitine on peripheral nerve function and vascular supply in experimental diabetes. *Metabolism: Clinical and Experimental*, 1995, 44/9

Acetyl-L-carnitine corrects the altered peripheral nerve function of experimental diabetes. *Metabolism: Clinical and Experimental*, 1995, 44/5

Diabetic neuropathy in the rat: 1. Alcar augments the reduced levels and axoplasmic transport of substance. *P. J. Neurosci. Res.*, 1995, 40/3 (414-419)

Hypothesis: the role of vitamin C in diabetic angiopathy. *Perspect. Biol. Med.,* 1974, 17/2 (210-217)

Treatment of symptomatic diabetic peripheral neuropathy with the anti-oxidant alpha- lipoic acid. A 3-week multicentre randomized controlled trial (Aladin Study). *Diabetologia* (Germany), 1995, 38/12 (1425-1433)

Alternative therapeutic principles in the prevention of microvascular and Neuropathic complications. *Diabetes Research and Clinical Practice* (Ireland), 1995, 28/Suppl

Effects of aminoguanidine on rat pancreatic islets in culture and on the pancreatic islet blood flow of anaesthetized rats. *Biochemical Pharmacology*, 1996, 51/12 (1711-1717)

Aminoguanidine prevents the decreased myocardial compliance produced by streptozotocin-induced diabetes mellitus in rats. *Circulation*, 1996, 93/10 (1905-1912)

Slowing of peripheral motor nerve conduction was ameliorated by aminoguanidine in streptozocin-induced diabetic rats. *European Journal of Endocrinology* (Norway), 1996, 134/4 (467-473)

Thiamine pyrophosphate and pyridoxamine inhibit the formation of antigenic advanced glycation end-products: Comparison with aminoguanidine. *Biochemical and Biophysical Research Communications*, 1996, 220/1

Advanced glycosylation end products in diabetic renal and vascular disease. *American Journal of Kidney Diseases*, 1995, 26/6 (875-888)

Aminoguanidine treatment inhibits the development of experimental diabetic retinopathy. *Proc. Natl Acad. Sci. U. S. A.*, 1991, 88/24 (11555-11558)

Aminoguanidine effects on nerve blood flow, vascular permeability, electrophysiology, and oxygen free radicals. *Proc. Natl Acad. Sci. U. S. A.*, 1991, 88/14 (6107-6111)

Diabetes Type II (Adult Onset Diabetes)

Effect of ginger (Zingiber officinale Rosc.) and fenugreek (Trigonella foenumgraecum L.) on blood lipids, blood sugar and platelet aggregation in patients with coronary artery disease. *Prostaglandins Leukot Essent Fatty Acids* 1997 May; 56(5):379-84

Effects of non-steroidal anti-inflammatory drugs on the in vivo synthesis of thromboxane and prostacyclin in humans. *Adv Prostaglandin Thromboxane Leukot Res* 1991;21A:153-6

alpha-Lipoic acid corrects neuropeptide deficits in diabetic rats via induction of trophic support. *Neurosci Lett* 1997 Feb 7;222(3):191-4

Biotin for diabetic peripheral neuropathy. *Biomed Pharmacother* 1990;44(10):511-4

The inhibition of sugar-induced structural alterations in collagen by aspirin and other compounds. *Biochem Biophys Res Commun* 1994 Mar 15;199(2):683-6

Combined high blood pressure and glucose in type 2 diabetes: double jeopardy. British trial shows clear effects of treatment, especially blood pressure reduction. *BMJ* 1998 Sep 12;317(7160):693-4

Meta-analysis of nicotinamide treatment in patients with recent-onset IDDM. The Nicotinamide Trialists. *Diabetes Care* 1996 Dec;19(12):1357-63

Acetyl-L-carnitine for symptomatic diabetic neuropathy. *Diabetologia* 1995 Jan;38(1):123

Inhibition of development of peripheral neuropathy in streptozotocin-induced diabetic rats with N-acetylcysteine. *Diabetologia* 1996 Mar;39(3):263-9

Carbohydrate feeding before exercise: effect of glycemic index. *Int J Sports Med* 1991 Apr;12(2):180-6

Effect of intensive blood-glucose control with metformin on complications in overweight patients with type 2 diabetes (UKPDS 34). *Lancet* 1998 Sep 12;352(9131):854-65. Published erratum appears in *Lancet* 1998 Nov 7;352(9139):1557

Recent progress on the biologic and clinical significance of advanced glycosylation end products. *J Lab Clin Med* 1994 Jul;124(1):19-30

The Deutsche Nicotinamide Intervention Study: an attempt to prevent type 1 diabetes. DENIS Group. *Diabetes* Jun 1998, 47 (6) p980-4

Prevention of type 2 diabetes in childhood. *Clinical Pediatrics,* 1998, 37/2 (123-130)

Prevention of juvenile diabetes (type 1): reality or fiction?]. *Bull Mem Acad R Med Belg* (Belgium) 1994, 149 (12) p435-43; discussion 443-4

Insulin-like effect of vanadyl ion on streptozotocin-induced diabetic rats. *J Endocrinol* (England) Sep 1990, 126 (3) p451-9

Pathogenesis of type 1 and type 2 diabetes mellitus. *Ann Acad Med Singapore* (Singapore) Jul 1990, 19 (4) p506-11

Taurine and kynureninase. *Advances in Experimental Medicine and Biology* 1996, 403/- (55-58)

Sulfur amino acid metabolism in juvenile-onset nonketotic and ketotic diabetic patients. *Metabolism: Clinical and Experimental* 1984, 33/5 (425-428)

The correlation between EDTA chelation therapy and improvement in cardiovascular function: a meta-analysis. *J Adv Med* 1993, 6, 139

Benefits of EDTA chelation therapy in arteriosclerosis: a retrospective study of 470 patients. *J Advancement in Medicine,* 1993 Fall, 6:3

Acetyl-L-carnitine effects on nerve conduction and glycemic regulation in experimental diabetes. *Endocrine Research,* 1997, 23/1-2 (27-36)

Age-related decreases in chromium levels in 51,665 hair, sweat, and serum samples from 40,872 patients - Implications for the prevention of cardiovascular disease and type II diabetes mellitus. *Metabolism: Clinical and Experimental,* 1997, 46/5 (469-473)

Lipoic acid (thioctic acid): Antioxidant properties and their clinical implications. *Diabetes und Stoffwechsel* (Germany), 1996, 5/3 Suppl. (98-101)

Effect of lipoic acid (thioctic acid) on peripheral nerve of experimental diabetic neuropathy. *Diabetes und Stoffwechsel* (Germany), 1996, 5/3 Suppl. (94-97)

Lipoic acid alpha-potential modulator of insulin sensitivity in patients with non-insulin-dependent diabetes mellitus. *Diabetes und Stoffwechsel* (Germany), 1996, 5/3 Suppl. (64-70)

Lipoic acid acutely ameliorates insulin sensitivity in obese subjects with type 2 diabetes. *Diabetes und Stoffwechsel* (Germany), 1996, 5/3 Suppl. (59-63)

Treatment of symptomatic diabetic peripheral neuropathy with alpha-lipoic acid. A 3-week multicentre randomized controlled trial (Aladin Study). *Diabetes und Stoffwechsel* (Germany), 1996, 5/3 Suppl. (102-110)

Effect of lipoic acid (thioctic acid) on glucose homeostasis and muscle glucose transporters in diabetic rats. *Diabetes und Stoffwechsel* (Germany), 1996, 5/3 Suppl. (50-54)

Altered 14C-deoxyglucose incorporation in rat brain following treatment with alpha-lipoic acid (thioctic acid). Clinical implications for diabetic neuropathy and neurodegenerative disorders. *Diabetes und Stoffwechsel* (Germany), 1996, 5/3 Suppl. (31-35)

Studies on the bioavailability of alpha lipoic acid in type I and type II diabetics with diabetic neuropathy. *Diabetes und Stoffwechsel* (Germany), 1996, 5/3 Suppl. (23-26)

On the pharmacokinetics of alpha-lipoic acid in patients with diabetic polyneuropathy. *Diabetes und Stoffwechsel* (Germany), 1996, 5/3 Suppl. (17-22)

Chromium oligopeptide activates insulin receptor tyrosine kinase activity. *Biochemistry,* 1997, 36/15 (4382-4385)

Effect of chromium nicotinic acid supplementation on selected cardiovascular disease risk factors. *Biological Trace Element Research,* 1996, 55/3 (297-305)

Modulation of cellular reducing equivalent homeostasis by alpha-lipoic acid. Mechanisms and implications for diabetes and ischemic injury. *Biochemical Pharmacology,* 1997, 53/3 (393-399)

Endothelial dysfunction: Clinical implications. *Progress in Cardiovascular Diseases,* 1997, 39/4 (287-324)

Effects of treatment with the antioxidant alpha-lipoic acid on cardiac autonomic neuropathy in Niddm patients: A 4-month randomized controlled multicenter trial (Dekan study). *Diabetes Care,* 1997, 20/3 (369-373)

alpha-Lipoic acid corrects neuropeptide deficits in diabetic rats via induction of trophic support. *Neuroscience Letters* (Ireland), 1997, 222/3 (191-194)

Chromium picolinate supplementation improves cardiac metabolism, but not myosin isoenzyme distribution in the diabetic heart. *Journal of Nutritional Biochemistry,* 1996, 7/11 (617-622)

Dehydroepiandrosterone and diseases of aging. *Drugs and Aging* (New Zealand), 1996, 9/4 (274-291)

Sex hormones and DHEA-SO4 in relation to ischemic heart disease mortality in diabetic subjects: The Wisconsin Epidemiologic Study of Diabetic Retinopathy. *Diabetes Care,* 1996, 19/10 (1045-1050)

The effects of acetyl-L-carnitine and sorbinil on peripheral nerve structure, chemistry, and function in experimental diabetes. *Metabolism: Clinical and Experimental,* 1996, 45/7 (902-907)

Acetyl-L-carnitine deficiency as a cause of altered nerve myo-inositol content, Na,K-ATPase activity, and motor conduction velocity in the streptozotocin-diabetic rat. *Metabolism: Clinical and Experimental,* 1996, 45/7 (865-872)

Unrecognized pandemic subclinical diabetes of the affluent nations: Causes, cost and prevention. *Journal of Orthomolecular Medicine* (Canada), 1996, 11/2 (95-99)

Evidence of a relationship between childhood-onset type I diabetes and low groundwater concentration of zinc. *Diabetes Care,* 1996, 19/8 (873-875)

Improved pallesthetic sensitivity of pudendal nerve in impotent diabetic patients treated with acetyl-L-carnitine. *Acta Urologica Italica* (Italy), 1996, 10/3 (185-187)

Primary preventive and secondary interventionary effects of acetyl-L- carnitine on diabetic neuropathy in the bio-breeding Worcester rat. *Journal of Clinical Investigation,* 1996, 97/8 (1900-1907)

Vitamin and mineral deficiencies which may predispose to glucose intolerance of pregnancy. *Journal of the American College of Nutrition,* 1996, 15/1 (14-20)

Antioxidant status in patients with uncomplicated insulin-dependent and non-insulin-dependent diabetes mellitus. *European Journal of Clinical Investigation* (UK), 1997, 27/6 (484-490)

Nutrient intake and food use in an Ojibwa-Cree community in Northern Ontario assessed by 24h dietary recall. *Nutrition Research,* 1997, 17/4 (603-618)

Effect of vitamin C supplementation on hepatic cytochrome P450 mixed-function oxidase activity in streptozotocin-diabetic rats. *Toxicology Letters* (Ireland), 1996, 89/3 (249-256)

The effect of dietary treatment on lipid peroxidation and antioxidant status in newly diagnosed noninsulin dependent diabetes. *Free Radical Biology and Medicine,* 1996, 21/5 (719-726)

Vitamin B6 alleviates the vascular complications of insulin-treated STZ-induced diabetic rats. *Nutritional Sciences Journal* (Taiwan), 1996, 21/3 (235-248)

Total vitamin C, ascorbic acid, and dehydroascorbic acid concentrations in plasma of critically ill patients. *American Journal of Clinical Nutrition,* 1996, 63/5 (760-765)

Clinical study of vitamin influence in diabetes mellitus. *Journal of the Medical Society of Toho University* (Japan), 1996, 42/6 (577-581)

Vitamins and metals: Potential dangers for the human being. *Schweizerische Medizinische Wochenschrift* (Switzerland), 1996, 126/15 (607-611)

Leukocyte lipid peroxidation, superoxide dismutase, glutathione peroxidase and serum and leukocyte vitamin C levels of patients with type II diabetes mellitus. *Clinica Chimica Acta* (Netherlands), 1996, 244/2 (221-227)

Erythrocyte and plasma antioxidant activity in type I diabetes mellitus. *Presse Medicale* (France), 1996, 25/5 (188-192)

Vitamin C improves endothelium-dependent vasodilation in patients with non-insulin-dependent diabetes mellitus. *Journal of Clinical Investigation,* 1996, 97/1 (22-28)

Effects of aspirin or basic amino acids on collagen cross-links and complications in Niddm. *Diabetes Care* May 1997, 20 (5) p832-5

Acute and chronic response to vanadium following two methods of streptozotocin-diabetes induction. *Can J Physiol Pharmacol* (Canada) Feb 1997, 75 (2) p83-90

[Comparison of metabolism of water-soluble vitamins in healthy children and in children with insulin-dependent diabetes mellitus depending upon the level of vitamins in the diet]. *Vopr Med Khim* (Russia) Apr-Jun 1996, 42 (2) p153-8

Spice constituents scavenging free radicals and inhibiting pentosidine formation in a model system. *Biosci Biotechnol Biochem* (Japan) Feb 1997, 61 (2) p263-6

L-Arginine reduces lipid peroxidation in patients with diabetes mellitus. *Free Radic Biol Med* 1997, 22 (1-2) p355-7

Short-term oral administration of L-arginine reverses defective endothelium-dependent relaxation and cGMP generation in diabetes. *Eur J Pharmacol* (Netherlands) Dec 19 1996, 317 (2-3) p317-20

A diet enriched in protein accelerates diabetes manifestation in NOD mice. *Acta Diabetol* (Germany) Sep 1996, 33 (3) p236-40

Metformin improves hemodynamic and rheological responses to L-arginine in Niddm patients. *Diabetes Care* Sep 1996, 19 (9) p934-9

Impairment of coronary blood flow regulation by endothelium-derived nitric oxide in dogs with alloxan-induced diabetes. *J Cardiovasc Pharmacol* Jul 1996, 28 (1) p60-7

Involvement of the L-arginine-nitric oxide pathway in hyperglycaemia-induced coronary artery dysfunction of isolated guinea pig hearts. *Eur J Clin Invest* (England) Aug 1996, 26 (8) p707-12

Deficient nitric oxide responsible for reduced nerve blood flow in diabetic rats: effects of L-Name, L-arginine, sodium nitroprusside and evening primrose oil. *Br J Pharmacol* (England) May 1996, 118 (1) p186-90

Interactions between essential fatty acid, prostanoid, polyol pathway and nitric oxide mechanisms in the neurovascular deficit of diabetic rats. *Diabetologia* (Germany) Feb 1996, 39 (2) p172-82

Effects of vanadyl sulfate on carbohydrate and lipid metabolism in patients with non-insulin-dependent diabetes mellitus. *Metabolism* Sep 1996, 45 (9) p1130-5

Contraction and relaxation of aortas from diabetic rats: effects of chronic anti-oxidant and aminoguanidine treatments. *Naunyn Schmiedebergs Arch Pharmacol* (Germany) Apr 1996, 353 (5) p584-91

[Erythrocyte and plasma antioxidant activity in diabetes mellitus type I]. Activite anti-oxydante erythrocytaire et plasmatique dans le diabete de type I. *Presse Med* (France) Feb 10 1996, 25 (5) p188-92

Hyperglycemia-induced latent scurvy and atherosclerosis: the scorbutic-metaplasia hypothesis. *Med Hypotheses* (England) Feb 1996, 46 (2) p119-29

Oral vanadyl sulfate improves insulin sensitivity in Niddm but not in obese nondiabetic subjects. *Diabetes* May 1996, 45 (5) p659-66

Homologous physiological effects of phenformin and chromium picolinate. *Med Hypotheses* (England) Oct 1993, 41 (4) p316-24

[The effect of chromium picolinate on the liver levels of trace elements] Efecto del picolinato de cromo en los niveles hepaticos de algunos elementos traza. *Nutr Hosp* (Spain) Nov-Dec 1995, 10 (6) p373-6

Anabolic effects of insulin on bone suggest a role for chromium picolinate in preservation of bone density. *Med Hypotheses* (England) Sep 1995, 45 (3) p241-6

Longevity effect of chromium picolinate—'rejuvenation' of hypothalamic function? *Med Hypotheses* (England) Oct 1994, 43 (4) p253-65

Thiamine pyrophosphate and pyridoxamine inhibit the formation of antigenic advanced glycation end-products: comparison with aminoguanidine. *Biochem Biophys Res Commun* Mar 7 1996, 220 (1) p113-9

Loss of glucose-induced insulin secretion and Glut2 expression in transplanted beta-cells. *Diabetes* Jan 1995, 44 (1) p75-9

Case report: amelioration of insulin resistance in diabetes with dehydroepiandrosterone. *Am J Med Sci* Nov 1993, 306 (5) p320-4

Therapeutic effects of dehydroepiandrosterone metabolites in diabetes mutant mice (C57BL/KsJ-db/db). *Endocrinology* Jul 1984, 115 (1) p239-43

The endocrine pancreas in pyridoxine deficient rats. *Medicine* (Japan) Jul 1981, 134 (3) p331-6

Vitamin B6 metabolism and diabetes. *Biochem Med Metab Biol* Jun 1994, 52 (1) p10-7

A deficiency of vitamin B6 is a plausible molecular basis of the retinopathy of patients with diabetes mellitus. *Biochem Biophys Res Commun* Aug 30 1991, 179 (1) p615-9

Erythrocyte O2 transport and metabolism and effects of vitamin B6 therapy in type II diabetes mellitus. *Diabetes* Jul 1989, 38 (7) p881-6

Diabetes and adrenal disease. *Baillieres Clin Endocrinol Metab* (England) Oct 1992, 6 (4) p829-47

[Preventive treatment of diabetic microangiopathy: blocking the pathogenic mechanisms]. *Diabete Metab* (France) 1994, 20 (2 Pt 2) p219-28

Alternative therapeutic principles in the prevention of microvascular and neuropathic complications. *Diabetes Res Clin Pract* (Ireland) Aug 1995, 28 Suppl pS201-7

Enhancement of glucose disposal in patients with type 2 diabetes by alpha-lipoic acid. *Arzneimittelforschung* (Germany) Aug 1995, 45 (8) p872-4

Inhibition with N-acetylcysteine of enhanced production of tumor necrosis factor in streptozotocin-induced diabetic rats. *Clin Immunol Immunopathol* Jun 1994, 71 (3) p333-7

Effects of acetyl- and proprionyl-L-carnitine on peripheral nerve function and vascular supply in experimental diabetes. *Metabolism* Sep 1995, 44 (9) p1209-14

Acetyl-L-carnitine for symptomatic diabetic neuropathy [letter]. *Diabetologia* (Germany) Jan 1995, 38 (1) p123

Peptide alterations in autonomic diabetic neuropathy prevented by acetyl-L-carnitine. *Int J Clin Pharmacol Res* (Switzerland) 1992, 12 (5-6) p225-30

Prevention of cardiovascular and renal pathology of aging by the advanced glycation inhibitor aminoguanidine. *Proc Natl Acad Sci U S A* Apr 30 1996, 93 (9) p3902-7

Prevention of long-term complications of non-insulin-dependent diabetes mellitus. *Clin Invest Med* (Canada) Aug 1995, 18 (4) p332-9

Secondary intervention with aminoguanidine retards the progression of diabetic retinopathy in the rat model. *Diabetologia* (Germany) Jun 1995, 38 (6) p656-60

Prevention of glomerular basement membrane thickening by aminoguanidine in experimental diabetes mellitus. *Metabolism* Oct 1991, 40 (10) p1016-9

Can metformin reduce insulin resistance in polycystic ovary syndrome? *Fertil Steril* May 1996, 65 (5) p946-9

Effects of diet and metformin administration on sex hormone-binding globulin, androgens, and insulin in hirsute and obese women. *J Clin Endocrinol Metab* Jul 1995, 80 (7) p2057-62

[The value of metformin in therapy of type 2 diabetes: effect on insulin resistance, diabetic control and cardiovascular risk factors]. *Wien Klin Wochenschr* (Austria) 1994, 106 (24) p793-802

Oral vanadyl sulfate improves hepatic and peripheral insulin sensitivity in patients with non-insulin-dependent diabetes mellitus. *J Clin Invest* Jun 1995, 95 (6) p2501-9

Toxicity studies on one-year treatment of non-diabetic and streptozotocin-diabetic rats with vanadyl sulphate. *Pharmacol Toxicol* (Denmark) Nov 1994, 75 (5) p265-73

Antidiabetic action of vanadyl in rats independent of in vivo insulin-receptor kinase activity. *Diabetes* Apr 1991, 40 (4) p492-8

Digestive Disorders

Hepatoprotective activity of polyphenolic compounds from Cynara scolymnus against CCl4 toxicity in isolated rat hepatocytes. *J Nat Prod*. 50: 612, 1987

Antidyspeptische und lipidsenkende Wirkungen von Artischockenextrakt. Ergebnisse klinischer Untersuchungen zur Wirksamkeit und Vertraglichkeit von Hepar SL Forte an 553 Patienten. *Z. Allg. Med*. 72:48, 1996

Therapeutic profile and mechanism of action of artichoke leaf extract: hypolipemic, antioxidant, hepatoprotective and choleretic properties. *Phytomed.* 1996. Suppl 1: 50

Uber die lipidsenkende Wirkung von Cynarin. *Subsidia Medica* 25 (3): 5, 1973

Artischockenblatterextrakt: In vitro Nachweis einer Hemmwirkung auf die cholesterin-Biosynthese. *Med. Welt* 46: 348-35-, 1995

Neue experimentelle Erkenntnisse zur Wirkung von Artischockenblatterextrakt. *Z Allg. Med.* 72: 20-23, 1996

Antioxidative and protective properties of extract from leaves of the artichoke (Cynara scolymnus L,) against hydro-peroxide-induced oxidative stress incultured rat hepatocytes. *Toxicol Appl Pharmacol* 144: 279-286, 1997

Inhibition of Cholesterol Biosynthesis in Primary Cultured Rat Hepatocytes by Artichoke (Cynara scolymnus L.) Extracts. *J Pharmacol Exp Ther* 286: 3, 1998

Polyphenols and flavonoids as antioxidant and hepatoprotective principles of artichoke extracts. *Cell Biology and Toxicology,* 1996

Scavenging of peroxinitrite by a phenolic/peroxidase system prevents oxidative damage to DNA. *FEBS Letters* 426(1): 24-8, 1998

Uber den Einfluss von cynarin auf hyperlipidamien unter besonderer Berucksichtigung des types II (hypercholesterinamie). *Wiener Med. Wschr.* 41: 601-605, 1973

Hammerl H, Pichler O: Uber eine moglichkeit der kausalen Behandlung von Erkrankungen der Gallenwege mit einem Artischockenpreparat. *Wiener Med. Wschr.* 107 (25/26): 545, 1957

Untersuchungen uber den Einfluss eines Artischockenextraktes auf die Serumlipide in Hinblick auf die Arterioskleroseprophylaxe. *Wiener Med. Wschr.* 109 (44): 853, 1959

Artischocke bei Gallenwegsdyskinesien. Neue Aspekte zur Therapie mit Choleretika. *Z. Klin. Med.* 47:92, 1992

Chlorogenic acid and synthetic chlorogenic acid derivatives: novel inhibitors of hepatic glucose-6-phosphate translocase. *J Medicinal Chemistry* 40(2): 137-45, 1997

Increase in choleresis by means of artichoke extract. Results of a randomized placebo-controlled double-blind study. *Phytomedicine* 1: 107, 1994

Effect of dietary caffeic and chlorogenic acids on in vivo xenobiotic enzyme systems. *Plant Foods for Human Nutrition* 45(3):287-98, 1994

The supression of the *N*-nitrosating reaction by chlorogenic acid. *Biochemical Journal* 312(Pt3): 947-53, 1995

Antioxidant activity of polyphenolics in diets. *Biochimica et Biophysica Acta* 1335(3): 335-42, 1997

Prufung der choleretischen Aktivitat eines pflanzlichen Cholagogums. *Z. Allg. Med.* (67): 1046, 1991

Choleretic and cholesterol lowering properties of two artichoke extracts. *Filoterapia* 48: 153,1977

Wirkungen der Cynara scolymnus-Extrakte auf die Regeneration der Rattenleber. *Arzneim-Forsch* 18: 184, 1966

Dicaffeoylquinic and dicaffeoyltartaric acids are selective inhibitors of human immunodeficiency virus type 1 integrase. *Antimicrob Agents Chemother* 42(1): 140-6, 1998

Inhibitory effect of chlorogenic acid on methylazoxymethanolacetate-induced carcinogenesis in large intestine and liver of hamsters. *Cancer Letters* 30(1):49-54, 1986

Regressive effects of various chemopreventive agents on azoxymethane-induced aberrant crypt foci in the rat colon. *Jpn J Cancer Res* 88: 815-20. 1997

Effects of artichoke leaf extract on lipoptotein metabolism in vitro and in vivo. *Atherosclerosis* 129: 147, 1997

Artichoke leaf extract for serum cholesterol reduction. *Perfusion* 11: 338-340, 1998

Dicaffeoylquinic acid inhibitors of human immunodeficiency virus integrase: inhibition of the core catalytic domain of human immunodeficiency virus integrase. *Molecular Pharmacology* 50(4): 846-55, 1996

The influence of 1,5-dicaffeoylquinic acid on serum lipids in the experimentally alcoholized rat. *Panminerva Med* 13(11): 87,1971

The action of herbs and roots of artichokes (Cynara scolymnus) and cardoon (Cynara cardunculus) on the development of experimental atherosclerosis in white rats. *Diss. Pharm.* 14: 115, 1962

Inhibition of 4-nitroquinoline-1-oxide- induced rat tongue carcinogenesis by the naturally occurring plant phenolics caffeic, ellagic, chlorogenic and ferulic acids. *Carcinogenesis* 14(7): 1321-5, 1993

Les actions physiologiques et therapeutique des Cynara Scolymnus. *Presse Med.* 44:880, 1939

Influence of an extract from artichoke (Cynara sclymnus) on the level of lipids in serum of aged men. *Herba Pol.* 27: 265, 1981

Effect of 1,5-dicaffeoylquinic acid on ethanol-induced hypertriglyceridemia. *Arzneim-Forsch / Drug Res.* 26 (11): 2047, 1976

Effects of 1,5-dicaffeoylquinic acid (cynarin) on cholesterol levels in serum and liver of acute ethanol-treated rats. *Drug Alcohol Dep.* 3: 143, 1978

British Medical Journal 1996 Feb 17;312(7028):421-5

The Healing Herbs: The Ultimate Guide to the Curative Power of Mature's Medicines. Sheldon Sault Hendler

Current Therapeutic Research, 1994, vol. 55, no. 5

The Artichoke—A Healing Plant With a History and a Future (eine Heilpflanze mit Geschichte und Zukunftsperspektive.) *Naturamed* 1995; 10:1

European Journal of Epidemiology 1998 Jan;14(1):1-8

Randomized controlled trial of silymarin treatment in patients with cirrhosis of the liver. *J Hepatol* 1989 Jul; 9(1):105-13

HPLC evaluation of the active constituents in the newly introduced strain of Cynara scolymus cultivated in Egypt. *Planta Med* 57 Supplement Issue 2, 1991:A119

Hepatology, 1996, vol. 23, no. 4

Herbs for Health, November/December 1998, p 22

Isolation and properties of raphanin, an antibacterial substance from radish seed. *Proc Soc Exp Biol Med* 1947; 66:625-31

Artichoke leaf extract: recent findings reflecting effect on lipid metabolism, liver, and gastrointestinal tracts. *Phytomedicine* 1997; 4(4):369-78

The Lawrence Review of Natural Products. St Louis MO: Lippincott Company, November 1992

Fire in the belly. *Time* 1999 (April 26):108

Two thousand years of artichoke (Zwei Jahrtausend Artischocke). *Austrian Pharmaceutical Magazine* 1965; 19:4

Scientific Validation of Herbal Remedies. USA: Keats Publishing, 1990

Herbal Tonic Therapies. USA: Keats Publishing, 1993

Nutrition 1998 May;14(5):452-7

Nutritive and Therapeutic Value of Fruit and Vegetables, 144, *Chem Abstr.* 1962; 57: 964

Planta Medica, 1984, vol. 50, no. 3

Immunomodulation par des produits natural, Note I: effect d'un extrait aqueux de Raphanus sativus niger sur l'infection grippale experimentale chez la souris. *Virologie* 1987; (Apr-Jun):38(2):115-20

Frequent heartburn should not be ignored in subjects who self-medicate with antacids. Oklahoma Foundation for Digestive Research, University of Arizona Health Sciences Center, Tucson. Presented May 20, 1996

Deutshe Apotheker Zeitung 1984; 124:1433-43

The Natural Guide to Medicinal Herbs and Plants. New York: Dorset Press, 1992

Herbal Medicine. Gothenburg: AB Arcanum, 1988; Beaconsfield England: Beaconsfield Publishers, 1988

References regarding digestive disorders in Europe: *British Medical Journal* 1996 Feb 17;312(7028):421-5

Annals of Rheumatk Disease (1947)

Relief of chronic arterial obstruction using intravenous brinase. A control study. *Scand J Thorac Cardiovasc Surg* 1979;13(3):327-32

Wayne, NJ; *Enzyme Nutrition: The Food Enzyme Concept.* Aver'Publishing Group, 1985 Percival M. *Nutritional Pearls* (vol 35)

Unique features and application of non-animal derived enzymes. *Clinical Nutrition Insights* 1997; 5(10)

Pancreatic enzyme replacement therapy: comparative effects of conventional and enteric-coated microspheric pancreatin and acid-stable fungal enzyme preparations on steatorrhoea in chronic pancreatitis. *Hepatogastroenterology* 1985 Apr;32(2):97-102

Digestive processes in the human colon. *Nutrition,* 1995, 11/1 (37-45)

The ileum and carbohydrate-mediated feedback regulation of postprandial pancreaticobiliary secretion in normal humans. *Pancreas*, 1991, 6/5 (495-505)

Factors influencing carbohydrate digestion: Acute and long-term consequences.*Diabetes Nutr. Metab. Clin. Exp.* (Italy), 1990, 3/3 (251-258): Two distinct adaptive responses in the synthesis of exocrine pancreatic enzymes to inverse changes in protein and carbohydrate in the diet. *Am. J. Physiol.*, 1984, 10/6 (G611-G616)

Carbohydrate absorption. *Med. Clin. N. Amer.*, 1974, 58/6 (1387-1395)

Dietary carbohydrates. Their indications and contraindications in clinical medicine. *Practitioner* (England), 1974, 212/1270 (448-453)

An analysis on fat digestion in the upper small intestine after intragastric infusion of a test meal in patients with exocrine pancreatic insufficiency. *Japanese Journal of Gastroenterology* (Japan), 1995, 92/8 (1169-1177)

Pancreatic triglyceride lipase and colipase: Insights into dietary fat digestion. *Gastroenterology,* 1994, 107/5 (1524-1536)

Role of nonpancreatic lipolytic activity in exocrine pancreatic insufficiency. *Gastroenterology,* 1987, 92/1 (125-129)

Rat lingual lipase: Effect of proteases, bile, and pH on enzyme stability Roberts I.M. *Am. J. Physiol.*, 1985, 12/4 (G496-G500)

Fat digestion by lingual lipase: Mechanism of lipolysis in the stomach and upper small intestine. *Pediatr. Res.*, 1984, 18/5 (402-409)

Fat digestion in the stomach: Stability of lingual lipase in the gastric environment. *Pediatr. Res.*, 1984, 18/3 (248-254)

Colipase and lipase secretion in childhood-onset pancreatic insufficiency. Delineation of patients with steatorrhea secondary to relative colipase deficiency. *Gastroenterology,* 1984, 86/1 (1-7)

New results about the role of lipase, colipase and bile acids in the fat digestion. *Dtsch. Z. Verdau.-Stoffwechselkr.* (Germany, East), 1980, 40/6 (246-252)

Lipases, bile salts and fat digestion: New insights. *Ital. J. Gastroenterol.* (Italy), 1980, 12/2 (140-145)

Congenital pancreatic lipase deficiency. *J. Pediatr.*, 1980, 96/3I (412-416)

Controlled, double-blind multicenter trial of alyophilized total pancreas preparation against placebo in functional digestive disorders. *France Med. Chir. Dig.* (France), 1987, 16/2 (137-141)

Down Syndrome

Effect of an aerobic training on magnesium, trace elements and antioxidant systems in a Down syndrome population. *Magnes Res* (England) Mar 1997, 10 (1) p65-71

Detection of apoptosis in peripheral blood cells of 31 subjects affected by Down syndrome before and after zinc therapy. *Ultrastruct Pathol* Sep-Oct 1997, 21 (5) p449-52

Treatment of functional decline in adults with Down syndrome using selective serotonin-reuptake inhibitor drugs. *J Geriatr Psychiatry Neurol* Jul 1997, 10 (3) p99-104

Screening for the aneuploid fetus. *Obstet Gynecol Clin North Am* Sep 1998, 25 (3) p573-95

Prenatal screening in the first trimester of pregnancy. *Prenat Diagn* (England) Jun 1998, 18 (6) p537-43

Cell-type-specific enhancement of amyloid-beta deposition in a novel presenilin-1 mutation (P117L). *J Neuropathol Exp Neurol* Sep 1998, 57 (9) p831-8

Total cavopulmonary anastomosis (Fontan) in children with Down's syndrome. *Ann Thorac Surg* Aug 1998, 66 (2) p523-6

Early-onset periodontitis associated with Down's syndrome—clinical interventional study. *Ann Periodontol* Jul 1998, 3 (1) p370-80

Morgagni's hernia in infants and children. *Eur J Surg* (Norway) Apr 1998, 164 (4) p275-9

Detection of chromosomal abnormalities, an outcome of ultrasound screening. The Eurofetus Team. *Ann N Y Acad Sci* Jun 18 1998, 847 p136-40

Acute myelogenous leukemia in Down's syndrome: report of a single pediatric institution using a BFM treatment strategy. *Leuk Res* (England) May 1998, 22 (5) p465-72

Fetal heart rate and nuchal translucency in detecting chromosomal abnormalities other than Down syndrome. *Obstet Gynecol* Jul 1998, 92 (1) p68-71

Intestinal atresia and stenosis: a 25-year experience with 277 cases. *Arch Surg* May 1998, 133 (5) p490-6; discussion 496-7

hCG and the free beta-subunit as screening tests for Down syndrome. *Prenat Diagn* (England) Mar 1998, 18 (3) p235-45

Antenatal screening for Down's syndrome. *Health Technol Assess* (England) 1998, 2 (1) pi-iv, 1-112

Antioxidant enzymes and fatty acid status in erythrocytes of Down's syndrome patients. *Clin Chem* May 1998, 44 (5) p924-9

An economic evaluation of first-trimester genetic sonography for prenatal detection of Down syndrome. *Obstet Gynecol* Apr 1998, 91 (4) p535-9

Prospective evaluation of prenatal maternal serum screening for trisomy 18. *Am J Obstet Gyne*col Mar 1998, 178 (3) p446-50

Subtle ultrasonographic anomalies: do they improve the Down syndrome detection rate? *Am J Obstet Gynecol* Mar 1998, 178 (3) p441-5

Prenatal detection of trisomy 21 and 18 from amniotic fluid by quantitative fluorescent polymerase chain reaction. *J Med Genet* (England) Feb 1998, 35 (2) p126-9

Insulin-like growth factor binding protein-3 in the detection of fetal Down syndrome pregnancies. *Obstet Gynecol* Feb 1998, 91 (2) p192-5

Factors in improved survival from paediatric cancer. *Drugs* (New Zealand), 1998, 56/5 (757-765)

Three-dimensional ultrasound evaluation of fetal tooth germs. *Ultrasound in Obstetrics and Gynecology* (UK), 1998, 12/4 (240-243)

Second-trimester maternal serum inhibin A levels in fetal trisomy 18 and Turner syndrome with and without hydrops. *Prenatal Diagnosis* (UK), 1998, 18/10 (1061-1067)

Trends and outcomes in educational placements for children with Down syndrome. *European Journal of Special Needs Education* (UK), 1998, 13/3 (225-237)

Screening for Down's syndrome by fetal nuchal translucency measurement in a high-risk population. *Ultrasound in Obstetrics and Gynecology* (UK), 1998, 12/3 (156-162)

Evolution of an inhibin A ELISA method: Implications for Down's syndrome screening. *Annals of Clinical Biochemistry* (UK), 1998, 35/5 (656-664)

Correlation between down's-syndrome and malformations of pediatric surgical interest. *Journal of Pediatric Surgery,* 1998, 33/9 (1380-1382)

The value of screening for Down's syndrome in a socioeconomically deprived area with a high ethnic population. *British Journal of Obstetrics and Gynaecology* (UK), 1998, 105/8 (855-859)

Congenital disorders sharing oxidative stress and cancer proneness as phenotypic hallmarks: Prospects for joint research in pharmacology. *Medical Hypotheses* (UK), 1998, 51/3 (253-266)

Glucose effects on cognition in adults with Down's syndrome. *Neuropsychology,* 1998, 12/3 (479-484)

The influence of maternal weight correction formulas in Asian Down syndrome screening using alpha-fetoprotein and free beta-human chorionic gonadotropin. *Journal of Maternal-Fetal Investigation*, 1998, 8/2 (66-70)

Rapid and simple prenatal DNA diagnosis of Down's syndrome. *Lancet* (UK), 1998, 352/9121 (9-12)

Atypical background somatic mutant frequencies at the HPRT locus in children and adults with Down syndrome. *Mutat Res* (Netherlands) Jul 17 1998, 403 (1-2) p35-43

Centromeric genotyping and direct analysis of nondisjunction in humans: Down syndrome. *Chromosoma* (Germany) Jun 1998, 107 (3) p166-72

Elucidating the mechanisms of paternal non-disjunction of chromosome 21 in humans. *Hum Mol Genet* (England) Aug 1998, 7 (8) p1221-7

The 'Severe Impairment Battery': assessing cognitive ability in adults with Down syndrome. *Br J Clin Psychol* (England) May 1998, 37 (Pt 2) p213-6

Prenatal diagnosis with use of fetal cells isolated from maternal blood: five-color fluorescent in situ hybridization analysis on flow-sorted cells for chromosomes X, Y, 13, 18, and 21. *Am J Obstet Gynecol* Jul 1998, 179 (1) p203-9

Adoption and fostering of babies with Down syndrome: a cohort of 593 cases. *Prenat Diagn* (England) May 1998, 18 (5) p437-45

New triple screen test for Down syndrome: combined urine analytes and serum AFP. *J Matern Fetal Med* May-Jun 1998, 7 (3) p111-4

Vitamin E and Alzheimer's disease in subjects with Down syndrome. *Journal of Mental Deficiency Research* 1988 Dec Vol 32(6) 479-484

Behavioral disorders, learning disabilities and megavitamin therapy. *Adolescence* 1987 Fal Vol 22(87) 729-738

Macrocytosis and cognitive decline in Down syndrome. *British Journal of Psychiatry* 1986 Dec Vol 149 797-798

Treatment approaches in Down syndrome: A review. *Australia & New Zealand Journal of Developmental Disabilities*

A double blind study of vitamin B_6 in Down syndrome infants: I. Clinical and biochemical results. *Journal of Mental Deficiency Research* 1985 Sep Vol 29(3) 233-240

A double blind study of vitamin B_6 in Down syndrome infants: II. Cortical auditory evoked potentials. *Journal of Mental Deficiency Research* 1985 Sep Vol 29(3) 241-246

Xylose absorption in Down syndrome. *Journal of Mental Deficiency Research* 1985 Jun Vol 29(2) 173-177

Nutritional aspects of Down syndrome with special reference to the nervous system. *British Journal of Psychiatry* 1984 Aug Vol 145 115-120

Children's mental retardation study is attacked: A closer look. *International Journal of Biosocial Research* 1982 Vol 3(2) 75-86

Effects of nutritional supplementation on IQ and certain other variables associated with Down syndrome. *American Journal of Mental Deficiency* 1983 Sep Vol 88(2) 214-217

Vitamin A and carotene values of institutionalized mentally retarded subjects with and without Down syndrome. *Journal of Mental Deficiency Research* 1977 Mar Vol 21(1) 63-74

Sodium-dependent glutamate binding in senile dementia. *Neurobiology of Aging* 1987 May-Jun Vol 8(3) 219-223

Alzheimer-like neurotransmitter deficits in adult Down syndrome brain tissue. *Journal of Neurology, Neurosurgery & Psychiatry* 1987 Jun Vol 50(6) 775-778

A report on phosphatidylcholine therapy in a Down Syndrome child. *Psychological Reports* 1986 Feb Vol 58(1) 207-217

Emphysema and Chronic Obstructive Pulmonary Disease

The effect of inhaled glucocorticosteroids in emphysema due to alpha1-antitrypsin deficiency. *Respir Med* (England) May 1997, 91 (5) p275-9

[Mechanism of short-term improvement in exercise tolerance after lung volume reduction surgery for severe emphysema] *Nihon Kokyuki Gakkai Zasshi* (Japan) Apr 1998, 36 (4) p323-9

Outcome of Medicare patients with emphysema selected for, but denied, a lung volume reduction operation. *Ann Thorac Surg* Aug 1998, 66 (2) p331-6

The effect of interleukin-8 and granulocyte macrophage colony stimulating factor on the response of neutrophils to formyl methionyl leucyl phenylalanine. *Biochim Biophys Acta* (Netherlands) Aug 14 1998, 1407 (2) p146-54

Nonuniformity of diffusing capacity from small alveolar gas samples is increased in smokers. *Can Respir J* (Canada) Mar-Apr 1998, 5 (2) p101-8

Prediction of individual response to postnatal dexamethasone in ventilator dependent preterm infants. *Arch Dis Child Fetal Neonatal Ed* (England) May 1998, 78 (3) pF199-203

Does lung transplantation prolong life? A comparison of survival with and without transplantation. *J Heart Lung Transplant* May 1998, 17 (5) p511-6

Preferential binding of lysozyme to elastic fibres in pulmonary emphysema. *Thorax* (England) Mar 1998, 53 (3) p193-6

Improved lung function and quality of life following increased elastic recoil after lung volume reduction surgery in emphysema. *Respir Med* (England) Apr 1998, 92 (4) p653-8

Lung volume reduction surgery for emphysema. A review. *J Cardiovasc Surg* (Torino) (Italy) Apr 1998, 39 (2) p237-43

Serial lung function and elastic recoil 2 years after lung volume reduction surgery for emphysema. *Chest* Jun 1998, 113 (6) p1497-506

Return to work after lung transplantation. *J Heart Lung Transplant* Apr 1998, 17 (4) p430-6

Bilateral thoracoscopic stapled volume reduction for bullous vs diffuse emphysema. *Surg Endosc* (Germany) Apr 1998, 12 (4) p338-41

The treatment of unrelated disorders in patients with chronic medical diseases [see comments] *N Engl J Med* May 21 1998, 338 (21) p1516-20

Lung volume reduction surgery: an analysis of hospital costs. *Chest* Apr 1998, 113 (4) p896-9

Comparison of short-term functional outcomes following unilateral and bilateral lung volume reduction surgery. *Chest* Apr 1998, 113 (4) p890-5

Treatment by VATS of giant bullous emphysema: results. *Eur J Cardiothorac Surg* (Netherlands) Jan 1998, 13 (1) p66-70

Lung Transplantation for COPD. *Chest* Apr 1998, 113 (4 Suppl) p269S-276S

Morphologic grading of the emphysematous lung and its relation to improvement after lung volume reduction surgery. *Ann Thorac Surg* Mar 1998, 65 (3) p793-9

Relation between preoperative inspiratory lung resistance and the outcome of lung-volume-reduction surgery for emphysema. *N Engl J Med* Apr 23 1998, 338 (17) p1181-5

Lobectomy combined with volume reduction for patients with lung cancer and advanced emphysema. *J Thorac Cardiovasc Surg* Mar 1998, 115 (3) p681-8

Rate of FEV1 change following lung volume reduction surgery. *Chest* Mar 1998, 113 (3) p652-9

MR analysis of lung volume and thoracic dimensions in patients with emphysema before and after lung volume reduction surgery. *AJR Am J Roentgenol* Mar 1998, 170 (3) p707-14

Lung reduction operation and resection of pulmonary nodules in patients with severe emphysema. *Ann Thorac Surg* Feb 1998, 65 (2) p314-8

Wild-type alpha 1-antitrypsin is in the canonical inhibitory conformation. *J Mol Biol* (England) Jan 23 1998, 275 (3) p419-25

Preoperative screening for lung volume reduction surgery: usefulness of combining thin-section CT with physiologic assessment. *AJR Am J Roentgenol* Feb 1998, 170 (2) p309-14

Lung resection in pediatric patients. *Pediatr Surg Int* (Germany) Jan 1998, 13 (1) p10-3

Lobectomy improves ventilatory function in selected patients with severe COPD. *Ann Thorac Surg* Sep 1998, 66 (3) p898-902

Safety and cost-effectiveness of MIDCABG in high-risk CABG patients. *Ann Thorac Surg* Sep 1998, 66 (3) p1002-7

The effects of nebulised isotonic saline and terbutaline on breathlessness in severe chronic obstructive pulmonary disease (COPD). *Aust N Z J Med* (Australia) Jun 1998, 28 (3) p322-6

Effects of theophylline and ipratropium bromide on exercise performance in patients with stable chronic obstructive pulmonary disease. *Thorax* (England) Apr 1998, 53 (4) p269-73

A multivariate model for predicting respiratory status in patients with chronic obstructive pulmonary disease. *J Gen Intern Med* Jul 1998, 13 (7) p462-8

Using nasal intermittent positive pressure ventilation on a general respiratory ward. *J R Coll Physicians Lond* (England) May-Jun 1998, 32 (3) p219-24

Determination of functional residual capacity (FRC) by multibreath nitrogen washout in a lung model and in mechanically ventilated patients. Accuracy depends on continuous dynamic compensation for changes of gas sampling delay time. *Intensive Care Med* May 1998, 24 (5) p487-93

[Knowledge about drugs used by adult patients with asthma for self-treatment] *Ned Tijdschr Geneeskd* (Netherlands) Mar 28 1998, 142 (13) p711-5

No effects of high-dose omeprazole in patients with severe airway hyperresponsiveness and (a)symptomatic gastro-oesophageal reflux. *Eur Respir J* (Denmark) May 1998, 11 (5) p1070-4

Domiciliary nocturnal intermittent positive pressure ventilation in patients with respiratory failure due to severe COPD: long-term follow up and effect on survival. *Thorax* (England) Jun 1998, 53 (6) p495-8

Randomised controlled trial of inhaled corticosteroids in patients with chronic obstructive pulmonary disease. *Thorax* (England) Jun 1998, 53 (6) p477-82

Effect of beta-blockade on mortality among high-risk and low-risk patients after myocardial infarctio [see comments] *N Engl J Med* Aug 20 1998, 339 (8) p489-97

Rehabilitation of patients admitted to a respiratory intensive care unit. *Arch Phys Med Rehabil* Jul 1998, 79 (7) p849-54

TQI in the Albuquerque Veterans Affairs Medical Center's long-term oxygen therapy program. *Jt Comm J Qual Improv* Apr 1998, 24 (4) p203-11

The need for acute, subacute and nonacute care at 105 general hospital sites in Ontario. Joint Policy and Planning Committee Non-Acute Hospitalization Project Working Group. *CMAJ* (Canada) May 19 1998, 158 (10) p1289-96

Pubovaginal sling using polypropylene mesh and Vesica bone anchors. *Urology* May 1998, 51 (5) p708-13

The self-inflating bulb to detect esophageal intubation during emergency airway management. *Anesthesiology* Apr 1998, 88 (4) p898-902

Effects of specialized community nursing care in patients with chronic obstructive pulmonary disease. *Heart Lung* Mar-Apr 1998, 27 (2) p109-20

Development of a shortened version of the Breathing Problems Questionnaire suitable for use in a pulmonary rehabilitation clinic: a purpose-specific, disease-specific questionnaire. *Qual Life Res* (England) Apr 1998, 7 (3) p227-33

Independent association between acute renal failure and mortality following cardiac surgery. *Am J Med* Apr 1998, 104 (4) p343-8

Multicenter review of preoperative risk factors for endarterectomy for asymptomatic carotid artery stenosis. *Stroke* Apr 1998, 29 (4) p750-3

Noninvasive mechanical ventilation in the weaning of patients with respiratory failure due to chronic obstructive pulmonary disease. A randomized, controlled trial. *Ann Intern Med* May 1 1998, 128 (9) p721-8

The accuracy of substituted judgments in patients with terminal diagnoses. *Ann Intern Med* Apr 15 1998, 128 (8) p621-9

Vitamin D binding protein variants and the risk of COPD. *Am J Respir Crit Care Med* Mar 1998, 157 (3 Pt 1) p957-61

[The importance of training intensity for improving endurance capacity of patients with chronic obstructive pulmonary disease] *Dtsch Med Wochenschr* (Germany) Feb 13 1998, 123 (7) p174-8

Clinical, physiological and radiological features of asthma with incomplete reversibility of airflow obstruction compared with those of COPD. *Canadian Respiratory Journal* (Canada), 1998, 5/4 (270-277)

Alteration in nutritional status and diaphragm muscle function. *Reproduction Nutrition Development* (France), 1998, 38/2 (175-180)

Muscle and serum magnesium in pulmonary intensive care unit patients. *Crit Care Med* Aug 1988, 16 (8) p751-60

Fluid and electrolyte considerations in diuretic therapy for hypertensive patients with chronic obstructive pulmonary disease. *Arch Intern Med* Jan 1986, 146 (1) p129-33

Safety and effectiveness of ticarcillin plus clavulanate potassium in treatment of lower respiratory tract infections. *Am J Med* Nov 29 1985, 79 (5B) p78-80

Frequently nebulized beta-agonists for asthma: effects on serum electrolytes. *Ann Emerg Med* Nov 1992, 21 (11) p1337-42

Effect of nebulized albuterol on serum potassium and cardiac rhythm in patients with asthma or chronic obstructive pulmonary disease. *Pharmacotherapy* Nov-Dec 1994, 14 (6) p729-33

The intrabronchial microbial flora in chronic bronchitis patients: a target for *N*-acetylcysteine therapy? *Eur Respir J* (Denmark) Jan 1994, 7 (1) p94-101

[The influence of *N*-acetylcysteine on chemiluminescence of granulocytes in peripheral blood of patients with chronic bronchitis]. *Pneumonol Alergol Pol* (Poland) 1993, 61 (11-12)

Effects of coenzyme Q10 administration on pulmonary function and exercise performance in patients with chronic lung diseases. *Clin Investig* (Germany) 1993, 71 (8 Suppl) pS162-6

Protection by *N*-acetylcysteine of the histopathological and cytogenetical damage produced by exposure of rats to cigarette smoke. *Cancer Lett* (Netherlands) Jun 15 1992, 64 (2) p123-31

Investigation of the protective effects of the antioxidants ascorbate, cysteine, and dapsone on the phagocyte-mediated oxidative inactivation of human alpha-1-protease inhibitor in vitro. *Am Rev Respir Dis* Nov 1985, 132 (5) p1049-54

The role of dornase alfa (Pulmozyme) in the treatment of cystic fibrosis. *Annals of Pharmacotherapy*, 1996, 30/6 (656-661)

Inhalation therapy with recombinant human deoxyribonuclease I Gonda I (Pulmozyme). *Advanced Drug Delivery Reviews* (Netherlands), 1996, 19/1 (37-46)

Aerosolized dornase alpha (rhDNase-Pulmozyme) in cystic fibrosis. *Journal of Clinical Pharmacy and Therapeutics* (UK), 1995, 20/6

New pharmacologic approaches: rhDNase. *Revue de Pneumologie Clinique* (France), 1995, 51/3 (193-200)

Taurine and serine supplementation modulates the metabolic response to tumor necrosis factor alpha in rats fed a low protein diet. *J. Nutr.*, 1992, 122/7 (1369-1375)

L-Carnitine and its role in medicine: A current consideration of its pharmacokinetics, its role in fatty acid metabolism and its use in ischaemic cardiac disease and primary and secondary *L-carnitine* deficiencies. *Epitheorese Klinikes Farmakologias kai Farmakokinetikes* (Greece), 1996, 14/1 (11-64)

Esophageal Reflux (Heartburn)

Research of non-specific hyperreactivity of upper airways in subjects with gastro-esophageal reflux (G.E.R.): preliminary reports. *Allergol Immunopathol* (Madr) (Spain) Nov-Dec 1997, 25 (6) p266-71

[Gastro-esophageal reflux successfully treated with transgastrostomal jejunal tube feeding]. *Nippon Ronen Igakkai Zasshi* (Japan) Jan 1997, 34 (1) p60-4

Esophageal reflux after total or proximal gastrectomy in patients with adenocarcinoma of the gastric cardia. *Am J Gastroenterol* Aug 1997, 92 (8) p1347-50

Assessment of non-acid esophageal reflux : comparison between long-term reflux aspiration test and fiberoptic bilirubin monitoring. *Dis Esophagus* (Scotland) Jan 1997, 10 (1) p24-8

Gastro-esophageal reflux in asthmatic patients. *Tuberculosis and Respiratory Diseases* (South Korea) 1997, 44/4 (836-843)

The medical treatment of gastro-esophageal reflux: Combining effectiveness, ethical considerations and cost. *Acta Endoscopica* (France) 1997, 27/3 (221-238)

Occurence of gastro-esophageal reflux and the efficiency of antireflux treatment in reactive airway diseases of children. *Medical Science Monitor* (Poland) 1997, 3/4 (485-488)

Prevalence and characteristics of gastro-esophageal reflux in asthmatic patients. *European Journal of Internal Medicine* (Italy) 1997, 8/2 (107-111)

Gastroesophageal reflux (I). Resistance factors in medical treatment of esophagitis by esophageal reflux. *Presse Medicale* (France) 1997, 26/25 (1216-1220)

Chronic laryngitis and gastro esophageal reflux. *Medizinische Welt (Med. Welt)* (Germany) 1997, 48/5 (183-185)

First line treatment with omeprazole provides an effective and superior alternative strategy in the management of dyspepsia compared to antacid/alginate liquid: a multicentre study in general practice. *Aliment Pharmacol Ther* (England) Feb 1998, 12 (2) p147-57

Esophageal impairment in adult celiac disease with steatorrhea. *Am J Gastroenterol* Aug 1998, 93 (8) p1243-9

Outcomes of atypical symptoms attributed to gastroesophageal reflux treated by laparoscopic fundoplication. *Surgery* Jul 1998, 124 (1) p28-32

Helicobacter pylori colonization does not influence the symptomatic response to prokinetic agents in patients with functional dyspepsia. *J Gastroenterol Hepatol* (Australia) May 1998, 13 (5) p500-4

Pneumatic balloon dilation in achalasia: a prospective comparison of balloon distention time. *Am J Gastroenterol* Jul 1998, 93 (7) p1064-7

Gastrin, cholecystokinin, and somatostatin in a laboratory experiment of patients with functional dyspepsia. *Psychosom Med* May-Jun 1998, 60 (3) p331-7

An analysis of operations for gastroesophageal reflux disease: identifying the important technical elements. *Arch Surg* Jun 1998, 133 (6) p600-6; discussion 606-7

Pharmacokinetic profile of cisapride 20 mg after once- and twice-daily dosing. *Clin Ther* Mar-Apr 1998, 20 (2) p292-8

The management of acid-related dyspepsia in general practice: a comparison of an omeprazole versus an antacid-alginate/ranitidine management strategy. Complete Research Group. *Aliment Pharmacol Ther* (England) Mar 1998, 12 (3) p263-71

The effects of low doses of ranitidine on intragastric acidity in healthy men. *Aliment Pharmacol Ther* (England) Mar 1998, 12 (3) p255-61

Is cholecystectomy effective treatment for symptomatic gallstones? Clinical outcome after long-term follow-up. *Ann R Coll Surg Engl* (England) Jan 1998, 80 (1) p25-32

One-week omeprazole treatment in the diagnosis of gastro-oesophageal reflux disease. *Scand J Gastroenterol* (Norway) Jan 1998, 33 (1) p15-20

Functional adaptation after extensive small bowel resection in humans. *European Journal of Gastroenterology and Hepatology* (UK) 1994, 6/3 (197-202)

Milk hypersensitivity: RAST studies using new antigens generated by pepsin hydrolysis of beta-lactoglobulin. *Annals of Allergy* 1980, 45/4 (242-245)

Racially determined abnormal essential fatty acid and prostaglandin metabolism and food allergies linked to autoimmune, inflammatory, and psychiatric disorders among Coastal British Columbia Indians. *Medical Hypotheses* (UK) 1988, 25/2 (103-109)

Adverse reactions to food constituents: Allergy, intolerance, and autoimmunity *Canadian Journal of Physiology and Pharmacology* (Canada) 1997, 75/4 (241-254)

Food allergies. I. Pathogenesis, clinical findings and diagnosis. *Schweizerische Medizinische Wochenschrift* (Switzerland) 1985, 115/41 (1428-1436)

Gastrointestinal defense mechanisms: Their role in the pathogenesis of food allergy *Immunology and Allergy Practice* 1983, 5/4 (116-123)

Prevention of esophageal cancer: the nutrition intervention trials in Linxian, China. Linxian Nutrition Intervention Trials Study Group. *Cancer Res.* 1994 Apr 1. 54(7 Suppl). p2029s-2031s

Effects of vitamin/mineral supplementation on the proliferation of esophageal squamous epithelium in Linxian, China. *Cancer Epidemiol Biomarkers Prev.* 1994 Apr-May. 3(3). P 277-9

[Preliminary report on the results of nutrition prevention trials of cancer and other common diseases among residents in Linxian, China] *Chung Hua Chung Liu Tsa Chih.* 1993 May. 15(3). p165-81

Chemoprevention of oral leukoplakia and chronic esophagitis in an area of high incidence of oral and esophageal cancer. *Ann Epidemiol.* 1993 May. 3(3). p225-34

[Clinical aspects, diagnosis and treatment of esophageal spasm] *Grud Serdechnososudistaia Khir.* 1991 Jun. (6). p57-60

Association of esophageal cytological abnormalities with vitamin and lipotrope deficiencies in populations at risk for esophageal cancer. *Anticancer Res.* (Greece), 1988, 8/4 (711-716)

The effect of gamma-linolenic acid on clinical status, red cell fatty acid composition and membrane microviscosity in infants with atopic dermatitis. SO:*Drugs Exp Clin Res.* 1994. 20(2). p77-84

Fatty acid compositions of plasma lipids in atopic dermatitis/asthma patients. SO: *Arerugi.* 1994 Jan. 43(1). p37-43

Possible immunologic involvement of antioxidants in cancer prevention. *Am J Clin Nutr.* 1995 Dec. 62 (6 Suppl). p1477S-1482S

Estrogen Replacement Therapy

See references under Female Hormone Modulation Therapy.

Female Hormone Modulation Therapy

Long-term longitudinal measurements of plasma dehydroepiandrosterone sulfate in normal men. *J Clin Endocrinol Metab* 1992 Oct;75(4):1002-4

Estrogenic effects on memory in women. *Ann N Y Acad Sci* Nov 14 1994, 743 p213-30; discussion 230-1

Serum gonadotropins and steroid hormones and the development of ovarian cancer. *JAMA* 1995 Dec 27;274(24):1926-30

Risks of menopausal androgen supplementation. *Semin Reprod Endocrinol* 1998, 16 (2) p145-52

Androgen metabolism and the menopause. *Semin Reprod Endocrinol* 1998, 16 (2) p111-5

Contribution of BRCA1 Mutations to Ovarian Cancer. *The New England Journal of Medicine*, April 17, 1997, Vol. 336, No. 16

Hormonal therapy in the management of premenstrual syndrome. *J Am Board Fam Pract* Sep-Oct 1998, 11 (5) p378-81

Cognitive therapy for premenstrual syndrome: a controlled trial. *J Psychosom Res* Oct 1998, 45 (4) p307-18

Premenstrual syndrome. *Psychiatr Clin North Am* Sep 1998, 21 (3) p577-90

Premenstrual syndrome: diagnosis and intervention. *Nurse Pract* Sep 1998, 23 (9) p40, 45, 49-52 passim

Insulin-like growth factor-1 and insulin-like growth factor-binding protein-3 in women with premenstrual syndrome. *Fertil Steril* Dec 1998, 70 (6) p1077-80

Premenstrual syndrome: diagnosis and treatment experiences. *J Womens Health* Sep 1998, 7 (7) p893-907

A double-blind trial of four medications to treat severe premenstrual syndrome. *Int J Gynaecol Obstet* Jul 1998, 62 (1) p63-7

Interactive case challenge. Dysphoric disorders in women: a case of premenstrual syndrome. *Medscape Womens Health* Oct 1998, 3 (5) p2

Differentiating between natural progesterone and synthetic progestins: clinical implications for premenstrual syndrome and perimenopause management. *Compr Ther* Jun-Jul 1998, 24 (6-7) p336-9

Calcium carbonate and the premenstrual syndrome: effects on premenstrual and menstrual symptoms. Premenstrual Syndrome Study Group. *Am J Obstet Gynecol* Aug 1998, 179 (2) p444-52

Coping with anger and the premenstrual syndrome. *Wien Klin Wochenschr* May 22 1998, 110 (10) p370-5

Citalopram increases pregnanolone sensitivity in patients with premenstrual syndrome: an open trial. *Psychoneuroendocrinology* Jan 1998, 23 (1) p73-88

Allopregnanolone in women with premenstrual syndrome. *Horm Metab Res* Apr 1998, 30 (4) p227-30

Pituitary-adrenal hormones and testosterone across the menstrual cycle in women with premenstrual syndrome and controls. *Biol Psychiatry* Jun 15 1998, 43 (12) p897-903

Treatment strategies for premenstrual syndrome. *Am Fam Physician* Jul 1998, 58 (1) p183-92, 197-8

Premenstrual syndrome: comparison between different methods to diagnose cyclicity using daily symptom ratings. *Acta Obstet Gynecol Scand* May 1998, 77 (5) p551-7

Luteal-phase estradiol relates to symptom severity in patients with premenstrual syndrome. *J Clin Endocrinol Metab* Jun 1998, 83 (6) p1988-92

Incidence of premenstrual syndrome and remedy usage: a national probability sample study. *Altern Ther Health Med* May 1998, 4 (3) p75-9

Circadian changes in body temperature during the menstrual cycle of healthy adult females and patients suffering from premenstrual syndrome. *Int J Clin Pharmacol Res* 1997, 17 (4) p155-64

Elevations of complex partial epileptic-like experiences during increased geomagnetic activity for women reporting "premenstrual syndrome." *Percept Mot Skills* Feb 1998, 86 (1) p240-2

Patients with premenstrual syndrome have a different sensitivity to a neuroactive steroid during the menstrual cycle compared to control subjects. *Neuroendocrinology* Feb 1998, 67 (2) p126-38

Differential behavioral effects of gonadal steroids in women with and in those without premenstrual syndrome [see comments] *N Engl J Med* Jan 22 1998, 338 (4) p209-16

Patients with premenstrual syndrome have reduced sensitivity to midazolam compared to control subjects. *Neuropsychopharmacology* Dec 1997, 17 (6) p370-81

Premenstrual syndrome: evidence for symptom stability across cycles. *Am J Psychiatry* Dec 1997, 154 (12) p1741-6

Sleep pattern changes in menstrual cycles of women with premenstrual syndrome: a preliminary study. *Am J Obstet Gynecol* Sep 1997, 177 (3) p554-8

Progesterone metabolite allopregnanolone in women with premenstrual syndrome. *Obstet Gynecol* Nov 1997, 90 (5) p709-14

Intermittent luteal phase sertraline treatment of dysphoric premenstrual syndrome. *J Clin Psychiatry* Sep 1997, 58 (9) p399-402

Effect of progesterone therapy on arginine vasopressin and atrial natriuretic factor in premenstrual syndrome. *Clin Invest Med* Aug 1997, 20 (4) p211-23

Menstrual migraines: etiology, treatment, and relationship to premenstrual syndrome. *Curr Opin Obstet Gynecol* Jun 1997, 9 (3) p154-9

Premenstrual syndrome: current perspectives on treatment and etiology. *Curr Opin Obstet Gynecol* Jun 1997, 9 (3) p147-53

Effects of a yeast-based dietary supplementation on premenstrual syndrome. A double-blind placebo-controlled study. *Gynecol Obstet Invest* 1997, 43 (2) p120-4

Perceptual and coping processes across the menstrual cycle: an investigation in a premenstrual syndrome clinic and a community sample. *Behav Med* Winter 1997, 22 (4) p152-9

Effect of positive reframing and social support on perception of perimenstrual changes among women with premenstrual syndrome. *Health Care Women Int* Mar-Apr 1997, 18 (2) p175-93

[Premenstrual syndrome in France: epidemiology and therapeutic effectiveness of 1000 mg of micronized purified flavonoid fraction in 1473 gynecological patients]. *Contracept Fertil Sex* Jan 1997, 25 (1) p85-90

Patients with premenstrual syndrome have decreased saccadic eye velocity compared to control subjects. *Biological Psychiatry*, 1998, 44/8 (755-764)

An update on the treatment of premenstrual syndrome. *American Journal of Managed Care*, 1998, 4/2 (266-274)

Clinical significance of premenstrual syndrome and its treatment possibilities. *Lege Artis Medicine* 1998, 8/7-8 (486-492)

Hormonal treatments for premenstrual syndrome. *Drugs of Today* 1998, 34/7 (603-610)

Anger coping and premenstrual syndrome. *Wiener Klinische Wochenschrift* 1998, 110/10 (370-375)

Exercise is linked to reductions in anxiety but not premenstrual syndrome in women with prospectively-assessed symptoms. *Psychology, Health and Medicine* 1998, 3/2 (211-222)

Variation in body weight and water during the menstrual cycle in patients with premenstrual syndrome. *Endocrinology and Metabolism* 1997, 4/2 (135-140)

The frequency of premenstrual syndrome in the rural region of Eskisehir. *Jinekoloji ve Obstetri Bulteni* 1997, 6/4 (157-162)

Psychological profile of a sample of women suffering from premenstrual syndrome. *Revista de Psiquiatria de la Facultad de Medicina de Barcelona* 1997, 24/5 (126-132)

Hormonal therapy in the management of premenstrual syndrome. *J Am Board Fam Pract* Sep-Oct 1998, 11 (5) p378-81

Role of androgens in surgical menopause. *Am J Obstet Gynecol* Mar 1999, 180 (3 Pt 2) p325-7

Psychosexual effects of menopause: role of androgens. *Am J Obstet Gynecol* Mar 1999, 180 (3 Pt 2) p319-24

Vasomotor flushes in menopausal women. *Am J Obstet Gynecol* Mar 1999, 180 (3 Pt 2) p312-6

Management of endometrial hyperplasia: a retrospective analysis. *J Med Assoc Thai* Jan 1999, 82 (1) p33-9

Isoflavones from red clover improve systemic arterial compliance but not plasma lipids in menopausal women. *J Clin Endocrinol Metab* Mar 1999, 84 (3) p895-8

Menopausal status and distensibility of the common carotid artery. *Arterioscler Thromb Vasc Biol* Mar 1999, 19 (3) p713-7

Socioeconomic status and determinants of hemostatic function in healthy women. *Arterioscler Thromb Vasc Biol* Mar 1999, 19 (3) p485-92

Hormone replacement therapy: can nurses help? *Presse Med* Feb 20 1999, 28 (7) p323-9

Hormonal therapy for menopause and ovarian cancer in a collaborative re-analysis of European studies. *Int J Cancer* Mar 15 1999, 80 (6) p848-51

Effect of lifetime occupational physical activity on indices of bone mineral status in healthy postmenopausal women. *Calcif Tissue Int* Feb 1999, 64 (2) p112-6,

The menopause. *Lancet* Feb 13 1999, 353 (9152) p571-80

Effect of menopause and different combined estradiol-progestin regimens on basal and growth hormone-releasing hormone-stimulated serum growth hormone, insulin-like growth factor-1, insulin-like growth factor binding protein (IGFBP)-1, and IGFBP-3 levels. *Fertil Steril* Feb 1999, 71 (2) p261-7

Osteoporosis: current modes of prevention and treatment. *J Am Acad Orthop Surg* Jan 1999, 7 (1) p19-31

Disappearance of endogenous luteinizing hormone is prolonged in postmenopausal women. *J Clin Endocrinol Metab* Feb 1999, 84 (2) p688-94

Estrogen supplementation attenuates glucocorticoid and catecholamine responses to mental stress in perimenopausal women. *J Clin Endocrinol Metab Feb* 1999, 84 (2) p606-10

Perimenopausal weight gain and progression of breast cancer precursors. *Cancer Detect* Prev 1999, 23 (1) p31-6

Memory functioning at menopause: impact of age in ovariectomized women. Gynecol *Obstet Invest* 1999, 47 (1) p29-36

Prospective study of factors influencing the onset of natural menopause. *J Clin Epidemiol* Dec 1998, 51 (12) p1271-6

Hormone replacement therapy: cardiovascular benefits for aging women. *Coron Artery Dis* 1998, 9 (12) p789-93

[An exploratory study of the association between lipid profile and bone mineral density in menopausal women in a Campinas reference hospital]. *Cad Saude Publica* Oct-Dec 1998, 14 (4) p779-86

The influence of sex hormones on obesity across the female life span. *J Womens Health* Dec 1998, 7 (10) p1247-56

Is there an association between hormone replacement therapy and breast cancer? *J Womens Health* Dec 1998, 7 (10) p1231-46

Declining fecundity and ovarian ageing in natural fertility populations. *Maturitas* Oct 12 1998, 30 (2) p127-36

Age at menopause as a marker of reproductive ageing. *Maturitas* Oct 12 1998, 30 (2) p119-25

Ovarian ageing and the general biology of senescence. *Maturitas* Oct 12 1998, 30 (2) p105-11

Premature ovarian failure. *Endocrinol Metab Clin North Am* Dec 1998, 27 (4) p989-1006

Women and menopause: beliefs, attitudes, and behaviors. The North American Menopause Society 1997 Menopause Survey. *Menopause Winter* 1998, 5 (4) p197-202

Menopausal status: subjectively and objectively defined. *J Psychosom Obstet Gynaecol* Sep 1998, 19 (3) p165-73

Hormone replacement therapy and urinary prostaglandins in postmenopausal women. *Maturitas* Sep 20 1998, 30 (1) p79-83

Relationship between dermato-physiological changes and hormonal status in pre-, peri-, and postmenopausal women. *Maturitas* Sep 20 1998, 30 (1) p55-62

Phyto-oestrogen excretion and rate of bone loss in postmenopausal women. *Eur J Clin Nutr* Nov 1998, 52 (11) p850-5

Body composition characteristics after menopause. *Coll Antropol* Dec 1998, 22 (2) p393-402

Cervical cytology in menopausal women at high risk for endometrial disease. *Eur J Cancer Prev* Apr 1998, 7 (2) p149-52

Hormone replacement therapy and breast cancer: revisiting the issues. *J Am Pharm Assoc* Nov-Dec 1998, 38 (6) p738-44; quiz 744-6

Menopause. Hormone substitution therapy and prevention of cardiovascular risk. *Minerva Ginecol* Jul-Aug 1998, 50 (7-8) p329-31

Estradiol as an antioxidant: incompatible with its physiological concentrations and function. *J Lipid Res* Nov 1998, 39 (11) p2111-8

Why has menopause become a public health problem? *Therapie* Jan-Feb 1998, 53 (1) p49-59

Biological bases of premature ovarian failure. *Reprod Fertil Dev* 1998, 10 (1) p73-8

Menopause: lessons from anthropology. *Psychosom Med* Jul-Aug 1998, 60 (4) p410-9

Postmenopausal sexual functioning: a case study. *Int J Fertil Womens Med* Mar-Apr 1998, 43 (2) p122-8

[Psychosexual problems in menopause]. *Minerva Ginecol* Mar 1998, 50 (3) p77-81

Risks of menopausal androgen supplementation. *Semin Reprod Endocrinol* 1998, 16 (2) p145-52

[Female sex hormones increase the risk of breast cancer]. *Tidsskr Nor Laegeforen* Aug 20 1998, 118 (19) p2969-74

Alternative aging. *AWHONN Lifelines* Jun 1998, 2 (3) p55-8

Menopause and tear function: the influence of prolactin and sex hormones on human tear production. *Cornea* Jul 1998, 17 (4) p353-8

A review of the effectiveness of Cimicifuga racemosa (black cohosh) for the symptoms of menopause. *J Womens Health* Jun 1998, 7 (5) p525-9

Usual consumption of plant foods containing phytoestrogens and sex hormone levels in postmenopausal women in Wisconsin. *Nutr Cancer* 1998, 30 (3) p207-12

Insulin-like growth factor-I and bone mineral density. *Bone Jul* 1998, 23 (1) p13-6

Association of diet and other lifestyle with onset of menopause in Japanese women. *Maturitas* Jun 3 1998, 29 (2) p105-13

Facial wrinkling in postmenopausal women. Effects of smoking status and hormone replacement therapy. *Maturitas* May 20 1998, 29 (1) p75-86

Methodological problems in the study of sexuality and the menopause. *Maturitas* May 20 1998, 29 (1) p51-60

Concentration of sex steroids in adipose tissue after menopause. *Steroids* May-Jun 1998, 63 (5-6) p319-21

[Treatment of neurovegetative menopausal symptoms with a phytotherapeutic agent]. *Minerva Ginecol* May 1998, 50 (5) p207-11

Alternative treatments for menopausal symptoms. Systematic review of scientific and lay literature [published erratum appears in *Can Fam Physician* 1998 Aug;44:1998]. *Can Fam Physician* Jun 1998, 44 p1299-308

Alternative treatments for menopausal symptoms. Qualitative study of women's experiences. *Can Fam Physician* Jun 1998, 44 p1271-6

"Natural" hormone replacement therapy and dietary supplements used in the treatment of menopausal symptoms. *Lippincotts Prim Care Pract* May-Jun 1998, 2 (3) p292-302

The controversy of hormone-replacement therapy in breast cancer survivors. *Oncol Nurs Forum* May 1998, 25 (4) p699-706; quiz 707-8

Relationship of serum sex steroid levels and bone turnover markers with bone mineral density in men and women: a key role for bioavailable estrogen. *J Clin Endocrinol Metab* Jul 1998, 83 (7) p2266-74

A new alternative to estrogen: raloxifene. *Health News* Jun 25 1998, 4 (8) p4

Estriol: safety and efficacy. *Altern Med Rev* Apr 1998, 3 (2) p101-13

Cognitive function in nondemented older women who took estrogen after menopause. *Neurology* Feb 1998, 50 (2) p368-73

[Conversion of androstenedione in the lymphocytes infiltrating the breast tumor tissue]. *Biull Eksp Biol Med* Oct 1997, 124 (10) p440-3

Why do women doctors in the UK take hormone replacement therapy? *J Epidemiol Community Health* Aug 1997, 51 (4) p373-7

Evidence for age-related differences in the fatty acid composition of human adipose tissue, independent of diet. *Eur J Clin Nutr* Sep 1997, 51 (9) p619-24

Estrogen replacement therapy and longitudinal decline in visual memory. A possible protective effect? *Neurology* Dec 1997, 49 (6) p1491-7

[Estrogen replacement therapy: myth or reality?] *Contracept Fertil Sex* (France) Oct 1997, 25 (10) p793-7

The effect of estrogen replacement therapy on cognitive function in women: a critical review of the literature. *J Clin Epidemiol* (England) Nov 1997, 50 (11) p1249-64

Estrogen replacement therapy and mortality among older women. The study of osteoporotic fractures. *Arch Intern Med* Oct 27 1997, 157 (19) p2181-7

Dietary soy protein and estrogen replacement therapy improve cardiovascular risk factors and decrease aortic cholesteryl ester content in ovariectomized cynomolgus monkeys. *Metabolism* Jun 1997, 46 (6) p698-705

Pharmacologic approaches to cognitive deficits in Alzheimer's disease. *J Clin Psychiatry* 1998, 59 Suppl 9 p22-7

Medical and interventional therapy of coronary artery disease in women. *J La State Med Soc* Feb 1998, 150 (2) p78-80

Osteoporosis: detection, prevention, and treatment in primary care. *Geriatrics* Aug 1998, 53 (8) p22-3, 27-8, 33

Management of osteoporosis. An overview. *Drugs Aging* (New Zealand) May 1998, 12 Suppl 1 p25-32

Growth hormone therapy in patients with Turner syndrome. *Hormone Research* (Switzerland) , 1998 , 49/Suppl. 2 (62-66)

Neuropsychiatric function and dehydroepiandrosterone sulfate in elderly women: a prospective study. *Biol Psychiatry* 1998 May 1;43(9):694-700

Effects of replacement dose of dehydroepiandrosterone in men and women of advancing age. Published erratum appears in *J Clin Endocrinol Metab* 1995 Sep;80(9):2799

Endogenous levels of dehydroepiandrosterone sulfate, but not other sex hormones, are associated with depressed mood in older women: the Rancho Bernardo Study. *Am Geriatr Soc* 1999 Jun;47(6):685-91

Elevated serum dehydroepiandrosterone sulfate levels in practitioners of the Transcendental Meditation (TM) and TM-Sidhi programs. *J Behav Med* 1992 Aug; 15(4):327-41

Effects of estrogen replacement therapy on dehydroepiandrosterone, dehydroepiandrosterone sulfate, and cortisol responses to exercise in postmenopausal women. Published erratum appears in *Fertil Steril* 1998 Mar;69(3):606

Endogenous androgens and carotid intimal-medial thickness in women. *J Clin Endocrinol Metab* 1999 Jun;84(6):2008-12

Dehydroepiandrosterone treatment of midlife dysthymia. *Biol Psychiatry* 1999 Jun 15;45(12):1533-41

Estrogen Replacement Therapy

Dietary soy protein and estrogen replacement therapy improve cardiovascular risk factors and decrease aortic cholesteryl ester content in ovariectomized cynomolgus monkeys. *Metabolism: Clinical and Experimental*, 1997, 46/6 (698-705)

Daidzein sulfoconjugates are potent inhibitors of sterol sulfatase (EC 3.1.6.2). *Biochemical and Biophysical Research Communications*, 1997, 233/3 (579-583)

Adrenal puberty or adrenarche. *Andrologie* (France), 1997, 7/2 (165-186)

Urinary steroids at time of surgery in postmenopausal women with breast cancer. *Breast Cancer Research and Treatment*, 1997, 44/1 (83-89)

Relation of serum levels of testosterone and dehydroepiandrosterone sulfate to risk of breast cancer in postmenopausal women. *American Journal of Epidemiology*, 1997, 145/11 (1030-1038)

Role of glucose-6-phosphate dehydrogenase inhibition in the antiproliferative effects of dehydroepiandrosterone on human breast cancer cells. *British Journal of Cancer* (UK), 1997, 75/4 (589-592)

Effects of soya consumption for one month on steroid hormones in premenopausal women: Implications for breast cancer risk reduction. *Cancer Epidemiology Biomarkers and Prevention*, 1996, 5/1 (63-70)

Chemoprevention by dietary dehydroepiandrosterone against promotion/progressi on phase of radiation-induced mammary tumorigenesis in rats. *Journal of Steroid Biochemistry and Molecular Biology* (UK), 1995, 54/1-2 (47-53)

Epidemiology of soy and cancer: Perspectives and directions. *Journal of Nutrition*, 1995, 125/3 Suppl. (709S-712S)

Prevention by dehydroepiandrosterone of the development of mammary carcinoma induced by 7,12-dimethyl-benz(a)anthracene (DMBA) in the rat. *Breast Cancer Res. Treat.*, 1994, 29/2 (203-217)

Serum sex hormone levels after menopause and subsequent breast cancer. *Journal of the National Cancer Institute*, 1996, 88/5 (291-296)

Relationship of serum dehydroepiandrosterone (DHEA), DHEA sulfate, and 5-androstene-3beta,17beta-diol to risk of breast cancer in postmenopausal women. *Cancer Epidemiology Biomarkers and Prevention*, 1997, 6/3 (177-181)

Effects of oestrogen and progesterone on age-related changes in arteries of postmenopausal women. *Clin Exp Pharmacol Physiol* (Australia) Jun 1997, 24 (6) p457-9

Hormone replacement therapy in postmenopausal women: urinary *N*-telopeptide of type I collagen monitors therapeutic effect and predicts response of bone mineral density. *Am J Med* Jan 1997, 102 (1) p29-37

Estrogen inhibits cuff-induced intimal thickening of rat femoral artery: effects on migration and proliferation of vascular smooth muscle cells. *Atherosclerosis* (Ireland) Apr 1997, 130 (1-2) p1-10

Ovarian aging and hormone replacement therapy. Hormonal levels, symptoms, and attitudes of African-American and white women. *J Gen Intern Med* Apr 1997, 12 (4) p230-6

In vivo estrogen regulation of epidermal growth factor receptor in human endometrium. *J Clin Endocrinol Metab* May 1997, 82 (5) p1467-71

The perimenopausal hot flash: epidemiology, physiology, and treatment. *Nurse Pract* Mar 1997, 22 (3) p55-6, 61-6

Effects of hormone replacement modalities on low density lipoprotein composition and distribution in ovariectomized cynomolgus monkeys. *Atherosclerosis* (Ireland) Apr 5 1996, 121 (2) p217-29

Cause-specific mortality in women receiving hormone replacement therapy. *Epidemiology* Jan 1997, 8 (1) p59-65

Hormone replacement therapy increases trabecular and cortical bone density in osteoporotic women. *Medicina* (B Aires) (Argentina) 1996, 56 (3) p247-51

DHEA: a hormone with multiple effects. *Curr Opin Obstet Gynecol* Oct 1996, 8 (5) p351-4

Mammographic changes in women on hormonal replacement therapy. *Maturitas* (Ireland) Aug 1996, 25 (1) p51-7

Androgen replacement therapy in women: myths and realities. *Int J Fertil Menopausal Stud* Jul-Aug 1996, 41 (4) p412-22

Sequential addition of low dose of medrogestone or medroxyprogesterone acetate to transdermal estradiol: a pilot study on their influence on the endometrium. *Eur J Obstet Gynecol Reprod Biol* (Ireland) Sep 1996, 68 (1-2) p137-41

Hormone replacement therapy: clinical benefits and side-effects. *Maturitas* (Ireland) May 1996, 23 Suppl pS31-6

Progestins. *Maturitas* (Ireland) May 1996, 23 Suppl pS13-8

Evidence for primary and secondary prevention of coronary artery disease in women taking oestrogen replacement therapy. *Eur Heart J* (England) Aug 1996, 17 Suppl D p9-14

Practical aspects of preventing and managing athersclerotic disease in post-menopausal women. *Eur Heart J* (England) Aug 1996, 17 Suppl D p32-7

Hormone replacement therapy is associated with improved arterial physiology in healthy post-menopausal women. *Clin Endocrinol* (Oxf) (England) Oct 1996, 45 (4) p435-41

An examination of the effect of combined cyclical hormone replacement therapy on lipoprotein(a) and other lipoproteins. *Atherosclerosis* (Ireland) Jan 26 1996, 119 (2) p215-22

Effects of estrogens and progestogens on the renin-aldosterone system and blood pressure. *Steroids* Apr 1996, 61 (4) p166-71

Effects of progestogens on haemostasis. *Maturitas* (Ireland) May 1996, 24 (1-2) p1-19

Effects of hormone therapy on bone mineral density: results from the postmenopausal estrogen/progestin interventions (PEPI) trial. *The Writing Group for the PEPI JAMA* Nov 6 1996, 276 (17) p1389-96

Transdermal estrogen replacement therapy in normal peri-menopausal women: effects on pituitary-ovarian function. *Gynecol Endocrinol* (England) Feb 1996, 10 (1) p49-53

The effects of androgens and other sex hormones on serum lipoproteins. *Lijec Vjesn* (Croatia) Mar 1996, 118 Suppl 1 p33-7

Hormonal and environmental factors affecting cell proliferation and neoplasia in the mammary gland. *Prog Clin Biol Res* 1996, 394 p211-53

The menopause and hormone replacement therapy: lipids, lipoproteins, coagulation and fibrinolytic factors. *Maturitas* (Ireland) Mar 1996, 23 (2) p209-16

Hormonal therapy and genital tract cancer. *Curr Opin Obstet Gynecol* Feb 1996, 8 (1) p38-41

Health consequences of short- and long-term postmenopausal hormone therapy. *Clin Chem* Aug 1996, 42 (8 Pt 2) p1342-4

Current concepts in postmenopausal hormone replacement therapy. *J Fam Pract* Jul 1996, 43 (1) p69-75

Regulation of estrogen/progestogen receptors in the endometrium. *Int J Fertil Menopausal Stud* Jan-Feb 1996, 41 (1)p16-21

Hormone replacement therapy and breast cancer risk. *Arch Fam Med* Jun 1996, 5 (6) p341-8

Hormone replacement therapy, hormone levels, and lipoprotein cholesterol concentrations in elderly women. *Am J Obstet Gynecol* Mar 1996, 174 (3) p897-902

Hormone replacement therapy as treatment of breast cancer—a phase II study of Org OD 14 (tibilone). *Br J Cancer* (England) May 1996, 73 (9) p1086-8

Postmenopausal hormone therapy and breast cancer. *Obstet Gynecol* Feb 1996, 87 (2 Suppl)

Future aspects of hormone-replacement therapy. *Acta Chirurgica Austriaca* (Austria), 1996, 28/5 (282-284)

Neuroendocrine aspects of the menopause and hormone replacement therapy. *Journal of Cardiovascular Pharmacology*, 1996, 28/Suppl. 5 (S58-S60)

Hormone therapy and phytoestrogens. *Journal of Clinical Pharmacy and Therapeutics* (UK), 1996, 21/2 (101-111)

The effects of hormone replacement therapy on plasma vitamin E levels in post-menopausal women. *European Journal of Obstetrics Gynecology and Reproductive Biology* (Ireland), 1996, 66/2 (151-154)

Effects of hormonal therapies and dietary soy phytoestrogens on vaginal cytology in surgically postmenopausal macaques. *Fertility and Sterility*, 1996, 65/5 (1031-1035)

Dietary and behavioral determinants of menopause. *Clinical Consultations in Obstetrics and Gynecology*, 1996, 8/1 (21-26)

A review of the clinical effects of phytoestrogens. *Obstetrics and Gynecology*, 1996, 87/5 II Suppl. (897-904)

Molecular effects of genistein on estrogen receptor mediated pathways. *Carcinogenesis* (UK), 1996, 17/2 (271-275)

Rationale for the use of genistein-containing soy matrices in chemoprevention trials for breast and prostate cancer. *Journal of Cellular Biochemistry*, 1995, 58/Suppl. 22

Dietary flour supplementation decreases post-menopausal hot flushes: Effect of soy and wheat. *Maturitas* (Ireland), 1995, 21/3 (189-195)

Soy and experimental cancer: Animal studies. *Journal of Nutrition*, 1995, 125/3 Suppl

Aromatase in bone cell: Association with osteoporosis in post-menopausal women. *Journal of Steroid Biochemistry and Molecular Biology* (UK), 1995, 53/1-6 (165-174)

Estrogen replacement therapy and fatal ovarian cancer. *Am J Epidemiol* May 1 1995

Inhibition of breast cancer cell growth by combined treatment with vitamin D3 analogueues and tamoxifen. *Cancer Res* Nov 1 1994, 54 (21) p5711-7

Melatonin modulation of estrogen-regulated proteins, growth factors, and proto-oncogenes in human breast cancer. *J Pineal Res* (Denmark) Mar 1995

Melatonin inhibition of MCF-7 human breast-cancer cells growth: influence of cell proliferation rate. *Cancer Lett* (Ireland) Jul 13 1995

Modulation of cancer endocrine therapy by melatonin: a phase II study of tamoxifen plus melatonin in metastatic breast cancer patients progressing under tamoxifen alone. *Br J Cancer* (England) Apr 1995

Modulation of estrogen receptor mRNA expression by melatonin in MCF-7 human breast cancer cells. *Mol Endocrinol* Dec 1994

Melatonin modulates growth factor activity in MCF-7 human breast cancer cells. *J Pineal Res* (Denmark) Aug 1994

Role of pineal gland in aetiology and treatment of breast cancer. *Lancet* (England) Oct 14 1978

3beta-hydroxysteroid dehydrogenase/isomerase and aromatase activity in primary cultures of developing zebra finch telencephalon: Dehydroepiandrosterone as substrate for synthesis of androstenedione and estrogens. *General and Comparative Endocrinology*, 1996, 102/3 (342-350)

Abnormal production of androgens in women with breast cancer. *Anticancer Res.* (Greece), 1994, 14/5 B (2113-2117)

Endogenous sex hormones: Impact on lipids, lipoproteins, and insulin. *Am. J. Med.*, 1995, 98/1 A (40S-47S)

Dehydroepiandrosterone antiestrogenic action through androgen receptor in MCF-7 human breast cancer cell line. *Anticancer Res.* (Greece), 1993, 13/6 A (2267-2272)

Effect of flax seed ingestion on the menstrual cycle. *J. Clin. Endocrinol. Metab.*, 1993, 77/5 (1215-1219)

Estrogen and nerve growth factor-related systems in brain. Effects on basal forebrain cholinergic neurons and implications for learning and memory processes and aging. *Ann. New York Acad. Sci.*, 1994, 743/- (165-199)

Postmenopausal estrogen replacement: A long-term cohort study. *Am. J. Med.*, 1994, 97/1 (66-77)

Impact of the menopause on the epidemiology and risk factors of coronary artery heart disease in women. *Exp. Gerontol.*, 1994, 29/3-4 (357-375)

Hormone therapy and endometrium cancer. *Reprod. Hum. Horm.* (France), 1994, 7/4 (137-139)

Progestin replacement in the menopause: Effects on the endometrium and serum lipids. *Curr. Opin. Obstet. Gynecol.*, 1994, 6/3 (284-292)

Effects of hormone replacement therapy on lipoprotein(a) and lipids in postmenopausal women. *Arterioscler. Thromb.*, 1994, 14/2 (275-281)

Aromatase in bone cell: Association with osteoporosis in postmenopausal women. *Journal of Steroid Biochemistry and Molecular Biology* (UK), 1995, 53/1-6 (165-174)

Transdermal estrogen replacement therapy in normal perimenopausal women: Effects on pituitary- ovarian function. *Gynecological Endocrinology* (UK), 1996, 10/1 (49-53)

Hormone replacement therapy, hormone levels, and lipoprotein cholesterol concentrations in elderly women. *American Journal of Obstetrics and Gynecology*, 1996, 174/3

Menopause

Menopause before the age of 40 years. *Journal De Gynecologie Obstetrique Et Biologie De La Reproduction* (France), 1997, 26/3 231-237

Endometrial cancer and hormone replacement therapy: Appropriate use of progestins to oppose endogenous and exogenous estrogen. *Endocrinology and Metabolism Clinics of North America,* 1997, 26/2 (399-412)

Women's hearts are different. *Current Problems in Obstetrics, Gynecology and Fertility*, 1997,20/3 (72-92)

Estrogen and the prevention and treatment of osteoporosis. *Journal of Clinical Rheumatology*, 1997, 3/2 Suppl. (S28-S33)

Neoadjuvant progesterone therapy for primary breast cancer: Rationale for a clinical trial. *Clinical Therapeutics*, 1997, 19/1 (56-61)

Cardiovascular pathophysiology of ovarian hormones. *Schweizerische Rundschau fur Medizin / Praxis* (Switzerland), 1997, 86/5 (138-144)

Hemostasis during hormone replacement therapy. *Infertility and Reproductive Medicine Clinics of North America*, 1997, 8/1 (35-48)

Androgens and the menopause; a study of 40-60-year-old women. *Clinical Endocrinology* (UK), 1996, 45/5 (577-587)

Cardiovascular effects of the ovarian hormones. *Archives des Maladies du Coeur et des Vaisseaux* (France), 1996, 89/SPEC.ISS. 7 (9-16)

The effect of hormones on the lower urinary tract. *Archives of STD / HIV Research*, 1996, 10/3 (145-150)

Hormone substances and their efficacy in hormonal replacement therapy. *Acta Chirurgica Austriaca* (Austria), 1996, 28/5 (259-262)

The effects of various hormone replacement therapy regimens on bone mineral density after 2 years of treatment. *Marmara Medical Journal* (Turkey), 1996, 9/4 (165-168)

A randomized, double-blind, placebo-controlled, crossover study on the effect of oral oestradiol on acute menopausal symptoms. *Maturitas* (Ireland), 1996, 25/2 (115-123)

The female brain hypoestrogenic continuum from the premenstrual syndrome to menopause: A hypothesis and review of supporting data. *Journal of Reproductive Medicine for the Obstetrician and Gynecologist*, 1996, 41/9 (633-639)

Treatments for oestoporosis. *Revue Francaise de Gynecologie et d'Obstetrique* (France), 1996, 91/6 (329-334)

Variations in steroid hormone receptor content throughout age and menopausal periods, and menstrual cycle in breast cancer patients. *Neoplasma* (Slovak Republic), 1996, 43/3 (163-169)

Hormone therapy and Phytoestrogens. *Journal of Clinical Pharmacy and Therapeutics* (UK), 1996,21/2 (101-111)

The menopause and hormone replacement therapy: Lipids, lipoproteins, coagulation and fibrinolytic factors. *Maturitas* (Ireland), 1996, 23/2 (209-216)

Prevention of cardiovascular disease by hormone replacement therapy in the ostmenopause. *Zentralblatt fur Gynakologie* (Germany), 1996, 118/4 (188-197)

Menopause and osteoporosis: The role of HRT. *Journal of the American Pharmaceutical Association*, 1996, 36/4 (234-242)

Characterization of reproductive hormonal dynamics in the perimenopause. *Journal of Clinical Endocrinology and Metabolism*, 1996, 81/4 (1495-1501)

Clinical evaluation of near-continuous oral micronized progesterone therapy in estrogenized postmenopausal women. *Gynecological Endocrinology* (UK), 1996, 10/1 (41-47)

The regulation of adipose tissue distribution in humans. *International Journal of Obesity* (UK), 1996, 20/4 (291-302)

Adrenal and gonadal steroid hormone deficiency in the etiopathogenesis of rheumatoid arthritis. *Journal of Rheumatology* (Canada), 1996, 23/Suppl. 44 (10-12)

Dietary and behavioral determinants of menopause. *Clinical Consultations in Obstetrics and Gynecology,* 1996, 8/1(21-26)

Alpha-tocopherol and hydroperoxide content in breast adipose tissue from patients with breast tumors. *Int J Cancer* Jul 17 1996, 67 (2) p170-5

A review of the clinical effects of phytoestrogens. *Obstet Gynecol* May 1996, 87 (5 Pt 2) p897-904

Value of micronutrient supplements in the prevention or correction of disturbances accompanying the menopause. *Rev. Fr. Gynecol. Obstet.* (France), 1990, 85/12 (702-705)

Effect of vitamin B-6 on plasma and red blood cell magnesium levels in premenopausal women. *Ann. Clin. Lab. Sci.*, 1981, 11/4 333-336

Effect of a natural and artificial menopause on serum, urinary and erythrocyte magnesium. *United Kingdom Clin. Sci.* (England), 1980, 58/3 (255-257)

Vitamins as therapy in the 1990s. *Journal of the American Board of Family Practice*, 1995, 8/3 (206-216)

Functional capacity of the tryptophan niacin pathway in the premenarchial phase and in the menopausal age. Egypt *Amer. J. Clin. Nutr.*, 1975, 28/1 (4-9)

Dehydroepiandrosterone sulphate as a source of steroids in menopause. *Acta Ginecologica* (Spain), 1995, 52/9 (279-284)

Distribution of glutathione *S*-transferase isoenzymes in human ovary. *J. Reprod. Fertil.* (UK), 1991, 93/2 (303-311)

Changes in circulating steroids with aging in postmenopausal women. *Obstet. Gynecol.*, 1981, 57/5 (624-628)

Adrenal and gonadal steroid hormone deficiency in the etiopathogenesis of rheumatoid arthritis. *Journal of Rheumatology* (Canada), 1996, 23/Suppl. 44 (10-12)

The effects of oral dehydroepiandrosterone on endocrine-metabolic parameters in postmenopausal women. *J. Clin. Endocrinol. Metab.*, 1990, 71/3 (696-704)

Catabolic effects and the influence on hormonal variables under treatment with Gynodian-Depot (Reg.trademark) or dehydroepiandrosterone (DHEA) oenanthate. *Sweden Maturitas* (Netherlands), 1981, 3/3-4 (225-234)

Nutrition and osteoporosis: An analysis of dietary intake in postmenopausal women. *Wiener Klinische Wochenschrift* (Austria), 1995, 107/14 (418-422)

Magnesium supplementation and osteoporosis. *Nutrition Reviews*, 1995, 53/3 (71-74)

Calcium, phosphorus and magnesium intakes correlate with bone mineral content in postmenopausal women. *Gynecol. Endocrinol.* (UK), 1994, 8/1 (55-58)

Incident pain caused by collapsed vertebrae in menopause. The logical background to a personal treatment protocol. *Italy Minerva Anestesiol.* (Italy), 1984, 50/11 (573-576)

Interaction of family history of breast cancer and dietary antioxidants with breast cancer risk (New York, United States). *Cancer Causes and Control* (UK), 1995, 6/5 (407-415)

Altered menstrual cycles in rhesus monkeys induced by lead. *Fundam. Appl. Toxicol.*, 1987, 9/4 (722-729)

Effect of glucocorticoids and calcium intake on bone density and bone, liver and plasma minerals in guinea pigs. *J. Nutr.*, 1979, 109/7 (1175-1188)

Relationships between usual nutrient intake and bone-mineral content of women 35-65 years of age: Longitudinal and cross-sectional analysis. *Am. J. Clin. Nutr.*, 1986, 44/6 (863-876)

Iron deficiency anemia in postmenopausal women. *J. Amer. Geriat. Soc.*, 1976, 24/12 (558-559)

Effect of menopause and estrogen substitutional therapy on magnesium metabolsim. *Denmark Miner. Electrolyte Metabol.* (Switzerland), 1984, 10/2 (84-87)

Value of micronutrient supplements in the prevention or correction of disturbances accompanying the menopause. *Rev. Fr. Gynecol. Obstet.* (France), 1990, 85/12 (702-705)

Effect of vitamin B-6 on plasma and red blood cell magnesium levels in premenopausal women. *Ann. Clin. Lab. Sci.*, 1981, 11/4 333-336)

Effect of a natural and artificial menopause on serum, urinary and erythrocyte magnesium. *United Kingdom Clin. Sci.* (England), 1980, 58/3 (255-257)

Vitamins as therapy in the 1990s. *Journal of the American Board of Family Practice*, 1995, 8/3 (206-216)

Functional capacity of the tryptophan niacin pathway in the premenarchial phase and in the menopausal age. Egypt *Amer. J. Clin. Nutr.*, 1975, 28/1 (4-9)

Dehydroepiandrosterone sulphate as a source of steroids in menopause. Sulfate de dehidro-epi-androsterona come fuente de esteroides en la menopausia (i). *Acta Ginecologica* (Spain), 1995, 52/9 (279-284)

Distribution of glutathione *S*-transferase isoenzymes in human ovary. *J. Reprod. Fertil.* (UK), 1991, 93/2 (303-311)

Changes in circulating steroids with aging in postmenopausal women. *Obstet. Gynecol.*, 1981, 57/5 (624-628)

Adrenal and gonadal steroid hormone deficiency in the etiopathogenesis of rheumatoid arthritis. *Journal Of Rheumatology* (Canada), 1996, 23/Suppl. 44 (10-12)

The effects of oral dehydroepiandrosterone on endocrine-metabolic parameters in postmenopausal women. *J. Clin. Endocrinol. Metab.*, 1990, 71/3 (696- 704)

Catabolic effects and the influence on hormonal variables under treatment with Gynodian-Depot (Reg.trademark) or dehydroepiandrosterone (DHEA) oenanthate. *Sweden Maturitas* (Netherlands), 1981, 3/3-4 (225- 234)

Nutrition and osteoporosis: An analysis of dietary intake in postmenopausal women. *Wiener Klinische Wochenschrift* (Austria), 1995, 107/14 (418-422)

Magnesium supplementation and osteoporosis. *Nutrition Reviews*, 1995, 53/3 (71-74)

Calcium, phosphorus and magnesium intakes correlate with bone mineral content in postmenopausal women. *Gynecol. Endocrinol.* (UK), 1994, 8/1 (55-58)

Incident pain caused by collapsed vertebrae in menopause. The logical background to a personal treatment protocol. *Italy Minerva Anestesiol.* (Italy), 1984, 50/11 (573-576)

Interaction of family history of breast cancer and dietary antioxidants with breast cancer risk (New York, United States). *Cancer Causes and Control* (UK), 1995, 6/5 (407-415)

Altered menstrual cycles in rhesus monkeys induced by lead. *Fundam. Appl. Toxicol.*, 1987, 9/4 (722-729)

Effect of glucocorticoids and calcium intake on bone density and bone, liver and plasma minerals in guinea pigs. *J. Nutr.*, 1979, 109/7 (1175-1188)

Relationships between usual nutrient intake and bone-mineral content of women 35-65 years of age: Longitudinal and cross-sectional analysis. *Am. J. Clin. Nutr.*, 1986, 44/6 (863-876)

Iron deficiency anemia in postmenopausal women. *J. Amer. Geriat. Soc.*, 1976, 24/12 (558-559)

Effect of menopause and estrogen substitutional therapy on magnesium metabolsim. *Denmark Miner. Electrolyte Metabol.* (Switzerland), 1984, 10/2 (84-87)

Menstrual Disorders (Premenstrual Syndrome)

Use of nomegestrol acetate in the treatment of menstrual disorders. Our experience of 56 patients. *Minerva Ginecologica* (Italy), 1997, 49/4 (181-185)

Oral contraception and other factors in relation to hospital referral for menstrual problems without known underlying cause: Findings in a large cohort study. *British Journal of Family Planning* (UK), 1997, 22/4 (166-169)

[Risk analysis of menstrual disorders in young women from urban population]. *Przegl Epidemiol* (Poland) 1996, 50 (4) p467-74

Severe vaginal bleeding associated with recombinant interferon beta-1B. *Ann Pharmacother* Jan 1997, 31 (1) p50-2

Prevalence of menstrual dysfunction in Norwegian long-distance runners participating in the Oslo Marathon games. *Scand J Med Sci Sports* (Denmark) Jun 1996, 6 (3) p164-71

Effect of vitamin B6 on the side effects of a low-dose combined oral contraceptive. *Contraception* Apr 1997, 55 (4) p245-8

Effects of a yeast-based dietary supplementation on premenstrual syndrome. A double-blind placebo-controlled study. *Gynecologic and Obstetric Investigation* (Switzerland), 1997, 43/2 (120-124)

Role of estrogen in postmenopausal depression. *Neurology*, 1997, 48/5 Suppl. 7 (S16-S20)

Reduced benzodiazepine sensitivity in patients with premenstrual syndrome: A pilot study. *Psychoneuroendocrinology* (UK), 1997, 22/1 (25-38)

Treatment of premenstrual syndrome (PMS) with lisuride maleate. *Ginecologia y Obstetricia de Mexico* (Mexico), 1996, 64/DEC. (556-560)

Premenstrual syndrome. *Trends in Endocrinology and Metabolism*, 1996, 7/5 (184-189)

Hormonal approaches to treatment for mood disorders. *Infertility and Reproductive Medicine Clinics of North America*, 1996, 7/2 (381-395)

Clinical and biochemical effects of nutritional supplementation on the premenstrual syndrome. *J. Reprod. Med.*, 1987, 32/6 (435-441)

Reduced bone mass in women with premenstrual syndrome. *Journal of Women's Health*, 1995, 4/2 (161-168)

Calcium-regulating hormones across the menstrual cycle: Evidence of a secondary hyperparathyroidism in women with PMS. *Journal of Clinical Endocrinology and Metabolism,* 1995, 80/7

Linolenic acid formulations for the treatment of premenstrual syndrome. *Curr. Opin. Ther. Pat.* (UK), 1992, 2/12 (2000-2002)

Calcium supplementation in premenstrual syndrome: A randomized crossover trial. *J. Gen. Intern. Med.*, 1989, 4/3 (183-189)

Plasma copper, zinc and magnesium levels in patients with premenstrual tension syndrome. *Acta Obstet. Gynecol. Scand.* (Denmark), 1994, 73/6 (452-455)

Use of a vitamin-mineral supplement in the management of premenstrual syndrome. *Br. J. Clin. Res.* (UK), 1993, 4/- (219-224)

Oral magnesium successfully relieves premenstrual mood changes. *Obstet. Gynecol.*, 1991, 78/2 (177-181)

Clinical and biochemical effects of nutritional supplementation on the premenstrual syndrome. *J. Reprod. Med.*, 1987, 32/6 (435-441)

Magnesium and the premenstrual syndrome. *Ann. Clin. Biochem.* (UK), 1986, 23/6 (667-670)

The role of essential fatty acids and prostaglandins in the premenstrual syndrome. *J. Reprod. Med.*, 1983, 28/7 (465-468)

Vitamin B6 in the treatment of the premenstrual syndrome - Review (1). *Br. J. Obstet. Gynaecol.* (UK), 1991, 98/3 (329-330), *Br. J. Clin. Pract.* (UK), 1988, 42/11 (448-452)

Fibrinogen and Cardiovascular Disease

Comparison of the effects of two low fat diets with different alpha-linolenic:linoleic acid ratios on coagulation and fibrinolysis. *Atherosclerosis* (Ireland), 1999, 142/1 (159-168)

Effect of niacin supplementation on fibrinogen levels in patients with peripheral vascular disease. *Am J Cardiol* Sep 1 1998, 82 (5) p697-9, A9

Effect of garlic (Allium sativum) on blood lipids, blood sugar, fibrinogen and fibrinolytic activity in patients with coronary artery disease. *Prostaglandins Leukot Essent Fatty Acids* (Scot) Apr 1998, 58 (4) p257-63

Factor XIIIa cross-links lipoprotein(a) with fibrinogen and is present in human atherosclerotic lesions. *Circ Res* Aug 10 1998, 83 (3) p264-9

Homocysteine and vitamins in cardiovascular disease. *Clin Chem* Aug 1998, 44 (8 Pt 2) p1833-43

The effect of minor constituents of olive oil on cardiovascular disease: new findings. *Nutr Rev* May 1998, 56 (5 Pt 1) p142-7

Serum ascorbic acid and cardiovascular disease prevalence in U.S. adults. *Epidemiology* May 1998, 9 (3) p316-21

[The effect of N-3 fatty acid administration on selected indicators of cardiovascular disease risk in patients with type 2 diabetes mellitus]. *Bratisl Lek Listy* (Slovakia) Jan 1998, 99 (1) p37-42

Dietary intakes among Siberian Yupiks of Alaska and implications for cardiovascular disease. *Int J Circumpolar Health* (Finland) Jan 1998, 57 (1) p4-17

Folic acid supplementation prevents deficient blood folate levels and hyperhomocysteinemia during longterm, low dose methotrexate therapy for rheumatoid arthritis: implications for cardiovascular disease prevention. *J Rheumatol* (Canada) Mar 1998, 25 (3) p441-6

Homocysteine and cardiovascular disease. *Annu Rev Med* 1998, 49 p31-62

Vitamins E plus C and interacting conutrients required for optimal health. A critical and constructive review of epidemiology and supplementation data regarding cardiovascular disease and cancer. *Biofactors* (Netherlands) 1998, 7 (1-2) p113-74

Homocysteine and cardiovascular disease. *Cardiovascular Reviews and Reports*, 1998, 19/8 (49-61)

Recent nutritional approaches to the prevention and therapy of cardiovascular disease. *Prog Cardiovasc Nurs* Summer 1997, 12 (3) p3-23

Association between plasma total homocysteine and parental history of cardiovascular disease in children with familial hypercholesterolemia. *Circulation* Sep 16 1997, 96 (6) p1803-8

Plasma homocysteine, a risk factor for cardiovascular disease, is lowered by physiological doses of folic acid. *QJM* (England) Aug 1997, 90 (8) p519-24

Does vegetable oil attenuate the beneficial effects of fish oil in reducing risk factors for cardiovascular disease? [see comments] *Am J Clin Nutr* Jul 1997, 66 (1) p89-96

Age-related decreases in chromium levels in 51,665 hair, sweat, and serum samples from 40,872 patients-implications for the prevention of cardiovascular disease and type II diabetes mellitus. *Metabolism* May 1997, 46 (5) p469-73

Potassium, blood pressure, and cardiovascular disease: An epidemiologic perspective. *Cardiology in Review*, 1997, 5/5 (255-260)

Infection, hemostatic factors and cardiovascular disease. *Fibrinolysis and Proteolysis* (UK), 1997, 11/Suppl. 1 (149-153)

Epidemiologic evidence on vitamin E in the prevention and treatment of cardiovascular disease. *Diabetes und Stoffwechsel* (Germany), 1997, 6/Suppl. 2 (38-40)

Novel tocotrienols of rice bran modulate cardiovascular disease risk parameters of hypercholesterolomic humans. *Journal of Nutritional Biochemistry*, 1997, 8/5 (290-298)

Omega3 fatty acids in the prevention-management of cardiovascular disease. *Canadian Journal of Physiology and Pharmacology* (Canada), 1997, 75/3 (234-239)

Interactions between dietary fat, fish, and fish oils and their effects on platelet function in men at risk of cardiovascular disease. *Arteriosclerosis, Thrombosis, and Vascular Biology*, 1997, 17/2 (279-286)

Nicotinic acid treatment shifts the fibrinolytic balance favourably and decreases plasma fibrinogen in hypertriglyceridaemic men. *J Cardiovasc Risk* 1997 Jun;4(3):165-71

A prospective study of fibrinogen and risk of myocardial infarction in the Physicians' Health Study. *J Am Coll Cardiol* 1999 Apr;33(5):1347-52

Effect of ciprofibrate on fibrinogen synthesis in vitro on hepatoma cells and in vivo in genetically obese Zucker rats. *Blood Coagul Fibrinolysis* 1999 Jul;10(5):239-44

Dietary (n-3) fatty acids increase superoxide dismutase activity and decrease thromboxane production in the rat heart. *Nutrition Research*, 1997, 17/1 (163-175)

Effects of n-3 fatty acids and fenofibrate on lipid and hemorrheological parameters in familial dysbetalipoproteinemia and familial hypertriglyceridemia. *Metabolism: Clinical and Experimental*, 1996, 45/10 (1305-1311)

Repeated fasting and refeeding with 20:5, n-3 Eicosapentaenoic Acid (EPA): A novel approach for rapid fatty acid exchanges and its effect on blood pressure, plasma lipids and hemostasis. *Journal of Human Hypertension* (UK), 1996, 10/Suppl. 3 (S135-S139)

Acute phase response and plasma carotenoid concentrations in older women: Findings from the nun study. *Nutrition*, 1996, 12/7-8 (475-478)

Epidemiology of coagulation factors, inhibitors and activation markers: The Third Glasgow MONICA Survey. II. Relationships to cardiovascular risk factors and prevalent cardiovascular disease. *Br J Haematol* (England) Jun 1997, 97 (4) p785-97

A long-term study on the effect of spontaneous consumption of reduced fat products as part of a normal diet on indicators of health. *Int J Food Sci Nutr* (England) Jan 1997, 48 (1) p19-29

Acute phase response and plasma carotenoid concentrations in older women: findings from the nun study. *Nutrition* Jul-Aug 1996, 12 (7-8) p475-8

Cadmium and atherosclerosis in the rabbit: reduced atherogenesis by superseding of iron? *Food Chem Toxicol* (England) Jul 1996, 34 (7) p611-21

Vitamin intake: A possible determinant of plasma homocyst(e)ine among middle-aged adults. *Annals of Epidemiology*, 1997, 7/4 (285-293)

Vitamin C blocks inflammatory platelet-activating factor mimetics created by cigarette smoking. *Journal of Clinical Investigation*, 1997, 99/10 (2358-2364)

V677 mutation of methylenetetrahydrofolate reductase and cardiovascular disease in Canadian Inuit (5). *Lancet* (UK), 1997, 349/9060 (1221-1222)

Dietary vitamin C, beta-carotene and 30-year risk of stroke: Results from the western electric study. *Neuroepidemiology* (Switzerland), 1997, 16/2 (69-77)

Beta-carotene, vitamin C, and vitamin E: The protective micronutrients. *Nutrition Reviews*, 1996, 54/11 II (S109-S114)

Alpha-2 adrenoceptor subtype causing nitric oxide-mediated vascular relaxation in rats. *Journal of Pharmacology and Experimental Therapeutics*, 1996, 278/3 (1235-1243)

Vitamin C and cardiovascular disease: A systematic review. *Journal of Cardiovascular Risk* (UK), 1996, 3/6 (513-521)

Position of the American Dietetic Association: Phytochemicals and functional foods. *Journal of Nutraceuticals, Functional and Medical Foods*, 1997, 1/1 (33-45)

The effect of hormone replacement therapy on vitamin E status in postmenopausal women. *Maturitas* (Ireland), 1997, 26/2 (121-124)

Vitamin E inhibits low-density lipoprotein-induced adhesion of monocytes to human aortic endothelial cells in vitro. *Arteriosclerosis, Thrombosis, and Vascular Biology*, 1997, 17/3 (429-436)

Endothelial dysfunction: Clinical implications. *Progress in Cardiovascular Diseases*, 1997, 39/4 (287-324)

Interactions between dietary fat, fish, and fish oils and their effects on platelet function in men at risk of cardiovascular disease. *Arteriosclerosis, Thrombosis, and Vascular Biology*, 1997, 17/2 (279-286)

The role of folic acid in deficiency states and prevention of disease. *Journal of Family Practice*, 1997, 44/2 (138-144)

Use of antioxidant vitamins in the cardiovascular disease. A review of epidemiological study and clinical trials. *Giornale Italiano di Farmacia Clinica* (Italy), 1996, 10/3 (155-162)

Intake of dietary fiber and risk of coronary heart disease in a cohort of Finnish men: The Alpha-Tocopherol, Beta-Carotene Cancer Prevention Study. *Circulation*, 1996, 94/11 (2720-2727)

alpha-Tocopherol inhibits aggregation of human platelets by a protein kinase C-dependent mechanism. *Circulation*, 1996, 94/10 (2434-2440)

Dietary and physiological studies involving magnesium homeostasis in the heart. *Annals of the New York Academy of Sciences*, 1996, 793/- (473-478)

Prevention of neural tube defects. *CNS Drugs* (New Zealand), 1996, 6/5 (399-412)

Neurally mediated cardiac effects of forskolin in conscious dogs. *American Journal of Physiology—Heart and Circulatory Physiology*, 1996, 271/4 40-4 (H1473-H1482)

Will an increased dietary folate intake reduce the incidence of cardiovascular disease? *Nutrition Reviews*, 1996, 54/7 (213-216)

Genetic polymorphism of methylenetetrahydrofolate reductase and myocardial infarction: A case-control study. *Circulation*, 1996, 94/8 (1812-1814)

The effect of dietary treatment on lipid peroxidation and antioxidant status in newly diagnosed noninsulin dependent diabetes. *Free Radical Biology and Medicine*, 1996, 21/5 (719-726)

Antioxidant properties of ethanolic and aqueous extracts of green tea compared to black tea. *Biochemical Society Transactions* (UK), 1996, 24/3 (390S)

Nutrition and women's health. *Current Problems in Obstetrics, Gynecology and Fertility*, 1996, 19/4 (112-166)

Smoking, plasma antioxidants and essential fatty acids before and after nutratherapy. *Canadian Journal of Cardiology* (Canada), 1996, 12/7 (665-670)

Relation of total homocysteine and lipid levels in children to premature cardiovascular death in male relatives. *Pediatric Research*, 1996, 40/1 (47-52)

Reduction of plasma peroxide levels by oral antioxidants. *Medical Science Research* (UK), 1996, 24/5 (357-359)

Changes in atherosclerotic aorta of rabbit fed with high cholesterol diet: The effect of vitamin E. Klinik. *Gelisim* (Turkey), 1996, 9/2 (4063-4068)

In vitro effects of a flavonoid-rich extract on LDL oxidation. *Atherosclerosis* (Ireland), 1996, 123/1-2 (83-91)

Folate status is the major determinant of fasting total plasma homocysteine levels in maintenance dialysis patients. *Atherosclerosis* (Ireland), 1996, 123/1-2 (193-202)

Dietary antioxidant vitamins and death from coronary heart disease in postmenopausal women. *New England Journal of Medicine*, 1996, 334/18 (1156-1162)

The cardiovascular protective role of docosahexaenoic acid. *European Journal of Pharmacology* (Netherlands), 1996, 300/1-2 (83-89)

Vitamins as homocysteine-lowering agents. *Journal of Nutrition*, 1996, 126/4 Suppl. (1276S-1280S)

The effect of modest vitamin E supplementation on lipid peroxidation products and other cardiovascular risk factors in diabetic patients. *Lipids*, 1996, 31/3 Suppl. (S87-S90)

Plasma ascorbic acid concentrations in the Republic of Karelia, Russia and in North Karelia, Finland. *European Journal of Clinical Nutrition* (UK), 1996, 50/2 (115-120)

Vegetable, fruit, and cereal fiber intake and risk of coronary heart disease among men. *Journal of the American Medical Association*, 1996, 275/6 (447-451)

Homocysteine: Relation with ischemic vascular diseases. *Revue de Medecine Interne* (France), 1996, 17/1 (34-45)

Effects of various fatty acids alone or combined with vitamin E on cell growth and fibrinogen concentration in the medium of HepG2 cells. *Thromb Res* Oct 1 1995, 80 (1) p75-83

[The role of platelets in the protective effect of a combination of vitamins A, E, C and P in thrombinemia]. *Gematol Transfuziol* (Russia) Sep-Oct 1995, 40 (5) p9-11

[Improvement of hemorheology with ginkgo biloba extract. Decreasing a cardiovascular risk factor]. *Fortschr Med* (Germany) May 10 1992, 110 (13) p247-50

On the pharmacology of bromelain: an update with special regard to animal studies on dose-dependent effects. *Planta Med* (Germany, West) Jun 1990, 56 (3) p249-53

Effects of various fatty acids alone or combined with vitamin E on cell growth and fibrinogen concentration in the medium of HepG2 cells. *Thromb Res* Oct 1 1995, 80 (1) p75-83

Protein/platelet interaction with an artificial surface: effect of vitamins and platelet inhibitors. *Thromb Res* Jan 1 1986, 41 (1) p9-22

[Preventive effects of green tea extract on lipid abnormalities in serum, liver and aorta of mice fed a atherogenic diet]. *Nippon Yakurigaku Zasshi* (Japan) Jun 1991, 97 (6) p329-37

Relationship between plasma essential fatty acids and smoking, serum lipids, blood pressure and haemostatic and rheological factors. *Prostaglandins Leukot Essent Fatty Acids* (Scotland) Aug 1994, 51 (2) p101-8

Omega-3 fatty acids in health and disease and in growth and development. *Am J Clin Nutr* Sep 1991, 54 (3) p438-63

Fibromyalgia

Recognizing and treating fibromyalgia. *Nurse Pract* Dec 1997, 22 (12) p18-26, 28, 31; quiz

A population study of the incidence of fibromyalgia among women aged 26-55 yr. *Br J Rheumatol* (England) Dec 1997, 36 (12) p1318-23

Psychosocial factors in fibromyalgia compared with rheumatoid arthritis: II. Sexual, physical, and emotional abuse and neglect. *Psychosom Med* Nov-Dec 1997, 59 (6) p572-7

Health status and disease severity in fibromyalgia: results of a six-center longitudinal study [see comments]. *Arthritis Rheum* Sep 1997, 40 (9) p1571-9

Increased concentrations of homocysteine in the cerebrospinal fluid in patients with fibromyalgia and chronic fatigue syndrome. *Scand J Rheumatol* (Norway) 1997, 26 (4) p301-7

Hypothalamic-pituitary-insulin-like growth factor-I axis dysfunction in patients with fibromyalgia. *J Rheumatol* (Canada) Jul 1997, 24 (7) p1384-9

Reactive oxygen species, antioxidant status and fibromyalgia. *Journal of Musculoskeletal Pain* 1997, 5/4 (5-15)

Thyroid status of 38 fibromyalgia patients: Implications for the etiology of fibromyalgia. *Clinical Bulletin of Myofascial Therapy* 1997, 2/1 (47-64)

Exercise training in treatment of fibromyalgia. *Journal of Musculoskeletal Pain* 1997, 5/1 (71-79)

Measuring the quality of life of women with fibromyalgia: A Hebrew version of the quality of life scale. *Journal of Musculoskeletal Pain* 1997, 5/1 (5-17)

Pain treatment of fibromyalgia by acupuncture [letter]. *Rheumatol Int* (Germany) 1998, 18 (1) p35-6

The detoxification enzyme systems. *Altern Med Rev* Jun 1998, 3 (3) p187-98

The effects of nutritional supplements on the symptoms of fibromyalgia and chronic fatigue syndrome. *Integr Physiol Behav Sci* Jan-Mar 1998, 33 (1) p61-71

Fibromyalgia and chronic fatigue: the holistic perspective. *Holist Nurs Pract* Apr 1998, 12 (3) p55-63

Treatment of fibromyalgia. *Zh Nevrol Psikhiatr Im S S Korsakova* (Russia) 1998, 98 (4) p40-3

Normal melatonin levelsin patients with fibromyalgia syndrome. *J Rheumatol* (Canada) Mar 1998, 25 (3) p551-5

Sleep disturbances, fibromyalgia and primary Sjogren's syndrome. *Clin Exp Rheumatol* (Italy) Jan-Feb 1997, 15 (1) p71-4

Effects of experimental muscle pain on muscle activity and coordination during static and dynamic motor function. *Electroencephalogr Clin Neurophysiol* (Ireland) Apr 1997, 105 (2) p156-64

Trigger points and tender points: one and the same? Does injection treatment help? *Rheum Dis Clin North Am* May 1996, 22 (2) p305-22

Fibromyalgia and migraine, two faces of the same mechanism. Serotonin as the common clue for pathogenesis and therapy. *Adv Exp Med Biol* 1996, 398 p373-9

Self-reported illness and health status among Gulf War veterans. A population-based study. The Iowa Persian Gulf Study Group. *Jama* Jan 15 1997, 277 (3) p238-45

[Fibromyalgia in dentistry]. *J Can Dent Assoc* (Canada) Nov 1996, 62 (11) p874-6, 879-80

Fibromyalgia, depression, and alcoholism: a family history study. *J Rheumatol* (Canada) Jan 1996, 23 (1) p149-54

Chronic regional muscular pain in women with precise manipulation work. A study of pain characteristics, muscle function, and impact on daily activities. *Scand J Rheumatol* (Norway) 1996, 25 (4) p213-23

The management of treatment-resistant depression in disorders on the interface of psychiatry and medicine. Fibromyalgia, chronic fatigue syndrome, migraine, irritable bowel syndrome, atypical facial pain, and premenstrual dysphoric disorder. *Psychiatr Clin North Am* Jun 1996, 19 (2) p351-69

Profile of patients with chemical injury and sensitivity. *Environmental Health Perspectives,* 1997, 105/Suppl. 2 (417-436)

The relationship between fibromyalgia and interstitial cystitis. *Journal of Psychiatric Research* (UK), 1997, 31/1 (125-131)

Pressure and heat pain thresholds and tolerances in patients with fibromyalgia. *Journal of Musculoskeletal Pain*, 1997, 5/2 (43-53)

Measuring change in fibromyalgic pain: The relevance of pain distribution. *Journal of Musculoskeletal Pain*, 1997, 5/2 (29-41)

Thyroid status of 38 fibromyalgia patients: Implications for the etiology of fibromyalgia. *Clinical Bulletin of Myofascial Therapy*, 1997, 2/1 (47-64)

A prospective long-term study of fibromyalgia syndrome. *Arthritis and Rheumatism*, 1996, 39/4 (682-685)

Oral *S*-adenosylmethionine in primary fibromyalgia? Double-blind clinical evaluation. *Scand J Rheumatol* (Sweden) 1991, 20 (4) p294-302

Cerebrospinal fluid *S*-adenosylmethionine in depression and dementia: effects of treatment with parenteral and oral *S*-adenosylmethionine. *J Neurol Neurosurg Psychiatry* (England) Dec 1990, 53 (12) p1096-8

The antidepressant potential of oral *S*-adenosyl-*L*-methionine. *Acta Psychiatr Scand* (Denmark) May 1990, 81 (5) p432-6

Oral *S*-adenosylmethionine in depression: a randomized, double-blind, placebo-controlled trial. *Am J Psychiatry* May 1990, 147 (5) p591-5

Disability and impairment in fibromyalgia syndrome: Possible pathogenesis and etiology. *Critical Reviews In Physical And Rehabilitation Medicine*, 1995, 7/3 (189-232)

Primary fibromyalgia is responsive to S-adenosyl-L-methionine. *Curr. Ther. Res. Clin. Exp.*, 1994, 55/7 (797-806)

S-adenosyl-L-methionine in Sjogren's syndrome and fibromyalgia. *Curr. Ther. Res. Clin. Exp.*, 1994, 55/6 (699-706)

Clinical evaluation of S-adenosyl-L-methionine versus transcutaneous electrical nerve stimulation in primary fibromyalgia. *Curr. Ther. Res. Clin. Exp.*, 1993, 53/2 (222-229)

Evaluation of S-adenosylmethionine in primary fibromyalgia. A double-blind crossover study. *Am. J. Med.*, 1987, 83/5 A (107-110)

S-adenosylmethionine blood levels in major depression: Changes with drug treatment. *Acta Neurol. Scand. Suppl.* (Denmark), 1994, 89/154 (15-18)

Psychological distress during puerperium: A novel therapeutic approach using S-adenosylmethionine. *Curr. Ther. Res. Clin. Exp.*, 1993, 53/6 (707-716)

Double blind, placebo-controlled study of S-adenosyl-L-methionine in depressed postmenopausal women. *Psychother. Psychosom.* (Switzerland), 1993, 59/1 (34-40)

S-adenosylmethionine treatment of depression: A controlled clinical trial. *Am. J. Psychiatry*, 1988, 145/9 (1110-1114)

Treatment of depression in rheumatoid arthritic patients. A comparison of S-adenosylmethionine (Samyr) and placebo in a double-blind study. *Clin. Trials J.* (UK), 1987, 24/4 (305-310)

Monitoring S-adenosyl-methionine blood levels and antidepressant effect. *Acta Neurol.* (Italy), 1980, 35/6 (488-495)

Evaluation of S-adenosylmethionine (SAMe) effectiveness on depression. *Curr. Ther. Res., Clin. Exp.*, 1980, 27/6II (908-918)

Gingivitis

Folate mouthwash: effects on established gingivitis in periodontal patients. *J Clin Periodontol* 1984 Oct;11(9):619-28

Effects of topical and systemic folic acid supplementation on gingivitis in pregnancy. *J Clin Periodontol* 1980 Oct;7(5):402-14

Effects of extended systemic and topical folate supplementation on gingivitis of pregnancy. *J Clin Periodontol* 1982 May;9(3):275-80

The effect of topical application of folic acid on gingival health. *J Oral Med* 1978 Jan-Mar;33(1):22-2

The effect of folic acid on gingival health. *J Periodontol* 1976 Nov;47(11):667-8

A controlled evaluation of an allopurinol mouthwash as prophylaxis against 5-fluorouracil-induced stomatitis. *Cancer* 1990 Apr 15;65(8):1879-82

Oral changes in a folic acid deficient patient precipitated by anticonvulsant drug therapy. *Journal of Periodontology* (J. Periodontol.), 1973, 44/- (645-650)

Effectiveness of the Sonicare sonic toothbrush on reduction of plaque, gingivitis, probing pocket depth and subgingival bacteria in adolescent orthodontic patients. *J Clin Dent* 1997; 8 (1 Spec No):15-9

The comparative efficacy of stabilized stannous fluoride dentifrice, peroxide/baking soda dentifrice and essential oil mouthrinse for the prevention of gingivitis. *J Clin Dent* 1997; 8 (2 Spec No):46-53

Effects of folate mouthwash on experimental gingivitis in man. *J Clin Periodontol* (Denmark) Aug 1986, 13 (7) p671-6

The effect of folic acid on experimentally produced gingivitis. *J Prev Dent* Jul-Aug 1978, 5 (4) p30-2

Epidemiological and biochemical studies of necrotizing ulcerative gingivitis and noma (cancrum oris) in Nigerian children. *Arch Oral Biol* (England) Sep 1972, 17 (9) p1357-71

[Effectivennes of Bactrim and Rovamycine in periodontitis]. *SSO Schweiz Monatsschr Zahnheilkd* (Switzerland) Jul 1973, 83 (7) p828-39

[Clinical study of a new bactericidal chemotherapeutic agent]. *Rev Odontostomatol Midi Fr* (France) 1971, 29 (2) p148-52

Inverse correlation between the proportion of salivary bacteria inhibiting Streptococcus mutans and the percentage of untreated carious teeth. *J Oral Pathol Med* (Denmark) Nov 1995, 24 (10) p462-7

[Effect of vitamins A, E and K on the indices of the glutathione antiperoxide system in gingival tissues in periodontosis]. *Vopr Pitan* (USSR) Jul-Aug 1985, (4) p54-6

Further characterization of Bacteroides endodontalis, an asaccharolytic black-pigmented Bacteroides species from the oral S cavity. *J Clin Microbiol* Jul 1985, 22 (1) p75-9

Effects of estradiol and progesterone on Bacteroides melaninogenicus and Bacteroides gingivalis. *Infect Immun* Jan 1982, 35 (1) p256-63

The effect of propolis and its components on eicosanoid production during the inflammatory response. *Prostaglandins Leukot Essent Fatty Acids* (Scotland) Dec 1996, 55 (6) p441-9

Local treatment of rheumatic diseases with propolis compounds (see comments]. *Orv Hetil* (Hungary) Jun 23 1996, 137 (25) p1365-70

Immunomodulatory action of propolis. VI. Influence of a water soluble derivative on complement activity in vivo. *J Ethnopharmacol* (Ireland) Jul 28 1995, 47 (3) p145-7

Mechanisms involved in the antiinflammatory effect of propolis extract. *Drugs Exp Clin Res* (Switzerland) 1993, 19 (5) p197-203

[Apiphytotherapeutic original preparations in the treatment of chronic marginal parodontopathies. A clinical and microbiological study]. *Rev Chir Oncol Radiol O R L Oftalmol Stomatol Ser Stomatol* (Romania) Apr-Jun 1989, 36 (2) p91-8

Effect of Propolis-gel in the treatment of gingival inflammation]. *Stomatol Vjesn* (Yugoslavia) 1985, 14 (3-4) p107-10

Properties and use of propolis. *Pol Tyg Lek* (Poland) Dec 13 1982, 37 (49) p1489-92

The inhibitory effect of funoran and eucalyptus extract-containing chewing gum on plaque formation. *J Oral Sci* (Japan) Sep 1998, 40 (3) p115-7

Antibacterial activity of Camellia sinensis extracts against dental caries. *Arch Pharm Res* (Korea) Jun 1998, 21 (3) p348-52

Simultaneous determination of catechins in human saliva by high-performance liquid chromatography. *J Chromatogr B Biomed Sci Appl*(Netherlands) Dec 5 1997,703(1-2)p253-8

Study on feasibility of Chinese green tea polyphenols (CTP) for preventing dental caries. *Chung Hua Kou Chiang Hsueh Tsa Chih* (China) Jul 1993,28(4)p197-9,254

Anticariogenic effects of green tea. *Fukuoka Igaku Zasshi* (Japan) Apr 1992, 83 (4) p174-80

Anticaries effects of polyphenolic compounds from Japanese green tea. *Caries Res* (Switzerland) 1991, 25 (6) p438-43

A pilot study of Japanese green tea as a medicament: antibacterial and bactericidal effects. *J Endod* Mar 1991, 17 (3) p122-4

Effect of tea polyphenols on glucan synthesis by glucosyltransferase from Streptococcus mutans. *Chem Pharm Bull* (Tokyo) (Japan) Mar 1990, 38 (3) p717-20

Triterpene alcohols from the flowers of compositae and their anti-inflammatory effects. *Phytochemistry* Dec 1996, 43 (6) p1255-60

[Anti-inflammatory action of a group of plant extracts]. *Vet Med Nauki* (Bulgaria) 1981, 18 (6) p87-94

Anti-calculus activity of a toothpaste with microgranules. *Oral Dis* (England) Sep 1998, 4 (3) p213-6

Effect of citric acid concentration on dentin demineralization, dehydration, and rehydration: atomic force microscopy study. *J Biomed Mater Res* Dec 15 1998, 42 (4) p500-7

The effectiveness of three irrigating solutions on root canal cleaning after hand and mechanical preparation. *Int Endod J* (England) Jan 1997, 30 (1) p51-7

Effect of citric acid clearance on the saturation with respect to hydroxyapatite in saliva. *Caries Res* (Switzerland) 1996, 30 (3) p213-7

Site specificity of citric acid retention after an oral rinse. *Caries Res* (Switzerland) 1995, 29 (6) p467-9

The effect of ultrasonic irrigation before and after citric acid treatment on collagen fibril exposure: an in vitro SEM study. *J Periodontol* Oct 1995, 66 (10) p887-91

Salivary clearance of citric acid after an oral rinse. *J Dent* (England) Aug 1995, 23 (4) p209-12

Comparison between 3 triclosan dentifrices on plaque, gingivitis and salivary microflora. *J Clin Periodontol* (Denmark) Jan 1995, 22 (1) p63-70

Antimicrobial activity of Pelargonium essential oils added to a quiche filling as a model food system. *Lett Appl Microbiol* (England) Oct 1998, 27 (4) p207-10

Factors that interact with the antibacterial action of thyme essential oil and its active constituents. *J Appl Bacteriol* (England) Jun 1994, 76 (6) p626-31

Vitamin C, oral scurvy and periodontal disease. *S Afr Med J* (South Africa) May 26 1984, 65 (21)

[Anticalculus dentifrices. A new era in preventive dentistry?]. *Ned Tijdschr Tandheelkd* (Netherlands) Dec 1989, 96 (12)

Effect of tea polyphenols on glucan synthesis by glucosyltransferase from Streptococcus mutans. *Chem Pharm Bull* (Tokyo) (Japan) Mar 1990, 38 (3)

Green Tea to Prevent Dental Cares. *Chung Hua Kou Chiang Hsueh Tsa Chih* (China) Jul 1993, 28 (4) p197-9 54

[Management of gingival inflammation with active ingredients in toothpaste] *Dtsch Zahnarztl Z* (Germany, West) Jun 1975, 30 (6) p382-4

Evidence for enhanced treatment of periodontal disease by therapy with coenzyme Q. *Int J Vitam Nutr Res* (Switzerland) Apr 1973, 43 (4) p537-48

Zinc in etiology of periodontal disease. *Med Hypotheses* (England) Mar Stomatological Clinic, Medical 1993, 40 (3) p182-5

Diabetes and periodontal diseases. Possible role of vitamin c deficiency: an hypothesis. *J Periodontol* May 1981, 52 (5) p251-4

Relationship of mineral status and intake to periodontal disease. *Am J Clin Nutr* Jul 1976, 29 (7)

Comparative In Vitro Activity of Sanguinarine Against Oral. *Antimicrobial Agents And Chemotheropy*, Apr. 1985, p. 663-65 Vol. 27, No. 4

MICs of sanguinarine were determined for 52 oral reference strains and 129 fresh isolates from human dental plaque. Sanguinarine was found to completely inhibit the growth of 98% of the isolates at a concentration of 16 mg/ml Zinc And Sanguinaria. *J Periodontol* 60(2):91-5, 1989)

Supplementation or loca1 application may reduce gingival exudate from inflammed and infected gums—which suggests improved tissue health. (Folate mouthwash appears to to be more effective than oral folate.) *J Clin Periodonlol* 14(6):315-9, 1987)

Effects on established gingivitis in periodontal patients. *J Clin Periodontol* 11:619-28, 1984)

Glaucoma

Medical management of glaucoma. *N Engl J Med* 1998 Oct 29;339(18):1298-307

Aqueous humour and serum zinc and copper concentrations of patients with glaucoma and cataract. *British Journal of Ophthalmology* (UK) 1990, 74/11 (661-662)

Analysis of the medical use of marijuana and its societal implications [see comments]. *J Am Pharm Assoc* (Wash) (U S) Mar-Apr 1998, 38 (2) p220-7

Glycerol: Biochemistry, pharmacokinetics and clinical and practical applications. *Sports Medicine* (New Zealand), 1998, 26/3 (145-167)

Medicinal marijuana: A comprehensive review. *Journal of Psychoactive Drugs*, 1998, 30/2 (137-147)

Vitamins Binf 1 and PP in treating glaucomatous patients (Russian). *Vestnik Oftalmologii* (Vestn. Oftalmol.) 1974, No.3/-(19-21)

Blood levels of thiamine and ascorbic acid in chronic open-angle glaucoma. *Ann Ophthalmol* Jul 1979, 11 (7) p1095-1100

Neurotransmitters and intraocular pressure. *Fundam. Clin. Pharmacol.* (France), 1988, 2/4 (305-325)

HP 663: A novel compound for the treatment of glaucoma. *Drug Dev. Res.*, 1988, 12/3-4 (197-209)

Intraocular pressure effects of multiple doses of drugs applied to glaucomatous monkey eyes. *Arch. Ophthalmol.*, 1987, 105/2 (249-252)

Laser-induced glaucoma in rabbits. *Exp. Eye Res.* (UK), 1986, 43/6 (885-894)

Regulation of aqueous flow by the adenylate cyclase receptor complex in the ciliary epithelium. *Am. J. Ophthalmol.*, 1985, 100/1 (194-198)

Forskolin suppresses sympathetic neuron function and causes ocular hypotension. *Curr. Eye Res.* (England), 1985, 4/2 (87-96)

Forskolin lowers intraocular pressure by reducing aqueous inflow. *Invest. Ophthalmol. Visual Sci.*, 1984, 25/3 (268-276)

Indomethacin and epinephrine effects on outflow facility and cyclic adenosine monophosphate formation in monkeys. *Investigative Ophthalmology and Visual Science*, 1996, 37/7 (1348-1359)

Hair Loss

See references under Baldness.

Hearing Loss

Attenuation of aminoglycoside-induced cochlear damage with the metabolic antioxidant alpha-lipoic acid. *Hear Res* (Netherlands) Feb 1999, 128 (1-2) p40-4

Effects of Ginkgo biloba extract on the cochlear damage induced by local gentamicin installation in guinea pigs. *J Korean Med Sci* (Korea) Oct 1998, 13 (5) p525-8

Changes in cochlear antioxidant enzyme activity after sound conditioning and noise exposure in the chinchilla. *Hear Res* (Netherlands) Mar 1998, 117 (1-2) p31-8

Role of glutathione in protection against noise-induced hearing loss. *Brain Res* (Netherlands) Feb 16 1998, 784 (1-2) p82-90

Vitamin E and lipoic acid, but not vitamin C improve blood oxygenation after high-energy IMPULSE noise (BLAST) exposure. *Biochem Biophys Res Commun* 1998 Dec 9;253(1):114-8

The efficacy of Lasix-vitamin therapy (L-V therapy) for sudden deafness and other sensorineural hearing loss. *Acta Otolaryngol Suppl* (Stockh) 1991;486:78-91

Thioctic (lipoic) acid: a therapeutic metal-chelating antioxidant? *Biochem Pharmacol* 1995 Jun 29;50(1):123-6

Dihydrolipoic acid—a universal antioxidant both in the membrane and in the aqueous phase. Reduction of peroxyl, ascorbyl and chromanoxyl radicals. *Biochem Pharmacol* 1992 Oct 20;44(8):1637-49

Interplay between lipoic acid and glutathione in the protection against microsomal lipid peroxidation. *Biochim Biophys Acta* 1988 Dec 16;963(3):558-61

Glutathione monoethyl ester: preparation, uptake by tissues, and conversion to glutathione. *Arch Biochem Biophys* 1985 Jun;239(2):538-48

Sulfhydryl compounds and antioxidants inhibit cytotoxicity to outer hair cells of a gentamicin metabolite in vitro. *Hear Res* 1994 Jun 15;77(1-2):75-80

alpha-Lipoic acid protects against reperfusion injury following cerebral ischemia in rats. *Brain Res* 1996 Apr 22;717(1-2):184-8

Automatic monitoring of mechano-electrical transduction in the guinea pig cochlea. *Hear Res* 1998 Nov;125(1-2):1-16

Uptake of amikacin by hair cells of the guinea pig cochlea and vestibule and ototoxicity: comparison with gentamicin. *Hear Res* 1995 Feb;82(2):179-83

Aminoglycoside ototoxicity and the medial efferent system: II. Comparison of acute effects of different antibiotics. *Audiology* 1998 May-Jun;37(3):162-73

[The influence on sound damages by an extract of ginkgo biloba]. *Arch Otorhinolaryngol* Jul 8, 1975, 209 (3) p203-15

[Hydergine in pathology of the inner ear]. *An Otorrinolaringol Ibero Am* (Spain) 1990, 17 (1) p85-98

[Ginkgo extract EGb 761 (tenobin)/HAES versus naftidrofuryl A randomized study of therapy of sudden deafness]. *Laryngorhinootologie* (Germany) Mar 1994, 73 (3) p149-52

[Therapeutic trial in acute cochlear deafness. A comparative study of Ginkgo biloba extract and nicergoline]. *Presse Med* (France) Sep 25 1986, 15 (31) p1559-61

[The influence on sound damages by an extract of ginkgo biloba]. *Arch Otorhinolaryngol* Jul 8 1975, 209 (3) p203-15

Results of combined low-power laser therapy and extracts of Ginkgo biloba in cases of sensorineural hearing loss and tinnitus. *Adv Otorhinolaryngol* (Switzerland) 1995, 49 p101-4

Trial of an extract of Ginkgo biloba (EGB) for tinnitus and hearing loss [letter]. *Clin Otolaryngol* (England) Dec 1988, 13 (6) p501-2

Hemochromatosis

Primary hemochromatosis and dietary iron. *Tidsskr Nor Laegeforen* (Norway) Oct 10 1997, 117 (24) p3506–7

The effect of withdrawal of food iron fortification in Sweden as studied with phlebotomy in subjects with genetic hemochromatosis. *Eur J Clin Nutr* (England) Nov 1997, 51 (11) p782–6

Noninvasive prediction of fibrosis in C282Y homozygous hemochromatosis. *Gastroenterology* Oct 1998, 115 (4) p929–36

Hemochromatosis: advances in molecular genetics and clinical diagnosis. *J Clin Gastroenterol* Jul 1998, 27 (1) p41–6

Defective iron metabolism in genetic hemochromatosis. [The mechanisms remain unknown in spite of genetic advances] *Lakartidningen* (Sweden) Aug 5 1998, 95 (32–33) p3430–35

Clinical characteristics of hereditary hemochromatosis patients who lack the C282Y mutation. *Hepatology* Aug 1998, 28 (2) p526–29

Haemochromatosis. *Clin Lab Haematol* (England) Apr 1998, 20 (2) p65–75

Classification and diagnosis of iron overload. *Haematologica* (Italy) May 1998, 83 (5) p447–55, 078

Hereditary haemochromatosis mutation frequencies in the general population. *J Med Screen* (England) 1998, 5 (1) p34–6

Factors affecting the rate of iron mobilization during venesection therapy for genetic hemochromatosis. *Am J Hematol* May 1998, 58 (1) p16–9

Heterogeneity of hemochromatosis in Italy. *Gastroenterology* May 1998, 114 (5) p996–1002

Hemochromatosis and iron needs. *Nutr Rev* Feb 1998, 56 (2 Pt 2) ps30–7; discussion s54–75

Understanding iron absorption and metabolism, aided by studies of hemochromatosis. *Ann Clin Lab Sci* Jan–Feb 1998, 28 (1) p30–3

Clinical trial on the effect of regular tea drinking on iron accumulation in genetic haemochromatosis. *Gut* (UK), 1998, 43/5 (699–704)

Does calcium interfere with iron absorption? *Am J Clin Nutr* 1998 Jul;68(1):3–4

Biological markers of oxidative stress induced by ethanol and iron overload in rat. *Int J Occup Med Environ Health* (Poland) 1994, 7 (4) p355–63

Antioxidant status and lipid peroxidation in hereditary haemochromatosis. *Free Radic Biol Med* Mar 1994, 16 (3)

Iron storage, lipid peroxidation and glutathione turnover in chronic anti-HCV positive hepatitis. *J Hepatol* (Denmark) Apr 1995, 22 (4) p449–56

Induction of oxidative single- and double-strand breaks in DNA by ferric citrate. *Free Radic Biol Med* Aug 1993

A unique rodent model for both the cardiotoxic and hepatotoxic effects of prolonged iron overload. *Lab Invest* Aug 1993, 69 (2) p217–22

Biochemical and biophysical investigations of the ferrocene-iron-loaded rat. An animal model of primary haemochromatosis. *Eur J Biochem* (Germany) Dec 5 1991, 202 (2) p405–10

Antioxidant and iron-chelating activities of the flavonoids catechin, quercetin and diosmetin on iron-loaded rat hepatocyte cultures. *Biochem. Pharmacol.* (UK), 1993

Iron absorption and phenolic compounds: Importance of different phenolic structures. *Europ. J. Clin. Nutr.* (UK), 1989

Inhibition of the tobacco-specific nitrosamine-induced lung tumorigenesis by compounds derived from cruciferous vegetables and green tea. *Ann. New York Acad. Sci.*, 1993, 686

The effects of caffeic acid and its related catechols on hydroxyl radical formation by 3-hydroxyanthranilic acid, ferric chloride, and hydrogen peroxide. *Arch. Biochem. Biophys.*, 1990, 276/1

A novel antioxidant flavonoid (IdB 1031) affecting molecular mechanisms of cellular activation. *Free Radic. Biol. Med.*, 1994, 16/5 (547–553)

Prevention of postischemic cardiac injury by the orally active iron chelator 1,2-dimethyl-3-hydroxy-4-pyridone (L1) and the antioxidant (+)-cyanidanol-3. *Circulation*, 1989, 80/1 (158–164)

Hepatotoxicity of menadione predominates in oxygen-rich zones of the liver lobule. *J. Pharmacol. Exp. Ther.*, 1989, 248/3 (1317–1322)

Iron-load increases the susceptibility of rat hearts to oxygen reperfusion damage. Protection by the antioxidant (+)-cyanidanol-3 and deferoxamine. *Circulation*, 1988, 78/2 (442–49)

Hepatocyte injury resulting from the inhibition of mitochondrial respiration at low oxygen concentrations involves reductive stress and oxygen activation. *Chemico-Biological Interactions* (Ireland), 1995, 98/1 (27–44)

Modulating hypoxia-induced hepatocyte injury by affecting intracellular redox state. *Biochimica et Biophysica Acta - Molecular Cell Research* (Netherlands), 1995, 1269/2 (153–161)

Protection of rat myocardial phospholipid against peroxidative injury through superoxide-(xanthine oxidase)-dependent, iron-promoted fenton chemistry by the male contraceptive gossypol. *Biochem. Pharmacol.* (UK), 1988, 37/17 (3335–3342)

Protective effect of tea polyphenol on rat myocardial injury induced by isoproterenol. *Chinese Traditional and Herbal Drugs* (China)(Apr) 1995

Effect of the interaction of tannins with coexisting substances. Part 2. reduction of heavy metal ions and solubilization of precipitates. *Journal of the Pharmaceutical Society of Japan* (Japan), V102, (8), 1982

Free radicals scavenging action and anti-enzyme activities of procyanidines from Vitis vinifera. A mechanism for their capillary protective action. *Arzneimittelforschung* (Germany) May 1994, 44 (5) p592–601

The inhibitory action of chlorogenic acid on the intestinal iron absorption in rats. *Acta Physiol Pharmacol Ther Latinoam* (Argentina) 1992, 42 (3)

Inhibition of tobacco-specific nitrosamine-induced lung tumorigenesis by compounds derived from cruciferous vegetables and green tea. *Ann N Y Acad Sci* May 28 1993, 686

Ascorbic acid prevents the dose-dependent inhibitory effects of polyphenols and phytates on nonheme-iron absorption. *Am J Clin Nutr* Feb 1991, 53 (2)

Phytic acid. A natural antioxidant. *J Biol Chem* Aug 25 1987, 262 (24)

[Effect of polyphenols of coffee pulp on iron absorption]. *Arch Latinoam Nutr* (Venezuela) Jun 1985, 35 (2)

Factors affecting the absorption of iron from cereals. *Br J Nutr* (England) Jan 1984, 51 (1) p37–46

The effect of red and white wines on nonheme-iron absorption in humans. *Am J Clin Nutr* Apr 1995

Prevention of iron deficiency. *Baillieres Clin Haematol* (England) Dec 1994, 7 (4)

Iron absorption and phenolic compounds: importance of different phenolic structures. *Eur J Clin Nutr* (England) Aug 1989, 43 (8) p547–57

Hepatitis B

[Chronic viral hepatitis—diagnosis, therapy and prognosis]. *Versicherungsmedizin* 1999 Mar 1;51(1):3–11

[Hepatitis B and C: current therapy]. *Schweiz Rundsch Med Prax* 1998 Oct 14;87(42):1408–12

[New antiviral agents in the treatment of chronic hepatitis B and C]. *Rev Esp Enferm Dig* 1998 Apr;90(4):291–304

Treatment of chronic viral hepatitis. *Antivir Chem Chemother* 1998 Nov;9(6):449–60Natural therapy of children with chronic persistent hepatitis B. Preliminary report. *Medical Science Monitor* (Poland) 1997, 3/4 (446–450)

Review article: glycyrrhizin as a potential treatment for chronic hepatitis C. *Aliment Pharmacol Ther* (England) Mar 1998, 12 (3) p199–205

Historical treatment of chronic hepatitis B and chronic hepatitis C. *Gut* (UK) 1993, 34/Suppl. 2 (S69–S73)

Therapeutic basis of glycyrrhizin on chronic hepatitis B. *Antiviral Res* 1996 May;30(2–3):171–7

Effects of glycyrrhizin on hepatitis B surface antigen: a biochemical and morphological study. *J Hepatol* 1994 Oct;21(4):601–9

[Treatment of chronic hepatitis B. Part 2: Effect of glycyrrhizic acid on the course of illness]. [Article in German] *Fortschr Med* 1992 Jul 30;110(21):395–8

Enhancement of interferon-gamma production in glycyrrhizin-treated human peripheral lymphocytes in response to concanavalin A and to surface antigen of hepatitis B virus. *Proc Soc Exp Biol Med* 1986 Feb;181(2):205–10

Interferon alfa for chronic hepatitis B infection: increased efficacy of prolonged treatment. *Hepatology* 1999 Jul;30(1):238–43

Plasma selenium levels and risk of hepatocellular carcinoma among men with chronic hepatitis virus infection. *Am J Epidemiol* 1999 Aug 15;150(4):367–74

Protective role of selenium against hepatitis B virus and primary liver cancer in Qidong. *Biol Trace Elem Res* 1997 Jan;56(1):117–24

Chemoprevention trial of human hepatitis with selenium supplementation in China. *Biol Trace Elem Res* 1989 Apr–May;20(1–2):15–22

Selenium chemoprevention of liver cancer in animals and possible human applications. *Biol Trace Elem Res* 1988 Jan–Apr;15:231–41

[Markers of chronic hepatitis B in children after completion of therapywith isoprinosine] *Pol Tyg Lek* (Poland) Mar 15–29 1993, 48 (11–13) p263–4

[Course of chronic virus hepatitis B in children and attempts at modifying its treatment] *Pol Tyg Lek* (Poland) Mar 15–29 1993, 48 (11–13) p258–60

Isoprinosine in the treatment of chronic active hepatitis type B. *Scand J Infect Dis* (Sweden) 1990, 22 (6) p645–8

[Evaluation of the treatment of chronic active hepatitis (HBsAg+) with isoprinosine. II. Immunological studies]. *Pol Tyg Lek* (Poland) Apr 16–30 1990, 45 (16–18) p347–51

In vitro studies on the effect of certain natural products against hepatitis B virus. *Indian J Med Res* (India) Apr 1990, 92 p133–8

Effects of glycyrrhizin on hepatitis B surface antigen: a biochemical and morphological study. *J Hepatol* (Denmark) Oct 1994, 21 (4) p601–9

Glycyrrhizin withdrawal followed by human lymphoblastoid interferon in the treatment of chronic hepatitis B. *Gastroenterol Jpn* (Japan) Dec 1991, 26 (6) p742–6

Combination therapy of glycyrrhizin withdrawal and human fibroblast Interferon for chronic hepatitis B. *Clin Ther* 1989, 11 (1) p161–9

Alpha-interferon combined with immunomodulation in the treatment of chronic hepatitis B. *J Gastroenterol Hepatol* (Australia) 1991, 6 Suppl 1 p13–4

Improvement of liver fibrosis in chronic hepatitis C patients treated with natural interferon alpha. *J Hepatol* (Denmark) Feb 1995, 22 (2) p135–42

Diagnosis and treatment of the major hepatotropic viruses. *Am J Med Sci* Oct 1993, 306 (4) p248–61

Treatment of chronic viral hepatitis. *J Antimicrob Chemother* (England) Jul 1993, 32 Suppl A p107–20

[Mechanisms of the effect of interferon (IFN) therapy in patients with type B and C chronic hepatitis]. *Hokkaido Igaku Zasshi* (Japan) May 1993, 68 (3) p297–309

A pilot study of ribavirin therapy for recurrent hepatitis C virus infection after liver transplantation. *Transplantation* May 27 1996, 61 (10) p1483–88

Ribavirin as therapy for chronic hepatitis C. A randomized, double-blind, placebo-controlled trial. *Ann Intern Med* Dec 15 1995, 123 (12) p897–903

Treatment with ribavirin+alpha interferon in HCV chronic active hepatitis non-responders to interferon alone: preliminary results. *J Chemother* (Italy) Feb 1995, 7 (1) p58–61

Combined treatment with interferon alpha-2b and ribavirin for chronic hepatitis C in patients with a previous non-response or non-sustained response to interferon alone. *J Med Virol* May 1995, 46 (1) p43–7

Increase in hepatic iron stores following prolonged therapy with ribavirin in patients with chronic hepatitis C. *J Hepatol* (Denmark) Dec 1994, 21 (6) p1109–12

Therapy for chronic hepatitis C. *Gastroenterol Clin North Am* Sep 1994, 23 (3) p603–13

Treatment of chronic viral hepatitis. *Baillieres Clin Gastroenterol* (England) Jun 1994, 8 (2) p233–53

Elevated serum iron predicts poor response to interferon treatment in patients with chronic HCV infection. *Dig Dis Sci* Nov 1995, 40 (11) p2431–3

Distribution of iron in the liver predicts the response of chronic hepatitis C infection to interferon therapy [published erratum appears in Am J Clin Pathol 1995 Aug;104(2):232]. *Am J Clin Pathol* Apr 1995, 103 (4) p419–24

Increased serum iron and iron saturation without liver iron accumulation distinguish chronic hepatitis C from other chronic liver diseases. *Dig Dis Sci* Dec 1994, 39 (12) p2656–9

Response related factors in recombinant interferon alfa-2b treatment of chronic hepatitis C. *Gut* (England) 1993, 34 (2 Suppl) pS139–40

Measurements of iron status in patients with chronic hepatitis. [see comments] *Gastroenterology* Jun 1992, 102 (6) p2108–13

[Effect of green tea on iron absorption in elderly patients with iron deficiency anemia]. *Nippon Ronen Igakkai Zasshi* (Japan) Sep 1990, 27 (5) p555–8

[Current knowledge in the treatment of chronic hepatitis C] Acquisitions recentes dans le traitement de l'hepatite C chronique. *Rev Med Liege* (Belgium) Dec 1995, 50 (12) p501-4

Hepatitis C

Effect of interferon-alpha and ribavirin therapy on serum GB virus C/hepatitis G virus (GBV-C/HGV) RNA levels in patients chronically infected with hepatitis C virus and GBV-C/HGV. *J Infect Dis* 1997 Aug;176(2):421-6

Interferon-ribavirin for chronic hepatitis C with and without cirrhosis: analysis of individual patient data of six controlled trials. Eurohep Study Group for Viral Hepatitis. *Gastroenterology* 1999 Aug;117(2):408-13

A randomized trial of ribavirin and interferon-alpha vs. interferon-alpha alone in patients with chronic hepatitis C who were non-responders to a previous treatment. *J Hepatol* 1999 Jul;31(1):1-7

Health-related quality of life in chronic hepatitis C: impact of disease and treatment response. *Hepatology* 1999 Aug;30(2):550-55

Combination therapy for chronic hepatitis C: interferon and ribavirin. *Hosp Med* 1999 May;60(5):357-61

Retreatment of non-responder or relapser chronic hepatitis C patients with interferon plus ribavirin vs interferon alone. *Ital J Gastroenterol Hepatol* 1999 Apr;31(3):211-15

[Experience with combined interferon alpha-2b and ribavirin in the therapy of chronic hepatitis C. Experience with one-year therapy of 100 patients. Multicenter study]. *Orv Hetil* 1999 May 30;140(22):1235-8

Changes in serum hepatitis C virus RNA in interferon nonresponders retreated with interferon plus ribavirin: a preliminary report. *J Clin Gastroenterol* 1999 Jun;28(4):313-6

Pilot study of triple antiviral therapy for chronic hepatitis C in interferon alpha non-responders. *Ital J Gastroenterol Hepatol* 1999 Mar;31(2):130-4

[Effectiveness of interferon, glycyrrhizin combination therapy in patients with chronic hepatitis C]. *Nippon Rinsho* 1994 Jul;52(7):1817-22

Plasma selenium levels and risk of hepatocellular carcinoma among men with chronic hepatitis virus infection. *Am J Epidemiol* 1999 Aug 15;150(4):367-74

Two cases of hepatitis C treated with herbs and supplements. *J Altern Complement Med* 1997 Spring;3(1):77-82

Ribavirin as therapy for chronic hepatitis C. A randomized, double-blind, placebo-controlled trial. *Ann Intern Med* Dec 15 1995, 123 (12) p897-903

Treatment with ribavirin+alpha interferon in HCV chronic active hepatitis non-responders to interferon alone: preliminary results. *J Chemother* (Italy) Feb 1995, 7 (1) p58-61

Combined treatment with interferon alpha-2b and ribavirin for chronic hepatitis C in patients with a previous non-response or non-sustained response to interferon alone. *J Med Virol* May 1995, 46 (1) p43-7

[Evaluation of the treatment of chronic active hepatitis (HBsAg+) with isoprinosine. II. Immunological studies]. *Pol Tyg Lek* (Poland) Apr 16-30 1990, 45 (16-18) p347-51

In vitro studies on the effect of certain natural products against hepatitis B virus. *Indian J Med Res* (India) Apr 1990, 92 p133-8

Effects of glycyrrhizin on hepatitis B. Surface antigen: a biochemical and morphological study. *J Hepatol* 1994 Oct;21(4):601-9

Glycyrrhizin withdrawal followed by human lymphoblastoid interferon in the treatment of chronic hepatitis B. *Gastroenterol Jpn* (Japan) Dec 1991, 26 (6) p742-6

Combination therapy of glycyrrhizin withdrawal and human fibroblast interferon for chronic hepatitis B. *Clin Ther* 1989, 11 (1) p161-9

Alpha-interferon combined with immunomodulation in the treatment of chronic hepatitis B. *J Gastroenterol Hepatol* (Australia) 1991, 6 Suppl 1 p13-4

Improvement of liver fibrosis in chronic hepatitis C patients treated with natural interferon alpha. *J Hepatol* (Denmark) Feb 1995, 22 (2) p135-42

Diagnosis and treatment of the major hepatotropic viruses. *Am J Med Sci* Oct 1993, 306 (4) p248-61

Treatment of chronic viral hepatitis. *J Antimicrob Chemother* (England) Jul 1993, 32 Suppl A p107-20

[Mechanisms of the effect of interferon (IFN) therapy in patients with type B and C chronic hepatitis]. *Hokkaido Igaku Zasshi* (Japan) May 1993, 68 (3) p297-309

A pilot study of ribavirin therapy for recurrent hepatitis C virus infection after liver transplantation. *Transplantation* May 27 1996, 61 (10) p1483-88

Therapy for chronic hepatitis C. *Gastroenterol Clin North Am* Sep 1994, 23 (3) p603-13

Treatment of chronic viral hepatitis. *Baillieres Clin Gastroenterol* (England) Jun 1994, 8 (2) p233-53

Elevated serum iron predicts poor response to interferon treatment in patients with chronic HCV infection. *Dig Dis Sci* Nov 1995, 40 (11) p2431-33

Distribution of iron in the liver predicts the response of chronic hepatitis C infection to interferon therapy [published erratum appears in Am J Clin Pathol 1995 Aug;104(2):232]. *Am J Clin Pathol* Apr 1995, 103 (4) p419-24

Increased serum iron and iron saturation without liver iron accumulation distinguish chronic hepatitis C from other chronic liver diseases. *Dig Dis Sci* Dec 1994, 39 (12) p2656-59

Response related factors in recombinant interferon alfa-2b treatment of chronic hepatitis C. *Gut* (England) 1993, 34 (2 Suppl) pS139-40

Measurements of iron status in patients with chronic hepatitis. *Gastroenterology* Jun 1992, 102 (6) p2108-13

[Markers of chronic hepatitis B in children after completion of therapy with isoprinosine]. *Pol Tyg Lek* (Poland) Mar 15-29 1993, 48 (11-13) p263-4

Course of chronic virus hepatitis B in children and attempts at modifying its treatment]. *Pol Tyg Lek* (Poland) Mar 15-29 1993, 48 (11-13) p258-60

Isoprinosine in the treatment of chronic active hepatitis type B. *Scand J Infect Dis* (Sweden) 1990, 22 (6) p645-8

Antioxidant and iron-chelating activities of the flavonoids catechin, quercetin and diosmetin on iron-loaded rat hepatocyte cultures. *Biochem. Pharmacol.* (UK), 1993

Iron absorption and phenolic compounds: Importance of different phenolic structures. *Europ. J. Clin. Nutr.* (UK), 1989

Inhibition of the tobacco-specific nitrosamine-induced lung tumorigenesis by compounds derived from cruciferous vegetables and green tea. *Ann. New York Acad. Sci.*, 1993, 686

The effects of caffeic acid and its related catechols on hydroxyl radical formation by 3-hydroxyanthranilic acid, ferric chloride, and hydrogen peroxide. *Arch. Biochem. Biophys.*, 1990, 276/1

A novel antioxidant flavonoid (IdB 1031) affecting molecular mechanisms of cellular activation. *Free Radic. Biol. Med.*, 1994, 16/5 (547-553)

Prevention of postischemic cardiac injury by the orally active iron chelator 1,2-dimethyl-3-hydroxy-4-pyridone (L1) and the antioxidant (+)-cyanidanol-3. *Circulation,* 1989, 80/1 (158-164)

Hepatotoxicity of menadione predominates in oxygen-rich zones of the liver lobule. *J. Pharmacol. Exp. Ther.*, 1989, 248/3 (1317-1322)

HIV Infection (AIDS)(Opportunistic Infections)

Association Between Vitamin A and E Levels and HIV-1 Disease Progression. *AIDS* 11: 613620,1997

Glutathione Deficiency is Asssociated with Impaired Survival in HIV Disease. *Proc Natl Acad Sci* 1997; 94:1967-1972

Nutritional Status and Immune Responses in Mice with Murine AIDS are Normalized by Vitamin E Supplementation. *J Nutr 124:2024-2032, 1994.*

Dietary Recommendations to Maintain Adequate Blood Nutrient Levels in Early HIV-1 Infection. *VIII International Conference ON AIDS*, Abstract # POB-3675, July 1992.

Systemic Glutathione Deficiency in Symptom-free HIV Seropositive Individuals. *The Lancet* 1989;11:1 294-297

Role of Cysteine and Glutathione in HIV Infection and Other Diseases Associated with Muscle Wasting and Immunological Dysfunctions. *FASEB J* 1997; 11:1077-1089.

Impairment of Intestinal Glutathione Synthesis in Patients with Inflammatory Bowel Disease. *Gut* 1998;42:485-92.

Oxidative Stress, HIV and AIDS. *Res. Immunol 1992*; 143: 145-48.

Low Concentration of Acid-soluble Thiol (cysteine) in the Blood Plasma of HIV-1-Infected Patients. *Biol Chem1989*, Hoppe-Selyer, 370, 101-108

Decreased Serum Dehydroepiandrosterone is Associated with an Increased Progression of Human Immunodeficiency Virus Infection in Men with CD4 Cell Counts of 200-499. *J. Infect Dis* (USA), 1991, 164/5 (864-868).

Dehydroepiandrosterone as a Predictor for Progression to AIDS in Asymptomatic Human Immunodeficiency Virus-Infected Men. *J. Infect Dis* (USA), 1992, 165/3 (413-418)

Inhibition of HIV 1 Latency Reactivation by Dehydroepiandrosterone (DHEA) and an Analog of DHEA. *AIDS Res. Hum. Retroviruses* (USA), 1994, 201/3 (1424-32).

Evidence for Changes in Adrenal and Testicular Steroids During HIV Infection. *J Acquired Immune Defic. Syndrome.* (USA), 1992, 5/8 (841-46)

Biochemistry of Pharmacology of *S*-Adenosyl-*L*-methionine and Rationale for Its Use in Liver Disease. *Drugs* (New Zealand), 1990, 40/Supp.3 (98-110)

S-Adenosyl-*L*-Methionine. A Review of Its Pharmacological Properties and Therapeutic Potential in Liver Dysfunction and Affective Disorders in Relation to Its Physiological Role in Cell Metabolism. *Drugs* (New Zealand), 1989, 38/3.

The Activities of Coenzyme Q10 and Vitamin B6 for Immune Responses. *Biochem Biophys Res Commun* (USA), 1993, 193/1 (88-92).

Coenzyme Q10 Increases T4/T8 Ratios of Lymphocytes in Ordinary Subjects and Relevance to Patients Having the AIDS Related Complex. *Biochem Biophys Res Commun* (USA), 1991, 176/2 (786-791).

Biochemical Deficiency of Coenzyme Q10 in HIV-Infection and Exploratory Treatment. *Biochem Biophys Res Commun* (USA), 1988, 153/2 (888-896).

Simultaneous Detection of Ubiquinol and Ubiquinone in Human Plasma as a Marker of Oxidative Stress. *Anal Biochem* 250:66-73, 1997

Comparative Study of the Anti-HIV Activities of Ascorbate and Thio-Containing Reducing Agents in Chronically HIV-Infected Cells. *Am J Clib Nutr* (United States) Dec 1991, 54 (6 Suppl) (1231S-1235S).

Beta Carotene in HIV Infection. *AIDS* 6:272-276, 1993

Vitamin B_{12} Abnormalities in HIV-Infected Patients. *Eur J Haematol* (Denmark), 1991, 47/1(60-64).

HIV-Infected Patients with Vitamin B_{12} Deficiency and Autoantibodies to Intrinsic Factor: Disease Pathogenesis and Therapy. *AIDS Patient Care* (USA), 1991, 5/3 (125-128)

"Curbing the Craving: Naltrexone and Alcohol," *Penn Health Magazine.* July/August 1995 Issue. Available on the University of Pennsylvania Health Systems website at http://www.med.upenn.edu/~recovery/cons/pnhealth.html

"Naltrexone for AIDS/ARC," *AIDS Treatment News* Archive. Article dated October 24, 1986, Issue 016. Available on the Immunet website at www.immunet.org.

"The Role of Free Radicals and Antioxidants in HIV Disease," *Beta.* December 1993.

Bihari, Bernard, MD, Treatment Newsletter. August 15, 1996. Self-published by Bernard Bihari, MD, 29 West 15 Street, New York, NY 10011.

Bihari, Bernard, MD, "Naltrexone Stops AIDS Progression: Press Release," *How to Reverse Immune Dysfunction,* Sixth Edition by Mark Konlee. West Allis, WI: Keep Hope Alive, 1997. pp. 28-29.

Bihari, Bernard, MD, and Aaron Bihari. "Multiple Prophylaxis For Opportunistic Infections: A Longitudinal Observation Study." Publication and publication date unknown

The Efficacy of Inosine Pranobex in Preventing the Acquired Immunodeficiency Syndrome in Patients with Human Immunodeficiency Virus Infection. *New Engl J Med* (USA), 1990, 322/25 (1757-63).

Isoprinosine and Imuthiol, Two Potentially Active Compounds in Patients with AIDS-Related Complex Symptoms. *Cancer Res* 1985a. *(Suppl.)*, 45, 4671s-4673s.

Invitro Inhibition of LAV/HTLV-111-Infected Lymphocytes by Dithiocarb and Inodine Pranobex. *The Lancet* 1985b,11, 1423

A Pilot Study of Diethyldithiocarbamate in Patients with Acquired Immune Deficiency Syndrome (AIDS) and the AIDS-Related Complex. *Life Science* 1989, 45, 2509-2520.

Randomized, Double-Blind Placebo-Controlled Trial of Dithiocarb Sodium ("Imuthiol") in Human Immunodeficiency Virus Infection. *The Lancet* 1988,11, 702-706.

Dithiocarb Sodium (Diethyldithiocarbamate) Therapy in Patients with Symptomatic HIV Infection and AIDS. *J. Amer. Med. Ass.,* 265, 1538-1544, 1991.

Inhibition of HIV Progression by Dithiocarb. *The Lancet* 1990, 335, 679-682.

Glucose, Glutamine, and Ketone Body Metabolism in Human Enterocytes. *Metabolism* 37 1998:602-609.

Glutamine Metabolism by the Intestinal Tract. *JPEN* 9, 1985;608-617.

Intestinal Glutamine Metabolism. *Metabolism* 38,1989;18-24

Effects of Glutamine-Supplemented Diets on Immunology of the Gut. *JPEN* 14,1990;1092S-113S.

Glutamine Metabolism in Lymphocytes: Its Biochemical, Physiological and Clinical Importance. *QJ Eper Physiol* 70, 1985;473-489

"A Study of the Olive Leaf Preparation 'Tincture OleFoliorum' in the Treatment of Infection Caused by HIV." Unpublished study, written September 9, 1994.

"Treatment Issue's Second Survey of Physicians' Treatment Practice," *GMHC* Gay Men's Health Crisis, *Treatment Issues.* Volume 12, Number 1, Winter 1997/98.

"Inactivation of DNA Polymerases of Murine Leukemia viruses by Calcium Elenolate," *Nature New Biology* 238:277-279, August 30, 1972.

Privitera, James R., MD, Olive Leaf Extract: A New/Old Healing Bonanza for Mankind. Covina, CA: NutriScreen, Inc., 1996. This paper is also available on the World Wide Web at various sites, including www.oliveleafextract.com.

"In Vitro Antiviral Activity of Calcium Elenolate," *Antimicrobial Agents and Chemotherapy.* 1970. pp. 167-168.

"Maintaining Immune Functioning During Chronic Stress With Implications For AIDS." Copyright 1996 James F. Ripka. Publication status unknown. Available on the World Wide Web at http://www.biosyna.com/resch- l .html.

Walker, Morton, DPM, Olive Leaf Extract. New York: Kensington Books,1997.

Efficacy and Safety of Buxus Sempervirens L. Preparations (SPV-30) in HIV-infected Asymptomatic Patients: A Multicenter, Randomized, Double-Blind, Placebo-Controlled Trial. *Phytomedicine; International Journal of Phytotherapy and Phytopharmacology* 1998, Vol. 5(1):1-10.

Rasnick D. HIV Protease and Its Inhibitors. March 1997. Available calling (415) 826-1241 and rasnick@mindspring.com

The Valley Advocate, "The Big 'Tease" February 20, 1997 HEAL-Los Angelos (Health-Education-AIDS Liason, Los Angelos chapter) What's Up with the Viral Load Theory? 1996. 11684 Ventura Blvd, Studio City, CA, 91604 Tel. (213) 896-8260.

Centers for Disease Control, HIV/AIDS Surveillance Report, Vol.8 No.2 Table 13 AIDS Case Fatality Rates.

HEAL-Los Angeles (Health-Education-AIDS Liason, Los Angeles chapter) The Truth Behind T-Cell Counts. 1996. 11684 Ventura Blvd, Studio City, CA,91604 Tel. (213) 896-8260

Jeffrey Baggish, M.D. *How Your Immune System Works.* Emeryville, CA, Ziff-Davis Press, 1994

A Critical Analysis of the HIV-T4- Cell *AIDS Hypothesis. Genetica* 1995; 95:5-24.

Reapprasing AIDS, The Group for the Scientific Reappraisal of the HIV/AIDS Hypothesis, La Jolla, CA, Tel. (810) 772-9926, *Reappraising AIDS*, Volume 4, Number 10, October 1996

Methemoglobulinemia from Sniffing Butyl Nitrite. *Am Int. Med.* 1979;91:417-418.

Fatal Methemoglobulinemia Resulting from Ingestion of Isobutyl Nitrite, a Room Odorizer Widely Used for Recreational Purposes. *Journal Forensic Science* 1981;26:5 87-593.

Tyler D, *The Mitochondrion in Health and Disease.* New York: VCH Publishing, 1992

Selenium and HIV in Pediatrics. *J. Nutr. Immunol.*, 1994, 3/1 (41-49)

N-Acetylcysteine enhances T cell functions and T cell growth in culture. *Int. Immunol.* (UK), 1993, 5/1 (97-101

Cysteine and glutathione deficiency in HIV-infected patients. The basis for treatment with *N*-acetyl-cysteine. *AIDS-Forschung* (Germany), 1992, 7/4 (197-199)

N-acetylcysteine (NAC) enhances interleukin-2 but suppresses interleukin-4 secretion from normal and HIV+ CD4+ T-cells. *Cell Mol Biol* (Noisy-le-grand) (France) 1995, 41 Suppl 1 pS35-40

N-acetylcysteine enhances antibody-dependent cellular cytotoxicity in neutrophils and mononuclear cells from healthy adults and human immunodeficiency virus-infected patients. *J Infect Dis* Dec 1995, 172 (6) p1492-502

Glutathione precursor and antioxidant activities of *N*-acetylcysteine and oxothiazolidine carboxylate compared in in vitro studies of HIV replication. *AIDS Res Hum Retroviruses* Aug 1994, 10 (8) p961-7

Role for oxygen radicals in self-sustained HIV-1 replication in monocyte-derived macrophages: enhanced HIV-1 replication by *N*-acetyl-*L*-cysteine. *J Leukoc Biol* Dec 1994, 56 (6) p702-7

Effects of glutathione precursors on human immunodeficiency virus replication. *Chem Biol Interact* (Ireland) Jun 1994, 91 (2-3) p217-24

Effect of glutathione depletion and oral *N*-acetyl-cysteine treatment on CD4+ and CD8+ cells. *Faseb J* Apr 1 1994, 8 (6) p448-51

N-acetylcysteine enhances T cell functions and T cell growth in culture. *Int Immunol* (England) Jan 1993, 5 (1) p97-101

Comparative study of the anti-HIV activities of ascorbate and thiol-containing reducing agents in chronically HIV-infected cells. *Am J Clin Nutr* Dec 1991, 54 (6 Suppl) p1231S-1235S

Role for oxygen radicals in self-sustained HIV-1 replication in monocyte-derived macrophages: Enhanced HIV-1 replication by *N*-acetyl-*L*-cysteine. *J. Leukocyte Biol.*, 1994, 56/6 (702-707)

Effects of glutathione precursors on human immunodeficiency virus replication. *Chem-Biol. Interact.* (Ireland), 1994, 91/2-3 (217-24)

Antioxidant status and lipid peroxidation in patients infected with HIV. *Chem.-Biol. Interact.* (Ireland), 1994, 91/2-3 (165-180)

N-acetylcysteine inhibits latent HIV expression in chronically infected cells. *Aids Res. Hum. Retroviruses*, 1991, 7/6 (563-67)

Selenium mediated inhibition of transcription factor NF-kappaB and HIV-1 LTR promoter activity. *Archives Of Toxicology* (Germany), 1996, 70/5 (277-83)

Release of nitric oxide from astroglial cells: A key mechanism in neuroimmune disorders. *Advances in Neuroimmunology* (UK), 1995, 5/4 (421-430)

Carnitine depletion in peripheral blood mononuclear cells from patients with AIDS: Effect of oral *L*-carnitine. *AIDS* (UK), 1994, 8/5 (655-660)

High dose *L*-carnitine improves immunologic and metabolic parameters in AIDS patients. *Immunopharmacol. Immunotoxicol.*, 1993, 15/1 (1-12)

Stress, Immunity and Ageing. A role for acetyl-*L*-carnitine: proceedings of the workshop. ICS844.

Vitamin B_{12} abnormalities in HIV-infected patients. *Eur. J. Haematol.* (Denmark), 1991, 47/1 (60-64)

HIV-infected patients with vitamin B_{12} deficiency and autoantibodies to intrinsic factor: Disease pathogenesis and therapy. *Aids Patient Care*, 1991, 5/3 (125-128)

One-year follow-up on the safety and efficacy of isoprinosine for human immunodeficiency virus infection. *J. Intern. Med.* (UK), 1992, 231/6 (607-15)

Immunotherapy of human immunodeficiency virus infection. *Trends Pharmacol. Sci.* (UK), 1991, 12/3 (107-111)

The efficacy of inosine pranobex in preventing the acquired immunodeficiency syndrome in patients with human immunodeficiency virus infection. *New Engl. J. Med.*, 1990, 322/25 (1757-1763)

The activities of coenzyme Q10 and vitamin B6 for immune responses. *Biochem. Biophys. Res. Commun.*, 1993, 193/1 (88-92)

Coenzyme Q10 increases T4/T8 ratios of lymphocytes in ordinary subjects and relevance to patients having the AIDS related complex. *Biochem. Biophys. Res. Commun.*, 1991, 176/2 (786-91)

Biochemical deficiencies of coenzyme Q_{10} in HIV-infection and exploratory treatment. *Biochem. Biophys. Res. Commun.*, 1988, 153/2 (888-96)

Coenzyme Q10 increases T4/T8 ratios of lymphocytes in ordinary subjects and relevance to patients having the AIDS related complex. *Biochem. Biophys. Res. Commun.*, 1991, 176/2 (786-91)

Relationship between sex steroid hormone levels and CD4 lymphocytes in HIV infected men. *Experimental and Clinical Endocrinology and Diabetes* (Germany),1996,104

Inhibition of 3'azido-3'deoxythymidine-resistant HIV-1 infection by dehydroepiandrosterone in vitro. *Biochem. Biophys. Res. Commun.*, 1994, 201/3 (1424-32)

Inhibition of HIV-1 latency reactivation by dehydroepiandrosterone (DHEA) and an analogue of DHEA. *Aids Res. Hum. Retroviruses*, 1993, 9/8 (747-54)

Evidence for changes in adrenal and testicular steroids during HIV infection. *J. Acquired Immune Defic. Syndr.*, 1992, 5/8 (841-46)

Dehydroepiandrosterone as predictor for progression to AIDS in asymptomatic human immunodeficiency virus-infected men. *J. Infect. Dis.*, 1992, 165/3 (413-418)

Decreased serum dehydroepiandrosterone is associated with an increased progression of human immunodeficiency virus infection in men with CD4 cell counts of 200-499. *J. Infect. Dis.*, 1991, 164/5 (864-868)

Homocysteine

Reduction of plasma homocyst(e)ine levels by breakfast cereal fortified with folic acid in patients with coronary heart disease. *N Engl J Med* 1998 Apr 9;338(15):1009-15

Vitamin B_{12}, vitamin B_6, and folate nutritional status in men with hyperhomocysteinemia. *Am J Clin Nutr* 1993 Jan;57(1):47-53

Hyperhomocysteinemia and low pyridoxal phosphate. Common and independent reversible risk factors for coronary artery disease. *Circulation* 1995 Nov 15;92(10):2825-30

Homocysteine metabolism and risk of myocardial infarction: relation with vitamins B6, B12, and folate. *Am J Epidemiol* 1996 May 1;143(9):845-59

Total serum homocysteine in senile dementia of Alzheimer type. *Int J Geriatr Psychiatry* 1998 Apr;13(4):235-39

Abnormal amino acid metabolism in patients with early stage Alzheimer dementia. *J Neural Transm* 1998;105 (2-3):287-94

Is metabolic evidence for vitamin B_{12} and folate deficiency more frequent in elderly patients with Alzheimer's disease? *J Gerontol A Biol Sci Med Sci* 1997 Mar;52(2):M76-79

Decreased methionine adenosyltransferase activity in erythrocytes of patients with dementia disorders. *Eur Neuropsycho Pharmacol* 1995 Jun;5(2):107-14

Homocysteine and arterial occlusive disease: a concise review. *Cardiologia* 1999 Apr;44(4):341-45

Homocysteine and short-term risk of myocardial infarction and stroke in the elderly: the Rotterdam Study. *Arch Intern Med* 1999 Jan 11;159(1):38-44

Vitamin intake: a possible determinant of plasma homocyst(e)ine among middle-aged adults. *Ann Epidemiol* 1997 May;7(4):285-93

Folic acid fortification of the food supply. Potential benefits and risks for the elderly population. *JAMA* 1996 Dec 18;276(23):1879-85

Hypertension (High Blood Pressure)

Dietary factors in the pathogenesis and treatment of hypertension. *Annals of Medicine* (UK), 1998, 30/2 (143-150)

Role of adequate dietary calcium intake in the prevention and management of salt-sensitive hypertension. *American Journal of Clinical Nutrition*, 1997, 65/2 Suppl. (712S-716S)

Effects of school-based aerobic exercise on blood pressure in adolescent girls at risk for hypertension. *Am J Public Health* Jun 1998, 88 (6) p949-51

[Nonpharmacologic approaches to hypertension. Weight, sodium, alcohol, exercise, and tobacco considerations. *Med Clin North Am* Nov 1997, 81 (6) p1289-303

The effects of aerobic physical training of short duration using upper limbs in paraplegic persons with mild hypertension. *Arq Bras Cardiol* (Brazil) Sep 1997, 69 (3) p169-73

Prospective study of nutritional factors, blood pressure, and hypertension among US women. *Hypertension* May 1996, 27 (5) p1065-72

[Non pharmacological therapy in hypertensive patients—effect of physical exercise on hypertension] *Nippon Rinsho* (Japan) Aug 1997, 55 (8) p2034-8

Vegetarian diet, hypertension and coronary heart disease. *Cahiers de Nutrition et de Dietetique* (France), 1997, 32/4 (261-266)

Onion extract in treatment of hypertension and hyperlipidemia: A preliminary communication, *Department of Preventive Medicine*, University of Medicine and Dentistry, New Jersey Medical School, Newark, NJ 07103 USA

Role of elements in pathophysiology of hypertension and antihypertensive drug development. *Acta Pharmacol Toxicol* (Copenh) (Denmark) 1986, 59 Suppl 7 p344-7

Effects of increased adrenomedullary activity and taurine in young patients with borderline hypertension. *Circulation* Mar 1987, 75 (3) p525-32

Zinc, cadmium, and hypertension in parturient women [see comments] *Am J Obstet Gynecol* Aug 1989, 161 (2) p437-40

A prospective study of nutritional factors and hypertension among US women. *Circulation* Nov 1989, 80 (5) p1320-27, 0009-7322

Hypertension prophylaxis with omega-3 fatty acids in heart transplant recipients. *J Am Coll Cardiol* May 1997, 29 (6) p1324-31

Nonpharmacologic interventions successfully treat hypertension in older persons. *Nutrition Reviews*, 1998, 56/11 (341-343)

Is Letigen contraindicated in hypertension? A double-blind, placebo controlled multipractice study of Letigen administered to normotensive and adequately treated patients with hypersensitivity] *Ugeskr Laeger* (Denmark) Jun 29 1998, 160 (27) p4073-75

Phytotherapy of hypertension and diabetes in oriental Morocco. *J Ethnopharmacol* (Ireland) Sep 1997, 58 (1) p45-54

Hypothalamic-pituitary-adrenocortical responses to psychological stress and caffeine in men at high and low risk for hypertension. *Psychosomatic Medicine*, 1998, 60/4 (521-27)

Summary of the NATO advanced research workshop on dietary omega 3 and omega 6 fatty acids: biological effects and nutritional essentiality. *J Nutr* Apr 1989, 119 (4) p521-28

Simopoulos AP. *J Nutr* Apr 1989, 119 (4) p521-28

Vasodilating agents and platelet function: intracellular free calcium concentration, cyclic nucleotides, and shape-change response. *J Cardiovasc Pharmacol* 1986, 8 Suppl 8 pS102-6

L-arginine restores dilator responses of the basilar artery to acetylcholine during chronic hypertension. *Hypertension* Apr 1996, 27 (4) p893-6

Prospective study of nutritional factors, blood pressure, and hypertension among US women. *Hypertension* May 1996, 27 (5) p1065-72

Association of macronutrients and energy intake with hypertension. *J Am Coll Nutr* Feb 1996, 15 (1) p21-35

Relations between magnesium, calcium, and plasma renin activity in black and white hypertensive patients. *Miner Electrolyte Metab* (Switzerland) 1995, 21 (6) p417-22

Effect of renal perfusion pressure on excretion of calcium, magnesium, and phosphate in the rat. *Clin Exp Hypertens* Nov 1995, 17 (8) p1269-85

Potassium depletion and salt-sensitive hypertension in Dahl rats: effect on calcium, magnesium, and phosphate excretions. *Clin Exp Hypertens* Aug 1995, 17 (6) p989-1008

Dietary *L*-arginine attenuates blood pressure in mineralocorticoid-salt hypertensive rats. *Clin Exp Hypertens* Oct 1995, 17 (7) p1009-24

Associations between blood pressure and dietary intake and urinary excretion of electrolytes in a Chinese population. *J Hypertens* (England) Jan 1995, 13 (1) p49-56

Concentration of free intracellular magnesium in the myocardium of spontaneously hypertensive rats treated chronically with calcium antagonist or angiotensin converting enzyme inhibitor. *Arch Mal Coeur Vaiss* (France) Aug 1994, 87 (8) p1041-45

Nonpharmacologic treatment of hypertension. *Curr Opin Nephrol Hypertens* Oct 1992, 1 (1) p85-90

Micronutrient effects on blood pressure regulation. *Nutr Rev* Nov 1994, 52 (11) p367-75

Role of magnesium and calcium in alcohol-induced hypertension and strokes as probed by in vivo television microscopy, digital image microscopy, optical spectroscopy, 31P-NMR, spectroscopy and a unique magnesium ion-selective electrode. *Alcohol Clin Exp Res* Oct 1994, 18 (5) p1057-68

Consequences of magnesium deficiency on the enhancement of stress reactions; preventive and therapeutic implications (a review). *J Am Coll Nutr* Oct 1994, 13 (5) p429-46

Dietary management of blood pressure. *J Assoc Acad Minor Phys* 1994, 5 (4) p147-51

Community-based prevention of stroke: nutritional improvement in Japan. *Health Rep* (Canada) 1994, 6 (1) p181-88

Effect of dietary magnesium supplementation on intralymphocytic free calcium and magnesium in stroke-prone spontaneously hypertensive rats. *Clin Exp Hypertens* May 1994, 16 (3) p317-26

Impact of increasing calcium in the diet on nutrient consumption, plasma lipids, and lipoproteins in humans. *Am J Clin Nutr* Apr 1994, 59 (4) p900-7

Electrolytes and hypertension: results from recent studies. *Am J Med Sci* Feb 1994, 307 Suppl 1 pS17-20

Calcium antagonists in pregnancy as an antihypertensive and tocolytic agent. *Wien Med Wochenschr* (Austria) 1993, 143 (19-20) p519-21

Augmentation of the renal tubular dopaminergic activity by oral calcium supplementation in patients with essential hypertension. *Am J Hypertens* Nov 1993, 6 (11 Pt 1) p933-37

Nutrition and diseases of women: cardiovascular disorders. *J Am Coll Nutr* Aug 1993, 12 (4) p417-25

The pathogenesis of eclampsia: the 'magnesium ischaemia' hypothesis. *Med Hypotheses* (England) Apr 1993, 40 (4) p250-56

Longitudinal changes during the development of hypertension in rats fed excess chloride and sodium. *Proc Soc Exp Biol Med* Jul 1993, 203 (3) p377-85

Salivary electrolytes in treated hypertensives at low or normal sodium diet. *Clin Exp Hypertens* Mar 1993, 15 (2) p245-56

Can guava fruit intake decrease blood pressure and blood lipids? *J Hum Hypertens* (England) Feb 1993, 7 (1) p33-38

Preventive nutrition: disease-specific dietary interventions for older adults. *Geriatrics* Nov 1992, 47 (11) p39-40, 45-9

Intracellular Mg2+, Ca2+, Na2+ and K+ in platelets and erythrocytes of essential hypertension patients: relation to blood pressure. *Clin Exp Hypertens* [A] 1992, 14 (6) p1189-209

A prospective study of nutritional factors and hypertension among US men. *Circulation* Nov 1992, 86 (5) p1475-84

The effects of nonpharmacologic interventions on blood pressure of persons with high normal levels. Results of the Trials of Hypertension Prevention, Phase I [published erratum appears in *JAMA* 1992 May 6;267(17):2330]. *JAMA* Mar 4 1992, 267 (9) p1213-20

Overview: studies on spontaneous hypertension-development from animal models toward man. *Clin Exp Hypertens* [A] 1991, 13 (5) p631-44

Electrolytes in the epidemiology, pathophysiology, and treatment of hypertension. *Prim Care* Sep 1991, 18 (3) p545-57

Effect of migration on blood pressure: the Yi People Study. *Epidemiology* Mar 1991, 2 (2) p88-97

Minerals and blood pressure. *Ann Med* (Finland) Aug 1991, 23 (3) p299-305

Renal function of cations excretion in children predisposed to essential hypertension. *Chung Hua Yu Fang I Hsueh Tsa Chih* (China) May 1991, 25 (3) p152-54

Nutrition and blood pressure among elderly men and women (Dutch Nutrition Surveillance System). *J Am Coll Nutr* Apr 1991, 10 (2) p149-55

The effect of Ca and Mg supplementation and the role of the opioidergic system on the development of DOCA-salt hypertension. *Am J Hypertens* Jan 1991, 4 (1 Pt 1) p72-75

Cellular mechanisms in hypertension and therapeutic implications in blacks. *Cardiovasc Drugs Ther* Mar 1990, 4 Suppl 2 p317-19

Experimental intervention of hypertension and cardiovascular diseases. *Clin Exp Hypertens* [A] 1990, 12 (5) p939-52

Attenuated vasodilator responses to Mg2+ in young patients with borderline hypertension. *Circulation* Aug 1990, 82 (2) p384-93

Dietary modulators of blood pressure in hypertension. *Eur J Clin Nutr* (England) Apr 1990, 44 (4) p319-27

Daily intake of macro and trace elements in the diet. 4. Sodium, potassium, calcium, and magnesium. *Ann Ig* (Italy) Sep-Oct 1989, 1 (5) p923-42

Fish oils modulate blood pressure and vascular contractility in the rat and vascular contractility in the primate. *Blood Press* (Norway) May 1995, 4 (3) p177-86

Vasorelaxant properties of n-3 polyunsaturated fatty acids in aortas from spontaneously hypertensive and normotensive rats. *J Cardiovasc Risk* (England) Jun 1994, 1 (1) p75-80

Effects of fish oil, nifedipine and their combination on blood pressure and lipids in primary hypertension. *J Hum Hypertens* (England) Feb 1993, 7 (1) p25-32

Effects of a combination of evening primrose oil (gamma linolenic acid) and fish oil (eicosapentaenoic + docahexaenoic acid) versus magnesium, and versus placebo in preventing preeclampsia. *Women Health* 1992, 19 (2-3) p117-31

Microbial infection or trauma at cardiovascular representation area of medulla oblongata as some of the possible causes of hypertension or hypotension. *Acupunct Electrother Res* 1988, 13 (2-3) p131-45

Garlic (Allium sativum)—a potent medicinal plant. *Fortschr Med* (Germany) Jul 20 1995, 113 (20-21) p311-15

A meta-analysis of the effect of garlic on blood pressure. *J Hypertens* (England) Apr 1994, 12 (4) p463-8

Patient preferences for novel therapy: an *N*-of-1 trial of garlic in the treatment for hypertension. *J Gen Intern Med* Nov 1993, 8 (11) p619-21

Can garlic lower blood pressure? A pilot study. *Pharmacotherapy* Jul-Aug 1993, 13 (4) p406-7

Hypertension and hyperlipidaemia: garlic helps in mild cases. *Br J Clin Pract Symp Suppl* (England) Aug 1990, 69 p3-6

Antithrombotic activity of garlic: its inhibition of the synthesis of thromboxane-B_2 during infusion of arachidonic acid and collagen in rabbits. *Prostaglandins Leukot Essent Fatty Acids* (Scotland) Oct 1990, 41 (2) p95-99

Garlic (Allium sativum) and onion (Allium cepa): a review of their relationship to cardiovascular disease. *Prev Med* Sep 1987, 16 (5) p670-85

Bulgarian traditional medicine: a source of ideas for phytopharmacological investigations. *J Ethnopharmacol* (Switzerland) Feb 1986, 15 (2) p121-32

Garlic as a natural agent for the treatment of hypertension: a preliminary report. *Cytobios* (England) 1982, 34 (135-36) p145-52

Plants and hypotensive, antiatheromatous and coronarodilatating action. *Am J Chin Med* Autumn 1979, 7 (3) p197-236

Treatment of essential hypertension with Coenzyme Q_{10}. *Mol Aspects Med* (England) 1994, 15 Suppl pS265-72

Coenzyme Q_{10} in essential hypertension. *Mol Aspects Med* (England) 1994, 15 Suppl ps257-63

Usefulness of Coenzyme Q_{10} in clinical cardiology: a long-term study. *Mol Aspects Med* (England) 1994, 15 Suppl ps165-75

Influence of Coenzyme Q_{10} on the hypotensive effects of enalapril and nitrendipine in spontaneously hypertensive rats. *Pol J Pharmacol* (Poland) Sep-Oct 1994, 46 (5) p457-61

Isolated diastolic dysfunction of the myocardium and its response to CoQ10 treatment. *Clin Investig* (Germany) 1993, 71 (8 Suppl) pS140-44

Muscle fibre types, ubiquinone content and exercise capacity in hypertension and effort angina. *Ann Med* (Finland) Aug 1991, 23 (3) p339-44

Effect of Coenzyme Q_{10} on structural alterations in the renal membrane of stroke-prone spontaneously hypertensive rats. *Biochem Med Metab Biol* Apr 1991, 45 (2) p216-26

Coenzyme Q_{10}: a new drug for cardiovascular disease. *J Clin Pharmacol* Jul 1990, 30 (7) p596-608

Coenzyme Q_{10}: a new drug for myocardial ischemia? *Med Clin North Am* Jan 1988, 72 (1) p243-58

Clinical study of cardiac arrhythmias using a 24-hour continuous electrocardiographic recorder (5th report)—antiarrhythmic action of coenzyme Q10 in diabetics. *Tohoku J Exp Med* (Japan) Dec 1983, 141 Suppl p453-63

Bioenergetics in clinical medicine. XVI. Reduction of hypertension in patients by therapy with coenzyme Q10. *Res Commun Chem Pathol Pharmacol* Jan 1981, 31 (1) p129-40

Prospects for nutritional control of hypertension. *Med Hypotheses* (England) Mar 1981, 7 (3) p271-83

Bioenergetics in clinical medicine XV. Inhibition of Coenzyme Q_{10} enzymes by clinically used adrenergic blockers of beta-receptors. *Res Commun Chem Pathol Pharmacol* May 1977, 17 (1) p157-64

Bioenergetics in clinical medicine. VIII. Adminstration of Coenzyme Q_{10} to patients with essential hypertension. *Res Commun Chem Pathol Pharmacol* Aug 1976, 14 (4) p721-7

Bioenergetics in clinical medicine. III. Inhibition of Coenzyme Q_{10} enzymes by clinically used anti-hypertensive drugs. *Res Commun Chem Pathol Pharmacol* Nov 1975, 12 (3) p533-40

Bioenergetics in clinical medicine. Studies on coenzyme Q10 and essential hypertension. *Res Commun Chem Pathol Pharmacol* Jun 1975, 11 (2) p273-88

Antioxidant status in controlled and uncontrolled hypertension and its relationship to endothelial damage. *J Hum Hypertens* (England) Nov 1994, 8 (11) p843-49

The role of antioxidants in the prevention of cardiovascular diseases. *Bratisl Lek Listy* (Slovakia) May 1994, 95 (5) p199-211

Prevention of cerebrovascular insults. *Schweiz Med Wochenschr* (Switzerland) Nov 12 1994, 124 (45) p1995-2004

A double-blind, placebo-controlled parallel trial of vitamin C treatment in elderly patients with hypertension. *Gerontology* (Switzerland) 1994, 40 (5) p268-72

Essential antioxidants in cardiovascular diseases—lessons for Europe. *Ther Umsch* (Switzerland) Jul 1994, 51 (7) p475-82

Antioxidant vitamin intake and coronary mortality in a longitudinal population study. *Am J Epidemiol* Jun 15 1994, 139 (12) p1180-89

The decline in stroke mortality. An epidemiologic perspective. *Ann Epidemiol* Sep 1993, 3 (5) p571-75

Can anti-oxidants prevent ischaemic heart disease? *J Clin Pharm Ther* (England) Apr 1993, 18 (2) p85-895

Antioxidant therapy in the aging process. *EXS* (Switzerland) 1992, 62 p428-37

Anthropometry, lipid- and vitamin status of 215 health-conscious Thai elderly. *Int J Vitam Nutr Res* (Switzerland) 1991, 61 (3) p215-23

Anti-oxidants show an anti-hypertensive effect in diabetic and hypertensive subjects. *Clin Sci* (Colch) (England) Dec 1991, 81 (6) p739-42

Calcium intake: covariates and confounders. *Am J Clin Nutr* Mar 1991, 53 (3) p741-4

Factors associated with age-related macular degeneration. An analysis of data from the first National Health and Nutrition Examination Survey. *Am J Epidemiol* Oct 1988, 128 (4) p700-10

Vitamin C deficiency and low linolenate intake associated with elevated blood pressure *J Hypertens Suppl* (England) Dec 1987, 5 (5) pS521-24

Relationship of magnesium intake and other dietary factors to blood pressure: the Honolulu heart study. *Am J Clin Nutr* Feb 1987, 45 (2) p469-75

Pathogenetic factors of aging macular degeneration. *Ophthalmology* May 1985, 92 (5) p628-35

Nutrition and the elderly: a general overview. *J Am Coll Nutr* 1984, 3 (4) p341-50

Blood pressure and nutrient intake in the United States. *Science* Jun 29 1984, 224 (4656) p1392-98

Nitric oxide and the regulation of blood pressure in the hypertension-prone and hypertension-resistant Sabra rat. *Hypertension* Sep 1996, 28 (3) p367-71

Serum calcium, magnesium, copper and zinc and risk of cardiovascular death. *Eur J Clin Nutr* (England) Jul 1996, 50 (7) p431-37

Vascular effects of metformin. Possible mechanisms for its antihypertensive action in the spontaneously hypertensive rat. *Am J Hypertens* Jun 1996, 9 (6) p570-76

Plasma ubiquinol-10 is decreased in patients with hyperlipi daemia. *Atherosclcrosis* (Ireland), 1997, 129/1 (119-126)

Role of exogenous *L*-arginine in hepatic ischemia-reperfusion injury. *Journal of Surgical Research*, 1997, 69/2 (429-434)

Effects of taurine and guanidinoethane sulfonate on toxicity of the pyrrolizidine alkaloid monocrotaline. *Biochemical Pharmacology*, 1996, 51/3 (321-29)

The Inuit diet. Fatty acids and antioxidants, their role in ischemic heart disease, and exposure to organochlorines and heavy metals. An international study. *Arctic Med Res* (Finland) 1996, 55 Suppl 1 p20-24

Renal denervation prevents intraglomerular platelet aggregation and glomerular injury induced by chronic inhibition of nitric oxide synthesis. *Nephron* (Switzerland) 1996, 73 (1) p34-40

Enhanced vasodilation to acetylcholine in athletes is associated with lower plasma cholesterol. *Am J Physiol* Jun 1996, 270 (6 Pt 2) pH2008-13

Central depressor action of nitric oxide is deficient in genetic hypertension. *Am J Hypertens* Mar 1996, 9 (3) p237-41

Cigarette smoking potentiates endothelial dysfunction of forearm resistance vessels in patients with hypercholesterolemia. Role of oxidized LDL. *Circulation* Apr 1 1996, 93 (7) p1346-53

Effect of salt intake and inhibitor dose on arterial hypertension and renal injury induced by chronic nitric oxide blockade. *Hypertension* May 1996, 27 (5) p1165-72

Role of nitric oxide in the maintenance of resting cerebral blood flow during chronic hypertension. *Life Sci* (England) 1996, 58 (15) p1231-38

Angiotensin II-mediated hypertension in the rat increases vascular superoxide production via membrane NADH/NADPH oxidase activation. Contribution to alterations of vasomotor tone. *J Clin Invest* Apr 15 1996, 97 (8) p1916-23

Endothelial function in deoxycorticosterone-NaCl hypertension: effect of calcium supplementation. *Circulation* Mar 1 1996, 93 (5) p1000-8

Can the kidney prevent cardiovascular diseases? *Clin Exp Hypertens* Apr-May 1996, 18 (3-4) p501-11

Vitamin C status and blood pressure. *J Hypertens* (England) Apr 1996, 14 (4) p503-8

[Evaluation of selected parameters of zinc metabolism in patients with primary hypertension]. *Pol Arch Med Wewn* (Poland) Mar 1996, 95 (3) p198-204

Acute sympathoinhibitory actions of metformin in spontaneously hypertensive rats. *Hypertension* Mar 1996, 27 (3 Pt 2) p619-25

[Overview—suppression effect of essential trace elements on arteriosclerotic development and its mechanism]. *Nippon Rinsho* (Japan) Jan 1996, 54 (1) p59-66

L-arginine prevents corticotropin-induced increases in blood pressure in the rat. *Hypertension* Feb 1996, 27 (2) p184-89

Improvement of cardiac output and liver blood flow and reduction of pulmonary vascular resistance by intravenous infusion of *L*-arginine during the early reperfusion period in pig liver transplantation. *Transplantation* May 15 1997, 63 (9) p1225-33

Hypertension, diabetes mellitus, and insulin resistance: the role of intracellular magnesium. *Am J Hypertens* Mar 1997, 10 (3) p346-55

Prevention of preeclampsia with calcium supplementation and its relation with the *L*-arginine:nitric oxide pathway. *Braz J Med Biol Res* (Brazil) Jun 1996, 29 (6) p731-41

[Guidelines on treatment of hypertension in the elderly, 1995—a tentative plan for comprehensive research projects on aging and health—Members of the Research Group for "Guidelines on Treatment of Hypertension in the Elderly", Comprehensive Research Projects on Aging and Health, the Ministry of Health and Welfare of Japan]. *Nippon Ronen Igakkai Zasshi* (Japan) Dec 1996, 33 (12) p945-75

Treatment of essential hypertension with Coenzyme Q_{10}. *Mol Aspects Med* (England) 1994, 15 Suppl

Coenzyme Q_{10} in essential hypertension. *Mol Aspects Med* (England) 1994, 15 Suppl

Usefulness of Coenzyme Q_{10} in clinical cardiology: a long-term study. *Mol Aspects Med* (England) 1994, 15 Suppl

Influence of Coenzyme Q_{10} on the hypotensive effects of enalapril and nitrendipine in spontaneously hypertensive rats. *Pol J Pharmacol* (Poland) Sep-Oct 1994, 46 (5) p457-61

Isolated diastolic dysfunction of the myocardium and its response to CoQ_{10} treatment. *Clin Investig* (Germany) 1993, 71 (8 Suppl)

Effect of coenzyme Q_{10} on structural alterations in the renal membrane of stroke-prone spontaneously hypertensive rats. *Biochem Med Metab Biol* Apr 1991

Coenzyme Q10: a new drug for cardiovascular disease. *J Clin Pharmacol* Jul 1990

Coenzyme Q10: a new drug for myocardial ischemia? *Med Clin North Am* Jan 1988

Bioenergetics in clinical medicine. XVI. Reduction of hypertension in patients by therapy with coenzyme Q10. *Res Commun Chem Pathol Pharmacol* Jan 1981

Bioenergetics in clinical medicine. VIII. Adminstration of coenzyme Q10 to patients with essential hypertension. *Res Commun Chem Pathol Pharmacol* Aug 1976

Bioenergetics in clinical medicine. III. Inhibition of Coenzyme Q_{10} enzymes by clinically used anti-hypertensive drugs. *Res Commun Chem Pathol Pharmacol* Nov 1975

Bioenergetics in clinical medicine. Studies on Coenzyme Q_{10} and essential hypertension. *Res Commun Chem Pathol Pharmacol* Jun 1975

[Garlic (Allium sativum)—a potent medicinal plant]. *Fortschr Med* (Germany) Jul 20 1995

A meta-analysis of the effect of garlic on blood pressure. *J Hypertens* (England) Apr 1994

Patient preferences for novel therapy: an *N*-of-1 trial of garlic in the treatment for hypertension. *J Gen Intern Med* Nov 1993

Can garlic lower blood pressure? A pilot study. *Pharmacotherapy* Jul-Aug 1993

Hypertension and hyperlipidaemia: garlic helps in mild cases. *Br J Clin Pract Symp Suppl* (England) Aug 1990

Defective renal adenylate cyclase response to prostaglandin E2 in spontaneously hypertensive rats. *J Hypertens* (England) Apr 1985, 3 (2)

Renal response to *L*-arginine in salt-sensitive patients with essential hypertension. *Hypertension* Mar 1996

L-arginine restores dilator responses of the basilar artery to acetylcholine during chronic hypertension. *Hypertension* Apr 1996

Vitamin C deficiency and low linolenate intake associated with elevated blood pressure: the Kuopio Ischaemic Heart Disease Risk Factor Study. *J Hypertens Suppl* (England) Dec 1987

Regulation of blood pressure by nitroxidergic nerve. *J Diabetes Complications* Oct-Dec 1995

[Endothelial function and arterial hypertension]. *Ann Ital Med Int* (Italy) Oct 1995, 10 Suppl

Contrasting effect of antihypertensive treatment on the renal response to *L*-arginine. *Hypertension* Dec 1995

Prospective study of nutritional factors, blood pressure, and hypertension among US women. *Hypertension* May 1996

[Overview—suppression effect of essential trace elements on arteriosclerotic development and it's mechanism]. *Nippon Rinsho* (Japan) Jan 1996

[Interrelationship between dietary intake of minerals and prevalence of hypertension]. *Vopr Pitan* (Russia) 1995, (6)

Potassium depletion and salt-sensitive hypertension in Dahl rats: effect on calcium, magnesium, and phosphate excretions. *Clin Exp Hypertens* Aug 1995

Consequences of magnesium deficiency on the enhancement of stress reactions; preventive and therapeutic implications (a review). *J Am Coll Nutr* Oct 1994

Relationship of magnesium intake and other dietary factors to blood pressure: the Honolulu heart study. *Am J Clin Nutr* Feb 1987

[Role of electrolytes in the development and maintenance of hypertension]. *Nippon Naibunpi Gakkai Zasshi* (Japan) May 20 1994

The decline in stroke mortality. An epidemiologic perspective. *Ann Epidemiol* Sep 1993

Antioxidant therapy in the aging process. *EXS* (Switzerland) 1992, 62

Antioxidants show an anti-hypertensive effect in diabetic and hypertensive subjects. *Clin Sci* (Colch) (England) Dec 1991

[Relation between vitamin C consumption and risk of ischemic heart disease] *Vopr Pitan* (USSR) Nov-Dec 1983

Blood pressure and nutrient intake in the United States. *Science* Jun 29 1984

Hypoglycemia

Effects of coca chewing on the glucose tolerance test. *Medicina* (B Aires) (Argentina) 1997, 57 (3) p261-4

Effect of melatonin on hypoglycemia and metoclopramide-stimulated arginine vasopressin secretion in normal men. *Neuropeptides* (Scotland) Aug 1997, 31 (4) p323-26

Oral administration of growth hormone (GH) releasing peptide-mimetic MK-677 stimulates the GH/insulin-like growth factor-I axis in selected GH-deficient adults. *J Clin Endocrinol Metab* Oct 1997, 82 (10) p3455-63

Alterations in circulating fatty acids and the compartmentation of selected metabolites in women with breast cancer. *Biochem Mol Biol Int* (Australia) Jan 1997, 41 (1) p1-10

Nutritional strategies to minimize fatigue during prolonged exercise: fluid, electrolyte and energy replacement. *J Sports Sci* (England) Jun 1997, 15 (3) p305-13

Metabolic response to lactitol and xylitol in healthy men. *Am J Clin Nutr* Apr 1997, 65 (4) p947-50

A metabolic complications of nutritional support. I. Carbohydrates, amino acids, fats, water, ions, trace elements. *Klinicka Biochemie a Metabolismus* (Czech Republic) 1997, 5/4 (251-57)

R. Paul St. Amand, M.D., Assistant Clinical Professor of Medicine Endocrinology, *Hypoglycemia,* U.C.L.A., 4560 Admiralty Way, Suite 355, Marina del Rey, CA 90292

John D. Kirschmann, Director; Lavon J. Dunne, *Nutrition Almanac / Nutrition Search, Inc. - 3rd ed.*, New York, NY: McGraw-Hill, Publishers Copyright 1990, p.182-83

Hypoglycemia Association, Inc (HAI), Box 165, Ashton, MD 20861-0165, (202) 544-4044

Preventing Hypoglycemia. *Anti-Aging News,* January 1982 Vo.2, No. 1 pg 6-7

Glutathione protects against hypoxic/hypoglycemic decreases in 2- deoxyglucose uptake and presynaptic spikes in hippocampal slices. *Eur J Pharmacol* (Netherlands) Jan 24 1995, 273 (1-2) p191-95

Glutathione protects against hypoxic/hypoglycemic decreases in 2-deoxyglucose uptake and presynaptic spikes in hippocampal slices. *Eur J Pharmacol* (Netherlands) Jan 24 1995, 273 (1-2) p191-95

Immune Enhancement

Treatment of systemic lupus erythematosus with dehydroepiandrosterone: 50 patients treated up to 12 months. *J Rheumatol,* 1998 Feb, 25:2, 285-89

Chemoprevention of rat prostate carcinogenesis by early and delayed administration of dehydroepiandrosterone. *Cancer Res* 1999 Jul 1;59(13):3084-89

Endogenous sex hormones and prostate cancer: a quantitative review of prospective studies. *Cancer Research* 1999 Jul 1;59(13):3084-89

Chemoprevention of hormone-dependent prostate cancer in the Wistar-Unilever rat. *Eur Urol* 1999;35(5-6):464-67

The relationship of serum dehydroepiandrosterone and its sulfate to subsequent cancer of the prostate. *Cancer Epidemiol Biomarkers Prev* 1993 May-Jun;2(3):219-21

Dehydroepiandrosterone in the treatment of erectile dysfunction: a prospective, double-blind, randomized, placebo-controlled study. *Urology* 1999 Mar;53(3):590-94; discussion 594-95

Androgens in patients with benign prostatic hyperplasia before and after prostatectomy. *J Clin Endocrinol Metab* 1976 Dec;43(6):1250-54

Micronutrient supplementation and immune function in the elderly. *Clinical Infectious Diseases* 1999, 28/4 (717-22)

Plant sterols and sterolins: a review of their immune-modulating properties. *Altern Med Rev* Jun 1999, 4 (3) p170-77

Role of cysteine and glutathione in signal transduction, immunopathology and cachexia. *Biofactors* 1998, 8 (1-2) p97-102

Zinc, iron, and magnesium status in athletes—influence on the regulation of exercise-induced stress and immune function. *Exerc Immunol Rev* 1998, 4 p2-21

Influence of systemic arginine-lysine on immune organ function: an electrophysiological study. *Brain Res Bull* Mar 15 1998, 45 (5) p437-41

Effects of growth hormone and insulin-like growth factor I binding to natural killer cells. *Acta Paediatr Suppl* Nov 1997, 423 p80-81

Adrenergic beta 1- and beta 1 + 2-receptor blockade suppress the natural killer cell response to head-up tilt in humans. *J Appl Physiol Nov* 1997, 83 (5) p1492-8

Chronic stress and natural killer cell activity after exposure to traumatic death. *Psychosom Med* Sep-Oct 1997, 59 (5) p467-76

Preoperative natural killer cell activity: correlation with distant metastases in curatively research colorectal carcinomas. *Int Surg* Apr-Jun 1997, 82 (2) p190-93

Role of cysteine and glutathione in HIV infection and other diseases associated with muscle wasting and immunological dysfunction. *FASEB J Nov* 1997, 11 (13) p1077-89

Oxidized low-density lipoproteins affect natural killer cell activity by impairing cytoskeleton function and altering the cytokine network. *Exp Cell Res* Nov 1 1997, 236 (2) p436-45

Enhancement of natural killer and antibody-dependent cytolytic activities of the peripheral blood mononuclear cells of HIV-infected patients by recombinant IL-15. *J Acquir Immune Defic Syndr Hum Retrovirol* Nov 1 1997, 16 (3) p137-45

Involvement of catecholamines and glucocorticoids in ethanol-induced suppression of splenic natural killer cell activity in a mouse model for binge drinking. *Alcohol Clin Exp Res* Sep 1997, 21 (6) p1030-36

Rapid immunologic reconstitution following transplantation with mobilized peripheral blood stem cells as compared to bone marrow. *Bone Marrow Transplant* Jan 1997, 19 (2) p161-72

Effect of alpha-interferon on natural killer cell activity and lymphocyte subsets in thalassemia patients with chronic hepatitis C. *Acta Haematol* 1997, 98 (2) p83-88

Interleukin-2-activated killer cell activity in colorectal tumor patients: evaluation of in vitro effects by prothymosin alpha1. *J Cancer Res Clin Oncol* 1997, 123 (8) p420-28

Long-term melatonin supplementation does not recover the impairment of natural killer cell activity and lymphocyte proliferation in aging mice. *Life Sci* 1997, 61 (9) p857-64

Natural killer cells in the late decades of human life. *Clin Immunol Immunopathol* Sep 1997, 84 (3) p269-75

Effects of purified bovine whey factors on cellular immune functions in ruminants. *Vet Immunol Immunopathol* May 1997, 56 (1-2) p85-96

Modulation of natural killer cell functional activity in athymic mice by beta-carotene, oestrone and their association. *Anticancer Res* Jul-Aug 1997, 17 (4A) p2523-27

Depressed natural killer cell activity due to decreased natural killer cell population in a vitamin E-deficient patient with Shwachman syndrome: reversible natural killer cell abnormality by alpha-tocopherol supplementation [see comments] *Eur J Pediatr* Jun 1997, 156 (6) p444-48

Interleukin (IL)-2 deficiency aggravates the defect of natural killer cell activity in AIDS patients. *Thymus* 1997, 24 (3) p147-56

Vitamin E supplementation decreases lung virus titers in mice infected with influenza. *J Infect Dis* Jul 1997, 176 (1) p273-76

Idiopathic hypoparathyroidism with fungal seminal vesiculitis. *Intern Med* Feb 1997, 36 (2) p113-17

Life events, frontal electroencephalogram laterality, and functional immune status after acute psychological stressors in adolescents. *Psychosom Med* Mar-Apr 1997, 59 (2) p178-86

Local inhibition of natural killer cell activity promotes the progressive growth of intraocular tumors. *Invest Ophthalmol Vis Sci* May 1997, 38 (6) p1277-82

Exercise immunology: practical applications. *Int J Sports Med* Mar 1997, 18 Suppl 1 pS91-100

Aging, exercise, training, and the immune system. *Exerc Immunol Rev* 1997, 3 p68-95

Effects of varying the type of saturated fatty acid in the rat diet upon serum lipid levels and spleen lymphocyte functions. *Biochim Biophys Acta* Apr 21 1997, 1345 (3) p223-36

The interaction of maintenance interferon with cytolytic cells in patients with multiple myeloma who responded to cytotoxic chemotherapy [published erratum appears in *Pharmacotherapy* 1997 May-Jun;17(3):634]. *Pharmacotherapy* Mar-Apr 1997, 17 (2) p248-55

Adverse effects of intraportal chemotherapy on natural killer cell activity in colorectal cancer patients. *J Surg Oncol* Apr 1997, 64 (4) p324-30

The natural killer gene complex: a genetic basis for understanding natural killer cell function and innate immunity. *Immunol Rev* Feb 1997, 155 p53-65

Enhanced human CD4+ T cell engraftment in beta2-microglobulin-deficient NOD-scid mice. *J Immunol* Apr 15 1997, 158 (8) p3578-86

Circadian immune measures in healthy volunteers: relationship to hypothalamic-pituitary-adrenal axis hormones and sympathetic neurotransmitters. *Psychosom Med* Jan-Feb 1997, 59 (1) p42-50

In vitro effects of echinacea and ginseng on natural killer and antibody-dependent cell cytotoxicity in healthy subjects and chronic fatigue syndrome or acquired immunodeficiency syndrome patients. *Immunopharmacology* Jan 1997, 35 (3) p229-35

Vitamin E-deficient diets enriched with fish oil suppress lethal Plasmodium yoelii infections in athymic and scid/bg mice. *Infect Immun* Jan 1997, 65 (1) p197-202

Dehydroepiandrosterone sulfate decreases the interleukin-2-mediated overactivity of the natural killer cell compartment in senile dementia of the Alzheimer type *Dementia and Geriatric Cognitive Disorders* 1999 , 10/1 (21-27)

Enhancement of human natural killer cytotoxic activity by vitamin C in pure and augmented formulations. *Journal of Nutritional and Environmental Medicine* 1997, 7/3 (187-195)

Nutrition and host defence. *Biotherapy* 1997, 11/4 (492-499)

Lipopolysaccharide-induced enhancement of natural killer cell cytotoxicity: Comparison of rats fed menhaden, safflower and essential fatty acid deficient diets. *Journal of Nutritional Immunology* 1997, 5/2 (47-56)

Alcohol and cancer. *Recent Dev Alcohol* 1998, 14 p67-95

Cytoprotective properties of melatonin: presumed association with oxidative damage and aging [see comments] *Nutrition* Sep 1998, 14 (9) p691-6

Improvement by several antioxidants of macrophage function in vitro. *Life Sci* 1998, 63 (10) p871-81

Comparative study of effects of three kinds of herbal mixture decoctions on improving immune senescence and free radical metabolism. *Chin Med J* Oct 1997, 110 (10) p750-4

Free radicals, exercise and antioxidant supplementation. *Proc Nutr Soc* Feb 1998, 57 (1) p9-13

Nutritional metabolic diseases of poultry and disorders of the biological antioxidant defence system. *Acta Vet Hung* 1997, 45 (3) p349-60

Exercise, free radical generation and vitamins. *Eur J Cancer Prev* Mar 1997, 6 Suppl 1 pS55-67

Essential fatty acids, immune function, and exercise. *Exerc Immunol* Rev 1997, 3 p1-31

Melatonin *Archives of Hellenic Medicine* 1998, 15/3 (281-306)

Trace elements that act as antioxidants in parenteral micronutrition. *Canada Journal of Nutritional Biochemistry* , 1998, 9/6 (304-307)

Immune function in aged women is improved by ingestion of vitamins C and E. *Can J Physiol Pharmacol* Apr 1998, 76 (4) p373-80

Prospects of the clinical utilization of melatonin. *Biol Signals Recept* Jul-Aug 1998, 7 (4) p195-219

Immunological hazards from nutritional imbalance in athletes. *Exerc Immunol Rev* 1998, 4 p22-48

Zinc and immune function: the biological basis of altered resistance to infection. *Am J Clin Nutr* Aug 1998, 68 (2 Suppl) p447S-463S

Selenium and immune function. *Z Ernahrungswiss* 1998, 37 Suppl 1 p50-6

Effect of antioxidative vitamins on immune function with clinical applications. *Int J Vitam Nutr Res* 1997, 67 (5) p312-20

Melatonin in relation to cellular antioxidative defense mechanisms. *Horm Metab Res* Aug 1997, 29 (8) p363-72

Effect of glutamine on immune function in the surgical patient. *Nutrition* Nov-Dec 1996, 12 (11-12 Suppl) pS82-4

The role of oxidative stress in HIV disease. *Free Radic Biol Med* Oct 1995, 19 (4) p523-8

Micronutrients in critical illness [published erratum appears in Crit Care Clin 1996 Oct;12(4):xi] *Crit Care Clin* Jul 1995, 11 (3) p651-73

Melatonin in edible plants identified by radioimmunoassay and by high performance liquid chromatography-mass spectrometry. *J Pineal Res* Jan 1995, 18 (1) p28-31

Exercise-induced changes in immune function: effects of zinc supplementation. *J Appl Physiol* Jun 1994, 76 (6) p2298-303

Dietary lipids and risk of autoimmune disease. *Clin Immunol Immunopathol* Aug 1994, 72 (2) p193-7

Longitudinal exposure of human T lymphocytes to weak oxidative stress suppresses transmembrane and nuclear signal transduction. *J Immunol* Dec 1 1994, 153 (11) p4880-9

Critical reappraisal of vitamins and trace minerals in nutritional support of cancer patients. *Support Care Cancer* Nov 1993, 1 (6) p295-7

Preventive nutrition: disease-specific dietary interventions for older adults. *Geriatrics* Nov 1992, 47 (11) p39-40, 45-9

Immunocompetence and oxidant defense during ascorbate depletion of healthy men. *Am J Clin Nutr* Dec 1991, 54 (6 Suppl) p1302S-1309S

Vitamin E and immune functions. *Basic Life Sci* 1988, 49 p615-20

Functional food science and the cardiovascular system *British Journal of Nutrition* 1998, 80/SUPPL. 1 (S113-S146)

Monounsaturated fats and immune function *Brazilian Journal of Medical and Biological Research* 1998, 31/4 (453-465)

Cancer chemopreventive and therapeutic activities of red ginseng. *Journal of Ethnopharmacology* 1998, 60/1 (71-78)

Nutrition and immune function: Overview *Journal of Nutrition* 1996, 126/10 Suppl. (2611S-2615S)

Vitamin E and immunomodulation for cancer and AIDS resistance *Expert Opinion on Investigational Drugs* 1996, 5/9 (1221-1225)

Vitamin E in humans: Demand and delivery *Annual Review of Nutrition* 1996, 16/- (321-347)

Vitamin E stimulation of disease resistance and immune function. *Expert Opinion on Investigational Drugs* 1995, 4/3 (201-211)

Nutritional support in critically ill patients. *Ann. Surg.* 1994, 220/5 (610-616)

Nutritional status and immune function in cocaine and heroin abusers and in methadone treated subjects. *Res. Common. Subst. Abuse* 1991, 12/4 (209-215)

Regulation of copper/ zinc and manganese superoxide dismutase by UVB irradiation, oxidative stress and cytokines. *J Photochem Photobiol B* Oct 1997, 40 (3) p288-93

Changes in cytokine production and T cell subpopulations in experimentally induced zinc-deficient humans. *Am J Physiol* Jun 1997, 272 (6 Pt 1) pE1002-7

Zinc deficiency: changes in cytokine production and T-cell subpopulations in patients with head and neck cancer and in noncancer subjects. *Proc Assoc Am Physicians* Jan 1997, 109 (1) p68-77

Zinc regulates DNA synthesis and IL-2, IL-6, and IL-10 production of PWM-stimulated PBMC and normalizes the periphere cytokine concentration in chronic liver disease. *Journal of Trace Elements in Experimental Medicine* 1997, 10/1 (19-27)

The effect of zinc and vitamin A supplementation on immune response in an older population. *J Am Geriatr Soc* Jan 1998, 46 (1) p19-26

Nutritional modulation of cytokine biology. *Nutrition* Jul-Aug 1998, 14 (7-8) p634-40

Beta-carotene-induced enhancement of natural killer cell activity in elderly men: an investigation of the role of cytokines. *Am J Clin Nutr* Jul 1998, 68 (1) p164-70

Does N-acetyl-L-cysteine influence cytokine response during early human septic shock? *Chest* Jun 1998, 113 (6) p1616-24

Pro- and anti-inflammatory cytokines in healthy volunteers fed various doses of fish oil for year. *Eur J Clin Invest* Dec 1997, 27 (12) p1003-8

Regulation of copper/zinc and manganese superoxide dismutase by UVB irradiation, oxidative stress and cytokines. *J Photochem Photobiol B* Oct 1997, 40 (3) p288-93

Distinct mechanisms for N-acetylcysteine inhibition of cytokine-induced E-selectin and VCAM-1 expression. *Am J Physiol* Aug 1997, 273 (2 Pt 2) pH817-26

Plasma levels of lipid and cholesterol oxidation products and cytokines in diabetes mellitus and cigarette smoking: effects of vitamin E treatment. *Atherosclerosis* Mar 21 1997, 129 (2) p169-76

Micronutrient supplementation and immune function in the elderly. *Clinical Infectious Diseases* 1999, 28/4 (717-722)

Metabolic and immune effects of dietary arginine, glutamine and omega-3 fatty acids supplementation in immunocompromised patients. *J Med Assoc Thai* 1998 May;81(5):334-43

Reversal of doxorubicin-induced cardiac metabolic damage by L-carnitine. *Pharmacol Res*, 39(4). 289-5 1999 Apr

Isoprinosine In The Treatment Of Genital Warts. *Cancer Detect Prev*; 12(1-6):497-501 1988

Summary of the NATO advanced research workshop on dietary omega 3 and omega 6 fatty acids: biological effects and nutritional essentiality. *J Nutr* Apr 1989, 119 (4) p521-8

Carnitine in human immunodeficiency virus type 1 infection/acquired immune deficiency syndrome. *J Child Neurol* Nov 1995, 10 Suppl 2 pS40-4

Utilization of intracellular acylcarnitine pools by mononuclear phagocytes. *Biochim Biophys Acta* (Netherlands) Nov 11 1994, 1201 (2) p321-7

Carnitine depletion in peripheral blood mononuclear cells from patients with AIDS: effect of oral L-carnitine. *AIDS* May 1994, 8 (5) p655-60

Nutritional factors in the pathogenesis and therapy of respiratory insufficiency in neuromuscular diseases. *Monaldi Arch Chest Dis* (Italy) Aug 1993, 48 (4) p327-30

Sudden infant death syndrome (SIDS): oxygen utilizat[illegible] energy production. *Med Hypotheses* (England) Jun 1993, [illegible] p364-6

High dose L-carnitine improves immunologic and metabolic parameters in AIDS patients. *Immunopharmacol Immunotoxicol* Jan 1993, 15 (1) p1-12

Effects of acetyl-L-carnitine oral administration on lymphocyte antibacterial activity and TNF-alpha levels in patients with active pulmonary tuberculosis. A randomized double blind versus placebo study. *Immunopharmacol Immunotoxicol* 1991, 13 (1-2) p135-46

Immunological parameters in aging: studies on natural immunomodulatory and immunoprotective substances. *Int J Clin Pharmacol Res* (Switzerland) 1990, 10 (1-2) p53-7

Carnitine deficiency with cardiomyopathy presenting as neonatal hydrops: successful response to carnitine therapy. *J Inherit Metab Dis* (Netherlands) 1990, 13 (1) p69-75

Medium-chain triglycerides—useful energy carriers in parenteral nutrition. *Wien Klin Wochenschr* (Austria) Apr 14 1989, 101 (8) p300-3

Rationales for micronutrient supplementation in diabetes. *Med Hypotheses* (England) Feb 1984, 13 (2) p139-51

Recent knowledge concerning the biochemistry and significance of ascorbic acid. *Z Gesamte Inn Med* (Germany, East) Jan 15 1984, 39 (2) p21-7

Reversibility by L-carnitine of immunosuppression induced by an emulsion of soya bean oil, glycerol and egg lecithin. *Arzneimittelforschung* (Germany, West) 1982, 32 (11) p1485-8

Vitamins and immunity: II. Influence of L-carnitine on the immune system. *Acta Vitaminol Enzymol* (Italy) 1982, 4 (1-2) p135-40

Suppression of tumor growth and enhancement of immune status with high levels of dietary vitamin B6 in BALB/c mice. *J Natl Cancer Inst* May 1987, 78 (5) p951-9

Ontogenetic analysis of immune amplification by thymus-derived cells in chickens. *Exp Hematol* (Denmark) Sep 1981, 9 (8) p856-64

The activities of coenzyme Q10 and vitamin B6 for immune responses. *Biochem Biophys Res Commun* May 28 1993, 193 (1) p88-92

Food uses and health effects of corn oil. *J Am Coll Nutr* Oct 1990, 9 (5) p438-70

A modified determination of coenzyme Q10 in human blood and CoQ10 blood levels in diverse patients with allergies. *Biofactors* (England) Dec 1988, 1 (4) p303-6

Biochemical deficiencies of coenzyme Q10 in HIV-infection and exploratory treatment. *Biochem Biophys Res Commun* Jun 16 1988, 153 (2) p888-96

Research on coenzyme Q10 in clinical medicine and in immunomodulation. *Drugs Exp Clin Res* (Switzerland) 1985, 11 (8) p539-45

The polypeptide composition of the mitochondrial NADH: ubiquinone reductase complex from several mammalian species. *Biochem J* (England) Sep 15 1985, 230 (3) p739-46

...position of bovine heart ... oxidoreductase by two- ... el electrophoresis. *Biochem J* ... 2) p435-43

...ce in mice and its reversal by coenzyme ... (Switzerland) Mar 1978, 7 (3) p189-97

... the severity of dextran-induced colitis in ... *Res* (Denmark) Aug 1995, 19 (1) p31-9

Melatonin affects proopiomelanocortin gene expression in the immune organs of the rat. *Eur J Endocrinol* (Norway) Dec 1995, 133 (6) p754-60

Immune effects of preoperative immunotherapy with high-dose subcutaneous interleukin-2 versus neuroimmunotherapy with low-dose interleukin-2 plus the neurohormone melatonin in gastrointestinal tract tumor patients. *J Biol Regul Homeost Agents* (Italy) Jan-Mar 1995, 9 (1) p31-3

Serial transplants of DMBA-induced mammary tumors in Fischer rats as model system for human breast cancer. IV. Parallel changes of biopterin and melatonin indicate interactions between the pineal gland and cellular immunity in malignancy. *Oncology* (Switzerland) Jul-Aug 1995, 52 (4) p278-83

Inhibitory effect of melatonin on production of IFN gamma or TNF alpha in peripheral blood mononuclear cells of some blood donors. *J Pineal Res* (Denmark) Nov 1994, 17 (4) p164-9

Specific binding of 2-[125I]iodomelatonin by rat splenocytes: characterization and its role on regulation of cyclic AMP production. *J Neuroimmunol* (Netherlands) Mar 1995, 57 (1-2) p171-8

Pineal-opioid system interactions in the control of immunoinflammatory responses. *Ann N Y Acad Sci* Nov 25 1994, 741 p191-6

Evidence for a direct action of melatonin on the immune system. *Biol Signals* (Switzerland) Mar-Apr 1994, 3 (2) p107-17

The immuno-reconstituting effect of melatonin or pineal grafting and its relation to zinc pool in aging mice. *J Neuroimmunol* (Netherlands) Sep 1994, 53 (2) p189-201

Multiple sclerosis: the role of puberty and the pineal gland in its pathogenesis. *Int J Neurosci* (England) Feb 1993, 68 (3-4) p209-25

Modulation of human lymphoblastoid interferon activity by melatonin in metastatic renal cell carcinoma. A phase II study. *Cancer* Jun 15 1994, 73 (12) p3015-9

Modulation of 2[125I]iodomelatonin binding sites in the guinea pig spleen by melatonin injection is dependent on the dose and period but not the time. *Life Sci* (England) 1994, 54 (19) p1441-8

Binding of [125I]-labelled iodomelatonin in the duck thymus. *Biol Signals* (Switzerland) Sep-Oct 1992, 1 (5) p250-6

Characteristics of 2-[125I]iodomelatonin binding sites in the pigeon spleen and modulation of binding by guanine nucleotides. *J Pineal Res* (Denmark) May 1993, 14 (4) p169-77

Pinealectomy ameliorates collagen II-induced arthritis in mice. *Clin Exp Immunol* (England) Jun 1993, 92 (3) p432-6

The immunoneuroendocrine role of melatonin. *J Pineal Res* (Denmark) Jan 1993, 14 (1) p1-10

2[125I]iodomelatonin binding sites in spleens of guinea pigs. *Life Sci* (England) 1992, 50 (22) p1719-26

Melatonin: a chronobiotic with anti-aging properties? *Med Hypotheses* (England) Apr 1991, 34 (4) p300-9

Effect of dose and time of melatonin injections on the diurnal rhythm of immunity in chicken. *J Pineal Res* (Denmark) Jan 1991, 10 (1) p30-5

The pineal neurohormone melatonin stimulates activated CD4+, Thy-1+ cells to release opioid agonist(s) with immunoenhancing and anti-stress properties. *J Neuroimmunol* (Netherlands) Jul 1990, 28 (2) p167-76

Alterations of pineal gland and of T lymphocyte subsets in metastatic cancer patients: preliminary results. *J Biol Regul Homeost Agents* Oct-Dec 1989, 3 (4) p181-3

Endocrine and immune effects of melatonin therapy in metastatic cancer patients. *Eur J Cancer Clin Oncol* (England) May 1989, 25 (5) p789-95

Replacement of DHEA in aging men and women. Potential remedial effects. *Ann N Y Acad Sci* Dec 29 1995, 774 p128-42

Dehydroepiandrosterone (DHEA) treatment reverses the impaired immune response of old mice to influenza vaccination and protects from influenza infection. *Vaccine* (England) 1995, 13 (15) p1445-8

Dehydroepiandrosterone modulation of lipopolysaccharide-stimulated monocyte cytotoxicity. *J Immunol* Jan 1 1996, 156 (1) p328-35

Dehydroepiandrosterone modulates the spontaneous and IL-6 stimulated fibrinogen production of human hepatoma cells. *Acta Microbiol Immunol Hung* (Hungary) 1995, 42 (2) p229-33

Administration of dehydroepiandrosterone reverses the immune suppression induced by high dose antigen in mice. *Immunol Invest* May 1995, 24 (4) p583-93

Effects of dehydroepiandrosterone in immunosuppressed adult mice infected with Cryptosporidium parvum. *J Parasitol* Jun 1995, 81 (3) p429-33

Relationship between dehydroepiandrosterone and calcitonin gene-related peptide in the mouse thymus. *Am J Physiol* Jan 1995, 268 (1 Pt 1) pE168-73

Dehydroepiandrosterone functions as more than an antiglucocorticoid in preserving immunocompetence after thermal injury. *Endocrinology* Feb 1995, 136 (2) p393-401

Pregnenolone and dehydroepiandrosterone as precursors of native 7-hydroxylated metabolites which increase the immune response in mice. *J Steroid Biochem Mol Biol* (England) Jul 1994, 50 (1-2) p91-100

In vitro potentiation of lymphocyte activation by dehydroepiandrosterone, androstenediol, and androstenetriol. *J Immunol* Aug 15 1994, 153 (4) p1544-52

Immune senescence and adrenal steroids: immune dysregulation and the action of dehydroepiandrosterone (DHEA) in old animals. *Eur J Clin Pharmacol* (Germany) 1993, 45 Suppl 1 pS21-3; discussion S43-4

Effects of dehydroepiandrosterone in immunosuppressed rats infected with Cryptosporidium parvum. *J Parasitol* Jun 1993, 79 (3) p364-70

Dehydroepiandrosterone protects mice inoculated with West Nile virus and exposed to cold stress. *J Med Virol* Nov 1992, 38 (3) p159-66

The relationship of serum DHEA-S and cortisol levels to measures of immune function in human immunodeficiency virus-related illness. *Am J Med Sci* Feb 1993, 305 (2) p79-83

Mobilization of cutaneous immunity for systemic protection against infections. *Ann N Y Acad Sci* Apr 15 1992, 650 p363-6

Dehydroepiandrosterone-induced reduction of Cryptosporidium parvum infections in aged Syrian golden hamsters. *J Parasitol* Jun 1992, 78 (3) p554-7

Dehydroepiandrosterone enhances IL2 production and cytotoxic effector function of human T cells. *Clin Immunol Immunopathol* Nov 1991, 61 (2 Pt 1) p202-11

Protection from glucocorticoid induced thymic involution by dehydroepiandrosterone. *Life Sci* (England) 1990, 46 (22) p1627-31

Regulation of murine lymphokine production in vivo. II. Dehydroepiandrosterone is a natural enhancer of interleukin 2 synthesis by helper T cells. *Eur J Immunol* (Germany, West) Apr 1990, 20 (4) p793-802

Biomarks in secondary osteoporosis. *Clin Rheumatol* (Belgium) Jun 1989, 8 Suppl 2 p89-94

Protection against acute lethal viral infections with the native steroid dehydroepiandrosterone (DHEA). *J Med Virol* Nov 1988, 26 (3) p301-14

Food intake reduction and immunologic alterations in mice fed dehydroepiandrosterone. *Exp Gerontol* (England) 1984, 19 (5) p297-304

Steroid induction of gonadotropin surges in the immature rat. I. Priming effects of androgens. *Endocrinology* Nov 1978, 103 (5) p1822-8

Effect of thyroxine and chicken growth hormone on immune function in autoimmune thyroiditis (obese) strain chicks. *Proc Soc Exp Biol Med* Jan 1992, 199 (1) p114-22

Binding and functional effects of thyroid stimulating hormone on human immune cells. *J Clin Immunol* Jul 1990, 10 (4) p204-10

The in vitro effect of a thymic polypeptidic extract on the function of T-cells and macrophages. *Endocrinologie* (Romania) Apr-Jun 1987, 25 (2) p83-9

Effect of immunization on functional state of thyroid gland and thyroxine binding in rat organs. *Biull Eksp Biol Med* (Ussr) Feb 1982, 93 (2) p46-8

Thyroid function and triiodothyronine and thyroxine kinetics in rabbits immunized with thyroid hormones. *Acta Endocrinol* (Copenh) (Denmark) Feb 1975, 78 (2) p276-88

Effect of isoprinosine on lymphocyte proliferation and natural killer cell activity following thermal injury. *Immunopharmacol Immunotoxicol* 1989, 11 (4) p631-44

Immunopharmacology of the immunotherapy of cancer, infection, and autoimmunity. *Fundam Clin Pharmacol* (France) 1987, 1 (4) p283-96

Immunorestoration in children with recurrent respiratory infections treated with isoprinosine. *Int J Immunopharmacol* (England) 1987, 9 (8) p947-9

A randomized double-blind study of inosiplex (isoprinosine) therapy in patients with alopecia totalis. *J Am Acad Dermatol* May 1987, 16 (5 Pt 1) p977-83

Isoprinosine abolishes the blocking factor-mediated inhibition of lymphocyte responses to Epstein-Barr virus antigens and phytohemagglutinin. *Int J Immunopharmacol* (England) 1986, 8 (1) p101-6

Isoprinosine as an immunopotentiator in an animal model of human osteosarcoma. *Int J Immunopharmacol* (England) 1981, 3 (4) p383-9

Determination of the antiinfectious activity of RU 41740 (Biostim) as an example of an immunomodulator. *Adv Exp Med Biol* 1992, 319 p165-74

Effect of an immunostimulatory substance of Klebsiella pneumoniae on inflammatory responses of human granulocytes, basophils and platelets. *Arzneimittelforschung* (Germany) Aug 1991, 41 (8) p815-20

Determination of the anti-infective action of an immunomodulator. Biostim as an example. *Allerg Immunol* (Paris) (France) Apr 1991, 23 (4) p145-52

The effect of Biostim (RU-41740) on the expression of cytokine mRNAs in murine peritoneal macrophages in vitro. *Toxicol Lett* (Netherlands) Oct 1990, 53 (3) p327-37

Immunotolerance of RU 41740. *Presse Med* (France) Jul 27 1988, 17 (28) p1458-60

Clinical immunopharmacology of RU 41740. *Presse Med* (France) Jul 27 1988, 17 (28) p1438-40

Effect of An Immunomodulator, RU 41740, On Experimental Infections. *Presse Med* (France) Jul 27 1988, 17 (28) p1430-2

The effect of the immunomodulator RU 41,740 (biostim) on the specific and nonspecific immunosuppression induced by thermal injury or protein deprivation. *Arch Surg* Feb 1988, 123 (2) p207-11

The effect of RU 41.740, an immune modulating compound, in the prevention of acute exacerbations in patients with chronic bronchitis. *Eur J Respir Dis* (Denmark) Oct 1986, 69 (4) p235-41

Activation of murine B lymphocytes by RU 41740, a glycoprotein extract from Klebsiella pneumoniae. *C R Acad Sci III* (France) 1984, 298 (6) p135-8

Influence of RU 41.740, a glycoprotein extract from Klebsiella pneumoniae, on the murine immune system. I. T-independent polyclonal B cell activation. *J Immunol* Feb 1984, 132 (2) p616-21

Vitamins and immunity: II. Influence of L-carnitine on the immune system. *Acta Vitaminol Enzymol* (Italy) 1982, 4 (1-2)

Suppression of tumor growth and enhancement of immune status with high levels of dietary vitamin B6 in BALB/c mice. *J Natl Cancer Inst* May 1987

The activities of coenzyme Q10 and vitamin B6 for immune responses. *Biochem Biophys Res Commun* May 28 1993, 193 (1)

Research on coenzyme Q10 in clinical medicine and in immunomodulation. *Drugs Exp Clin Res* (Switzerland) 1985, 11 (8) p539- 45

Immunoenhancing effect of flavonoid compounds on lymphocyte proliferation and immunoglobulin synthesis. *Int J Immunopharmacol* (England) 1984, 6 (3) p205-15

Immunological senescence in mice and its reversal by coenzyme Q10. *Mech Ageing Dev* (Switzerland) Mar 1978, 7 (3)

Immune effects of preoperative immunotherapy with high-dose subcutaneous interleukin-2 versus neuroimmunotherapy with low-dose interleukin-2 plus the neurohormone melatonin in gastrointestinal tract tumor patients. *J Biol Regul Homeost Agents* (Italy) Jan-Mar 1995, 9 (1) p31-3

Pineal-opioid system interactions in the control of immunoinflammatory responses. *Ann N Y Acad Sci* Nov 25 1994

Evidence for a direct action of melatonin on the immune system. *Biol Signals* (Switzerland) Mar-Apr 1994

The immuno-reconstituting effect of melatonin or pineal grafting and its relation to zinc pool in aging mice. *Neuroimmunol* (Netherlands) Sep 1994

The immunoneuroendocrine role of melatonin. *J Pineal Res* (Denmark) Jan 1993, 14 (1) p1-10

The pineal neurohormone melatonin stimulates activated CD4+, Thy-1+ cells to release opioid agonist(s) with immunoenhancing and anti-stress properties. *J Neuroimmunol* (Netherlands) Jul 1990, 28 (2)

Endocrine and immune effects of melatonin therapy in metastatic cancer patients. *Eur J Cancer Clin Oncol* (England) May 1989

Dehydroepiandrosterone (DHEA) treatment reverses the impaired immune response of old mice to influenza vaccination and protects from influenza infection. *Vaccine* (England) 1995, 13 (15) p1445-8

Dehydroepiandrosterone modulation of lipopolysaccharide-stimulated monocyte cytotoxicity. *J Immunol* Jan 1 1996, 156 (1)

Administration of dehydroepiandrosterone reverses the immune suppression induced by high dose antigen in mice. *Immunol Invest* May 1995

Pregnenolone and dehydroepiandrosterone as precursors of native 7-hydroxylated metabolites which increase the immune response in mice. *J Steroid Biochem Mol Biol* (England) Jul 1994

The relationship of serum DHEA-S and cortisol levels to measures of immune function in human immunodeficiency virus-related illness. *Am J Med Sci* Feb 1993

Dehydroepiandrosterone enhances IL2 production and cytotoxic effector function of human T cells. *Clin Immunol Immunopathol* Nov 1991

Protection from glucocorticoid induced thymic involution by dehydroepiandrosterone. *Life Sci* (England) 1990, 46 (22)

Immune development in young-adult C.RF-hyt mice is affected by congenital and maternal hypothyroidism. *Proc Soc Exp Biol Med* Oct 1993

Binding and functional effects of thyroid stimulating hormone on human immune cells. *J Clin Immunol* Jul 1990

Immunorestoration in children with recurrent respiratory infections treated with isoprinosine. *Int J Immunopharmacol* (England) 1987, 9 (8)

The effect of Biostim (RU-41740) on the expression of cytokine mRNAs in murine peritoneal macrophages in vitro. *Toxicol Lett* (Netherlands) Oct 1990

Isoprinosine (Inosine Pranobex Ban, INPX) in the treatment of Aids and other acquired immunodeficiencies of importance. *Cancer Detect Prev Suppl;* 1:597-609 1987

Immunological effests of Isoprinosine as a pulse immunotherapy in melanoma and ARC patients in melanoma and ARC patients. *Cancer Detect Prev Suppl*; 1:457-62 1987

A modified determination of coenzyme Q10 in human blood and CoQ10 blood levels in diverse patients with allergies. *Biofactors* (England) Dec 1988, 1 (4)

Carnitine in human immunodeficiency virus type 1 infection/ acquired immune deficiency syndrome. *J Child Neurol* Nov 1995, 10 Suppl

Oxidative damage and mitochondrial decay in aging. *Proc Natl Acad Sci U S A* Nov 8 1994

Carnitine depletion in peripheral blood mononuclear cells from patients with AIDS: effect of oral L-carnitine. *AIDS* May 1994, 8 (5) p655-60

Immunological parameters in aging: studies on natural immunomodulatory and immunoprotective substances. *Int J Clin Pharmacol Res* (Switzerland) 1990, 10 (1- 2)

Influenza Virus (Flu)

The use of the Multi-Tabs vitamin and mineral complex to prevent influenza. *Lik Sprava* (Ukraine) May 1998, (3) p107-9

Prophylactic effect of black tea extract as gargle against influenza. *Kansenshogaku Zasshi* (Japan) Jun 1997, 71 (6) p487-94

Attenuation of influenza -like symptomatology and improvement of cell-mediated immunity with long-term *N*-acetylcysteine treatment. *Eur Respir J* (Denmark) Jul 1997, 10 (7) p1535-41

The effect of DHEAS on influenza vaccination in aging adults. *J Am Geriatr Soc* Jun 1997, 45 (6) p747-51

Prevention and treatment of influenza in immunocompromised patients. *American Journal of Medicine*, 1997, 102/3 A (55-60)

The value of the dehydroepiandrosterone-annexed vitamin C infusion treatment in the clinical control of chronic fatigue syndrome (CFS). II. Characterization of CFS patients with special reference to their response to a new vitamin C infusion treatment. *In Vivo* (Greece) Nov-Dec 1996, 10 (6) p585-96

Inhibitory effects of recombinant manganese superoxide dismutase on influenza virus infections in mice. *Antimicrob Agents Chemother* Nov 1996, 40 (11) p2626-31

Influenza. More than mom and chicken soup. *J Fla Med Assoc* Jan 1996, 83 (1) p19-22

[Drugs active against respiratory viruses]. *Rev Prat* (France) Mar 15 1997, 47 (6) p646-51

Oxidant stress responses in influenza virus pneumonia: Gene expression and transcription factor activation. *American Journal of Physiology—Lung Cellular and Molecular Physiology*, 1996, 271/3 15-3 (L383-L391)

Antiviral activity of influenza virus M1 zinc finger peptides. *Journal of Virology*, 1996, 70/12 (8639-8644)

Viral and atypical pneumonias. *Primary Care—Clinics in Office Practice*, 1996, 23/4 (837-848)

In vivo anti-influenza virus activity of a zinc finger peptide. *Antimicrobial Agents and Chemotherapy*, 1997, 41/3 (687-692)

Efficacy and safety of aerosolized ribavirin in young children hospitalized with influenza: a double-blind, multicenter, placebo-controlled trial. *J Pediatr* Jul 1994

Antivirals for the chemoprophylaxis and treatment of influenza. *Semin Respir Infect* Mar 1992

Utilization of pulse oximetry for the study of the inhibitory effects of antiviral agents on influenza virus in mice. *Antimicrob Agents Chemother* Feb 1992

Further studies with short duration ribavirin aerosol for the treatment of influenza virus infection in mice and respiratory syncytial virus infection in cotton rats. *Antiviral Res* (Netherlands) Jan 1992

High dose-short duration ribavirin aerosol treatment—a review. *Bull Int Union Tuberc Lung Dis* (France) Jun-Sep 1991

Molecular mechanisms of action of ribavirin. *Rev Infect Dis* Nov-Dec 1990

Ribavirin aerosol treatment of influenza. *Infect Dis Clin North Am* Jun 1987

Comparative activities of several nucleoside analogues against influenza A,B, and C viruses in vitro. *Antimicrob Agents Chemother* Jun 1988

Ribavirin aerosol in the elderly. *Chest* Jun 1988

Favorable outcome after treatment with amantadine and ribavirin in a pregnancy complicated by influenza pneumonia. A case report. Department of Obstetrics and Gynecology, Baylor College of Medicine, Houston, TX 77030

Oral ribavirin treatment of influenza A and B. *Antimicrob Agents Chemother* Aug 1987

Ribavirin: a clinical overview. *Eur J Epidemiol* (Italy) Mar 1986

Ribavirin small-particle aerosol treatment of infections caused by influenza virus strains A/Victoria/7/83 (H1N1) and B/Texas/1/84. *Antimicrob Agents Chemother* Mar 1985

Effect of ribavirin triphosphate on primer generation and elongation during influenza virus transcription in vitro. *Antiviral Res* (Netherlands) Feb 1985, 5 (1) p39-48

Ribavirin aerosol treatment of influenza B virus infection. *Trans Assoc Am Physicians* 1983, 96

Treatment of influenza A (H1N1) virus infection with ribavirin aerosol. *Antimicrob Agents Chemother* Aug 1984

Immune modulating properties of root extracts of different Echinacea species. *Zeitschrift fur Phytotherapie* (Germany), 1995, 16/3 (157-162+165-166)

Echinacea Pharm. J. (UK), 1994, 253/6806 (342-343)

Echinacea combinations; efficacy and acceptability in 'flu' and nasopharyngeal inflammations. *Dtsch. Apoth.-Ztg* (Germany, West), 1987, 127/16 (853-854)

Papilloma virus infections of the skin. *Breisgau* (Germany, West)

Direct characterization of caffeoyl esters with antihyaluronidase activity in crude extracts from Echinacea angustifolia roots by fast atom bombardment tandem mass spectrometry. *Farmaco* (Italy), 1993, 48/10 (1447-1461)

Anti-inflammatory activity of Echinacea angustifolia fractions separated on the basis of molecular weight. *Pharmacol. Res. Commun.* (UK), 1988, 20/Suppl. 5 (87-90)

In vitro activity of Mercurius cyanatus against relevant pathogenic bacteria isolates. *Arzneimittel-Forschung / Drug Research* (Germany), 1995, 45/9 (1018-1020)

Mechanisms of propolis water extract antiherpetic activity. II. Activity of propolis water extract lectines. *Rev. Roum. Virol.* (Romania), 1993, 44/1-2 (49-54)

Comparison of the anti-herpes simplex virus activities of propolis and 3- methyl-but-2-enyl caffeate. *J. Nat. Prod. Lloydia*, 1994, 57/5 (644-647)

Synergistic effect of flavones and flavonols against herpes simplex virus type 1 in cell culture. Comparison with the antiviral activity of propolis. *J. Nat. Prod. Lloydia*, 1992, 55/12 (1732-1740)

Recent advances in the chemotherapy of herpes virus infections. *Rev. Roum. Med.* (Rumania), 1981, 32/1 (57-77)

Anti-influenza virus effect of some propolis constituents and their analogueues (esters of substituted cinnamic acids). *J. Nat. Prod. Lloydia*, 1992, 55/3 (294-297)

The effect of an aqueous propolis extract, of rutin and of a rutin-quercetin mixture on experimental influenza virus infection in mice. *Rev. Roum. Med.* (Rumania), 1981, 32/3 (213-215)

Insomnia

The relation between cigarette smoking and sleep disturbance. *Prev Med* 1994 May;23(3):328-34

Narcolepsy and cataplexy. Clinical features, treatment and cerebrospinal fluid findings. *Quarterly Journal of Medicine* 1974, 43/172 (525-536)

Melatonin replacement therapy of elderly insomniacs. *Sleep*, 1995, 18/7 (598-603)

Improvement of sleep equality in elderly people by controlled-release melatonin. *Lancet* (UK), 1995, 346/8974 (541-544)

Sleep-inducing effects of low doses of melatonin ingested in the evening. *Clinical Pharmacology and Therapeutics*, 1995, 57/5 (552-558)

Light, melatonin and the sleep-wake cycle. *J. Psychiatry Neurosci.* (Canada), 1994, 19/5 (345-353)

Melatonin rhythms in night shift workers. *Sleep*, 1992, 15/5 (434-441)

Effect of melatonin replacement on serum hormone rhythms in a patient lacking endogenous melatonin. *Brain Res. Bull.*, 1991, 27/2 (181-185)

Melatonin administration in insomnia. *Neuropsychopharmacology,* 1990, 3/1 (19-23)

Melatonin replacement therapy of elderly insomniacs. *Sleep* Sep 1995, 18 (7) p598-603

Melatonin replacement corrects sleep disturbances in a child with pineal tumor. *Neurology,* 1996, 46/1 (261-263)

Use of melatonin in circadian rhythm disorders and following phase shifts. *Acta Neurobiologiae Experimentalis* (Poland), 1996, 56/1 (359-362)

Treatment of delayed sleep phase syndrome. *General Hospital Psychiatry,* 1995, 17/5 (335-345)

Nutritional factors in the etiology of the premenstrual tension syndromes. *J Reprod Med* Jul 1983, 28 (7) p446-64

Effects of intravenously administered vitamin B12 on sleep in the rat. *Physiol Behav* Jun 1995, 57 (6) p1019-24

Treatment of persistent sleep-wake schedule disorders in adolescents with methylcobalamin (vitamin B12). *Sleep* Oct 1991, 14 (5) p414-8

Vitamin B12 treatment for sleep-wake rhythm disorders. *Sleep* Feb 1990, 13 (1) p15-23

[Folate and the nervous system (author's transl)] Folates et systeme nerveux. *Sem Hop* (France) Sep 18-25 1979, 55 (31-32) p1383-7

The effects of nicotinamide upon sleep in humans. *Biol Psychiatry* Feb 1977, 12 (1) p139-43

Jet Lag

[Role of the pharmacopoeia in the prevention of jet-lag]. *Bull Soc Pathol Exot* 1997;90(4):291-2

Efficacy of melatonin treatment in jet lag, shift work, and blindness. *J Biol Rhythms* 1997 Dec;12(6):604-17

[Phototherapy of jet lag, night work and sleep disorders]. *Tidsskr Nor Laegeforen* 1997 Jun 30;117(17):2489-92

A double-blind trial of Melatonin as a treatment for jet lag in international cabin crew. *Biol Psychiatry* Apr 1 1993

Melatonin and jet lag: confirmatory result using a simplified protocol. *Biol Psychiatry* Oct 15 1992, 32 (8) p705-11

[Role of biological clock in human pathology]. *Presse Med* (France) Jun 17 1995, 24 (22) p1041-6

Melatonin marks circadian phase position and resets the endogenous circadian pacemaker in humans. *Ciba Found Symp* (Netherlands) 1995, 183 p303-17; discussion 317-21

The role of pineal gland in circadian rhythms regulation. *Bratisl Lek Listy* (Slovakia) Jul 1994, 95 (7) p295- 303

Light, melatonin and the sleep-wake cycle. *J Psychiatry Neurosci* (Canada) Nov 1994, 19 (5) p345-53

Circadian rhythms, jet lag, and chronobiotics: an overview. *Chronobiol Int* Aug 1994, 11 (4) p253-65

[Chronobiological sleep disorders and their treatment possibilities]. *Ther Umsch* (Switzerland) Oct 1993, 50 (10) p704-8

Chronopharmacological actions of the pineal gland. *Drug Metabol Drug Interact* (England) 1990, 8 (3-4) p189-201

Some effects of Melatonin and the control of its secretion in humans. *Ciba Found Symp* (Netherlands) 1985, 117 p266-83

Kidney Disease

Polycystic kidney disease: an unrecognized emerging infectious disease? *Emerg Infect Dis* 1997 Apr-Jun;3(2):113-27

Potassium-magnesium citrate is an effective prophylaxis against recurrent calcium oxalate nephrolithiasis. *J Urol* 1997 Dec;158(6):2069-73

Effect of mineral water containing calcium and magnesium on calcium oxalate urolithiasis risk factors. *Urol Int* 1997; 58(2):93-9

PKD2, a gene for polycystic kidney disease that encodes an integral membrane protein. *Science* 1996 May 31;272(5266):1339-42

Gene therapy for kidney disease. *Adv Nephrol Necker Hosp* 1997;26:73-80

Gene transfer into kidney tubules and vasculature by adenoviral vectors. *Exp Nephrol* 1997 Mar-Apr;5(2):137-43

DNA diagnosis and clinical manifestations of autosomal dominant polycystic kidney disease. *Folia Biol* (Praha) (Czech Republic) 1997, 43 (5) p201-4

Autosomal dominant polycystic kidney disease: clinical and genetic aspects. *J Nephrol* (Italy) Nov-Dec 1997, 10 (6) p295-310

Mechanisms of progression in autosomal dominant polycystic kidney disease. *Kidney Int Suppl* Dec 1997, 63 pS93-7

Neonatal presentation of autosomal dominant polycystic kidney disease with a maternal history of tuberous sclerosis. *Nephrol Dial Transplant* (England) Nov 1997, 12 (11) p2284-8

Ambulatory blood pressure in hypertensive patients with autosomal dominant polycystic kidney disease. *Nephrol Dial Transplant* (England) Oct 1997, 12 (10) p2075-80

Renal vascular resistance in autosomal dominant polycystic kidney disease. Evaluation with color Doppler ultrasound. *Acta Radiol* (Denmark) Sep 1997, 38 (5) p840-6

Left ventricular hypertrophy in autosomal dominant polycystic kidney disease. *J Am Soc Nephrol* Aug 1997, 8 (8) p1292-7

Recent advances in the understanding of polycystic kidney disease. *Curr Opin Nephrol Hypertens* Jul 1997, 6 (4) p377-83

Kidney stone clinic: Ten years of experience. *Nederlands Tijschrift voor de Klinische Chemie* (Netherlands), 1996, 21/1

Magnesium in the physiopathology and treatment of renal calcium stones. *Presse Med.* (France), 1987, 16/1 (25-27)

Urinary factors of kidney stone formation in patients with Crohn's disease. *Klin. Wochenschr.* (Germany, Federal Republic of), 1988, 66/3 (87-91)

Renal stone formation in patients with inflammatory bowel disease. *Scanning Microsc.*, 1993, 7/1 (371-380)

Calcium and calcium magnesium carbonate specimens submitted as urinary tract stones. *J. Urol.*, 1993, 149/2 (244-249)

Etiology and treatment of urolithiasis. *Am. J. Kidney Dis.*, 1991, 18/6 (624-637)

Pathogenesis of nephrolithiasis post-partial ileal bypass surgery: Case-control study. *Kidney Int.*, 1991, 39/6 (1249-1254)

The effect of glucose intake on urine saturation with calcium oxalate, calcium phosphate, uric acid and sodium urate. *Int. Urol. Nephrol.* (Netherlands), 1988, 20/6

Magnesium metabolism in health and disease. *Dis. Mon.*, 1988, 34/4 (166-218)

Prophylaxis of recurring urinary stones: hard or soft mineral water. *Minerva Med.* (Italy), 1987, 78/24 (1823-1829)

Urothelial injury to the rabbit bladder from various alkaline and acidic solutions used to dissolve kidney stones. *J. Urol.* (Baltimore), 1986, 136/1 (181-183)

Kidney stones, magnesium and spa treatment. *Presse Therm. Clim.* (France), 1983, 120/1 (33-35)

Learning Disorders

Refer *to references under Attention Deficit Disorder (ADD) or Age Associated Mental Impairment (Brain Aging).*

Leukemia-Lymphoma (and non-Hodgkin's Disease)

Telomerase inhibition, telomere shortening, and senescence of cancer cells by tea catechins. *Biochem Biophys Res Commun* Aug 19 1998, 249 (2) p391-6

Natural retinoids and beta-carotene: From food to their actions on gene expression. *Journal of Nutritional Biochemistry,* 1998, 9/8 (446-456)

[Clinical observation on 112 cases with non-Hodgkin's lymphoma treated by Chinese herbs combined with chemotherapy] *Chung Kuo Chung Hsi I Chieh Ho Tsa Chih* (China) Jun 1997, 17 (6) p325-7

The role of interferon as maintenance therapy in malignant lymphoma. *Med Oncol* (England) Sep-Dec 1997, 14 (3-4) p153-7

Medical history risk factors for non-Hodgkin's lymphoma in older women. *Journal of the National Cancer Institute* (UK) 1997, 89/4 (314-318)

Thrombotic complications in acute promyelocytic leukemia during all-trans-retinoic acid therapy. *Acta Haematol* (Switzerland) 1997, 97 (4) p228-30

Secondary cytogenetic changes in acute promyelocytic leukemia—prognostic importance in patients treated with chemotherapy alone and association with the intron 3 breakpoint of the PML gene: a Cancer and Leukemia Group B study. *J Clin Oncol* May 1997, 15 (5) p1786-95

Thrombosis in patients with acute promyelocytic leukemia treated with and without all-trans retinoic acid. *Leuk Lymphoma* (Switzerland) Feb 1996, 20 (5-6) p435-9

The in vitro effects of all-trans-retinoic acid and hematopoietic growth factors on the clonal growth and self-renewal of blast stem cells in acute promyelocytic leukemia. *Leuk Res* (England) Apr 1997, 21 (4) p285-94

All-trans retinoic acid in hematological malignancies, an update. GER (GruppoEmatologico Retinoidi). *Haematologica* (Italy) Jan-Feb 1997, 82 (1) p106-21

Molecular genetics of acute leukaemia. *Lancet* (England) Jan 18 1997, 349 (9046) p196-200

All-trans retinoic acid (Tretinoin). *Gan To Kagaku Ryoho* (Japan) Apr 1997, 24 (6) p741-6

A case of acute eosinophilic granulocytic leukemia with PML-RAR alpha fusion gene expression and response to all-trans retinoic acid. *Leukemia* (England) Apr 1997, 11 (4) p609-11

Effects of receptor class- and subtype-selective retinoids and an apoptosis-inducing retinoid on the adherent growth of the NIH:OVCAR-3 ovarian cancer cell line in culture. *Cancer Lett* (Ireland) May 1 1997, 115 (1) p1-7

All-trans retinoic acid (ATRA) in the treatment of acute promyelocytic leukemia (APL). *Hematol Oncol* (England) Sep 1996, 14 (3) p147-54

Inhibition of proliferation by retinoic acid on adult T cell leukemia cells. *Nihon Rinsho Meneki Gakkai Kaishi* (Japan) Oct 1996, 19 (5) p477-87

Curcumin, an antioxidant and anti-tumor promoter, induces apoptosis in human leukemia cells. *Biochim Biophys Acta* (Netherlands) Nov 15 1996, 1317 (2) p95-100

All-trans and 9-cis retinoic acid enhance 1,25-dihydroxyvitamin D3-induced monocytic differentiation of U937 cells. *Leuk Res* (England) Aug 1996, 20 (8) p665-76

Experience in administration low dose all-trans retinoic acid for a child with acute promyelocytic leukemia. *Rinsho Ketsueki* (Japan) Feb 1996, 37 (2) p129-33

Down-regulation of bcl-2 in AML blasts by all-trans retinoic acid and its relationship to CD34 antigen expression. *Br J Haematol* (England) Sep 2 1996, 94 (4) p671-5

Induction therapy with all-trans retinoic acid for acute promyelocytic leukemia: a clinical study of 10 cases, including a fatal [correction of fetal] case with thromboembolism. *Intern Med* (Japan) Jan 1996, 35 (1) p10-4

Effect of the protein tyrosine kinase inhibitor genistein on normal and leukaemic haemopoietic progenitor cells. *Br J Haematol* (England) Jun 1 1996, 93 (3) p551-7

Differentiating therapy in acute myeloid leukemia. *Leukemia* (England) Jun 1996, 10 Suppl 2 ps33-8

Expression of Retinoid X Receptor alpha is increased upon monocytic cell differentiation. *Biochem Biophys Res Commun* Mar 18 1996, 220 (2) p315-22

In vivo and in vitro characterization of the B1 and B2 zinc-binding domains from the acute promyelocytic leukemia protooncoprotein PML. *Proc Natl Acad Sci U S A* Feb 20 1996, 93 (4) p1601-6

All-trans retinoic acid combined with interferon-alpha effectively inhibits granulocyte-macrophage colony formation in chronic myeloid leukemia. *Leuk Res* (England) Mar 1996, 20 (3) p243-8

Expression of the p53 tumor suppressor gene induces differentiation and promotes induction of differentiation by 1,25-dihydroxycholecalciferol in leukemic U-937 cells. *Blood* Feb 1 1996, 87 (3) p1064-74

Retinoids and carcinogenesis. *Biotherapy* (Japan), 1997, 11/4 (512-517)

Combination of a potent 20-epi-vitamin D3 analogueue (KH 1060) with 9- cis-retinoic acid irreversibly inhibits clonal growth, decreases bcl-2 expression, and induces apoptosis in HL-60 leukemic cells. *Cancer Research*, 1996, 56/15 (3570-3576)

Monocytic differentiation modulates apoptotic response to cytotoxic anti-Fas antibody and tumor necrosis factor alpha in human monoblast U937 cells. *Journal of Leukocyte Biology*, 1996, 60/6 (778-783)

Myeloma cell growth arrest, apoptosis, and interleukin-6 receptor modulation induced by EB1089, a vitamin D3 derivative, alone or in association with dexamethasone. *Blood*, 1996, 88/12 (4659-4666)

Mutation in the ligand-binding domain of the retinoic acid receptor alpha in HL-60 leukemic cells resistant to retinoic acid and with increased sensitivity to vitamin D3 analogues. *Leukemia Research* (UK), 1996, 20/9 (761-769)

Selection of myeloid progenitors lacking BCR/ABL mRNA in chronic myelogenous leukemia patients after in vitro treatment with the tyrosine kinase inhibitor genistein. *Blood*, 1996, 88/8 (3091-3100)

Influence of dietary components on occurrence of and mortality due to neoplasms in male F344 rats. *Aging—Clinical and Experimental Research* (Italy), 1996, 8/4 (254-262)

The activities of tyrosine protein kinase and phosphotyrosine protein phosphatase by two differentiation inducers in HL-60 cells. *Chinese Journal of Clinical Oncology* (China), 1996, 23/2 (84-88)

Retinoids in cancer treatment. *J Clin Pharmacol*. 1992 Oct. 32(10). P 868-88

Induction of differentiation and enhancement of vincristine sensitivity of human erythroleukemia HEL cells by vesnarinone, a positive inotropic agent. *Exp Hematol*. 1996 Jan. 24(1). P 37-42

1,25-dihydroxyvitamin D3 primes acute promyelocytic cells for TPA-induced monocytic differentiation through both PKC and tyrosine phosphorylation cascades. *Exp Cell Res*. 1996 Jan 10. 222(1). P 61-9

Probing the pathobiology of response to all-trans retinoic acid in cute promyelocytic leukemia: premature chromosome condensation/fluorescence in situ hybridization analysis. *Blood*. 1996 Jan 1. 87(1). P 218-26

Acute renal failure associated with the retinoic acid syndrome in acute promyelocytic leukemia. *Am J Kidney Dis*. 1996 Jan. 27(1). P 134-7

[Synthesis of retinoids with a modified polar group and their antitumor activity. Report I]. *Bioorg Khim*. 1995 Dec. 21(12). P 941-9

Induction of differentiation in murine erythroleukemia cells by 1 alpha,25-dihydroxy vitamin D3. *Cancer Lett*. 1995 Apr 14. 90(2). P 225-30

Synergistic differentiation of U937 cells by all-trans retinoic acid and 1 alpha, 25-dihydroxyvitamin D3 is associated with the expression of retinoid X receptor alpha. *Biochem Biophys Res Commun*. 1994 Aug 30. 203(1). P 272-80

1,25(OH)2-16ene-vitamin D3 is a potent antileukemic agent with low potential to cause hypercalcemia. *Leuk Res* (1994 Jun) 18(6):453-63

Genistein enhances the ICAM-mediated adhesion by inducing the expression of ICAM-1 and its counter-receptors. *Biochem Biophys Res Commun* (1994 Aug 30) 203(1):443-9

Induction of differentiation and dna breakage in human hl-60 and k-562 leukemia cells by genistein. *Proc Annu Meet Am Assoc Cancer Res* (1990) 31:A2605

Tretinoin. A review of its pharmacodynamic and pharmacokinetic properties and use in the management of acute promyelocytic leukaemia. *Drugs*. 1995 Nov. 50(5). P 897-923

[Treatment of acute promyelocytic leukemia with trans-retinoic acid. Experience of the Santa Maria Hospital, Medical School of Lisbon]. *Acta Med Port*. 1994 Dec. 7(12). P 717-24

Vitamin A preserves the cytotoxic activity of adriamycin while counteracting its peroxidative effects in human leukemic cells in vitro. *Biochem Mol Biol Int*. 1994 Sep. 34(2). P 329-35

In vitro all-trans retinoic acid (ATRA) sensitivity and cellular retinoic acid binding protein (CRABP) levels in relapse leukemic cells after remission induction by ATRA in acute promyelocytic leukemia. *Leukemia*. 1994 Jun. 8(6). P 914-7

Mechanisms of protection of hematopoietic stem cells from irradiation. *Leuk Lymphoma*. 1994 Mar. 13(1-2). P 27-32

Treatment of mucositis with vitamin E during administration of neutropenic antineoplastic agents. *Ann Med Interne* (Paris). 1994. 145(6). P 405-8

Effects of sodium ascorbate (vitamin C) and 2-methyl-1,4-naphthoquinone (vitamin K3) treatment on human tumor cell growth in vitro. II. Synergism with combined chemotherapy action. *Anticancer Res*. 1993 Jan-Feb. 13(1). P 103-6

[Remission of acute promyelocytic leukemia after all-trans-retinoic acid]. *Harefuah*. 1992 Dec 1. 123(11). P 445-8, 507

Abnormal vitamin B6 status in childhood leukemia. *Cancer*. 1990 Dec 1. 66(11). P 2421-8

In vitro all-trans retinoic acid (ATRA) sensitivity and cellular retinoic acid binding protein (CRABP) levels in relapse leukemic cells after remission induction by ATRA in acute promyelocytic leukemia. *Leukemia*. 1994. 8 Suppl 2P S16-9

Liver Cirrhosis

Antioxidants in the treatment of cholelithiasis patients]. *Vestn Khir Im I I Grek* (Russia) 1997, 156 (1) p36-9

Trace elements and chronic liver diseases. *J Trace Elem Med Biol* (Germany) Nov 1997, 11 (3) p158-61

Erythrocyte membrane lipids and serum selenium in post-viral and alcoholic cirrhosis. *Clinica Chimica Acta* (Netherlands), 1998, 270/2 (139-150)

Alcohol consumption and micronutrient intake as risk factors for liver cirrhosis: a case-control study. The Provincial Group for the study of Chronic Liver Disease. *Ann Epidemiol* Apr 1998, 8 (3) p154-9

Anemias in Thai patients with cirrhosis. *Int J Hematol* (Ireland) Jun 1997, 65 (4) p365-73

Cirrhotic liver expresses low levels of the full-length and truncated growth hormone receptors. *Journal of Clinical Endocrinology and Metabolism*, 1998, 83/7 (2532-2538)

Growth hormone-stimulated insulin-like growth factor (IGF) I and IGF- binding protein-3 in liver cirrhois. *Journal of Hepatology* (Denmark), 1997, 27/5 (796-802)

S-adenosil-L-methionine is able to reverse the immunosuppressive effects of chenodeoxycholic acid in vitro. *International Journal of Immunopharmacology* (UK), 1997, 19/3 (157-165)

Plasma vitamin K1 level is decreased in primary biliary cirrhosis. *Am J Gastroenterol* Nov 1997, 92 (11) p2059-61

Cholastasis: Therapeutic options. *Therapeutische Umschau* (Switzerland), 1998, 55/2 (97-103)

Vitamin A concentration in the liver decreases with age in patients with cystic fibrosis. *J Pediatr Gastroenterol Nutr* Mar 1997, 24 (3) p264-70

Dark adaptation in early primary biliary cirrhosis. *United Kingdom Eye* (UK), 1998, 12/3 A (419-426)

Therapy of hepatitis C: Other options. *Hepatology*, 1997, 26/3 Suppl. (143S-151S)

Blood amino acid levels in sarin poisoning patients. *Rinsho Byori* (Japan) Aug 1997, 45 (8) p785-9

Long-term (12 months) treatment with an anti-oxidant drug (silymarin) is effective on hyperinsulinemia, exogenous insulin need and malondialdehyde levels in cirrhotic diabetic patients. *J Hepatol* (Denmark) Apr 1997, 26 (4) p871-9

Influence of Legalon (R) 140 on the metabolism of collagen in patients with chronic liver disease - Review by measurement of PIIINP-values. *Zeitschrift fur Allgemeinmedizin* (Germany), 1998, 74/11-12 (577-584)

Wine and heart. *Rev Esp Cardiol* (Spain) Jun 1998, 51 (6) p435-49

Chaparral-associated hepatotoxicity. *Arch Intern Med* Apr 28 1997, 157 (8) p913-9

Alpha-lipoic acid in liver metabolism and disease. *Free Radical Biology and Medicine*, 1998, 24/6 (1023-1039)

Hepatic tocopherol content in primary hepatocellular carcinoma and liver metastases. *Hepatology*, 1997, 26/1 (67-72)

Coffee consumption and decreased serum gamma-glutamyltransferase and aminotransferase activities among male alcohol drinkers. *International Journal of Epidemiology* (UK), 1998, 27/3 (438-443)

Determination of hepatic zinc content in chronic liver disease due to hepatitis B virus. *Hepatogastroenterology* (Greece) Mar-Apr 1998, 45 (20) p472-6

Oral L-ornithine-L-aspartate therapy of chronic hepatic encephalopathy: results of a placebo-controlled double-blind study. *J Hepatol* (Denmark) May 1998, 28 (5) p856-64

Zinc supplementation improves glucose disposal in patients with cirrhosis. *Metabolism* Jul 1998, 47 (7) p792-8

[Pre- and postoperative correction of hyposiderosis in surgical treatment of portal hypertension]. *Khirurgiia (Mosk)* (Russia) 1998, (5) p18-20

[Frequent chemolipiodolization and prostaglandin E1 administration for hepatocellular carcinoma with advanced liver cirrhosis]. *Nippon Shokakibyo Gakkai Zasshi* (Japan) Apr 1998, 95 (4) p311-6

Effects of supplementation with unsaturated fatty acids on plasma and membrane lipid composition and platelet function in patients with cirrhosis and defective aggregation. *J Hepatol* (Denmark) Apr 1998, 28 (4) p654-61

Effects of L-arginine on the systemic, mesenteric, and hepatic circulation in patients with cirrhosis. *Hepatology* Feb 1998, 27 (2) p377-82

Consequences of cholestasis from the hepatologist's viewpoint. *Schweiz Med Wochenschr* (Switzerland) May 10 1997, 127 (19) p821-8

Ursodeoxycholic acid in the treatment of liver diseases. *Postgrad Med J* (England) Feb 1997, 73 (856) p75-80

Lamivudine treatment of chronic hepatitis B. *Reviews in Medical Virology* (UK), 1998, 8/3 (153-159)

Ursodeoxycholic acid, new approach to the treatment of gravidic cholestasis? Three case reports. *Journal de Gynecologie Obstetrique et Biologie de la Reproduction* (France), 1998, 27/6 (617-621)

Spontaneous pulsatility and pharmacokinetics of growth hormone in liver cirrhotic patients. *Journal of Hepatology* (Denmark), 1998, 29/4 (559-564)

A pregnancy complicated with intrahepatic cholestasis managed by ursodeoxycholic acid. *Jinekoloji ve Obstetri Bulteni* (Turkey), 1998, 7/3 (120-123)

Pharmacological management of chronic viral hepatitis. *Journal of Pharmaceutical Care in Pain and Symptom Control*, 1998, 6/3 (41-62)

Hepatitis B and C: Current treatment. *Schweizerische Rundschau fur Medizin / Praxis* (Switzerland), 1998, 87/42 (1408-1412)

Zinc deficiency in liver cirrhosis: Curiosity or problem? *Annali Italiani di Medicina Interna* (Italy), 1998, 13/3 (157-162)

Effects of ribavirin on hepatitis C-associated nephrotic syndrome in four liver transplant recipients. *Kidney International*, 1998, 54/4 (1311-1319)

Ursodeoxycholic acid therapy for primary biliary cirrhosis. A 10-year British single-centre population-based audit of efficacy and survival. *Postgraduate Medical Journal* (UK), 1998, 74/874 (482-485)

Colchicine: 1998 update. *Seminars in Arthritis and Rheumatism*, 1998, 28/1 (48-59)

Heavy and moderate drinking: Risks and benefits. *Journal of the Irish Colleges of Physicians and Surgeons* (Ireland), 1998, 27/3 (161-176)

Antioxidants: A therapy of the future?. *Nutricion Hospitalaria* (Spain), 1997, 12/3 (108-120)

Zinc therapy in gastroenterology. *Medizinische Welt* (Germany), 1998, 49/2 (78-83)

Malnutrition and bacterial infections in hepatic cirrhosis. *GED—Gastrenterologia Endoscopia Digestiva* (Brazil), 1997, 16/6 (226-230)

Nutritional intervention in the alimentary tract diseases. *Gastroenterologia Polska* (Poland), 1997, 4/5 (501-515)

Disruption of the diurnal rhythm of plasma melatonin in liver cirrhosis. *Wiener Klinische Wochenschrift* (Austria), 1997, 109/18 (741-746)

Antacids. *SENDROM* (Turkey), 1997, 9/8 (20-27)

Zinc regulates DNA synthesis and IL-2, IL-6, and IL-10 production of PWM-stimulated PBMC and normalizes the periphere cytokine concentration in chronic liver disease. *Journal of Trace Elements in Experimental Medicine*, 1997, 10/1 (19-27)

Nutritional considerations and management of the child with liver disease. *Nutrition*, 1997, 13/3 (177-184)

Effects of extra-carbohydrate supplementation in the late evening on energy expenditure and substrate oxidation in patients with liver cirrhosis. *Journal of Parenteral and Enteral Nutrition*, 1997, 21/2 (96-99)

[Antioxidants in the treatment of cholelithiasis patients]. *Vestn Khir Im I I Grek* 1997;156(1):36-9.

Anemias in Thai patients with cirrhosis. *International Journal of Hematology* (Ireland), 1997, 65/4 (365-373)

Therapeutic efficacy of L-ornithine-L-aspartate infusions in patients with cirrhosis and hepatic encephalopathy: Results of a placebo-controlled, double-blind study. *Hepatology*, 1997, 25/6 (1351-1360)

The use of methotrexate, colchicine, and other immunomodulatory drugs in the treatment of primary biliary cirrhosis. *Seminars in Liver Disease*, 1997, 17/2 (129-136)

Inhibition by green tea extract of diethylnitrosamine-initiated but not choline-deficient, L-amino acid-defined diet-associated development of putative preneoplastic, glutathione S-transferase placental form-positive lesions in rat liver. *Japanese Journal of Cancer Research* (Japan), 1997, 88/4 (356-362)

Chronic alcoholism in the absence of Wernicke-Korsakoff syndrome and cirrhosis does not result in the loss of serotonergic neurons from the median raphe nucleus. *Metabolic Brain Disease*, 1996, 11/3 (217-228)

Iron in liver diseases other than hemochromatosis. *Seminars in Liver Disease*, 1996, 16/1 (65-82)

Antioxidant defenses in metal-induced liver damage. *Seminars in Liver Disease*, 1996, 16/1 (39-46)

Vitamins and metals: Potential dangers for the human being. *Schweizerische Medizinische Wochenschrift* (Switzerland), 1996, 126/15 (607-611)

Effects of hepatic stimulator substance, herbal medicine, selenium/vitamin E, and ciprofloxacin on cirrhosis in the rat. *Gastroenterology*, 1996, 110/4 (1150-1155)

Hepatic encephalopathy. *Pathogenesis and therapy. Infezioni in Medicina* (Italy), 1997, 5/1 (14-19)

Long-term (12 months) treatment with an anti-oxidant drug (silymarin) is effective on hyperinsulinemia, exogenous insulin need and malondialdehyde levels in cirrhotic diabetic patients. *Journal of Hepatology* (Denmark), 1997, 26/4 (871-879)

Comparative effects of colchicine and silymarin on CCl4-chronic liver damage in rats. *Archives of Medical Research* (Mexico), 1997, 28/1 (11-17)

Properties and medical use of flavonolignans (Silymarin) from Silybum marianum. *Phytotherapy Research* (UK), 1996, 10/Suppl. 1 (S25-S26)

Phytotherapy in Germany: Its role in self-medication and in medical prescribing. *Natural Medicines* (Japan), 1996, 50/4 (259-264)

Reliable phytotherapy in chronic liver diseases. *Therapiewoche* (Germany), 1996, 46/17 (916+918-919)

Oral supplementation with branched-chain amino acids improves transthyretin turnover in rats with carbon tetrachloride-induced liver cirrhosis. *Journal of Nutrition*, 1996, 126/5 (1412-1420)

Inhibition by acetylsalicylic acid, a cyclo-oxygenase inhibitor, and p-bromophenacylbromide, a phospholipase A2 inhibitor, of both cirrhosis and enzyme-altered nodules caused by a choline-deficient, L-amino acid-defined diet in rats. *Carcinogenesis* (UK), 1996, 17/3 (467-475)

Overview of randomized clinical trials of oral branched-chain amino acid treatment in chronic hepatic encephalopathy. *Journal of Parenteral and Enteral Nutrition*, 1996, 20/2 (159-164)

Leucine metabolism in rats with cirrhosis. *J Hepatol* (Denmark) Feb 1996, 24 (2) p209-16

Renal and pressor effects of aminoguanidine in cirrhotic rats with ascites. *J Am Soc Nephrol* Dec 1996, 7 (12) p2694-9

Nutrient-induced thermogenesis and protein-sparing effect by rapid infusion of a branched chain-enriched amino acid solution to cirrhotic patients. *J Med* 1996, 27 (3-4) p176-82

Serum amino acid changes in rats with thioacetamide-induced liver cirrhosis. *Toxicology* (ireland) Jan 8 1996, 106 (1-3) p197-206

Vitamin A concentration in the liver decreases with age in patients with cystic fibrosis. *J Pediatr Gastroenterol Nutr* Mar 1997, 24 (3) p264-70

The prolyl 4-hydroxylase inhibitor HOE 077 prevents activation of Ito cells, reducing procollagen gene expression in rat liver fibrosis induced by choline-deficient L-amino acid-defined diet. *Hepatology* Apr 1996, 23 (4) p755-63

Glutathione kinetics in normal man and in patients with liver cirrhosis. *J Hepatol* (Denmark) Mar 1997, 26 (3) p606-13

Proton magnetic resonance spectroscopy of the brain in symptomatic and asymptomatic patients with liver cirrhosis. *Gastroenterology* May 1997, 112 (5) p1610-6

Effect of branched chain amino acid infusions on body protein metabolism in cirrhosis of liver. *Gut* (1986 Nov) 27 Suppl 1:96-102

Severe recurrent hepatic encephalopathy that responded to oral branched chain amino acids. *American Journal of Gastroenterology*, 1996, 91/6 (1266-1268)

[Branched-chain amino acids in the treatment of latent porto-systemic encephalopathy. A placebo-controlled double-blind cross-over study]. *Z Ernahrungswiss*. 1986 Mar. 25(1). P 9-28

A prospective, randomized, double-blind, controlled trial. *J Parenter Enteral Nutr.* 1985 May-Jun. 9(3). P 288- 95

Prevention of CCL4-induced liver cirrhosis by silymarin. *Fundam Clin Pharmacol* (1989) 3(3):183-91

Free radicals in tissue damage in liver diseases and therapeutic approach. *Tokai J Exp Clin Med* (1986) 11 Suppl:121-34

Serum neutral amino acid concentrations in cirrhotic patients with impaired carbohydrate metabolism. *Acta Med Okayama.* 1983 Aug. 37(4). P 381-4

Is intravenous administration of branched chain amino acids effective in the treatment of hepatic encephalopathy? A multicenter study. *Hepatology.* 1983 Jul-Aug. 3(4). P 475-80

Branched-chain amino acid-enriched elemental diet in patients with cirrhosis of the liver. A double blind crossover trial. *Gastroenterol.* 1983 Nov. 21(11). P 644-50

Effect of euglycemic insulin infusion on plasma levels of branched- chain amino acids in cirrhosis. *Hepatology.* 1983 Mar-Apr. 3(2). P 184-7

Effect of glucose and/or branched chain amino acid infusion on plasma amino acid imbalance in chronic liver failure. *J Parenter Enteral Nutr.* 1981 Sep-Oct. 5(5). P 414-9

A comparison of the effects of intravenous infusion of individual branched-chain amino acids on blood amino acid levels in man. *Clin Sci* (Colch). 1981 Jan. 60(1). P 95-100

[Pathogenesis of hepatic encephalopathy (author's transl)]. *Leber Magen Darm.* 1977 Aug. 7(4). P 241-54

Clearance rate of plasma branched-chain amino acids correlates significantly with blood ammonia level in patients with liver cirrhosis. *International Hepatology Communications* (Ireland), 1995, 3/2 (91-96)

Nutritional treatment of liver cirrhosis with branched chain amino acids. (BCAA) Nutritional support in organ failure: proceedings of the International Symposium, 1990

Branched-chain amino acids - A highly effective substrate of parenteral nutrition for critically ill children with Reye's syndrome. *Clin. Nutr.*, 1987, 6/2 (101-104)

Ammonia detoxification by accelerated oxidation of branched chain amino acids in brains of acute hepatic failure rats. *Biochem. Med. Metab. Biol.*, 1986, 35/3 (367- 375)

Branched chain amino acids in the treatment of latent portosystemic encephalopathy. A double-blind placebo-controlled crossover study. *Gastroenterology,* 1985, 88/4 (887-895)

L-leucine prevent ammonia-induced changes in glutamate receptors in the brain and in visual evoked potentials in the rabbit. *J. Parenter. Enter. Nutr.*, 1984, 8/6 (700-704)

Effects of amino acid infusions on liver regeneration after partial hepatectomy in the rat. *J. Parenter. Enter. Nutr.*, 1986, 10/1 (17-20)

A comparison of the effects of intravenous infusion of individual branched-chain amino acids on blood amino acid levels in man. *Clin Sci* (England) Jan 1981, 60 (1) p95-100

The role of insulin and glucagon in the plasma aminoacid imbalance of chronic hepatic encephalopathy. *Z Gastroenterol* (Germany, West) Jul 1979, 17 (7) p469-76

Drug metabolism in cirrhosis. Selective changes in cytochrome P-450 isozymes in the choline-deficient rat model. *Biochem Pharmacol* (England) Jun 1 1986, 35 (11) p1817-24

Action of curcumin on the cytochrome P450-system catalyzing the activation of aflatoxin B1. *Chem Biol Interact* (Ireland) Mar 8 1996, 100 (1) p41-51

Inhibition of lipid peroxidation and cholesterol levels in mice by curcumin. *Indian J Physiol Pharmacol* (India) Oct 1992, 36 (4) p239-43

Induction of glutathione S-transferase activity by curcumin in mice. *Arzneimittelforschung* (Germany) Jul 1992, 42 (7) p962-4

Effect of polyene phosphatidylcholine (Essentiale forte, cps.) in the treatment of steatosis of the liver, focused on the ultrasonographic finding—Preliminary investigation. *Cas. Lek. Cesk.* (Czech Republic), 1994, 133/12 (366- 369)

Relationship between liver cirrhosis death rate and nutritional factors in 38 countries. *Int. J. Epidemiol.* (UK), 1988, 17/2 (414-418)

Vitamin B6 status in cirrhotic patients in relation to apoenzyme of serum alanine aminotransferase. *Clin. Biochem.* (Canada), 1988, 21/6 (367-370)

Vitamin B6 concentrations in patients with chronic liver disease and hepatocellular carcinoma. *Br. Med. J.* (UK), 1986, 293/6540 (175)

Choline and human nutrition. *Annu. Rev. Nutr.*, 1994, 14/- (269-296)

Prostaglandin E2 production by hepatic macrophages and peripheral monocytes in liver cirrhosis patients. *Life Sci.*, 1993, 53/4 (323-331)

Biochemistry of pharmacology of S-adenosyl-L-methionine and rationale for its use in liver disease. *Drugs* (New Zealand), 1990, 40/Suppl. 3 (98-110)

Choline may be an essential nutrient in malnourished patients with cirrhosis. *Gastroenterology,* 1989, 97/6 (1514-1520)

Use of polyunsaturated phosphatidyl choline in HBsAg negative chronic active hepatitis: Results of prospective double-blind controlled trial. *Liver* (Denmark), 1982, 2/2 (77-81)

Acetyl-L-carnitine increases cytochrome oxidase subunit I mRNA content in hypothyroid rat liver. *Febs Lett.* (Netherlands), 1990, 277/1-2 (191-193)

S-Adenosyl-L-methionine. A review of its pharmacological properties and therapeutic potential in liver dysfunction and affective disorders in relation to its physiological role in cell metabolism. *Drugs* (New Zealand), 1989, 38/3

Lupus

Refer to references under Autoimmune Diseases.

Macular Degeneration (Dry)

Age-related macular degeneration: a review of experimental treatments. *Surv Ophthalmol* (Netherlands) Sep-Oct 1998, 43 (2) p134-46

[Dynamics of accumulation and degradation of lipofuscin in retinal pigment epithelium in senile macular degeneration]. *Klin Monatsbl Augenheilkd* (Germany) Jul 1998, 213 (1) p32-7

[Autofluorescence characteristics of lipofuscin components in different forms of late senile macular degeneration]. *Klin Monatsbl Augenheilkd* (Germany) Jul 1998, 213 (1) p23-31

Cigarette smoking and age-related macular degeneration. *Optom Vis Sci* Jul 1998, 75 (7) p476-84

Genetic association of apolipoprotein E with age-related macular degeneration. *Am J Hum Genet* Jul 1998, 63 (1) p200-6

Age-related macular degeneration. Can we stem this worldwide public health crisis? *Postgrad Med* May 1998, 103 (5) p153-6, 161-4

Moderate wine consumption is associated with decreased odds of developing age-related macular degeneration in NHANES-1 [see comments]. *J Am Geriatr Soc* Jan 1998, 46 (1) p1-7

Treatment of macular degeneration, according to Bangerter. *Eur J Med Res* (Germany) Oct 30 1997, 2 (10) p445-54

[Radiotherapy and age-related macular degeneration: a review of the literature]. *Cancer Radiother* (France) 1997, 1 (3) p208-12

Sun exposure and age-related macular degeneration. An Australian case-control study. *Ophthalmology* May 1997, 104 (5) p770-6

[Antioxidants and angiogenetic factor associated with age-related macular degeneration (exudative type)]. *Nippon Ganka Gakkai Zasshi* (Japan) Mar 1997, 101 (3) p248-51

Oxidative protector enzymes in the macular retinal pigment epithelium of aging eyes and eyes with age-related macular degeneration. *Transactions of the American Ophthalmological Society* 1998, 96/- (635-689)

Alternative therapies in exudative age related macular degeneration. *British Journal of Ophthalmology* (UK) 1998, 82/12 (1441-1443)

Zinc as a treatment for age-related macular degeneration. *Journal of Trace Elements in Experimental Medicine* 1998, 11/2-3 (137-145).

Photodynamic therapy with verteporfin for choroidal neovascularization caused by age-related macular degeneration: Results of a single treatment in a phase 1 and 2 study. *Archives of Ophthalmology* 1999, 117/9 (1161-1173)

Treatment of senile macular degeneration with Ginkgo biloba extract. A preliminary double-blind, drug versus placebo study. *Presse Med.* (France), 1986, 15/31 (1556-1558)

Hydergine—a new promise in neuro-retinal disorders. *Afro-Asian J. Ophthalmol.* (India), 1989, 8/1

Inhibition of glutathione reductase by flavonoids. A structure-activity study. *Biochem. Pharmacol.* (UK), 1992, 44/8

Flavonoids, a class of natural products of high pharmacological potency. *Biochem. Pharmacol.* (England), 1983, 32/7

Results with anthocyanosides from Vaccinium myrtillus equivalent to 25% of anthocyanidines in the treatment of haemorrhagic diathesis due to defective primary haemostasis. *Gazz. Med. Ital.* (Italy), 1981, 140/10 (445-449)

Studies on vaccinium myrtillus anthocyanosides. I. Vasoprotective and antiinflammatory activity. *Arzneimittel-Forsch.* (Germany, West), 1976, 26/5

Atrophic macular degeneration. Rate of spread of geographic atrophy and visual loss. *Ophthalmology,* 1989, 96/10

Study of aging macular degeneration in China. *Jpn. J. Ophthalmol.* (Japan), 1987, 31/3

Subretinal neovascularization in senile macular degeneration. *Am. J. Ophthalmol.*, 1984, 97/2

Delayed macular choriocapillary circulation in age related macular. *International Ophthalmology* (Netherlands), 1995, 19/1

Cystoid macular degeneration in experimental branch retinal vein occlusion. *Ophthalmology,* 1988, 95/10

The clinical picture of retinal thrombosis. *Klin. Monatsbl. Augenheilkd.* (Germany, West), 1977, 170/2

Results of fluorescence angiography of the posterior pole of the eye. *Ber. Dtsch. Ophthal. Gesellsch.* (Germany, West), 1975, vol 73

The evoked cortical potential in macular degeneration. *J .Amer. Geriat. Soc.*, 1974, 22/12

The development of neovascularization of senile disciform macular degeneration. *Amer. J. Ophthal.*, 1973, 76/1

Macular Degeneration (Wet)

Age-related macular degeneration: a review of experimental treatments. *Surv Ophthalmol* (Netherlands) Sep-Oct 1998, 43 (2) p134-46

Dynamics of accumulation and degradation of lipofuscin in retinal pigment epithelium in senile macular degeneration]. *Klin Monatsbl Augenheilkd* (Germany) Jul 1998, 213 (1) p32-7

Autofluorescence characteristics of lipofuscin components in different forms of late senile macular degeneration]. *Klin Monatsbl Augenheilkd* (Germany) Jul 1998, 213 (1) p23-31

Cigarette smoking and age-related macular degeneration. *Optom Vis Sci* Jul 1998, 75 (7) p476-84

Genetic association of apolipoprotein E with age-related macular degeneration. *Am J Hum Genet* Jul 1998, 63 (1) p200-6

Age-related macular degeneration. Can we stem this worldwide public health crisis? *Postgrad Med* May 1998, 103 (5) p153-6, 161-4

Moderate wine consumption is associated with decreased odds of developing age-related macular degeneration in NHANES-1 [see comments]. *J Am Geriatr Soc* Jan 1998, 46 (1) p1-7

Treatment of macular degeneration, according to Bangerter. *Eur J Med Res* (Germany) Oct 30 1997, 2 (10) p445-54

[Radiotherapy and age-related macular degeneration: a review of the literature]. *Cancer Radiother* (France) 1997, 1 (3) p208-12

Sun exposure and age-related macular degeneration. An Australian case-control study. *Ophthalmology* May 1997, 104 (5) p770-6

[Antioxidants and angiogenetic factor associated with age-related macular degeneration (exudative type)]. *Nippon Ganka Gakkai Zasshi* (Japan) Mar 1997, 101 (3) p248-51

Oxidative protector' enzymes in the macular retinal pigment epithelium of aging eyes and eyes with age-related macular degeneration. *Transactions of the American Ophthalmological Society* 1998, 96/- (635-689)

Alternative therapies in exudative age related macular degeneration. *British Journal of Ophthalmology* (UK) 1998, 82/12 (1441-1443)

Zinc as a treatment for age-related macular degeneration. *Journal of Trace Elements in Experimental Medicine* 1998, 11/ 2-3 (137-145).

Photodynamic therapy with verteporfin for choroidal neovascularization caused by age-related macular degeneration: Results of a single treatment in a phase 1 and 2 study. *Archives of Ophthalmology* 1999, 117/9 (1161-1173)

Dietary carotenoids, vitamins A, C, and E, and advanced age-related macular degeneration. Eye Disease Case-Control Study Group. *JAMA* Nov 9 1994

Evidence by in vivo and in vitro studies that binding of pycnogenols to elastin affects its rate of degradation by elastases. *Biochem. Pharmacol.* (England), 1984

Studies on the mechanism of early onset macular degeneration in cynomolgus monkeys. II. Suppression of metallothionein synthesis in the retina in oxidative stress. *Experimental Eye Research* (UK), 1996, 62/4 (399-408)

Antioxidant enzymes of the human retina: Effect of age on enzyme activity of macula and periphery. *Current Eye Research* (UK), 1996, 15/3 (273-278)

Low glutathione reductase and peroxidase activity in age-related macular degeneration. *Br. J. Ophthalmol.* (UK), 1994, 78/10 (791-794)

Antioxidant enzymes in RBCs as a biological index of age related macular degeneration. *Acta Ophthalmol.* (Denmark), 1993, 71/2 (214-218)

Oxidative effects of laser photocoagulation. *Free Radic. Biol. Med.*, 1991, 11/3 (327-330)

Antioxidant status and neovascular age-related macular degeneration. *Arch. Ophthalmol.*, 1993, 111/1 (104-109)

Nutrition in the elderly. *Ann. Intern. Med.*, 1988, 109/11 (890-904)

Male Hormone Modulation Therapy

1. [Sexual hormones in ageing males]. *Aktuelle Gerontol* 1976 Feb;6(2):61-7
2. Hypophyseal-gonadal system during male aging. *Arch Gerontol Geriatr* 1985 Apr;4(1):13-9
3. Age variation of the 24-hour mean plasma concentrations of androgens, estrogens, and gonadotropins in normal adult men. *J Clin Endocrinol Metab* 1982 Mar;54(3):534-8
4. Age-related changes of plasma steroids in normal adult males. *J Steroid Biochem* 1982 Dec;17(6):683-7
5. Changes in the pituitary-testicular system with age. *Clin Endocrinol* (Oxf) 1976 Jul;5(4):349-72
6. Androgen and estrogen production in elderly men with gynecomastia and testicular atrophy after mumps orchitis. *J Clin Endocrinol Metab* 1980 Feb;50(2):380-6
7. Effects of testosterone supplementation in the aging male. *Journal of Clinical Endocrinology & Metabolism* 75 (4): p 1092-1098 1992
8. [Endocrine environment of benign prostatic hyperplasia—relationships of sex steroid hormone levels with age and the size of the prostate]. *Nippon Hinyokika Gakkai Zasshi* 1992 May;83(5):664-71
9. Therapeutic effects of an androgenic preparation on myocardial ischemia and cardiac function in 62 elderly male coronary heart disease patients. *Chin Med J* (Engl) 1993 Jun;106(6):415-8
10. The influence of aging on plasma sex hormones in men: the Telecom Study. *Am J Epidemiol* 1992 Apr 1;135(7):783-91
11. Serum 5alpha-dihydrotestosterone and testosterone changes with age in man. *Acta Endocrinol* (Copenh) 1976 Jun;82(2):444-8
12. Sex hormones and age: a cross-sectional study of testosterone and estradiol and their bioavailable fractions in community-dwelling men. *Am J Epidemiol* 1998 Apr 15;147(8):750-4
13. Steroid hormones, memory and mood in a healthy elderly population. *Psychoneuroendocrinology* 1998 Aug;23(6):583-603
14. Estrogen-androgen levels in aging men and women: therapeutic considerations. *J Am Geriatr Soc* 1976 Apr;24(4):173-8
15. The effect of testosterone aromatization on high-density lipoprotein cholesterol level and postheparin lipolytic activity. *Metabolism* 1993 Apr;42(4):446-50
16. Evidence that brain aromatization regulates LH secretion in the male dog. *Am J Physiol* 1981 Sep;241(3):E246-50
17. Origin of estrogen in normal men and in women with testicular feminization. *J Clin Endocrinol Metab* 1979 Dec;49(6):905-16
18. Familial gynecomastia with increased extraglandular aromatization of plasma carbon19-steroids. *J Clin Invest* 1985 Jun;75(6):1763-9
19. The pharmacokinetics of intravenous testosterone in elderly men with coronary artery disease. *J Clin Pharmacol* 1998 Sep;38(9):792-7
20. Testosterone pharmacokinetics after application of an investigational transdermal system in hypogonadal men. *J Clin Pharmacol* 1997 Dec;37(12):1139-45
21. The effect of supraphysiologic doses of testosterone on fasting total homocysteine levels in normal men. *Atherosclerosis* 1997 Apr;130(1-2):199-202
22. [Therapeutic efficacy of testolactone (aromatase inhibitor) to oligozoospermia with high estradiol/testosterone ratio]. *Nippon Hinyokika Gakkai Zasshi* 1991 Feb;82(2):204-9
23. Familial effects on plasma sex-steroid content in man: testosterone, estradiol and Sex-hormone-binding globulin. *Metabolism* 1982 Jan;31(1):6-9
24. Conversion of androgens to estrogens in cirrhosis of the liver. *J Clin Endocrinol Metab* 1975 Jun;40(6):1018-26

25. Alteration in the plasma testosterone: estradiol ratio: an alternative to the inhibin hypothesis. *Ann N Y Acad Sci* 1982;383:295-306

26. Which testosterone replacement therapy? *Clin Endocrinol (Oxf)* 1984 Aug;21(2):97-107

27. Conversion of androgens to estrogens in idiopathic hemochromatosis: comparison with alcoholic liver cirrhosis. *J Clin Endocrinol Metab* 1985 Jul;61(1):1-6

28. Sublingual administration of testosterone-hydroxypropyl-beta-cyclodextrin inclusion complex simulates episodic androgen release in hypogonadal men. *J Clin Endocrinol Metab* 1991 May;72(5):1054-9

29. The association of hyperestrogenemia with coronary thrombosis in men. *Arterioscler Thromb Vasc Biol* 1996 Nov;16(11):1383-7

30. Lower androgenicity is associated with higher plasma levels of prothrombotic factors irrespective of age, obesity, body fat distribution, and related metabolic parameters in men. *Metabolism* 1997 Nov;46(11):1287-93

31. Endogenous testosterone, fibrinolysis, and coronary heart disease risk in hyperlipidemic men. *J Lab Clin Med* 1993 Oct;122(4):412-20

32. Effects of androgens on haemostasis. *Maturitas* 1996 Jul;24(3):147-55

33. Plasminogen activator inhibitor in plasma is related to testosterone in men. *Metabolism* 1989 Oct;38(10):1010-5

34. Testosterone increases human platelet thromboxane A2 receptor density and aggregation responses [see comments] *Circulation* Jun 1 1995, 91 (11) p2742-7

35. Endocrine environment of benign prostatic hyperplasia: prostate size and volume are correlated with serum estrogen concentration. *Scand J Urol Nephrol* 1995 Mar;29(1):65-8

36. A prospective study of plasma hormone levels, nonhormonal factors, and development of benign prostatic hyperplasia. *Prostate* 1995 Jan;26(1):40-9

37. Estrogen formation in human prostatic tissue from patients with and without benign prostatic hyperplasia. *Prostate* 1986;9(4):311-8

38. Expression of estrogen receptor in diseased human prostate assessed by non-radioactive in situ hybridization and immunohistochemistry. *Prostate* 1995 Dec;27(6):304-13

39. Roles of estrogen and SHBG in prostate physiology. *Prostate* 1996 Jan;28(1):17-23

40. [The role of tissue steroids in benign hyperplasia and prostate cancer] *Urologe [A]* 1987 Nov;26(6):349-57

41. Estradiol causes the rapid accumulation of cAMP in human prostate. *Proc Natl Acad Sci U S A* 1994 Jun 7;91(12):5402-5

42. The effect of extracts of the roots of the stinging nettle (Urtica dioica) on the interaction of SHBG with its receptor on human prostatic membranes. *Planta Med* 1995 Feb;61(1):31-2

43. Effects of stinging nettle root extracts and their steroidal components on the Na+,K(+)-ATPase of the benign prostatic hyperplasia. *Planta Med* 1994 Feb;60(1):30-3

44. The inhibiting effects of Urtica dioica root extracts on experimentally induced prostatic hyperplasia in the mouse. *Planta Med* 1997 Aug;63(4):307-10

45. Severe sexual impairment produced by morbid obesity. Report of a case. *Int J Obes* (England) 1988, 12 (3) p185-9

46. Shippen and Fryer *The Testosterone Syndrome* New York, NY: M. Evans and Company 1998.

47. Endocrine aspects of ageing in the male. *Mol Cell Endocrinol* 1998 Oct 25;145(1-2):153-9

48. [Sexual hormones in ageing males (author's transl)] Kley HK; Nieschlag E; Wiegelmann W; Kruskemper HL *Aktuelle Gerontol* (Germany, West) Feb 1976, 6 (2) p61-7

49. Direct effects of estrogens on the endocrine function of the mammalian testis. *Can J Physiol Pharmacol* 1980 Sep;58(9):1011-22

50. Direct inhibitory effect of estrogen on the human testis in vitro. *Arch Androl* 1988;20(2):131-5

51. The acute effect of estrogens on testosterone production appears not to be mediated by testicular estrogen receptors. *Mol Cell Endocr* 31 (1). 1983. 105-116.

52. The effect of testosterone aromatization on high-density lipoprotein cholesterol level and postheparin lipolytic activity. *Metabolism* (United States) Apr 1993, 42 (4) p446-50,

53. Effects of estradiol administration in vivo on testosterone production in two populations of rat Leydig cells. *Biochemical and Biophysical Research Communications (Biochem. Biophys. Res. Commun.)* 1982, 107/4 (1340-1348)

54. Tetrahydroisoquinoline alkaloids mimic direct but not receptor-mediated inhibitory effects of estrogens and phytoestrogens on testicular endocrine function. Possible significance for Leydig cell insufficiency in alcohol addiction. *Life Sci* 1991;49(18):1319-29

55. Levels of sex hormone-binding globulin and corticosteroid-binding globulin mRNAs in corpus luteum of human subjects: correlation with serum steroid hormone levels. *Gynecol Endocrinol* 1999 Apr;13(2):82-8

56. Effects of ethinyloestradiol on plasma levels of pituitary gonadotrophins, testicular steroids and sex hormone binding globulin in normal men. *Clin Endocrinol (Oxf)* 1981 Mar;14(3):237-43

57. Changes in testosterone muscle receptors: effects of an androgen treatment on physically trained rats. *Cell Mol Biol* (Noisy-le-grand) 1994 May;40(3):291-4

58. Steroid hormones and neurotrophism: relationship to nerve injury. *Metab Brain Dis* Mar 1988, 3 (1) p1-18

59. Androgen deficiency and aging in men. *West J Med* 1993 Nov;159(5):579-85

60. Androgens and aging in men. *Exp Gerontol* 1993 Jul-Oct;28(4-5):435-46

61. Transdermal dihydrotestosterone treatment of 'andropause'. *Ann Med* 1993 Jun;25(3):235-41

62. Testosterone replacement therapy. *Arch Androl* 1998 Sep-Oct;41(2):79-90

63. Effect of androgens on the brain and other organs during development and aging. *Psychoneuroendocrinology* 1992 Aug;17(4):375-83

64. Endogenous sex steroids and bone mineral density in older women and men: the Rancho Bernardo Study. *J Bone Miner Res* 1997 Nov;12(11):1833-43

65. Endocrine aspects of ageing in the male. *Mol Cell Endocrinol* 1998 Oct 25;145(1-2):153-9

66. The effects of testosterone treatment on body composition and metabolism in middle-aged obese men. *Int J Obes Relat Metab Disord* 1992 Dec;16(12):991-7

67. Effects of testosterone supplementation in the aging male. *J Clin Endocrinol Metab* 1992 Oct;75(4):1092-8

68. Predictors of skeletal muscle mass in elderly men and women. *Mech Ageing Dev* 1999 Mar 1;107(2):123-36

69. Testosterone injection stimulates net protein synthesis but not tissue amino acid transport. *Am J Physiol* 1998 Nov;275(5 Pt 1):E864-71

70. Testosterone administration to elderly men increases skeletal muscle strength and protein synthesis. *Am J Physiol* 1995 Nov;269(5 Pt 1):E820-6

71. Testosterone deficiency in young men: marked alterations in whole body protein kinetics, strength, and adiposity. *J Clin Endocrinol Metab* 1998 Jun;83(6):1886-92

72. Androgen administration to aging men. *Endocrinol Metab Clin North Am* 1994 Dec;23(4):877-92

73. Endocrine aspects of ageing in the male. *Mol Cell Endocrinol* 1998 Oct 25;145(1-2):153-9

74. Therapeutic role of androgens in the treatment of osteoporosis in men. *Baillieres Clin Endocrinol Metab* 1998 Oct;12(3):453-70

75. Clinical experience using the Androderm testosterone transdermal system in hypogonadal adolescents and young men with beta-thalassemia major. J Pediatr Endocrinol Metab 1998;11 Suppl 3:891-900

76. Insulin resistance, body fat distribution, and sex hormones in men. *Diabetes* 1994 Feb;43(2):212-9

77. Decreased testosterone and dehydroepiandrosterone sulfate concentrations are associated with increased insulin and glucose concentrations in nondiabetic men. *Metabolism* 1994 May;43(5):599-603

78. Effects of acute hyperinsulinemia on testosterone serum concentrations in adult obese and normal-weight men. *Metabolism* 1997 May;46(5):526-9

79. Testosterone and regional fat distribution. *Obes Res* 1995 Nov;3 Suppl 4:609S-612S

80. Androgen treatment of middle-aged, obese men: effects on metabolism, muscle and adipose tissues. *Eur J Med* 1992 Oct;1(6):329-36

81. Androgen and estrogen-androgen hormone replacement therapy: a review of the safety literature, 1941 to 1996. *Clin Ther* 1997 May-Jun;19(3):383-404; discussion 367-8

82. Testosterone inhibits the immunostimulant effect of thymosin fraction 5 on secondary immune response in mice. *Int J Immunopharmacol* (England) Feb 1992, 14 (2) p263-8

83. Testosterone inhibits immunoglobulin production by human peripheral blood mononuclear cells. *Clin Exp Immunol* (England) Nov 1996, 106 (2) p410-5

84. Sex hormones and bone mineral density in elderly men. *Bone Miner* 1993 Feb;20(2):133-40

85. Does hypogonadism contribute to the occurrence of a minimal trauma hip fracture in elderly men? *J Am Geriatr Soc* 1991 Aug;39(8):766-71

86. Relations of endogenous anabolic hormones and physical activity to bone mineral density and lean body mass in elderly men. *Clin Endocrinol* (Oxf) 1994 May;40(5):653-61

87. Effect of castration on the morphology of the motor endplates of the rat levator ani muscle. *Eur J Cell Biol* 1982 Feb;26(2):284-8

88. Electrophysiological and contractile properties of the levator ani muscle after castration and testosterone administration. *Pflugers Arch* 1977 Mar 11;368(1-2):105-9

89. The influence of testosterone on neuromuscular transmission in hormone sensitive mammalian skeletal muscles. *Muscle Nerve* 1982 Mar;5(3):232-7

90. Role of striated penile muscles in penile reflexes, copulation, and induction of pregnancy in the rat. *J Reprod Fertil* 1982 Nov;66(2):433-43

91. Stephen B. Strum, *Anemia of Androgen Deprivation (AAD) in patients receiving combination hormonal blockade response to erythropoietin*. Culver City, & Whittier, California

92. Anaemia associated with androgen deprivation in patients with prostate cancer receiving combined hormone blockade. *Br J Urol* (England) Jun 1997, 79 (6) p933-41

93. [No title available]. *Pol Arch Med Wewn* 1998 Sep;100(3):212-21

94. Testosterone and depression in aging men. *Am J Geriatr Psychiatry* 1999 Winter;7(1):18-33

95. Bioavailable testosterone and depressed mood in older men: the Rancho Bernardo Study. *J Clin Endocrinol Metab* 1999 Feb;84(2):573-7

96. Testosterone, gonadotropin, and cortisol secretion in male patients with major depression. *Psychosom Med* 1999 May-Jun;61(3):292-6

97. Testosterone therapy for human immunodeficiency virus-positive men with and without hypogonadism. *J Clin Psychopharmacol* Feb 1999, 19 (1) p19-27

98. Biological actions of androgens. *Endocr Rev* 1987 Feb;8(1):1-28

99. The effects of exogenous testosterone on sexuality and mood of normal men. *J Clin Endocrinol Metab* 1992 Dec;75(6):1503-7

100. Hormonal replacement and sexuality in men. *Clin Endocrinol Metab* 1982 Nov;11(3):599-623

101. Male hormone replacement therapy including 'andropause'. *Endocrinology and Metabolism Clinics of North America (Endocrinol. Metab. Clin. North Am.)* 1998, 27/4 (969-987)

102. Transdermal testosterone therapy in the treatment of male hypogonadism. *J Clin Endocrinol Metab* 1988 Mar;66(3):546-51

103. Evidence for hyperestrogenemia as the link between diabetes mellitus and myocardial infarction. *Am J Med* 1984 Jun;76(6):1041-8

104. Abnormalities in sex hormones are a risk factor for premature manifestation of coronary artery disease in South African Indian men. *Atherosclerosis* 1990 Aug;83(2-3):111-7

105. Relationship between serum sex hormones and glucose, insulin and lipid abnormalities in men with myocardial infarction. *Proc Natl Acad Sci U S A* 1977 Apr;74(4):1729-33

106. Relationship between sex hormones, myocardial infarction, and occlusive coronary disease. *Arch Intern Med* 1982 Jan;142(1):42-4

107. Estradiol, testosterone, apolipoproteins, lipoprotein cholesterol, and lipolytic enzymes in men with premature myocardial infarction and angiographically assessed coronary occlusion. *Artery* 1983;12(1):1-23

108. The association of hypotestosteronemia with coronary artery disease in men. *Arterioscler Thromb* 1994 May;14(5):701-6

109. Testosterone induces dilation of canine coronary conductance and resistance arteries in vivo. *Circulation* 1996 Nov 15;94(10):2614-9

110. Testosterone causes direct relaxation of rat thoracic aorta. *J Pharmacol Exp Ther* 1996 Apr;277(1):34-9

111. Testosterone relaxes rabbit coronary arteries and aorta. *Circulation* 1995 Feb 15;91(4):1154-60

112. Effect of acute testosterone on myocardial ischemia in men with coronary artery disease. *Am J Cardiol* 1999 Feb 1;83(3):437-9, A9

113. Acute anti-ischemic effect of testosterone in men with coronary artery disease. *Circulation* 1999 Apr 6;99(13): 1666-70

114. Effect of testosterone replacement therapy on lipids and lipoproteins in hypogonadal and elderly men. *Atherosclerosis* 1996 Mar;121(1):35-43

115. Regulation of atrial natriuretic peptide, thromboxane and prostaglandin production by androgen in elderly men with coronary heart disease. *Chin Med Sci J* 1993 Dec;8(4): 207-9

116. [Antianginal and lipid lowering effects of oral androgenic preparation (Andriol) on elderly male patients with coronary heart disease]. *Chung Hua Nei Ko Tsa Chih* 1993 Mar;32(4):235-8

117. Aromatization of androstenedione to estrogen by benign prostatic hyperplasia, prostate cancer and expressed prostatic secretions. *Urol Res* 1987;15(3):165-7

118. Endocrine therapy for benign prostatic hyperplasia in the 90's. *J Urol* (Paris) 1995;101(1):22-5

119. [Physiopathological aspects of the treatment of benign prostatic hypertrophy. Role of prostatic stroma and estrogens]. *J Urol* (Paris) 1993;99(6):303-6

120. Estrogen receptor-beta: implications for the prostate gland. *Prostate* 1999 Jul 1;40(2):115-24

121. The monkey and human uridine diphosphate-glucuronosyltransferase UGT1A9, expressed in steroid target tissues, are estrogen-conjugating enzymes. *Endocrinology* 1999 Jul;140(7):3292-302

122. Imprinting by Neonatal Sex Steroids on the Structure and Function of the Mature Mouse Prostate. *Biol Reprod* 1999 Jul;61(1):200-208

123. Mitogen-activated protein kinase kinase kinase 1 activates androgen receptor-dependent transcription and apoptosis in prostate cancer. *Mol Cell Biol* 1999 Jul;19(7):5143-54

124. Neonatal estrogen exposure alters the transforming growth factor-beta signaling system in the developing rat prostate and blocks the transient p21(cip1/waf1) expression associated with epithelial differentiation. *Endocrinology* 1999 Jun;140(6):2801-13

125. Expression of pepsinogen II with androgen and estrogen receptors in human prostate carcinoma. *Pathol Int* 1999 Mar;49(3):203-7

126. Phosphorylation/dephosphorylation of androgen receptor as a determinant of androgen agonistic or antagonistic activity. Biochem Biophys Res Commun 1999 May 27;259(1):21-8

127. The estrogen receptor beta subtype: a novel mediator of estrogen action in neuroendocrine systems. *Front Neuroendocrinol* 1998 Oct;19(4):253-86

128. The novel estrogen receptor-beta subtype: potential role in the cell- and promoter-specific actions of estrogens and anti-estrogens. *FEBS Lett* 1997 Jun 23;410(1):87-90

129. Identification of a splice variant of the rat estrogen receptor beta gene. *Mol Cell Endocrinol* 1997 Sep 19;132(1-2):195-9

130. Therapeutic potential of selective estrogen receptor modulators. *Curr Opin Chem Biol* 1998 Aug;2(4):508-11

131. Estrogen receptor in human benign prostatic hyperplasia. *J Urol* 1983 Jul;130(1):183-7

132. Estrogen receptors in human prostate: evidence for multiple binding sites. J Clin Endocrinol Metab 1983 Jul;57(1):166-76

133. Steroid hormone receptors in prostatic hyperplasia and prostatic carcinoma. Med J Malaya 1990 Jun;45(2):148-53

134. Estrogen receptors and clinical correlations with human prostatic disease. Urology 1982 Apr;19(4):399-403

135. Inhibitory effect of selenomethionine on the growth of three selected human tumor cell lines. *Cancer Lett* 1998 Mar 13;125(1-2):103-10

136. Vitamins E plus C and interacting conutrients required for optimal health. A critical and constructive review of epidemiology and supplementation data regarding cardiovascular disease and cancer. *Biofactors* 1998;7(1-2):113-74

137. Serum and tissue lycopene and biomarkers of oxidation in prostate cancer patients: a case-control study. *Nutr Cancer* 1999;33(2):159-64

138. Chemoprevention for prostate cancer. *Cancer* (Philadelphia) 75 (7 Suppl.):p1783-1789 1995

139. Chemoprevention of prostate cancer: concepts and strategies. *Eur Urol* 1999;35(5-6):342-50

140. Diet, micronutrients, and the prostate gland. *Nutr Rev* 1999 Apr;57(4):95-103

141. Lower prostate cancer risk in men with elevated plasma lycopene levels: results of a prospective analysis. *Cancer Res* 1999 Mar 15;59(6):1225-30

142. Lycopene in association with alpha-tocopherol inhibits at physiological concentrations proliferation of prostate carcinoma cells. *Biochem Biophys Res Commun* 1998 Sep 29;250(3):582-5

143. Study of prediagnostic selenium level in toenails and the risk of advanced prostate cancer. *J Natl Cancer Inst* 1998 Aug 19;90(16):1219-24

144. Chemoprevention of prostate cancer: The prostate cancer prevention trial. *Prostate* 33 (3):p217-221 Nov. 1, 1997

145. Effect of the lipidosterolic extract of Serenoa repens (Permixon) and its major components on basic fibroblast growth factor-induced proliferation of cultures of human prostate biopsies. *Eur Urol* 1998;33(3):340-7

146. Efficacy and acceptability of tadenan (Pygeum africanum extract) in the treatment of benign prostatic hyperplasia (BPH): a multicentre trial in central Europe. *Curr Med Res Opin* (England) 1998, 14 (3) p127-39

147. Review of recent placebo-controlled trials utilizing phytotherapeutic agents for treatment of BPH. *Prostate (Prostate)* 1998, 37/3 (187-193)

148. Clinical relevance of growth factor antagonists in the treatment of benign prostatic hyperplasia. *European Urology (Eur. Urol.)* (Switzerland) 1997, 32/Suppl. 1 (28-31)

149. Cellular and molecular aspects of bladder hypertrophy. *European Urology (Eur. Urol.)* (Switzerland) 1997, 32/ Suppl. 1 (15-21)

150. Phytotherapy of benign prostatic hyperplasia (BPH) with Cucurbita, Hypoxis, Pygeum, Urtica and Sabal serrulata (Serenoa repens). *Phytotherapy Research (Phytother. Res.)* (UK) 1996, 10/Suppl. 1 (S141-S143)

151. Pygeum africanum extract for the treatment of patients with benign prostatic hyperplasia: A review of 25 years of published experience. *Current Therapeutic Research—Clinical and Experimental (Curr. Ther. Res. Clin. Exp.)* 1995, 56/8 (796-817)

152. Inhibition of bFGF and EGF-induced proliferation of 3T3 fibroblasts by extract of Pygeum africanum (Tadenan(R)). *Biomedicine and Pharmacotherapy (Biomed. Pharmacother.)* (France) 1994, 48/Suppl. 1 (43S-47S)

153. Quantitative-comparative histology of prostatic adenomas in medically and surgically treated patients. *International Urology and Nephrology (Int. Urol. Nephrol.)* (Hungary) 1994, 26/4 (455-460)

154. Effect of Pygeum africanum extract on A23187-stimulated production of lipoxygenase metabolites from human polymorphonuclear cells. *Journal of Lipid Mediators and Cell Signalling (J. Lipid Mediators Cell Signal.)* (Netherlands) 1994, 9/3 (285-290)

155. Combined extracts of Urtica dioica and Pygeum africanum in the treatment of benign prostatic hyperplasia: Double-blind comparison of two doses. *Clinical Therapeutics (Clin. Ther.)* 1993, 15/6 (1011-1020)

156. Efficacy of Pygeum africanum extract in the treatment of micturitional disorders due to benign prostatic hyperplasia. Evaluation of objective and subjective parametes. A multicentre, randomized, double-blind trial. *Wiener Klinische Wochenschrift (Wien. Klin. Wochenschr.)* (Austria) 1990, 102/22 (667-673)

157. Binding of permixon, a new treatment for prostatic benign hyperplasia, to the cytosolic androgen receptor in the rat prostate. *Journal of Steroid Biochemistry (J. Steroid Biochem.)* (UK) 1984, 20/1 (521-523)

158. An urodynamic study of patients with benign prostatic hypertrophy treated conservatively with phytotherapy or testosterone. *Wiener Klinische Wochenschrift (Wien. Klin. Wochenschr.)* (Austria) 1979, 91/18 (622-627)

159. Saw palmetto extracts potently and noncompetitively inhibit human alpha1-adrenoceptors in vitro. *Prostate* Feb 15 1999, 38 (3) p208-15

160. Urtica dioica L. *Fitoterapia (Fitoterapia)* (Italy) 1997, 68/5 (387-402)

161. Aromatase inhibitors from Urtica dioica roots. *Planta Medica (Planta Med.)* (Germany) 1995, 61/2 (138-140)

162. Effects of stinging nettle root extracts and their steroidal components on the Na^+, K^+-ATPase of the benign prostatic hyperplasia. *Planta Medica* (Germany) 1994, 60/1 (30-33)

163. Antiproliferative effect of Pygeum africanum extract on rat prostatic fibroblasts. *J Urol*; 157(6):2381-7 1997

164. Role of Mepartricin in the treatment of benign prostatic adenoma. *Arch Sci Med* (Torino); 135(1):95-98 1978

165. Influence of V-1326 extract of Pygeum-Africanum on pituitary gonadal adrenal axis of the rat. *Therapie* (Paris) 32 (1). 1977 99-110.

166. Soy, disease prevention, and prostate cancer. *Semin Urol Oncol* 1999 May;17(2):97-102

167. Does high soy milk intake reduce prostate cancer incidence? The Adventist Health Study. *Cancer Causes Control* 1998 Dec;9(6):553-7

168. Genistein, a component of soy, inhibits the expression of the EGF and ErbB2/Neu receptors in the rat dorsolateral prostate. *Prostate* 1998 Sep 15;37(1):36-43

169. Genistein inhibits the growth of human-patient BPH and prostate cancer in histoculture. *Prostate* 1998 Feb 1;34(2):75-9

170. Genistein-induced apoptosis of prostate cancer cells is preceded by a specific decrease in focal adhesion kinase activity. *Mol Pharmacol* 1997 Feb;51(2):193-200

171. Treatment with finasteride preserves usefulness of prostate-specific antigen in the detection of prostate cancer: results of a randomized, double-blind, placebo-controlled clinical trial. PLESS Study Group. Proscar Long-term Efficacy and Safety Study. *Urology* 1998 Aug;52(2):195-201; discussion 201-2

172. Differential effect of finasteride on the tissue androgen concentrations in benign prostatic hyperplasia. *Clin Endocrinol* (Oxf) 1997 Feb;46(2):137-44

173. [Effect of finasteride on the percentage of free PSA: implications in the early diagnosis of prostatic cancer] *Actas Urol Esp* 1998 Nov-Dec;22(10):835-9

174. Effect of finasteride and/or terazosin on serum PSA: results of VA Cooperative Study #359. *Prostate* 1999 Jun 1;39(4):234-9

175. Androgen metabolism in the prostate of the finasteride-treated, adult rat: a possible explanation for the differential action of testosterone and 5 alpha-dihydrotestosterone during development of the male urogenital tract. *Endocrinology* 1997 Mar;138(3):871-7

176. [Benign prostatic hyperplasia--the outcome of age-induced alteration of androgen-estrogen balance?] *Urologe A* 1997 Jan;36(1):3-9

177. Influence of finasteride on free and total serum prostate specific antigen levels in men with benign prostatic hyperplasia. *J Urol* 1998 Feb;159(2):449-53

178. The effect of finasteride on the prostate gland in men with elevated serum prostate-specific antigen levels. *Br J Cancer* 1998 Aug;78(3):413-8

179. Finasteride: A Clinical Review. *Biomedicine and Pharmacotherapy (Biomed. Pharmacother.)* (France) 1995, 49/7-8 (319-324)

180. Comparison of finasteride (Proscar(R)), a 5alpha reductase inhibitor, and various commercial plant extracts in in vitro and in vivo 5alpha reductase inhibition. *Prostate (Prostate)* 1993, 22/1 (43-51)

181. Evaluation of men on finasteride. *Semin Urol Oncol*; 14(3):139-44 1996

182. (A) The effect of finasteride in men with benign prostatic hyperplasia. The Finasteride Study Group . *N Engl J Med*; 327(17):1185-91 1992

182. (B) Estrogen suppression as a pharmacotherapeutic strategy in the medical treatment of benign prostatic hyperplasia: evidence for its efficacy from studies with mepartricin. *Wien Klin Wochenschr* 1998 Dec 11;110(23):817-23

183. Aromatase in hyperplasia and carcinoma of the human prostate. *Prostate* 1997 May 1;31(2):118-24

184. Aromatase mRNA levels in benign prostatic hyperplasia and prostate cancer. *Int J Urol* 1996 Jul;3(4):292-6

185. Effect of exogenous testosterone replacement on prostate-specific antigen and prostate-specific membrane antigen levels in hypogonadal men. *J Surg Oncol* 1995 Aug;59(4):246-50

186. Longitudinal evaluation of serum androgen levels in men with and without prostate cancer. *Prostate* 1995 Jul;27(1):25-31

187. The role of sex steroids in the pathogenesis and maintenance of benign prostatic hyperplasia. J Androl 1989 May-Jun;10(3):240-7

188. Endogenous sex hormones and prostate cancer: a quantitative review of prospective studies.*Br J Cancer* 1999 Jun;80(7):930-4

189. Relationships of serum androgens and estrogens to prostate cancer risk: results from a prospective study in Finland.*Cancer Epidemiol Biomarkers Prev* 1998 Dec;7(12):1069-74

190. 5 alpha-reductase activity and prostate cancer: a case-control study using stored sera. *Cancer Epidemiol Biomarkers Prev* 1997 Jan;6(1):21-4

191. Prediagnostic serum hormones and the risk of prostate cancer. Cancer Res 1988 Jun 15;48(12):3515-7

192. Physical characteristics and factors related to sexual development and behaviour and the risk for prostatic cancer. *Eur J Cancer Prev* 1992 Apr;1(3):239-45

193. Serum steroids in relation to prostate cancer risk in a case-control study (Greece). *Cancer Causes Control* 1997 Jul;8(4):632-6

194. Serological precursors of cancer: serum hormones and risk of subsequent prostate cancer. *Cancer Epidemiol Biomarkers Prev* 1993 Jan-Feb;2(1):27-32

195. Peripheral hormone levels in controls and patients with prostatic cancer or benign prostatic hyperplasia: results from the Dutch-Japanese case-control study. *Cancer Res* 1991 Jul 1;51(13):3445-50

196. Testicular and adrenocortical function in men with prostatic cancer and in healthy age-matched controls. *Br J Urol* 1997 Mar;79(3):427-31

197. Dihydrotestosterone and testosterone levels in men screened for prostate cancer: a study of a randomized population. *Br J Urol* 1996 Mar;77(3):433-40

198. Familial factors affecting prostatic cancer risk and plasma sex-steroid levels. *Prostate* 1985;6(2):121-8

199. A prospective, population-based study of androstenedione, estrogens, and prostatic cancer. *Cancer Res* 1990 Jan 1;50(1):169-73

200. Serum pituitary and sex steroid hormone levels in the etiology of prostatic cancer--a population-based case-control study. *Br J Cancer* 1993 Jul;68(1):97-102

201. Pretreatment plasma levels of testosterone and sex hormone binding globulin binding capacity in relation to clinical staging and survival in prostatic cancer patients. *Prostate* 1988;12(4):325-32

202. Serum hormone levels among patients with prostatic carcinoma or benign prostatic hyperplasia and clinic controls. *Prostate* 1987;11(2):171-82

203. Plasma estradiol, free testosterone, sex hormone binding globulin binding capacity, and prolactin in benign prostatic hyperplasia and prostatic cancer. *Prostate* 1983;4(3):223-9

204. Familial prostatic cancer risk and low testosterone. *J Clin Endocrinol* Metab 1982 Jun;54(6):1104-8

205. Carcinoma of the prostate: relationship of pretreatment hormone levels to survival. *Eur J Cancer Clin Oncol* 1984 Apr;20(4):477-82

206. Occult prostate cancer in men with low serum testosterone levels. *JAMA* 1996 Dec 18;276(23):1904-6

207. Pretreatment hormone levels in prostatic cancer. *Scand J Urol Nephrol Suppl* 1988;110:137-43

208. Results of a study to correlate serum prostate specific antigen and reproductive hormone levels in patients with localized prostate cancer. *J Natl Med Assoc* 1995 Nov;87(11):813-9

209. Production, clearance, and metabolism of testosterone in men with prostatic cancer. *Prostate* 1987;10(1):25-31

210. Endocrine profiles during administration of the new non-steroidal anti-androgen Casodex in prostate cancer. *Clin Endocrinol* (Oxf) 1994 Oct;41(4):525-30

211. Responses of serum levels of testicular steroid hormones to hCG stimulation in patients with prostatic cancer and benign prostatic hypertrophy. *Prostate Suppl* 1981;1:19-26

212. Androgens in serum and the risk of prostate cancer: a nested case-control study from the Janus serum bank in Norway. *Cancer Epidemiol Biomarkers Prev* 1997 Nov;6(11):967-9

213. Serum androgens and prostate cancer. *Cancer Epidemiol Biomarkers Prev* 1996 Aug;5(8):621-5

214. Prospective study of sex hormone levels and risk of prostate cancer. *J Natl Cancer Inst* 1996 Aug 21;88(16):1118-26

215. Estradiol and testosterone metabolism and production in men with prostatic cancer. *J Steroid Biochem* 1989 Jul;33(1):19-24

216. Serum androgens: associations with prostate cancer risk and hair patterning. *J Androl* 1997 Sep-Oct;18(5):495-500

217. Dramatic rise in prostate-specific antigen after androgen replacement in a hypogonadal man with occult adenocarcinoma of the prostate. *Urology* 1999 Feb;53(2):423-4

218. Smith Kline Beecham, *Androderm Testosterone Transdermal System*. U.S. Prescribing Information 1997

219. Androgen-behavior correlations in hypogonadal men and eugonadal men. II. Cognitive abilities. *Horm Behav* 1998 Apr;33(2):85-94

220. Decreased serum testosterone in men with acute ischemic stroke. *Arterioscler Thromb Vasc Biol* Jun 1996, 16 (6) p749-54

221. Hyposomatomedinemia and hypogonadism in hemiplegic men who live in nursing homes. *Arch Phys Med Rehabil* May 1994, 75 (5) p594-9

222. Hormonal changes in cerebral infarction in the young and elderly. *J Neurol Sci* (Netherlands) Sep 1990, 98 (2-3) p235-43

223. Circulating testosterone in pure motor stroke. *Funct Neurol* (Italy) Jan-Mar 1991, 6 (1) p29-34

224. Prognostic factors in survival free of progression after androgen deprivation therapy for treatment of prostate cancer. *J Urol* 1989 May;141(5):1139-42

225. Low serum testosterone and a younger age predict for a poor outcome in metastatic prostate cancer. *Am J Clin Oncol* 1997 Dec;20(6):605-8

226. Prognostic factors in patients with advanced prostate cancer. *Urology* 1989 May;33(5 Suppl):53-6

227. Serum testosterone as a prognostic factor in patients with advanced prostatic carcinoma. *Scand J Urol Nephrol Suppl* 1994;157:41-7

228. A prognostic index for the clinical management of patients with advanced prostatic cancer: a British Prostate Study Group investigation. *Prostate 1985;7(2):131-41*

229. The importance of prognostic factors in advanced prostate cancer. *Cancer* 1990 Sep 1;66(5 Suppl):1017-21

230. Sex hormone-binding protein, hyperinsulinemia, insulin resistance and noninsulin-dependent diabetes. *Horm Res* 1996;45(3-5):233-7

231. Sex hormone levels in young Indian patients with myocardial infarction. *Arteriosclerosis* 1986 Jul-Aug;6(4):418-21

232. Androgen receptors mediate hypertrophy in cardiac myocytes. *Circulation* 1998 Jul 21;98(3):256-61

233. The relationship of natural androgens to coronary heart disease in males: a review. *Atherosclerosis* (Ireland) Aug 23 1996, 125 (1) p1-13

234. Induction of circadian rhythm of feeding activity by testosterone implantations in arrhythmic Japanese quail males. *J Biol Rhythms* Aug 1998, 13 (4) p278-87

235. Androgen receptors in experimentally induced colon carcinogenesis. *Journal of Cancer Research and Clinical Oncology (J. Cancer Res. Clin. Oncol.)* (Germany) 1986, 112/1 (39-46)

236. Effects of androgen manipulations on chemically induced colonic tumours and on macroscopically normal colonic mucosa in male Sprague-Dawley rats. *Circulation* 1998 Jul 21;98(3):256-61

237. Androgens and abdominal obesity. *Baillieres Clin Endocrinol Metab* 1998 Oct;12(3):441-51

238. Increased estrogen production in obese men. *J Clin Endocrinol Metab* 48 (4). 1979. 633-638.

239. Lower endogenous androgens predict central adiposity in men. *Ann Epidemiol* Sep 1992, 2 (5) p675-82

240. Enhanced conversion of androstenedione to estrogens in obese males. *J Clin Endocrinol Metab* 1980 Nov;51(5): 1128-32

241. Relationship of plasma sex hormones to different parameters of obesity in male subjects. *Metabolism* 1980 Oct;29(11):1041-5

242. The relationship between aromatase activity and body fat distribution. *Steroids* Jul-Sep 1987, 50 (1-3) p61-72

243. Effects of a fat-containing meal on sex hormones in men. *Metabolism* 1990 Sep;39(9):943-6

244. Phytosterol feeding induces alteration in testosterone metabolism in rat tissues. *Journal of Nutritional Biochemistry* 9 (12): p 712-717 Dec., 1998

245. 24 Hour profiles of circulating androgens and estrogens in male puberty with and without gynecomastia. *Clin Endocrinology* 11 (5). 1979. 505-522.

246. The association between moderate alcoholic beverage consumption and serum estradiol and testosterone levels in normal postmenopausal women: relationship to the literature. *Alcohol Clin Exp Res* Feb 1992, 16 (1) p87-92

247. Dietary zinc deficiency alters 5-alpha-reduction and aromatization of testosterone and androgen and estrogen receptors in rat liver. *Journal of Nutrition* 126 (4): p 842-848 1996

248. Classification of obese patients and complications related to the distribution of surplus fat. *Bjorntorp P, Nutrition* Mar-Apr 1990, 6 (2) p131-7

249. Sex steroids and bone mass in older men. Positive associations with serum estrogens and negative associations with androgens. *J Clin Invest* 1997 Oct 1;100(7):1755-9

250. Biotransformation of oral dehydroepiandrosterone in elderly men: significant increase in circulating estrogens. *J Clin Endocrinol Metab* 1999 Jun;84(6):2170-6

251. Lignans from the roots of Urtica dioica and their metabolites bind to human sex hormone binding globulin (SHBG). *Planta Med* 1997 Dec;63(6):529-32

252. Plant constituents interfering with human sex hormone-binding globulin. Evaluation of a test method and its application to Urtica dioica root extracts. *Z Naturforsch [C]* 1995 Jan-Feb;50(1-2):98-104

253. Testosterone metabolism in primary cultures of human prostate epithelial cells and fibroblasts. *J Steroid Biochem Mol Biol* (England) Dec 1995, 55 (3-4) p375-83

254. Effect of exogenous testosterone on prostate volume, serum and semen prostate specific antigen levels in healthy young men. *J Urol* 1998 Feb;159(2):441-3

255. The effect of exogenous testosterone on total and free prostate specific antigen levels in healthy young men. *J Urol* 1996 Aug;156(2 Pt 1):438-41; discussion 441-2

256. Prostate-specific antigen and prostate gland size in men receiving exogenous testosterone for male contraception. *Int J Androl* 1993 Feb;16(1):35-40

257. Prostate size in hypogonadal men treated with a nonscrotal permeation-enhanced testosterone transdermal system. *Urology* 1997 Feb;49(2):191-6

258. Effect of oral androstenedione on serum testosterone and adaptations to, resistance training in young men: a randomized controlled trial. *JAMA* 1999 Jun 2;281(21):2020-8

259. Severe sexual impairment produced by morbid obesity. Report of a case. *Int J Obes* (England) 1988, 12 (3) p185-9

260. Shippen and Fryer *The Testosterone Syndrome*. 1998 M. Evans and Company New York, NY

261. Sex hormones and coronary artery disease. *Am J Med* 1987 Nov;83(5):853-9

262. Serum estrogen levels in men with acute myocardial infarction. *Am J Med* 1982 Dec;73(6):872-81

263. Variability in plasma oestrogen concentrations in men with a myocardial Infarction. *Dan Med Bull* 1990 Dec;37(6):552-6

264. Relationships of plasminogen activator inhibitor activity and lipoprotein(a) with insulin, testosterone, 17 beta-estradiol, and testosterone binding globulin in myocardial infarction patients and healthy controls. *J Clin Endocrinol Metab* 1995 Jun;80(6):1794-8

265. Sex hormones, insulin, lipids, and prevalent ischemic heart disease. *Am J Epidemiol* 1987 Oct;126(4):647-57

266. The determination of serum estradiol, testosterone and progesterone in acute myocardial infarction. *Jpn Heart J* 1986 Nov;27(6):825-37

267. Serum estradiol and testosterone levels following acute myocardial infarction in men. *Indian J Physiol Pharmacol* 1998 Apr;42(2):291-4

268. Oestradiol levels in diabetic men with and without a previous myocardial infarction. *Q J Med* 1987 Jul;64(243):617-23

269. Sex hormones and hemostatic risk factors for coronary heart disease in men with hypertension. *J Hypertens* 1993 Jul;11(7):699-702

270. [Plasma testosterone, free testosterone fraction LH and FSH in males during the early stage of acute myocardial infarction]. *Z Kardiol* 1979 Nov;68(11):776-83

271. Current status of testosterone replacement therapy in men. *Arch Fam Med* 1999 May-Jun;8(3):257-63

272. Direct effects of estrogens on the endocrine function of the mammalian testis. *Can J Physiol Pharmacol* 1980 Sep;58(9):1011-22

273. Direct inhibitory effect of estrogen on the human testis in vitro. *Arch Androl* 1988;20(2):131-5

274. The acute effect of estrogens on testosterone production appears not to be mediated by testicular estrogen receptors. *Mol Cell Endocr* 31 (1). 1983. 105-116.

275. The effect of testosterone aromatization on high-density lipoprotein cholesterol level and postheparin lipolytic activity. *Metabolism* (United States) Apr 1993, 42 (4) p446-50

276. Effects of estradiol administration in vivo on testosterone production in two populations of rat Leydig cells. *Res. Commun.* (United States) 1982, 107/4 (1340-1348)

277. Tetrahydroisoquinoline alkaloids mimic direct but not receptor-mediated inhibitory effects of estrogens and phytoestrogens on testicular endocrine function. Possible significance for Leydig cell insufficiency in alcohol addiction. *Life Sci* 1991;49(18):1319-29

278. Fat tissue a steroid reservoir and site of steroid metabolism. *J Clin Endocrinol Metab* 61 (3). 1985. 564-570.

279. Treatment of men with idiopathic oligozoospermic infertility using the aromatase inhibitor, testolactone. Results of a double-blinded, randomized, placebo-controlled trial with crossover. *Mt Sinai J Med* 1997 Jan;64(1):20-5

280. Clinical utility of sex hormone-binding globulin measurement. *Horm Res* 1996;45(3-5):148-55

281. Sex hormone binding globulin: origin, function and clinical significance. *Ann Clin Biochem* 1990 Nov;27 (Pt 6):532-41

282. Androgens, estrogens, and sex hormone-binding globulin in middle-aged men. *J Clin Endocrinol Metab* 1990 Dec;71(6):1442-6

283. Sex hormone changes in male epileptics. *Clin Endocrinol (Oxf)* 1980 Apr;12(4):391-5

284. Age, disease, and changing sex hormone levels in middle-aged men: results of the Massachusetts Male Aging Study. *J Clin Endocrinol Metab* 1991 Nov;73(5):1016-25

285. The influence of age, alcohol consumption, and body build on gonadal function in men. *J Clin Endocrinol Metab* 1980 Sep;51(3):508-12

286. Serum testosterone and sex hormone-binding globulin concentrations and the risk of prostate carcinoma: a longitudinal study. *Cancer* 1999 Jul 15;86(2):312-5

287. Effect of testosterone treatment on body composition and muscle strength in men over 65 years of age. *J Clin Endocrinol Metab* 1999 Aug;84(8):2647-53

288. Approaches to prostatic cancer chemotherapy using the Dunning R3327H prostatic adenocarcinoma. *Prostate* 1985;6(2):129-43

289. [No Title] *Endocrine News*;1996, Vol 21, No. 3, p-2

Meningitis

Refer to references under Viral Meningitis.

Menopause

Refer to references under Female Hormone Modulation Therapy.

Menstrual Disorders (Premenstrual Syndrome)

Refer to references under Female Hormone Modulation Therapy.

Migraine

High-dose riboflavin as a prophylactic treatment of migraine: Results of an open pilot study. *Cephalalgia* (Norway), 1994, 14/5 (328-329)

Herbal medicinals: selected clinical considerations focusing on known or potential drug-herb interactions. *Arch Intern Med* Nov 9 1998, 158 (20) p2200-11

Herbal 'health' products: what family physicians need to know [see comments]. *Am Fam Physician* Oct 1 1998, 58 (5) p1133-40

Herbal products begin to attract the attention of brand-name drug companies [see comments]. *CMAJ* (Canada) Jul 15 1996, 155 (2) p216-9 Comment in *Can Med Assoc J* 1996 Nov 1;155(9):1236

Feverfew and vascular smooth muscle: extracts from fresh and dried plants show opposing pharmacological profiles, dependent upon sesquiterpene lactone content. *Planta Med* (Germany) Feb 1993, 59 (1) p20-5

Inhibition of 5-lipoxygenase and cyclo-oxygenase in leukocytes by feverfew. Involvement of sesquiterpene lactones and other components. *Biochem Pharmacol* (England) Jun 9 1992, 43 (11) p2313-20

A comparison of the effects of an extract of feverfew and parthenolide, a component of feverfew, on human platelet activity in-vitro. *J Pharm Pharmacol* (England) Aug 1990, 42 (8) p553-7

Compounds extracted from feverfew that have anti-secretory activity contain an alpha-methylene butyrolactone unit. *J Pharm Pharmacol* (England) Sep 1986, 38 (9) p709-12

Chromosomal aberrations and sister chromatid exchanges in lymphocytes and urine mutagenicity of migraine patients: a comparison of chronic feverfew users and matched non-users. *Hum Toxicol* (England) Mar 1988, 7 (2) p145-52

Randomised double-blind placebo-controlled trial of feverfew in migraine prevention. *Lancet* (England) Jul 23 1988, 2 (8604) p189-92

Efficacy of feverfew as prophylactic treatment of migraine. *Br Med J* (Clin Res Ed) (England) Aug 31 1985, 291 (6495) p569-73

Feverfew (Tanacetum parthenium) as a prophylactic treatment for migraine: A double-blind placebo-controlled study. *Phytotherapy Research* (UK) 1997, 11/7 (508-511)

The essential oil of Tanacetum parthenium (L.) Schultz-Bip. *Flavour and Fragrance Journal* (UK) 1996, 11/6 (367-371)

Herbal therapy for migraine: An unconventional approach. *Postgraduate Medicine* 1987, 82/1 (197-198)

Pathogenesis of migraine. *Semin Neurol* 1997, 17 (4) p335-41

Platelet ionized magnesium, cyclic AMP, and cyclic GMP levels in migraine and tension-type headache. *Headache* Oct 1997, 37 (9) p561-4

Visual evoked potentials and serum magnesium levels in juvenile migraine patients. *Headache* Jun 1997, 37 (6) p383-5

Omega- 3: Essential for good health. *American Druggist* 1997, 214/7 (52-53)

Pathophysiology of the migraine aura. *Bollettino - Lega Italiana contro l'Epilessia* (Italy) 1997, -/99 (359-362)

Food and headache. *Headache Quarterly* 1997, 8/4 (319-329)

Migraine treatment. *Seminars in Neurology* 1997, 17/4 (325-333)

Trigeminal afferents to cerebral arteries and forehead are not divergent axon collaterals in cat. *Neurosci Lett* (Netherlands) Sep 16 1985, 60 (1) p63-8

Perivascular meningeal projections from cat trigeminal ganglia: possible pathway for vascular headaches in man. *Science* Jul 10 1981, 213 (4504) p228-30

In search of the ideal treatment for migraine headache. *Med Hypotheses* (England) Jan 1998, 50 (1) p1-7

Diet and migraine. *Rev Neurol* (Spain) May 1996, 24 (129) p534-8

Multiple sclerosis and possible relationship to cocoa: a hypothesis. *Ann Allergy* Jul 1987, 59 (1) p76-9

Dietary factors in migraine precipitation: The physicians' view. *Headache* 1985, 25/4 (184-187)

Migraine. A homoeopathic aproach. *British Homeopathic Journal* (UK) 1984, 73/1 (1-10)

Role of magnesium in the pathogenesis and treatment of migraines. *Clin Neurosci* 1998;5(1):24-7

Feverfew—an antithrombotic drug?. *Folia Haematol Int Mag Klin Morphol Blutforsch* 1988;115(1-2):181-4.

In vivo administration of propranolol decreases exaggerated amounts of serum TNF-alpha in patients with migraine without aura. Possible mechanism of action. *Acta Neurol* (Napoli); 14(4-6):313-9 1992

Concurrent use of antidepressants and propranolol: case report and theoretical considerations. *Biol Psychiatry*; 18(2):237-41 1983

Nocturnal melatonin excretion is decreased in patients with migraine without aura attacks associated with menses. *Cephalalgia* (Norway), 1995, 15/2 (136-139)

Urinary melatonin excretion throughout the ovarian cycle in menstrually related migraine. *Cephalalgia* (Norway), 1994

Nocturnal plasma melatonin levels in migraine: A preliminary report. *Headache* Apr 1989, 29 (4) p242-5

Octopamine and some related noncatecholic amines in invertebrate nervous systems. *Int.Rev.Neurobiol.*, 1976, Vol.19 (173-224)

Nocturnal melatonin excretion is decreased in patients with migraine without aura attacks associated with menses. *Cephalalgia* (Norway) Apr 1995, 15 (2) p136-9; discussion 79

The co-occurrence of multiple sclerosis and migraine headache: the serotoninergic link. *Int J Neurosci* (England) Jun 1994, 76 (3-4) p249-57

Urinary melatonin excretion throughout the ovarian cycle in menstrually related migraine [see comments]. *Cephalalgia* (Norway) Jun 1994, 14 (3) p205-9

The influence of the pineal gland on migraine and cluster headaches and effects of treatment with picoTesla magnetic fields. *Int J Neurosci* (England) Nov-Dec 1992, 67 (1-4) p145-71

Nocturnal plasma melatonin levels in migraine: a preliminary report. *Headache* Apr 1989, 29 (4) p242-5

Is migraine due to a deficiency of pineal melatonin? *Ital J Neurol Sci* (Italy) Jun 1986, 7 (3) p319-23

Melatonin in humans physiological and clinical studies. *J Neural Transm Suppl* (Austria) 1978, (13) p289-310

Multiple Sclerosis (MS)

NMSS B the National Multiple Sclerosis Society, 733 Third Avenue, New York, NY 10017

The Mayo Clinic, Rochester, MN

Swank M.S. Clinic, 13655 SW Jekins Rd, Beaverton, Oregon 97005

[The use of alternative medicine by multiple sclerosis patients—patient characteristics and patterns of use]. *Fortschr Neurol Psychiatr* (Germany) Dec 1997, 65 (12) p555-61

Multiple sclerosis: The lipid relationship. *American Journal of Clinical Nutrition* 1988, 48/6 (1387-1393)

Exogenous lipids in myelination and myelination. *Kao Hsiung I Hsueh Ko Hsueh Tsa Chih* (Taiwan) Jan 1997, 13 (1) p19-29

Nutritional factors in the aetiology of multiple sclerosis: A case-control study in Montreal, Canada. *International Journal of Epidemiology (Int. J. Epidemiol.)* (UnitedKingdom) 1998, 27/5 (845-852)

Vitamin D and multiple sclerosis. *Proc Soc Exp Biol Med* Oct 1997, 216 (1) p21-7

Trace metals in multiple sclerosis. *Neurology Psychiatry and Brain Research* (Germany) 1995, 3/3 (149-154)

Vitamin B12 metabolism and massive-dose methyl vitamin B12 therapy in Japanese patients with multiple sclerosis. *Intern Med* (Japan) Feb 1994, 33 (2) p82-6

Vitamin B12 and its relationship to age of onset of multiple sclerosis. *Int J Neurosci* (England) Jul-Aug 1993, 71 (1-4) p93-9

Homocysteine and vitamin B12 in multiple sclerosis. *Biogenic Amines* (Netherlands) 1995, 11/6 (479-485)

Measurement of low-molecular-weight antioxidants, uric acid, tyrosine and tryptophan in plaques and white matter from patients with multiple sclerosis. *Eur Neurol* (Switzerland) 1992, 32 (5) p248-52

Dietary polyunsaturated fatty acids and depression: When cholesterol does not satisfy. *American Journal of Clinical Nutrition*, 1995, 62/1 (1-9)

Health implications of fatty acids. *Arzneim.-Forsch. Drug Res.* (Germany), 1994, 44/8 (976-981)

Lipids and neurological diseases. *Med. Hypotheses* (UK), 1991, 34/3 (272-274)

Plasma lipids and their fatty acid composition in multiple sclerosis. *Acta Neurol. Scand.* (Denmark), 1988, 78/2 (152-157)

Relevance of essential fatty acids in medicine and nutrition. *Aktuel. Endokrinol. Stoffwechsel* (Germany, West), 1986, 7/1 (18-27)

Essential fatty acids in perspective. *Hum. Nutr. Clin. Nutr.* (England), 1984, 38/4 (245-260)

Essential fatty acids in the serum and cerebrospinal fluid of multiple sclerosis patients. *Acta Neurol. Scand.* (Denmark), 1983, 67/3 (151-163)

Polyunsaturated (essential) fatty acids and their importance in pathogenesis, diagnosis and therapy of multiple sclerosis. *Forstschr. Neurol. Psychiatr.* (Germany, West), 1982, 50/6 (173-189)

Clinical trials of unsaturated fatty acids in multiple sclerosis. *Ircs Med. Sci.* (England), 1981, 9/12 (1081)

Essential fatty acids in serum and cerebrospinal fluid of patients during multiple sclerosis. *Nervenarzt* (Germany, West), 1981, 52/2 (100-107)

Abnormality of fatty acid composition of plasma lipid in multiple sclerosis. *Brain Nerve* (Tokyo) (Japan), 1979, 31/8 (797-801)

The pineal and regulation of fibrosis: pinealectomy as a model of primary biliary cirrhosis: Roles of melatonin and prostaglandins in fibrosis and regulation of T lymphocytes. *Med. Hypotheses* (England), 1979, 5/4 (403-414)

Multiple sclerosis: The rational basis for treatment with colchicine and evening primrose oil. *Med. Hypotheses* (England), 1979, 5/3 (365-378)

Fat deficiency in rats during development of the central nervous system and susceptibility to experimental allergic encephalomyelitis. *J. Nutr.*, 1975, 105/3 (288-300)

Dietary intake of linoleic acid in multiple sclerosis and other diseases. *J. Neurol. Neurosurg. Psychiat.* (England), 1973, 36/4 (668-673)

Fatty acid patterns of serum lipids in multiple sclerosis and other diseases. *Biochem. Soc. Trans.* (England), 1973, 1/1 (141-143)

Magnesium concentration in brains from multiple sclerosis patients. *Acta Neurol. Scand.* (Denmark), 1990, 81/3 (197-200)

Zinc, copper and magnesium concentration in serum and CSF of patients with neurological disorders. *Acta Neurol. Scand.* (Denmark), 1989, 79/5 (373-378)

The susceptibility of the centrocecal scotoma to electrolytes, especially in multiple sclerosis. *Ideggyog. Szle* (Hungary), 1973, 26/7 (307-312)

Evaluation of a nutrition education programme for people with multiple sclerosis. J. *Hum. Nutr. Diet.* (UK), 1993, 6/2 (131-147)

Multiple sclerosis: A diathesis? *Gazz. Sanit.* (Milano) (Italy), 1973, 22/1 (37-39)

Arachidonic and docosahexanoic acid content of bovine brain myelin: Implications for the pathogenesis of multiple sclerosis. *Neurochem. Res.*, 1990, 15/1 (7-11)

On the causes of multiple sclerosis. *Med. Hypotheses* (UK), 1993, 41/2 (93-96)

Multiple sclerosis: vitamin D and calcium as environmental determinants of prevalence (a viewpoint). I.: Sunlight, dietary factors and epidemiology. *Int. J. Environ. Stud.* (England), 1974, 6/1 (19-27)

Biological effects of fish oils in relation to chronic diseases. *Lipids* Dec 1986, 21 (12) p731-2

Supplementation of polyunsaturated fatty acids in multiple sclerosis. *Ital J Neurol Sci* (Italy) Jun 1992, 13 (5) p401-7

Essential fatty acid and lipid profiles in plasma and erythrocytes in patients with multiple sclerosis. *Am J Clin Nutr* Oct 1989, 50 (4) p801-6

Reduction by linoleic acid of the severity of experimental allergic encephalomyelitis in the guinea pig. *J Neurol Sci* (Netherlands) Feb 1978, 35 (2-3) p291-308

Red blood cell and adipose tissue fatty acids in mild inactive multiple sclerosis. *Acta Neurol Scand* (Denmark) Jul 1990, 82 (1) p43-50

Multiple sclerosis: effect of gamma linolenate administration upon membranes and the need for extended clinical trials of unsaturated fatty acids. *Eur Neurol* (Switzerland) 1983, 22 (1) p78-83

The nutritional regulation of T lymphocyte function. *Med Hypotheses* (England) Sep 1979, 5 (9) p969-85

Polyunsaturated fatty acids in treatment of acute remitting multiple sclerosis. *Br Med J* (England) Nov 18 1978, 2 (6149) p1390-1

Effect of prolonged ingestion of gamma-linolenate by MS patients. *Eur Neurol* (Switzerland) 1978, 17 (2) p67-76

Experimental and clinical studies on dysregulation of magnesium metabolism and the aetiopathogenesis of multiple sclerosis. *Magnes Res* (England) Dec 1992, 5 (4) p295-302

Measurement of low-molecular-weight antioxidants, uric acid, tyrosine and tryptophan in plaques and white matter from patients with multiple sclerosis. *Eur Neurol* (Switzerland) 1992, 32 (5) p248-52

Clinical trials of unsaturated fatty acids in multiple sclerosis. *Ircs Med. Sci.* (England), 1981, 9/12 (1081)

Dietary polyunsaturated fatty acids and depression: When cholesterol does not satisfy. *American Journal of Clinical Nutrition*, 1995, 62/1 (1-9)

Expression and regulation of brain metallothionein. *Neurochem Int* (England) Jul 1995, 27 (1) p1-22

Indirect evidence for nitric oxide involvement in multiple sclerosis by characterization of circulating antibodies directed against conjugated S-nitrosocysteine. *J Neuroimmunol* (Netherlands) Jul 1995, 60 (1-2) p117-24

Isoprenoid (coQ10) biosynthesis in multiple sclerosis. *Acta Neurol Scand* (Denmark) Sep 1985, 72 (3) p328-35

Abnormality of fatty acid composition of plasma lipid in multiple sclerosis. *Brain Nerve* (Tokyo) (Japan), 1979, 31/8 (797-801)

The pineal and regulation of fibrosis: pinealectomy as a model of primary biliary cirrhosis: Roles of melatonin and prostaglandins in fibrosis and regulation of T lymphocytes. *Med. Hypotheses* (England), 1979, 5/4 (403-414)

Fatty acid patterns of serum lipids in multiple sclerosis and other diseases. *Biochem. Soc. Trans.* (England), 1973, 1/1 (141-143)

Alternate usages for medications update. *Journal of Neurological and Orthopaedic Medicine and Surgery,* 1995 16/3 (167-172)

Magnesium concentration in plasma and erythrocytes in MS. *Acta Neurologica Scandinavica* (Denmark), 1995, 92/1 (109-111)

Comparative findings on serum IMg2+ of normal and diseased human subjects with the Nova and Kone Ise's for Mg2+. *Scand. J. Clin. Lab. Invest. Suppl.* (UK), 1994, 54/217

Magnesium concentration in brains from multiple sclerosis patients. *Acta Neurol. Scand.* (Denmark), 1990, 81/3 (197-200)

Zinc, copper and magnesium concentration in serum and CSF of patients with neurological disorders. *Acta Neurol. Scand.* (Denmark), 1989, 79/5 (373-378)

Multiple sclerosis: Decreased relapse rate through dietary supplementation with calcium, magnesium and vitamin D. *Med. Hypotheses* (UK), 1986, 21/2 (193-200)

Painful tonic seizures in multiple sclerosis. Clinical and electromyographic aspects. *Med. Clin.* (Barcelona) (Spain), 1981, 76/10 (454- 456)

On the ion concentration in the cerebrospinal fluid in multiple sclerosis. *Psychiatr. Neurol. Med. Psychol.* (Germany, East), 1977, 29/8 (482-489)

Evaluation of a nutrition education programme for people with multiple sclerosis. *J. Hum. Nutr. Diet.* (UK), 1993, 6/2 (131-147)

Mineral composition of brains of normal and multiple sclerosis victims. *Proc. Soc. Exp. Biol. Med.*, 1980, 165/2 (327- 329)

Multiple sclerosis: A diathesis? *Gazz. Sanit.* (Milano) (Italy), 1973, 22/1 (37-39)

On the causes of multiple sclerosis. *Med. Hypotheses* (UK), 1993, 41/2 (93-96)

Dietary polyunsaturated fatty acids and depression: when cholesterol does not satisfy. *Am J Clin Nutr* Jul 1995, 62 (1) p1-9

Lipids and neurological diseases. *Med Hypotheses* (England) Mar 1991, 34 (3) p272-4

Essential fatty acid and lipid profiles in plasma and erythrocytes in patients with multiple sclerosis. *Am J Clin Nutr* Oct 1989, 50 (4) p801-6

Plasma lipids and their fatty acid composition in multiple sclerosis. *Acta Neurol Scand* (Denmark) Aug 1988, 78 (2) p152-7

The effect of nutritional counselling on diet and plasma EFA status in multiple sclerosis patients over 3 years. *Hum Nutr Appl Nutr* (England) Oct 1987, 41 (5) p297- 310

[Metabolic aspects of multiple sclerosis]. *Wien Med Wochenschr* (Austria) Jan 31 1985, 135 (1-2) p20-2

Essential fatty acids in the serum and cerebrospinal fluid of multiple sclerosis patients. *Acta Neurol Scand* (Denmark) Mar 1983, 67 (3) p151-63

Multiple sclerosis: some epidemiological clues to etiology. *Acta Neurol Latinoam* (Uruguay) 1975, 21 (1-4) p66-85

Red blood cell and adipose tissue fatty acids in mild inactive multiple sclerosis. *Acta Neurol Scand* (Denmark) Jul 1990, 82 (1) p43-50

Multiple sclerosis: effect of gamma linolenate administration upon membranes and the need for extended clinical trials of unsaturated fatty acids. *Eur Neurol* (Switzerland) 1983, 22 (1) p78-83

The nutritional regulation of T lymphocyte function. *Med Hypotheses* (England) Sep 1979, 5 (9) p969-85

Polyunsaturated fatty acids in treatment of acute remitting multiple sclerosis. *Br Med* J (England) Nov 18 1978, 2 (6149) p1390-1

Effect of prolonged ingestion of gamma-linolenate by MS patients. *Eur Neurol* (Switzerland) 1978, 17 (2) p67-76

Multiple sclerosis patients express increased levels of beta-nerve growth factor in cerebrospinal fluid. *Neurosci Lett* (Netherlands) Nov 23 1992, 147 (1) p9- 12

Experimental and clinical studies on dysregulation of magnesium metabolism and the aetiopathogenesis of multiple sclerosis. *Magnes Res* (England) Dec 1992, 5 (4) p295-302

Muscle Building

Blunting by chronic phosphatidylserine administration of the stress-induced activation of the hypothalamo-pituitary-adrenal axis in healthy men. *Eur J Clin Pharmacol*, 42(4):385-8 1992

Effects of phosphatidylserine on the neuroendocrine response to physical stress in humans. *Neuroendocrinology*, 52(3):243-8 1990 Sep

Conversion of beta-methylbutyric acid to beta-hydroxy-beta-methylbutyric acid by Galactomyces reessii. *Appl Environ Microbiol*, 63(11):4191-5 1997 Nov

Effect of leucine metabolite beta-hydroxy-beta-methylbutyrate on muscle metabolism during resistance-exercise training. *J Appl Physiol*, 81(5):2095-104 1996 Nov

Elevation of creatine in resting and exercised muscle of normal subjects by creatine supplementation. *Clin Sci (Colch)*, 83(3):367-74 1992 Sep

Carbohydrate ingestion augments creatine retention during creatine feeding in humans. *Acta Physiol Scand*, 158(2):195-202 1996 Oct

Supplementary creatine as a treatment for gyrate atrophy of the choroid and retina. *N Engl J Med* Apr 9 1981, 304 (15) p867-70

The effects of creatine supplementation on high-intensity exercise performance in elite performers. *Eur J Appl Physiol* (Germany) Aug 1998, 78 (3) p236-40

Effects of creatine supplementation on body composition, strength, and sprint performance. *Med Sci Sports Exerc* Jan 1998, 30 (1) p73-82

Effects of creatine supplementation on repetitive sprint performance and body composition in competitive swimmers. *Int J Sport Nutr* Dec 1997, 7 (4) p330-46

A randomized, controlled trial of creatine monohydrate in patients with mitochondrial cytopathies. *Muscle Nerve* Dec 1997, 20 (12) p1502-9

Guanidino compounds in guanidinoacetate methyltransferase deficiency, a new inborn error of creatine synthesis. *Metabolism* Oct 1997, 46 (10) p1189-93

Effect of oral creatine supplementation on jumping and running performance. *Int J Sports Med* (Germany) Jul 1997, 18 (5) p369-72

Creatine supplementation enhances intermittent work performance. *Res Q Exerc Sport* Sep 1997, 68 (3) p233-40

Creatine ingestion increases anaerobic capacity and maximum accumulated oxygen deficit. *Can J Appl Physiol* Jun 1997, 22 (3) p231-43

Creatine supplementation enhances muscular performance during high-intensity resistance exercise. *J Am Diet Assoc* Jul 1997, 97 (7) p765-70

Guanidinoacetate methyltransferase deficiency: a newly recognized inborn error of creatine biosynthesis. *Wien Klin Wochenschr* (Austria) Feb 14 1997, 109 (3) p86-8

Creatine replacement therapy in guanidinoacetate methyltransferase deficiency, a novel inborn error of metabolism. *Lancet* (England) Sep 21 1996, 348 (9030) p789-90

Creatine deficiency in the brain: a new, treatable inborn error of metabolism. *Pediatr Res* Sep 1994, 36 (3) p409-13

The nutritional biochemistry of creatine. *Journal of Nutritional Biochemistry* 1997, 8/11 (610-618)

Evaluation of a casein and a whey hydrolysate for treatment of cow's-milk-sensitive enteropathy. *European Journal of Pediatrics (Eur. J. Pediatr.)* (Germany) 1989, 149/1 (68-71)

Initiation of cure in kwashiorkor patients by means of a whey milk product: A comparison with cow's milk. *South African Medical Journal (S. Afr. Med. J.)* (South Africa) 1983, 64/18 (710-712)

Dehydroepiandrosterone reduces serum low density lipoprotein levels and body fat but does not alter insulin sensitivity in normal men. *J Clin Endocrinol Metab* Jan 1988, 66 (1) p57-61

The role of dehydroepiandrosterone in AIDS. *Annals of Pharmacotherapy* 1997, 31/5 (639-642)

Replacement of DHEA in aging men and women. Potential remedial effects. *Annals of the New York Academy of Sciences* 1995, 774/- (128-142)

Coenzyme Q10 treatment in mitochondrial encephalomyopathies. Short-term double-blind, crossover study. *Eur Neurol* (Switzerland) 1997, 37 (4) p212-8

Effects of L-carnitine on the pyruvate dehydrogenase complex and carnitine palmitoyl transferase activities in muscle of endurance athletes. *FEBS Lett* (Netherlands) Mar 14 1994, 341 (1) p91-3

Plasma lipid concentrations in hyperlipidemic patients consuming a high-fat diet supplemented with pyruvate for 6 wk. *Am J Clin Nutr* Nov 1992, 56 (5) p950-4

Enhanced leg exercise endurance with a high-carbohydrate diet and dihydroxyacetone and pyruvate. *J Appl Physiol* Nov 1990, 69 (5) p1651-6

Fat metabolism in exercise. *Advances in Experimental Medicine and Biology* 1998, 441/- (147-156)

Coenzyme Qinf 1inf 0 treatment in mitochondrial encephalomyopathies. Short-term double-blind, crossover study. *European Neurology* (Eur. Neurol.) (Switzerland) 1997, 37/4 (212-218)

Low plasma glutamine in combination with high glutamate levels indicate risk for loss of body cell mass in healthy individuals: the effect of N-acetyl-cysteine. *J Mol Med* (Germany) Jul 1996, 74 (7) p393-400

Glutamine metabolism and transport in skeletal muscle and heart and their clinical relevance. *J Nutr* Apr 1996, 126 (4 Suppl) p1142S-9S

Lung glutamine flux following open heart surgery. *J Surg Res* Jul 1991, 51 (1) p82-6

Absorption and metabolic effects of enterally administered glutamine in humans. *Am J Physiol* May 1991, 260 (5 Pt 1) pG677-82

Role of glutamine and its analogs in posttraumatic muscle protein and amino acid metabolism. *JPEN J Parenter Enteral Nutr* (U S) Jul-Aug 1990, 14 (4 Suppl) p125S-129S

Influence of enterectomy on peripheral tissue glutamine efflux in critically ill patients. *Surgery* Mar 1990, 107 (3) p321-6

Addition of glutamine to total parenteral nutrition after elective abdominal surgery spares free glutamine in muscle, counteracts the fall in muscle protein synthesis and improves nitrogen balance. *Ann Surg* Apr 1989, 209 (4) p455-61

Glutamine: a major energy source for cultured mammalian cells. *Fed Proc* Jan 1984, 43 (1) p121-5

Glutamine: Effects on the immune system, protein metabolism and intestinal function. *Wiener Klinische Wochenschrift* (Austria)1996,108/21 (669-676)

Bioavailability of glutamine and effects of glutamine on protein metabolism. *Nutrition Clinique et Metabolisme (Nutr. Clin. Metab.)* (France) 1994, 8/4 (231-240)

The effect of glutamine on the gastrointestinal tract. *Rivista Italiana di Nutrizione Parenterale ed Enterale* (Italy) 1992, 10/1 (1-6)

Glutamine metabolism by the intestinal tract. *Journal of Parenteral and Enteral Nutrition* 1985, 9/5 (608-617)

Antagonistic effects of glutamine and histamine on in vitro lysozyme activity. *Enzyme (Enzyme)* 1974, 18/3-4 (253-256)

Calcium beta-hydroxy-beta-methylbutyrate. 1. Potential role as a phosphate binder in uremia: in vitro study. *Nephron (Switzerland)* 1996, 72 (3) p391-4

Nutritional role of the leucine metabolite beta-hydroxy beta-methylbutyrate (HMB). *Journal of Nutritional Biochemistry* 1997, 8/6 (300-311)

Ornithine alpha-ketoglutarate in nutritional support. *Nutrition* Sep-Oct 1991, 7 (5) p313- 22

Anabolic effects of insulin-like growth factor-I (IGF-I) and an IGF-I variant in normal female rats. *J Endocrinol* (England) Jun 1993, 137 (3) p413-21

Arginine needs, physiological state and usual diets. A reevaluation. *J Nutr* Jan 1986, 116 (1) p36-46

Effects of dietary chromium picolinate supplementation on growth, carcass characteristics, and accretion rates of carcass tissues in growing-finishing swine. *J Anim Sci* Nov 1995, 73 (11)

Anabolic effects of insulin on bone suggest a role for chromium picolinate in preservation of bone density. *Med Hypotheses* (England) Sep 1995, 45 (3) p241-6

Effect of chromium picolinate on growth, body composition, and tissue accretion in pigs. *J Anim Sci* Jul 1995, 73 (7) p2033-42

Longevity effect of chromium picolinate—'rejuvenation' of hypothalamic function? *Med Hypotheses* (England) Oct 1994, 43 (4) p253-65

Effects of chromium picolinate on beginning weight training students. *Int J Sport Nutr* Dec 1992, 2 (4) p343-50

Modulation of immune function and weight loss by L-arginine in obstructive jaundice in the rat. *Br J Surg* (England) Aug 1994, 81 (8) p1199-201

Nutritional ergogenic aids: chromium, exercise, and muscle mass. *Int J Sport Nutr* Sep 1991, 1 (3) p289-93

Efficacy of chromium supplementation in athletes: emphasis on anabolism. *Int J Sport Nutr* Jun 1992, 2 (2) p111-22

Dietary supplements: Alternatives to anabolic steroids? *Physician Sportsmed.*, 1992, 20/3 (189-193+196+198)

Direct anabolic effects of thyroid hormone on isolated mouse heart. *Am. J. Physiol.*, 1983, 14/3 (C328-C333)

Feeding conjugated linoleic acid to animals partially overcomes catabolic responses due to endotoxin injection. *Biochem Biophys Res Commun* Feb 15 1994, 198 (3 p1107-12)

Muscular Dystrophy

Early onset, autosomal recessive muscular dystrophy with Emery-Dreifuss phenotype and normal emerin expression. *Neurology* Oct 1998, 51 (4) p1116-20

Clinical, pathological, and genetic features of limb-girdle muscular dystrophy type 2A with new calpain 3 gene mutations in seven patients from three Japanese families. *Muscle Nerve* Nov 1998, 21 (11) p1493-501

Deletion analysis & calpain status for carrier detection in a family with Duchenne muscular dystrophy. *Indian J Med Res* (India) Sep 1998, 108 p93-7

Congenital muscular dystrophy with complete lamnin-alpha2-deficiency, cortical dysplasia, and cerebral white-matter changes in children. *J Child Neurol* Jun 1998, 13 (6) p253-6

The psychosocial and cognitive impact of Duchenne's muscular dystrophy. *Semin Pediatr Neurol* Jun 1998, 5 (2) p116-23

Pilot study of myoblast transfer in the treatment of Becker muscular dystrophy. *Neurology* Aug 1998, 51 (2) p589-92

Congenital muscular dystrophy with partial merosin deficiency and late onset epilepsy. *Eur Neurol* (Switzerland) Jul 1998, 40 (1) p37-45

Molecular characterisation of Duchenne muscular dystrophy and phenotypic correlation. *J Neurol Sci* (Netherlands) May 7 1998, 157 (2) p179-86

Role of dystrophin isoforms and associated proteins in muscular dystrophy (review). *Int J Mol Med* (Greece) Dec 1998, 2 (6) p639-48

Surgery of the spine in Duchenne's muscular dystrophy]. *Rev Chir Orthop Reparatrice Appar Mot* (France) May 1998, 84 (3) p224-30

Effects of iron deprivation on the pathology and stress protein expression in murine X-linked muscular dystrophy. *Biochem Pharmacol* (England) Sep 15 1998, 56 (6) p751-7

Mosaic expression of two dystrophins in a boy with progressive muscular dystrophy. *Muscle Nerve* Oct 1998, 21 (10) p1317-20

[Myocardial involvement in carrier states for Duchenne muscular dystrophy. A rare cause of supraventricular arrhythmia]. *Dtsch Med Wochenschr* (Germany) Jul 31 1998, 123 (31-32) p930-5

Nine-year follow-up study of heart rate variability in patients with Duchenne-type progressive muscular dystrophy. *Am Heart J* Aug 1998, 136 (2) p289-96

Spinal instrumentation for Duchenne's muscular dystrophy: experience of hypotensive anaesthesia to minimise blood loss [see comments]. *J Pediatr Orthop* Nov-Dec 1997, 17 (6) p750-3

Duchenne muscular dystrophy: a model for studying the contribution of muscle to energy and protein metabolism. *Reprod Nutr Dev* (France) Mar-Apr 1998, 38 (2) p181-6

The molecular basis of activity-induced muscle injury in Duchenne muscular dystrophy. *Mol Cell Biochem* (Netherlands) Feb 1998, 179 (1-2) p111-23

Social adjustment in adult males affected with progressive muscular dystrophy. *Am J Med Genet* Feb 7 1998, 81 (1) p4-12

Genetic diagnosis of Duchenne/Becker muscular dystrophy; clinical application and problems]. *No To Hattatsu* (Japan) Mar 1998, 30 (2) p141-7

Detection of mutation in dystrophin gene in Duchenne muscular dystrophy—multiplex PCR and Southern blot analysis]. *Nippon Rinsho* (Japan) Dec 1997, 55 (12) p3126-30

Scoliosis in Duchenne muscular dystrophy: aspects of orthotic treatment. *Prosthet Orthot Int* (Denmark) Dec 1997, 21 (3) p202-9

Challenges in Duchenne muscular dystrophy. *Neuromuscul Disord* (England) Dec 1997, 7 (8) p482-6

Problems and potential for gene therapy in Duchenne muscular dystrophy. *Neuromuscul Disord* (England) Jul 1997, 7 (5) p319-24

Improved adenoviral vectors for gene therapy of Duchenne muscular dystrophy. *Neuromuscul Disord* (England) Jul 1997, 7 (5) p277-83

Two successful double-blind trials with coenzyme Q10 (vitamin Q10) on muscular dystrophies and neurogenic atrophies. *Biochim Biophys Acta* (Netherlands) May 24 1995

Biochemical rationale and the cardiac response of patients with muscle disease to therapy with coenzyme Q10. *Proc Natl Acad Sci U S A* Jul 1985

[Efficiency of ubiquinone and p-oxybenzoic acid in prevention of E- hypovitaminosis-induced development of muscular dystrophy]. *Ukr Biokhim Zh* (USSR) Sep-Oct 1981, 53 (5) p73-9

Effect of coenzyme Q on serum levels of creatine phosphokinase in preclinical muscular dystrophy. *Proc Natl Acad Sci U S A* May 1974

[Some indices of energy metabolism in the tissues of mice with progressive muscular dystrophy under the action of ubiquinone]. *Vopr Med Khim* (USSR) May 1974, 20 (3) p276-84

Free radicals, lipid peroxides and antioxidants in blood of patients with myotonic dystrophy. *J Neurol*. 1995 Feb. 242(3). p 119-22

Myasthenia Gravis

Recent studies on traditional Chinese medicinal plants. *Drug Development Research* 1996, 39/2 (147-157)

Humoral and cellular immunity to intrinsic factor in myasthenia gravis. *Scand J Haematol* (Denmark) Nov 1979, 23 (5) p442-8

[Myasthenia and pernicious anemia or Biermer's (author's transl)]. *Rev Neurol* (Paris) (France) Oct 1979, 135 (8-9) p605-14

Neurological complications of pregnancy and anaesthesia. *Clinics in Obstetrics and Gynaecology* (UK) 1982, 9/2 (333-350)

Study of megavitamin therapy on experimental myasthenia gravis in Guinea pigs by electromyographic monitoring. *Journal of Applied Nutrition* 1980, 32/1 (37-43)

Diagnosis and treatment of eye muscle palsies Huber A. *Klinische Monatsblatter fur Augenheilkunde* (Germany) 1978, 172/2 (138-140)

Effects of thiamine, ascorbic acid and alpha tocopherol on neuronal and muscular function. *Journal of Applied Nutrition* 1975, 27/1 (51-63).

Humoral and cellular immunity to intrinsic factor in myasthenia gravis. *Scand J Haematol*; 23(5):442-448 1979

Dietary precursors and brain neurotransmitter formation. *Annu Rev Med* 1981, 32 p413-25

[The role of nutrition in the synthesis of neurotransmitters and in cerebral functions: clinical implications]. *Schweiz Med Wochenschr* (Switzerland) Sep 26 1981, 111 (39)

Myofascial Syndrome

See references under Fibromyalgia.

Nails

Biotin in the treatment of idiopathic brittle nails. *Giornale Italiano di Dermatologia e Venereologia* (Italy) 1993, 128/12 (699-702)

Comparing the mechanism of action of different active ingredience in treatment of brittle nails. *H+G Zeitschrift fur Hautkrankheiten (H G Z. Hautkr.)* (Germany) 1993, 68/8 (517-520)

Brittle nails: Response to daily biotin supplementation. *Cutis (Cutis)* 1993, 51/4 (303-305)

Treatment of brittle fingernails and onychoschizia with biotin: Scanning electron microscopy. *Journal of the American Academy of Dermatology* (U S) 1990, 23/6 I (1127-1132)

Treatment of brittle finger nails with biotin. *H+G Zeitschrift fur Hautkrankheiten (H G Z. Hautkr.)* (Germany) 1989, 64/1 (41-48)

Acquired Acrodermatitis enteropathica: A case report. *Chronica Dermatologica (Chron. Dermatol.)* (Italy) 1997, 7/5 (693-698)

[Gelatin-cystine, keratogenesis and structure of the hair]. *Boll Soc Ital Biol Sper* (Italy) Jan 31 1983, 59 (1)

Nutrition — Miscellanea; Health — Miscellanea. *Better Nutrition for Today's Living*, Sep94, Vol. 56 Issue 9, p8, 1p, 1c

Food — Health aspects. *Better Nutrition for Today's Living*, Sep 94, Vol. 56 Issue 9, p8, 1p, 1c

Cosmetics — Marketing. *Environmental Nutrition*, Mar 96, Vol. 19 Issue 3, p1, 2p

Silica — Physiological Effect. *Better Nutrition For Today's Living*, Dec 95, Vol. 57 Issue 12, p30, 1p, 1c

Biotin — Therapeutic use. *Prevention*, Dec 94, Vol. 46 Issue 12, p122, 3p, 2c

Neuropathy

Ginkgo biloba extract and folic acid in the therapy of changes caused by autonomic neuropathy]. *Acta Med Austriaca* (Austria) 1989, 16 (2) p35-7

Hypothesis on the pathogenesis of vacuolar myelopathy, dementia, and peripheral neuropathy in AIDS. *J Neurol Neurosurg Psychiatry* (England) Jul 1998, 65 (1) p23-8

The biochemical basis of the neuropathy in cobalamin deficiency. *Baillieres Clin Haematol* (England) Sep 1995, 8 (3) p479-97

Epidemic optic neuropathy in Cuba—clinical characterization and risk factors. The Cuba Neuropathy Field Investigation Team [see comments]. *N Engl J Med* Nov 2 1995, 333 (18) p1176-82

Folate responsive neuropathy. *Presse Med* (France) Jan 29 1994, 23 (3) p131-7

Peptide alterations in autonomic diabetic neuropathy prevented by acetyl-L-carnitine. *Int J Clin Pharmacol Res* (Switzerland) 1992, 12 (5-6) p225-30

CSF enkephalins in diabetic neuropathy. *Neuropeptides* (Scotland) Jun 1992, 22 (2) p125-8

Methionine in the treatment of nitrous-oxide-induced neuropathy and myeloneuropathy. *J Neurol* (Germany) Aug 1992, 239 (7) p401-3

The roles of oxidative stress and antioxidant treatment in experimental diabetic neuropathy. *Diabetes* Sep 1997, 46 Suppl 2 pS38-42

Inhibition of development of peripheral neuropathy in streptozotocin-induced diabetic rats with N-acetylcysteine. *Diabetologia* (Germany) Mar 1996, 39 (3) p263-9

Lipoic acid improves nerve blood flow, reduces oxidative stress, and improves distal nerve conduction in experimental diabetic neuropathy. *Diabetes Care* Aug 1995, 18 (8) p1160-7

Low-dose glutathione administration in the prevention of cisplatin-induced peripheral neuropathy in rats. *Neurotoxicology* Fall 1994, 15 (3) p701-4

Potential use of glutathione for the prevention and treatment of diabetic neuropathy in the streptozotocin-induced diabetic rat. *Diabetologia* (Germany) Sep 1992, 35 (9) p813-7

Oxidative stress and antioxidant treatment in diabetic neuropathy. *Neuroscience Research Communications* (UK) 1997, 21/1 (41-48)

Effect of lipoic acid (thioctic acid) on peripheral nerve of experimental diabetic neuropathy. *Diabetes und Stoffwechsel* (Germany) 1996, 5/3 Suppl. (94-97)

Biotin for diabetic peripheral neuropathy. *Biomed Pharmacother* (France) 1990, 44 (10) p511-4

Review of the symptomatic treatment of diabetic neuropathy. *Pharmacotherapy* Nov-Dec 1994, 14 (6) p689-97

Topical capsaicin in painful diabetic neuropathy. Controlled study with long-term follow-up [see comments]. *Diabetes Care* Jan 1992, 15 (1) p8-14

Topical capsaicin in painful diabetic neuropathy. Effect on sensory function. *Diabetes Care* Jan 1992, 15 (1) p15-8

Capsaicin: a therapeutic option for painful diabetic neuropathy. *Henry Ford Hosp Med J* 1991, 39 (2) p138-40

A double-blind comparison of topical capsaicin and oral amitriptyline in painful diabetic neuropathy. *Advances in Therapy* 1995, 12/2 (111-120)

A monthly critical overview of current medicine: Hot peppers for painful diabetic neuropathy? *Hospital Practice* 1992, 27/2 (165-166)

[Chronic neuropathy, a high level of protein in cerebrospinal fluid, and vitamin B1 and folate deficiency in a patient with normal-pressure hydrocephalus]. *Nippon Ronen Igakkai Zasshi* (Japan) Jun 1997, 34 (6) p521-8

[Folic acid deficiency with leukoencephalopathy and chronic axonal neuropathy of sensory predominance]. *Rev Neurol* (Paris) (France) Jun 1997, 153 (5) p351-3

Folate-responsive optic neuropathy. *J Neuroophthalmol* Sep 1994, 14 (3) p163-9

[Patients with type-II diabetes mellitus and neuropathy have no deficiency of vitamins A, E, beta-carotene, B1, B2, B6, B12 and folic acid]. *Med Klin* (Germany) Aug 15 1993, 88 (8) p453-7

Peripheral neuropathy and folate deficiency as the first sign of Crohn's disease. *J Clin Gastroenterol* Aug 1991, 13 (4) p442-4

Dementia-peripheral neuropathy during combined deficiency of vitamin B12 and folate. Light microscopy and ultrastructural study of sural nerve. *Ital J Neurol Sci* (Italy) Oct 1986, 7 (5) p545-52

Vitamin B-12 and folate function in chronic alcoholic men with peripheral neuropathy and encephalopathy. *J Nutr* Mar 1989, 119 (3) p416-24

Brain atrophy, peripheral neuropathy and folic acid deficiency. *Ital J Neurol Sci* (Italy) Apr 1983, 4 (1) p113-5

The role of folate deficiency in electrophysiological neuropathy of experimental hepatoma of the rats. *Acta Neurol Scand* (Denmark) Dec 1981, 64 (6) p446-51

Relapsing neuropathy, cerebral atrophy and folate deficiency. A close association. *Appl Neurophysiol* (Switzerland) 1979, 42 (3) p171-83

Serum cobalamin and folate in the optic neuropathy associated with tobacco smoking. *Can J Ophthalmol* (Canada) Apr 1978, 13 (2) p105-9

Optic neuropathy associated with vitamin B12 deficiency. *Am J Ophthalmol* Apr 1977, 83 (4) p465-8

Folate-responsive neuropathy: report of 10 cases. *Br Med J* (England) May 15 1976, 1 (6019) p1176-8

Peripheral neuropathy and lipid-lowering therapy. *South Med J* Jul 1998, 91 (7) p667-8

Evaluation of the efficacy of thiamine and pyridoxine in the treatment of symptomatic diabetic peripheral neuropathy. *East Afr Med J* (Kenya) Dec 1997, 74 (12) p803-8

[Vitamin status in diabetic neuropathy (thiamine, riboflavin, pyridoxin, cobalamin and tocopherol)]. *Z Ernahrungswiss* (Germany, West) Mar 1980, 19 (1) p1-13

Peripheral neuropathy and myopathy. An experimental study of rats on alcohol and variable dietary thiamine. *Virchows Arch A Pathol Pathol Anat* (Germany, West) Aug 23 1979, 383 (3) p241-52

Supplemental therapy in isolated vitamin E deficiency improves the peripheral neuropathy and prevents the progression of ataxia. *J Neurol Sci* (Netherlands) Apr 1 1998, 156 (2) p177-9

Lack of tocopherol in peripheral nerves of vitamin E-deficient patients with peripheral neuropathy. *N Engl J Med* Jul 30 1987, 317 (5) p262-5

Arrest of neuropathy and myopathy in abetalipoproteinemia with high-dose vitamin E therapy. *Can Med Assoc J* (Canada) Jan 1 1985, 132 (1) p41-4

Therapeutic affect of zinc sulfate on central scotoma due to optic neuropathy of alcohol and tobacco abuse]. *J Fr Ophtalmol* (France) 1983, 6 (3) p237-42

Motonuclear changes after cranial nerve injury and regeneration. *Arch Ital Biol* 1997 Sep;135(4):343-51

Acetyl-L-carnitine effects on nerve conduction and glycemic regulation in experimental diabetes. *Endocr Res* 1997 Feb-May;23(1-2):27-36

Polyol pathway hyperactivity is closely related to carnitine deficiency in the pathogenesis of diabetic neuropathy of streptozotocin-diabetic rats. *J Pharmacol Exp Ther* 1998 Dec;287(3):897-902

Peripheral neuropathy with nucleoside antiretrovirals: risk factors, incidence and management. *Drug Saf* 1998 Dec;19(6): 481-94

Diabetic polyneuropathy: New therapy plan from alpha lipoic acid. *Therapiewoche* (Germany), 1995, 45/36 (2118)

Oral alpha lipoic acid preparation proves good bioavailability in diabetic polyneuropathy. *Frankfurt am Main Germany Therapiewoche* (Germany), 1995, 45/23 (1367- 1370)

Therapy with high dose alpha lipoic acid improves the long-term prognosis in diabetic polyneuropathy. *Tw Neurol. Psychiatr.* (Germany), 1994, 8/12 (699-700)

High dose alpha lipoic acid improves the long-term prognosis in diabetic polyneuropathy. *Therapiewoche* (Germany), 1994, 44/38 (2247-2248)

Alpha-lipoic acid: A versatile drug which is proved Alpha lipoic acid. Avoidance and therapy of polyneuropathy in diabetes. *Z. Allgemeinmed.* (Germany), 1993, 69/17 (492-494)

Alternative therapeutic principles in the prevention of microvascular and neuropathic complications. *Diabetes Res Clin Pract* (Ireland) Aug 1995, 28 Suppl pS201-7

[Preventive treatment of diabetic microangiopathy: blocking the pathogenic mechanisms]. *Diabete Metab* (France) 1994, 20 (2 Pt 2) p219-28

[Diabetes mellitus—a free radical-associated disease. Results of adjuvant antioxidant supplementation]. *Z Gesamte Inn Med* (Germany) May 1993, 48 (5)

[Treatment of diabetic neuropathy with oral alpha-lipoic acid]. *MMW Munch Med Wochenschr* (Germany, West) May 30 1975

Comparison of the effects of evening primrose oil and triglycerides containing gamma-linolenic acid on nerve conduction and blood flow in diabetic rats. *J Pharmacol Exp Ther* Apr 1995

The effects of gamma-linolenic acid on breast pain and diabetic neuropathy: possible non-eicosanoid mechanisms. *Prostaglandins Leukot Essent Fatty Acids* (Scotland) Jan 1993

The use of gamma-linolenic acid in diabetic neuropathy. *Agents Actions Suppl* (Switzerland) 1992, 37 p120-44

Structural and biochemical effects of essential fatty acid deficiency on peripheral nerve. *J Neuropathol Exp Neurol* Nov 1980, 39 (6)

Treatment of diabetic neuropathy with gamma-linolenic acid. *Diabetes Care*, 1993, 16/1 (8-15)

The effects of gamma-linolenic acid on breast pain and diabetic neuropathy: Possible non-eicosanoid mechanisms. *Prostaglandins Leukotrienes Essen Fatty Acids* (UK), 1993, 8/1

The use of gamma-linolenic acid in diabetic neuropathy. *Agents Actions* (Switzerland), 1992, 37/Suppl. (120-144)

Structural and biochemical effects of essential fatty acid deficiency on peripheral nerve. *J. Neuropathol. Exp. Neurol.*, 1980, 39/6 (683-691)

Primary preventive and secondary interventionary effects of acetyl-L-carnitine on diabetic neuropathy in the bio-breeding Worcester rat. *J Clin Invest* Apr 15 1996, 97 (8) p1900-7

Altered neuroexcitability in experimental diabetic neuropathy: effect of acetyl-L-carnitine. *Int J Clin Pharmacol Res* (Switzerland) 1992, 12 (5-6)

Acetyl-L-carnitine corrects the altered peripheral nerve function of experimental diabetes. *Metabolism: Clinical and Experimental*, 1995, 44/5 (677-680)

Diabetic neuropathy in the rat: 1. Alcar augments the reduced levels and axoplasmic transport of substance *RES.*, 1995, 40/3

Neural dysfunction and metabolic imbalances in diabetic rats: Prevention by acetyl-L-carnitine. *Diabetes*, 1994, 43/12 (1469-1477)

Acetyl-L-carnitine prevents substance P loss in the sciatic nerve and lumbar spinal cord of diabetic animals. *Int. J. Clin. Pharmacol. Res.* (Switzerland), 1992, 12/5-6 (243-246)

Altered neuroexcitability in experimental diabetic neuropathy: Effect of acetyl-L-carnitine. *Int. J. Clin. Pharmacol. Res.* (Switzerland), 1992, 12/5-6 (237-241)

Acetyl-L-carnitine effect on nerve conduction velocity in streptozotocin-diabetic rats. *Arzneim.-Forsch. Drug Res.* (Germany), 1993, 43/3 (343-346)

Differential effects of acetyl-L-carnitine, L-carnitine and gangliosides on nerve Na+,K+-ATPase impairment in experimental diabetes. *Diabetes Nutr. Metab. Clin. Exp.* (Italy), 1992, 5/1 (31-36)

Treatment of symptomatic diabetic peripheral neuropathy with the anti-oxidant alpha-lipoic acid. A 3-week multicentre randomized controlled trial. *Diabetologia* (Germany), 1995, 38/12 (1425-1433)

Peptide alterations in autonomic diabetic neuropathy prevented by acetyl-L-carnitine. *Int J Clin Pharmacol Res* (Switzerland) 1992, 12 (5-6)

Obesity

Conjugated linoleic acid modulates hepatic lipid composition in mice. *Lipids* 1997 Feb;32(2):199-204

Opposite effects of linoleic acid and conjugated linoleic acid on human prostatic cancer in SCID mice. *Anticancer Res* 1998 May-Jun;18(3A):1429-34

Proliferative responses of normal human mammary and MCF-7 breast cancer cells to linoleic acid, conjugated linoleic acid and eicosanoid synthesis inhibitors in culture. *Anticancer Res* 1997 Jan-Feb;17(1A):197-203

Dietary conjugated linoleic acid normalizes impaired glucose tolerance in the Zucker diabetic fatty fa/fa rat. *Biochem Biophys Res Commun* 1998 Mar 27;244(3):678-82

Retention of conjugated linoleic acid in the mammary gland is associated with tumor inhibition during the post-initiation phase of carcinogenesis. *Carcinogenesis* 1997 Apr;18(4):755-9

Conjugated linoleic acid and linoleic acid are distinctive modulators of mammary carcinogenesis. *Nutr Cancer* 1997;27(2):131-5

Review of the effects of trans fatty acids, oleic acid, n-3 polyunsaturated fatty acids, and conjugated linoleic acid on mammary carcinogenesis in animals. *Am J Clin Nutr* 1997 Dec;66(6 Suppl):1523S-1529S

Production of conjugated linoleic acid by dairy starter cultures. *J Appl Microbiol* 1998 Jul;85(1):95-102

Conjugated linoleic acid and atherosclerosis in rabbits. *Atherosclerosis* 1994 Jul;108(1):19-25

Conjugated linoleic acid decreases hepatic stearoyl-CoA desaturase mRNA expression. *Biochem Biophys Res Commun* 1998 Jul 30;248(3):817-21

Conjugated linoleic acids alter bone fatty acid composition and reduce ex vivo prostaglandin E2 biosynthesis in rats fed n-6 or n-3 fatty acids. *Lipids* 1998 Apr;33(4):417-25

Conjugated linoleic acid modulation of phorbol ester-induced events in murine keratinocytes. *Lipids* 1997 Jul;32(7):725-30

Conjugated linoleic acid reduces arachidonic acid content and PGE2 synthesis in murine keratinocytes. *Cancer Lett* 1998 May 15;127(1-2):15-22

Dietary conjugated linoleic acid reduces plasma lipoproteins and early aortic atherosclerosis in hypercholesterolemic hamsters. *Artery* 1997;22(5):266-77

Effect of conjugated linoleic acid on body composition in mice. *Lipids* 1997 Aug;32(8):853-8

Toxicological evaluation of dietary conjugated linoleic acid in male Fischer 344 rats. *Food Chem Toxicol* 1998 May;36(5):391-5

Conjugated linoleic acid modulates tissue levels of chemical mediators and immunoglobulins in rats. *Lipids* 1998 May;33(5):521-7

Morphological and biochemical status of the mammary gland as influenced by conjugated linoleic acid: implication for a reduction in mammary cancer risk. *Cancer Res* 1997 Nov 15;57(22):5067-72

Conjugated linoleic acid suppresses the growth of human breast adenocarcinoma cells in SCID mice. *Anticancer Res* 1997 Mar-Apr;17(2A):969-73

Influence of long-chain polyunsaturated fatty acids on oxidation of low density lipoprotein. *Prostaglandins Leukot Essent Fatty Acids* 1998 Aug;59(2):143-51

Effects of conjugated linoleic acid on body fat and energy metabolism in the mouse. *Am J Physiol* 1998 Sep;275(3 Pt 2):R667-72

Effects of dietary conjugated linoleic acid on lymphocyte function and growth of mammary tumors in mice. *Anticancer Res* 1997 Mar-Apr;17(2A):987-93

Dietary effect of conjugated linoleic acid on lipid levels in white adipose tissue of Sprague-Dawley rats. *Biosci Biotechnol Biochem* 1999 Jun;63(6):1104-6

Hypocholesterolemic action of chitosans with different viscosity in rats. *Lipids* 1988 Mar;23(3):187-91

Mechanism for the inhibition of fat digestion by chitosan and for the synergistic effect of ascorbate. *Biosci Biotechnol Biochem* 1995 May;59(5):786-90

A 54-month evaluation of a popular very low calorie diet program. *J Fam Pract* 1995 Sep;41(3):231-6

Secular trends in diet and risk factors for cardiovascular disease: the Framingham Study. *J Am Diet Assoc* 1995 Feb;95(2):171-9

Severe obesity: expensive to society, frustrating to treat, but important to confront. *South Med J* 1995 Sep;88(9):895-902

Weight control practices of U.S. adults trying to lose weight. *Ann Intern Med* 1993 Oct 1;119(7 Pt 2):661-6

[Inhibition by chitosan of productive infection of T-series bacteriophages in the Escherichia coli culture]. *Mikrobiologiia* 1995 Mar-Apr;64(2):211-5

[Phytotherapeutic aspects of diseases of the circulatory system. 4. Chitin and chitosan]. *Ceska Slov Farm* 1995 Aug;44(4):190-5

Chitosan—as a biomaterial. *Biomater Artif Cells Artif Organs* 1990;18(1):1-24

Comparative effects of chitosan and cholestyramine on lymphatic absorption of lipids in the rat. *Am J Clin Nutr* 1983 Aug;38(2):278-84

Some effects of chitosan on liver function in the rat. *Endocrinology* 1993 Mar;132(3):1078-84

Body weight and mortality among women. *N Engl J Med* 1995 Sep 14;333(11):677-85

Obesity: adverse effects on health and longevity. *Am J Clin Nutr* 1979 Dec;32(12 Suppl):2723-33

Abdominal obesity and mortality risk among men in nineteenth-century North America. *Int J Obes Relat Metab Disord* 1994 Oct;18(10):686-91

Sudden death as a result of heart disease in morbid obesity. *Am Heart J* 1995 Aug;130(2):306-13

[Abdominal obesity and coronary heart disease. Pathophysiology and clinical significance]. *Herz* 1995 Feb;20(1):47-55

Dietary treatment of hypercholesterolemia. *Tex Med* 1990 Apr;86(4):31-7

Pre-morbid body size and the prognosis of women with breast cancer. *Int J Cancer* 1994 Nov 1;59(3):363-8

The fattening of America. *JAMA* 1994 Jul 20;272(3):238-9

Increasing prevalence of overweight among US adults. The National Health and Nutrition. Examination Surveys, 1960 to 1991. *JAMA* 1994 Jul 20;272(3):205-11

Sedentary lifestyle and state variation in coronary heart disease mortality. *Public Health Rep* 1995 Jan-Feb;110(1):100-2

A prospective study of effects of weight cycling on cardiovascular risk factors. *Arch Intern Med* 1995 Jul 10;155(13):1416-22

Interaction of dietary fiber with lipids—mechanistic theories and their limitations. *Adv Exp Med Biol* 1990;270:67-82

A novel use of chitosan as a hypocholesterolemic agent in rats. *Am J Clin Nutr* 1980 Apr;33(4):787-93

Effect of chitin and chitosan on nutrient digestibility and plasma lipid concentrations in broiler chickens. *Br J Nutr* 1994 Aug;72(2):277-88

Effect of modest weight loss on changes in cardiovascular risk factors: are there differences between men and women or between weight loss and maintenance?. *Int J Obes Relat Metab Disord* 1995 Jan;19(1):67-73

Fluvastatin efficacy and tolerability in comparison and in combination with cholestyramine. *Eur J Clin Pharmacol* 1994;46(5):445-9

Interrelated effects of dietary fiber and fat on lymphatic cholesterol and triglyceride absorption in rats. *J Nutr* 1989 Oct;119(10):1383-7

A comparison of the lipid-lowering and intestinal morphological effects of cholestyramine, chitosan, and oat gum in rats. *Proc Soc Exp Biol Med* 1988 Oct;189(1):13-20

Interaction of bile acids, phospholipids, cholesterol and triglyceride with dietary fibers in the small intestine of rats. *J Nutr* 1989 Aug;119(8):1100-6

Effect of chitosan feeding on intestinal bile acid metabolism in rats. *Lipids* 1991 May;26(5):395-9

[Comprehensive obesity therapy program]. *Versicherungsmedizin* 1995 Feb 1;47(1):23-6

Epidemiology of obesity and its link to heart disease. *Metabolism* 1995 Sep;44(9 Suppl 3):1-3

Human body composition and the epidemiology of chronic disease. *Obes Res* 1995 Jan;3(1):73-95

The role of gastric surgery in the multidisciplinary management of severe obesity. *Am J Surg* 1995 Mar;169(3):361-7

Determinants of body mass index: a study from northern Italy. *Int J Obes Relat Metab Disord* 1994 Jul;18(7):497-502

Is there a role for dietary fish oil in the treatment of hypertension? *J Hum Hypertens* 1994 Dec;8(12):895-905

Weight and osteoarthritis. *J Rheumatol Suppl* 1995 Feb;43:7-9

Food consumption habits in Germany—the clinician's point of view. *Metabolism* 1995 Feb;44(2 Suppl 2):14-7

Prevalence of obesity among patients admitted for elective orthopaedic surgery. *Int J Obes Relat Metab Disord* 1994 Oct;18(10):709-13

Cholesterol-related counseling by registered dietitians in northern California. *Prev Med* 1992 Nov;21(6):746-53

Primary prevention of hypertension: a challenge for occupational health nurses. *AAOHN J* 1995 Jun;43(6):306-12

Obesity: a move from traditional to more patient-oriented management. *J Am Board Fam Pract* 1995 Mar-Apr;8(2):99-108

Database marketing targets existing patients. *Healthc Financ Manage* 1990 Jun;44(6):72, 74-5

Computerized system offers quality at less cost. *Health Manag Technol* 1994 Jan;15(1):31-3

Energy restriction reduces metabolic rate in adult male Fisher-344 rats. *J Nutr* 1993 Jan;123(1):90-7

The rate of DNA damage and aging. *EXS* 1992;62:20-30

The contribution of lipids to coronary heart disease in diabetes mellitus. *J Intern Med Suppl* 1994;736:41-6

The relation of parental cardiovascular disease to risk factors in children and young adults. The Bogalusa Heart Study. *Circulation* 1995 Jan 15;91(2):365-71

Four-week supplementation with a natural dietary compound produces favorable changes in body composition. *Adv Ther* 1998 Sep-Oct;15(5):305-14

Effect of supplementation with chromium picolinate on antibody titers to 5-hydroxymethyl uracil. *Eur J Epidemiol* 1998 Sep;14(6):621-6

[Effect of chromium yeast and chromium picolinate on body composition of obese, non-diabetic patients during and after a formula diet]. *Acta Med Austriaca* 1997;24(5):185-7

Drug therapy for obesity in the elderly. *Drugs Aging* 1997 Nov;11(5):338-51

Chromium and exercise training: effect on obese women. *Med Sci Sports Exerc* 1997 Aug;29(8):992-8

Effects of chromium picolinate on body composition. *J Sports Med Phys Fitness* 1995 Dec;35(4):273-80

Management of dietary essential metals (iron, copper, zinc, chromium and manganese) by Wistar and Zucker obese rats fed a self-selected high-energy diet. *Biometals* 1994 Apr;7(2):117-29

The Binding Of Micellar Lipids To Chitosan. *Lipids* 18 (10). 1983. 714-719.

Decreasing Effect of Chitosan on the Apparent Fat Digestibility by Rats Fed on a High-fat Diet. *Bioscience Biotechnology and Biochemistry* 58 (9):p1613-1616 1994

Effect of the viscosity or deacetylation degree of chitosan on fecal fat excreted from rats fed on a high-fat diet. *Biosci Biotechnol Biochem* (Japan) May 1995, 59 (5) p781-5

Increasing Effect of a Chitosan and Ascorbic Acid Mixture on Fecal Dietary Fat Excretion. *Bioscience Biotechnology and Biochemistry* 58 (9):p1617-1620 1994

Dietary fiber and intestinal adaptation: effects on lipid absorption and lymphatic transport in the rat. *Am J Clin Nutr* Feb 1988, 47 (2) p201-6

Non-soluble dietary fiber effects on lipid absorption and blood serum lipid patterns. *Lipids* Nov 1985, 20 (11) p802-7

Dietary Fiber And Lipid Absorption. *Lab. Nutrition Chem.*, Kyushu Univ. Sch. Agric. 46-09, Fukuoka 812, Japan. 1993

Effects of dietary fiber on carbohydrate and amino-acid absorption and on tri glyceride and phospho lipid metabolism in rat intesting. *Gastroenterology* 78 (5 Part 2). 1980. 1256.

[Use of liquid sorbents based on chitosan for treatment of diffuse forms of peritonitis]. *Patol Fiziol Eksp Ter* (Russia) Jul-Sep 1994, (3) p49-50.

Modification of chitosan to improve its hypocholesterolemic capacity. *Biosci Biotechnol Biochem* (Japan) May 1999, 63 (5) p833-9

Hypocholesterolemic effect of chitosan in adult males. *Bioscience Biotechnology and Biochemistry* 57 (9):p1439-1444 1993

Effects Of Dietary Chitin And Chitosan On Growth And Abdominal Fat Deposition In Chicks. *Japanese Poultry Science* 28 (2). 1991. 88-94.

Effects of chitosan hydrolysates on lipid absorption and on serum and liver lipid concentration in rats. *Journal of Agricultural and Food Chemistry* 41 (3):p431-435 1993

Effect of Chitosan of Serum and Liver Cholesterol Levels in Cholesterol Fed Rats. *Nutrition Reports International* 19 (3). 1979. 327-334

A comparison of standard height-weight indices and algorithmic ElectroLipoGraphy in the clinical Diagnosis of Obesity. Syracuse Medical Center, 1994.

Fat binder as a weight reducer in patients with moderate Obesity. *ARS Medicina*, Helsinki, 1994 Aug-October.

The Hypolipidemic Activity of Chitosan and other Polysaccharides in Rats. *Nutrition Reports International*, volume 20 No. 5, 1979.

Compartive effects of Chitosan and Cholestramine on lymphatic absorption on lipids in rats. *The American Journal of Clinical Nutrition*, 1993, pp. 278-284.

Physician's and dietitian's role in obese care. *Journal of Flordia Medical Association*, 1992 Jun.

Are there effective treatments for severly obese? *Journal of Louisiana State Medical Society*, 1994 Aug.

Calorie Control Council Survey 1995.

Clinical Market Analysis, Computers in Healthcare 1987. Ronn Kelsey

Computerized treatment protocols developed by Intelligent Health. *Healthcare Forum Journal,* 1993. November/December

Group Practice Journal, 1994. March/April . RR. Kelsey, E Hanks

Intelligent Health, Polysaccharides, Weight Management and Health, 1995.

Health Trends. R. Coile. Aspen Publishing, 1995.

The New Medicine. R. Kelsey. 1994 & 1995.

Food Labeling: Health Claims and Label Statements: Dietary Fiber and Cardiovascular Disease, vol 58, no.3 Rules and Regulations 1993, Food and Drug Adminstration FDA.

World Health Organization (WHO), BioSis Database 1995, CDC. Mortality and Morbidity (MMRW) Database. 1995.

Clinical Report. Dovre Medical Centre, Fjellhammer, Norway, May 1991.

Magnesium and carbohydrate metabolism. *Therapie* (France), 1994, 49/1 (1-7)

Disorders of magnesium metabolism. *Endocrinology and Metabolism Clinics of North America*, 1995, 24/3

Magnesium deficiency produces insulin resistance and increased thromboxane synthesis. *Hypertension*, 1993, 21/6 II (1024-1029)

Magnesium and glucose homeostasis. *Diabetologia* (Germany, Federal Republic of), 1990, 33/9 (511-514)

Effect of thyroxine supplementation on the response to perfluoro-n-decanoic acid (PFDA) in rats. *J. Toxicol. Environ. Health*, 1988, 24/4 (491- 498)

The role of thyroid hormones and insulin in the regulation of energy metabolism. *Am. J. Clin. Nutr.*, 1983, 38/6 (1006-1017)

The effect of triiodothyronine on weight loss and nitrogen balance of obese patients on a very low calorie liquid formula diet. *Int. J. Obesity* (England), 1981, 5/3 (279-282)

The effect of a low-calorie diet alone and in combination with triiodothyronine therapy on weight loss and hypophyseal thyroid function in obesity. *Int. J. Obesity* (England), 1983, 7/2 (123-131)

The effect of triiodothyronine on weight loss, nitrogen balance and muscle protein catabolism in obese patients on a very low calorie diet. *Nutr. Rep. Int.,* 1981, 24/1 (145-151)

Effect of triiodothyronine on some metabolic responses of obese patients. *Amer. J. Clin. Nutr.*, 1973, 26/7 (715-721)

The variability of weight reduction during fasting: Predictive value of thyroid hormone measurements. *Int. J. Obesity* (England), 1982, 6/1 (101-111)

The effects of triiodothyronine on energy expenditure, nitrogen balance and rates of weight and fat loss in obese patients during prolonged caloric restriction. *Int. J. Obesity* (EN), 1985, 9/6 (433-442)

Desiccated thyroid in a nutritional supplement. *J. Fam. Pract.*, 1994, 38/3 (287-288)

Factors determining energy expenditure during very-low-calorie diets. *Am. J. Clin. Nutr.*, 1992, 56/1 Suppl. (224S-229S)

Resting metabolic rate, body composition and thyroid hormones. Short term effects of very low calorie diet. *Horm. Metab. Res.* (Germany, Federal Republic of), 1990, 22/12 (632- 635)

Decrease in resting metabolic rate during rapid weight loss is reversed by low dose thyroid hormone treatment. *Metab. Clin. Exp.*, 1986, 35/4 (289-291)

Relationship between the changes in serum thyroid hormone levels and protein status during prolonged protein supplemented caloric deprivation. *Clin. Endocrinol. (Oxford)* (England), 1985, 22/1 (1-15)

Thyroid hormone changes in obese subjects during fasting and a very-low-calorie diet. *Int. J. Obesity* (England), 1981, 5/3 (305-311)

The role of T_3 and its receptor in efficient metabolisers receiving very-low-calorie diets. *Int. J. Obesity* (England), 1981, 5/3 (283-286)

Effects of total fasting in obese women. III. Response of serum thyroid hormones to thyroxine and triiodothyronine administration. *Endokrinologie* (Germany, East), 1979, 73/2 (221-226)

Thyroidal hormone metabolism in obesity during semi-starvation. *Clin. Endocrinol.* (Oxford) (England), 1978, 9/3 (227-231)

Clinical characteristics of hyperthyroidism. A study of 100 patients. *Rev.Cuba.Med.* (Cuba), 1973, 12/1 (39-52)

The effect of triiodothyronine (T_3) on protein turnover and metabolic rate. *Int. J. Obesity* (England), 1985, 9/6 (459-463)

Soy protein, thyroid regulation and cholesterol metabolism. *Journal Of Nutrition*, 1995, 125/3 Suppl.

Overview of proposed mechanisms for the hypocholesterolemic effect of soy. *Journal of Nutrition*, 1995, 125/3 Suppl.

Endocrinological response to soy protein and fiber in mildly hypercholesterolemic men. *Nutr. Res.*, 1993, 13/8 (873-884)

Response of hormones modulating plasma cholesterol to dietary casein or soy protein in minipigs. *J. Nutr.*, 1990, 120/11 (1387-1392)

Dietary protein effects on cholesterol and lipoprotein concentrations: A review. *J. Am. Coll. Nutr.*, 1986, 5/6 (533-549)

Comparison of dietary casein or soy protein effects on plasma lipids and hormone concentrations in the gerbil (Meriones unguiculatus). *J. Nutr.*, 1986, 116/7 (1165-1171)

Hypolipidemic effect of casein vs. soy protein in the hyperlipidemic hypothyroid chick model. *Nutr. Rep. Int.*, 1980, 21/4 (497-503)

Characterization of the insulin resistance of glucose utilization in adipocytes from patients with hyper- and hypothyroidism. *Acta Endocrinol* (Copenh) (Denmark) Oct 1988

Thyroid hormone action on intermediary metabolism. Part I: respiration, thermogenesis and carbohydrate metabolism. *Klin Wochenschr* (Germany, West) Jan 2 1984

Relative roles of the thyroid hormones and noradrenaline on the thermogenic activity of brown adipose tissue in the rat. *J Endocrinol* (England) Jun 1995, 145

Age-related differences in body weight loss in response to altered thyroidal status. *Exp Gerontol* (England) 1990, 25 (1)

Long-term weight regulation in treated hyperthyroid and hypothyroid subjects. *Am J Med* Jun 1984, 76 (6)

Chromium improves insulin response to glucose in rats. *Metabolism* Oct 1995, 44 (10)

Enhancing central and peripheral insulin activity as a strategy for the treatment of endogenous depression—an adjuvant role for chromium picolinate? *Med Hypotheses* (England) Oct 1994, 43 (4)

Homologous physiological effects of phenformin and chromium picolinate. *Med Hypotheses* (England) Oct 1993, 41 (4)

Chromium in human nutrition: a review. *J Nutr* Apr 1993, 123 (4)

Use of the artificial beta cell (ABC) in the assessment of peripheral insulin sensitivity: effect of chromium supplementation in diabetic patients. *Gen Pharmacol* (England) 1984, 15 (6)

Obsessive Compulsive Disorder

Treatment of obsessive compulsive neurosis: pharmacological approach. *Psychosomatics* 1976, 17/4 (180-184)

Effect of kava extract and individual kavapyrones on neurotransmitter levels in the nucleus accumbens of rats. *Progress in Neuro-Psychopharmacology and Biological Psychiatry* 1998, 22/7 (1105-1120)

In vivo effects of the kavapyrones (+)-dihydromethysticin and (+/-)- kavain on dopamine, 3,4-dihydroxyphenylacetic acid, serotonin and 5- hydroxyindoleacetic acid levels in striatal and cortical brain regions. *Planta Medica* (Germany) 1998, 64/6 (507-510)

Influence of genuine kavapyrone enantiomers on the GABA(A) binding site. *Planta Medica* (Germany) 1998, 64/6 (504-506)

Contribution to the quantitative and enantioselective determination of kavapyrones by high-performance liquid chromatography on ChiraSpher NT material. *Journal of Chromatography B: Biomedical Applications* (Netherlands) 1997, 702/1-2 (240-244)

Piper methysticum: Enantiomeric separation of kavapyrones by high performance liquid chromatography. *Planta Medica* (Germany) 1997, 63/1 (63-65)

Kavapyrone enriched extract from Piper methysticum as modulator of the GABA binding site in different regions of rat brain. *Psychopharmacology* (Germany) 1994, 116/4 (469-474)

[Kava-kava preparations—alternative anxiolytics]. *Pol Merkuriusz Lek* (Poland) Mar 1998, 4 (21) p179-180a

Tolerability of kava-kava extract WS 1490 on anxiety disorders (Multicentric Brazilian study). *Revista Brasileira de Medicina* (Brazil) 1999, 56/4 (280-284)

Over-the-counter psychotropics: A review of melatonin, St John's wort, valerian, and kava-kava. *Journal of American College Health* 1998, 46/6 (271-276)

Piper methysticum Forst: A new antianxiety agents. *Revista Brasileira de Farmacia* (Brazil) 1997, 78/2 (44-48)

Psychopharmacological treatment of anxiety disorders. *Therapeutische Umschau* (Switzerland) 1997, 54/10 (595-599)

Actions of kavain and dihydromethysticin on ipsapirone-induced field potential changes in the hippocampus. *Human Psychopharmacology* (UK) 1997, 12/3 (265-270)

Effects of kawain and dihydromethysticin on field potential changes in the hippocampus. *Progress in Neuro-Psychopharmacology and Biological Psychiatry* 1997, 21/4 (697-706)

Kava-kava and kavain. Herbal anxiolytic—A critical review of clinical trials. *Munchener Medizinische Wochenschrift* (Germany) 1997, 139/4 (42-46)

Clinical efficacy of a kava extrakt in patients with anxiety syndrome. Double-blind placebo controlled study over 4 weeks. *Arzneimittel-Forschung / Drug Research* (Germany) 1991, 41/6 (584-588)

Neurovegetative dystonia in the female climacteric. Studies on the clinical efficacy and tolerance of kava extract WS 1490. *Fortschritte der Medizin* (Germany) 1991, 109/4 (65-71)

Parameters of kava used as a challenge to alcohol. *Australian and New Zealand Journal of Psychiatry* (Australia) 1986, 20/1 (70-76)

Piper methysticum (kava kava). *Altern Med Rev* Dec 1998, 3 (6) p458-60

Kava-kava extract in anxiety disorders: an outpatient observational study. *Adv Ther* 1998 Jul-Aug;15(4):261-9

Herbal medicines in Hawaii from tradition to convention. *Hawaii Med J* 1998 Jan;57(1):382-6

L-tryptophan in neuropsychiatric disorders: a review. *Int J Neurosci* (England) Nov-Dec 1992, 67 (1-4) p127-44

Serotonin activity in anorexia and bulimia nervosa:relationship to the modulation of feeding and mood. *J Clin Psychiatry* Dec 1991, 52 Suppl p41-8

Can hypoglycaemia cause obsessions and ruminations?. *Med Hypotheses* (England) Sep 1984, 15 (1) p3-13

Dietary treatment of chronic obsessional ruminations. *Br J Clin Psychol* (England) Nov 1983, 22 (Pt 4) p314-6

Sequential administration of augmentation strategies in treatment-resistant obsessive-compulsive disorder : preliminary findings. *Int Clin Psychopharmacol* (England) Mar 1996, 11 (1) p37-44

Plasma melatonin and cortisol circadian patterns in patients with obsessive- compulsive disorder before and after fluoxetine treatment. *Psychoneuroendocrinology* (England) 1995, 20 (7) p763-70

Neuroendocrine responses to intravenous L-tryptophan in obsessive compulsive disorder. *J Affect Disord* (Netherlands) Oct 1994, 32 (2) p97-104

Tryptophan depletion in patients with obsessive-compulsive disorder who respond to serotonin reuptake inhibitors. *Arch Gen Psychiatry* Apr 1994, 51 (4) p309-17

Circadian rhythms of melatonin, cortisol and prolactin in patients with obsessive-compulsive disorder. *Acta Psychiatr Scand* (Denmark) Jun 1994, 89 (6) p411-5

Biological approaches to treatment-resistant obsessive compulsive disorder. *J Clin Psychiatry* Jun 1993, 54 Suppl p16-26

Pharmacotherapy of obsessive compulsive disorder. *J Clin Psychiatry* Apr 1992, 53 Suppl p29-37

Plasma tryptophan levels and plasma tryptophan/neutral amino acids ratio in patients with mood disorder, patients with obsessive- compulsive disorder, and normal subjects. *Psychiatry Res* (Ireland) Nov 1992, 44 (2) p85-91

Melatonin and cortisol secretion in patients with primary obsessive-compulsive disorder. *Psychiatry Res* (Ireland) Dec 1992, 44 (3) p217-25

Role of serotonin in obsessive-compulsive disorder. *Br J Psychiatry Suppl* (England) 1998, (35) p13-20

Psychiatric manifestations of homocystinuria due to cystathionine beta-synthase deficiency: prevalence, natural history, and relationship to neurologic impairment and vitamin B6-responsiveness. *Am J Med Genet* Apr 1987, 26 (4) p959-69

Alphainf 2-adrenoreceptor status in obsessive- compulsive disorder. *Biological Psychiatry* 1990, 27/10 (1083-1093)

Vitamin Binf 1inf 2 and folic acid serum levels in obsessive compulsive disorder. *Acta Psychiatrica Scandinavica* (Denmark) 1988, 78/1 (8-10)

Controlled trials of inositol in psychiatry. *Eur Neuropsycho Pharmacol* (Netherlands) May 1997, 7 (2) p147-55

Inositol treatment of obsessive-compulsive disorder. *Am J Psychiatry* Sep 1996, 153 (9) p1219-21

Role of inositol in the treatment of psychiatric disorders. Basic and clinical aspects. *CNS Drugs* (New Zealand) 1997, 7/1 (6-16)

Lithium and tryptophan augmentation in clomipramine-resistant obsessive-compulsive disorder. *Am J Psychiatry* Oct 1984, 141 (10) p1283-5

Vitamin B12 and folic acid serum levels in obsessive compulsive disorder. *Acta Psychiatr Scand* (Denmark) Jul 1988, 78 (1) p8-10

Obsessive compulsive disorder arising in a 75-year-old woman. *International Journal of Geriatric Psychiatry* (UK) 1992, 7/2 (139-142)

Lithium augments fluoxetine treatment of obsessive compulsive disorder. *Lithium* (UK) 1992, 3/1 (69-71)

WS 1490 (kava extract) in the treatment of anxiety neurosis. *Fortschritte der Medizin* (Germany) 1992, 110/9 (86)

Inhibition of platelet MAO-B by kava pyrone-enriched extract from Piper methysticum Forster (kava-kava). *Pharmacopsychiatry* 1998 Sep;31(5):187-92.

Organic Brain Syndrome

Refer to references under Alzheimer's Disease.

Osteoporosis

Effects of cyclical etidronate combined with calcitriol versus cyclical etidronate alone on spine and femoral neck bone mineral density in postmenopausal osteoporotic women. *Ann Rheum Dis* (England) Jun 1998, 57 (6) p346-9

Alendronate does not block the anabolic effect of PTH in postmenopausal osteoporotic women. *J Bone Miner Res* Jun 1998, 13 (6) p1051-5

Development and evaluation of the osteoporosis Self-Efficacy Scale. *Res Nurs Health* Oct 1998, 21 (5) p395-403

A placebo-controlled, single-blind study to determine the appropriate alendronate dosage in postmenopausal Japanese patients with osteoporosis. The Alendronate Research Group. *Endocr J* (Japan) Apr 1998, 45 (2) p191-201

[Why regular physical activity favors longevity (editorial)]. *Minerva Med* (Italy) Jun 1998, 89 (6) p197-201

Prevention of estrogen deficiency-related bone loss with human parathyroid hormone-(1-34): a randomized controlled trial. *JAMA* Sep 23-30 1998, 280 (12) p1067-73

Biochemical markers of bone turnover. *Int J Clin Pract* (England) Jun 1998, 52 (4) p255-6

Educating patients about the benefits and drawbacks of hormone replacement therapy. *Drugs Aging* (New Zealand) Jul 1998, 13 (1) p33-41

Markers of bone remodelling in metabolic bone disease. *Drugs Aging* (New Zealand) 1998, 12 Suppl 1 p9-14

Management of osteoporosis. An overview. *Drugs Aging* (New Zealand) 1998, 12 Suppl 1 p25-32

[NTx—a sensitive laboratory parameter of bone resorption]. *Bratisl Lek Listy* (Slovakia) Jun 1998, 99 (6) p327-30

Treatment of osteoporosis with bisphosphonates. *Endocrinol Metab Clin North Am* Jun 1998, 27 (2) p419-39

The role of calcitonin in the prevention of osteoporosis. *Endocrinol Metab Clin North Am* Jun 1998, 27 (2) p411-8

The roles of calcium and vitamin D in the prevention of osteoporosis. *Endocrinol Metab Clin North Am* Jun 1998, 27 (2) p389-98

The roles of exercise and fall risk reduction in the prevention of osteoporosis. *Endocrinol Metab Clin North Am* Jun 1998, 27 (2) p369-87

[Ipriflavone]. *Nippon Rinsho* (Japan) Jun 1998, 56 (6) p1537-43

[Vitamin K2]. *Nippon Rinsho* (Japan) Jun 1998, 56 (6) p1525-30

[Treatment of osteoporosis by active vitamin D]. *Nippon Rinsho* (Japan) Jun 1998, 56 (6) p1505-10

Exercise is medicine: health benefits of regular physical activity. *J La State Med Soc* Jul 1998, 150 (7) p319-23

Osteoporosis: detection, prevention, and treatment in primary care. *Geriatrics* Aug 1998, 53 (8) p22-3, 27-8, 33

Dissociation of bone formation from resorption during 2-week treatment with human parathyroid hormone-related peptide-(1-36) in humans: potential as an anabolic therapy for osteoporosis. *J Clin Endocrinol Metab* Aug 1998, 83 (8) p2786-91

Daily oral magnesium supplementation suppresses bone turnover in young adult males. *J Clin Endocrinol Metab* Aug 1998, 83 (8) p2742-8

Clodronate is effective in preventing corticosteroid-induced bone loss among asthmatic patients. *Bone* May 1998, 22 (5) p577-82

Management of postmenopausal osteoporosis for primary care. *Menopause* 1998 Summer;5(2):123-31

[Reduced serum dehydroepiandrosterone levels in postmenopausal osteoporosis]. *Ceska Gynekol* (Czech Republic) Apr 1998, 63 (2) p110-3

Avoidance of vertebral fractures in men with idiopathic osteoporosis by a three year therapy with calcium and low-dose intermittent monofluorophosphate. *Osteoporos Int* (England) 1998, 8 (1) p47-52

Glucocorticoid-induced osteoporosis: prevention and treatment. *Steroids* May-Jun 1998, 63 (5-6) p344-8

Effect of ipriflavone—a synthetic derivative of natural isoflavones—on bone mass loss in the early years after menopause. *Menopause* Spring 1998, 5 (1) p9-15

Alendronate for the prevention and treatment of glucocorticoid-induced osteoporosis. Glucocorticoid-Induced osteoporosis Intervention Study Group. *N Engl J Med* Jul 30 1998, 339 (5) p292-9

Aminoterminal propeptide of type I procollagen (PINP) correlates to bone loss and predicts the efficacy of antiresorptive therapy in pre- and post-menopausal non-metastatic breast cancer patients. *Br J Cancer* (Scotland) Jul 1998, 78 (2) p240-5

Combining herbal supplements with prescription drugs. *Adv Nurse Pract* May 1998, 6 (5) p28

Relationship between exercise and bone mineral density among over 5,000 women aged 40 years and above. *J Epidemiol* (Japan) Mar 1998, 8 (1) p28-32

Alendronate for osteoporosis. Safe and efficacious nonhormonal therapy. *Can Fam Physician* (Canada) Feb 1998, 44 p327-32

Bone marker and bone density responses to dopamine agonist therapy in hyperprolactinemic males. *J Clin Endocrinol Metab* Mar 1998, 83 (3) p807-13

Clinical report on long-term bone density after short-term EMF application. *Bioelectromagnetics* 1998, 19 (2) p75-8

Epidemiology of medication-related falls and fractures in the elderly. *Drugs Aging* (New Zealand) Jan 1998, 12 (1) p43-53

Risedronate increases bone mass in an early postmenopausal population: two years of treatment plus one year of follow-up. *J Clin Endocrinol Metab* Feb 1998, 83 (2) p396-402,

Alendronate prevents postmenopausal bone loss in women without osteoporosis. A double-blind, randomized, controlled trial. Alendronate osteoporosis Prevention Study Group [see comments]. *Ann Intern Med* Feb 15 1998, 128 (4) p253-61

Prevention of bone loss with alendronate in postmenopausal women under 60 years of age. Earlytion Cohort Study Group. *N Engl J Med* Feb 19 1998, 338 (8) p485-92

Quantitative bone SPECT in young males with delayed puberty and hypogonadism: implications for treatment of low bone mineral density. *J Nucl Med* Jan 1998, 39 (1) p104-7

Annual Spring Meeting of the European Working Group on Cardiac Rehabilitation and Exercise Physiology, 22-23 May 1998, Bern Switzerland: Cardiac rehabilitation: Where are we going? *European Heart Journal* (UK), 1998, 19/Suppl. O (O5-O12)

Efficacy and tolerability of calcitonin in the prevention and treatment of osteoporosis. *BioDrugs* (New Zealand), 1998, 10/4 (295-300)

The estrogen receptor beta subtype: A novel mediator of estrogen action in neuroendocrine s. *Frontiers in Neuroendocrinology,* 1998, 19/4 (253-286)

Growth, development and differentiation: A functional food science approach. *British Journal of Nutrition* (UK), 1998, 80/Suppl. 1 (S5-S45)

Risks, benefits and costs of HRT in menopausal women. *Revue Medicale de Liege* (Belgium), 1998, 53/5 (298-304)

Bone-specific treatments of postmenopausal osteoporosis: Pharmaco- economic aspects. *Revue Medicale de Liege* (Belgium), 1998, 53/5 (290-293)

Osteoporosis as a candidate for disease management: Epidemiological and cost-of-illness considerations. *Disease Management and Health Outcomes* (New Zealand), 1998, 3/5 (207-214)

Osteoporosis in rheumatoid arthritis—Loss of bone mass in the early stage of the disease and the possibility to influence it by calcium and vitamin D. *Ceska Revmatologie* (Czech Republic), 1998, 6/2 (39-47)

Selective oestrogen receptor modulation: An alternative to conventional oestrogen. *Current Obstetrics and Gynaecology* (UK), 1998, 8/2 (96-101)

Hormone replacement therapy in women with diabetes mellitus: A survey of knowledge of risks and benefits. *Practical Diabetes International* (UK), 1998, 15/3 (78-81)

Prevention and therapy by hormone replacement therapy (HRT). *Fortschritt und Fortbildung in der Medizin* (Germany), 1998 1999, 22/- (27-34+329)

The effectiveness of exercises on treatment of postmenopausal osteoporosis. *Fizik Tedavi Rehabilitasyon Dergisi* (Turkey), 1997, 21/1 (20-24)

The BsmI vitamin D receptor restriction fragment length polymorphism (bb) influences the effect of calcium intake on bone mineral density. *Journal of Bone and Mineral Research,* 1997, 12/7 (1049-1057)

The effect of 1,25(OH)2 vitamin D3 on CD4+/CD8+ subsets of T lymphocytes in postmenopausal women. *Life Sciences*, 1997, 61/2 (147-152)

Acute changes in serum calcium and parathyroid hormone circulating levels induced by the oral intake of five currently available calcium salts in healthy male volunteers. *Clinical Rheumatology* (Belgium), 1997, 16/3 (249-253)

1-alpha-hydroxyvitamin D3 treatment decreases bone turnover and modulates calcium-regulating hormones in early postmenopausal women. *Bone,* 1997, 20/6 (557-562)

Nonestrogen management of menopausal symptoms. *Endocrinology and Metabolism Clinics of North America*, 1997, 26/2 (379-390)

Role of dietary lipid and antioxidants in bone metabolism. *Nutrition Research*, 1997, 17/7 (1209-1228)

The response to calcitriol therapy in postmenopausal osteoporotic women is a function of initial calcium absorptive status. *Calcified Tissue International,* 1997, 61/1 (6-9)

Bone mineral density changes during lactation: Maternal, dietary, and biochemical correlates. *American Journal of Clinical Nutrition*, 1997, 65/6 (1738-1746)

Postprandial parathyroid hormone response to four calcium-rich foodstuffs. *American Journal of Clinical Nutrition,* 1997, 65/6 (1726-1730)

Complementary medical treatment for Colles' fracture: A comparative, randomized, longitudinal study. *Calcified Tissue International*, 1997, 60/6 (567-570)

Treatment of postmenopausal osteoporosis: Spoilt for choice? Part 1—Foundations for an individually adapted management concept. *Munchener Medizinische Wochenschrift* (Germany), 1997, 139/20 (33-34+37-38)

Calcium and vitamin D in the prevention and treatment of osteoporosis. *Journal of Clinical Rheumatology,* 1997, 3/2 Suppl. (S52-S56)

Calcium intake and fracture risk: Results from the study of osteoporotic fractures. *American Journal of Epidemiology,* 1997, 145/10 (926-934)

Bone loss and turnover after cardiac transplantation. *Journal of Clinical Endocrinology and Metabolism*, 1997, 82/5 (1497-1506)

Effect of dietary calcium on urinary oxalate excretion after oxalate loads. *American Journal of Clinical Nutrition*, 1997, 65/5 (1453-1459)

1alpha-Hydroxyvitamin D2 partially dissociates between preservation of cancellous bone mass and effects on calcium homeostasis in ovariectomized rats. *Calcified Tissue International*, 1997, 60/5 (449-456)

What's hip in diet and osteoporosis? *Scandinavian Journal of Nutrition / Naringsforskning* (Sweden), 1997, 41/1 (2-8+12)

Prevention and management of osteoporosis. Current trends and future prospects. *Drugs* (New Zealand), 1997, 53/5 (727-735)

A high dietary calcium intake is needed for a positive effect on bone density in Swedish postmenopausal women. *Osteoporosis International* (UK), 1997, 7/2 (155-161)

Stress injury to bone in the female athlete. *Clinics in Sports Medicine*, 1997, 16/2 (197-224)

Amelioration of hemiplegia-associated osteopenia more than 4 years after stroke by 1alpha-hydroxyvitamin D3 and calcium supplementation. *Stroke,* 1997, 28/4 (736-739)

Effects of growth hormone (GH) replacement on bone metabolism and mineral density in adult onset of GH deficiency: Results of a double-blind placebo-controlled study with open follow-up. *European Journal of Endocrinology* (Norway), 1997, 136/3 (282-289)

Experimental study of glucocorticoid-induced rabbit osteoporosis. *Chinese Pharmacological Bulletin* (China), 1996, 12/6 (540-542)

Decreased serum IGF-I and dehydroepiandrosterone sulphate may be risk factors for the development of reduced bone mass in postmenopausal women with endogenous subclinical hyperthyroidism. *European Journal of Endocrinology* (Norway), 1997, 136/3 (277-281)

The usefulness of bone turnover in predicting the response to transdermal estrogen therapy in postmenopausal osteoporosis. *Journal of Bone and Mineral Research*, 1997, 12/4 (624-631)

Osteoporotic vertebral fractures in postmenopausal women. *American Family Physician*, 1997, 55/4 (1315-1322)

Proteins and bone health. *Pathologie Biologie* (France), 1997, 45/1 (57-59)

Osteoporosis: Prevention, diagnosis, and management. *American Journal of Medicine*, 1997, 102/1 A (35S-39S)

Serum vitamin D metabolites and calcium absorption in normal young and elderly free-living women and in women living in nursing homes. *American Journal of Clinical Nutrition*, 1997, 65/3 (790-797)

Long-term vegetarian diet and bone mineral density in postmenopausal Taiwanese women. *Calcified Tissue International*, 1997, 60/3 (245-249)

Effect of 1,25(OH)2 vitamin D3 on circulating insulin-like growth factor-I and beta2 microglobulin in patients with osteoporosis. *Calcified Tissue International*, 1997, 60/3 (236-239)

Influence of the vitamin D receptor gene alleles on bone mineral density in postmenopausal and osteoporotic women. *Journal of Bone and Mineral Research*, 1997, 12/2 (241-247)

Connections between phospho-calcium metabolism and bone turnover. Epidemiologic study on osteoporosis (second part). *Minerva Medica* (Italy), 1996, 87/12 (565-576)

Treatment of post-menopausal osteoporosis with recombinant human growth hormone and salmon calcitonin: A placebo controlled study. *Clinical Endocrinology* (UK), 1997, 46/1 (55-61)

Calcium regulation and bone mass loss after total gastrectomy in pigs. *Annals of Surgery,* 1997, 225/2 (181-192)

Management of osteoporosis in the elderly. *Journal of Geriatric Drug Therapy,* 1996, 11/1 (5-16)

Osteoporosis and bone mineral metabolism disorders in cirrhotic patients referred for orthotopic liver transplantation. *Calcified Tissue International*, 1997, 60/2 (148-154)

Effect of hormone replacement therapy on bone mineral content and fractures. *Ugeskrift for Laeger* (Denmark), 1997, 159/5 (570-576)

Effect of measuring bone mineral density on calcium intake. *Japanese Journal of Geriatrics* (Japan), 1996, 33/11 (840-846)

Estrogen therapy and osteoporosis: Principles and practice. *American Journal of the Medical Sciences,* 1997, 313/1 (2-12)

Alternatives to estrogen replacement therapy for preventing osteoporosis. *Journal of the American Pharmaceutical Association*, 1996,36/12 (707-715)

Osteoporosis: Its pediatric causes and prevention opportunities. *Primary Care Update for Ob / Gyns,* 1997, 4/1 (15-20)

Estimated dietary calcium intake and food sources for adolescent females: 1980-92. *Journal of Adolescent Health*, 1997, 20/1 (20-26)

The importance of genetic and nutritional factors in responses to vitamin D and its analogues in osteoporotic patients. *Calcified Tissue International*, 1997, 60/1 (119-123)

The pathogenesis of age-related osteoporotic fracture: Effects of dietary calcium deprivation. *Journal of Clinical Endocrinology and Metabolism*, 1997, 82/1 (260-264)

Increased catabolism of 25-hydroxyvitamin D in patients with partial gastrectomy and elevated 1,25-dihydroxyvitamin D levels. Implications for metabolic bone disease. *Journal of Clinical Endocrinology and Metabolism*, 1997, 82/1 (209-212)

Can the fast bone loss in osteoporotic and osteopenic patients be stopped with active vitamin D metabolites? *Calcified Tissue International*, 1997, 60/1 (115-118)

Is there a differential response to alfacalcidol and vitamin D in the treatment of osteoporosis? *Calcified Tissue International*, 1997, 60/1 (111-114)

Rationale for active vitamin D analogue therapy in senile osteoporosis. *Calcified Tissue International*, 1997, 60/1 (100-105)

Efficacy and safety of long-term, open-label treatment of calcitriol in postmenopausal osteoporosis: A retrospective analysis. *Current Therapeutic Research—Clinical and Experimental*, 1996, 57/11 (857-868)

Osteoporosis prevention and treatment. Pharmacological management and treatment implications. *Drugs and Aging* (New Zealand), 1996, 9/6 (472-477)

Magnesium deficiency: Possible role in osteoporosis associated with gluten-sensitive enteropathy. *Osteoporosis International* (UK), 1996, 6/6 (453-461)

Effects of vitamin B12 on cell proliferation and cellular alkaline phosphatase activity in human bone marrow stromal osteoprogenitor cells and UMR106 osteoblastic cells. *Metabolism: Clinical and Experimental,* 1996, 45/12 (1443-1446)

Calcium metabolism in the elderly. *Giornale di Gerontologia* (Italy), 1996, 44/2 (91-96)

Hormones, vitamins, and growth factors in cancer treatment and prevention: A critical appraisal. *Cancer,* 1996, 78/11 (2264-2280)

Therapy of osteoporosis: Calcium, vitamin D, and exercise. *American Journal of the Medical Sciences*, 1996, 312/6 (278-286)

Pathophysiology of osteoporosis. *American Journal of the Medical Sciences*, 1996, 312/6 (251-256)

Involutional osteoporosis in the elderly. *Giornale di Gerontologia* (Italy), 1996, 44/2 (85-89)

Osteoporosis and hormone replacement therapy. *Acta Chirurgica Austriaca* (Austria), 1996, 28/5 (263-265)

The effect of season and latitude on in vitro vitamin D formation by sunlight in South Africa. *South African Medical Journal* (South Africa), 1996, 86/10 (1270-1272)

Risk for osteoporosis in black women. *Calcified Tissue International*, 1996, 59/6 (415-423)

Age considerations in nutrient needs for bone health: Older adults. *Journal of the American College of Nutrition*, 1996, 15/6 (575-578)

Osteoporosis in lung transplantation candidates with end-stage pulmonary disease. *American Journal of Medicine*, 1996, 101/3 (262-269)

Dietary calcium intake and its relation to bone mineral density in patients with inflammatory bowel disease. *Journal of Internal Medicine* (UK), 1996, 240/5 (285-292)

Development of clinical practice guidelines for prevention and treatment of osteoporosis. 1 (S30-S33) *Calcified Tissue International*, 1996, 59/Suppl.

Harmonization of clinical practice guidelines for the prevention and treatment of osteoporosis and osteopenia in Europe: A difficult challenge. *Calcified Tissue International*, 1996, 59/Suppl. 1 (S24-S29)

Clinical practice guidelines for the diagnosis and management of osteoporosis. *Canadian Medical Association Journal* (Canada), 1996, 155/8 (1113-1129)

Current and potential future drug treatments for osteoporosis. *Annals of the Rheumatic Diseases* (UK), 1996, 55/10 (700-714)

Osteoporosis of the lumbar spine. *Schweizerische Rundschau fur Medizin / Praxis* (Switzerland), 1996, 85/43 (1354-1359)

Common polymorphism of the vitamin D receptor gene is associated with variation of peak bone mass in young Finns. *Calcified Tissue International*, 1996, 59/4 (231-234)

Diminished effect of etidronate in vitamin D deficient osteopenic postmenopausal women. *European Journal of Clinical Pharmacology* (Germany), 1996, 51/2 (145-147)

Vitamin D metabolites and analogues in the treatment of osteoporosis. *Canadian Medical Association Journal* (Canada), 1996, 155/7 (955-961)

Calcium nutrition and osteoporosis. *Canadian Medical Association Journal* (Canada), 1996, 155/7 (935-939)

Interrelationships of food, nutrition, diet and health: The national association of state universities and land grant colleges white paper. *Journal of the American College of Nutrition*, 1996, 15/5 (422-433)

Osteoporosis of Crohn's disease: A critical review. *Canadian Journal of Gastroenterology* (Canada), 1996, 10/5 (317-321)

Effect of Vitamin D receptor gene polymorphism on vitamin D therapy for postmenopausal bone loss. *Acta Obstetrica et Gynaecologica Japonica* (Japan), 1996, 48/9 (799-805)

The preparation and stability of compound active calcium tablets. *Chinese Pharmaceutical Journal* (China), 1996, 31/8 (474-477)

Immunosuppression: Tightrope walk between iatrogenic side effects and therapy. *Schweizerische Medizinische Wochenschrift* (Switzerland), 1996, 126/38 (1603-1609)

Secondary osteoporosis in rheumatic diseases. *Ceska Revmatologie* (Czech Republic), 1996, 4/2 (51-57)

Does lactose intolerance predispose to low bone density? A population-based study of perimenopausal Finnish women. *Bone*, 1996, 19/1 (23-28)

Glucocorticoid-induced osteoporosis. *Medecine et Hygiene* (Switzerland), 1996, 54/2127 (1490-1495)

Relation of common allelic variation at vitamin D receptor locus to bone mineral density and postmenopausal bone loss: Cross sectional and longitudinal population study. *British Medical Journal* (UK), 1996, 313/7057 (586-590)

Nutrition and women's health. *Current Problems in Obstetrics, Gynecology and Fertility,* 1996, 19/4 (112-166)

Systemic osteoporosis in rheumatoid arthritis. Pathogenetic mechanisms and therapeutic approaches. *Zeitschrift fur Rheumatologie* (Germany), 1996, 55/3 (149-157)

Current treatment options for osteoporosis. *Journal of Rheumatology* (Canada), 1996, 23/Suppl. 45 (11-14)

Treatments for oestoporosis. *Revue Francaise de Gynecologie et d'Obstetrique* (France), 1996, 91/6 (329-334)

Estrogen replacement may be an alternative to parathyroid surgery for the treatment of osteoporosis in elderly postmenopausal women presenting with primary hyperparathyroidism: A preliminary report. *Osteoporosis International* (UK), 1996, 6/4 (329-333)

A comparison of the effects of alfacalcidol treatment and vitamin D2 supplementation on calcium absorption in elderly women with vertebral fractures. *Osteoporosis International* (UK), 1996, 6/4 (284-290)

The effect of calcium supplementation and Tanner Stage on bone density, content and area in teenage women. *Osteoporosis International* (UK), 1996, 6/4 (276-283)

Corticosteroid induced osteoporosis. *Journal of Rheumatology* (Canada), 1996, 23/Suppl. 45 (19-22)

The role of vitamin D in the pathogenesis and treatment of osteoporosis. *Journal of Rheumatology* (Canada), 1996, 23/ Suppl. 45 (15-18)

Review: Treatment of primary biliary cirrhosis. *Journal of Gastroenterology and Hepatology* (Australia),1996, 11/7 (605-609)

Osteoporosis. *Physical Medicine and Rehabilitation Clinics of North America*, 1996, 7/3 (583-599)

Nutritional and biochemical studies on vitamin D and its active derivatives. *Yakugaku Zasshi* (Japan), 1996, 116/6 (457-472)

Osteoporosis and calcium ingest. *Progresos en Obstetricia y Ginecologia* (Spain), 1996, 39/4 (289-292)

Lower serum 25-hydroxyvitamin D is associated with increased bone resorption markers and lower bone density at the proximal femur in normal females: A population-based study. *Experimental and Clinical Endocrinology and Diabetes* (Germany), 1996, 104/3 (289-292)

Hormone therapy and phytoestrogens. *Journal of Clinical Pharmacy and Therapeutics* (UK), 1996, 21/2 (101-111)

Recent progress in treatment of osteoporosis. *Japanese Journal of Geriatrics* (Japan), 1996, 33/4 (240-244)

Vitamin D and calcium in the prevention of corticosteroid induced osteoporosis: A 3 year followup. *Journal of Rheumatology* (Canada), 1996, 23/6 (995-1000)

Novelties and issues in the drug market 1995. *Ricerca e Pratica* (Italy), 1996, 12/68 (63-71)

Influence of life style in the MEDOS study. *Scandinavian Journal of Rheumatology, Supplement* (Norway), 1996, 25/103 (112)

Roles of diet and physical activity in the prevention of osteoporosis. *Scandinavian Journal of Rheumatology, Supplement* (Norway), 1996, 25/103 (65-74)

The problem: Health impact of osteoporosis. *Scandinavian Journal of Rheumatology, Supplement* (Norway), 1996, 25/103 (3-5)

Vitamin D in the treatment of osteoporosis revisited. *Proceedings of the Society for Experimental Biology and Medicine*, 1996, 212/2 (110-115)

Prevention of bone loss in cardiac transplant recipients: A comparison of biphosphonates and vitamin D. *Transplantation*, 1996, 61/10 (1495-1499)

Prophylaxis of osteoporosis with calcium, estrogens and/or eelcatonin: Comparative longitudinal study of bone mass. *Maturitas* (Ireland), 1996, 23/3 (327-332)

Open-label, controlled study on the metabolic and absorptiometric effects of calcitriol in involutional osteoporosis. *Clinical Drug Investigation* (New Zealand), 1996, 11/5 (270-277)

Nutritional prevention of aging osteoporosis. *Cahiers de Nutrition et de Dietetique* (France), 1996, 31/2 (98-101)

Effects of 2 years' treatment of osteoporosis with 1alpha-hydroxy vitamin D3 on bone mineral density and incidence of fracture: A placebo-controlled, double-blind prospective study. *Endocrine Journal* (Japan), 1996, 43/2 (211-220)

Osteoporotic fractures: Background and prevention strategies. *Maturitas* (Ireland), 1996, 23/2 (193-207)

Energy and nutrient intake in patients with CF. *Monatsschrift fur Kinderheilkunde* (Germany), 1996, 144/4 (396-402)

Current and future nonhormonal approaches to the treatment of osteoporosis. *International Journal of Fertility and Menopausal Studies*, 1996, 41/2 (148-155)

Dietary protein intake and bone mass in women. *Calcified Tissue International*, 1996, 58/5 (320-325)

1,25-Dihydroxyvitamin D3 enhances the enzymatic activity and expression of the messenger ribonucleic acid for aromatase cytochrome P450 synergistically with dexamethasone depending on the vitamin D receptor level in cultured human osteoblasts. *Endocrinology*, 1996, 137/5 (1860-1869)

Effects of hormonal therapies and dietary soy phytoestrogens on vaginal cytology in surgically postmenopausal macaques. *Fertility and Sterility*, 1996, 65/5 (1031-1035)

Transient osteoporosis of the hip. Case report and review of the literature. *Acta Orthopaedica Belgica* (Belgium), 1996, 62/1 (56-59)

Osteomalacia and osteoporosis in a woman with ankylosing spondylitis. *Journal of Bone and Mineral Research*, 1996, 11/5 (697-703)

Evaluation of acceptability, tolerance and observance of a new calcium-vitamine D combination. *Rhumatologie* (France), 1996, 48/2 (37-42)

Sequential effects of chronic human PTH (1-84) treatment of estrogen-deficiency osteopenia in the rat. *Journal of Bone and Mineral Research*, 1996, 11/4 (430-439)

Effects of vitamin K on bone mass and bone metabolism. *Journal of Nutrition*, 1996, 126/4 Suppl. (1187S-1191S)

Calcium and vitamin D nutritional needs of elderly women. *Journal of Nutrition*, 1996, 126/4 Suppl. (1165S-1167S)

Vitamin D and bone health. *Journal of Nutrition*, 1996, 126/4 Suppl. (1159S-1164S)

Influence of ovariectomy on bone metabolism in very old rats. *Calcified Tissue International*, 1996, 58/4 (256-262)

Heated oyster shell-seaweed calcium (AAA Ca) on osteoporosis. *Calcified Tissue International*, 1996, 58/4 (226-230)

Age-related factors in the pathogenesis of senile (type II) femoral neck fractures: An integrated view. *American Journal of Orthopedics*, 1996, 25/3 (198-204)

Protein consumption and bone fractures in women. *American Journal of Epidemiology*, 1996, 143/5 (472-479)

The epidemiology of osteoporosis: The oriental perspective in a world context. *Clinical Orthopaedics and Related Research*, 1996, /323 (65-74)

Comparison of nonrandomized trials with slow-release sodium fluoride with a randomized placebo-controlled trial in postmenopausal osteoporosis. *Journal of Bone and Mineral Research,* 1996, 11/2 (160-168)

Stimulation of the growth of femoral trabecular bone in ovariectomized rats by the novel parathyroid hormone fragment, hPTH-(1-31)NH2 (Ostabolin). *Calcified Tissue International,* 1996, 58/2 (81-87)

The lack of influence of long-term potassium citrate and calcium citrate treatment in total body aluminum burden in patients with functioning kidneys. *Journal of the American College of Nutrition*, 1996, 15/1 (102-106)

Kidney stone clinic: Ten years of experience. *Nederlands Tijschrift voor de Klinische Chemie* (Netherlands), 1996, 21/1 (8-10)

Calcium deficiency in fluoride-treated osteoporotic patients despite calcium supplementation. *Journal of Clinical Endocrinology and Metabolism*, 1996, 81/1 (269-275)

Endocrinology. *Medecine et Hygiene* (Switzerland), 1996, 54/2100 (85-95)

Dietary soybean protein prevents bone loss in an ovariectomized rat model of osteoporosis. *Journal of Nutrition*, 1996, 126/1 (161-167)

Bone density in children and adolescents with cystic fibrosis. *Journal of Pediatrics*, 1996, 128/1 (28-34)

Axial bone mass in older women. *Annals of Internal Medicine*, 1996, 124/2 (187-196)

Bone mineral density in mother-daughter pairs: Relations to lifetime exercise, lifetime milk consumption, and calcium supplements. *American Journal of Clinical Nutrition*, 1996, 63/1 (72-79)

Is postmenopausal osteoporosis related to pineal gland functions? *Int J Neurosci* (England) Feb 1992, 62 (3-4) p215-25

Glucocorticoid-induced osteoporosis: mechanisms for bone loss; evaluation of strategies for prevention. *J Gerontol* Sep 1990, 45 (5) pM153-8

Progesterone as a bone-trophic hormone. *Endocr Rev* May 1990, 11 (2) p386-98

Osteocalcin and its message: relationship to bone histology in magnesium-deprived rats. *Am J Physiol* Jul 1992, 263 (1 Pt 1) pE107-14

[Influence of active vitamine D3 on bones]. *Nippon Seikeigeka Gakkai Zasshi* (Japan) Dec 1979, 53 (12) p1823-37

Relation of magnesium to osteoporosis and calcium urolithiasis. *Magnes Trace Elem* (Switzerland) 92 1991, 10 (2-4) p281-6

Role of vitamin D, its metabolites, and analogues in the management of osteoporosis. *Rheum Dis Clin North Am* Aug 1994, 20 (3) p759-75

Anabolic steroids in corticosteroid-induced osteoporosis. *Wien Med Wochenschr* (Austria) 1993, 143 (14-15) p395-7

Osteocalcin and its message: relationship to bone histology in magnesium-deprived rats. *Am J Physiol* Jul 1992, 263 (1 Pt 1) pE107-14

Glucocorticoid-induced osteoporosis: mechanisms for bone loss; evaluation of strategies for prevention. *J Gerontol* Sep 1990, 45 (5) pM153-8

Nutritional insurance supplementation and corticosteroid toxicity. *Med Hypotheses* (England) Aug 1982, 9 (2) p145-56

Effects of recombinant human growth hormone (GH) on bone and intermediary metabolism in patients receiving chronic glucocorticoid treatment with suppressed endogenous GH response to GH-releasing hormone. *J Clin Endocrinol Metab* Jan 1995, 80 (1) p122-9

Human marrow stromal osteoblast-like cells do not show reduced responsiveness to in vitro stimulation with growth hormone in patients with postmenopausal osteoporosis. *Calcif Tissue Int* Jan 1994, 54 (1) p1-6

Growth hormone and bone. *Horm Metab Res* (Germany) Jul 1993, 25 (7) p335-43

Growth hormone and bone. *Horm Res* (Switzerland) 1991, 36 Suppl 1 p49-55

Aromatase in bone cell: association with osteoporosis in postmenopausal women. *J Steroid Biochem Mol Biol* (England) Jun 1995, 53 (1-6) p165-74

Biological properties and clinical application of propolis. VIII. Experimental observation on the influence of ethanol extract of propolis (EEP) on the regeneration of bone tissue. *Arzneim.-Forsch.* (Germany, West), 1978, 28/1 (35-37)

Pain

Enhancement of a kappa-opioid receptor agonist-induced analgesia by L-tyrosine and L-tryptophan. *Eur J Pharmacol* (Netherlands) Jun 13 1994, 258 (3) p173-8

L-Tyrosine-induced antinociception in the mouse: involvement of central delta-opioid receptors and bulbo-spinal noradrenergic system. *Eur J Pharmacol* (Netherlands) Mar 23 1993, 233 (2-3) P255-60

L-dopa induces opposing effects on pain in intact rats: (-)-sulpiride, SCH 23390 or alpha-methyl-DL-p-tyrosine methylester hydrochloride reveals profound hyperalgesia in large antinociceptive doses. *J Pharmacol Exp Ther* Nov 1992, 263 (2) p470-9

Dietary influences on neurotransmission. *Adv Pediatr* 1986, 33 p23-47

Pancreatic Cancer

See references under Cancer.

Parathyroid (Hyperparathyroidism)

Analgesic effect of L-arginine in patients with persistent pain. *Eur Neuropsychopharmacol* (Netherlands) Dec 1991, 1 (4) p529-33

Mood, performance, and pain sensitivity: changes induced by food constituents. *J Psychiatr Res* (England) 83 1982, 17 (2) p135-45

Studies of the analgesic effects of L-arginine on chronic pain. *Journal of the Medical Society of Toho University* (Japan) 1997, 43/5 (554-559)

Vitamin D3 and calcium to prevent hip fractures in the elderly women. *N Engl J Med* 1992 Dec 3;327(23):1637-42

Effect of hormone replacement therapy on bone mineral density in postmenopausal women with mild primary hyperparathyroidism. A randomized, controlled trial. *Ann Intern Med.* 1996 Sep 1;125(5):360-8.

Hyperparathyroidism. *Otolaryngol Clin North Am* 1996 Aug;29(4):663-79

Estrogen replacement may be an alternative to parathyroid surgery for the treatment of osteoporosis in elderly postmenopausal women presenting with primary hyperparathyroidism: a preliminary report. *Osteoporos Int* 1996;6(4):329-33

Vitamin D supplementation, 25-hydroxyvitamin D concentrations, and safety. *Am J Clin Nutr* 1999 May;69(5):842-56

Long-term treatment with calcium-alpha-ketoglutarate corrects secondary hyperparathyroidism. *Miner Electrolyte Metab* 1996;22(1-3):196-9

Ultraviolet irradiation corrects vitamin D deficiency and suppresses secondary hyperparathyroidism in the elderly. *J Bone Miner Res* Aug 1998, 13 (8) p1238-42

Calcium and vitamin D are effective in preventing fractures in elderly people by reversing senile secondary hyperparathyroidism. *Osteoporosis International* (UK), 1998, 8/Suppl. 2 (S1-S2)

Clinical profile of primary hyperparathyroidism in adolescents and young adults. *Clin Endocrinol* (Oxf) (England) Apr 1998, 48 (4) p435-43

Different effects of PTH on erythrocyte calcium influx. *Italian Journal of Mineral and Electrolyte Metabolism* (Italy), 1996, 10/3-4 (149-152)

Hypercalcemia due to constitutive activity of the parathyroid hormone (PTH)/PTH-related peptide receptor: Comparison with primary hyperparathyroidism. *Journal of Clinical Endocrinology and Metabolism*, 1996, 81/10 (3584-3588)

Osteoclast cytomorphometry in patients with femoral neck fracture. *Pathology Research and Practice* (Germany), 1996, 192/6 (573-578)

Combined therapy with salmon calcitonin and high doses of active vitamin D3 metabolites in uremic hyperparathyroidism. *Polskie Archiwum Medycyny Wewnetrznej* (Poland), 1996, 96/1 (23-31)

The PTH-calcium relationship curve in secondary hyperparathyroidism, an index of sensitivity and suppressibility of parathyroid glands. *Nephrology Dialysis Transplantation* (UK), 1996, 11/Suppl. 3 (136-141)

Severe acute pancreatitis as a first symptom of primary hyperparathyroid adenoma: A case report. *Journal of Laryngology and Otology* (UK), 1996, 110/6 (602-603)

24,25 dihydroxyvitamin D supplementation corrects hyperparathyroidism and improves skeletal abnormalities in X-linked hypophosphatemic rickets —A clinical research center study. *Journal of Clinical Endocrinology and Metabolism*, 1996, 81/6 (2381-2388)

1-alpha-hydroxyvitamin D3 treatment decreases bone turnover and modulates calcium-regulating hormones in early postmenopausal women. *Bone,* 1997, 20/6 (557-562)

Role of parathyroid hormone-related peptide (PTHrP) in hypercalcemia of malignancy and the development of osteolytic metastases. *Journal of Clinical Rheumatology,* 1997, 3/2 Suppl. (S109-S113)

Experimental study of glucocorticoid-induced rabbit osteoporosis. *Chinese Pharmacological Bulletin* (China), 1996, 12/6 (540-542)

Medical parathyroidectomy—The value of vitamin D. *Acta Chirurgica Austriaca* (Austria), 1996, 28/Suppl. 124 (8-10)

Oral vitamin D or calcium carbonate in the prevention of renal bone disease? *Current Opinion in Nephrology and Hypertension*

Estrogen replacement may be an alternative to parathyroid surgery for the treatment of osteoporosis in elderly postmenopausal women presenting with primary hyperparathyroidism: A preliminary report. *Osteoporosis International* (UK), 1996, 6/4 (329-333)

A comparison of the effects of alfacalcidol treatment and vitamin D2 supplementation on calcium absorption in elderly women with vertebral fractures. *Osteoporosis International* (UK), 1996, 6/4 (284-290)

Comparison of effects of calcitriol and calcium carbonate on secretion of interleukin-1beta and tumour necrosis factor-alpha by uraemic peripheral blood mononuclear cells. *Nephrology Dialysis Transplantation* (UK), 1996, 11/Suppl. 3 (15-21)

Hyperparathyroidism. *Otolaryngologic Clinics of North America*, 1996, 29/4 (663-679)

Intradialytic calcium balances with different calcium dialysate levels. Effects on cardiovascular stability and parathyroid function. *Nephron* (Switzerland), 1996, 72/4 (530-535)

Influence of ovariectomy on bone metabolism in very old rats. *Calcified Tissue International*, 1996, 58/4 (256-262)

Biochemical effects of calcium and vitamin D supplementation in elderly, institutionalized, vitamin D-deficient patients. *Revue du Rhumatisme* (English Edition) (France), 1996, 63/2 (135-140)

Long-term treatment with calcium-alpha-ketoglutarate corrects secondary hyperparathyroidism. *Mineral and Electrolyte Metabolism* (Switzerland), 1996, 22/1-3 (196-199)

Long-term effect of intravenous calcitriol on the treatment of severe hyperparathyroidism, parathyroid gland mass and bone mineral density in haemodialysis patients. *Am J Nephrol* (Switzerland) 1997, 17 (2) p118-23

Calcitriol in the management of secondary hyperparathyroidism of renal failure. *Pharmacotherapy* Jul-Aug 1996, 16 (4) p619-30

Parathyroid hormone increases bone formation and improves mineral balance in vitamin D-deficient female rats. *Endocrinology* Jun 1997, 138 (6) p2449-57

Effects on bone mineral density of low-dosed oral contraceptives compared to and combined with physical activity. *Contraception* Feb 1997, 55 (2) p87-90

The importance of genetic and nutritional factors in responses to vitamin D and its analogues in osteoporotic patients. *Calcif Tissue Int* Jan 1997, 60 (1) p119-23

Effective suppression of parathyroid hormone by 1 alpha-hydroxy-vitamin D2 in hemodialysis patients with moderate to severe secondary hyperparathyroidism. *Kidney Int* Jan 1997, 51 (1) p317-23

The rise and fall of primary hyperparathyroidism: a population-based study in Rochester, Minnesota, 1965-1992. *Ann Intern Med* Mar 15 1997, 126 (6) p433-40

Effects of 12 months of growth hormone (GH) treatment on calciotropic hormones, calcium homeostasis, and bone metabolism in adults with acquired GH deficiency: a double blind, randomized, placebo-controlled study. *J Clin Endocrinol Metab* Sep 1996, 81 (9) p3352-9

Acute biochemical effects of growth hormone treatment compared with conventional treatment in familial hypophosphataemic rickets. *Clin Endocrinol* (Oxf) (England) Jun 1996, 44 (6) p687-96

Calcium, phosphate, vitamin D, and the parathyroid. *Pediatric Nephrology* (Germany), 1996, 10/3 (364-367)

Vitamin D metabolism in chronic childhood hypoparathyroidism: Evidence for a direct regulatory effect of calcium. *J. Pediatr.*, 1990, 116/2 (252-257)

Determinants for serum 1,25-dihydroxycholecalciferol in primary hyperparathyroidism. *Bone Miner.* (Netherlands), 1989, 5/3 (279-290)

Magnesium hormonal regulation and metabolic interrelations. *Presse Med.* (France), 1988, 17/12 (584-587)

Treatment with active vitamin D (alphacalcidol) in patients with mild primary hyperparathyroidism. *Acta Endocrinol.* (Denmark), 1989, 120/2 (250-256)

Intravenous 1,25(OH)2 vitamin D3 therapy in haemodialysis patients: Evaluation of direct and calcium-mediated short-term effects on serum parathyroid hormone concentration.

Calcium, phosphate, vitamin D, and the parathyroid. *Pediatric Nephrology* (Germany), 1996, 10/3 (364-367)

Vitamin D metabolism in chronic childhood hypoparathyroidism: Evidence for a direct regulatory effect of calcium. *J. Pediatr.*, 1990, 116/2 (252-257)

Determinants for serum 1,25-dihydroxycholecalciferol in primary hyperparathyroidism. *Bone Miner.* (Netherlands), 1989, 5/3 (279-290)

Magnesium hormonal regulation and metabolic interrelations. Regulation hormonale et interrelations metaboliques du magnesium. *Presse Med.* (France), 1988, 17/12 (584-587)

Treatment with active vitamin D (alphacalcidol) in patients with mild primary hyperparathyroidism. *Acta Endocrinol.* (Denmark), 1989, 120/2 (250-256)

Intravenous 1,25(OH)2 vitamin D3 therapy in haemodialysis patients: Evaluation of direct and calcium-mediated short-term effects on serum parathyroid hormone concentration. *Nephrol. Dial. Transplant.* (Germany, Federal Republic of), 1990, 5/6 (457-460)

Parkinson's Disease

Cerebrospinal fluid carnitine levels in patients with Parkinson's disease. *J Neurol Sci* Feb 12 1997, 145 (2) p183-5

Further insights into the influence of L-cysteine on the oxidation chemistry of dopamine: reaction pathways of potential relevance to Parkinson' s disease. *Chem Res Toxicol* Jun 1996, 9 (4) p751-63

A significant reduction of putative transmitter amino acids in cerebrospinal fluid of patients with Parkinson's disease and spinocerebellar degeneration. *Neurosci Lett* May 27 1991, 126 (2) p155-8

Clinical pharmacodynamics of acetyl-L-carnitine in patients with Parkinson's disease. *Int J Clin Pharmacol Res* 1990, 10 (1-2) p139-43

Alteration of amino acids in cerebrospinal fluid from patients with Parkinson's disease and spinocerebellar degeneration. *Acta Neurol Scand* Feb 1986, 73 (2) p105-10

Irreversible inhibition of mitochondrial complex I by 7-(2-aminoethyl)- 3,4-dihydro-5-hydroxy-2H-1,4-benzothiazine-3-carboxylic acid (DHBT-1): A putative nigral endotoxin of relevance to Parkinson's disease. *Journal of Neurochemistry* 1997, 69/4(1530-1541)

Octacosanol in parkinsonism [letter] *Ann Neurol* Dec 1984, 16 (6) p723

L-tryptophan supplementation in Parkinson's disease. *Int J Neurosci* Apr 1989, 45 (3-4) p215-9

Effect of a controlled low- protein diet on the pharmacological response to levodopa and on the plasma levels of L-dopa and amino acids in patients with Parkinson's disease] *Arch Neurobiol* Nov-Dec 1991, 54 (6) p296-302

Dietary modification of Parkinson's disease. *Eur J Clin Nutr* May 1991, 45 (5) p263-6

On-off phenomenon in Parkinson's disease: relationship between dopa and other large neutral amino acids in plasma. *Neurology* Aug 1988, 38 (8) p1245-8

Amount and distribution of dietary protein affects clinical response to levodopa in Parkinson's disease. *Neurology* Apr 1989, 39 (4) p552-6

Practical application of a low- protein diet for Parkinson's disease. *Neurology* Jul 1988, 38 (7) p1026-31

Protein intake and treatment of Parkinson's disease with levodopa. *New England Journal of Medicine* 1975, 292/3(181-184)

Decreased cerebrospinal fluid levels of neutral and basic amino acids in patients with Parkinson's disease. *J Neurol Sci* Sep 10 1997, 150 (2) p123-7

Striatal dopamine depletion, dopamine receptor stimulation, and GABA metabolism: Implications for the therapy of Parkinson's disease. *Annals of Neurology* 1986, 19/2

Brain neurotransmitters and neuropeptides in Parkinson's disease *Acta Physiologica et Pharmacologica Latinoamericana* 1984, 34/3 (287-299)

Effects of oral L- tyrosine administration on CSF tyrosine and homovanillic acid levels in patients with Parkinson's disease. *Life Sci* Mar 8 1982 , 30 (10) p827-32

L-tryptophan supplementation in Parkinson's disease. *Int J Neurosci* Apr 1989, 45 (3-4) p215-9

L-tryptophan: a rational anti-depressant and a natural hypnotic? *Aust N Z J Psychiatry* (Australia) Mar 1988, 22 (1) p83-97

L-dopa-induced psychoses and their treatment with L-tryptophan] *Fortschr Med* Apr 30 1986, 104 (17) p360-2

Tryptophan deficiency stupor--a new psychiatric syndrome. *Acta Psychiatr Scand Suppl* 1982, 300 p1-57

L-dopa competes with tyrosine and tryptophan for human brain uptake. *Nutr Metab* 1980, 24 (6) p417-23

L-tryptophan administration in L-dopa-induced hallucinations in elderly Parkinsonian patients. *Gerontology* 1977, 23 (6) p438-44

Normalization of brain serotonin by L-tryptophan in levodopa-treated rats. *Neurology* Sep 1975, 25 (9) p861-5

L-tryptophan in the treatment of levodopa induced psychiatric disorders. *Disease of the Nervous System* 1974, 35/1 (20-23)

Rotations induced by L-dopa in parkinsonian rats are reduced by an ingestion of amino acids. *J Neural Transm Park Dis Dement Sect* 1993, 6 (3) p211-4

Bioavailability of levodopa after consumption of Vicia faba seedlings by parkinsonian patients and control subjects. *Clinical Neuropharmacology* 1994, 17/2 (138-146)

Long-term efficacy and safety of deprenyl (selegiline) in advanced Parkinson's disease. *Neurology* 1989, 39/8 (1109-1111)

Effect of chronic levodopa treatment on pyridoxine metabolism. *Neurology* Mar 1975, 25 (3) p263-6

Treatment of obsessive compulsive neurosis: pharmacological approach. *Psychosomatics* 1976, 17/4 (180-184)

Vitamins, neuroleptics, and antiparkinsonian drugs in catecholamine excretion. *Biological Psychiatry* 1976, 11/3 (363-366)

Involuntary movements induced by levodopa. *Schweizerische Medizinische Wochenschrift* 1975, 105/4 (121-124)

Interactions between levodopa and other drugs: significance in the treatment of Parkinson's disease. *Drugs*1973, 6/5-6 (364-388)

Antiparkinsonian therapies and brain mitochondrial complex I activity. *Mov Disord* May 1995, 10 (3) p312-7

Letter: Ascorbic acid in levodopa therapy. *Lancet* Mar 1 1975, 1 (7905) p527

Ascorbic acid in levodopa therapy. *Lancet* 1975, I/7905 (527)

[Treatment of complicated Parkinson disease with a solution of levodopa-carbidopa and ascorbic acid]. *Neurologia* Jun-Jul 1995, 10 (6) p220-3

Case-control study of early life dietary factors in Parkinson's disease. *Arch Neurol* Dec 1988, 45 (12) p1350-3

Raised cerebrospinal-fluid copper concentration in Parkinson's disease. *Lancet* Aug 1 1987, 2 (8553) p238-41

The cerebrospinal-fluid copper concentration, measured by Genetic and environmental risk factors in Parkinson's disease. *Clin Neurol Neurosurg* Mar 1998, 100 (1) p15-26

Environmental antecedents of young-onset Parkinson's disease. *Neurology* Jun 1993, 43 (6) p1150-8

[Mortality from Parkinson's disease in Spain (1980-1985). Distribution by age, sex and geographic areas]. *Neurologia* 1992, 7 (3) p89-93

[Parkinson's disease and environmental factors] *Rev Epidemiol Sante Publique* 1991, 39 (4) p373-87

A rationale for monoamine oxidase inhibition as neuroprotective therapy for Parkinson's disease. *Mov Disord* 1993, 8 Suppl 1 pS1-7

Neuromelanin-containing neurons of the substantia nigra accumulate iron and aluminum in Parkinson's disease: a LAMMA study. *Brain Res* Oct 16 1992, 593 (2) p343-6

Iron in brain function and dysfunction with emphasis on Parkinson's disease. *Eur Neurol* 1991, 31 Suppl 1 p34-40

Depletion of nigrostriatal and forebrain tyrosine hydroxylase by S-adenosylmethionine: a model that may explain the occurrence of depression in Parkinson's disease. *Life Sci* 1997, 61 (5) p495-502

Parkinson's disease-like effects of S-adenosyl-L- methionine: effects of L-dopa. *Pharmacol Biochem Behav* Oct 1992, 43 (2) p423-31

Diet and Parkinson's disease II: A possible role for the past intake of specific nutrients. Results from a self-administered food-frequency questionnaire in a case-control study *Neurology* 1996, 47/3 (644-650)

L-dopa treatment and Parkinson's disease. *Quarterly Journal of Medicine* 1986,59/230 (535-547)

Results of treatment of Parkinson's disease with carbidopa and levodopa. *Rev. Fac. Cienc. Med. Univ. Cordoba* 1974, 32/2 (161-174)

Oxidative stress and antioxidant therapy in Parkinson's disease. *Prog Neurobiol* Jan 1996, 48 (1) p1-19

Treatment of Parkinson's disease. From theory to practice. *Postgrad Med* Apr 1994, 95 (5) p52-4, 57-8, 61-4

Neuroprotection by anti-oxidant strategies in Parkinson's disease. *Eur Neurol* 1993, 33 Suppl 1 p24-30

Concentrations of vitamins A, C and E in elderly patients with Parkinson's disease. *Postgrad Med J* Aug 1992, 68 (802) p634-7

Detection of subclinical ascorbate deficiency in early Parkinson's disease. *Public Health* Sep 1992, 106 (5) p393-5

Oxidative stress as a cause of nigral cell death in Parkinson's disease and incidental Lewy body disease. *Ann Neurol* 1992, 32 Suppl pS82-7

Vitamin E therapy in Parkinson's disease. *Adv Neurol* 1990, 53 p457-61

Cerebrospinal fluid choline levels are decreased in Parkinson's disease [see comments]. *Ann Neurol* Jun 1990, 27 (6) p683-5

Brain muscarinic receptor subtypes are differently affected in Alzheimer's disease and Parkinson's disease. *Brain Res* Apr 3 1989, 483 (2) p402-6

GABAA receptor but not muscarinic receptor density was decreased in the brain of patients with Parkinson's disease. *Jpn J Pharmacol* Nov 1988, 48 (3) p331-9

Clinical trial on the use of cytidine diphosphate choline in Parkinson's disease. *Clin Ther* 1988, 10 (6) p664-71

Neurochemical basis of dementia in Parkinson's disease. *Can J Neurol Sci* Feb 1984, 11 (1 Suppl) p185-90

Lecithin in Parkinson's disease. *J Neural Transm Suppl* 1980, (16) p187-93

Vitamin E and Parkinson's. *Neurologia* 1998, 13/6 (292-296)

Treatment of Parkinson's syndrome. *Fortschritte der Medizin* 1986, 104/44 (41-47)

Co-dergocrine (Hydergine) regulates striatal and hippocampal acetylcholine release through D-2 receptors. *Neuroreport* 5 (6):p674-676 1994

Co-dergocrine (Hydergine) regulates striatal and hippocampal acetylcholine release through D-2 receptors. *Neuroreport* 5 (6):p674-676 1994

Absorption, tolerability, and effects on mitochondrial activity of oral coenzyme Q10 in parkinsonian patients. *Neurology* 50: 793-795, Mar 1998.1 March 1998 (19980301)

Coenzyme Q-10 levels correlated with the activities of complexes I and II/III in mitochondria from Parkinsonian and nonparkinsonian subjects. *Annals of Neurology* 42 (2):p261-264 1997

Neuroprotective strategies for treatment of lesions produced by mitochondrial toxins: Implications for neurodegenerative diseases. *Neuroscience* 71 (4):p1043-1048 1996

Coenzyme Q-10 and nicotinamide and a free radical spin trap protect against MPTP neurotoxicity. *Experimental Neurology* 132 (2):p279-283 1995

Different control mechanisms of growth hormone (GH) secretion between gamma-amino- and gamma-hydroxy-butyric acid: Neuroendocrine evidence in Parkinson's disease. *Psychoneuroendocrinology* 22 (7):p531-538 Oct., 1997

Distinction of idiopathic Parkinson's disease from multiple-system atrophy by stimulation of growth-hormone release with clonidine. *Lancet* 349 (9069):p1877-1881 1997

A study of dopaminergic sensitivity in Parkinson's disease: Comparison in "de novo" and levodopa-treated patients. *Clinical Neuropharmacology* 19 (5):p420-427 1996

Corticotropin-releasing factor receptors: Physiology, pharmacology, biochemistry and role in central nervous system and immune disorders. *Psychoneuroendocrinology* 20 (8):p789-819 1995

Psychotic and depressive symptoms in Parkinson's disease: A study of the growth hormone response to apomorphine. *British Journal of Psychiatry* 167 (4):p522-526 1995

Lack of ACTH/cortisol and GH responses to intravenously-infused substance P in Parkinson's disease. *Journal of Neural Transmission Parkinson's Disease and Dementia* Section 6 (2):p99-107 1993

Beta-Adrenoceptor expression on circulating mononuclear cells of idiopathic Parkinson's disease and autonomic failure patients before and after reduction of central sympathetic outflow by clonidine. *Neurology* 43 (6):p1181-1187 1993

Somatostatin In Alzheimer's Disease And Depression. *Life Sci* 51 (18). 1992. 1389-1410.

Plasma Profiles Of Acth Cortisol Growth Hormone And Prolactin In Patients With Untreated Parkinson's Disease. *J Neurol* 238 (1). 1991. 19-22.

Effects Of Cytidine 5'-Diphosphocholine Administration On Basal And Growth Hormone-Releasing Hormone-Induced Growth Hormone Secretion In Elderly Subjects. *Acta Endocrinol* 124 (5). 1991. 516-520.

Neuroendocrinological Effects Of L Threo-3 4 Dihydroxyphenylserine Dops A Putative Norepinephrine Precursor On Healthy Volunteers. *Japanese Journal of Psychiatry and Neurology* 44 (1). 1990. 73-78.

Neuroendocrinological Function In Alzheimer's Disease. *Neuroendocrinology* 48 (4). 1988. 367-370.

Clinical And Biochemical Features Of Depression In Parkinson's Disease *Am J Psychiatry* 143 (6). 1986. 756-759.

Effect Of L Dopa On Fracture Healing Of Rat Fibula *Journal of Catholic Medical College* 39 (1). 1986. 169-178

Corticoliberin Somatocrinin And Amine Contents In Normal And Parkinsonian Human Hypothalamus. *Neuroscience Letters* 56 (2). 1985. 217-222.

Neuroendocrinological Studies Of Parkinson Disease. *Hiroshima Journal of Medical Sciences* 33 (3). 1984 (RECD. 1985). 323-330.

Thyrotropin And Prolactin Responses To Trh In Patients With Parkinsons Disease. *Acta Endocrinol* 99 (3). 1982. 344-351

The thyrotropin (TSH) and prolactin (Prl)-releasing effects of Growth Hormone And Prolactin Stimulation By Madopar In Parkinson's Disease. *Journal of Neurology Neurosurgery and Psychiatry* 44 (12). 1981 (RECD. 1982). 1116-1123

Effects Of L Deprenyl On Human Growth Hormone Secretion *Journal of Neural Transmission* 51 (3-4). 1981. 223-232

Spontaneous Nocturnal Plasma Prolactin And Growth Hormone Secretion In Patients With Parkinsons Disease And Huntingtons Chorea. *Eur Neurol* 19 (3). 1980. 198-206.

Failure Of Melanocyte Stimulating Hormone Inhibiting Factor To Affect Behavioral Responses In Patients With Parkinson's Disease Under L Dopa Therapy. *Psychopharmacology* 63 (3). 1979. 217-222.

Plasma dopa and growth hormone in parkinsonism oscillations in symptoms. *Neurology* 29 (2). 1979. 194-200

Plasma Pituitary Hormones In Patients With Parkinson's disease treated with Bromocriptine. *Journal of Neural Transmission* 42 (2). 1978 151-158

Plasma Dopa Levels And Growth Hormone Response To L Dopa In Parkinsonism. *Journal of Neurology Neurosurgery and Psychiatry* 40 (2). 1977 162-167

Treatment Of Parkinsons Disease With Aporphines Possible Role Of Growth Hormone. *New England Journal of Medicine* 294 (11). 1976 567-572

Endocrinological study of long-term administration of pergolide mesilate in Parkinson's disease. *Rinsho Iyaku* 10: 1215-1220, No. 5, 1994.1 January 1994 (19940101)

A study of dopaminergic sensitivity in Parkinson's disease: comparison in de novo and Levodopa-treated patients. *Clinical*

Neuropharmacology 19: 420-427, Oct 1996.1 October 1996 (19961001)

Effects of terguride on anterior pituitary function in parkinsonian patients treated with L-dopa: a double-blind study versus placebo. *Clinical Neuropharmacology* 19:72-80, Feb 1996.1 February 1996 (19960201)

Defective 5-HT1-receptor-mediated neurotransmission in the control of growth hormone secretion in Parkinson's disease. *Neuropsychobiology* 35 (2):p79-83 1997

A controlled trial of Lazabemide (RO19-6327) in untreated Parkinson's disease. *Annals of Neurology* 33 (4):p350-356 1993

Changes in endocrine function after adrenal medullary transplantation to the central nervous system. *J. Clin. Endocrinol. Metab.*, 1990, 71/3

Co-dergocrine (Hydergine) regulates striatal and hippocampal acetylcholine release through D2 receptors. *Neuroreport* (UK), 1994, 5/6 (674-676)

Ergot alkaloids and central monoaminergic receptors. *J. Pharmacol.* (France), 1985, 16/Suppl. 3 (21-27)

Dementia in the aged. *Psychiatr. Clin. North Am.*, 1982, 5/1 (67-86)

Alterations of electroencephalographic patterns after intravenous administration of hydergine (dihydroergotoxine). *Arg. Neuro-Psiquiat.* (S.Paulo) (Brazil), 1973, 31/2

Phospholipid in Parkinson's disease: Biochemical and clinical data. *Italy Prog. Clin. Biol. Res.*, 1980, Vol.39 (205-214)

Efficacy and tolerability of amantadine sulfate in the treatment of Parkinson's disease. *Nervenheilkunde* (Germany), 1995, 14/2 (76-82)

Bromocriptine lessens the incidence of mortality in L-Dopa-treated parkinsonian patients: Prado-study discontinued. *Eur. J. Clin. Pharmacol.* (Germany), 1992, 43/4 (357-363)

Nicotinamidadenindinucleotide (NADH): The new approach in the therapy of Parkinson's disease. *Ann. Clin. Lab. Sci.*, 1989, 19/1 (38-43)

Levodopa and dopamine agonists in the treatment of Parkinson's disease: Advantages and disadvantages. *Eur. Neurol.* (Switzerland), 1994, 34/Suppl. 3 (20-28)

Plasma profiles of adrenocorticotropic hormone, cortisol, growth hormone and prolactin in patients with untreated Parkinson's disease. *J. Neurol.* (Germany, Federal Republic of), 1991, 238/1

Hypothalamo-pituitary function and dopamine dependence in untreated parkinsonian patients. *Acta Neurol. Scand.* (Denmark), 1991, 83/3 (145-150)

Effect of dopamine, dimethoxyphenylethylamine, papaverine, and related compounds on mitochondrial respiration and complex I activity. *Journal of Neurochemistry*, 1996, 66/3 (1174-1181)

Treatment of Parkinson's disease: From theory to practice. *Usa Postgrad. Med.*, 1994, 95/5

In vitro oxidation of vitamin E, vitamin C, thiols and cholesterol in rat brain mitochondria incubated with free radicals. *USA Neurochemistry International* (UK), 1995, 26/5 (527-535)

Dietary intake and plasma levels of antioxidant vitamins in health and disease: A hospital-based case-control study. *India Journal of Nutritional and Environmental Medicine* (UK) 1995, 5/3 (235-242)

Oxidative stress and antioxidant therapy in Parkinson's disease. *Progress in Neurobiology* (UK), 1996, 48/1 (1-19)

Clinical pharmacodynamics of acetyl-L-carnitine in patients with Parkinson's disease. *Int J Clin Pharmacol Res.* 1990. 10(1-2). P 139-43

The significance of eye blink rate in parkinsonism: a hypothesis. *Int J Neurosci.* 1990 Mar. 51(1-2). P 99-103

Mechanisms of action of ECT in Parkinson's disease: possible role of pineal melatonin. *Int J Neurosci.* 1990 Jan. 50(1-2). P 83-94

Pineal melatonin functions: possible relevance to Parkinson's disease. *Int J Neurosci.* 1990 Jan. 50(1-2). P 37-53

Locus coeruleus-pineal melatonin interactions and the pathogenesis of the "on-off" phenomenon associated with mood changes and sensory symptoms in Parkinson's disease. *Int J Neurosci.* 1989 Nov. 49(1-2). P 95-101

Pineal melatonin and sensory symptoms in Parkinson disease. *Ital J Neurol Sci.* 1989 Aug. 10(4). P 399-403

[Neuroendocrine and psychopharmacologic aspects of the pineal function. Melatonin and psychiatric disorders]. *Acta Psiquiatr Psicol Am Lat.* 1989 Jan-Jun. 35(1-2). P 71-9

Impact of deprenyl and tocopherol treatment on Parkinson's disease in Datatop patients requiring levodopa. Parkinson Study Group. *Ann Neurol.* 1996 Jan. 39(1). P 37-45

In vivo generation of hydroxyl radicals and MPTP-induced dopaminergic toxicity in the basal ganglia. *Ann N Y Acad Sci.* 1994 Nov 17. 738P 25-36

Antioxidant mechanism and protection of nigral neurons against MPP+ toxicity by deprenyl (selegiline). *Ann N Y Acad Sci.* 1994 Nov 17. 738P 214-21

Parkinson's disease: a chronic, low-grade antioxidant deficiency? *Med Hypotheses.* 1994 Aug. 43(2). P 111-4

Free radicals in brain metabolism and pathology. *Br Med Bull.* 1993 Jul. 49(3). P 577-87

Free radicals and their scavengers in Parkinson's disease. *Eur Neurol.* 1993. 33 Suppl 1P 60-8

Phospholipid in Parkinson's disease: Biochemical and clinical data. *Italy Prog. Clin. Biol. Res.*, 1980, VOL.39 (205-214)

Efficacy and tolerability of amantadine sulfate in the treatment of Parkinson's disease. *Nervenheilkunde* (Germany), 1995, 14/2 (76-82)

Bromocriptine lessens the incidence of mortality in L-Dopa-treated parkinsonian patients: Prado-study discontinued. *Eur. J. Clin. Pharmacol.* (Germany), 1992, 43/4 (357- 363)

Nicotinamidadenindinucleotide (NADH): The new approach in the therapy of Parkinson's disease. *Ann. Clin. Lab. Sci.*, 1989, 19/1 (38-43)

Levodopa and dopamine agonists in the treatment of Parkinson's disease: Advantages and disadvantages. *Eur. Neurol.* (Switzerland), 1994, 34/Suppl. 3 (20- 28)

Plasma profiles of adrenocorticotropic hormone, cortisol, growth hormone and prolactin in patients with untreated Parkinson's disease. *J. Neurol.* (Germany, Federal Republic of), 1991, 238/1

Hypothalamo-pituitary function and dopamine dependence in untreated parkinsonian patients. *Acta Neurol. Scand.* (Denmark), 1991, 83/3 (145-150)

Effect of dopamine, dimethoxyphenylethylamine, papaverine, and related compounds on mitochondrial respiration and complex I activity. *Journal of Neurochemistry,* 1996, 66/3 (1174-1181)

Treatment of Parkinson's disease: From theory to practice. *USA Postgrad. Med.*, 1994, 95/5

In vitro oxidation of vitamin E, vitamin C, thiols and cholesterol in rat brain mitochondria incubated with free radicals. *USA Neurochemistry International* (UK), 1995, 26/5 (527-535)

Dietary intake and plasma levels of antioxidant vitamins in health and disease: A hospital-based case-control study. *India Journal of Nutritional and Environmental Medicine* (UK) 1995, 5/3 (235-242)

Oxidative stress and antioxidant therapy in Parkinson's disease. *Progress in Neurobiology* (UK), 1996, 48/1 (1-19)

Co-dergocrine (Hydergine) regulates striatal and hippocampal acetylcholine release through D2 receptors. *Neuroreport* (UK), 1994, 5/6 (674-676)

Ergot alkaloids and central monoaminergic receptors. *J. Pharmacol.* (France), 1985, 16/Suppl. 3 (21-27)

Dementia in the aged. *Psychiatr. Clin. North Am.*, 1982, 5/1 (67-86)

Changes in endocrine function after adrenal medullary transplantation to the central nervous system. *J. Clin. Endocrinol. Metab.*, 1990, 71/3

Phenylalinine and Tyrosine Precautions

[Differential diagnosis and therapy of various forms of hyperphenylalaninemia: facts and fiction] *Wien Klin Wochenschr* 1992, 104 (16) p503-9

Retrospective approach to explain growth retardation and urolithiasis in a child with long-term nutritional acid loading. *Z Ernahrungswiss* Jun 1992, 31 (2) p121-9

[The analgesic action of d-phenylalanine in combination with morphine or methadone]. *Pharmazie* Dec 1991, 46 (12) p875-7

Biochemical and developmental features of experimental phenylketonuria induced by L-ethionine in suckling rats. *Biochem Med Metab Biol* Jun 1989, 41 (3) p201-11

The phenylalanine stress test in the classification of patients with phenylketonuria] *Klin Padiatr* (Germany, West) May-Jun 1989, 201 (3) p163-6

Treatment of hyperactive children with D- phenylalanine. *Am J Psychiatry* Jun 1987, 144 (6) p792-4

Extracorporeal enzyme reactors for depletion of phenylalanine in phenylketonuria. *Ann Intern Med* Apr 1987, 106 (4) p531-7

Characterization of experimental phenylketonuria. Augmentation of hyperphenylalaninemia with alpha-methylphenylalanine and p-chlorophenylalanine. *Biochim Biophys Acta* (Netherlands) Jan 17 1980, 627 (2) p144-56

[Des-phe-insulin-containing intermediary insulin compared with usual commercial preparations (author's transl)]. *Dtsch Med Wochenschr* (Germany, West) Mar 5 1982, 107 (9) p332-5

Long-term effects of a new ketoacid-amino acid supplement in patients with chronic renal failure. *Kidney Int* Jul 1982, 22 (1) p48-53

Use of aspartame by apparently healthy children and adolescents. *J Toxicol Environ Health* Nov 1976, 2 (2) p401-15

Clinical evaluation of peptichemio. *Cancer Treat Rep* Mar 1979, 63 (3) p385-9

Distribution of phenylalanine hydroxylase (EC 1.14.3.1) in liver and kidney of vertebrates. *J Exp Zool* May 1979, 208 (2) p161-7

Practical aspects on the determination of serum alkaline phosphatase isoenzymes using L-phenylalanine and urea. *Clin Chim Acta* (Netherlands) Oct 1 1975, 64 (1) p95-100

Studies on the analgetic effectiveness of D-phenylalanine in combination with morphine or methadone. *Pharmazie* (Germany) 1991, 46/12 (875-877)

Sampling and analytical method for workplace monitoring of aspartame in air. *Applied Industrial Hygiene* 1989, 4/9 (217-221)

The phenylalanine loading test and the classification of phenylketonuric patients. *Klinische Padiatrie* (Germany) 1989, 201/3 (163-166)

Brain development in experimental hyperphenylalaninaemia: Disturbed proliferation and reduced cell numbers in the cerebellum. *Neuropediatrics* (Germany) 1983, 14/1 (12-19)

D-phenylalanine in the treatment of endogenous depression. *IRCS Medical Science* (UK) 1980, 8/2 (116)

Experimental and clinical application of amino acid imbalance for the treatment of malignant diseases, with special reference to phenylalanine imbalance. *Acta Medica* (Japan) 1977, 47/4 (195-294)

Rescue from methotrexate toxicity. *Lancet* (UK) 1978, 2/8092 (737)

Narcolepsy and cataplexy. Clinical features, treatment and cerebrospinal fluid findings. *Quarterly Journal of Medicine* 1974, 43/172 (525-536)

[Brain-derived growth factor: current aspects] *Rev Neurol* (Spain) Jun 1998, 26 (154) p1027-32

Albinism in a Suffolk sheep. *J Hered* Jan-Feb 1993, 84 (1) p67-9

[L-tyrosine: a long term treatment of Parkinson's disease] *C R Acad Sci Iii* (France) 1989, 309 (2) p43-7

L-dopa competes with tyrosine and tryptophan for human brain uptake. *Nutr Metab* 1980, 24 (6) p417-23

Effects of precursors on brain neurotransmitter synthesis and brain functions. *Diabetologia* (Germany, West) Mar 1981, 20 Suppl p281-9

Dietary precursors and brain neurotransmitter formation. *Annu Rev Med* 1981, 32 p413-25

Pyridoxine, the pill and depression. *Journal of Pharmacotherapy* (UK) 1980, 3/1 (20-29)

Elevation of plasma tyrosine after a single oral dose of L-tyrosine. *Life Sciences* 1979, 25/3 (265-272)

Phobias

Piper methysticum (kava kava). *Altern Med Rev* 1998 Dec;3(6):458-60

Effect of kava extract and individual kavapyrones on neurotransmitter levels in the nucleus accumbens of rats. *Progress in Neuro-Psychopharmacology and Biological Psychiatry* 1998, 22/7 (1105-1120)

In vivo effects of the kavapyrones (+)-dihydromethysticin and (+/-)- kavain on dopamine, 3,4-dihydroxyphenylacetic acid, serotonin and 5- hydroxyindoleacetic acid levels in striatal and cortical brain regions. *Planta Medica* (Germany) 1998, 64/6 (507-510)

Influence of genuine kavapyrone enantiomers on the GABA(A) binding site. *Planta Medica* (Germany) 1998, 64/6 (504-506)

Contribution to the quantitative and enantioselective determination of kavapyrones by high-performance liquid chromatography on ChiraSpher NT material. *Journal of Chromatography B: Biomedical Applications* (Netherlands) 1997, 702/1-2 (240-244)

Kavapyrone enriched extract from Piper methysticum as modulator of the GABA binding site in different regions of rat brain. *Psychopharmacology* (Germany) 1994, 116/4 (469-474)

[Kava-kava preparations—alternative anxiolytics]. *Pol Merkuriusz Lek* (Poland) Mar 1998, 4 (21) p179-180a

Tolerability of kava-kava extract WS 1490 on anxiety disorders (Multicentric Brazilian study). *Revista Brasileira de Medicina* (Brazil) 1999, 56/4 (280-284)

Over-the-counter psychotropics: A review of melatonin, St John's wort, valerian, and kava-kava. *Journal of American College Health* 1998, 46/6 (271-276)

Psychopharmacological treatment of anxiety disorders. *Therapeutische Umschau* (Switzerland) 1997, 54/10 (595-599)

Actions of kavain and dihydromethysticin on ipsapirone-induced field potential changes in the hippocampus. *Human Psychopharmacology* (UK) 1997, 12/3 (265-270)

Effects of kawain and dihydromethysticin on field potential changes in the hippocampus. *Progress in Neuro-Psychopharmacology and Biological Psychiatry* 1997, 21/4 (697-706)

Kava-kava and kavain. Herbal anxiolytic—A critical review of clinical trials. *Munchener Medizinische Wochenschrift* (Germany) 1997, 139/4 (42-46)

Clinical efficacy of a kava extrakt in patients with anxiety syndrome. Double-blind placebo controlled study over 4 weeks. *Arzneimittel-Forschung / Drug Research (Arzneim.-Forsch. Drug Res.)* (Germany) 1991, 41/6 (584-588)

Neurovegetative dystonia in the female climacteric. Studies on the clinical efficacy and tolerance of kava extract WS 1490. *Fortschritte der Medizin* (Germany) 1991, 109/4 (65-71)

Parameters of kava used as a challenge to alcohol. *Australian and New Zealand Journal of Psychiatry* (Australia) 1986, 20/1 (70-76)

Inhibition of platelet MAO-B by kava pyrone-enriched extract from Piper methysticum Forster (kava-kava). *Pharmacopsychiatry* 1998 Sep;31(5):187-92

Kava-kava extract in anxiety disorders: an outpatient observational study., *Adv Ther* 1998 Jul-Aug;15(4):261-9

Herbal medicines in Hawaii from tradition to convention. *Hawaii Med J* 1998 Jan;57(1):382-6

Structure-activity relationships in kynurenine, diazepam and some putative endogenous ligands of the benzodiazepine receptors. *Neuroscience and Biobehavioral Reviews* 1983, 7/2 (107-118)

[Interaction of GABA-ergic component of NAD with benzodiazepine receptors during epileptogenesis]. *Ukr Biokhim Zh* (Ukraine) Mar-Apr 1997, 69 (2) p46-50

[Effect of withdrawal of phenazepam and nicotinamide on the status of the system of reception of benzodiazepines and NAD]. *Ukr Biokhim Zh* (Ukraine) Sep-Oct 1996, 68 (5) p20-5

gamma-Aminobutyric acid modulation of benzodiazepine receptor binding in vitro does not predict the pharmacologic activity of all benzodiazepine receptor ligands. *Neurosci Lett* (Netherlands) Mar 15 1985, 54 (2-3) p173-7

[Pharmacotherapy of the hyperventilation syndrome]. *Ann Med Psychol* (Paris) (France) Sep-Oct 1983, 141 (8) p859-74

Biological substrates of anxiety: benzodiazepine receptors and endogenous ligands. *Encephale* (France) 1982, 8 (2) p131-44

[Cross tolerance when benzodiazepines are administered with other substances]. *Biull Eksp Biol Med* (USSR) Jun 1981, 91 (6) p687-9

[Benzodiazepines, receptor affinity, their endogenous ligands and the modeling of new psychotropic preparations]. *Vestn Akad Med Nauk SSSR* (USSR) 1984, (11) p13-20

[Mg2+-ATPase activity of brain mitochondria fractions in chronic stress and its correction by psychotropic agents]. *Ukr Biokhim Zh* (USSR) Nov-Dec 1984, 56 (6) p637-41

[Nootropic and anxiolytic properties of endogenous ligands of benzodiazepine receptors and their structural analogs]. *Biull Eksp Biol Med* (USSR) Feb 1984, 97 (2) p174-

[Pharmacological properties of nicotinamide—possible ligand of benzodiazepine receptors]. *Farmakol Toksikol* (USSR) Nov-Dec 1981, 44 (6) p680-3

Temporal trends in drug use in one UK region, revealed by chemical group matching. *Pharmacoepidemiology and Drug Safety* (UK) 1997, 6/2 (93-100)

Nicotinic acid effectiveness in the treatment of benzodiazepine withdrawal. *Current Therapeutic Research—Clinical and Experimental* 1987, 41/6 (1017-1021)

[Mechanism of the tranquilizing action of electron structural analogs of nicotinamide]. *Biull Eksp Biol Med* (USSR) Mar 1986, 101 (3) p329-31

Central effects of nicotinamide and inosine which are not mediated through benzodiazepine receptors. *Br J Pharmacol* (England) Mar 1985, 84 (3) p689-96

Unwanted effects of psychotropic drugs. IV. Drugs for anxiety. *Practitioner* (UK) 1977, 219/1309 (117-121)

Distributional pattern and targets of GABA-containing neurons in the porcine small and large intestine. *European Journal of Morphology* (Netherlands) 1998, 36/3 (133-142)

delta-Guanidinovaleric acids as an endogenous and specific GABA-receptor antagonist: Electroencephalographic study. *Epilepsy Research* (Netherlands) 1987, 1/2 (114-120)

5-Hydroxytryptophan: a clinically-effective serotonin precursor., *Altern Med Rev* 1998 Aug;3(4):271-80

[Beta-blocking drugs and anxiety. A proven therapeutic value] Medications beta-bloquantes et anxiete. Un interet therapeutique certain. *Encephale* (France) Sep-Oct 1991, 17 (5) p481-92

Effect of beta-receptor blockade on anxiety with reference to the three-systems model of phobic behavior. *Neuropsychobiology* (Switzerland) 1985, 13 (4) p187- 93

The treatment of social phobia. Real-life rehearsal with nonprofessional therapists. *J Nerv Ment Dis* Mar 1981, 169 (3) p180-4

Polymyalgia and Rheumatica

Polyarthralgia disclosing hyperthyroidism: Report of two cases. *Presse Medicale* (France), 1998, 27/26 (1324-1326)

A 67-year-old woman with polymyalgia rheumatica and left hemispatial neglect. *Journal of Neuroimaging*, 1998, 8/4 (222-227)

Effects of glucocorticoids on bone mass in patients with polymyalgia rheumatica. A longitudinal study [4]. *Clinical and Experimental Rheumatology* (Italy), 1998, 16/5 (623)

Polymyalgia rheumatica in biopsy proven giant cell arteritis does not constitute a different subset but differs from isolated polymyalgia rheumatica. *Journal of Rheumatology* (Canada), 1998, 25/9 (1750-1755)

A case of anterior ischemic optic neuropathy associated with polymyalgia rheumatica. *Folia Ophthalmologica Japonica* (Japan), 1998, 49/8 (720-725)

Polymyalgia rheumatica and giant cell arteritis. *Clinics in Geriatric Medicine*, 1998, 14/3 (455-473)

Epidemiology and optimal management of polymyalgia rheumatica. *Drugs and Aging* (New Zealand), 1998, 13/2 (109-118)

Systemic corticosteroid therapy in rheumatology: Benefit-risk ratio. *Schweizerische Rundschau fur Medizin / Praxis* (Switzerland), 1998, 87/33 (1024-1027)

Ophthalmoplegia in treated polymyalgia rheumatica and healed giant cell arteritis. *Strabismus* (Netherlands), 1998, 6/2 (71-75)

Polymyalgia rheumatica in a patient with acute tubulointerstitial nephritis due to Sjogren's syndrome. *Journal of Internal Medicine* (UK), 1998, 244/1 (83-86)

Distal musculoskeletal manifestations in polymyalgia rheumatica: A prospective followup study. *Arthritis and Rheumatism*, 1998, 41/7 (1221-1226)

Anticardiolipin antibodies in giant cell arteritis and polymyalgia rheumatica: A study of 40 cases. *British Journal of Rheumatology* (UK), 1998, 37/2 (208-210)

An initially double-blind controlled 96 week trial of depot methylprednisolone against oral prednisolone in the treatment of polymyalgia rheumatica. *British Journal of Rheumatology* (UK), 1998, 37/2 (189-195)

The deleterious effects of low-dose corticosteroids on bone density in patients with polymyalgia rheumatica. *British Journal of Rheumatology* (UK), 1998, 37/3 (292-299)

Cytokines and adhesion molecules in patients with polymyalgia rheumatica. *British Journal of Rheumatology* (UK), 1998, 37/7 (766-769)

A 24-year-old man with symptoms and signs of polymyalgia rheumatica. *Journal of Family Practice*, 1998, 47/1 (68-71)

Deltoid muscle in patients with polymyalgia rheumatica. *Journal of Rheumatology* (Canada), 1998, 25/7 (1344-1351)

Polyarthritis associated with myelodysplastic syndromes: 5 cases. *European Journal of Internal Medicine* (Italy), 1998, 9/1 (57-60)

Clinical outcome of 149 patients with polymyalgia rheumatica and giant cell arteritis. *Journal of Rheumatology* (Canada), 1998, 25/1 (99-104)

Large vessel vasculitides. *Current Opinion in Rheumatology*, 1998, 10/1 (18-28)

Diagnosis and management of polymyalgia rheumatica/giant cell arteritis. *BioDrugs* (New Zealand), 1998, 9/1 (25-32)

Adverse outcomes of antiinflammatory therapy among patients with polymyalgia rheumatica. *Arthritis and Rheumatism*, 1997, 40/10 (1873-1878)

The sequential analysis of T lymphocyte subsets and interleukin-6 in polymyalgia rheumatica patients as predictors of disease remission and steroid withdrawal. *British Journal of Rheumatology* (UK), 1997, 36/9 (976-980)

Polymyalgia rheumatica—Therapy, course of disease, complications. *Geriatrie Forschung* (Germany), 1997, 7/1 (13-18)

Antibodies against Chlamydia pneumoniae, cytomegalovirus, enteroviruses and respiratory syncytial virus in patients with polymyalgia rheumatica. *Clinical and Experimental Rheumatology* (Italy), 1997, 15/3 (299-302)

False diagnosis: A common occurrence in autoimmune diseases. *Schweizerische Medizinische Wochenschrift* (Switzerland), 1997, 127/9 (349-354)

Risk factors and predictive models of giant cell arteritis in polymyalgia rheumatica. *American Journal of Medicine*, 1997, 102/4 (331-336)

Premenstrual Syndrome

Refer to references under Female Hormone Modulation Therapy.

Prevention Protocols

Vitamin E and coronary artery disease [see comments]. *Arch Intern Med* Jun 28 1999, 159 (12) p1313-20

Toward a new recommended dietary allowance for vitamin C based on antioxidant and health effects in humans. *Am J Clin Nutr* Jun 1999, 69 (6) p1086-107

Primary prevention of CHD: nine ways to reduce risk. *Am Fam Physician* Mar 15 1999, 59 (6) p1455-63, 1466

Carotenoids: 2. Diseases and supplementations studies. *Annales de Biologie Clinique* (France) 1999, 57/3 (273-282)

Reduction of cardiovascular disease risk factors by French maritime pine bark extract. *Cardiovascular Reviews and Reports* 1999, 20/6 (326-329)

Wine and polyphenols related to platelet aggregation and atherothrombosis. *Drugs under Experimental and Clinical Research* (Switzerland) 1999, 25/2-3 (125-131)

Vitamin D deficiency one of the causes of bone changes in chronic pancreatitis. *Vnitrni Lekarstvi* (Czech Republic) 1999, 45/5 (281-283)

MRC/BHF Heart Protection Study of cholesterol-lowering therapy and of antioxidant vitamin supplementation in a wide range of patients at increased risk of coronary heart disease death: Early safety and efficacy experience. *European Heart Journal* (UK) 1999, 20/10 (725-741)

Emphasizing and promoting overall health and nontraditional treatments after a prostate cancer diagnosis. *Seminars in Urologic Oncology* 1999, 17/2 (119-124)

Vitamin remedies, natural supplements in the prevention of heart disease in women. *Infertility and Reproductive Medicine Clinics of North America* 1999, 10/2 (259-275)

Dietary antioxidant vitamins intake and incidence of coronary heart disease. *Chinese Journal of Cardiology* (China) 1999, 27/1 (17-21)

Prevention of oral diseases by polyphenols (review). *In Vivo* (Greece) 1999, 13/2 (155-171)

Selected phenolic compounds in cultivated plants: Ecologic functions, health implications, and modulation by pesticides. *Environmental Health Perspectives* 1999, 107/Suppl. 1 (109-114)

The effect of antioxidant therapy on cell-mediated immunity following burn injury in an animal model. *Burns.* 1999 Mar;25(2):113-8.

[Primary preventive medicine and laboratory medicine]. *Rinsho Byori.* 1999 Feb;47(2):101-8. Review. Japanese.

Intake of vitamins B6 and C and the risk of kidney stones in women. *J Am Soc Nephrol* Apr 1999, 10 (4) p840-5

Vitamin and calcium supplement use is associated with decreased adenoma recurrence in patients with a previous history of neoplasia. *Dis Colon Rectum* Feb 1999, 42 (2) p212-7

High doses of multiple antioxidant vitamins: essential ingredients in improving the efficacy of standard cancer therapy. *J Am Coll Nutr* Feb 1999, 18 (1) p13-25

Demonstration of rapid onset vascular endothelial dysfunction after hyperhomocysteinemia: an effect reversible with vitamin C therapy. *Circulation* Mar 9 1999, 99 (9) p1156-60

Dietary carotenoids and vitamins A, C, and E and risk of breast cancer. *J Natl Cancer Inst* Mar 17 1999, 91 (6) p547-56

Prospective cohort study of antioxidant vitamin supplement use and the risk of age-related maculopathy. *Am J Epidemiol* Mar 1 1999, 149 (5) p476-84

Calcineurin inhibitors enhance low-density lipoprotein oxidation in transplant patients. *Kidney International, Supplement* 1999, 56/71 (S137-S140)

Ascorbic acid maintenance in HaCaT cells prevents radical formation and apoptosis by UV-B. *Free Radical Biology and Medicine* 1999, 26/9-10 (1172-1180)

Determination of factors responsible for the declining incidence of colorectal cancer. *Diseases of the Colon and Rectum* 1999, 42/6 (741-752)

Influence of diet on skin cancer. *Mature Medicine Canada* (Canada) 1999, 2/2 (102-104)

Cardiology update 1998. *Casopis Lekaru Ceskych* (Czech Republic) 1999, 138/8 (249-252)

Diet and brain cancer in adults: A case-control study in northeast China. *International Journal of Cancer* 1999, 81/1 (20-23)

Micronutrients and pregnancy outcome: A review of the literature. *Nutrition Research (Nutr. Res.)* 1999, 19/1 (103-159)

Smoking, plasma vitamins C, E, retinol, and carotene, and fatal prostate cancer: Seventeen-year follow-up of the prospective Basel study. *Prostate* 15 FEB 1999, 38/3 (189-198)

Dietary flavonols protect diabetic human lymphocytes against oxidative damage to DNA. *Diabetes* 1999, 48/1 (176-181)

Antioxidant effect of short-term hormonal treatment in postmenopausal women. *Maturitas* (Ireland) Jan 4 1999, 31 (2) p137-42

Activities of DNA turnover and free radical metabolizing enzymes in cancerous human prostate tissue [see comments]. *Cancer Invest* 1999, 17 (5) p314-9

The pineal secretory product melatonin reduces hydrogen peroxide-induced DNA damage in U-937 cells. *J Pineal Res* (Denmark) May 1999, 26 (4) p227-35

Plasma levels of antioxidant vitamins and cholesterol in a large population sample in central-northern Italy. *Eur J Nutr* (Germany) Apr 1999, 38 (2) p90-8

Additional information to the in vitro antioxidant activity of Ginkgo biloba L. *Phytother Res* (England) Mar 1999, 13 (2) p160-2

Protection of low density lipoprotein oxidation by the antioxidant agent IRFI005, a new synthetic hydrophilic vitamin E analogue. *Free Radic Biol Med* Apr 1999, 26 (7-8) p858-68

Comparison of the apoptotic pathways induced by L-amino acid oxidase and hydrogen peroxide. *J Biochem* (Tokyo) (Japan) Feb 1999, 125 (2) p305-9

Enhanced in vivo lipid peroxidation at elevated plasma total homocysteine levels. *Arterioscler Thromb Vasc Biol* May 1999, 19 (5) p1263-6

Dietary flavonoid intake and risk of cardiovascular disease in postmenopausal women. *Am J Epidemiol* May 15 1999, 149 (10) p943-9

Pharmacologic management of Alzheimer disease, Part II: Antioxidants, antihypertensives, and ergoloid derivatives. *Ann Pharmacother* Feb 1999, 33 (2) p188-97

Micronutrients, vitamins, and cancer risk. *Vitam Horm* 1999;57:1-23

Hydrogen peroxide suppresses U937 cell death by two different mechanisms depending on its concentration. *Exp Cell Res* May 1 1999, 248 (2) p430-8

Involvement of N-acetylcysteine sensitive pathways in ricin-induced apoptotic cell death in U937 cells. *Biosci Biotechnol Biochem* (Japan) Feb 1999, 63 (2) p341-8

Antioxidant therapy in the prevention of organ dysfunction syndrome and infectious complications after trauma: early results of a prospective randomized study. *Am Surg* 1999 May;65(5):478-83

Impact of trace elements and vitamin supplementation on immunity and infections in institutionalized elderly patients: a randomized controlled trial. MIN. VIT. AOX. geriatric network. *Arch Intern Med* Apr 12 1999, 159 (7) p748-54

Prevention of recurrent pancreatitis in familial lipoprotein lipase deficiency with high-dose antioxidant therapy. *J Clin Endocrinol Metab* Apr 1999, 84 (4) p1203-5

Ascorbate prevents prooxidant effects of urate in oxidation of human low density lipoprotein. *FEBS Lett* 1999 Mar 12;446(2-3):305-8

Anti-oxidant effect of flavonoids on hemoglobin glycosylation. *Pharm Acta Helv* 1999 Feb;73(5):223-6

Inhibition of copper-induced LDL oxidation by vitamin C is associated with decreased copper-binding to LDL and 2-oxo-histidine formation. *Free Radic Biol Med* Jan 1999, 26 (1-2) p90-8

Lower prostate cancer risk in men with elevated plasma lycopene levels: results of a prospective analysis. *Cancer Res* Mar 15 1999, 59 (6) p1225-30

NSAIDs and butyrate sensitize a human colorectal cancer cell line to TNF-alpha and Fas ligation: the role of reactive oxygen species. *Biochim Biophys Acta* (Netherlands) Jan 11 1999, 1448 (3) p425-38

Manganese superoxide dismutase (MnSOD) genetic polymorphisms, dietary antioxidants, and risk of breast cancer. *Cancer Res* 1999 Feb 1;59(3):602-6

Docosahexaenoic acid is an antihypertensive nutrient that affects aldosterone production in SHR. *Proc Soc Exp Biol Med* May 1999, 221 (1) p32-8

Prevention of sudden cardiac death by dietary pure omega-3 polyunsaturated fatty acids in dogs. *Circulation* May 11 1999, 99 (18) p2452-7

Dietary n-3 PUFA increases the apoptotic response to 1,2-dimethylhydrazine, reduces mitosis and suppresses the induction of carcinogenesis in the rat colon. *Carcinogenesis* 1999 Apr;20(4):645-50

Photoprotection. *Revue Francaise d'Allergologie et d'Immunologie Clinique* (France) 1999, 39/4 (311-323)

Effect of saturated, omega-3 and omega-6 polyunsaturated fatty acids on myocardial infarction. *Journal of Nutritional Biochemistry* 1999, 10/6 (338-344)

Serotonin-induced endothelial cell proliferation is blocked by omega-3 fatty acids. *Prostaglandins Leukotrienes and Essential Fatty Acids* (UK) 1999, 60/2 (115-123)

Effects of eicosapentaenoic acid on the contraction of intact, and spontaneous contraction of chemically permeabilized mammalian ventricular myocytes. *Journal of Molecular and Cellular Cardiology* (UK) 1999, 31/4 (733-743)

Omega-3 fatty acids in adipose tissue and risk of myocardial infarction: The EURAMIC study. *Arteriosclerosis, Thrombosis, and Vascular Biology* 1999, 19/4 (1111-1118)

Procoagulant activity and cytokine expression in whole blood cultures from patients with atherosclerosis supplemented with omega-3 fatty acids. *Thrombosis and Haemostasis* (Germany) 1999, 81/4 (566-570)

Antithrombotic effects of (n-3) polyunsaturated fatty acids in rat models of arterial and venous thrombosis. *Thrombosis Research* (UK) 01 Jan 1999, 93/1 (9-16)

PUFA and aging modulate cardiac mitochondrial membrane lipid composition and Ca^{2+} activation of PDH. *American Journal of Physiology - Heart and Circulatory Physiology* 1999, 276/1 45-1 (H149-H158)

Possibilities of fish oil application for food products enrichment with omega-3 PUFA. *International Journal of Food Sciences and Nutrition* (UK) 1999, 50/1 (39-49)

Fish oil supplementation prevents diabetes-induced nerve conduction velocity and neuroanatomical changes in rats. *Journal of Nutrition* 1999, 129/1 (207-213)

Cardiovasoprotective foods and nutrients: possible importance of magnesium intake. *Magnes Res* (England) Mar 1999, 12 (1) p57-61

Stimulation of cell division in the rat by NaCl, KCl, $MgCl_2$, and $CaCl_2$, and inhibition of the sodium chloride effect on the glandular stomach by ascorbic acid and beta-carotene. *J Cancer Res Clin Oncol* (Germany) 1999, 125 (3-4) p209-13

Lifestyle modifications to prevent and control hypertension. 1. Methods and an overview of the Canadian recommendations. Canadian Hypertension Society, Canadian Coalition for High Blood Pressure Prevention and Control, Laboratory Centre for Disease Control at Health Canada, Heart and Stroke Foundation of Canada. *CMAJ (Canada)* May 4 1999, 160 (9 Suppl) pS1-6

Prevention of eclampsia. *Semin Perinatol* Feb 1999, 23 (1) p65-78

Coronary microvascular protection with mg^{2+}: effects on intracellular calcium regulation and vascular function. *Am J Physiol* Apr 1999, 276 (4 Pt 2) pH1124-30

Thromboxane Ainf 2 fails to induce proliferation of smooth muscle cells enriched with eicosapentaenoic acid and docosahexaenoic acid. *Prostaglandins Leukotrienes and Essential Fatty Acids* (UK) 1999, 60/4 (275-281)

Fish oil-enriched nutritional supplement attenuates progression of the acute-phase response in weight-losing patients with advanced pancreatic cancer. *Journal of Nutrition* 1999, 129/6 (1120-1125)

Choline deficiency-induced apoptosis in PC12 cells is associated with diminished membrane phosphatidylcholine and sphingomyelin, accumulation of ceramide and diacylglycerol, and activation of a caspase. *FASEB J* Jan 1999, 13 (1) p135-42

Functional relationship between age-related immunodeficiency and learning deterioration. *Eur J Neurosci* (France) Dec 1998, 10 (12) p3869-75

Protection against developmental retardation in apolipoprotein E-deficient mice by a fatty neuropeptide: implications for early treatment of Alzheimer's disease. *J Neurobiol* Sep 1997, 33 (3) p329-42

The influence of DHEA on serum lipids, insulin and sex hormone levels in rabbits with induced hypercholesterolemia. *Gynecol Endocrinol* (England) Mar 1995, 9 (1) p23-8

The effect of administration of estradiol and testosterone on body growth of young male rats. *Physiol Res* (Czechoslovakia) 1992, 41 (5) p387-92

Homocysteine, a new crucial element in the pathogenesis of uremic cardiovascular complications. *Miner Electrolyte Metab* (Switzerland) Jan-Apr 1999, 25 (1-2) p95-9

Dietary folate from vegetables and citrus fruit decreases plasma homocysteine concentrations in humans in a dietary controlled trial. *J Nutr* Jun 1999, 129 (6) p1135-9

[Folic acid supplementation by 200 microgram per day during the periconceptional period: a necessary public health approach to reducing incidence of spina bifida]. *Contracept Fertil Sex* (France) Mar 1999, 27 (3) p238-42

American College of Preventive Medicine public policy statement. Folic acid fortification of grain products in the U.S. to prevent neural tube defects. *Am J Prev Med* (Netherlands) Apr 1999, 16 (3) p264-7

Knowledge and use of folic acid by women of childbearing age—United States, 1995 and 1998. *Morb Mortal Wkly Rep* Apr 30 1999, 48 (16) p325-7

Leptin prevents respiratory depression in obesity. *Am J Respir Crit Care Med* May 1999, 159 (5 Pt 1) p1477-84

Calcium supplements for the prevention of colorectal adenomas. Calc. Polyp Prev. Study Group. *N Engl J Med* Jan 14 1999, 340 (2) p101-7

The effect of hypertension treatment on the prevention of coronary artery disease events in the elderly. *American Journal of Geriatric Cardiology* 1998, 7/1 (28-34)

Prevention of ischaemic stroke. *Revue du Praticien* (France) 15 Jan 1998, 48/2 (165-170)

Lecithin-bound superoxide dismutase in the prevention of neutrophil- induced damage of corneal tissue. *Investigative Ophthalmology and Visual Science* 1998, 39/1 (30-35)

Carvedilol update IV: Prevention of oxidative stress, cardiac remodeling and progression of congestive heart failure. *Drugs of Today* (Spain) 1998, 34/Suppl. B (1-23)

Endocrine effects of IGF-I on normal and transformed breast epithelial cells: Potential relevance to strategies for breast cancer treatment and prevention. *Breast Cancer Research and Treatment* 1998, 47/3 (209-217)

Primary short-term and long-term prevention of first manifestations of allergic disease with dietary intervention—A meta-analysis with a moderately hydrolysed infant formula. *Allergologie* (Germany) 1998, 21/1 (3-23)

Combination hepatitis A-hepatitis B vaccine: Dual prevention of viral hepatitis. *Drugs and Therapy Perspectives* (New Zealand) 02 MAR 1998, 11/4 (1-4)

Gastroprotective agents for the prevention of NSAID-induced gastropathy. *Current Pharmaceutical Design* (Netherlands) 1998, 4/1 (17-36)

Cancer prevention studies: Past, present and future directions. *Nutrition* 1998, 14/2 (197-210)

Chronic active Crohn's disease: An update on prevention and treatment. *Research and Clinical Forums* (UK) 1998, 20/1 (169-177)

Primary and secondary prevention of stroke. *Hong Kong Practitioner* (Hong Kong) 1998, 20/2 (67-77)

Cholesterol, statins, and cardiovascular prevention: Resolved and unresolved issues. *Medecine et Hygiene* (Switzerland) 21 JAN 1998, 56/2193 (131-136)

A comparison of sucralfate and ranitidine for the prevention of upper gastrointestinal bleeding in patients requiring mechanical ventilation. *New England Journal of Medicine* 19 MAR 1998, 338/12 (791-797)

Vitamin D and its metabolites in the prevention and treatment of osteoporosis. *Revue Medicale de la Suisse Romande* (Switzerland) 1998, 118/3 (267-277)

Selenium in cancer prevention, recurrence prevention and cancer therapy. *Zeitschrift fur Onkologie* (Germany) 1998, 30/1 (6-12)

Prevention of hypertensive disorders of pregnancy. *Journal of Obstetrics and Gynaecology* (UK) 1998, 18/2 (123-126)

Once weekly azithromycin therapy for prevention of Mycobacterium avium complex infection in patients with AIDS: A randomized, double-blind, placebo-controlled multicenter trial. *Clinical Infectious Diseases* 1998, 26/3 (611-619)

Patients with nonvalvular atrial fibrillation at low risk of stroke during treatment with aspirin: Stroke prevention in atrial fibrillation III study. *Journal of the American Medical Association* 22 APR 1998, 279/16 (1273-1277)

From the field—Evaluation of mechanical methods for prevention of deep venous thrombosis. *Clinical Kinesiology* 1998, 52/1 (4-11)

beta-Fibrinogen gene polymorphism ($C_{148}T$) is associated with carotid atherosclerosis: Results of the Austrian stroke prevention study. *Arteriosclerosis, Thrombosis, and Vascular Biology* 1998, 18/3 (487-492)

The prevention of anthracycline cardiomyopathy. *Progress in Pediatric Cardiology* (Ireland) 1998, 8/3 (97-108)

Which drugs benefit diabetic patients for secondary prevention of myocardial infarction? *Diabetic Medicine* (UK) 1998, 15/4 (282-289)

Thrombosis prevention trial. *Cardiovascular Reviews and Reports* 1998, 19/7 (12-16)

Hormone replacement therapy and postmenopausal prevention of cardiovascular disease. *Annales de Cardiologie et d'Angeiologie* (France) 1998, 47/7 (481-487)

Prevention of maternal-fetal blood group incompatibility with traditional Chinese herbal medicine. *Chinese Medical Journal* (China) 1998, 111/7 (585-587)

Role of postmenopausal estrogen therapy in the prevention of coronary heart disease. *Turk Kardiyoloji Dernegi Arsivi* (Turkey) 1998, 26/5 (299-303+263)

Prevention of glucorticoid-induced osteoporosis. *Revue de Medecine Interne* (France) 1998, 19/7 (492-500)

Cutaneous photoimmunosuppression: Role of the UVA and prevention by sunscreens. *Nouvelles Dermatologiques* (France) 1998, 17/5 (326-329)

Acyclovir for the prevention of recurrent herpes simplex virus eye disease. *New England Journal of Medicine* 30 JUL 1998, 339/5 (300-306)

Sunscreens for primary prevention of malignant melanoma. *H+G Zeitschrift fur Hautkrankheiten* (Germany) 1998, 73/7-8 (467-473)

Vitamin D supplementation for prevention of osteoporosis in elderly people and the role of the pharmacist. *Pharmaceutisch Weekblad* (Netherlands) 04 SEP 1998, 133/36 (1368-1370)

Hormone supplementation on the rise. New developments in treatment and prevention of age-related disorders in women. *Pharmaceutisch Weekblad* (Netherlands) 04 SEP 1998, 133/36 (1355-1361)

Lectins: From basic science to clinical application in cancer prevention. *Expert Opinion on Investigational Drugs* (UK) 1998, 7/9 (1389-1403)

Prevention in the child through nutrition during pregnancy and lactation? *Monatsschrift fur Kinderheilkunde* (Germany) 1998, 146/8 Suppl. 1 (S73-S87).

Management 1997 of chronic obstructive pulmonary disease. Working Group of the Swiss Society of Pneumology. *Schweiz Med Wochenschr* (Switzerland) May 3 1997, 127 (18) p766-82

Chemoprevention of colorectal tumors: role of lactulose and of other agents. *Scand J Gastroenterol Suppl* (Norway) 1997, 222 p72-5

Biochemical basis of selenomethionine-mediated inhibition during 2-acetylaminofluorene-induced hepatocarcinogenesis in the rat. *Eur J Cancer Prev* (England) Dec 1996, 5 (6) p455-63

Application of molecular epidemiology to lung cancer chemoprevention. *J Cell Biochem Suppl* 1996, 25 p63-8

Effects of dietary vitamin C and E supplementation on the copper mediated oxidation of HDL and on HDL mediated cholesterol efflux. *Atherosclerosis* (Ireland) Nov 15 1996, 127 (1) p19-26

Antioxidant actions of beta-carotene in liposomal and microsomal membranes: role of carotenoid-membrane incorporation and alpha-tocopherol. *Arch Biochem Biophys* Feb 15 1997, 338 (2) p244-50

Comparative study of the effect of 21-aminosteroid and alpha-tocopherol on models of acute oxidative renal injury. *Free Radic Biol Med* 1996, 21 (5) p691-7

Possible prevention of postangioplasty restenosis by ascorbic acid. *Am J Cardiol* Dec 1 1996, 78 (11) p1284-6

Effectiveness of antioxidants (vitamin C and E) with and without sunscreens as topical photoprotectants. *Acta Derm Venereol* (Norway) Jul 1996, 76 (4) p264-8

Curcumin protects against 4-hydroxy-2-trans-nonenal-induced cataract formation in rat lenses. *Am J Clin Nutr* Nov 1996, 64 (5) p761-6

Prevention of asthma. *Eur Respir J* (Denmark) Jul 1996, 9 (7) p1545-55

Role of oxidant stress in the adult respiratory distress syndrome: evaluation of a novel antioxidant strategy in a porcine model of endotoxin-induced acute lung injury. *Shock* 1996, 6 Suppl 1 pS23-6

The new paradigm for coronary artery disease: altering risk factors, atherosclerotic plaques, and clinical prognosis. *Mayo Clin Proc* Oct 1996, 71 (10) p957-65

Synergism between N-acetylcysteine and doxorubicin in the prevention of tumorigenicity and metastasis in murine models. *Int J Cancer* Sep 17 1996, 67 (6) p842-8

Prevention of dopamine-induced cell death by thiol antioxidants: possible implications for treatment of Parkinson's disease. *Exp Neurol* Sep 1996, 141 (1) p32-9

Effect of flavonoids on the outcome of myocardial mitochondrial ischemia/reperfusion injury. *Res Commun Mol Pathol Pharmacol* Jan 1996, 91 (1) p65-75

[The dose-dependent effects of a combination of different classes of antioxidants exemplified by dibunol and beta-carotene]. *Izv Akad Nauk Ser Biol* (Russia) Mar-Apr 1996, (2) p147-52

Oxidative damage and defense. *Am J Clin Nutr* Jun 1996, 63 (6) p985S-990S

Dietary fiber and the chemopreventive modelation of colon carcinogenesis. *Mutat Res* (Netherlands) Feb 19 1996, 350 (1) p185-97

Selenium: a quest for better understanding. *Altern Ther Health Med* Jul 1996, 2 (4) p59-62, 65-7

[The Mediterranean diet in the prevention of arteriosclerosis]. *Recenti Prog Med* (Italy) Apr 1996, 87 (4) p175-81

Change for coronary artery disease. What to tell patients. *Postgrad Med* Feb 1996, 99 (2) p89-92, 95-6, 102-6

Population nutrient intake approaches dietary recommendations: 1991 to 1995 Framingham Nutrition Studies. *J Am Diet Assoc* Jul 1997, 97 (7) p742-9

The antioxidant potential of the Mediterranean diet. *Eur J Cancer Prev* (England) Mar 1997, 6 Suppl 1 pS15-9

[Atherogenic factors in the diet of the Costa Rican population, 1991]. *Arch Latinoam Nutr* (Venezuela) Mar 1996, 46 (1) p27-32

Vitamin C intake and cardiovascular disease risk factors in persons with non-insulin-dependent diabetes mellitus. From the Insulin Resistance Atherosclerosis Study and the San Luis Valley Diabetes Study. *Prev Med* May-Jun 1997, 26 (3) p277-83

The effect of dietary fat, antioxidants, and pro-oxidants on blood lipids, lipoproteins, and atherosclerosis. *J Am Diet Assoc* Jul 1997, 97 (7 Suppl) pS31-41

Reliability of a food frequency questionnaire to assess dietary antioxidant intake. *Ophthalmic Epidemiol* (Netherlands) Mar 1997, 4 (1) p33-9

Oxidative stress hypothesis in Alzheimer's disease. *Free Radic Biol Med* 1997, 23 (1) p134-47

Alcohol, ischemic heart disease, and the French paradox. *Clin Cardiol* May 1997, 20 (5) p420-4

Dietary antioxidants and Parkinson disease. The Rotterdam Study. *Arch Neurol* Jun 1997, 54 (6) p762-5

Anti-oxidants and coronary heart disease [letter]. *S Afr Med J* (South Africa) Jan 1997, 87 (1 Suppl) p103

Randomised trial of alpha-tocopherol and beta-carotene supplements on incidence of major coronary events in men with previous myocardial infraction. *Lancet* (England) Jun 14 1997, 349 (9067) p1715-20

Anti-oxidant therapy for ischaemic heart disease: where do we stand? *Lancet* (England) Jun 14 1997, 349 (9067) p1710-1

Lower ischemic heart disease incidence and mortality among vitamin supplement users. *Can J Cardiol* (Canada) Oct 1996, 12 (10) p930-4

Association of serum vitamin levels, LDL susceptibility to oxidation, and autoantibodies against MDA-LDL with carotid atherosclerosis. A case-control study. The ARIC Study Investigators. Atherosclerosis Risk in Communities. *Arterioscler Thromb Vasc Biol* Jun 1997, 17 (6) p1171-7

Validity of diagnoses of major coronary events in national registers of hospital diagnoses and deaths in Finland. *Eur J Epidemiol* (Netherlands) Feb 1997, 13 (2) p133-8

Vitamin C and cardiovascular disease: a systematic review. *J Cardiovasc Risk* (England) Dec 1996, 3 (6) p513-21

Biochemical basis of selenomethionine-mediated inhibition during 2-acetylaminofluorene-induced hepatocarcinogenesis in the rat. *Eur J Cancer Prev* (England) Dec 1996, 5 (6) p455-63

Glutathione transferases catalyse the detoxication of oxidized metabolites (o-quinones) of catecholamines and may serve as an antioxidant system preventing degenerative cellular processes. *Biochem J* (England) May 15 1997, 324 (Pt 1) p25-8

Nutrition and newly emerging viral diseases: an overview. *J Nutr* May 1997, 127 (5 Suppl) p948S-950S

Pathogenesis and treatment of liver fibrosis in alcoholics: 1996 update. *Dig Dis* (Switzerland) Jan-Apr 1997, 15 (1-2) p42-66

Adenocarcinomas of the esophagus and gastric cardia: the role of diet. *Nutr Cancer* 1997, 27 (3) p298-309

Vitamin C, neutrophil function, and upper respiratory tract infection risk in distance runners: the missing link. *Exerc Immunol Rev* 1997, 3 p32-5

Equine degenerative myeloencephalopathy. *Vet Clin North Am Equine Pract* Apr 1997, 13 (1) p43-52

Intake of fatty acids and risk of coronary heart disease in a cohort of Finnish men. The Alpha-Tocopherol, Beta-Carotene Cancer Prevention Study. *Am J Epidemiol* May 15 1997, 145 (10) p876-87

Functional effects of food components and the gastrointestinal system: chicory fructooligosaccharides. *Nutr Rev* Nov 1996, 54 (11 Pt 2) pS38-42

[Coronary heart disease—a free radical associated disease? What is the value of antioxidant substances?]. *Med Monatsschr Pharm* (Germany) Mar 1997, 20 (3) p66-70

Antioxidant flavonols and ischemic heart disease in a Welsh population of men: the Caerphilly Study. *Am J Clin Nutr* May 1997, 65 (5) p1489-94

[Vitamin E as a possible aid in the control of disease problems on pig farms: a field test]. *Tijdschr Diergeneeskd* (Netherlands) Apr 1 1997, 122 (7) p190-2

Antioxidants and dementia. *Lancet* (England) Apr 26 1997, 349 (9060) p1189-90

[Is supplemental vitamin E for prevention of coronary heart disease ov value?]. *Internist* (Berl) (Germany) Feb 1997, 38 (2) p168-76; discussion 176

The 'diet heart' hypothesis in secondary prevention of coronary heart disease. *Eur Heart J* (England) Jan 1997, 18 (1) p13-8

Tea and health: a historical perspective. *Cancer Lett* (Ireland) Mar 19 1997, 114 (1-2) p315-7

[Prevalence and risk factors in the population of Graz (Austrian Stroke Prevention Study)]. *Wien Med Wochenschr* (Austria) 1997, 147 (2) p36-40

Beta-2-agonists have antioxidant function in vitro. 2. The effect of beta-2-agonists on oxidant-mediated cytotoxicity and on superoxide anion generated by human polymorphonuclear leukocytes. *Respiration* (Switzerland) 1997, 64 (1) p23-8

Antioxidant vitamins and cardiovascular disease: current perspectives and future directions [editorial]. *Eur Heart J* (England) Feb 1997, 18 (2) p177-9

Protective effects of silymarin against photocarcinogenesis in a mouse skin model. *J Natl Cancer Inst* Apr 16 1997, 89 (8) p556-66

Which changes in diet prevent coronary heart disease? A review of clinical trials of dietary fats and antioxidants. *Acta Cardiol* (Belgium) 1996, 51 (6) p467-90

Antioxidants in the prevention of atherosclerosis. *Curr Opin Lipidol* Dec 1996, 7 (6) p374-80

[Cardio-protective effect of red wine as reflected in the literature]. *Orv Hetil* (Hungary) Mar 16 1997, 138 (11) p673-8

Tea and heart disease [letter]. *Lancet* (England) Mar 8 1997, 349 (9053) p735

Application of molecular epidemiology to lung cancer chemoprevention. *J Cell Biochem Suppl* 1996, 25 p63-8

Cancer risk factors for selecting cohorts for large-scale chemoprevention trials. *J Cell Biochem Suppl* 1996, 25 p29-36

Protection against induction of mouse skin papillomas with low and high risk of conversion to malignancy by green tea polyphenols. *Carcinogenesis* (England) Mar 1997, 18 (3) p497-502

Effects of dietary vitamin C and E supplementation on the copper mediated oxidation of HDL and on HDL mediated cholesterol efflux. *Atherosclerosis* (Ireland) Nov 15 1996, 127 (1) p19-26

Efficacy of a dentifrice and oral rinse containing sanguinaria extract in conjunction with initial periodontal therapy. *Aust Dent J* (Australia) Feb 1997, 42 (1) p47-51

The impact of zinc supplementation on Schistosoma mansoni reinfection rate and intensities: a randomized, controlled trial among rural Zimbabwean schoolchildren. *Eur J Clin Nutr* (England) Jan 1997, 51 (1) p33-7

Methylenetetrahydrofolate reductase polymorphism, dietary interactions, and risk of colorectal cancer. *Cancer Res* Mar 15 1997, 57 (6) p1098-102

Nutrition in women. Assessment and counseling. *Prim Care* Mar 1997, 24 (1) p37-51

Hypertension and borderline isolated systolic hypertension increase risks of cardiovascular disease and mortality in male physicians. *Circulation* Mar 4 1997, 95 (5) p1132-7

Bronchial reactivity and dietary antioxidants. *Thorax* (England) Feb 1997, 52 (2) p166-70

Effects of bisaramil on coronary-occlusion-reperfusion injury and free-radical-induced reactions. *Pharmacol Res* (England) Jun 1996, 33 (6) p327-36

Whole-grain consumption and chronic disease: protective mechanisms. *Nutr Cancer* 1997, 27 (1) p14-21

Dietary manipulation of plasma carotenoid concentrations of squirrel monkeys (Saimiri sciureus). *J Nutr* Jan 1997, 127 (1) p122-9

Mechanisms of spontaneous human cancers. *Environ Health Perspect* May 1996, 104 Suppl 3 p633-7

Molecular epidemiology in environmental carcinogenesis. *Environ Health Perspect* May 1996, 104 Suppl 3 p441-3

Vitamin C intake and susceptibility to the common cold. *Br J Nutr* (England) Jan 1997, 77 (1) p59-72

Antioxidant actions of beta-carotene in liposomal and microsomal membranes: role of carotenoid-membrane incorporation and alpha-tocopherol. *Arch Biochem Biophys* Feb 15 1997, 338 (2) p244-50

[Alcohol and free radicals: from basic research to clinical prospects]. *Ann Gastroenterol Hepatol* (Paris) (France) May-Jun 1996, 32 (3) p128-33; discussion 133-4

Melatonin reduces mortality from Aleutian disease in mink (Mustela vison). *J Pineal Res* (Denmark) Nov 1996, 21 (4) p214-7

Exercise causes blood glutathione oxidation in chronic obstructive pulmonary disease: prevention by O2 therapy. *J Appl Physiol* Nov 1996, 81 (5) p2198-202

Comparative study of the effect of 21-aminosteroid and alpha-tocopherol on models of acute oxidative renal injury. *Free Radic Biol Med* 1996, 21 (5) p691-7

Prospective study of moderate alcohol consumption and risk of peripheral arterial disease in US male physicians. *Circulation* Feb 4 1997, 95 (3) p577-80

Oxidized low-density lipoprotein and atherosclerosis. *Int J Clin Lab Res* (Germany) 1996, 26 (3) p178-84

Serum levels of antioxidant vitamins in relation to coronary artery disease: a case control study of Koreans. *Biomed Environ Sci* Sep 1996, 9 (2-3) p229-35

Antioxidants in food and chronic degenerative diseases. *Biomed Environ Sci* Sep 1996, 9 (2-3) p117-23

Randomized trials of dietary antioxidants in cardiovascular disease prevention and treatment. *J Cardiovasc Risk* (England) Aug 1996, 3 (4) p368-71

Basic research in antioxidant inhibition of steps in atherogenesis. *J Cardiovasc Risk* (England) Aug 1996, 3 (4) p352-7

General background on diet and cancer. ECP (UK) Headquarters, Lady Sobell GI Unit, Wexham Park Hospital 1996, 5 (5) p 413-4

Oxidative susceptibility of low-density lipoproteins—influence of regular alcohol use. *Alcohol Clin Exp Res* Sep 1996, 20 (6) p980-4

Molecular epidemiology and retinoid chemoprevention of head and neck cancer. *J Natl Cancer Inst* Feb 5 1997, 89 (3) p199-211

Do hydroxy-carotenoids prevent coronary heart disease? A comparison between Belfast and Toulouse. *Int J Vitam Nutr Res* (Switzerland) 1996, 66 (2) p113-8

Role of dietary phyto-oestrogens in the protection against cancer and heart disease. *Biochem Soc Trans* (England) Aug 1996, 24 (3) p795-800

Role of dietary flavonoids in protection against cancer and coronary heart disease. *Biochem Soc Trans* (England) Aug 1996, 24 (3) p785-9

Can carotenoids reduce oxidation-induced cataract? *Biochem Soc Trans* (England) Aug 1996, 24 (3) p385S

Rationale and design of a large study to evaluate the renal and cardiovascular effects of an ACE inhibitor and vitamin E in high-risk patients with diabetes. The MICRO-HOPE Study. Microalbuminuria, cardiovascular, and renal outcomes. Heart Outcomes Prevention Evaluation. *Diabetes Care* Nov 1996, 19 (11) p1225-8

Vitamin E ameliorates renal injury in an experimental model of immunoglobulin A nephropathy. *Pediatr Res* Oct 1996, 40 (4) p620-6

Demonstration of organotropic effects of chemopreventive agents in multiorgan carcinogenesis models. *Iarc Sci Publ* (France) 1996, (139) p143-50

The Leon Golberg Memorial Lecture. Antioxidants and disease prevention. *Food Chem Toxicol* (England) Oct 1996, 34 (10) p1013-20

Effect of nicotine on antioxidant defence mechanisms in rats fed a high-fat diet. *Pharmacology* (Switzerland) Mar 1996, 52 (3) p153-8

New carotenoid values for foods improve relationship of food frequency questionnaire intake estimates to plasma values. *Cancer Epidemiol Biomarkers Prev* Nov 1996, 5 (11) p907-12

Wheat kernel ingestion protects from progression of muscle weakness in mdx mice, an animal model of Duchenne muscular dystrophy. *Pediatr Res* Sep 1996, 40 (3) p444-9

Effects of the 21-amino steroid tirilazad mesylate (U-74006F) on brain damdema after perinatal hypoxia-ischemia in the rat. *Pediatr Res* Sep 1996, 40 (3) p399-403

What dose of vitamin E is required to reduce susceptibility of LDL to oxidation? *Aust N Z J Med* (Australia) Aug 1996, 26 (4) p496-503

Preliminary studies on the isolation and characterization of predominant prostatic proteins. *Department of Veterans Affairs Medical Center, Bay Pines Flo* Dec 1996, 2 9 (6) p381-5

Cardioprotective effects of individual conjugated equine estrogens through their possible modulation of insulin resistance and oxidation of low-density lipoprotein. *Fertil Steril* Jan 1997, 67 (1) p57-62

Antioxidants in cardiovascular disease: randomized trials. *Nutrition* Sep 1996, 12 (9) p583-8

Possible prevention of postangioplasty restenosis by ascorbic acid. *Am J Cardiol* Dec 1 1996, 78 (11) p1284-6

Does coronary artery screening by electron beam computed tomography motivate potentially beneficial lifestyle behaviors? [see comments]. *Am J Cardiol* Dec 1 1996, 78 (11) p1220-3, Comment in *Am J Cardiol* 1996 Dec 1;78(11):1265-6

Inhibition of steroid-induced cataract in rat eyes by administration of vitamin-E ophthalmic solution. *Ophthalmic Res* (Switzerland) 1996, 28 Suppl 2 p64-71

Anticataract action of vitamin E: its estimation using an in vitro steroid cataract model. *Ophthalmic Res* (Switzerland) 1996, 28 Suppl 2 p16-25

[Effect of antioxidants on the relative risk of coronary heart disease]. *Harefuah* (Israel) Nov 15 1996, 131 (10) p408-12

Randomized trial of antioxidants in the primary prevention of Alzheimer disease warranted? *Alzheimer Dis Assoc Disord* Fall 1996, 10 Suppl 1 p45-9

Effectiveness of antioxidants (vitamin C and E) with and without sunscreens as topical photoprotectants. *Acta Derm Venereol* (Norway) Jul 1996, 76 (4) p264-8

Human nutrition and its discontents: a personal view. *Perspect Biol Med* Autumn 1996, 40 (1) p1-6

Inhibitory effect of a traditional Chinese medicine, Juzen-taiho-to, on progressive growth of weakly malignant clone cells derived from murine fibrosarcoma. *Jpn J Cancer Res* (Japan) Oct 1996, 87 (10) p1039-44

Diet and the prevention and treatment of breast cancer. *Altern Ther Health Med* Nov 1996, 2 (6) p32-8

Beyond cholesterol reduction in coronary heart disease: is vitamin E the answer? *Heart* (England) Oct 1996, 76 (4) p293-4

Influence of heat shock protein 70 and metallothionein induction by zinc-bis-(DL-hydrogenaspartate) on the release of inflammatory mediators in a porcine model of recurrent endotoxemia. *Biochem Pharmacol* (England) Oct 25 1996, 52 (8) p1201-10

Intake of dietary fiber and risk of coronary heart disease in a cohort of Finnish men. The Alpha-Tocopherol, Beta-Carotene Cancer Prevention Study. *Circulation* Dec 1 1996, 94 (11) p2720-7

The hypocholesterolemic and antiatherogenic effects of topically applied phosphatidylcholine in rabbits with heritable hypercholesterolemia. *Artery* 1996, 22 (1) p1-23

Curcumin protects against 4-hydroxy-2-trans-nonenal-induced cataract formation in rat lenses. *Am J Clin Nutr* Nov 1996, 64 (5) p761-6

Delayed tumor onset in transgenic mice fed an amino acid-based diet supplemented with red wine solids. *Am J Clin Nutr* Nov 1996, 64 (5) p748-56

Study design and baseline characteristics of the study to evaluate carotid ultrasound changes in patients treated with ramipril and vitamin E: SECURE. *Am J Cardiol* Oct 15 1996, 78 (8) p914-9

Ascorbic acid and atherosclerotic cardiovascular disease. *Subcell Biochem* (England) 1996, 25 p331-67

Increased pancreatic metallothionein and glutathione levels: protecting against cerulein- and taurocholate-induced acute pancreatitis in rats. *Pancreas* Aug 1996, 13 (2) p173-83

Inhibition of LDL oxidation by cocoa [letter]. *Lancet* (England) Nov 30 1996, 348 (9040) p1514

Alpha-Tocopherol and beta-carotene supplements and lung cancer incidence in the alpha-tocopherol, beta-carotene cancer prevention study: effects of base-line characteristics and study compliance [see comments]. *J Natl Cancer Inst* Nov 6 1996, 88 (21) p1560-70

Risk factors for lung cancer and for intervention effects in Caret, the Beta-Carotene and Retinol Efficacy Trial [see comments]. *J Natl Cancer Inst* Nov 6 1996, 88 (21) p1550-9

Inhibition of phagocyte-endothelium interactions by oxidized fatty acids: a natural anti-inflammatory mechanism? *J Lab Clin Med* Jul 1996, 128 (1) p27-38

Effect of a mediterranean type of diet on the rate of cardiovascular complications in patients with coronary artery disease. Insights into the cardioprotective effect of certain nutriments [see comments]. *J Am Coll Cardiol* Nov 1 1996, 28 (5) p1103-8

Lipid peroxidation and antioxidant vitamins C and E in hypertensive patients. *Ir J Med Sci* (Ireland) Jul-Sep 1996, 165 (3) p210-2

[Alcohol, lipid metabolism and coronary heart disease]. *Herz* (Germany) Aug 1996, 21 (4) p217-26

Prevention of asthma. *Eur Respir J* (Denmark) Jul 1996, 9 (7) p1545-55

Epidemiological evidence for beta-carotene in prevention of cancer and cardiovascular disease. *Eur J Clin Nutr* (England) Jul 1996, 50 Suppl 3 pS57-61

Selenium as a risk factor for cardiovascular diseases. *J Cardiovasc Risk* (England) Feb 1996, 3 (1) p42-7

Role of oxidant stress in the adult respiratory distress syndrome: evaluation of a novel antioxidant strategy in a porcine model of endotoxin-induced acute lung injury. *Shock* 1996, 6 Suppl 1 pS23-6

Zinc administration prevents wasting in stressed mice. *Arch Med Res* (Mexico) Autumn 1996, 27 (3) p319-25

Vitamin E in humans: demand and delivery. *Annu Rev Nutr* 1996, 16 p321-47

The resistance of low density lipoprotein to oxidation promoted by copper and its use as an index of antioxidant therapy. *Atherosclerosis* (Ireland) Jan 26 1996, 119 (2) p169-79

[Selenium, glutathione peroxidase, peroxides and platelet functions]. *Ann Biol Clin* (Paris) (France) 1996, 54 (5) p181-7

Is there a fountain of youth? A review of current life extension strategies. *Pharmacotherapy* Mar-Apr 1996, 16 (2) p183-200

Pathogenic mechanisms in familial amyotrophic lateral sclerosis due to mutation of Cu, Zn superoxide dismutase. *Pathol Biol* (Paris) (France) Jan 1996, 44 (1) p51-6

Update on dietary antioxidants and cancer. *Pathol Biol* (Paris) (France) Jan 1996, 44 (1) p42-5

Antioxidants in cardiovascular disease: randomized trials. *Nutr Rev* Jun 1996, 54 (6) p175-7

Advances in diagnosis and treatment of cancer and cardiovascular disease as well as increased understanding of the mechanisms of the diseases have provided and will certainly continue to provide enormous benefit to affected individuals. At the same time, interventions that may prevent common cancers or atherosclerosis from developing in healthy people could, at least in theory, afford even greater benefits to society as a whole. (The new paradigm for coronary artery disease: altering risk factors, atherosclerotic plaques, and clinical prognosis). *Mayo Clin Proc* Oct 1996, 71 (10) p957-65

Deliberations and evaluations of the approaches, endpoints and paradigms for selenium and iodine dietary recommendations. *J Nutr* Sep 1996, 126 (9 Suppl) p2427S-2434S

Antioxidants in health and disease [see comments]. *J Am Optom Assoc* Jan 1996, 67 (1) p50-7

Multicenter ophthalmic and nutritional age-related macular degeneration study—part 2: antioxidant intervention and conclusions. *J Am Optom Assoc* Jan 1996, 67 (1) p30-49

Multicenter ophthalmic and nutritional age-related macular degeneration study—part 1: design, subjects and procedures. *J Am Optom Assoc* Jan 1996, 67 (1) p12-29

Vegetables, fruit, and cancer prevention: a review. *J Am Diet Assoc* Oct 1996, 96 (10) p1027-39

Synergism between N-acetylcysteine and doxorubicin in the prevention of tumorigenicity and metastasis in murine models. *Int J Cancer* Sep 17 1996, 67 (6) p842-8

Chemoprevention of stomach cancer. *Iarc Sci Publ* (France) 1996, (136) p35-9

Prevention of dopamine-induced cell death by thiol antioxidants: possible implications for treatment of Parkinson's disease. *Exp Neurol* Sep 1996, 141 (1) p32-9

Effect of flavonoids on the outcome of myocardial mitochondrial ischemia/reperfusion injury. *Res Commun Mol Pathol Pharmacol* Jan 1996, 91 (1) p65-75

The Inuit diet. Fatty acids and antioxidants, their role in ischemic heart disease, and exposure to organochlorines and heavy metals. *An internatedersen. Arctic Med Res* (Finland) 1996, 55 Suppl 1 p20-4

All vitamins, cancer, and cardiovascular disease [letter]. *N Engl J Med* Oct 3 1996, 335 (14) p1066-7

Antioxidant vitamins, cancer, and cardiovascular disease [letter]. *N Engl J Med* Oct 3 1996, 335 (14) p1065-6

[The dose-dependent effects of a combination of different classes of antioxidants exemplified by dibunol and beta-carotene]. *Izv Akad Nauk Ser Biol* (Russia) Mar-Apr 1996, (2) p147-52

Nutritional support to prevent and treat multiple organ failure. *World J Surg* May 1996, 20 (4) p474-81

Oxidative damage and defense. *Am J Clin Nutr* Jun 1996, 63 (6) p985S-990S

Do antioxidant micronutrients protect against the development and progression of knee osteoarthritis? *Arthritis Rheum* Apr 1996, 39 (4) p648-56

Beta-carotene, carotenoids, and disease prevention in humans. *Faseb J* May 1996, 10 (7) p690-701

Vegetable, fruit, and cereal fiber intake and risk of coronary heart disease among men [see comments]. *JAMA* Feb 14 1996, 275 (6) p447-51

Dietary non-tocopherol antioxidants present in extra virgin olive oil increase the resistance of low density lipoproteins to oxidation in rabbits. *Atherosclerosis* (Ireland) Feb 1996, 120 (1-2) p15-23

Antioxidants, Helicobacter pylori and stomach cancer in Venezuela. *Eur J Cancer Prev* (England) Feb 1996, 5 (1) p57-62

Dietary fiber and the chemopreventive modelation of colon carcinogenesis. *Mutat Res* (Netherlands) Feb 19 1996, 350 (1) p185-97

Antioxidant vitamins, cancer, and cardiovascular disease [editorial; comment]. *N Engl J Med* May 2 1996, 334 (18) p1189-90, 10/L/184

Effects of a combination of beta carotene and vitamin A on lung cancer and cardiovascular disease [see comments]. *N Engl J Med* May 2 1996, 334 (18) p1150-5

Lack of effect of long-term supplementation with beta carotene on the incidence of malignant neoplasms and cardiovascular disease [see comments]. *N Engl J Med* May 2 1996, 334 (18) p1145-9

Ascorbic acid protects against male infertility in a teleost fish. *Experientia* (Switzerland) Feb 15 1996, 52 (2) p97-100

Clinical evaluation of in-feed zinc bacitracin for the control of porcine intestinal adenomatosis in growing/fattening pigs. *Vet Rec* (England) May 18 1996, 138 (20) p489-92

The effect of modest vitamin E supplementation on lipid peroxidation products and other cardiovascular risk factors in diabetic patients. *Lipids* Mar 1996, 31 Suppl pS87-90

The role of oxidized lipoproteins in atherogenesis. *Free Radic Biol Med* (United States) 1996, 20 (5) p707-27

Inhibition of naphthalene cataract in rats by aldose reductase inhibitors. *Curr Eye Res* (England) Apr 1996, 15 (4) p423-32

Selenium: a quest for better understanding. *Altern Ther Health Med* Jul 1996, 2 (4) p59-62, 65-7

Primary and secondary prevention of myocardial infarction. *Clin Exp Hypertens* Apr-May 1996, 18 (3-4) p547-58

Tuberculosis in Siberia: 2. Diagnosis, chemoprophylaxis and treatment. *Tuber Lung Dis* (Scotland) Aug 1996, 77

Antioxidants, oxidants and free radical stress in cardiovascular disease. *J Assoc Physicians India* (India) Jan 1996, 44 (1) p43-8

Lipid peroxidation: a review of causes, consequences, measurement and dietary influences. *Int J Food Sci Nutr* (England) May 1996, 47 (3) p233-61

Female lung cancer. *Annu Rev Public Health* 1996, 17 p97-114

The role of metals in ischemia/reperfusion injury of the liver. *Semin Liver Dis* Feb 1996, 16 (1) p31-8

[Bronchopulmonary dysplasia]. *Rev Mal Respir* (France) Jul 1996, 13 (3) p243-9

[LDL oxidation in homozygous familial hypercholesterolemia: effects of selective LDL-apheresis treatment]. *Cardiologia* (Italy) May 1996, 41 (5) p435-9

Dietary antioxidants in disease prevention. *Nat Prod Rep* (England) Aug 1996, 13 (4) p265-73

Oxidative stress as a mechanism of cardiac failure in chronic volume overload in canine model. *J Mol Cell Cardiol* (England) Feb 1996, 28 (2) p375-85

Vascular incorporation of alpha-tocopherol prevents endothelial dysfunction due to oxidized LDL by inhibiting protein kinase C stimulation. *J Clin Invest* Jul 15 1996, 98 (2) p386-94

[The significance of ixidized low density lipoprotein in atherosclerosis]. *Ugeskr Laeger* (Denmark) May 6 1996, 158 (19) p2706-10

Nutrition and immunity with emphasis on infection and autoimmune disease. *Nutr Health* (England) 1996, 10 (4) p285-312

In vivo antioxidant treatment suppresses nuclear factor-kappa B activation and neutrophilic lung inflammation. *J Immunol* Aug 15 1996, 157 (4) p1630-7

Effect of radiation on red cell membrane and intracellular oxidative defense systems. *Free Radic Res* (Switzerland) Mar 1996, 24 (3) p199-204

Oxidatively modified LDL and atherosclerosis: an evolving plausible scenario. *Crit Rev Food Sci Nutr* Apr 1996, 36 (4) p341-55

The effects of alpha tocopherol supplementation on monocyte function. Decreased lipid oxidation, interleukin 1 beta secretion, and monocyte adhesion to endothelium. *J Clin Invest* Aug 1 1996, 98 (3) p756-63

Metallopanstimulin as a novel tumor marker in sera of patients with various types of common cancers: implications for prevention and therapy. *Anticancer Res* (Greece) Jul-Aug 1996, 16 (4B) p2177-85

Antioxidants and age-related eye disease. Current and future perspectives. *Ann Epidemiol* Jan 1996, 6 (1) p60-6

Hyperlipidemia. When does treatment make a difference? *Postgrad Med* Jul 1996, 100 (1) p138-49

[Free radicals in the central nervous system]. *Cesk Fysiol* (Czech Republic) Mar 1996, 45 (1) p4-12

[Can vitamin E prevent development of coronary heart disease?]. *Tidsskr Nor Laegeforen* (Norway) Mar 30 1996, 116 (9) p1109-13

Protection by multiple antioxidants against lipid peroxidation in rat liver homogenate. *Lipids* Jan 1996, 31 (1) p47-50

Effect of selenium on 1,2-dimethylhydrazine-induced intestinal cancer in rats. *Dis Colon Rectum* Jun 1996, 39 (6) p628-31

[The Mediterranean diet in the prevention of arteriosclerosis]. *Recenti Prog Med* (Italy) Apr 1996, 87 (4) p175-81

Serum high density lipoprotein cholesterol, alcohol, and coronary mortality in male smokers [see comments]. *BMJ* (England) May 11 1996, 312 (7040) p1200-3

Lifestyle change for coronary artery disease. What to tell patients. *Postgrad Med* Feb 1996, 99 (2) p89-92, 95-6, 102-6

Inhibition of Ca2+-pump ATPase and the Na+/K+-pump ATPase by iron-generated free radicals. Protection by 6,7-dimethyl-2,4-DI-1-pyrrolidinyl-7H-pyrrolo[2,3-d] pyrimidine sulfate (U-89843D), a potent, novel, antioxidant/free radical scavenger. *Biochem Pharmacol* (England) Feb 23 1996, 51 (4) p471-6

Long-term oral vitamin E supplementation in cystic fibrosis patients: RRR-alpha-tocopherol compared with all-rac-alpha-tocopheryl acetate preparations. *Am J Clin Nutr* May 1996, 63 (5) p722-8

The HOPE (Heart Outcomes Prevention Evaluation) Study: the design of a large, simple randomized trial of an angiotensin-converting enzyme inhibitor (ramipril) and vitamin E in patients at high risk of cardiovascular events. The HOPE study investigators. *Can J Cardiol* (Canada) Feb 1996, 12 (2) p127-37

Dietary antioxidant vitamins and death from coronary heart disease in postmenopausal women [see comments]. *N Engl J Med* May 2 1996, 334 (18) p1156-62

Mortality associated with low plasma concentration of beta carotene and the effect of oral supplementation. *JAMA* Mar 6 1996, 275 (9) p699-703

Effect of vitamin E and beta carotene on the incidence of angina pectoris. A randomized, double-blind, controlled trial. *JAMA* Mar 6 1996, 275 (9) p693-8

[Overview--suppression effect of essential trace elements on arteriosclerotic development and its mechanism]. *Nippon Rinsho* (Japan) Jan 1996, 54 (1) p59-66

Prevention of doxorubicin induced cardiotoxicity by catechin. *Cancer Lett* (Ireland) Jan 19 1996, 99 (1) p1-6

Relative resistance of the hamster to aortic atherosclerosis in spite of prolonged vitamin E deficiency and dietary hypercholesterolemia. Putative effect of increased HDL? *Biochim Biophys Acta* (Netherlands) Jan 19 1996, 1299 (2) p216-22

Gastroprotective activity of melatonin and its precursor, L-tryptophan, against stress-induced and ischaemia-induced lesions is mediated by scavenge of oxygen radicals. *Scand J Gastroenterol* (Norway) May 1997, 32 (5) p433-8

Comparison between dietary soybean protein and casein of the inhibiting effect on atherogenesis in the thoracic aorta of hypercholesterolemic (ExHC) rats treated with experimental hypervitamin D. *Biosci Biotechnol Biochem* (Japan) Mar 1997, 61 (3) p514-9

Melatonin: media hype or therapeutic breakthrough? *Nurse Pract* Feb 1997, 22 (2) p66-7, 71-2, 77

[Guidelines of drug therapies for Parkinson's disease]. *Nippon Rinsho* (Japan) Jan 1997, 55 (1) p52-7

Myocardium-protective effects of Ginkgo biloba extract (EGb 761) in old rats against acute isobaric hypoxia. An electron microscopic morphometric study. II. Protection of microvascular endothelium. *Exp Toxicol Pathol* (Germany) Jan 1996, 48 (1) p81-6

Myocardium-protective effects of Ginkgo biloba extract (EGb 761) in old rats against acute isobaric hypoxia. An electron microscopic morphometric study. I. Protection of cardiomyocytes. *Exp Toxicol Pathol* (Germany) Jan 1996, 48 (1) p33-9

The effect of coenzyme Q10 on infarct size in a rabbit model of ischemia/reperfusion. *Cardiovasc Res* (Netherlands) Nov 1996, 32 (5) p861-8

Prevention of cytokine-induced hypotension in cancer patients by the pineal hormone melatonin. *Support Care Cancer* (Germany) Jul 1996, 4 (4) p313-6

Protection by coenzyme Q10 of tissue reperfusion injury during abdominal aortic cross-clamping. *J Cardiovasc Surg* (Torino) (Italy) Jun 1996, 37 (3) p229-35

A review of the clinical effects of phytoestrogens. *Obstet Gynecol* May 1996, 87 (5 Pt 2) p897-904

Protection by multiple antioxidants against lipid peroxidation in rat liver homogenate. *Lipids* Jan 1996, 31 (1) p47-50

The making of a user friendly MAOI diet. *J Clin Psychiatry* Mar 1996, 57 (3) p99-104

Neuroprotective strategy for Alzheimer disease: intranasal administration of a fatty neuropeptide. *Proc Natl Acad Sci U S A* Jan 9 1996, 93 (1) p427-32

Effects of green tea catechins (Polyphenon 100) on cerulein-induced acute pancreatitis in rats. *Pancreas* Apr 1997, 14 (3) p276-9

Characterization of early pulmonary hyperproliferation and tumor progression and their inhibition by black tea in a 4-(methylnitrosamino)-1-(3-pyridyl)-1-butanone-induced lung tumorigenesis model with A/J mice. *Cancer Res* May 15 1997, 57 (10) p1889-94

Tea and health: a historical perspective. *Cancer Lett* (Ireland) Mar 19 1997, 114 (1-2) p315-7

[Cardio-protective effect of red wine as reflected in the literature]. *Orv Hetil* (Hungary) Mar 16 1997, 138 (11) p673-8

Delayed tumor onset in transgenic mice fed an amino acid-based diet supplemented with red wine solids. *Am J Clin Nutr* Nov 1996, 64 (5) p748-56

[Alcohol, lipid metabolism and coronary heart disease]. *Herz* (Germany) Aug 1996, 21 (4) p217-26

Oxidative damage and defense. *Am J Clin Nutr* Jun 1996, 63 (6) p985S-990S

Chemopreventive effects of green and black tea on pulmonary and hepatic carcinogenesis. *Fundam Appl Toxicol* Feb 1996, 29 (2) p244-50

Increased brain damage after stroke or excitotoxic seizures in melatonin-deficient rats. *FASEB Journal*, 1996, 10/13 (1546-1551)

Oxidative damage caused by free radicals produced during catecholamine autoxidation: Protective effects of O-methylation and melatonin. *Free Radical Biology and Medicine*, 1996, 21/2 (241-249)

Oxidative processes and antioxidative defense mechanisms in the aging brain. *FASEB Journal*, 1995, 9/7 (526-533)

Melatonin, hydroxyl radical-mediated oxidative damage, and aging: A hypothesis. *J. Pineal Res.* (Denmark), 1993, 14/4 (151-168)

Neuroimmunotherapy of human cancer with interleukin-2 and the neurohormone melatonin: Its efficacy in preventing hypotension. *Anticancer Res.* (Greece), 1990, 10/6 (1759-1761)

Loss of delta-6-desaturase activity as a key factor in aging. *Med. Hypotheses* (England), 1981, 7/9 (1211-1220)

Betaine:homocysteine methyltransferase—A new assay for the liver enzyme and its absence from human skin fibroblasts and peripheral blood lymphocytes. *Clin. Chim. Acta* (Netherlands), 1991, 204/1-3 (239-250)

Dimethylglycine and chemically related amines tested for mutagenicity under potential nitrosation conditions. *Mutat. Res.* (Netherlands), 1989, 222/4 (343-350)

Homocystinuria due to cystathionine beta-synthase deficiency—The effects of betaine treatment in pyridoxine-responsive patients. *Metab. Clin. Exp.*, 1985, 34/12 (1115-1121)

Prevention of strychnine-induced seizures and death by the N-methylated glycine derivatives betaine, dimethylglycine and sarcosine. *Pharmacol. Biochem. Behav.*, 1985, 22/4 (641-643)

Serenoa repens (Permixon (R)). A review of its pharmacology and therapeutic efficacy in benign prostatic hyperplasia. *Drugs and Aging* (New Zealand), 1996, 9/5 (379-395)

The extract of serenoa repens in the treatment of benign prostatic hyperplasia: A multicenter open study. *Curr. Ther. Res. Clin. Exp.*, 1994, 55/7 (776-785)

Influence of dietary components on occurrence of and mortality due to neoplasms in male F344 rats. *Aging—Clinical and Experimental Research* (Italy), 1996, 8/4 (254-262)

Soy isoflavonoids and cancer prevention: Underlying biochemical and pharmacological issues. *Advances in Experimental Medicine and Biology*, 1996, 401/-(87-100)

A review of the clinical effects of phytoestrogens. *Obstetrics and Gynecology*, 1996, 87/5 II Suppl. (897-904)

Perspectives on soy protein as a nonpharmacological approach for lowering cholesterol. *Journal of Nutrition*, 1995, 125/3 Suppl. (675S-678S)

Overview: Dietary approaches for reducing cardiovascular disease risks. *Journal of Nutrition*, 1995, 125/3 Suppl. (656S-665S)

Protective effects of soy protein on the peroxidizability of lipoproteins in cerebrovascular diseases. *Journal of Nutrition*, 1995, 125/3 Suppl. (639S-646S)

Modern applications for an ancient bean: Soybeans and the prevention and treatment of chronic disease. *Journal of Nutrition*, 1995, 125/3 Suppl. (567S-569S)

Green tea consumption and serum lipid profiles: A cross-sectional study in Northern Kyushu, Japan. *Prev. Med.*, 1992, 21/4 (526-531)

Use of soya-beans for the dietary prevention and management of malnutrition in Nigeria. *Acta Paediatr. Scand. Suppl.* (Sweden), 1991, 80/374 (175-182)

Increasing use of soyfoods and their potential role in cancer prevention. *J. Am. Diet. Assoc.*, 1991, 91/7 (836-840)

Diet and serum lipids in vegan vegetarians: A model for risk reduction. *J. Am. Diet. Assoc.*, 1991, 91/4 (447-453)

Nutritional contributors to cardiovascular disease in the elderly. *J. Am. Geriatr. Soc.*, 1986, 34/1 (27-36)

Human and laboratory studies on the causes and prevention of gastrointestinal cancer. *Scand. J. Gastroenterol. Suppl.* (Norway), 1984, 19/104 (15-26)

Preventive nutrition: Disease-specific dietary interventions for older adults. *Geriatrics*, 1992, 47/11 (39-49)

Significance of active and passive prevention of cancer, arteriosclerosis and senility. *Minerva Med.* (Italy), 1982, 73/41 (2867-2872)

Increased brain damage after stroke or excitotoxic seizures in melatonin-deficient rats. *FASEB Journal*, 1996, 10/13 (1546-1551)

Oxidative processes and antioxidative defense mechanisms in the aging brain. *FASEB Journal,* 1995, 9/7 (526-533)

Partial restoration of choline acetyltransferase activities in aging and AF64A-lesioned rat brains by vitamin *E. Neurochem. Int.* (UK), 1993, 22/5 (487-491)

Do antioxidant micronutrients protect against the development and progression of knee osteoarthritis? *Arthritis and Rheumatism*, 1996, 39/4 (648-656)

Dietary flavonoids, antioxidant vitamins, and incidence of stroke: The Zutphen study. *Archives of Internal Medicine*, 1996, 156/6 (637-642)

Free radicals, oxidative stress, oxidized low density lipoprotein (LDL), and the heart: Antioxidants and other strategies to limit cardiovascular damage. *Connecticut Medicine*, 1995, 59/10 (579-588)

Causes and prevention of premature aging. *Geriatrika* (Spain), 1994, 10/7 (19-24)

Antioxidant vitamins and disease—Risks of a suboptimal supply. *Ther. Umsch.* (Switzerland), 1994, 51/7 (467-474)

Tracking the daily supplement. *Today's Life Sci.* (Australia), 1994, 6/3 (24-31)

Preventive nutrition: Disease-specific dietary interventions for Older adults. *Geriatrics,* 1992, 47/11 (39-49)

Experimental approaches to nutrition and cancer: Fats, calories, vitamins and minerals. *Med. Oncol. Tumor Pharmacother.* (UK), 1990, 7/2-3 (183-192)

Vitamin D requirements for the elderly. *Clin. Nutr.*, 1986, 5/3 (121-129)

Vitamin D deficiency and hip fractures. *Tijdschr. Gerontol. Geriatr.* (NT), 1985, 16/6 (239-245)

The physiologic and pharmacologic factors protecting the lens transparency and the update approach to the prevention of experimental cataracts: A review. *Metab. Pediatr. Syst. Ophthalmol.*, 1983, 7/2 (115-124)

Prostate Cancer (Adjuvant Therapy)

Prevention of radioinduced cystitis by orgotein: a randomized study. *Anticancer Res* 16:2025-2028, 1996.

Dietary phytoestrogens and prostate cancer. *Proc Annu Meet Am Assoc Cancer Res* 36:687, 1995.

Pathological features of hereditary prostate cancer. *J Urol* 153:987-992, 1995.

Hereditary prostate cancer: epidemiologic and clinical features. *J Urol* 150:797-802, 1993.

Familial risk factors for prostate cancer. *Cancer Surv* 11:5, 1991.

Mendelian inheritance of familial prostate cancer. *Proc Natl Acad Sci* 89:3367, 1992.

Genetic epidemiology of prostate cancer in the Utah Mormon Genealogy. *Cancer Surv* 1:47-69, 1982.

Family history and the risk of prostate cancer. *Prostate* 17:337-347, 1990.

Familial patterns of prostate cancer: a case control analysis. *J Urol* 146:1305-1307, 1991.

Familial clustering of cancers of the breast and prostate in a population-based sample of postmenopausal women. *Proc Annu Meet Am Assoc Cancer Res* 35:A1724, 1994.

The Anti-Oxidant Revolution. Thomas Nelson Publisher. 1994.

Enter the Zone. Regan Books, 1995.

The Anti-Aging Zone. Regan Books, 1999.

Inhibition of arachidonate 5-lipoxygenase triggers massive apoptosis in human prostate cancer cells. *Proc Natl Acad Sci* 95:13182-13187, 1998.

Induction of cyclo-oxygenase-2 mRNA by prostaglandin E2 in human prostatic carcinoma cells. *Br J Cancer* 75:1111-8, 1997.

Prostate cancer and supplementation with alpha-tocopherol and beta-carotene: incidence and mortality in a controlled trial. *J Natl Cancer Inst* 90:440-6, 1998.

Vitamin E inhibits the high-fat diet promoted growth of established human prostate LNCaP tumor in nude mice. *J Urol* 161:1651-1654, 1999.

Effects of selenium supplementation for cancer prevention in patients with carcinoma of the skin. *JAMA* 276:1957-1963, 1996.

Inhibitory effects of selenium on the growth of DU-145 human prostate carcinoma cells in vitro. *Biochem Biophys Res Commun* 130:603-609, 1985.

Natural vitamin E (gamma-tocopherol) demonstrates greater inhibition of growth on a human prostate cancer cell line than synthetic vitamin E. (in press)

Genistein inhibits proliferation and in vitro invasive potential of human prostatic cancer cell lines. *Anticancer Res* 17:1199-204, 1997.

Genistein and biochanin A inhibit the growth of human prostate cancer cells but not epidermal growth factor receptor tyrosine autophosphorylation. *Prostate* 22:335-45, 1993.

Antiproliferative effect of Pygeum africanum extract on rat prostatic fibroblasts. *J Urol* 157:2381-7, 1997.

A flavonoid antioxidant, silymarin, inhibits activation of erbB1 signaling and induces cyclin-dependent kinase inhibitors, G1 arrest, and anticarcinogenic effects in human prostate carcinoma DU145 cells. *Cancer Res* 58:1920-9, 1998.

Inhibition of epidermal growth factor receptor (EGFr) tyrosine kinase activity by silymarin, a polyphenolic antioxidant and potent cancer chemopreventive agent. *Proc Annu Meet Am Assoc Cancer Res* 38:A1766, 1997.

Protective and therapeutic effect of silymarin on the development of latent liver damage. *Radiats Biol Radioecol* 38:411-5, 1998.

Protection against tumor promotion in mouse skin by silymarin (Meeting abstract). *Proc Annu Meet Am Assoc Cancer Res* 36:A3534, 1995.

Agarwal R Protective effects of silymarin against photocarcinogenesis in a mouse skin model. *J Natl Cancer Inst* 89:556-66, 1997.

Prostate Cancer (Early Stage)

Staging of early prostate cancer: a proposed tumor volume-based prognostic index. *Urology* 41:403-11, 1993.

Tumor volume and prostate specific antigen: implications for early detection and defining a window of curability. *J Urol* 154:1808-12, 1995.

Recent advances on PSA and cancer growth. *International Symposium on Recent Advances in Diagnosis and Treatment of Prostate Cancer,* September 21-23, 1995, Quebec City, p. 14, 1995.

PC: The development of human benign prostatic hyperplasia with age. *Walsh J Urol* 132:474-479, 1984.

Longitudinal evaluation of Prostate-Specific Antigen levels in men with and without prostate cancer. *JAMA* 267:2215-2220, 1992.

Prostate specific antigen progression rates after radical prosatectomy or radiation therapy for localized prostate cancer. *Surgery* 116:302-306, 1994.

Prostate specific antigen regression and progression after androgen deprivation for localized and metastatic prostate cancer. *J Urol* 153:1860-1865, 1995.

Early stage prostate cancer treated with radiation therapy: stratifying an intermediate risk group. *Int J Radiat Oncol Biol Phys* 38: 569-73, 1997.

Prostate specific antigen and Gleason grade: an immunohistochemical examination of prostate cancer. *J. Urol.* 151:1558-1564, 1994.

Prostate cancer volume adds significantly to prostate-specific antigen in the prediction of early biochemical failure after external beam radiation therapy *Int J Radiation Oncology Biol Phys* 35:273-279, 1996.

Calculated prostate predictor of actual cancer volume: the optimal volume and pathological stage *Urology* 49: 385-391, 1997.

Morphometry of the prostate: I. Distribution of tissue components in hyperplastic glands. *Urology* 44:486-92, 1994.

Inhibition of Kupffer cell functions as an explanation for the hepatoprotective properties of silibinin. *Hepatology* 23:749-54, 1996.

Anaemia associated with androgen deprivation in patients with prostate cancer receiving combined hormone blockade. *Br J Urol* 79: 933-41, 1997.

Anemia associated with androgen deprivation(AAAD) due to combination hormone blockade (CHB) responds to recombinant human erythropoietin (r hu-EPO). *J Urol* 157:232A 1997.

Improved survival in patients with locally advanced prostate cancer treated with radiotherapy and goserelin. *N Engl J Med* 337:295-300, 1997.

Predictors of improved outcome for patients with localized prostate cancer treated with neoadjuvant androgen ablation therapy and three-dimensional conformal radiotherapy. *J Clin Oncol* 16:3380-3385, 1998.

Stage T1-2 prostate cancer with pretreatment prostate-specific antigen level < or = 10 ng/ml: radiation therapy or surgery? *Int J Radiat Oncol Biol Phys* 38: 723-9, 1997.

Bilateral orchiectomy with or without flutamide for metastatic prostate cancer. *N Engl J Med* 339: 1036-42, 1998.

Major advantages of "early" administration of endocrine combination therapy in advanced prostate cancer. *Clin. Invest. Med.* 16:6 493-498, 1993.

Maximal androgen blockade: final analysis of EORTC Phase III Trial 30853. *Eur Urol* 33:144-151, 1998.

Treatment with Finasteride Following Radical Prostatectomy for Prostate Cancer, *Urology,* 45: 491-497, 1995.

Finasteride and flutamide as potency-sparing androgen-ablative therapy for advanced adenocarcinoma of the prostate. *Urology* 49: 913-920, 1997.

Intermittent androgen deprivation (IAD) with finasteride (F) during induction and maintenance permits prolonged time off IAD in localized prostate cancer (LPC). *J Urol* 161:156A, 1999.

A case for synchronous reduction of testicular androgen, adrenal androgen and prolactin for the treatment of advanced carcinoma of the prostate. *Eur J Cancer* 31A: 871-875, 1995.

Effects of protein kinase and phosphatase inhibitors on the growth of human prostatic cancer cells. *Medical Science Research* (UK), 1997, 25/5 (353-354)

Phyto-oestrogens and Western diseases. *Annals of Medicine* (UK), 1997, 29/2 (95-120)

Genistein inhibits proliferation and in vitro invasive potential of human prostatic cancer cell lines. *Anticancer Research* (Greece), 1997, 17/2 A (1199-1204)

Soy and rye diets inhibit the development of Dunning R3327 prostatic adenocarcinoma in rats. *Cancer Letters* (Ireland), 1997, 114/1-2 (313-314)

Measurement and metabolism of isoflavonoids and lignans in the human male. *Cancer Letters* (Ireland), 1997, 114/1-2 (145-151)

Inhibition of N-methyl-N-nitrosourea-induced mammary tumors in rats by the soybean isoflavones. *Anticancer Research* (Greece), 1996, 16/6 A (3293-3298)

Genistein-induced apoptosis of prostate cancer cells is preceded by a specific decrease in focal adhesion kinase activity. *Molecular Pharmacology,* 1997, 51/2 (193-200)

Genistein-stimulated adherence of prostate cancer cells is associated with the binding of focal adhesion kinase to beta-1-integrin. *Clinical and Experimental Metastasis* (UK), 1996, 14/4 (389-398)

Quantification of genistein and genistin in soybeans and soybean products. *Food and Chemical Toxicology* (UK), 1996, 34/5 (457-461)

Molecular effects of genistein on estrogen receptor mediated pathways. *Carcinogenesis* (UK), 1996, 17/2 (271-275)

Effects of soya consumption for one month on steroid hormones in premenopausal women: Implications for breast cancer risk reduction. *Cancer Epidemiology Biomarkers and Prevention,* 1996, 5/1 (63-70)

Early di. An update. *Medecine Biologie Environnement* (Italy), 1996, 24/2 (139-152)

Prostate-specific antigen as a screening test for prostate cancer: The United States experience. *Urologic Clinics of North America*, 1997, 24/2 (299-306)

Prostate cancer screening: The controversy. *Revue Medicale Libanaise* (Lebanon), 1996, 8/3 (152-154)

Clinical utility of measurements of free and total prostate-specific. *Prostate*, 1996, 29/Suppl. 7 (64-69)

Detection of human papillomavirus DNA and p53 gene mutations in human prostate cancer. *Prostate*, 1996, 28/5 (318-324)

Effects of potent vitamin D3 analogues on clonal proliferation of human prostate cancer cell lines. *Prostate*, 1997, 31/2 (77-83)

1,25-Dihydroxyvitamin D3 and 9-cis-retinoic acid act synergistically to inhibit the growthcause accumulation of cells in G1. *Endocrinology,* 1997, 138/4 (1491-1497)

Vitamin D receptor content and transcriptional activity do not fully predict antiproliferative effects of vitamin D in human prostate cancer cell lines. *Molecular and Cellular Endocrinology* (Ireland), 1997, 126/1 (83-90)

A preliminary report on the use of transfer factor for treating stage D3 hormone-unr metastatic prostate cancer. *Biotherapy* (Netherlands), 1996, 9/1-3 (123-132)

The role of vitamin D in normal prostate growth and differentiation. *Cell Growth and Differentiation,* 1996, 7/11 (1563-1570)

Effects of 1,25 dihydroxyvitamin D3 and its analogueues on induction of apoptosis in breast cancer cells. *Journal of Steroid Biochemistry and Molecular Biology* (UK), 1996, 58/4 (395-401)

Vitamin D receptor expression is required for growth modulation by 1alpha,25-dihydroxyvitamin D3 in the human prostatic carcinoma cell line ALVA-31. *Journal of Steroid Biochemistry and Molecular Biology* (UK), 1996, 58/3 (277-288)

Induction of transforming growth factor-beta autocrine activity by all-trans-retinoic acid and 1alpha,25-dihydroxyvitamin D3 in NRP-152 rat prostatic epithelial cells. *Journal of Cellular Physiology,* 1996, 166/1 (231-239)

Biologically active acylglycerides from the berries of saw-palmetto (Serenoa repens). *Journal of Natural Products*, 1997, 60/4 (417-418)

Effects of the lipidosterolic extract of Serenoa repens (Permixon (R)) on human prostatic cell lines. *Prostate*, 1996, 29/4 (219-230)

Comparison of in vitro effects of the pure antiandrogens OH-flutamide, casodex, and nilutamide on androgen-sensitive parameters. *Urology,* 1997, 49/4 (580-589)

Casodex (R) (Bicalutamide): Overview of a new antiandrogen developed for the treatment of prostate cancer. *European Urology* (Switzerland), 1997, 31/Suppl. 2 (30-39)

Recommended dose of flutamide with LH-RH agonist therapy in patients with advanced prostate cancer. *International Journal of Urology* (Japan), 1996, 3/6 (468-471)

Bicalutamide (Casodex). *Expert Opinion on Investigational Drugs* (UK), 1996, 5/12 (1707-1722)

U.S. Drug and biologic approvals in 1994-1995. *Drug Development Research*, 1996, 37/4 (197-207)

Cryosurgery of prostate cancer. Use of adjuvant hormonal therapy and temperature monitoring—A one year follow-up. *Anticancer Research* (Greece), 1997, 17/3 A (1511-1515)

The potential role of lycopene for human health. *Journal of the American College of Nutrition,* 1997, 16/2 (109-126)

Lycopene: A biologically important carotenoid for humans? *Archives of Biochemistry and Biophysics*, 1996, 336/1 (1-9)

cis-trans lycopene isomers, carotenoids, and retinol in the human prostate. *Cancer Epidemiology Biomarkers and Prevention*, 1996, 5/10 (823-833)

How is individual risk for prostate cancer assessed? *Hematology / Oncology Clinics of North America*, 1996, 10/3 (537-548)

A tomato a day for preventing prostate cancer? Diet may be key. *Geriatrics*, 1996, 51/2 (21)

Intake of carotenoids and retinol in relation to risk of prostate cancer. *Journal of the National Cancer Institute,* 1995, 87/23 (1767-1776)

Whatever happened to beta carotene? *Journal of the National Cancer Institute*, 1995, 87/23 (1739-1741)

Vegetable and fruit consumption in relation to prostate cancer risk in Hawaii: A reevaluation of the effect of dietary beta-carotene. *Am. J. Epidemiol.*, 1991, 133/3 (215-219)

Serologic precursors of cancer. Retinol, carotenoids, and tocopherol and risk of prostate cancer. *J. Natl. Cancer Inst.*, 1990, 82/11 (941-946)

Carcinogenicity of oral cadmium in the male Wistar (WF/NCr) rat: Effect of chronic dietary zinc deficiency. *Fundam. Appl. Toxicol.*, 1992, 19/4 (512-520)

Nutrition and prostate cancer: A case-control study. *Prostate,* 1985, 6/1 (7-17)

Zinc, vitamin A and prostatic cancer. *Br. J. Urol.* (England), 1983, 55/5 (525-528)

Influence of isoflavones in soy protein isolates on development of induced prostate-related cancers in L-W rats. *Nutrition and Cancer,* 1997, 28/1 (41-45)

Peptide growth factors: Clinical and therapeutic strategies. *Minerva Urologica e Nefrologica* (Italy), 1997, 49/2 (63-72)

Cancer risk factors for selecting cohorts for large-scale chemoprevention trials. *Journal of Cellular Biochemistry,* 1996, 63/Suppl. 25 (29-36)

Inhibition of liposomal lipid peroxidation by isoflavonoid type phyto-oestrogens from soybeans of different countries of origin. *Biochemical Society Transactions* (UK), 1996, 24/3 (392S)

Phytoestrogens: Epidemiology and a possible role in cancer protection. *Environmental Health Perspectives*, 1995, 103/Suppl. 7 (103-112)

Differential sensitivity of human prostatic cancer cell lines to the effects of protein kinase and phosphatase inhibitors. *Cancer Letters* (Ireland), 1995, 98/1 (103-110):

Genetic damage and the inhibition of 7,12-dimethylbenz(a)anthracene-induc ed genetic damage by the phytoestrogens, genistein and daidzein, in female ICR mice. *Cancer Letters* (Ireland), 1995, 95/1-2 (125-133)

Rationale for the use of genistein-containing soy matrices in chemoprevention trials for breast and prostate cancer. *Journal of Cellular Biochemistry*, 1995, 58/Suppl. 22 (181-187)

A simplified method to quantify isoflavones in commercial soybean diets and human urine after legume consumption. *Cancer Epidemiology Biomarkers and Prevention*, 1995, 4/5 (497-503)

Rapid HPLC analysis of dietary phytoestrogens from legumes and from human urine. *Proc. Soc. Exp. Biol. Med.*, 1995, 208/1 (18-26)

Soy intake and cancer risk: A review of the in vitro and in vivo data. *Nutr. Cancer*, 1994, 21/2 (113-131)

Plasma concentrations of phyto-oestrogens in Japanese men. *Lancet* (UK), 1993, 342/8881 (1209-1210)

Genistein is an effective stimulator of sex hormone-binding globulin production in hepatocarcinoma human liver cancer cells and suppresses proliferation of these cells in culture. *Steroids*, 1993, 58/7 (301-304)

Genistein and biochanin A inhibit the growth of human prostate cancer cells but not epidermal growth factor receptor tyrosine autophosphorylation. *Prostate*, 1993, 22/4 (335-345)

Surrogate endpoint biomarkers for phase II cancer chemoprevention trials. *J. Cell. Biochem.*, 1994, 56/Suppl. 19 (1-9)

The 16-ene vitamin D analogues. *Current Pharmaceutical Design* (Netherlands), 1997, 3/1 (99-123)

Signal transduction inhibitors as modifiers of radiation therapy in human prostate carcinoma xenografts. *Radiation Oncology Investigations*, 1996, 4/5 (221-230)

Calcium regulation of androgen receptor expression in the human prostate cancer cell line LNCaP. *Endocrinology*, 1995, 136/5 (2172-2178)

The role of calcium, pH, and cell proliferation in the programmed (apoptotic) death of androgen-independent prostatic cancer cells induced by thapsigarin. *Cancer Res.*, 1994, 54/23 (6167-6175)

Programmed cell death as a new target for prostatic cancer therapy. *Cancer Surv.*, 1991, 11/- (265-277):

Hyperparathyroidism in metastases of prostatic carcinoma: A biochemical, hormonal and histomorphometric study. *Eur. Urol.* (Switzerland), 1990, 17/1 (35-39)

In vitro studies of human prostatic epithelial cells: Attempts to identify distinguishing features of malignant cells. *Growth Factors* (UK), 1989, 1/3 (237-250)

Hypocalcemia associated with estrogen therapy for metastatic adenocarcinoma of the prostate. *J. Urol.*, 1988, 140/5 PART I (1025-1027)

Hypercalcemia in carcinoma of the prostate: Case report and review of the literature. *J. Urol.* (Baltimore), 1987, 137/2 (309-311)

Calcium excretion in metastatic prostatic carcinoma. *Br. J. Urol.* (England), 1984, 56/6 (687-689)

Osteomalacia associated with prostatic cancer and osteoblastic metastases. *Urology*, 1983, 21/1 (65-67)

Carcinoma of the prostate: The treatment of bone metastases by radiophosphorus. *Clin. Radiol.* (Scotland), 1981, 32/6 (695-697)

Management of cancer of the prostate. *Brit. J. Hosp. Med.* (England), 1974, 11/3 (357-372)

Intracavitary irradiation of prostate carcinomas. *Rev. Med. Suisse Romande* (Switzerland), 1980, 100/9

Epidemiology of prostatic cancer: A case-control study. *Prostate*, 1990, 17/3 (189-206)

Demonstration of specifically sensitized lymphocytes in patients treated with an aqueous mistletoe extract (Viscum album L.). *Klin. Wochenschr.* (Germany), 1991, 69/9 (397-403)

An urodynamic study of patients with benign prostatic hypertrophy treated conservatively with phytotherapy or testosterone. *Wien. Klin. Wochenschr.* (Austria), 1979, 91/18 (622-627)

Rationale for the use of genistein-containing soy matrices in chemoprevention trials for breast and prostate cancer. *Journal of Cellular Biochemistry*, 1995, 58/Suppl. 22

Phytoestrogens are partial estrogen agonists in the adult male mouse. *Environmental Health Perspectives*, 1995, 103/Suppl. 7

Urinary excretion of lignans and isoflavonoid phytoestrogens in Japanese men and women consuming a traditional Japanese diet. *Am. J. Clin. Nutr.*, 1991, 54/6

How is individual risk for prostate cancer assessed? *Hematology / Oncology Clinics of North America*, 1996, 10/3

Control of LNCaP proliferation and differentiation: Actions and interactions of androgens, 1alpha,25-dihydroxycholecalciferol, all-trans retinoid acid, 9-cis retinoic acid, and phenylacetate. *Prostate,* 1996, 28/3 (182-194)

1,25-Dihydroxy-16-ene-23-yne-vitamin D3 and prostate cancer cell proliferation in vivo. *Urology*, 1995, 46/3 (365-369)

Recent advances in hormonal therapy for cancer. *Current Opinion in Oncology*, 1995, 7/6

Endocrine control of prostate cancer. *Cancer Surveys*, 1995, 23/- (43-62)

Vitamin D and prostate cancer. *Advances in Experimental Medicine,* 1995, 375/-

Actions of vitamin D3 analogues on human prostate cancer cell lines: Comparison with 1,25-dihydroxyvitamin D3. *Endocrinology*, 1995, 136/1 (20-26)

Vitamin D and cancer. *Rev. Fr. Endocrinol. Clin. Nutr. Metab.* (France), 1994, 35/4-5

Human prostate cancer cells: Inhibition of proliferation by vitamin D analogues. *Anticancer Res.* (Greece), 1994, 14/3 A (1077-1081)

Vitamin D and prostate cancer: 1,25 Dihydroxyvitamin D3 receptors and actions in human prostate cancer cell lines. *Endocrinology*, 1993, 132/5 (1952-1960)

Is vitamin D deficiency a risk factor for prostate cancer? (hypothesis). *Anticancer Res.* (Greece), 1990, 10/5 A (1307-1312)

The in vitro response of four antisteroid receptor agents on the hormone-responsive prostate cancer cell line LNCaP. Oncology Reports (Greece), 1995, 2/2 (295-298)

Combination treatment in M1 prostate cancer. *Cancer,* 1993, 72/12 Suppl. (3880-3885)

Antiandrogenic drugs. *Cancer,* 1993, 71/3 Suppl. (1046-1049)

The effects of flutamide on total DHT and nuclear DHT levels in the human prostate. *Prostate*, 1981, 2/3 (309-314)

Endocrine profiles during administration of the new non-steroidal anti-androgen Casodex in prostate cancer. *Clin. Endocrinol.* (UK), 1994, 41/4 (525-530)

Antiandrogenic drugs. *Cancer,* 1993, 71/3 Suppl. (1046-1049)

Prostate Cancer (Late/Metastasized Stage)

Also refer to Cancer Overview.

Extensive personal experience: Combination of screening and preoperative endocrine therapy: the potential for an important decrease in prostate cancer mortality. *J Clin Endocrinol Metab* 80:2002-2013, 1995.

Diagnosis of advanced or noncurable prostate cancer can be practically eliminated by prostate-specific antigen. *Urology* 47: 212-217, 1996.

Evaluation of ProstaSure index in the detection of prostate cancer: a preliminary report. *Urology* 51:132-136, 1998.

Prostate cancer detection in men with serum PSA concentrations of 2.6 to 4.0 ng/mL and benign prostate examination. Enhancement of specificity with free PSA measurements [see comments]. *JAMA* 277:1452-5, 1997.

Prospective longitudinal evaluation of men with initial prostate specific antigen levels of 4.0 ng./ml. or less [see comments]. *J Urol* 157:1740-3, 1997.

Systematic 5 region prostate biopsy is superior to sextant method for diagnosing carcinoma of the prostate. 157: 199-203, 1997.

Heterogeneity of prostate cancer in radical prostatectomy samples. *Urology* 43:60-4, 1994.

Brawn PN: The dedifferentiation of prostate cancer. *Cancer* 52:246-51, 1983.

A model to study c-myc and v-H-ras induced prostate cancer progression in the Copenhagen rat. *Cell Mol Biol* 44:949-59, 1998.

Oncogene overexpression in human prostate cancer cell lines. *Proc Annu Meet Am Assoc Cancer Res* 34:A2309, 1993.

Expression of the proto-oncogene bcl-2 in the prostate and its association with emergence of androgen-independent prostate cancer. *Cancer Res* 52:6940-4, 1992.

p53 is mutated in a subset of advanced-stage prostate cancers. *Cancer Res* 53:3369-73, 1993.

Mutation of the androgen receptor gene in metastatic androgen-independent prostate cancer. *N Engl J Med* 332:1393-8, 1995.

A mutation in the ligand binding domain of the androgen receptor of human LNCaP cells affects steroid binding characteristics and response to anti-androgens. *Biochem Biophys Res Commun* 173:534-40, 1990.

Plasma testosterone and androstenedione after orchiectomy in prostatic adenocarcinoma. *Clin Endocrinol* 2:101-109, 1973.

Adrenal androgens predict for early progression to flutamide withdrawal in patients with androgen-independent prostate carcinoma. *Proc Am Soc Clin Oncol* 13:237, 1994.

Flutamide withdrawal syndrome: its impact on clinical trials in hormone-refractory prostate cancer. *J Clin Oncol* 11:1566-72, 1993.

Prostate specific antigen decline following discontinuation of flutamide in patients with stage D2 prostate cancer. *Am J Med* 98:412-14, 1995.

The antiandrogen withdrawal syndrome: Experience in a large cohort of unselected advanced prostate cancer patients. *Cancer* 76:1428-34, 1995.

Prostate-specific antigen decline after Casodex withdrawal: Evidence for an antiandrogen withdrawal syndrome. *Urology* 43:408-10, 1994.

A double-blind assessment of antiandrogen withdrawal from Casodex (C) or Eulexin (E) therapy while continuing luteinizing hormone releasing hormone analogue (LHRH-A) therapy for patients (Pts) with stage D2 prostate cancer (PCA). *Proc Am Soc Clin Oncol* 15:255A, 1996.

Dramatic PSA decline in response to discontinuation of megestrol acetate in advanced prostate cancer; expansion of the antiandrogen withdrawal syndrome. *J Urol* 153:1956-7, 1995.

Complete remission of hormone refractory adenocarcinoma of the prostate in response to withdrawal of diethylstilbestrol. *J Urol* 153:1944-5, 1995.

Mutant androgen receptor detected in an advanced-stage prostatic carcinoma is activated by adrenal androgens and progesterone. *Mol Endocr* 7:1541, 1993.

Mutation of the androgen receptor gene in metastatic androgen-independent prostate cancer. *N Engl J Med* 332:1393-8, 1995.

Anti-androgen activation of mutant androgen receptors from androgen-independent prostate cancer. *Clin Cancer Res* 3:1383, 1997.

The proliferative effect of "anti-androgens" on the androgen-sensitive human prostate tumor cell line LNCaP. *Endocrinology* 126:1457, 1990.

High dose bicalutamide for androgen independent prostate cancer: Effect of prior hormonal therapy. *J Urol* 159:149-53, 1998.

A novel and rapid treatment for advanced prostatic cancer. *J Urol* 130:152-3, 1983.

Synergistic effect of ketoconazole and anti-neoplastic agents in hormone-independent prostatic cancer cells. *Clin Invest Med* 12:363-6, 1989.

A possible direct cytotoxic effect on prostate carcinoma cells. *J Urol* 141:190-1,1989.

Ketoconazole effectively reverses multi-drug resistance in highly resistant KB cells. *J Urol* 151:485-491, 1994.

Long-term experience with high dose ketoconazole therapy in patients with stage D2 prostatic carcinoma. *J Urol* 137:902-4,1987.

Optimal dosing of ketoconazole (Keto) and hydrocortisone (HC) leads to long responses in hormone refractory prostate cancer. *Proc Am Soc Clin Oncol* 13:229A, 1994.

Ketoconazole retains activity in advanced prostate cancer patients with progression despite flutamide withdrawal. *J Urol* 157:1204-7, 1997.

Simultaneous antiandrogen withdrawal and treatment with ketoconazole and hydrocortisone in patients with advanced "prostate carcinoma." *Cancer* 80:1755-9, 1997.

Phase II study of ketoconazole combined with weekly doxorubicin in patients with androgen-independent prostate cancer. *J Clin Oncol* 12: 683-688, 1994.

Phase II trial of alternating weekly chemohormonal therapy for patients with androgen-independent prostate cancer. *Clinical Cancer Research* 3: 2371-2376, 1997.

Effects of an acidic beverage (Coca-Cola) on absorption of ketoconazole. *Antimicr Agents and Chemother* 39:1671-5, 1995.

Treatment of metastatic prostate cancer with low dose prednisone: Evaluation of pain and quality of life as pragmatic indices of response. *J Clin Oncol* 7:590-7, 1989.

Chemotherapy with mitoxantrone plus prednisone or prednisone alone for symptomatic hormone-resistant prostate cancer: A Canadian Randomized Trial with palliative end points. *J Clin Oncol* 14:1756-64, 1996.

Response of hormone resistant prostate cancer to dexamethasone (dex) by weekly intravenous (IV) injection: Improvement in performance status (PS), bone pain and reduction in prostate specific antigen (PSA). *Proc Am Soc Clin Oncol 1*3:255A, 1994.

Prostate specific antigen levels and clinical response to low-dose dexamethasone for hormone refractory prostate carcinoma. *Proc Am Soc Clin Oncol* 13: 235A, 1994.

The contribution of hydrocortisone to the observed response proportions of suramin. *Proc Am Soc Clin Oncol* 13:A710, 1994.

The in vitro localization of ^{3}H-estradiol in human prostatic carcinoma. *Cancer* 31:682-8, 1973.

Hormonal effects in vitro on ribonucleic acid polymerase in nuclei isolated from human prostatic tissue. *J Endocrinol* 59:367-368, 1973.

Metabolism and action of steroid hormones on human benign prostatic hyperplasia and prostatic carcinoma grown in organ culture. *J Steroid Biochem* 11:625-630, 1979.

The Veterans' Administrative Cooperative Urological Research Group's studies of cancer of the prostate. *Cancer* 32:1126-30, 1973.

The Veterans' Administrative Cooperative Urological Research Group studies of carcinoma of the prostate: a review. *Cancer Chemother Rep* 59(Part 1):225-7, 1975.

Comparison of diethylstilbestrol, cyproterone acetate, and medroxyprogesterone acetate in the treatment of advanced prostate cancer: final analysis of a randomizaed phase III trial of the European Organization for Research on the Treatment of Cancer Urological group. *J Urol* 136:624-30, 1986.

Haemostatic changes during hormone manipulation in advanced prostate cancer: a comparison of DES 3mg/day and Goserelin 3.6 mg/month. *Eur J Cancer* 26:315-9, 1990.

Hormone therapy for prostate cancer: results of the Veterans Administrative Cooperative Urological Research Group studies. *NCI Monogr* 7:165-70, 1988.

Hormonal therapy of prostatic cancer. *Cancer* 47(7 suppl):1929-36, 1980.

Clinical efficacy of Diethylstilbestrol treatment in post-orchiectomy progressive prostate cancer. *Proc Am Assoc Cancer Res* 35:233A, 1994.

A Phase II trial of oral diethylstilbestrol as a second-line hormonal agent in advanced prostate cancer. *Urology* 52:257-60, 1998.

Clinical trial of massive stilboestrol diphosphate therapy in advanced carcinoma of the prostate. *Br J Urol* 33:171, 1961.

The effect of stilboestrol and testosterone on the incorporation of selenomethionine^{75} by prostatic carcinoma cells. *Br J Urol* 62:166-72, 1988.

Bioavailability, distribution and pharmokinetics of diethylstilbestrol. *J Urol* 128:1336-9, 1982.

High dose intravenous estrogen therapy in advanced prostatic carcinoma: Use of prostate specific antigen as a serum marker. *Urology* 24:134-8, 1989.

High-dose continuous-infusion fosfestrol in hormone-resistant prostate cancer. *Cancer* 71:1123-30, 1993.

Use of intravenous stilbestrol diphosphate in patients with prostatic carcinoma refractory to conventional hormonal manipulation. *Urol Clin North Am* 18:139-42, 1991.

Prostate Cancer (Anticancer Properties and Activity of PC Spes)

Trends in alternative medicine use in the United States, 1990-1997 *JAMA* 280:1569-1575, 1998.

Cancer patients use of nonproven therapy: a 5-year follow-up study. *J Clin Oncol* 16:6-12, 1998.

Unconventional medicine in the United States: prevalence, costs, and patterns of use. *N Engl J Med* 328:246-52, 1993.

PC SPES. Pending united States patent number 08/697.920. "Herbal composition for treating prostate cancer."

Maximize Your Healthspan with Antioxidants. 1995. Keats publishing, New Canaan, Conn.

The anti-inflammatory activity of Scutellaria rivularis extracts and its active components. baicalin, baicalein and wogonin. *Am J Chin Med* 24:31-36, 1996.

Effects of baicalein and esculetin on transduction signals and growth factors expression in T-lymphoid leukemia cells. *Eur J Pharmacol* 268:73-78, 1994.

Antitumor effects of saikosaponins, baicalin and baicalein on human hepatoma cell lines. *Cancer Lett* 86: 91-95, 1994.

Anti-growth effects with components of Sho-saiko-to (TJ-9) on cultured human hepatoma cells. *Eur J Cancer Prev* 2:169-75, 1993.

The herbal medicine sho-saiko-to inhibits proliferation of cancer cell lines by inducing apoptosis and arrest at the Go/G1 phase. *Cancer Research* 54:448-454, 1994.

Free radical scavenging action of baicalein. *Arch Biochem Biophys* 306:261-266, 1993.

Effects of baicalein and alpha-tocopherol on lipid peroxidation, free radical scavenging activity and 12-0-tetradecanoylphorbol acetate-induced ear edema. *Eur J Pharmacol* 221:193- 198, 1992.

Testosterone metabolism in primary cultures of human prostate epithelial cell and fibroblasts. *J Steroid Biochem Molec Biol.* 55:375-383, 1995.

Regulation of androgen receptor (AR) and prostate specific antigen (PSA) expression in the androgen-responsive human prostate cell LNCaP cells by ethanolic extracts of the Chinese herbal preparation, PC SPES. *Biochem and Molec Biol Internl* 42:535-544, 1997.

Apoptosis and cell cycle effects induced by extracts of the Chinese herbal preparation PC SPES. *Int J Oncol* 11:437- 448, 1997.

Clinical and biologic activity of an estrogenic herbal combination (PC SPES) in prostate cancer. *N Engl J Med* 339:785-91, 1998.

A phase ll study of PC-SPES, an herbal compound, for the treatment. of advanced prostate cancer (PCa). *Proc Am Soc Clin Oncol* 18:320a, 1999.

PC-SPES: an active agent in patients with androgen-independent prostate cancer (AIPC). To be submitted for publication.

De la Taille A. et al., Effects of PC-SPES in prostate cancer: a preliminary investigation on human cell lines and patients. *Br J Urol* In press.

Kamada H. et al., A phase II study of PC-SPES, an herbal compound, for the treatment of advanced prostate cancer (abstract). Am. Assoc. Clin. Oncol Conference, Atlanta, GA (1999).

Moyad MA, Alternative therapies for advanced prostate cancer. What should I tell my patients? *Urol Clin North Am* 1999; 26: 413-17.

Small EJ, PC-SPES in prostate cancer. *New Engl J Med* 1999; 340:566-67.

Hsieh T. et al., Regulation of androgen receptor (AR) and prostate-specific antigen (PSA) expression in the androgen responsive human prostate LNCaP cells by ethanolic extracts of the Chinese herbal preparation PC-SPES. *Biochem Mol Biol Int* 1997; 42:535-44.

Geliebter J, Tiwari R, and Wu JM, PC-SPES in prostate cancer. *New Engl J Med* 1999; 340:567.

Dipole RS, Hiatt WN, and Gallo MA, PC-SPES in prostate cancer. *New Engl J Med* 1999; 340:567.

Tiwari RK et al., Antitumor effects of PC-SPES, an herbal formulation in prostate cancer. *Int J Oncol* 1999; 14:713-19.

Wang G et al., Antitumor active polysaccharides from the Chinese mushroom *Songshan linghzhi,* the fruiting body from Ganoderma tsughae. *Biosci Biotechnol Biochem* 1993; 57:894-900.

Chen WC et al., Effects of *ganoderma lucidum* and krestin on subset T cells in spleen of gamma irradiated mice. *Am Clin Med* 1995; 23: 289-98.

Ma MZ and Yao BY, Progress in indirubin treatment of chronic myelocytic leukemia. *J Trad Clin Med* 1983 3:245-48.

Liu JZ, Fang FD, and Zuo J, Studies on the mechanisms of indirubin action in the treatment of chronic granulocytic leukemia. V. Binding between indirubin and DNA and identification of the type of binding. *Sci Sin B* 1982; 25:1071-79.

Muan KC, *The Pharmacology of Chinese Herbs*. CRC Press, Boca Raton, FL, Raton, 1993.

Delos S et al., Testosterone metabolism in primary cultures of human prostate epithelial cell and fibroblasts. *J Steroid Biochem. Mol Biol* 1995; 55:375-83.

Wilt, TJ et al., Saw palmetto extracts for treatment of benign prostate hyperplasia: a systematic review. *JAMA* 1998; 280:1604-09.

Strauch G et al., Comparison of finestride (Proscar) and Serenoa repens (Permoxon)in the inhibition of 5-alpha reductase in healthy male volunteers. *Eur J Urol* 1994; 26:247-52.

Champault G et al., A double-blind trial of an extract of a plant, *Serenoa repens,* in benign prostatic hyperplasia. *Br J Clin Pharmacol* 1984; 18:461-62.

Prostate Cancer (Chemotherapy)

Major advantages of "early" administration of endocrine combination therapy in advanced prostate cancer. *Clin. Invest. Med.* 16:6 493-498, 1993.

Maximal androgen blockade: final analysis of EORTC Phase III Trial 30853. *Eur Urol* 33:144-151, 1998.

Treatment with Finasteride Following Radical Prostatectomy for Prostate Cancer, *Urology,* 45: 491-497, 1995.

Finasteride and flutamide as potency-sparing androgen-ablative therapy for advanced adenocarcinoma of the prostate. *Urology* 49: 913-920, 1997.

Intermittent androgen deprivation (IAD) with finasteride (F) during induction and maintenance permits prolonged time off IAD in localized prostate cancer (LPC). *J Urol* 161:156A, 1999.

A case for synchronous reduction of testicular androgen, adrenal androgen and prolactin for the treatment of advanced carcinoma of the prostate. *Eur J Cancer* 31A: 871-875, 1995.

The Androgen Deprivation Syndrome: the incidence and severity in prostate cancer patients receiving hormone blockade. Accepted for poster presentation at the ASCO meeting May 19th, 1998, Los Angeles, CA. *Proc Amer Soc Clin Oncol.* 17: 316A, 1998.

Prevention of radioinduced cystitis by orgotein: a randomized study. *Anticancer Res* 16:2025-2028, 1996.

Dietary phytoestrogens and prostate cancer. *Proc Annu Meet Am Assoc Cancer Res* 36:687, 1995.

Pathological features of hereditary prostate cancer. *J Urol* 153:987-992, 1995.

Hereditary prostate cancer: epidemiologic and clinical features. *J Urol* 150:797-802, 1993.

Familial risk factors for prostate cancer. *Cancer Surv* 11:5, 1991.

Mendelian inheritance of familial prostate cancer. *Proc Natl Acad Sci* 89:3367, 1992.

Genetic epidemiology of prostate cancer in the Utah Mormon Genealogy. *Cancer Surv* 1:47-69, 1982.

Family history and the risk of prostate cancer. *Prostate* 17:337-347, 1990.

Familial patterns of prostate cancer: a case control analysis. *J Urol* 146:1305-1307, 1991.

Familial clustering of cancers of the breast and prostate in a population-based sample of postmenopausal women. *Proc Annu Meet Am Assoc Cancer Res* 35:A1724, 1994.

The Anti-Oxidant Revolution. Thomas Nelson Publisher. 1994.

Enter the Zone. Regan Books, 1995.

The Anti-Aging Zone. Regan Books, 1999.

Inhibition of arachidonate 5 -lipoxygenase triggers massive apoptosis in human prostate cancer cells. *Proc Natl Acad Sci* 95:13182-13187, 1998.

Induction of cyclo-oxygenase-2 mRNA by prostaglandin E2 in human prostatic carcinoma cells. *Br J Cancer* 75:1111-8, 1997.

Prostate cancer and supplementation with alpha-tocopherol and beta-carotene: incidence and mortality in a controlled trial. *J Natl Cancer Inst* 90:440-6, 1998.

Vitamin E inhibits the high-fat diet promoted growth of established human prostate LNCaP tumor in nude mice. *J Urol* 161:1651-1654, 1999.

Effects of selenium supplementation for cancer prevention in patients with carcinoma of the skin. *JAMA* 276:1957-1963, 1996.

Inhibitory effects of selenium on the growth of DU-145 human prostate carcinoma cells in vitro. *Biochem Biophys Res Commun* 130:603-609, 1985.

Natural vitamin E (gamma-tocopherol) demonstrates greater inhibition of growth on a human prostate cancer cell line than synthetic vitamin E. (in press)

Genistein inhibits proliferation and in vitro invasive potential of human prostatic cancer cell lines. *Anticancer Res* 17:1199-204, 1997.

Genistein and biochanin A inhibit the growth of human prostate cancer cells but not epidermal growth factor receptor tyrosine autophosphorylation. *Prostate* 22:335-45, 1993.

Antiproliferative effect of Pygeum africanum extract on rat prostatic fibroblasts. *J Urol* 157:2381-7, 1997.

A flavonoid antioxidant, silymarin, inhibits activation of erbB1 signaling and induces cyclin-dependent kinase inhibitors, G1 arrest, and anticarcinogenic effects in human prostate carcinoma DU145 cells. *Cancer Res* 58:1920-9, 1998.

Inhibition of epidermal growth factor receptor (EGFr) tyrosine kinase activity by silymarin, a polyphenolic antioxidant and potent cancer chemopreventive agent. *Proc Annu Meet Am Assoc Cancer Res* 38:A1766, 1997.

Protective and therapeutic effect of silymarin on the development of latent liver damage. *Radiats Biol Radioecol* 38:411-5, 1998.

Protection against tumor promotion in mouse skin by silymarin (Meeting abstract). *Proc Annu Meet Am Assoc Cancer Res* 36:A3534, 1995.

Agarwal R Protective effects of silymarin against photocarcinogenesis in a mouse skin model. *J Natl Cancer Inst* 89:556-66, 1997.

Genistein inhibits the growth of human-patient BPH and prostate cancer in histoculture. *Prostate* 34:75-9, 1998.

Treatment of early recurrent prostate cancer with 1,25-dihydroxyvitamin D3. *J Urol.* 159:2035-2039, 1998.

19-nor-hexafluoride analogs of vitamin D3: A novel class of potent inhibitors of proliferation and induction of p27/Kip1 in human breast cancer cell lines. *Proc Annu Meet Am Assoc Cancer Res* 38:A579, 1997.

The effect of calcium supplementation on the circadian rhythm of bone resorption. *J Clin Endocrinol Metab* 79: 730-735, 1994.

Why drinking green tea could prevent cancer. *Nature* 387:561, 1997.

Overexpression of uPA by the MatLyLu rat prostatic cancer cell line results in enhanced tumor angiogenesis. *Proc Annu Meet Am Assoc Cancer Res* 38:A3518, 1997.

Green tea polyphenols inhibit growth of PC xenograft cwr-22 and decrease ornithine decarboxylase activity: implications for PC chemoprevention. *J Urol* 155: 510A, 1996.

Selective inhibition of steroid 5 _-reductase [5AR] by tea epicatechin-3-gallate and epigallocatechin-3-gallate. *Biochemical and Biophysical Research Communications*; 214:833-838,1995.

Growth inhibition and regression of human prostate and breast tumors in athymic mice by tea epigallocatechin gallate. *Cancer Letters* 96:239-243, 1995.

Intake of carotenoids and retinol in relation to risk of prostate cancer. *J Natl Cancer Inst* 87:1767-1776, 1995.

Effects of lycopene on spontaneous mammary tumour development in SHN virgin mice. *Anticancer Res* 15:1173-8, 1995.

Lycopene supplementation in men with prostate cancer (PCa) reduces grade and volume of preneoplasia (PIN) and tumor, decreases serum PSA and modulates biomarkers of growth and differentiation. *[No Journal cited]*

Identification of tricyclic analogs related to ellagic acid as potent/selective tyrosine protein kinase inhibitors. *J Med Chem* 37:2224-31, 1994.

Ellagic acid induces transcription of the rat glutathione S-transferase-Ya gene. *Carcinogenesis* 16:665-8, 1995.

Extensive personal experience: Combination of screening and preoperative endocrine therapy: the potential for an important decrease in prostate cancer mortality. *J Clin Endocrinol Metab* 80:2002-2013, 1995.

Diagnosis of advanced or noncurable prostate cancer can be practically eliminated by prostate-specific antigen. *Urology* 47: 212-217, 1996.

Evaluation of ProstaSure index in the detection of prostate cancer: a preliminary report. *Urology* 51:132-136, 1998.

Prostate cancer detection in men with serum PSA concentrations of 2.6 to 4.0 ng/mL and benign prostate examination. Enhancement of specificity with free PSA measurements [see comments]. *JAMA* 277:1452-5, 1997.

Prospective longitudinal evaluation of men with initial prostate specific antigen levels of 4.0 ng./ml. or less [see comments]. *J Urol* 157:1740-3, 1997.

Systematic 5 region prostate biopsy is superior to sextant method for diagnosing carcinoma of the prostate. 157: 199-203, 1997.

Heterogeneity of prostate cancer in radical prostatectomy samples. *Urology* 43:60-4, 1994.

Brawn PN: The dedifferentiation of prostate cancer. *Cancer* 52:246-51, 1983.

A model to study c-myc and v-H-ras induced prostate cancer progression in the Copenhagen rat. *Cell Mol Biol* 44:949-59, 1998.

Oncogene overexpression in human prostate cancer cell lines. *Proc Annu Meet Am Assoc Cancer Res* 34:A2309, 1993.

Expression of the proto-oncogene bcl-2 in the prostate and its association with emergence of androgen-independent prostate cancer. *Cancer Res* 52:6940-4, 1992.

p53 is mutated in a subset of advanced-stage prostate cancers. *Cancer Res* 53:3369-73, 1993.

Mutation of the androgen receptor gene in metastatic androgen-independent prostate cancer. *N Engl J Med* 332:1393-8, 1995.

A mutation in the ligand binding domain of the androgen receptor of human LNCaP cells affects steroid binding characteristics and response to anti-androgens. *Biochem Biophys Res Commun* 173:534-40, 1990.

Plasma testosterone and androstenedione after orchiectomy in prostatic adenocarcinoma. *Clin Endocrinol* 2:101-109, 1973.

Adrenal androgens predict for early progression to flutamide withdrawal in patients with androgen-independent prostate carcinoma. *Proc Am Soc Clin Oncol* 13:237, 1994.

Flutamide withdrawal syndrome: its impact on clinical trials in hormone-refractory prostate cancer. *J Clin Oncol* 11:1566-72, 1993.

Prostate specific antigen decline following discontinuation of flutamide in patients with stage D2 prostate cancer. *Am J Med* 98:412-14, 1995.

The antiandrogen withdrawal syndrome: Experience in a large cohort of unselected advanced prostate cancer patients. *Cancer* 76:1428-34, 1995.

Prostate-specific antigen decline after Casodex withdrawal: Evidence for an antiandrogen withdrawal syndrome. *Urology* 43:408-10, 1994.

A double-blind assessment of antiandrogen withdrawal from Casodex (C) or Eulexin (E) therapy while continuing luteinizing hormone releasing hormone analogue (LHRH-A) therapy for patients (Pts) with stage D2 prostate cancer (PCA). *Proc Am Soc Clin Oncol* 15:255A, 1996.

Dramatic PSA decline in response to discontinuation of megestrol acetate in advanced prostate cancer; expansion of the antiandrogen withdrawal syndrome. *J Urol* 153:1956-7, 1995.

Complete remission of hormone refractory adenocarcinoma of the prostate in response to withdrawal of diethylstilbestrol. *J Urol* 153:1944-5, 1995.

Mutant androgen receptor detected in an advanced-stage prostatic carcinoma is activated by adrenal androgens and progesterone. *Mol Endocr* 7:1541, 1993.

Mutation of the androgen receptor gene in metastatic androgen-independent prostate cancer. *N Engl J Med* 332:1393-8, 1995.

Anti-androgen activation of mutant androgen receptors from androgen-independent prostate cancer. *Clin Cancer Res* 3:1383, 1997.

The proliferative effect of "anti-androgens" on the androgen-sensitive human prostate tumor cell line LNCaP. *Endocrinology* 126:1457, 1990.

High dose bicalutamide for androgen independent prostate cancer: Effect of prior hormonal therapy. *J Urol* 159:149-53, 1998.

A novel and rapid treatment for advanced prostatic cancer. *J Urol* 130:152-3, 1983.

Synergistic effect of ketoconazole and anti-neoplastic agents in hormone-independent prostatic cancer cells. *Clin Invest Med* 12:363-6, 1989.

a possible direct cytotoxic effect on prostate carcinoma cells. *J Urol* 141:190-1,1989.

Ketoconazole effectively reverses multi-drug resistance in highly resistant KB cells. *J Urol* 151:485-491, 1994.

Long-term experience with high dose ketoconazole therapy in patients with stage D2 prostatic carcinoma. *J Urol* 137:902-4,1987.

Optimal dosing of ketoconazole (Keto) and hydrocortisone (HC) leads to long responses in hormone refractory prostate cancer. *Proc Am Soc Clin Oncol* 13:229A, 1994.

Ketoconazole retains activity in advanced prostate cancer patients with progression despite flutamide withdrawal. *J Urol* 157:1204-7, 1997.

Simultaneous antiandrogen withdrawal and treatment with ketoconazole and hydrocortisone in patients with advanced "prostate carcinoma. *Cancer* 80:1755-9, 1997.

Phase II study of ketoconazole combined with weekly doxorubicin in patients with androgen-independent prostate cancer. *J Clin Oncol* 12: 683-688, 1994.

Phase II trial of alternating weekly chemohormonal therapy for patients with androgen-independent prostate cancer. *Clinical Cancer Research* 3: 2371-2376, 1997.

Effects of an acidic beverage (Coca-Cola) on absorption of ketoconazole. *Antimicr Agents and Chemother* 39:1671-5, 1995.

Treatment of metastatic prostate cancer with low dose prednisone: Evaluation of pain and quality of life as pragmatic indices of response. *J Clin Oncol* 7:590-7, 1989.

Chemotherapy with mitoxantrone plus prednisone or prednisone alone for symptomatic hormone-resistant prostate cancer: A Canadian Randomized Trial with palliative end points. *J Clin Oncol* 14:1756-64, 1996.

Response of hormone resistant prostate cancer to dexamethasone (dex) by weekly intravenous (IV) injection: Improvement in performance status (PS), bone pain and reduction in prostate specific antigen (PSA). *Proc Am Soc Clin Oncol 1*3:255A, 1994.

Prostate specific antigen levels and clinical response to low-dose dexamethasone for hormone refractory prostate carcinoma. *Proc Am Soc Clin Oncol* 13: 235A, 1994.

The contribution of hydrocortisone to the observed response proportions of suramin. *Proc Am Soc Clin Oncol* 13:A710, 1994.

The in vitro localization of ^{3}H-estradiol in human prostatic carcinoma. *Cancer* 31:682-8, 1973.

Hormonal effects in vitro on ribonucleic acid polymerase in nuclei isolated from human prostatic tissue. *J Endocrinol* 59:367-368, 1973.

Metabolism and action of steroid hormones on human benign prostatic hyperplasia and prostatic carcinoma grown in organ culture. *J Steroid Biochem* 11:625-630, 1979.

The Veterans' Administrative Cooperative Urological Research Group's studies of cancer of the prostate. *Cancer* 32:1126-30, 1973.

The Veterans' Administrative Cooperative Urological Research Group studies of carcinoma of the prostate: a review. *Cancer Chemother Rep* 59(Part 1):225-7, 1975.

Comparison of diethylstilbestrol, cyproterone acetate, and medroxyprogesterone acetate in the treatment of advanced prostate cancer: final analysis of a randomizaed phase III trial of the European Organization for Research on the Treatment of Cancer Urological group. *J Urol* 136:624-30, 1986.

Haemostatic changes during hormone manipulation in advanced prostate cancer: a comparison of DES 3mg/day and Goserelin 3.6 mg/month. *Eur J Cancer* 26:315-9, 1990.

Hormone therapy for prostate cancer: results of the Veterans Administrative Cooperative Urological Research Group studies. *NCI Monogr* 7:165-70, 1988.

Hormonal therapy of prostatic cancer. *Cancer* 47(7 suppl):1929-36, 1980.

Clinical efficacy of Diethylstilbestrol treatment in post-orchiectomy progressive prostate cancer. *Proc Am Assoc Cancer Res* 35:233A, 1994.

A Phase II trial of oral diethylstilbestrol as a second-line hormonal agent in advanced prostate cancer. *Urology* 52:257-60, 1998.

Clinical trial of massive stilboestrol diphosphate therapy in advanced carcinoma of the prostate. *Br J Urol* 33:171, 1961.

The effect of stilboestrol and testosterone on the incorporation of selenomethionine^{75} by prostatic carcinoma cells. *Br J Urol* 62:166-72, 1988.

Bioavailability, distribution and pharmokinetics of diethylstilbestrol. *J Urol* 128:1336-9, 1982.

High dose intravenous estrogen therapy in advanced prostatic carcinoma: Use of prostate specific antigen as a serum marker. *Urology* 24:134-8, 1989.

High-dose continuous-infusion fosfestrol in hormone-resistant prostate cancer. *Cancer* 71:1123-30, 1993.

Use of intravenous stilbestrol diphosphate in patients with prostatic carcinoma refractory to conventional hormonal manipulation. *Urol Clin North Am* 18:139-42, 1991.

Trends in alternative medicine use in the United States, 1990-1997 *JAMA* 280:1569-1575, 1998.

Cancer patients use of nonproven therapy: a 5-year follow-up study. *J Clin Oncol* 16:6-12, 1998.

Unconventional medicine in the United States: prevalence, costs, and patterns of use. *N Engl J Med* 328:246-52, 1993.

PC SPES. Pending united States patent number 08/697.920. "Herbal composition for treating prostate cancer."

Maximize Your Healthspan with Antioxidants. 1995. Keats publishing, New Canaan, Conn.

The anti-inflammatory activity of Scutellaria rivularis extracts and its active components. baicalin, baicalein and wogonin. *Am J Chin Med* 24:31-36, 1996.

Effects of baicalcin and esculetin on transduction signals and growth factors expression in T-lymphoid leukemia cells. *Eur J Pharmacol* 268:73-78, 1994.

Antitumor effects of saikosaponins, baicalin and baicalein on human hepatoma cell lines. *Cancer Lett* 86: 91-95, 1994.

Anti-growth effects with components of Sho-saiko-to (TJ-9) on cultured human hepatoma cells. *Eur J Cancer Prev* 2:169-75, 1993.

The herbal medicine sho-saiko-to inhibits proliferation of cancer cell lines by inducing apoptosis and arrest at the Go/G1 phase. *Cancer Research* 54:448-454, 1994.

Free radical scavenging action of baicalein. *Arch Biochem Biophys* 306:261-266, 1993.

Effects of baicalein and alpha-tocopherol on lipid peroxidation, free radical scavenging activity and 12-0-tetradecanoylphorbol acetate-induced ear edema. *Eur J Pharmacol* 221:193- 198, 1992.

Testosterone metabolism in primary cultures of human prostate epithelial cell and fibroblasts. *J Steroid Biochem Molec Biol*. 55:375-383, 1995.

Regulation of androgen receptor (AR) and prostate specific antigen (PSA) expression in the androgen-responsive human prostate cell LNCaP cells by ethanolic extracts of the Chinese herbal preparation, PC SPES. *Biochem and Molec Biol Internl* 42:535-544, 1997.

Apoptosis and cell cycle effects induced by extracts of the Chinese herbal preparation PC SPES. *Int J Oncol* 11:437- 448, 1997.

Clinical and biologic activity of an estrogenic herbal combination (PC SPES) in prostate cancer. *N Engl J Med* 339:785-91, 1998.

A phase II study of PC-SPES, an herbal compound, for the treatment. of advanced prostate cancer (PCa). *Proc Am Soc Clin Oncol* 18:320a, 1999.

PC-SPES: an active agent in patients with androgen-independent prostate cancer (AIPC). To be submitted for publication.

Acid phosphatase: defining a role in androgen-independent prostate cancer. *Urology* 47:719-26, 1996.

Doxorubicin and dose-escalated cyclophosphamide with granulocyte colony-stimulating factor for the treatment of hormone-resistant prostate cancer. *JCO* 14(5):1617-1625, 1996.

Continuous infusion 5-Fluorouracil (5-FU) and weekly doxorubicin for hormone resistant prostate cancer. *Proc Am Soc Clin Oncol* 11:A641, 1992.

Phase II study of ketoconazole combined with weekly doxorubicin in patients with androgen-independent prostate cancer. *J Clin Oncol* 12: 683-688, 1994.

Phase II trial of alternating weekly chemohormonal therapy for patients with androgen-independent prostate cancer. *Clinical Cancer Research* 3: 2371-2376, 1997.

Combined hormone-chemotherapy for metastatic prostate carcinoma. *Urology* 30:352-355, 1987.

Cyclophosphamide (NSC 26271) versus the combination of Adriamycin (NSC 123127), 5-Fluorouracil (NSC 19893), and cyclophosphamide in the treatment of metastatic prostatic cancer. A randomized trial. *Cancer* 42:2546-2552, 1978.

The effects of African-American race on response and survival in phase II trials of patients with hormone-refractory prostate cancer. *Proc Amer Soc Clin Oncol* 15: A605, 1996.

N, N-diethyl-2-[4-(phenylmethyl)phenoxy]ethanamine in combination with cyclophosphamide: an active, low-toxicity regimen for metastatic hormonally unresponsive prostate cancer. *JCO* 13:1398-403, 1995.

Treatment of hormone refractory prostate cancer with ketoconazole, hydrocortisone and cyclophosphamide. *Proc Amer Soc Clin Oncol* 15: A698, 1996.

Ketoconazole retains activity in advanced prostate cancer patients with progression despite flutamide withdrawal. *J. Urol.* 157:1204-1207, 1997.

Simultaneous antiandrogen withdrawal and treatment with ketoconazole and hydrocortisone in patients with advanced prostate cancer. *Cancer* 80:1755-9, 1997.

Navelbine(NVB) single agent or in combination as first line chemotherapy in hormone refractory prostate cancer(HRPC). *Proc Am Soc Clin Oncol* 18:321A, 1999.

Oral estramustine and oral etoposide for hormone-refractory prostate cancer. *Urology* 50(5): 754-758, 1997.

Phase II oral estramustine and oral etoposide in hormone-refractory adenocarcinoma of the prostate. *Proc Am Soc Clin Oncol* 17:329A, 1998.

Platinum-based chemotherapy for patients with poorly differentiated hormone-refractory prostate cancers (HRPC): response and pathologic correlations. *Proc Amer Soc Clin Oncol* 14:232, 1995.

Estramustine and vinblastine: use of prostate specific antigen as a clinical trial end point for hormone refractory prostate cancer. *J. Urol.* 147:931-934, 1992.

Weekly paclitaxel by 3-hour infusion plus oral estramustine (EMP) in metastatic hormone refractory prostate cancer(HRPC*). Proc Am Soc Clin Oncol* 18:340A, 1999.

Paclitaxel (T), estramustine (E) and carboplatin(C) in patients (pts) with advanced prostate cancer (PC). *J Urol* 161:177A, 1999.

Activity of docetaxel (D) + estramustine (E) after dexamethasone (Dex) treatment in patients (pts) with androgen insensitive prostate cancer (AIP). *Proc Am Soc Clin Oncol* 17:343A, 1998.

Phase II trial of 96-hour paclitaxel plus oral estramustine phosphate in metastatic hormone-refractory prostate cancer. *JCO* 15:3156-163, 1997.

Phase I/II trial of estramustine (E) with taxotere (T) or vinorelbine (V) in patients (pts) with metastatic hormone-refractory prostate cancer (HRPC). *Proc Am Soc Clin Oncol* 17:338a, 1998.

Phase I/II trial of estramustine (E) and taxotere (T) in patients with metastatic hormone-refractory prostate cancer (HRPC). *Proc Am Soc Clin Oncol* 18:348A, 1999.

Phase I trial of docetaxel with estramustine in androgen-independent prostate cancer. *J Clin Oncol* 17:958-67, 1999.

A phase II study of docetaxel, estramustine, and low dose hydrocortisone in hormone refractory prostate cancer: preliminary results of CALGB 9780, *Proc Am Soc Clin Oncol* 18:321a, 1999.

Phase II study of estramustine (E) combined with docetaxel (D) in patients with androgen-independent prostate cancer (AIPCa). Proc *Am Soc Clin Oncol* 18:355A, 1999.

A phase II trial of docetaxel in patients with hormone refractory prostate cancer(HRPC): long term results. *Proc Am Soc Clin Oncol* 18:314a, 1999.

Clinical efficacy of Diethylstilbestrol treatment in post-orchiectomy progressive prostate cancer. *Proc AACR*, 35:233, 1994.

A phase II trial of oral diethylstilbestrol as a second-line hormonal agent in advanced prostate cancer. *Urology* 52:257-260, 1998.

Hydrocortisone and stilboestrol in combination for castration-relapsed prostate cancer. *Proc Am Soc Clin Oncol* 17:325a, 1998.

5-Fluorouracil and low-dose recombinant interferon-a-2a in patients with hormone-refractory adenocarcinoma of the prostate. *Prostate* 35:56-62, 1998.

Prostate Cancer (PSA Parameters and Heredity Factors)

Dietary phytoestrogens and prostate cancer. *Proc Annu Meet Am Assoc Cancer Res* 36:687, 1995.

Pathological features of hereditary prostate cancer. *J Urol* 153:987-992, 1995.

Hereditary prostate cancer: epidemiologic and clinical features. *J Urol* 150:797-802, 1993.

Familial risk factors for prostate cancer. *Cancer Surv* 11:5, 1991.

Mendelian inheritance of familial prostate cancer. *Proc Natl Acad Sci* 89:3367, 1992.

Genetic epidemiology of prostate cancer in the Utah Mormon Genealogy. *Cancer Surv* 1:47-69, 1982.

Family history and the risk of prostate cancer. *Prostate* 17:337-347, 1990.

Familial patterns of prostate cancer: a case control analysis. *J Urol* 146:1305-1307, 1991.

Extensive personal experience: Combination of screening and preoperative endocrine therapy: the potential for an important decrease in prostate cancer mortality. *J Clin Endocrinol Metab* 80:2002-2013, 1995.

Diagnosis of advanced or noncurable prostate cancer can be practically eliminated by prostate-specific antigen. *Urology* 47: 212-217, 1996.

Evaluation of ProstaSure index in the detection of prostate cancer: a preliminary report. *Urology* 51:132-136, 1998.

Prostate cancer detection in men with serum PSA concentrations of 2.6 to 4.0 ng/mL and benign prostate examination. Enhancement of specificity with free PSA measurements [see comments]. *JAMA* 277:1452-5, 1997.

Prospective longitudinal evaluation of men with initial prostate specific antigen levels of 4.0 ng./ml. or less [see comments]. *J Urol* 157:1740-3, 1997.

Systematic 5 region prostate biopsy is superior to sextant method for diagnosing carcinoma of the prostate. 157: 199-203, 1997.

Prostate Enlargement (Benign Prostatic Hypertrophy)

Efficacy and acceptability of tadenan (Pygeum africanum extract) in the treatment of benign prostatic hyperplasia (BPH): a multicentre trial in central Europe. *Curr Med Res Opin* 1998, 14 (3) p127-39

Review of recent placebo-controlled trials utilizing phytotherapeutic agents for treatment of BPH. *Prostate* Nov 1 1998, 37 (3) p187-93

Genistein inhibits the growth of human-patient BPH and prostate cancer in histoculture. *Prostate* Feb 1 1998, 34 (2) p75-9

Phytotherapy of BPH with pumpkin seeds—A multicentric clinical trial. *Zeitschrift fur Phytotherapie* 1998 , 19/2 (71-76)

Multicenter open trial for phytotherapy in benign prostate hyperplasia stage I and II. Sabal fruit and urtica reduces the residual urine and increases the urinary flow. *Therapie und Erfolg Urologie Nephrologie*, 1998 , 10/1-2 (48-51)

Saw Palmetto, African prune and stinging nettle for *Benign Prostatic Hyperplasia (BPH) Canadian Pharmaceutical Journal*, 1997, 130/9 (37-44+62)

Comparison of androgen-independent growth and androgen-dependent growth in BPH and cancer tissue from the same radical prostatectomies in sponge-gel matrix histoculture. *Prostate* Jun 1 1997, 31 (4) p250-4

Alpha-1 adrenoceptor subtypes (high, low) in human benign prostatic hypertrophy tissue according to the affinities for prazosin. *Prostate* Jun 1 1997, 31 (4) p216-22

[Urethral opening pressure: its clinical significance in prostatic obstruction]. *Nippon Hinyokika Gakkai Zasshi* (Japan) Apr 1997, 88 (4) p496-502

Free and total serum PSA values in patients with prostatic intraepithelial neoplasia (PIN), prostate cancer and BPH. Is F/T PSA a potential probe for dormant and manifest cancer? *Anticancer Res* (Greece) May-Jun 1997, 17 (3A) p1531-4

Optimising the medical management of benign prostatic hyperplasia. *Br J Clin Pract* (England) Mar 1997, 51 (2) p116-8

[Inferior vena cava obstruction syndrome caused by urinary retention]. *Arch Esp Urol* (Spain) Jan-Feb 1997, 50 (1) p61-2

[Diagnostic efficacy of free SPA/total PSA ratio in the diagnosis of prostatic carcinoma]. *Arch Ital Urol Androl* (Italy) Feb 1997, 69 Suppl 1 p93-5

[Laser-assisted endoscopic resection: a new surgical technique for the treatment of benign prostatic hypertrophy. Preliminary results of a study involving 100 patients]. *Arch Ital Urol Androl* (Italy) Feb 1997, 69 (1) p15-21

Blood haemoglobin and the long-term incidence of acute myocardial infarction after transurethral resection of the prostate. *Eur Urol (Switzerland)* 1997, 31 (2) p199-203

Insulin-like growth factor-binding protein-2 in patients with prostate carcinoma and benign prostatic hyperplasia. *Clin Endocrinol* (Oxf) (England) Feb 1997, 46 (2) p145-54

[Ureteral jet in patients with benign prostatic hypertrophy: prognostic evaluation during single and combined therapy]. *Arch Ital Urol Androl* (Italy) Dec 1996, 68 (5 Suppl) p175-8

[Laser treatment of benign prostatic hypertrophy: the correlation of histologic results to nuclear magnetic resonance imaging]. *Ann Urol* (Paris) (France) 1997, 31 (1) p19-26

[Laser-tissue interactions in urology]. *Ann Urol* (Paris) (France) 1997, 31 (1) p11-8

Effect of Serenoa repens extract (Permixon) on estradiol/testosterone-induced experimental prostate enlargement in the rat. *Pharmacol Res* (England) Sep-Oct 1996, 34 (3-4) p171-9

Immunohistochemical analysis of beta-tubulin isotypes in human prostate carcinoma and benign prostatic hypertrophy. *Prostate* Mar 1 1997, 30 (4) p263-8

[LH-RH agonists as therapeutic alternative in patients with benign prostatic hyperplasia (BPH) and surgical contraindication. Long term follow up]. *Arch Esp Urol* (Spain) Nov 1996, 49 (9) p923-7

c-erbB-2 oncoprotein: a potential biomarker of advanced prostate cancer. *Prostate* Feb 15 1997, 30 (3) p195-201

Role of m1 receptor-G protein coupling in cell proliferation in the prostate. *Life Sci* (England) 1997, 60 (13-14) p963-8

Transurethral prostatectomy—new trends. *Geriatr Nurs* Mar-Apr 1997, 18 (2) p78-80

[Sabal serrulata extract in the management of symptoms of prostatic hypertrophy]. *Orv Hetil* (Hungary) Feb 16 1997, 138 (7) p419-21

[Comparative effects of transurethral incision (TUIP) and the combination of TUIP and LHRH agonists in the treatment of benign prostatic hypertrophy]. *J Urol* (Paris) (France) 1996, 102 (3) p111-6

Immunochemical detection of 5 alpha-reductase in human serum. *Steroids* Nov 1996, 61 (11) p651-6

Nd:YAG laser transurethral evaporation of the prostate (TUEP) for urinary retention. *Lasers Surg Med* 1996, 19 (4) p480-6

Possible mechanisms of action of transurethral needle ablation of the prostate on benign prostatic hyperplasia symptoms: a neurohistochemical study. *J Urol* Mar 1997, 157 (3) p894-9

Histopathologic evaluation of the canine prostate following electrovaporization. *J Urol* Mar 1997, 157 (3) p1144-8

Transurethral vaporization of the prostate: a promising new technique. *Br J Urol* (England) Feb 1997, 79 (2) p186-9

Early experience with high-intensity focused ultrasound for the treatment of benign prostatic hypertrophy. *Br J Urol* (England) Feb 1997, 79 (2) p172-6

Detection of bladder tumor by urine cytology in cases of prostatic hypertrophy. Diagn *Cytopathol* Dec 1996, 15 (5) p409-11

Quantification and distribution of alpha 1-adrenoceptor subtype mRNAs in human prostate: comparison of benign hypertrophied tissue and non-hypertrophied tissue. *Br J Pharmacol* (England) Nov 1996, 119 (5) p797-803

Prostate-specific antigen and age. Is there a correlation? And why does it seem to vary? *Eur Urol* (Switzerland) 1996, 30 (3) p296-300

Colocalization of immunoglobulin binding factor and prostate specific antigen in human prostate gland. *Arch Androl* Nov-Dec 1996, 37 (3) p149-54

A study of the efficacy and safety of transurethral needle ablation (TUNA) treatment for benign prostatic hyperplasia. *Neurourol Urodyn* 1996, 15 (6) p619-28

[Diagnostic values and limitations of conventional urodynamic studies (uroflowmetry.residual urine measurement.cystometry) in benign prostatic hypertrophy]. *Nippon Hinyokika Gakkai Zasshi* (Japan) Dec 1996, 87 (12) p1321-3

Alpha 1a-adrenoceptor polymorphism: pharmacological characterization and association with benign prostatic hypertrophy. *Br J Pharmacol* (England) Jul 1996, 118 (6) p1403-8

[Double-blind evaluation of mepartricin 150.000 U (40 mg) compared with placebo in benign prostatic hypertrophy]. *Minerva Urol Nefrol* (Italy) Dec 1996, 48 (4) p207-11

[Alternative treatment of benign prostatic hypertrophy]. *Minerva Urol Nefrol* (Italy) Dec 1996, 48 (4) p177-82

Transition zone ratio and prostate-specific antigen density: the index of response of benign prostatic hypertrophy to an alpha blocker. *Int J Urol* (Japan) Sep 1996, 3 (5) p361-6

[A case of prostate cancer diagnosed one and half year after retropubic prostatectomy for benign prostatic hypertrophy]. *Hinyokika Kiyo* (Japan) Nov 1996, 42 (11) p907-9

The use of alpha-adrenoceptor antagonists in the pharmacological management of benign prostatic hypertrophy: an overview. *Pharmacol Res* (England) Mar 1996, 33 (3) p145-60

Clinical application of basic arginine amidase in human male urine. *Biol Pharm Bull* (Japan) Aug 1996, 19 (8) p1083-5

Free to total prostate-specific antigen (PSA) ratio is superior to total-PSA in differentiating benign prostate hypertrophy from prostate cancer. *Prostate Suppl* 1996, 7 p30-4

Clinical study on estramustine binding protein (EMBP) in human prostate. *Prostate* Sep 1996, 29 (3) p169-76

Three-year followup of patients treated with lower energy microwave thermotherapy. *J Urol* Dec 1996, 156 (6) p1959-63

Detection of Chlamydia trachomatis in the prostate by in-situ-hybridization and by transmission electron microscopy. *Int J Androl* (England) Apr 1996, 19 (2) p109-12

Breast and prostate cancer in the relatives of men with prostate cancer. *Br J Urol* (England) Oct 1996, 78 (4) p552-6

Effect of finasteride on free and total serum prostate-specific antigen in men with benign prostatic hyperplasia. *Br J Urol* (England) Sep 1996, 78 (3) p405-8

The safety of finasteride used in benign prostatic hypertrophy: a non-interventional observational cohort study in 14,772 patients. *Br J Urol* (England) Sep 1996, 78 (3) p379-84

[Transurethral thermotherapy with microwaves in patients with benign prostatic hypertrophy and urinary retention: comparative study between high energy (25) and standard energy (2.0)]. *Arch Esp Urol* (Spain) May 1996, 49 (4) p337-46

Detection of alpha 1-adrenoceptor subtypes in human hypertrophied prostate by insituhybridization. *Histochem J* (England) Apr 1996, 28 (4) p283-8

Safety profile of 3 months' therapy with alfuzosin in 13,389 patients suffering from benign prostatic hypertrophy. *Eur Urol* (Switzerland) 1996, 29 (1) p29-35

Estramustine-binding protein in carcinoma and benign hyperplasia of the human prostate. *Eur Urol* (Switzerland) 1996, 29 (1) p106-10

Surface-epitope masking and expression cloning identifies the human prostate carcinoma tumor antigen gene PCTA-1 a member of the galectin gene family. *Proc Natl Acad Sci U S A* Jul 9 1996, 93 (14) p7252-7

[The significance of free-type PSA and complex-type PSA in patients with prostatic carcinoma—the characteristics of ACS-PSA method compared with that of Delfia- and Eiken-PSA method]. *Rinsho Byori* (Japan) Apr 1996, 44 (4) p345-50

The Oxford Laser Prostate Trial: a double-blind randomized controlled trial of contact vaporization of the prostate against transurethral resection; preliminary results. *Br J Urol* (England) Mar 1996, 77 (3) p382-5

A case-control study of cancer of the prostate in Somerset and east Devon. *Br J Cancer* (England) Aug 1996, 74 (4) p661-6

Usefulness of PSA density and PSA excess in the differential diagnosis between prostate cancer and benign prostatic hypertrophy. *Int J Biol Markers* (Italy) Jan-Mar 1996, 11 (1) p12-7

[Detection of prostate cancer in urological practice: clinical establishment of serum PSA reference values by age]. *Nippon Hinyokika Gakkai Zasshi* (Japan) Mar 1996, 87 (3) p702-9

Free-to-total prostate specific antigen ratio as a single test for detection of significant stage T1c prostate cancer. *J Urol* Sep 1996, 156 (3) p1042-7; discussion 1047-9

[Transurethral thermotherapy with microwaves in symptomatic prostatic benign hypertrophy: comparison between the high-energy (2.5) protocol and the standard protocol (2.0)]. *Arch Esp Urol* (Spain) Mar 1996, 49 (2) p99-109

Two-dimensional outcome analysis as a guide for quality assurance of prostatectomy. *Int J Qual Health Care* (England) Feb 1996, 8 (1) p67-73

Alpha blockers: a reassessment of their role in therapy. *Am Fam Physician* Jul 1996, 54 (1) p263-6

Effect of prostatic growth factor, basic fibroblast growth factor, epidermal growth factor, and steroids on the proliferation of human fetal prostatic fibroblasts. *Prostate* Jun 1996, 28 (6) p352-8

The impact of prostate-specific antigen density in predicting prostate cancer when serum prostate-specific antigen levels are less than 10 ng/ml. *Eur Urol* (Switzerland) 1996, 29 (2) p189-92

Usefulness of prostate-specific antigen density as a diagnostic test of prostate cancer. *Tumour Biol* (Switzerland) 1996, 17 (1) p20-6

The extract of serenoa repens in the treatment of benign prostatic hyperplasia: A multicenter open study. *Curr. Ther. Res. Clin. Exp.*, 1994, 55/7 (776- 785)

Prostaserene (R). Treatment for *Bph. Drugs Future* (Spain), 1994, 19/5 (452-453)

The effect of Permixon on androgen receptors. *Acta Obstet. Gynecol. Scand.* (Sweden), 1988, 65/6

Pharmacological combinations in the treatment of benign prostatic hypertrophy. *J. Urol.* (France), 1993, 99/6 (316-320)

Inhibition of androgen metabolism and binding by a liposterolic extract of 'Serenoa repens B' in human foreskin fibroblasts. *J. Steroid Biochem.* (England), 1984, 20/1 (515-519)

Testosterone metabolism in primary cultures of human prostate epithelial cells and fibroblasts. *J Steroid Biochem Mol Biol* (England) Dec 1995, 55 (3-4) p375-83

The effect of Permixon on androgen receptors. *Acta Obstet Gynecol Scand* (Sweden) 1988, 67 (5) p397-9

Binding of Permixon, a new treatment for prostatic benign hyperplasia, to the cytosolic androgen receptor in the rat prostate. *J Steroid Biochem* (England) Jan 1984, 20 (1) p521-3

Inhibition of androgen metabolism and binding by a liposterolic extract of Serenoa repens B in human foreskin fibroblasts. *J Steroid Biochem* (England) Jan 1984, 20 (1) p515-9

Testosterone metabolism in primary cultures of human prostate epithelial cells and fibroblasts. *Journal of Steroid Biochemistry and Molecular Biology* (UK), 1995, 55/3-4 (375-383)

Human prostatic steroid 5alpha-reductase isoforms—A comparative study of selective inhibitors. *Journal of Steroid Biochemistry and Molecular Biology* (UK) 1995, 54/5-6 (273-279)

The lipidosterolic extract from Serenoa repens interferes with prolactin receptor signal. *Journal of Biomedical Science* (Switzerland), 1995, 2/4 (357-365)

Lack of effects of a lyposterolic extract of Serenoa repens on plasma levels of testosterone, follicle-stimulating hormone, and luteinizing hormone. *Clin. Ther.*, 1988, 10/5 (585-588)

Serenoa repens capsules: A bioequivalence study. *Acta Toxicol. Ther.* (Italy), 1994, 15/1 (21-39)

Rectal bioavailability and pharmacokinetics in healthy volunteers of serenoa repens new formulation. *Arch. Med. Interna* (Italy), 1994, 46/2 (77-86)

Clinical controlled trial on therapeutical bioequivalence and tolerability of Serenoa repens oral capsules 160 mg or rectal capsules 640 mg. *Arch. Med. Interna* (Italy), 1994, 46/2 (61-75)

Evidence that serenoa repens extract displays an antiestrogenic activity in prostatic tissue of benign prostatic hypertrophy patients. *Eur. Urol.* (Switzerland), 1992, 21/4 (309-314)

Liposterolic extract of Serenoa Repens in management of benign prostatic hypertrophy. *Urologia* (Italy), 1988, 55/5 (547-552)

Binding of permixon, a new treatment for prostatic benign hyperplasia, to the cytosolic androgen receptor in the rat prostate. *J. Steroid Biochem.* (England), 1984, 20/1 (521-523)

Effect of Pygeum africanum extract on A23187-stimulated production of lipoxygenase metabolites from human polymorphonuclear cells. *J Lipid Mediat Cell Signal.* 1994 May. 9(3). P 285-90.

Combined extracts of Urtica dioica and Pygeum africanum in the treatment of benign prostatic hyperplasia: double-blind comparison of two doses. *Clin Ther.* 1993 Nov-Dec. 15(6). P 1011-20

[Urological and sexual evaluation of treatment of benign prostatic disease using Pygeum africanum at high doses]. *Arch Ital Urol Nefrol Androl.* 1991 Sep. 63(3). P 341-5

[Efficacy of Pygeum africanum extract in the medical therapy of urination disorders due to benign prostatic hyperplasia: evaluation of objective and subjective parameters. A placebo-controlled double-blind multicenter study]. *Wien Klin Wochenschr.* 1990 Nov 23. 102(22). P 667-73

Pulmonary Insufficiencies

Refer to references under Emphysema and Chronic Obstructive Pulmonary Disease.

Raynaud's Syndrome

Increased susceptibility to oxidation of low-density lipoproteins isolated from patients with systemic sclerosis. *Arthritis Rheum* Aug 1995, 38 (8) p1060-7

Fish-oil fatty acid supplementation in mixed cryoglobulinemia: a preliminary report. *Clin Exp Rheumatol* (Italy) Sep-Oct 1994, 12 (5) p509-13

Medical literature as a potential source of new knowledge. *Bull Med Libr Assoc* Jan 1990, 78 (1) p29-37

Raynaud's phenomenon. *Curr Opin Rheumatol* Dec 1989, 1 (4) p490-8

Fish-oil dietary supplementation in patients with Raynaud' s phenomenon: a double-blind, controlled, prospective study. *Am J Med* Feb 1989, 86 (2) p158-64

Fish oil, Raynaud's syndrome, and undiscovered public knowledge. *Perspect Biol Med* Autumn 1986, 30 (1) p7-18

Evening primrose oil (Efamol) in the treatment of Raynaud's phenomenon: a double blind study. *Thromb Haemost* (Germany, West) Aug 30 1985, 54 (2) p490-4

Sjogren's syndrome and the sicca syndrome: the role of prostaglandin E1 deficiency. Treatment with essential fatty acids and vitamin C. *Med Hypotheses* (England) Mar 1980, 6 (3) p225-32

[Cryoglobulinemia, its clinical significance and its relation to fat metabolism]. *Z Gesamte Inn Med* (Germany, East) Aug 15 1970, 25 (16) p760-5

ABC of rheumatology. Raynaud's phenomenon, scleroderma, and overlap syndromes. *British Medical Journal* (UK) 1995, 310/6982 (795-798)

Raynaud's phenomenon. *H+G Zeitschrift fur Hautkrankheiten* (Germany) 1994, 69/9 (585-589)

Managing Raynaud's phenomenon: A practical approach. *American Family Physician* 1993, 47/4 (823-829)

Medical treatment of peripheral vascular disease: Are there new perspectives? *Vasa—Journal of Vascular Diseases* (Switzerland) 1992, 21/Suppl. 34 (20-24)

Raynaud's phenomenon a vasospastic disorder. *Current Practice in Surgery* (UK) 1991, 3/3 (170-175)

Pharmacotherapy of Raynaud's phenomenon. *Drugs* (New Zealand) Nov 1996, 52 (5) p682-95

Quantitative thermal imaging to assess inositol nicotinate treatment for Raynaud's syndrome. *J Int Med Res* (England) 1981, 9 (6) p393-400

An experimentally controlled evaluation of the effect of inositol nicotinate upon the digital blood flow in patients with Raynaud's phenomenon. *J Int Med Res* (England) 1979, 7 (6) p473-83

Quantitative thermographic assessment of inositol nicotinate therapy in Raynaud's phenomena. *J Int Med Res* (England) 1977, 5 (4) p217-22, Journal Code: E62

Raynaud's phenomenon. *Critical Ischaemia* (UK) 1997, 6/3 (68-73)

Retrospective comparison of iloprost with other treatments for secondary Raynaud's phenomenon. *Annals of the Rheumatic Diseases* (UK) 1991, 50/6 (359-361)

The effect of inositol nicotinate (Hexopal) in patients with Raynaud's phenomenon. A placebo-controlled study. *Clinical Trials Journal* (UK) 1985, 22/6 (521-529)

Raynaud's syndrome: Current trends. *British Journal of Rheumatology* (UK) 1983, 22/1 (50-55)

Clinical diagnosis found in patients with Raynaud's phenomenon: a multicentre study. *Rheumatol Int* (Germany) 1998, 18 (1) p17-20

Anatomoclinical meeting: polyneuritis, hepato-splenomegaly, hypothyroidism and Raynaud's disease (clinical conference)]. *Medicina* (B Aires) (Argentina) 1996, 56 (5 Pt 1) p499-508

Immune-related disease and normal-tension glaucoma. A case-control study [see comments]. *Arch Ophthalmol* Apr 1992, 110 (4) p500-2

Remission of Raynaud's phenomenon after L-thyroxine therapy in a patient with hypothyroidism. *J Endocrinol Invest* (Italy) Jan 1992, 15 (1) p49-51

Hypothyroidism, Raynaud's phenomenon, and acute myocardial infarction in a young woman. *Clin Cardiol* Jun 1983, 6 (6) p304-6

Raynaud's phenomenon and thyroid deficiency. *Arch Intern Med* Jun 1980, 140 (6) p832-3

Raynaud's phenomenon in hypothyroidism. *Angiology* Jan 1976, 27 (1) p19-25

Raynaud's phenomenon as the initial manifestation of hypothyroidism. *Journal of Clinical Rheumatology* 1998, 4/5 (270-273)

Drug options for vasospastic disease. *Drug Therapy* 1992, 22/10 (45-48+53-56)

Effect of magnesium sulfate infusion on circulating levels of noradrenaline and neuropeptide-Y-like immunoreactivity in patients with primary Raynaud's phenomenon. *Angiology (Angiology)* 1994, 45/7 (637-645)

Thromboxane metabolite excretion in patients with hand-arm vibration syndrome. *Clin Physiol* (England) Jul 1996, 16 (4) p361-7

Raynaud's phenomenon: State of the art 1998. *Scandinavian Journal of Rheumatology* (Norway) 1998, 27/5 (319-322)

Plasma catecholamines during behavioral treatments for Raynaud's disease. *Psychosom Med* Jul-Aug 1991, 53 (4) p433-9

Quantitative measurements of finger blood flow during behavioral treatments for Raynaud's disease. *Psychophysiology* Jul 1989, 26 (4) p437-41

The behavioral treatment of Raynaud's disease: a review. *Biofeedback Self Regul* Dec 1987, 12 (4) p257-72

Bringing the feet in from the cold: thermal biofeedback training of foot-warming in Raynaud's syndrome. *Biofeedback Self Regul* Dec 1984, 9 (4) p431-8

Behavioral treatment of Raynaud's phenomenon in scleroderma. *J Behav Med* Dec 1984, 7 (4) p343-53

Biofeedback, autogenic training, and progressive relaxation in the treatment of Raynaud's disease: a comparative study. *J Appl Behav Anal* Spring 1980, 13 (1) p3-11

Behavioral approaches to Raynaud's disease. *Psychother Psychosom* (Switzerland) 1981, 36 (3-4) p224-45

A 1-year follow-up of Raynaud's patients treated with behavioral therapy techniques. *J Behav Med* Dec 1979, 2 (4) p385-91

Behavioral treatment of Raynaud's disease. *J Behav Med* Sep 1978, 1 (3) p323-35

Long-term effectiveness of behavioral treatments for Raynaud's disease. *Behavior Therapy* 1987, 18/4 (387-399)

Biofeedback training in clinical cardiovascular disease. *Primary Cardiology* 1980, 6/9 (34-48)

[Esophageal motor abnormalities, gastroesophageal reflux and duodenogastric reflux in patients with Raynaud's disease]. *Clin Ter* (Italy) Dec 31 1989, 131 (6) p373-80

[Clinical studies on various therapy for the intractable trauma of toes and fingers in cases of diabetes mellitus and peripheral ischemic diseases]. *Nippon Geka Gakkai Zasshi* (Japan) May 1988, 89 (5) p763-70

'Phenomenon of hyperbaric accumulation of venous partial pressure of oxygen' concerning the hyperbaric therapy and lumbosacral sympathetic ganglionectomy L_2 and L_3 for healing of incurable wounding in patients with periphery circulatory disturbances. *Acta Medica Kinki University* (Japan) 1976, VOL. 1/- (1-16)

Micronutrient antioxidant status in patients with primary Raynaud's phenomenon and systemic sclerosis. *J Rheumatol* (Canada) Aug 1994, 21 (8) p1477-83

[Thermographic assessment of Raynaud's phenomenon in childhood mixed connective tissue disease]. *Ryumachi* (Japan) Dec 1994, 34 (6) p955-60

Is vitamin E involved in the autoimmune mechanism? *Cutis* Mar 1978, 21 (3) p321-5

Comparative double-blind trial of dl-alpha-tocopheryl nicotinate on vibration disease. *Tohoku J Exp Med* (Japan) Sep 1977, 123 (1) p67-75

[The effect of dimethyl sulfoxide on the thromboelastographic indices and the microcirculation in patients with rheumatic diseases]. *Ter Arkh* (USSR) 1989, 61 (12) p106-9

Pathophysiology of capillary circulation: Raynaud's disease. *Angiology* Jan 1978, 29 (1) p48-52

Vasodilator drugs in peripheral vascular disease. *New England Journal of Medicine* 1979, 300/13 (713-717)

Treatment of the Raynaud's phenomenon with piracetam. *Arzneimittelforschung* (Germany) May 1993, 43 (5) p526-35

Comprehensive management of Raynaud's syndrome. *Clinics in Plastic Surgery* 1997, 24/1 (133-160)

Raynaud's phenomenon in the emergency department. *Journal of Emergency Medicine* 1995, 13/3 (369-378).

Retinopathy

Therapeutic effect of liposomal superoxide dismutase in an animal model of retinopathy of prematurity. *Neurochem Res* 1997 May;22(5):597-605

Oxidative protein damage in human diabetic eye: evidence of a retinal participation. *Eur J Clin Invest* 1997 Feb;27(2):141-7

Antioxidant nutrient intake and diabetic retinopathy: the San Luis Valley Diabetes Study. *Ophthalmology* Dec 1998, 105 (12) p2264-70

Retinal changes mimicking diabetic retinopathy in two nondiabetic, growth hormone-treated patients. *J Clin Endocrinol Metab* Jul 1998, 83 (7) p2380-3

Reducing lipid peroxidation stress of erythrocyte membrane by alpha-tocopherol nicotinate plays an important role in improving blood rheological properties in type 2 diabetic patients with retinopathy. *Diabet Med* (England) May 1998, 15 (5) p380-5.

A deficiency of vitamin B6 is a plausible molecular basis of the retinopathy of patients with diabetes mellitus. *Biochem Biophys Res Commun.* 1991 Aug 30. 179(1). P 615-9

Pharmacological prevention of diabetic microangiopathy. *Mecanismes Pathogeniques, Diabete Metabol.* (France), 1994, 20/2 BIS (219-228)

Clinical study of vitamin influence in diabetes mellitus. *Journal of the Medical Society of Toho University* (Japan), 1996, 42/6

Erythrocyte and plasma antioxidant activity in type I diabetes mellitus. *Presse Medicale* (France), 1996, 25/5 (188-192)

Lipid peroxidation in insulin-dependent diabetic patients with early retina degenerative lesions: Effects of an oral zinc supplementation. *European Journal of Clinical Nutrition* (UK), 1995, 49/4 (282-288)

Angioid streaks associated with abetalipoproteinemia. *Ophthalmic Genet.* (Netherlands), 1994, 15/3-4 (151-159)

Comparison of gamma-glutamyl transpeptidase in retina and cerebral cortex, and effects of antioxidant therapy. *Curr. Eye Res.* (UK), 1994, 13/12 (891-896)

Status of antioxidants in patients with diabetes mellitus with and without late complications. *Aktuel. Ernahr.Med. Klin. Prax.* (Germany), 1994, 19/3 (155-159)

Vitamins for seeing. *Compr. Ther.*, 1990, 16/4 (62)

The regional distribution of vitamins E and C in mature and premature human retinas. *Invest. Ophthalmol. Visual Sci.*, 1988, 29/1 (22-26)

Oral vitamin E supplements can prevent the retinopathy of abetalipoproteinaemia. *Br. J. Ophthalmol.* (UK), 1986, 70/3 (166-173)

The role of taurine in developing rat retina. *Ophtalmologie* (France), 1995, 9/3 (283-286)

Taurine: Review and therapeutic applications (Part I). *J. Farm. Clin.* (Spain), 1990, 7/7 (580-600)

Supplemental taurine in diabetic rats: Effects on plasma glucose and triglycerides. *Biochem. Med. Metab. Biol.*, 1990, 43/1 (1-9+8)

Taurine deficiency retinopathy in the cat. *J. Small Anim. Pract.* (England), 1980, 21/10 (521- 534)

[Clinical experimentation with pyridoxylate in treatment of various chorioretinal degenerative disorders (50 cases)]. *Bull Soc Ophtalmol Fr.* 1969 Dec. 69(12). P 1145-50

Rationales for micronutrient supplementation in diabetes. *Med Hypotheses.* 1984 Feb. 13(2). P 139-51

Magnesium and potassium in diabetes and carbohydrate metabolism. Review of the present status and recent results. *Magnesium.* 1984. 3(4-6). P 315-23

Scleroderma

Linear scleroderma in children. *Int J Dermatol* May 1996, 35 (5) p330-6

Nodular scleroderma: focally increased tenascin expression differing from that in the surrounding scleroderma skin. *J Dermatol* (Japan) Apr 1995, 22 (4) p267-71

[Pathogenesis of anemia in systemic scleroderma]. *Klin Med (Mosk)* (Russia) 1994, 72 (3) p44-6

Lack of ocular changes with dimethyl sulfoxide therapy of scleroderma. *Pharmacotherapy* 1989, 9 (3) p165-8

[Effect of combined treatment with nicotinic acid and DMSO on microcirculatory disorders in systemic scleroderma]. *Ter Arkh* (USSR) 1978, 50 (9) p105-7

[A case of scleroderma associated with total medullary aplasia]. *Ateneo Parmense [Acta Biomed]* (Italy) 1977, 48 (5) p499-504

Effect of piascledine treatment of scleroderma]. *Przegl Dermatol* (Poland) Jul-Aug 1975, 62 (4) p555-8

[Clinical and biological study of the application of alpha-tocopheryl-quinone for 5 years of primary and secondary muscular diseases and for 1 case of scleroderma]. *Sem Hop* (France) Apr 26 1968, 44 (20) p1375-9

[Use of vitamin B12 in scleroderma]. *Vrach Delo* (USSR) Jun 1965, 6 p136

Enhanced lipid peroxidation in systemic scleroderma. *Zeitschrift fur Dermatologie* (Germany) 1996, 182/3 (124+126-128)

FDA Arthritis Advisory Committee meeting: Methotrexate; guidelines for the clinical evaluation of antiinflammatory drugs; DMSO in scleroderma. *Arthritis and Rheumatism* 1986, 29/10 (1289-1290)

Effect of the combined therapy with nicotinic acid and DMSO on microcirculatory disorders in systemic scleroderma. *Terapevticheskii Arkhiv* (Russia) 1978, 50/9 (105-107)

Scleroderma and bone marrow aplasia. *Acta Biomedica de l'Ateneo Parmense* (Italy) 1977, 48/5 (499-504)

Three recurrent abruptions of the placenta in a patient with scleroderma. *Proceedings of the Rudolf Virchow Medical Society in the City of New York* 1972, Vol.28/- (65-68)

Enterocyte function in progressive systemic sclerosis as estimated by the deconjugation of pteroyltriglutamate to folic acid. *Gut* (England) Apr 1987, 28 (4) p435-8

Gastrointestinal function in patients with progressive systemic sclerosis. *Clin Rheumatol* (Belgium) Dec 1985, 4 (4) p441-8

Improvement of progressive systemic sclerosis (PSS) with estriol treatment. *Acta Derm Venereol* (Sweden) 1984, 64 (2) p168-71

Cyclofenil versus placebo in progressive systemic sclerosis. A one-year double-blind crossover study of 27 patients. *Acta Medica Scandinavica* (Sweden) 1981, 210/5 (419-428)

Silicone-associated rheumatic disease: an unsupported myth. *Plast Reconstr Surg* Apr 1997, 99 (5) p1362-7

Modulation of collagen gene expression: its relation to fibrosis in systemic sclerosis and other disorders. *Ann Intern Med* Jan 1 1995, 122 (1) p60-2

[Pulmonary involvement in sclerodermia]. *Minerva Med* (Italy) Jun 1994, 85 (6) p293-300

Demonstration of silicon in sites of connective-tissue disease in patients with silicone-gel breast implants [see comments]. *Arch Dermatol* Jan 1993, 129 (1) p63-8

Early undifferentiated connective tissue disease: III. Outcome and prognostic indicators in early scleroderma (systemic sclerosis). *Ann Intern Med* Apr 15 1993, 118 (8) p602-9

Pulmonary manifestations of the collagen vascular diseases. *Clin Chest Med* Dec 1989, 10 (4) p677-722

Vasculitis in the lung. *J Thorac Imaging* Jan 1988, 3 (1) p33-48

[Fasciitis and Shulman's syndrome. A nosologic discussion]. *Rev Rhum Mal Osteoartic* (France) Feb 1987, 54 (2) p121-7

Role of inflammation in the lung disease of systemic sclerosis: comparison with idiopathic pulmonary fibrosis. *J Lab Clin Med* Mar 1986, 107 (3) p253-60

Reduced zinc in peripheral blood cells from patients with inflammatory connective tissue diseases. *Inflammation* Jun 1985, 9 (2) p189-99

[Morphology of immune inflammation in rheumatic diseases]. *Arkh Patol* (USSR) 1983, 45 (11) p44-50

Pathogenesis and staging of scleroderma. *Acta Derm Venereol* (Sweden) 1976, 56 (2) p83-92

The role of free oxygen radicals and trimetazidine in the pathogenesis of ischemic heart disease in patients with scleroderma. *Hellenic Journal of Cardiology* (Greece) 1995, 36/5 (528-532)

Cytokines in rheumatic diseases. *Biotherapy* (Netherlands) 1994, 8/2 (99-111)

Autoimmune connective tissue disease and connective tissue disease-like illnesses after silicone gel augmentation mammoplasty. *Journal of the American Academy of Dermatology* 1994, 31/4 (626-642)

Pulmonary involvements in progressive systemic sclerosis. *Minerva Medica* (Italy) 1994, 85/6 (293-300)

When the lungs are involved by connective tissue disease. *Postgraduate Medicine* 1993, 94/5 (147-158)

Dysphagia in systemic disease. *Dysphagia* 1993, 8/4 (368-383)

Medical use of dimethyl sulfoxide (DMSO). *Reviews in Clinical and Basic Pharmacology* (UK) 1985, 5/1-2 (1-33)

Cutaneous and systemic manifestations of auto-immune disorders. *International Journal of Dermatology* 1982, 21/7 (365-372)

Morphologic changes in the digital arteries of patients with progressive systemic sclerosis (scleroderma) and Raynaud phenomenon. *Medicine* 1980, 59/6 (393-408)

The microcirculation of the skin in collagen diseases and generalized vasculitis. *Medizinische Welt* 1975, 26/23 (1126-1128)

E.N.T. diseases in scleroderma. Subglottic localizations. *J. Franc. Oto Rhino Laryng.* 1975, 24/4 (261-275)

Mixed connective tissue disease. A newly created pathologic concept for a combination of different collagen diseases. *H+G Zeitschrift fur Hautkrankheiten* 1975, 50/2 (83-95)

[Observation on blood flow changes in 34 cases of progressive systemic scleroderma treated with Chinese herbal medicine]. *Chung Kuo Chung Hsi I Chieh Ho Tsa Chih* (China) Feb 1994, 14 (2) p86-8, 68

Vitamin D metabolites in generalized scleroderma. Evidence of a normal cutaneous and intestinal supply with vitamin D. *Acta Derm Venereol* (Sweden) 1985, 65 (4) p343-5

Procollagen gene expression by scleroderma fibroblasts in culture. Inhibition of collagen production and reduction of pro alpha 1(I) and pro alpha 1(III) collagen messenger RNA steady-state levels by retinoids. *Arthritis Rheum* Apr 1987, 30 (4) p404-11

Essential fatty acid metabolism in diseases of connective tissue with special reference to scleroderma and to Sjogren's syndrome. *Med Hypotheses* (England) Jul 1984, 14 (3) p233-47

Parathyroid hormone and calcium metabolism in generalized scleroderma. Increased PTH level and secondary hyperparathyroidism in patients with aberrant calcifications. Prophylactic treatment of calcinosis. *Arch Dermatol Res* (Germany, West) 1984, 276 (2) p91-5

Tryptophan metabolism "via" nicotimic acid in patients with scleroderma. *Acta Vitaminol Enzymol* (Italy) 1976, 30 (4-6) p134-9

Scleroderma-like disorders. *Seminars in Cutaneous Medicine and Surgery* 1998, 17/1 (65-76)

Management of localized scleroderma. *Seminars in Cutaneous Medicine and Surgery* 1998, 17/1 (34-40)

Lymphoproliferative responses to Borrelia burgdorferi in circumscribed scleroderma. *British Journal of Dermatology* (UK) 1996, 134/2 (285-291)

A case of localized scleroderma treated with Sairei-to. *Acta Dermatologica—Kyoto* (Japan) 1995, 90/1 (109-112)

Southwestern Internal Medicine Conference: The many faces of scleroderma. *American Journal of the Medical Sciences* 1992, 304/5 (319-333)

Localized scleroderma—response to 1,25-dihydroxyvitamin Dinf 3. *Clinical and Experimental Dermatology* (UK) 1990, 15/5 (396-398)

Stimulating circulation to end statis in scleroderma. *Chinese Medical Journal* (China) 1981, 94/2 (85-93)

Scleroderma. *Practitioner* (UK) 1977, 219/1314 (820-825)

A mixture of aliphatic alcohols, tocopherol and phytosterols ('piascledine') in treatment of scleroderma. Preliminary report (Polish). *Przeglad Dermatologiczny* 1974, 61/4 (525-527)

Ascorbic acid absorption in patients with systemic sclerosis. *J Rheumatol* (Canada) Dec 1997, 24 (12) p2353-7

Clinical aspects of the use of gamma linolenic acid in systemic sclerosis. *Acta Derm Venereol* (Norway) Mar 1996, 76 (2) p144-6

Dietary intake of micronutrient antioxidants in relation to blood levels in patients with systemic sclerosis. *J Rheumatol* (Canada) Apr 1996, 23 (4) p650-3

Increased susceptibility to oxidation of low-density lipoproteins isolated from patients with systemic sclerosis. *Arthritis Rheum* Aug 1995, 38 (8) p1060-7

Micronutrient antioxidant status in patients with primary Raynaud's phenomenon and systemic sclerosis. *J Rheumatol* (Canada) Aug 1994, 21 (8) p1477-83

Dietary intake and nutritional status in patients with systemic sclerosis. *Ann Rheum Dis* (England) Oct 1992, 51 (10) p1143-8

Essential fatty acid and prostaglandin metabolism in Sjogren's syndrome, systemic sclerosis and rheumatoid arthritis. *Scand J Rheumatol Suppl* (Sweden) 1986, 61 p242-5

Environmental and iatrogenic factors in systemic sclerosis and related conditions: Review of the literature. *Revue de Medecine Interne* (France) 1997, 18/3 (219-229)

Systemic sclerosis in the elderly. *Clinical Rheumatology* (Belgium) 1992, 11/4 (483-485)

Progressive systemic sclerosis: Pseudoscleroderma. *Clinics in Rheumatic Diseases* 1979, 5/1 (243-261)

Clastogenic activity in the plasma of scleroderma patients: a biomarker of oxidative stress. *Dermatology* (Switzerland) 1997, 194 (2) p140-6

Evidence of free radical-mediated injury (isoprostane overproduction) in scleroderma. *Arthritis Rheum* Jul 1996, 39 (7) p1146-50

Antimyenteric neuronal antibodies in scleroderma. *J Clin Invest* Aug 1994, 94 (2) p761-70

[A clinico-immunological assessment of the efficacy of combined methods of treating patients with different immunopathological forms of focal scleroderma]. *Vestn Dermatol Venerol* (USSR) 1990, (2) p47-50

Avian scleroderma: evidence for qualitative and quantitative T cell defects. *J Autoimmun* (England) Jun 1992, 5 (3) p261-76

[The cyclic nucleotide system of patients with focal scleroderma]. *Vestn Dermatol Venerol* (USSR) 1990, (3) p35-8

D-penicillamine therapy and interstitial lung disease in scleroderma. A long-term followup study. *Arthritis Rheum* Jun 1987, 30 (6) p643-50

Failure of dimethyl sulfoxide in the treatment of scleroderma. *Arch Dermatol* Oct 1977, 113 (10) p1398-402

D penicillamine in the treatment of rheumatoid arthritis and progressive systemic sclerosis. *British Journal of Dermatology* 1976, 94/6 (705-711)

Elevated plasma superoxide dismutase activity in patients with systemic sclerosis. *J Dermatol Sci* (Ireland) Mar 1996, 11 (3) p196-201

[Myasthenia gravis induced by D-penicillamine in a patient with progressive systemic sclerosis]. *Arq Neuropsiquiatr* (BRAZIL) Dec 1984, 42 (4) p380-3

The thymus in systemic sclerosis. *J Pathol* (England) May 1973, 110 (1) p97-100

Treatment of systemic sclerosis. *Curr Opin Rheumatol* Nov 1993, 5 (6) p792-801

Penicillamine in systemic sclerosis: a reappraisal. *Clin Rheumatol* (Belgium) Dec 1990, 9 (4) p517-22

Progressive systemic sclerosis: Management. Part IV: Colchicine. *Clinics in Rheumatic Diseases* 1979, 5/1 (294-302)

Fish-oil dietary supplementation in patients with Raynaud's phenomenon: a double-blind, controlled, prospective study. *Am J Med* Feb 1989, 86 (2) p158-64

Retrospective studies in scleroderma: effect of potassium para-aminobenzoate on survival. *J Clin Epidemiol* (England) 1988, 41 (2) p193-205

Lipodermatosclerosis is characterized by elevated expression and activation of matrix metalloproteinases: implications for venous ulcer formation. *J Invest Dermatol* Nov 1998, 111 (5) p822-7

Pathogenesis of scleroderma (systemic sclerosis). *J Invest Dermatol* Jul 1982, 79 Suppl 1 p87s-89s,

Cutaneous vitamin D3 formation in progressive systemic sclerosis. *J Rheumatol* (Canada) Aug 1991, 18 (8) p1196-8

Treatment of scleroderma with oral 1, 25- dihydroxyvitamin D3: evaluation of skin involvement using non-invasive techniques. Results of an open prospective trial. *Acta Derm Venereol* (Sweden) Dec 1993, 73 (6) p449-51

Localized scleroderma—response to 1, 25-dihydroxyvitamin D3. *Clin Exp Dermatol* (England) Sep 1990, 15 (5) p396-8

Isolation and structural identification of 1, 25- dihydroxyvitamin D3 produced by cultured alveolar macrophages in sarcoidosis. *J Clin Endocrinol Metab* May 1985, 60 (5) p960-6

Treatment of generalized systemic sclerosis. *Rheum Dis Clin North Am* Feb 1990, 16 (1) p217-41

[The effect of dimethyl sulfoxide on the thromboelastographic indices and the microcirculation in patients with rheumatic diseases]. *Ter Arkh* (USSR) 1989, 61 (12) p106-9

Double-blind, multicenter controlled trial comparing topical dimethyl sulfoxide and normal saline for treatment of hand ulcers in patients with systemic sclerosis. *Arthritis Rheum* Mar 1985, 28 (3) p308-14

The effect of percutaneous dimethyl sulfoxide on cutaneous manifestations of systemic sclerosis. *Ann N Y Acad Sci* 1983, 411 p120-30

DMSO revisited. *Canadian Pharmaceutical Journal* (Canada) 1994, 127/5 (248-249+255)

Control trials of dimethyl sulfoxide in rheumatoid and collagen diseases. *Annals of the New York Academy of Sciences* 1983, Vol. 411/- (309-315)

Experimental and clinical evaluation of topical dimethyl sulfoxide in venous disorders of the extremities. *Annals of the New York Academy of Sciences* 1975, Vol. 243/- (403-407)

Medical management of diseases of the small intestine. *Current Opinion in Gastroenterology* (UK) 1992, 8/2 (224-231)

Slides of lumbogluteal sclerodermas induced by intramuscular injections of vitamin K1. *Marseille Med.* 1975, 112/7-8 (419)

Glucose intolerance in patients with chronic inflammatory diseases is normalized by glucocorticoids. *Acta Med Scand* (Sweden) 1983, 213 (5) p351-5

Vitamin K1-induced localized scleroderma (morphea) with linear deposition of IgA in the basement membrane zone. *J Am Acad Dermatol* Feb 1998, 38 (2 Pt 2) p322-4

Inhibition of collagen production by traditional Chinese herbal medicine in scleroderma fibroblast cultures. *Intern Med* (Japan) Aug 1994, 33 (8) p466-71

Chloracne, palmoplantar keratoderma and localized scleroderma in a weed sprayer. *Clin Exp Dermatol* (England) May 1994, 19 (3) p264-7

[Studies on stimulating circulation to end stasis in scleroderma]. *Chung Hsi I Chieh Ho Tsa Chih* (China) Jan 1989, 9 (1) p19-21, 5

Lymphocyte subpopulations and reactivity to mitogens in patients with scleroderma. *Clin Exp Immunol* (England) Oct 1981, 46 (1) p70-6

Lymphocyte reactivity to mitogens in subjects with systemic lupus erythematosus, rheumatoid arthritis and scleroderma. *Clin Exp Immunol* (England) Jan 1977, 27 (1) p92-9

Pattern of gastric emptying in patients with systemic sclerosis. *Clin Nucl Med* May 1996, 21 (5) p379-82

Overlap syndrome of progressive systemic sclerosis and polymyositis: report of 40 cases. *Chin Med Sci J* (England) Jun 1991, 6 (2) p107-9

Antiphospholipid syndrome associated with progressive systemic sclerosis. *J Dermatol* (Japan) May 1996, 23 (5) p347-51

Progressive systemic sclerosis (PSS): Review of the pathophysiological, clinical and pharmacological aspects of the syndrome. *Lakartidningen* (Sweden) 1979, 76/4 (207-210)

Topical lithium succinate ointment (Efalith) in the treatment of AIDS-related seborrhoeic dermatitis. *Clin Exp Dermatol* (England) Sep 1997, 22 (5) p216-9

Topical calcipotriene for morphea/linear scleroderma. *J Am Acad Dermatol* Aug 1998, 39 (2 Pt 1) p211-5

Management of severe scleroderma with long-term extracorporeal photopheresis. *Dermatology* (Switzerland) 1998, 196 (3) p309-15

Successful treatment of scleroderma with PUVA therapy. *J Dermatol* (Japan) Jul 1996, 23 (7) p455-9

Effects of calcitriol on fibroblasts derived from skin of scleroderma patients. *Dermatology* (Switzerland) 1995, 191 (3) p226-33

Effects of tumor necrosis factor-alpha on connective tissue metabolism in normal and scleroderma fibroblast cultures. *Arch Dermatol Res* (Germany) 1993, 284 (8) p440-4

[Treatment of severe Raynaud syndrome in scleroderma or thromboangiitis obliterans with prostacyclin (prostaglandin I2)]. *Z Rheumatol* (Germany) Jan-Feb 1991, 50 (1) p16-20

A double-blind randomized controlled trial of ketotifen versus placebo in early diffuse scleroderma. *Arthritis Rheum* Mar 1991, 34 (3) p362-6

Factor XIII in scleroderma: in vitro studies. *Br J Dermatol* (England) Mar 1990, 122 (3) p371-82

5-fluorouracil in the treatment of scleroderma: a randomised, double blind, placebo controlled international collaborative study. *Ann Rheum Dis* (England) Nov 1990, 49 (11) p926-8

Systemic scleroderma. Clinical and pathophysiologic aspects. *J Am Acad Dermatol* Mar 1988, 18 (3) p457-81

[Treatment of systemic scleroderma using plasma exchange. A study of 19 cases]. *Ann Med Interne* (Paris) (France) 1988, 139 Suppl 1 p20-2

Captopril in the treatment of scleroderma renal crisis. *Arch Intern Med* Apr 1984, 144 (4) p733-5

Renal scleroderma: comparison of different modalities of treatment. *South Med J* May 1980, 73 (5) p657-9

Treatment of progressive systemic sclerosis (scleroderma, PSS) with a new drug influencing connective tissue. *Acta Med Scand* (Sweden) 1977, 201 (3) p203-6

Barium impaction as a complication of gastrointestinal scleroderma. *JAMA* Apr 19 1976, 235 (16) p1715-7

Physiatrics for deforming linear scleroderma. *Arch Dermatol* Jul 1976, 112 (7) p995-7

Cyclophosphamide therapy for scleroderma. *Current Opinion in Rheumatology* 1998, 10/6 (579-583)

Treatment of systemic scleroderma patients with calcitonin: Report on ten years experience. *H+G Zeitschrift fur Hautkrankheiten* (Germany) 1993, 68/7 (437-442)

Laser-Doppler-flowmetry in prostaglandin Einf 1-therapy of scleroderma. *H+G Zeitschrift fur Hautkrankheiten* (Germany) 1991, 66/6 (533-535)

Treatment of generalized scleroderma with connective tissue inhibitors (Danish). *Ugeskr.Laeg.* 1976, 138/22 (1325-1329)

Extracorporeal photochemotherapy in progressive systemic sclerosis: a follow-up study. *Int J Dermatol* May 1997, 36 (5) p380-5

Extracorporeal photochemotherapy in progressive systemic sclerosis. *Int J Dermatol* Jun 1993, 32 (6) p417-21

Visceral improvement following combined plasmapheresis and immunosuppressive drug therapy in progressive systemic sclerosis. *Scand J Rheumatol* (Sweden) 1988, 17 (5) p313-23

Effects of prostaglandin E1 on microvascular haemodynamics in progressive systemic sclerosis. *Br Med J (Clin Res Ed)* (England) Dec 11 1982, 285 (6356) p1688-90

Progressive systemic sclerosis: Management. Part II: D-Penicillamine. *Clinics in Rheumatic Diseases* 1979, 5/1 (277-288)

Thymus-dependent (T) lymphocyte deficiency in progressive systemic sclerosis. *Br J Dermatol* (England) Nov 1976, 95 (5) p469-73

Monocytes of patients with systemic sclerosis (scleroderma) spontaneously release in vitro increased amounts of superoxide anion. *J Invest Dermatol* Jan 1998, 112 (1) p78-84

The value of the Health Assessment Questionnaire and special patient-generated scales to demonstrate change in systemic sclerosis patients over time. *Arthritis Rheum* Nov 1997, 40 (11) p1984-91

Hematopoietic stem cell transplantation in rheumatic diseases other than systemic sclerosis and systemic lupus erythematosus. *J Rheumatol Suppl* (Canada) May 1997, 48 p94-7

Treatment of systemic sclerosis. *Curr Opin Rheumatol* Nov 1994, 6 (6) p637-41

Cardiopulmonary hemodynamics in systemic sclerosis and response to nifedipine and captopril. *Am J Med* May 1991, 90 (5) p541-6

Effects of immunomodulating therapy in systemic sclerosis. *Clin Rheumatol* (Belgium) Sep 1990, 9 (3) p319-24

The effect of captopril on thallium 201 myocardial perfusion in systemic sclerosis. *Clin Pharmacol Ther* Apr 1990, 47 (4) p483-9

Benoxaprofen in treatment of systemic sclerosis. *Acta Derm Venereol* (Sweden) 1986, 66 (2) p177-9

Lack of clinical benefit after treatment of systemic sclerosis with total lymphoid irradiation. *J Rheumatol* (Canada) Aug 1989, 16 (8) p1050-4

Recombinant interferon-gamma in the treatment of systemic sclerosis. *Am J Med* Sep 1989, 87 (3) p273-7

Isotretinoin in the treatment of systemic sclerosis. *Br J Dermatol* (England) Sep 1989, 121 (3) p367-74

Treatment of progressive systemic sclerosis with plasma exchange. Seven cases. *Int J Artif Organs* (Italy) Nov 1983, 6 (6) p315-8

Penicillamine therapy in systemic sclerosis. *Proc R Soc Med* (England) 1977, 70 Suppl 3 p82-8

Interferon-gamma in the treatment of systemic sclerosis: A randomized controlled multicentre trial. *British Journal of Dermatology* (UK) 1998, 139/4 (639-648)

Intravenous Lipo-PGE1 (Eglandin(R)) therapy in peripheral vascular diseases secondary to systemic lupus erythematosus and systemic sclerosis. *Journal of Korean Society for Clinical Pharmacology and Therapeutics* (South Korea) 1996, 4/1 (29-34)

Influence of calcitonin on eicosanoid serum levels in the treatment of patients with systemic sclerosis. *Journal of the European Academy of Dermatology and Venereology* (Netherlands) 1996, 7/2 (139-148)

Cyclosporin in the treatment of systemic sclerosis. *Przeglad Dermatologiczny* (Poland) 1995, 82/5 (459-464)

Interferon-gamma therapy for systemic sclerosis. *Allergologie* (Germany) 1994, 17/8 (389-392)

Soluble and cellular markers of immune activation in patients with systemic sclerosis. *Clin Immunol Immunopathol* 1990 Aug;56(2):259-70 .

Seasonal Affective Disorder (SAD)

Morning vs evening light treatment of patients with winter depression. *Arch Gen Psychiatry* 1998 Oct;55(10):890-6

A controlled trial of timed bright light and negative air ionization for treatment of winter, depression. *Arch Gen Psychiatry* 1998 Oct;55(10):875-82

Dawn simulation vs. lightbox treatment in winter depression: a comparative study. *Acta Psychiatr Scand* 1998 Jul;98(1):73-80

Seasonal affective disorder. *Lancet* 1998 Oct 24;352(9137):1369-74

Efficacy of light versus tryptophan therapy in seasonal affective disorder. *J Affect Disord* 1998 Jul;50(1):23-7

Effects of tryptophan depletion in fully remitted patients with seasonal affective disorder during summer. *Psychol Med* 1998 Mar;28(2):257-64

Vitamin D3 enhances mood in healthy subjects during winter. *Psychopharmacology* (Berl) 1998 Feb;135(4):319-23

Side effects of short-term 10,000-lux light therapy. *Am J Psychiatry* 1998 Feb;155(2):293-4

Cluster headache and periodic affective illness: common chronobiological features. *Funct Neurol* (Italy) Jul-Sep 1998, 13 (3) p263-72

Natural bright light exposure in the summer and winter in subjects with and without complaints of seasonal mood variations. *Biol Psychiatry* Oct 1 1998, 44 (7) p622-8

Bright light treatment of winter depression: a placebo-controlled trial [see comments]. *Arch Gen Psychiatry* Oct 1998, 55 (10) p883-9

Greater improvement in summer than with light treatment in winter in patients with seasonal affective disorder. *Am J Psychiatry* Nov 1998, 155 (11) p1614-6

[Melatonin and seasonal depression]. *Recenti Prog Med* (Italy) Jul-Aug 1998, 89 (7-8) p395-403

Light treatment for nonseasonal depression: speed, efficacy, and combined treatment. *J Affect Disord* (Netherlands) May 1998, 49 (2) p109-17

Platelet serotonergic functions and light therapy in seasonal affective disorder. *Psychiatry Res* (Ireland) May 8 1998, 78 (3) p163-72

Disorders of the sleep-wake cycle in adults. *Postgrad Med J* (England) Mar 1998, 74 (869) p134-8

Extrapineal melatonin and exogenous serotonin in seasonal affective disorder. *Medical Hypotheses* (UK) 1998, 51/5 (441-442)

Pharmacological treatment of seasonal affective disorder - The role of hypericum extract. *Psychopharmakotherapie, Supplement* (Germany) 1998, 5/8 (21-25)

L-tryptophan augmentation of light therapy in patients with seasonal affective disorder. *Can J Psychiatry* (Canada) Apr 1997, 42 (3) p303-6

Prediction of acute and late responses to light therapy from vocal (pitch) and self-rated activation in seasonal affective disorder. *J Affect Disord* (Netherlands) Feb 1997, 42 (2-3) p117-26

A controlled trial of light therapy for the treatment of pediatric seasonal affective disorder. *J Am Acad Child Adolesc Psychiatry* Jun 1997, 36 (6) p816-21

Effects of tryptophan depletion on drug-free patients with seasonal affective disorder during a stable response to bright light therapy. *Arch Gen Psychiatry* Feb 1997, 54 (2) p133-8

Sunny hospital rooms expedite recovery from severe and refractory depressions. *J Affect Disord* (Netherlands) Sep 9 1996, 40 (1-2) p49-51

The importance of full summer remission as a criterion for the diagnosis of seasonal affective disorder. *Psychopathology* (Switzerland), 1996, 29 (4) p230-5

Light therapy in bulimia nervosa: a double-blind, placebo-controlled study. *Psychiatry Res* (Ireland) Feb 28 1996, 60 (1) p1-9

Predictors of response and nonresponse to light treatment for winter depression. *Am J Psychiatry* Nov 1996, 153 (11) p1423-9

'Natural' light treatment of seasonal affective disorder. *J Affect Disord* (Netherlands) Apr 12 1996, 37 (2-3) p109-20

[Phototherapy in psychiatry: clinical update and review of indications]. *Encephale* (France) Mar-Apr 1996, 22 (2) p143-8

Seasonal affective disorder and season-dependent abnormalities of melatonin suppression by light. *Lancet* (1990 Sep 22) 336(8717):703-6.

(For additional references on treating seasonal affective disorder, refer to Depression, above.)

Shingles

A contribution to our knowledge of Leonurus L., i-mu-ts'ao, the Chinese motherwort. *Am J Chin Med* Autumn 1976, 4 (3) p219-37

Effect of Ganoderma lucidum on postherpetic neuralgia. *Am J Chin Med* 1998;26(3-4):375-81

Antinociceptive components of Ganoderma lucidum. *Planta Med* 1997 Jun;63(3):224-7

Antiviral drug therapy. *Am Fam Physician* 1991 Jan;43(1):197-204

Promising new antiviral drugs. *J Am Acad Dermatol* 1988 Jan;18(1 Pt 2):212-8

Clinical review of ribavirin. *Infect Control* 1987 May;8(5):215-8

Recent advances in antiviral therapy. *Clin Pharm* 1986 Dec;5(12):961-76

Ribavirin and inosiplex: a review of their present status in viral diseases. *Drugs* 1981 Aug;22(2):111-28

Antiviral agents. *Mayo Clin Proc* 1983 Apr;58(4):217-22

Antiviral agents. *Mayo Clin Proc* 1977 Nov;52(11):683-6

Skin Aging

Inhibition of 7,12-dimethylbenz(a)anthracene-induced skin papillomas and carcinomas by dehydroepiandrosterone and 3-beta-methylandrost-5-en-17-one in mice. *Cancer Res* 1985 Jan;45(1):164-6

High bioavailability of dehydroepiandrosterone administered percutaneously in the rat. *J Endocrinol* 1996 Sep;150 Suppl:S107-18

Sex hormones and skin collagen content in postmenopausal women. *Br Med J* (Clin Res Ed) 1983 Nov 5;287(6402):1337-8

Suppression of UV-induced erythema by topical treatment with melatonin (N-acetyl-5-methoxytryptamine). Influence of the application time point. *Dermatology* 1997;195(3):248-52

A diurnal variation in the tumorigenic response of mouse epidermis to a single application of the strong short-acting chemical carcinogen methylnitrosourea. A dose-response study of 1, 2 and 10 mg. *In Vivo* 1995 Mar-Apr;9(2):117-32

Dehydroepiandrosterone reduces progressive dermal ischemia caused by thermal injury. *J Surg Res* 1995 Aug;59(2):250-62

Hypothalamic neuroendocrine correlates of cutaneous burn injury in the rat: I. Scanning electron microscopy. *Brain Res Bull* 1986 Sep;17(3):367-78

A double-blind randomized clinical trial on the effectiveness of a daily glycolic acid 5% formulation in the treatment of photoaging. *Dermatol Surg* May 1998, 24 (5) p573-7; discussion 577-8

Cutaneous and psychosocial benefits of alpha hydroxy acid use. *Percept Mot Skills* Feb 1998, 86 (1) p137-8

Synergistic effect of glycolic acid on the antioxidant activity of alpha-tocopherol and melatonin in lipid bilayers and in human skin homogenates. *Biochem Mol Biol Int* (Australia) Sep 1997, 42 (6) p1093-102

Citric acid increases viable epidermal thickness and glycosaminoglycan content of sun-damaged skin. *Dermatol Surg* Aug 1997, 23 (8) p689-94

Cosmetic use of alpha-hydroxy acids. *Cleve Clin J Med* Jun 1997, 64 (6) p327-9

A peat of paleozoic origin as a multifunctional ingredient for skin care. *Journal of Applied Cosmetology* (Italy), 1998, 16/3 (73-80)

Adverse effects of sunlight on skin. *Nederlands Tijdschrift voor Geneeskunde* (Netherlands), 1998, 142/12 (620-625)

The effect of glycolic acid on cultured human skin fibroblasts: Cell proliferative effect and increased collagen synthesis. *Journal of Dermatology* (Japan), 1998, 25/2 (85-89)

Does estrogen prevent skin aging?: Results from the first national health and nutrition examination survey (NHANES I). *Archives of Dermatology,* 1997, 133/3 (339-342)

Sunscreen sensitization: A 5-year study. *Acta Dermato-Venereologica (Acta Derm.—Venereol.)* (Norway) 1999, 79/3 (211-213)

Do people who apply sunscreens, re-apply them? *Australas J Dermatol* (Australia) May 1999, 40 (2) p79-82

Sun-related behaviour and melanoma awareness among Swedish university students. *Eur J Cancer Prev* (England) Feb 1999, 8 (1) p27-34

Sun awareness in school teachers. *Br J Dermatol* (England) Aug 1998, 139 (2) p280-4

Sunscreen use, wearing clothes, and number of nevi in 6- to 7-year-old European children. *J Natl Cancer Inst* Dec 16 1998, 90 (24) p1873-80

Phenotypic markers, sunlight-related factors and sunscreen use in patients with cutaneous melanoma: an Austrian case-control study. *Melanoma Res* (England) Aug 1998, 8 (4) p370-8

Moles and melanoma. *Curr Opin Pediatr* Aug 1998, 10 (4) p398-404

[Skin cancers and environmental factors]. *Rev Med Brux* (Belgium) Sep 1998, 19 (4) pA346-50

Pediatric sun exposure. *Nurse Pract* Jul 1998, 23 (7) p67-8, 71-8, 83-6

The prevalence and predictors of solar protection use among adolescents. *Prev Med* May-Jun 1998, 27 (3) p391-9

Sun-protection behaviors used by adults for their children—United States, 1997. *Morb Mortal Wkly Rep* Jun 19 1998, 47 (23) p480-2

Melanoma and sunscreen use: need for studies representative of actual behaviours. *Melanoma Res* (England) Aug 1997, 7 Suppl 2 pS115-20

How well are sunscreen users protected? *Photodermatol Photoimmunol Photomed* (Denmark) Oct-Dec 1997, 13 (5-6) p186-8

Approaches to the prevention and control of skin cancer. *Cancer Metastasis Rev* Sep-Dec 1997, 16 (3-4) p309-27

The case for sunscreens. A review of their use in preventing actinic damage and neoplasia [see comments]. *Arch Dermatol* Sep 1997, 133 (9) p1146-54

Sun behaviour and perceptions of risk for melanoma among 21-year-old New Zealanders. *Aust N Z J Public Health* (Australia) Jun 1997, 21 (3) p329-34

Trends in sun exposure knowledge, attitudes, and behaviors: 1986 to 1996. *J Am Acad Dermatol* Aug 1997, 37 (2 Pt 1) p179-86

Skin cancer prevention: a time for action. *J Community Health* Jun 1997, 22 (3) p175-83

Summer sun exposure: knowledge, attitudes, and behaviors of Midwest adolescents. *Prev Med* May-Jun 1997, 26 (3) p364-72

A study of the impact of Sun Awareness Week 1995. *Br J Dermatol* (England) May 1997, 136 (5) p719-24

Teaching children about skin cancer: the draw-and-write technique as an evaluation tool. *Pediatr Dermatol* Jan-Feb 1997, 14 (1) p6-12

Trunk malignant melanoma. *Revista del Instituto Nacional de Cancerologia* (Mexico) 1998, 44/4 (205-209)

Could a national skin cancer primary prevention campaign in Australia be worthwhile? An economic perspective. *Health Promotion International* (UK) 1999, 14/1 (73-82)

Skin cancer of the head and neck. *Medical Clinics of North America* 1999, 83/1 (261-282)

Prevention of malignant melanoma: An overview of existing certainties. *Zeitschrift fur Dermatologie* (Germany) 1998, 184/2 (82-85)

Skin Precancer. *Cancer Surveys* 1998, 32/- (69-113)

Ultraviolet radiation: Human exposure and health risks. *Journal of Environmental Health* 1998, 61/2 (9-15)

Sunscreens for primary prevention of malignant melanoma. *H+G Zeitschrift fur Hautkrankheiten* (Germany) 1998, 73/7-8 (467-473)

Do sunscreens prevent skin cancer? *Drug and Therapeutics Bulletin* (UK) 1998, 36/7 (49-51)

UVA, malignant melanoma, sunscreen products—A controversy? *Journal of Dermatological Treatment* (UK) 1998, 9/ Suppl. 2 (17-21)

An estimate of the annual direct cost of treating cutaneous melanoma. *Journal of the American Academy of Dermatology* 1998, 38/5 I (669-680)

Care of the skin at midlife: Diagnosis of pigmented lesions. *Geriatrics* 1997, 52/8 (56-68)

The aging skin. *International Journal of Fertility and Women's Medicine* 1997, 42/2 (57-66)

American College of Preventive Medicine practice policy statement: Skin protection from ultraviolet light exposure. *American Journal of Preventive Medicine* 1998, 14/1 (83-86)

A clinical review of the evidence for the role of ultraviolet radiation in the etiology of cutaneous melanoma. *Cancer Investigation* 1997, 15/6 (561-567)

Chemoprevention of ultraviolet radiation-induced skin cancer. *Environmental Health Perspectives* 1997, 105/Suppl. 4 (981-984)

Should subjects who used psoralen suntan activators be screened for melanoma? *Annals of Oncology* (Netherlands) 1997, 8/5 (435-437)

Sunlight and cancer. *Cancer Causes and Control* (UK) 1997, 8/3 (271-283)

Cancer of the skin in the older patient. *Clinics in Geriatric Medicine* 1997, 13/2 (339-361)

Erythema, skin cancer risk, and sunscreens. *Archives of Dermatology* 1997, 133/3 (373-375)

Non-melanoma skin cancer and solar keratoses II analytical results of the South Wales Skin. *Br J Cancer* (Scotland) Oct 1996, 74 (8) p1308-12

Predictors of sun exposure in adolescents in a southeastern U.S. population [see comments]. *J Adolesc Health* Dec 1996, 19 (6) p409-15

Sunburn, sunscreen, and melanoma. *Curr Opin Oncol* Mar 1996, 8 (2) p159-66

[Is the sun our friend?]. *Cas Lek Cesk* (Czech Republic) Jul 26 1996, 135 (13) p403-4

Sun exposure, sunscreens, and skin cancer prevention: a year-round concern. *Ann Pharmacother* Jun 1996, 30 (6) p662-73

Children and exposure to the sun: relationships among attitudes, knowledge, intentions, and behavior. *Psychol Rep* Dec 1995, 77 (3 Pt 2) p1136-8

The epidemiology of non-melanoma skin cancer: who, why and what can we do about it. *J Dermatol* (Japan) Nov 1995, 22 (11) p853-7

Protection of children against sunburn: a survey of parental practice in Leicester. *Br J Dermatol* (England) Aug 1995, 133 (2) p264-6

Melanoma and use of sunscreens: an Eortc case-control study in Germany, Belgium and France. *Int J Cancer* Jun 9 1995, 61 (6) p749-55

Cutaneous melanoma in women. I. Exposure to sunlight, ability to tan, and other risk factors related to ultraviolet light. *Am J Epidemiol* May 15 1995, 141 (10) p923-33

Is the use of sunscreens a risk factor for malignant melanoma? [see comments]. *Melanoma Res* (England) Feb 1995, 5 (1) p59-65

[Effect of sunlight on the skin—what have we learned?]. *Nord Med* (Sweden) 1995, 110 (3) p85-7

Melanoma awareness and sun exposure in Leicester [see comments]. *Br J Dermatol* (England) Feb 1995, 132 (2) p251-6

Sun exposure of young children while at day care. *Pediatr Dermatol* Dec 1994, 11 (4) p304-9

Knowledge, beliefs, and sun protection behaviors of Alberta adults. *Prev Med* Mar 1994, 23 (2) p160-6

Effect of sunscreens on UV radiation-induced enhancement of melanoma growth in mice. *J Natl Cancer Inst* Jan 19 1994, 86 (2) p99-105

Rising trends in melanoma. An hypothesis concerning sunscreen effectiveness. *Ann Epidemiol* Jan 1993, 3 (1) p103-10

Changes in sun-related attitudes and behaviours, and reduced sunburn prevalence in a population at high risk of melanoma. *Eur J Cancer Prev* (England) Nov 1993, 2 (6) p447-56

Melanoma and skin cancer: evaluation of a health education programme for secondary schools. *Br J Dermatol* (England) Apr 1993, 128 (4) p412-7

Beneficial effects of sun exposure on cancer mortality. *Prev Med* Jan 1993, 22 (1) p132-40

Melanoma prevention: behavioral and nonbehavioral factors in sunburn among an Australian urban population. *Prev Med* Sep 1992, 21 (5) p654-69

Adolescence and sun protection. *N Z Med J* (New Zealand) Oct 14 1992, 105 (943) p401-3

Sun exposure and sunscreen use following a community skin cancer screening. *Prev Med* May 1992, 21 (3) p302-10

Case-control study of melanoma and dietary vitamin D: implications for advocacy of sun protection and sunscreen use. *J Invest Dermatol* May 1992, 98 (5) p809-11

Sun protection in childhood [corrected and republished article originally printed in *Clin Pediatr* (Phila) 1991 Jul;30(7):412-21]. *Clin Pediatr* (Phila) Dec 1991, 30 (12) p676-81

Sunscreen: one weapon against melanoma. *Dermatol Clin* Oct 1991, 9 (4) p789-93

Dysplastic nevi and malignant melanoma. *Am Fam Physician* Aug 1990, 42 (2) p372-85

Analysis of the effect of a sunscreen agent on the suppression of natural killer cell activity induced in human subjects by radiation from solarium lamps. *J Invest Dermatol* Mar 1987, 88 (3) p271-6

Harmful effects of ultraviolet radiation. Council on Scientific Affairs. *JAMA* Jul 21 1989, 262 (3) p380-4

The association of solar ultraviolet and skin melanoma incidence among caucasians in the United States. *Cancer Invest* 1987, 5 (4) p275-83

Risk reduction for nonmelanoma skin cancer with childhood sunscreen use. *Arch Dermatol* May 1986, 122 (5) p537-45

Efficacy of topical sunscreen preparations on the human skin: combined indoor-outdoor study. *Isr J Med Sci* (Israel) Jul 1984, 20 (7) p569-77

Predictors of sunbathing and sunscreen use in college undergraduates. *Journal of Behavioral Medicine (J. Behav. Med.)* 1996, 19/6 (543-561)

Protecting skin and preventing melanoma. *Manufacturing Chemist* (UK) 1996, 67/10 (79-81)

Photoprotection: An active shield against exposure to sunlight health information for the public. *Aktuelle Dermatologie* (Germany) 1996, 22/Suppl. 2 (93-96)

Relevance of in vitro melanocytic cell studies to the understanding of melanoma. *Cancer Surveys* 1995, 26/- (71-88)

Prevention and control of melanoma: The public health approach. *Ca-A Cancer Journal for Clinicians* 1996, 46/4 (199-216)

News in photoprotection. *Nouvelles Dermatologiques* (France) 1996, 15/5 (349-353)

Sun-induced skin damage. *Aktuelle Dermatologie* (Germany) 1996, 22/Suppl. 1 (2-6)

Chronic sunlight exposure-induced skin damage and skin cancer: Cutaneous manifestations, prevention, and treatment. *Aktuelle Dermatologie* (Germany) 1996, 22/Suppl. 1 (7-12)

Sunscreens: The ounce of prevention. *American Family Physician* 1996, 53/5 (1713-1719)

Prevention and early detection strategies for melanoma and skin cancer: Current status. *Archives of Dermatology* 1996, 132/4 (436-442)

Preventive strategies and research for ultraviolet-associated cancer. *Environmental Health Perspectives* 1995, 103/Suppl. 8 (255-257)

Overview of ultraviolet radiation and cancer: What is the link? How are we doing? *Environmental Health Perspectives* 1995, 103/Suppl. 8 (251-254)

Genotoxicity, mutagenicity, and carcinogenicity of UVA and UVB. *H+G Zeitschrift fur Hautkrankheiten* (Germany) 1995, 70/12 (877-881)

Environmental skin injuries in children. *Current Opinion in Pediatrics* 1995, 7/4 (423-430)

Cancer of the skin in the next century. *International Journal of Dermatology* (Canada) 1995, 34/7 (445-447)

Predictors of sunscreen use in childhood. *Archives of Pediatrics and Adolescent Medicine* 1995, 149/7 (804-807)

Self screening for risk of melanoma: Validity of self mole counting by patients in a single general practice. *British Medical Journal* (UK) 1995, 310/6984 (912-916)

Xeroderma pigmentosum. *Dermatologic Clinics* 1995, 13/1 (169-209)

Children and photoprotection. *Nouvelles Dermatologiques* (France) 1994, 13/6 (415-422)

Daily sun protection. *Dermatosen in Beruf und Umwelt* (Germany) 1994, 42/3 (107-110)

Melanoma: 1. Clinical characteristics. *Hospital Practice* 1994, 29/6 (37-40+43-44+47-48+50)

Melanocytic nevi in Turner syndrome. *Pediatric Dermatology* 1994, 11/2 (120-124)

Temporal changes in the incidence of malignant melanoma: Explanation from action spectra. *Mutation Research—Fundamental and Molecular Mechanisms of Mutagenesis* (Netherlands) 1994, 307/1 (365-374)

Effects of topical tretinoin on dysplastic nevi. *Journal of Clinical Oncology* 1994, 12/5 (1028-1035)

UV carcinogenesis: Epidemiology and risk models. *Aktuelle Dermatologie* (Germany) 1993, 19/12 (368-371)

Study of sunbathing habits in children and adolescents: Application to the prevention of melanoma. *Dermatology* (Switzerland) 1993, 186/2 (94-98)

Solar radiation protection for outdoor workers. *Journal of Occupational Health and Safety Australia and New Zealand* (Australia) 1992, 8/6 (479-485)

Multidisciplinary treatment of facial skin cancer. *Texas Medicine* 1991, 87/12 (64-69)

Sun protection in newborns: A comparison of educational methods. *American Journal of Diseases of Children* 1991, 145/10 (1125-1129)

Malignant melanoma: Aetiological importance of individual pigmentation and sun exposure. *British Journal of Dermatology* (UK) 1990, 122/1 (43-51)

Sunscreens: Topical and systemic approaches for protection of human skin against harmful effects of solar radiation. *Journal of the American Academy of Dermatology* 1982, 7/3 (285-314)

Inhibition of cyclobutane pyrimidine dimer formation in epidermal p53 gene of UV-irradiated mice by alpha-tocopherol. *Nutr Cancer* 1997, 29 (3) p205-11

Sunscreens protect from UV-promoted squamous cell carcinoma in mice chronically irradiated with doses of UV radiation insufficient to cause edema. *Photochem Photobiol* Jul 1996, 64 (1) p188-93

Cell survival and shuttle vector mutagenesis induced by ultraviolet A and ultraviolet B radiation in a human cell line. *J Invest Dermatol* Apr 1996, 106 (4) p721-8

Sun protection and sunscreen use after surgical treatment of basal cell carcinoma. *Photodermatol Photoimmunol Photomed* (Denmark) Aug 1995, 11 (4) p140-2

A prospective study of incident squamous cell carcinoma of the skin in the nurses' health study. *J Natl Cancer Inst* Jul 19 1995, 87 (14) p1061-6

High sun protection factor sunscreens in the suppression of actinic neoplasia. *Arch Dermatol* Feb 1995, 131 (2) p170-5

The Nambour Skin Cancer and Actinic Eye Disease Prevention Trial: design and baseline characteristics of participants. *Control Clin Trials* Dec 1994, 15 (6) p512-22

Photodamage, photoaging and photoprotection of the skin. *Am Fam Physician* Aug 1994, 50 (2) p327-32, 334

Reduction of solar keratoses by regular sunscreen use. *N Engl J Med* Oct 14 1993, 329 (16) p1147-51

Minimising the risks of PUVA treatment. *Drug Saf* (New Zealand) May 1993, 8 (5) p340-9

Effect of immunosuppressive agents and sunscreens on UV carcinogenesis in the hairless mouse. *Aust J Exp Biol Med Sci* (Australia) Dec 1985, 63 (Pt 6) p655-65

Sunscreen protection for lip mucosa: a review and update. *J Am Dent Assoc* Oct 1985, 111 (4) p617-21

Psoralen-containing sunscreen is tumorigenic in hairless mice. *J Am Acad Dermatol* Jun 1983, 8 (6) p830-6

Sunscreens for delay of ultraviolet induction of skin tumors. *J Am Acad Dermatol* Aug 1982, 7 (2) p194-202

Eyelid cancers. *Current Opinion in Ophthalmology (Curr. Opin. Ophthalmol.)* 1998, 9/5 (49-53)

Axillary basal cell cacrinoma: A need for full cutaneous examination. *American Family Physician* 15 APR 1998, 57/8 (1860-1864)

Sunlight and carcinogenesis: Expression of p53 and pyrimidine dimers in human skin following UVA I, UVA I + II and solar simulating radiations. *International Journal of Cancer* 13 APR 1998, 76/2 (201-206)

Long-term efficacy and safety of Jessner's solution and 35% trichloroacetic acid vs 5% fluorouracil in the treatment of widespread facial actinic keratoses. *Dermatologic Surgery* 1997, 23/3 (191-196)

Nonmelanoma skin cancer: Risks, treatment options, and tips on prevention. *Postgraduate Medicine* 1995, 98/6 (39-40+45-46+48+55-56+58)

Basal cell carcinoma: Choosing the best method of treatment for a particular lesion. *Postgraduate Medicine* 1993, 93/8 (101-111)

International poster parade: Sight bites from the 18th World Congress of Dermatology. *Cutis* 1992, 50/3 (217-220)

Sun-related skin diseases. *Postgraduate Medicine* 1991, 89/8 (51-54+59-61+64-66)

Photocarcinogenesis is retarded by a partly photodegraded solution of para-aminobenzoic acid. *Photodermatology* (Denmark) 1989, 6/6 (263-267)

[Use of photoprotective measures in relation to actual exposure to solar rays]. *Med Pregl* (Yugoslavia) Nov-Dec 1998, 51 (11-12) p555-8

A review of sunscreen safety and efficacy. *Photochem Photobiol* Sep 1998, 68 (3) p243-56

A novel in vivo model for evaluating agents that protect against ultraviolet A-induced photoaging. *J Invest Dermatol* Apr 1998, 110 (4) p343-7

Complications of laser resurfacing. Methods of prevention and management. *Dermatol Surg* Jan 1998, 24 (1) p91-9

Effectiveness of antioxidants (vitamin C and E) with and without sunscreens as topical photoprotectants. *Acta Derm Venereol* (Norway) Jul 1996, 76 (4) p264-8

Synergistic topical photoprotection by a combination of the iron chelator 2-furildioxime and sunscreen. *J Am Acad Dermatol* Oct 1996, 35 (4) p546-9

A review of skin ageing and its medical therapy. *Br J Dermatol* (England) Dec 1996, 135 (6) p867-75

Sun exposure and skin disease. *Annu Rev Med* 1996, 47 p181-91

Current concepts. Photoprotection. *Arch Fam Med* May 1996, 5 (5) p289-95

The effects of chronic sunscreen use on the histologic changes of dermatoheliosis. *J Am Acad Dermatol* Dec 1995, 33 (6) p941-6

Effect of a conjugated oestrogen (Premarin) cream on ageing facial skin. A comparative study with a placebo cream. *Maturitas* (Ireland) Oct 1994, 19 (3) p211-23

Sunbathing: college students' knowledge, attitudes, and perceptions of risks. *J Am Coll Health* Jul 1993, 42 (1) p21-6

Photoaging and the skin. The effects of tretinoin. *Dermatol Clin* Jan 1993, 11 (1) p97-105

In vivo evaluation of photoprotection against chronic ultraviolet-A irradiation by a new sunscreen Mexoryl SX. *Photochem Photobiol* (England) Apr 1992, 55 (4) p549-60

Photoprotective effects of sunscreens in cosmetics on sunburn and Langerhans cell photodamage. *Photodermatol Photoimmunol Photomed* (Denmark) Jun 1992, 9 (3) p113-20

Experience with tretinoin therapy in temperate regions. *Br J Dermatol* (England) Sep 1992, 127 Suppl 41 p51-3

Facial moisturizers and wrinkles. *Dermatol Nurs* Jun 1992, 4 (3) p205-7

Sunscreens with low sun protection factor inhibit ultraviolet B and A photoaging in the skin of the hairless albino mouse. *Photodermatol Photoimmunol Photomed* (Denmark) Feb 1991, 8 (1) p12-20

Time-dependent decrease in sunscreen protection against chronic photodamage in UVB-irradiated hairless mouse skin. *J Photochem Photobiol B* (Switzerland) Jun 1991, 9 (3-4) p323-34

Sunscreens and the prevention of skin aging. *J Dermatol Surg Oncol* Oct 1990, 16 (10) p936-8

Photosensitivity in the elderly. *Br J Dermatol* (England) Apr 1990, 122 Suppl 35 p29-36

Senescence and sunscreens [see comments]. *Br J Dermatol* (England) Apr 1990, 122 Suppl 35 p111-4

Drug treatment of photoaged skin. *Drugs and Aging (Drugs Aging)* (New Zealand) 1999, 14/4 (289-301)

Molecular mechanisms of cutaneous aging: Connective tissue alterations in the dermis. *Journal of Investigative Dermatology Symposium Proceedings* 1998, 3/1 (41-44)

The role of cosmetology and the aesthetic within dermatology in Spain. *Nouvelles Dermatologiques* (France) 1998, 17/4 (249-252)

The study on the ultraviolet-B blocking effect of sunscreens in the epidermal Langerhans cells of hairless mice. *Annals of Dermatology* (South Korea) 1995, 7/4 (288-294)

Awarness tophotodamage versus the actual use of sun protection methods by young adults. *Journal of the European Academy of Dermatology and Venereology* (Netherlands) 1995, 4/3 (260-266)

Skin photosensitizing agents and the role of reactive oxygen species in photoaging. *J. Photochem. Photobiol. B Biol.* (Switzerland), 1992, 14/1-2 (105-124)

An in vitro model to test relative antioxidant potential: Ultraviolet- induced lipid peroxidation in liposomes. *Arch. Biochem. Biophys.*, 1990, 283/2 (234-240)

Diminished stimulation of hyaluronic acid synthesis by PDGF, IGF-I or serum in the senescence phase of skin fibroblasts in vitro. *Z. Gerontol.* (Germany), 1994, 27/3 (177-181)

Ultrastructural study of hyaluronic acid before and after the use of a pulsed electromagnetic field, electrorydesis, in the treatment of wrinkles. *Int. J. Dermatol.* (Canada), 1994, 33/9 (661-663)

Hyaluronic acid in cutaneous intrinsic aging. *Int. J. Dermatol.* (Canada), 1994, 33/2 (119-122)

Stimulation of cell proliferation by hyaluronidase during in vitro aging of human skin fibroblasts. *Exp. Gerontol.*, 1993, 28/1 (59-68)

Topical retinoic acid treatment of photoaged skin: Its effects on hyaluronan distribution in epidermis and on hyaluronan and retinoic acid in suction blister fluid. *Acta Derm.—Venereol.* (Norway), 1992, 72/6 (423-427)

Werner's syndrome: Biochemical and cytogenetic studies. *Arch. Dermatol.*, 1985, 121/5 (636-641)

Urinary acidic glycosaminoglycans in Werner's syndrome. *Experientia* (Switzerland), 1982, 38/3 (313-314)

Non-enzymatic degradation of acid-soluble calf skin collagen by superoxide ion: Protective effect of flavonoids. *Biochem. Pharmacol.* (England), 1983, 32/1 (53-58)

In vitro cytotoxic effects of enzymatically induced oxygen radicals in human fibroblasts: Experimental procedures and protection by radical scavengers. *Toxicol. Vitro* (UK), 1989, 3/2 (103-109)

Antiviral activity of plant components. 1st Communication: flavonoids. *Arzneim.-Forsch.* (Germany, West), 1978, 28/3 (347-350)

Therapy of radiation damage in mice with O (L hydroxyethyl) rutoside. *Strahlentherapie* (Germany, West), 1973, 145/6 (731-734)

Anti-ageing active principals by the oral route. Myth or reality? *Nouv. Dermatol.* (France), 1994, 13/6 (423-425)

Topical 8% glycolic acid and 8% L-lactic acid creams for the treatment of photodamaged skin: A double-blind vehicle-controlled clinical trial. *Archives of Dermatology*, 1996, 132/6 (631-636)

Alpha hydroxy acids in the cosmetic treatment of photo-induced skin ageing. *Journal of Applied Cosmetology* (Italy), 1996, 14/1 (1-8)

Effects of alpha-hydroxy acids on photoaged skin: A pilot clinical, histologic, and ultrastructural study. *Journal of the American Academy of Dermatology*, 1996, 34/2 I (187- 195)

Topical gelatin-glycine and alpha-hydroxy acids for photoaged skin. *J. Appl. Cosmetol.* (Italy), 1994, 12/1 (1-10)

Antioxidants, fat and skin cancer. *Skin Cancer* (Portugal), 1995, 10/2 (97-101)

An in vitro model to test relative antioxidant potential: Ultraviolet-induced lipid peroxidation in liposomes. *Arch. Biochem. Biophys.*, 1990, 283/2 (234-240)

Photoprotective effect of superoxide scavenging antioxidants against ultraviolet radiation-induced chronic skin damage in the hairless mouse. *Photodermatology Photoimmunology Photomedicine* (Denmark), 1990, 7/2 (56-62)

Impairment of enzymic and nonenzymic antioxidants in skin by UVB irradiation. *J. Invest. Dermatol.*, 1989, 93/6 (769-773)

Low levels of essential fatty acids are related to impaired delayed skin hypersensitivity in malnourished chronically ill elderly people. *Eur. J. Clin. Invest.* (UK), 1994, 24/9 (615-620)

Two concentrations of topical tretinoin (retinoic acid) cause similar improvement of photoaging but different degrees of irritation: A double-blind, vehicle-controlled comparison of 0.1% and 0.025% tretinoin creams. *Archives Of Dermatology*, 1995, 131/9 (1037-1044)

Topical tretinoin (retinoic acid) treatment for liver spots associated with photodamage. *New Engl. J. Med.*, 1992, 326/6 (368-374)

The effects of an abrasive agent on normal skin and on photoaged skin in comparison with topical tretinoin. *Br. J. Dermatol.* (UK), 1990, 123/4 (457-466)

Aging and the skin. *Postgrad. Med.*, 1989, 86/1 (131-144)

Topical tretinoind and photoaged skin. *Cutis*, 1989, 43/5 (476-482)

Stress

Refer to references under Anxiety.

Stroke (Hemorrhagic)

Antioxidant vitamin intake and coronary mortality in a longitudinal population study. *Am J Epidemiol* 1994 Jun 15;139(12):1180-9

Vitamin B-12, vitamin B-6, and folate nutritional status in men with hyperhomocysteinemia. *Am J Clin Nutr* 1993 Jan;57(1):47-53

Association between plasma homocysteine concentrations and extracranial carotid-artery stenosis. *N Engl J Med* 1995 Feb 2;332(5):286-91

Vitamin requirements for the treatment of hyperhomocysteinemia in humans. *J Nutr* 1994 Oct;124(10):1927-33

Serum carotenoids and coronary heart disease. The Lipid Research Clinics Coronary Primary. *JAMA* 1994 Nov 9;272(18):1439-41

Double-blind trial of vitamin C in elderly hypertensives. *J Hum Hypertens* 1993 Aug;7(4):403-5

Effect of combined supplementation with alpha-tocopherol, ascorbate, and beta carotene on low-density lipoprotein oxidation. *Circulation* 1993 Dec;88(6):2780-6

A comparison of the efficacy and toxic effects of sustained- vs immediate-release niacin in hypercholesterolemic patients. *JAMA* 1994 Mar 2;271(9):672-7

Thiamin status, diuretic medications, and the management of congestive heart failure. *J Am Diet Assoc* 1995 May;95(5):541-4

Effect of vitamin E and beta carotene on the incidence of angina pectoris. A randomized, double-blind, controlled trial. *JAMA* 1996 Mar 6;275(9):693-8, Published erratum appears in *JAMA* 1998 May 20;279(19):1528

Randomised controlled trial of vitamin E in patients with coronary disease: Cambridge Heart Antioxidant Study. *Lancet* 1996 Mar 23;347(9004):781-6

Ascorbic acid and plasma lipids. *Epidemiology* 1994 Jan;5(1):19-26

Flavonoid intake and coronary mortality in Finland: a cohort study. *BMJ* 1996 Feb 24;312(7029):478-81

Usefulness of antioxidant vitamins in suspected acute myocardial infarction (the Indian experiment of infarct survival-3). *Am J Cardiol* 1996 Feb 1;77(4):232-6

Vitamin E and vitamin C supplement use and risk of all-cause and coronary heart disease mortality in older persons: the

Established Populations for Epidemiologic Studies of the Elderly. *Am J Clin Nutr* 1996 Aug;64(2):190-6

Homocysteine metabolism and risk of myocardial infarction: relation with vitamins B6, B12, and folate. *Am J Epidemiol* 1996 May 1;143(9):845-59

Vitamin supplementation and other variables affecting serum homocysteine and methylmalonic acid concentrations in elderly men and women. *J Am Coll Nutr* 1996 Aug;15(4):364-76

Effectiveness of low-dose crystalline nicotinic acid in men with low high-density lipoprotein cholesterol levels. *Arch Intern Med* 1996 May 27;156(10):1081-8

Plasma homocysteine levels and mortality in patients with coronary artery disease. *N Engl J Med* 1997 Jul 24;337(4):230-6

Vitamin C deficiency and risk of myocardial infarction: prospective population study of men from eastern Finland. *BMJ* 1997 Mar 1;314(7081):634-8

Vitamin C status and blood pressure. *J Hypertens* 1996 Apr;14(4):503-8

Putaminal and thalamic hemorrhage in ethnic chinese living in Hong Kong. *Surg Neurol* Nov 1996, 46 (5) p441-5

Diet and heart disease. The role of fat, alcohol, and antioxidants. *Cardiol Clin* Feb 1996, 14 (1) p69-83,.777

[Effect of piracetam on inorganic phosphates and phospholipids in the blood of patients with cerebral infarction in the earliest period of the disease]. *Neurol Neurochir Pol* (Poland) Nov-Dec 1991, 25 (6)

Effect of piracetam on recovery and rehabilitation after stroke: A double- blind, placebo-controlled study. *Clin. Neuropharmacol.* (USA, 1994, 17/4 (320-331)

Ergoloids (Hydergine) and ischaemic strokes; Efficacy and mechanism of action. *Journal of International Medical Research* (UK), 1995, 23/3 (154-160)

Satellite symposium 'Piracetam and acute stroke : Pass' within the framework of the 3rd International Conference on stroke, 18-21 October 1995 in Prague satelliten-symposium 'Piracetam and acute stroke: Pass' im rahmen der 3. International Conference on stroke, 18.-21. Oktober 1995, Prag. *Nervenheilkunde* (Germany, 1996, 15/1

The nootropic agent piracetam in the treatment of acute stroke. Nootropika. Piracetam Beim Akuten Schlaganfall. *TW Neurologie Psychiatrie* (Germany, 1996, 10/1-2 (81)

Cerebroprotective effect of piracetam: The acute and chronic administrations of piracetam during short-term and long-term transient ischaemia. *Turkish Journal of Medical Sciences* (Turkey), 1995, 24/Suppl.(39)

Stroke (Thrombotic)

Coffee consumption in hypertensive men in older middle-age and the risk of stroke: the Honolulu Heart Program. *J Clin Epidemiol* (England) Jun 1998, 51 (6) p487-94

The white blood cell and plasma fibrinogen in thrombotic stroke. A significant correlation. *Int Angiol* (Italy) Jun 1998, 17 (2) p120-4

Elevated serum glycosaminoglycans with hypomagnesemia in patients with coronary artery disease & thrombotic stroke. *Indian J Med Res* (India) Mar 1995, 101 p115-9

Serum lipids and lipoprotein abnormalities in patients with thrombotic stroke—with exploring the protective role of HDL subfractions. *Proc Natl Sci Counc Repub China [B]* (Taiwan) Oct 1985, 9 (4) p298-304

Effect of piracetam on recovery and rehabilitation after stroke: a double-blind, placebo-controlled study. *Clin Neuropharmacol* 1994 Aug;17(4):320-31

The role of piracetam in the treatment of acute and chronic aphasia. *Pharmacopsychiatry* 1999 Mar;32 Suppl 1:38-43

The clinical safety of high-dose piracetam—its use in the treatment of acute stroke. De Reuck J., *Pharmacopsychiatry* 1999 Mar;32 Suppl 1:33-7

Neuroprotective therapy. *Semin Neurol* 1998;18(4):485-92

Acute treatment of stroke. PASS group. Piracetam Acute Stroke Study. *Lancet* 1998 Jul 25;352(9124):326

[Piracetam treatment in ischemic stroke]. *Neurol Neurochir Pol* 1997 Nov-Dec;31(6):1101-9

Treatment of acute ischemic stroke with piracetam. Members of the Piracetam in Acute Stroke Study (PASS) Group. *Stroke* 1997 Dec;28(12):2347-52

[Factors influencing the prescribing of nootropic drugs. Results of a representative inquiry in Lower Saxony]. *Dtsch Med Wochenschr* 1995 Nov 24;120(47):1614-9

tPA in acute ischemic stroke: United States experience and issues for the future. *Neurology* 1998 Sep;51(3 Suppl 3):S53-5

Secondary stroke prevention with low-dose aspirin, sustained release dipyridamole alone and in combination. *Thromb Res* 1998 Sep 15;92(1 Suppl 1):S1-6

Diminished production of malondialdehyde after carotid artery surgery as a result of vitamin administration. *Medical Science Research* (UK), 1996, 24/11 (777-780)

Spermine partially normalizes in vivo antioxidant defense potential in certain brain regions in transiently hypoperfused rat brain. *Neurochemical Research*, 1996, 21/12 (1497-1503)

Positron-labeled antioxidant 6-deoxy-6-(18F)fluoro-L-ascorbic acid: Increased uptake in transient global ischemic rat brain. *Nuclear Medicine and Biology*, 1996, 23/4 (479-486)

Stroke is an emergency. *Disease-a-Month*, 1996, 42/4 (202-264)

Antithrombotic agents in cerebral ischemia. *American Journal of Cardiology*, 1995, 75/6 (34B-38B)

Platelet activity and stroke severity. *J. Neurol. Sci.* (Netherlands), 1992, 108/1 (1-6)

The use of antithrombotic drugs in artery disease. *Clin. Haematol.* (UK), 1986, 15/2 (509-559)

Medical management in the endovascular treatment of carotid-cavernous aneurysms. *Journal of Neurosurgery*, 1996, 84/5 (755-761)

Mechanism of hydrogen peroxide and hydroxyl free radical-induced intracellular acidification in cultured rat cardiac myoblasts. *Circulation Research*, 1996, 78/4 (564-572)

Thrombolysis of the cervical internal carotid artery before balloon angioplasty and stent placement: Report of two cases. *Neurosurgery,* 1996, 38/3 (620-624)

Aspirin at any dose above 30 mg offers only modest protection after cerebral ischaemia. *Journal of Neurology Neurosurgery and Psychiatry* (UK), 1996, 6 0/2 (197-199)

Mild hyperhomocysteinemia and hemostatic factors in patients witharterial vascular diseases. *Thromb Haemost* (Germany) Mar 1997, 77 (3) p466-71

Vitamin E plus aspirin compared with aspirin alone in patients with transient ischemic attacks. *American Journal of Clinical Nutrition*, 1995, 62/6 Suppl.

Poor plasma status of carotene and vitamin C is associated with higher mortality from ischemic heart disease and stroke: Basel Prospective Study. *Clin. Invest.* (Germany), 1993, 71/1 (3-6)

The treatment of acute cerebral ischemia. Ginkgo: Free radical scavenger and PAF antagonist. *Therapiewoche* (Germany), 1994, 44/24 (1394-1396)

Efficiency of ginkgo biloba extract (EGb 761) in antioxidant protection against myocardial ischemia and reperfusion injury. *Biochemistry and Molecular Biology International* (Australia), 1995, 35/1 (125-134)

Magnesium content of erythrocytes in patients with vasospastic angina. *Cardiovasc. Drugs Ther.*, 1991, 5/4 (677-680)

Neuroprotective properties of Ginkgo biloba—Constituents. *Z. Phytother.* (Germany), 1994, 15/2 (92-96)

Variant angina due to deficiency of intracellular magnesium. *Clin. Cardiol.*, 1990, 13/9 (663-665)

Magnesium and sudden death. *S. Afr. Med. J.* (South Africa), 1983, 64/18 (697-698)

Magnesium deficiency produces spasms of coronary arteries: Relationship to etiology of sudden death ischemic heart disease. *Science*, 1980, 208/4440 (198-200)

Effect of vitamin E on hydrogen peroxide production by human vascular endothelial cells after hypoxia/reoxygenation. *Free Radical Biology and Medicine*, 1996, 20/1 (99-105)

On the mechanism of the anticlotting action of vitamin E quinone. *Proceedings of the National Academy of Sciences of the United States of America*, 1995, 92/18 (8171-8175)

Vitamin E may enhance the benefits of aspirin in preventing stroke. *American Family Physician*, 1995, 51/8 (1977

Antioxidant vitamins and disease—Risks of a suboptimal supply. *Ther. Umsch.* (Switzerland), 1994, 51/7 (467-474)

Vitamin E consumption and the risk of coronary disease in women. *New Engl. J. Med.*, 1993, 328/20 (1444-1449)

Increased risk of cardiovascular disease at suboptimal plasma concentrations of essential antioxidants: An epidemiological update with special attention to carotene and vitamin C. *Am. J. Clin. Nutr.*, 1993, 57/5 Suppl. (787S-797S)

Lipid peroxide, phospholipids, glutathione levels and superoxide dismutase activity in rat brain after ischaemia: Effect of ginkgo biloba extract. *Pharmacological Research* (UK), 1995, 32/5 (273-278)

Protection of hypoxia-induced ATP decrease in endothelial cells by ginkgo biloba extract and bilobalide. *Biochemical Pharmacology* (UK), 1995, 50/7 (991-999)

Lipid peroxidation in experimental spinal cord injury. Comparison of treatment with Ginkgo biloba, TRH and methylprednisolone. *Research in Experimental Medicine* (Germany), 1995, 195/2 (117-123)

Effects of natural antioxidant Ginkgo biloba extract (EGb 761) on myocardial ischemia-reperfusion injury. *Free Radic. Biol. Med.*, 1994, 16/6 (789-794)

Experimental model of cerebral ischemia. Preventive activity of Ginkgo biloba extract. *SEM. HOP.* (France), 1979, 55/43-44 (2047-2050)

On brain protection of co-dergocrine mesylate (Hydergine (R)) against hypoxic hypoxidosis of different severity: Double-blind placebo-controlled quantitative EEG and psychometric studies. *Int. J. Clin. Pharmacol. Ther. Toxicol.* (Germany, Federal Republic of), 1990, 28/12 (510-524)

Pharmacodynamics of the cerebral circulation. Effects of ten drugs on cerebral blood flow and metabolism in cerebrovascular insufficiency. *Path.Biol.* (Paris) (France), 1974, 22/9 (815-825)

Effects of ionic and nonionic contrast media on clot structure, platelet function and thrombolysis mediated by tissue plasminogen activator in plasma clots. *Haemostasis* (Switzerland), 1995, 25/4 (172-181)

Thrombolytic therapy: Recent advances. Treatment of myocardial infarction. *Appl. Cardiopulm. Pathophysiol.* (Netherlands), 1991/92, 4/3 (193-204)

Selective decrease in lysis of old thrombi after rapid administration of tissue-type plasminogen activator. *J. Am. Coll. Cardiol.*, 1989, 14/5 (1359-1364)

Antioxidant Curcuma extracts decrease the blood lipid peroxide levels of human subjects. *Age,* 1995, 18/4 (167-169)

Inhibition of tumor necrosis factor by curcumin, a phytochemical. *Biochemical Pharmacology* (UK), 1995, 49/11 (1551-1556)

Inhibitory effect of curcumin, an anti-inflammatory agent, on vascular smooth muscle cell proliferation. *Eur. J. Pharmacol.* (Netherlands), 1992, 221/2-3 (381-384)

Change of fatty acid composition, platelet aggregability and RBC function in elderly subjects with administration of low dose fish oil concentrate and comparison with those in younger subjects. *Jpn. J. Geriatr.* (Japan), 1994, 31/8 (596-603)

Premature Carotid Atherosclerosis: Does It Occur in Both Familial Hypercholesterolemia and Homocystinuria? Ultrasound Assessment of Arterial Intima-Media Thickness and Blood Flow Velocity. *Stroke*, May 1994;25(5):943-950.

Fibrinogen, Arterial Risk Factor in Clinical Practice. *Clinical Hemorrheology,* 1994;14(6):739-767

Fibrinogen and Cardiovascular Disorders. *Quarterly Journal of Medicine*, 1995;88:155-165.

Can Lowering Homocysteine Levels Reduce Cardiovascular Risk? *The New England Journal of Medicine*, February 2, 1995;332(5):328-329.

Fibrinogen, Arterial Risk Factor in Clinical Practice. *Clinical Hemorrheology,* 1994;14(6):739-767

The Lipoprotein(a). Significance and Relation to Atherosclerosis. *ACTA Clinica Belgica*, 1991;46(6):371-383.

Surgical Precautions

Refer to references under Anesthesia and Surgical Precautions.

Thrombosis

Homocysteine: update on a new risk factor. *Cleve Clin J Med* Nov-Dec 1997, 64 (10) p543-9

Total plasma antioxidant capacity predicts thrombosis-prone status in NIDDM patients. *Diabetes Care* Oct 1997, 20 (10) p1589-93

Effects of dietary fat quality and quantity on postprandial activation of blood coagulation factor VII. *Arterioscler Thromb Vasc Biol* Nov 1997, 17 (11) p2904-9

Hyperhomocysteinaemia in black patients with cerebral thrombosis. *QJM* (England) Oct 1997, 90 (10) p635-9

High antibody levels to prothrombin imply a risk of deep venous thrombosis and pulmonary embolism in middle-aged men--a nested case-control study. *Thromb Haemost* (Germany) Oct 1997, 78 (4) p1178-82

Plasminogen activator inhibitor-1, the acute phase response and vitamin C. *Atherosclerosis* (Ireland) Aug 1997, 133 (1) p71-6

Hyperhomocysteinemia and thrombosis: acquired conditions. *Thromb Haemost* (Germany) Jul 1997, 78 (1) p527-31

Hyperhomocysteinemia as a risk factor for arterial and venous disease. A review of evidence and relevance. *Thromb Haemost* (Germany) Jul 1997, 78 (1) p520-2

Homocysteine in Greenland Inuits. *Thromb Res* May 15 1997, 86 (4) p333-5

Homocysteine, oxidative stress, and vascular disease [see comments]. *Hosp Pract* (Off Ed) Jun 15 1997, 32 (6) p81-2, 85

Hyperhomocysteinemia and venous thromboembolic disease. *Haematologica* (Italy) Mar-Apr 1997, 82 (2) p211-9

Diet and haemostasis: time for nutrition science to get more involved. *Br J Nutr* (England) May 1997, 77 (5) p671-84

Homocyst(e)ine: an important risk factor for atherosclerotic vascular disease. *Curr Opin Lipidol* Feb 1997, 8 (1) p28-34

High plasma homocysteine: A risk factor for arterial and venous thrombosis in patients with normal coagulation profiles. *Clinical and Applied Thrombosis/Hemostasis*, 1997, 3/4 (239-244)

Influence of n-6 versus n-3 polyunsaturated fatty acids in diets low in saturated fatty acids on plasma lipoproteins and hemostatic factors. *Arteriosclerosis, Thrombosis, and Vascular Biology*, 1997, 17/12 (3449-3460)

Fatty acids, triglycerides and syndromes of insulin resistance. *Prostaglandins Leukotrienes and Essential Fatty Acids* (UK), 1997, 57/4-5 (379-385)

Hyperhomocysteinemia: A risk factor for arterial and venous thrombosis. *Annali Italiani di Medicina Interna* (Italy), 1997, 12/3 (160-165)

Dietary fatty acids and arteriosclerosis. *Biomedicine and Pharmacotherapy* (France), 1997, 51/8 (333-336)

Relation of plaque lipid composition and morphology to the stability of human aortic plaques. *Arteriosclerosis, Thrombosis, and Vascular Biology*, 1997, 17/7 (1337-1345)

Antioxidants and atherosclerotic heart disease. *New England Journal of Medicine*, 1997, 337/6 (408-416)

The effect of short-term diets rich in fish, red meat, or white meat on thromboxane and prostacyclin synthesis in humans. *Lipids*, 1997, 32/6 (635-644)

Purple grape juice has a significant platelet inhibitory effect. *American Family Physician*, 1997, 55/7 (2507-2508)

Dietary fatty acids in human thrombosis and hemostasis. *American Journal of Clinical Nutrition*, 1997, 65/5 Suppl. (1687S-1698S)

[How do we manage the hemorrhagic risk on hypovitaminosis K and treatments with antivitamin K]. *Ann Fr Anesth Reanim* (France) 1998, 17 Suppl 1 p14s-17s

A double-blind randomized comparison of combined aspirin and ticlopidine therapy versus aspirin or ticlopidine alone on experimental arterial thrombogenesis in humans. *Blood* Sep 1 1998, 92 (5) p1518-25

The use of aspirin in polycythaemia vera and primary thrombocythaemia. *Blood Rev* (Scotland) Mar 1998, 12 (1) p12-22

Thrombosis and coronary disease: neutrophils, nitric oxide and aspirin. *Rev Esp Cardiol* (Spain) Mar 1998, 51 (3) p171-7

Prophylaxis for deep vein thrombosis with aspirin or low molecular weight dextran in Korean patients undergoing total hip replacement. A randomized controlled trial. *Int Orthop* (Germany) 1998, 22 (1) p6-10

Effect of supplementation with different doses of DHA on the levels of circulating DHA as non-esterified fatty acid in subjects of Asian Indian background. *J Lipid Res* Feb 1998, 39 (2) p286-92

Hyperhomocysteinemia and venous thrombosis: A meta-analysis. *Thrombosis and Haemostasis* (Germany), 1998, 80/6 (874-877)

Effect of breakfast fat content on glucose tolerance and risk factors of atherosclerosis and thrombosis. *British Journal of Nutrition* (UK), 1998, 80/4 (323-331)

High prevalence of hyperhomocysteinemia in patients with inflammatory bowel disease: A pathogenic link with thromboembolic complications? *Thrombosis and Haemostasis* (Germany), 1998, 80/4 (542-545)

Health aspects of fish and n-3 polyunsaturated fatty acids from plant and marine origin. *European Journal of Clinical Nutrition* (UK), 1998, 52/10 (749-753)

Functional food science and the cardiovascular system. *British Journal of Nutrition* (UK), 1998, 80/Suppl. 1

Vitamin supplementation reduces blood homocysteine levels: A controlled trial in patients with venous thrombosis and healthy volunteers. *Arteriosclerosis, Thrombosis, and Vascular Biology,* 1998, 18/3 (356-361)

Homocysteine and vascular diseases. *Hematologie* (France), 1998, 4/1 (7-16)

Coffee consumption in hypertensive men in older middle-age and the risk of stroke: the Honolulu Heart Program. *J Clin Epidemiol* (England) Jun 1998, 51 (6) p487-94

Lipids and stroke: Neglect of a useful preventive measure? *Cardiovascular Research* (Netherlands), 1998, 40/2 (265-271)

Thyroid Deficiency

The thyroid, magnesium and calcium in major depression. *Biol Psychiatry.* 1996 Sep 1;40(5):428-9.

Vitamin E and coenzyme Q concentrations in the thyroid tissues of patients with various thyroid disorders. *Am J Med Sci* 1998 Apr;315(4):230-2

[A simple health control for the elderly. Screening for vitamin B12 deficiency and thyroid disease]. *Lakartidningen* 1997 Nov 19;94(47):4329-32

Selected micronutrient intake and thyroid carcinoma risk. *Cancer* 1997 Jun 1;79(11):2186-92

Regelson William, Colman Carol, *The Superhormone Promise,* Simon& Schuster 1996, pp(190-202).

Induction of manganese superoxide dismutase by thyroid stimulating hormone in rat thyroid cells. *FEBS Lett*, 416(1):69-71 1997 Oct 13

The effect of manganese supply on thyroid hormone metabolism in the offspring of manganese-depleted dams. *Biol Trace Elem Res*, 55(1-2):137-45 1996 Oct-Nov

Forskolin stimulation of adenylate cyclase in human thyroid membranes. *Acta Endocrinol* (Copenh) 1985 Feb;108(2):200-5

The influence of dietary vitamin A on triiodothyronine, retinoic acid, and glucocorticoid receptors in liver of hypothyroid rats. *Br J Nutr* 1996 Aug;76(2):295-306

Sodium selenite therapy and thyroid-hormone status in cystic fibrosis and congenital hypothyroidism. *Biol Trace Elem Res* 1994 Mar;40(3):247-53

[Effects of the combined deficiency of selenium and iodine on thyroid function]. *Ann Ist Super Sanita* 1998;34(3):349-55

Influence of zinc and selenium deficiency on parameters relating to thyroid hormone metabolism. *Horm Metab Res* 1996 May;28(5):223-6

Low selenium status in the elderly influences thyroid hormones. *Clin Sci* (Colch) 1995 Dec;89(6):637-42

[Changes in the thyroid gland of the rat after increasing the amount of manganese in its food]. *Gig Sanit* 1969 Jan;34(1):113-4

Cyclic AMP-stimulated protein kinase prepared from bovine thyroid glands. *Metabolism* 1972 Feb;21(2):150-8

Protein tyrosine phosphorylation influences adhesive junction assembly and follicular organization of cultured thyroid epithelial cells. *Endocrinology,* 1997, 138/6 (2315-2324)

An extract of soy flour influences serum cholesterol and thyroid hormones in rats and hamsters. *Journal of Nutrition,* 1996, 126/12 (3046-3053)

Identification of hormonogenic tyrosines in fragment 1218-1591 of bovine thyroglobulin by mass spectrometry. Hormonogenic acceptor Tyr-1291 and donor Tyr-1375. *Journal of Biological Chemistry,* 1997, 272/1 (639-646)

Selectivity in tyrosyl iodination sites in human thyroglobulin. *Archives of Biochemistry and Biophysics,* 1996, 334/2 (284-294)

Soy protein concentrate and isolated soy protein similarly lower blood serum cholesterol but differently affect thyroid hormones in hamsters. *Journal of Nutrition,* 1996, 126/8 (2007-2011)

Involvement of tyrosine phosphorylation in the regulation of 5'-deiodinases in FRTL-5 rat thyroid cells and rat astrocytes. *Endocrinology,* 1996, 137/4 (1313-1318)

Characterization of a melanosomal transport system in murine melanocytes mediating entry of the melanogenic substrate tyrosine. *Journal of Biological Chemistry,* 1996, 271/8 (4002-4008)

Influence of the thyroid hormone status on tyrosine hydroxylase in central and peripheral catecholaminergic structures. *Neurochemistry International* (UK), 1996, 28/3 (277-281)

Soy protein, thyroid regulation and cholesterol metabolism. *Journal of Nutrition,* 1995, 125/3 Suppl. (619S-623S)

Comparative pharmacology of the thyroid hormones. *Ann. Thorac. Surg.,* 1993, 56/1 Suppl. (S2-S8)

Primary hypothyroidism in an adult patient with protein-calorie malnutrition: A study of its mechanism and the effect of amino acid deficiency. *Metab. Clin. Exp.,* 1988, 37/1 (9-14)

Preferential formation of triiodothyronine residues in newly synthesized (14C)tyrosine-labeled thyroglobulin molecules in follicles reconstructed in a suspension culture of hog thyroid cells. *Mol. Cell. Endocrinol.* (Ireland), 1988, 59/1-2 (117-124)

Importance of the content and localization of tyrosine residues for thyroxine formation within the N-terminal part of human thyroglobulin den. *European Journal of Endocrinology* (Norway), 1995, 132/5 (611-617)

Melatonin and the endocrine role of the pineal organ. Argentina *Curr. Topics Exp. Endocrin.,* 1974, Vol. 2 (107-128)

Brief report: Circadian melatonin, thyroid-stimulating hormone, prolactin, and cortisol levels in serum of young adults with autism. *Israel Journal of Autism and Developmental Disorders,* 1995, 25/6 (641-654)

Effects of melatonin and thyroxine replacement on thyrotropin, luteinizing hormone, and prolactin in male hypothyroid hamsters. *Endocrinology,* 1985, 117/6 (2402-2407)

Influence of phytogenic substances with thyreostatic effects in combination with iodine on the thyroid hormones and somatomedin level in pigs. *Exp. Clin. Endocrinol.* (Germany, East), 1985, 85/2 (183-190)

Tinnitus

The use of Ginkgo Biloba extract associated with magnesium and arginyne in patients with tinnitus of a vascular origin. *Riv-*

ista Italiana di Otorinolaringologia Audiologia e Foniatria (Italy), 1998, 18/1 (37-39)

Clinical improvement of memory and other cognitive functions by Ginkgo biloba: Review of relevant literature. *Advances in Therapy,* 1998, 15/1 (54-65)

Effect of traditional Chinese acupuncture on severe tinnitus: a double-blind, placebo-controlled, clinical investigation with open therapeutic control. *Br J Audiol* (England) Jun 1998, 32 (3) p197-204

Effect of melatonin on tinnitus. *Laryngoscope* Mar 1998, 108 (3) p305-10

Physiology, pathophysiology, and anthropology/epidemiology of human earcanal secretions. *J Am Acad Audiol* (Canada) Dec 1997, 8 (6) p391-400

Attenuation of salicylate-induced tinnitus by Ginkgo biloba extract in rats. *Audiology and Neuro-Otology* (Germany), 1997, 2/4 (197-212)

Tinnitus rehabilitation in sensorineural hearing loss. Based on 400 patients. *Otorinolaringologia* (Italy), 1994, 44/5 (227-229)

The value of rheological, vasoactive and metabolically active substances in the initial treatment of acute acoustic trauma. *HNO* (Germany, West), 1986, 34/10 (424-428)

Trental and Cavinton in the therapy of cochleovestibular disorders. *Cesk. Otolaryngol.* (Czechoslovakia), 1984, 33/4 (264-267)

Prospects of using Cavinton in Meniere's disease. *Vestn. Otorinolaringol.* (USSR), 1980, 42/3 (18-22)

Results of combined low-power laser therapy and extracts of Ginkgo biloba in cases of sensorineural hearing loss and tinnitus. In: *Adv Otorhinolaryngol* (1995) 49:101-4

[Hydergine in pathology of the inner ear] Hydergina en patologia del oido interno. *An Otorrinolaringol Ibero Am* (1990) 17(1):85-98 (Published in Spanish)

Trauma

Metabolic and immune effects of dietary arginine, glutamine and omega-3 fatty acids supplementation in immunocompromised patients. *J Med Assoc Thai* (Thailand) May 1998, 81 (5) p334-43

Changes in the plasma concentrations of retinol, alpha-tocopherole and beta-carotene in polytraumatized patients and in patients with osteitis in dependence on the outcome of injury. *Zentralblatt fur Chirurgie* (Germany), 1998, 123/11 (1277-1283)

Aphthous ulcers and vitamin B12 deficiency. *Netherlands Journal of Medicine,* 1998, 53/4 (172-175)

Essential fatty acids predict metabolites of serotonin and dopamine in cerebrospinal fluid among healthy control subjects, and early- and late-onset alcoholics. *Biological Psychiatry,* 1998, 44/4 (235-242)

Treatment of hyperpathia/allodinia in CRPS, earlier called RSDS, a metabolic approach. *Pain Clinic,* 1998, 10/4 (261-274)

Influence of arginine, omega-3 fatty acids and nucleotide-supplemented enteral support on systemic inflammatory resp. syndrome and multiple organ failure in patients after severe trauma. *Nutrition,* 1998, 14/2 (165-172)

Impact of supplemented enteral nutrition in patients with multiple trauma. *Unfallchirurg* (Germany), 1998, 101/2 (105-114)

Diets and infection: Composition and consequences. *World Journal of Surgery* (United States), 1998, 22/2 (209-212)

[Nutritional support for the large burn patient]. *Nutr Hosp* (Spain) May-Jun 1997, 12 (3) p121-33

Effects of intravenously infused fish oil on platelet fatty acid phospholipid composition and on platelet function in postoperative trauma. *J Parenter Enteral Nutr* Sep-Oct 1997, 21 (5) p296-301

The effect of nutritional support on the perioperative course in patients after extensive surgical procedures. *Wiad Lek* (Poland) 1997, 50 Su 1 Pt 2 p447-51

Vitamins Q and E, extracorporal circulation and hemolysis. *Mol Cell Biochem* (Netherlands) Aug 1997, 173 (1-2) p33-41

Metabolic response to injury and sepsis: changes in protein metabolism. *Nutrition* Sep 1997, 13 (9 Suppl) p52S-57S

Carotenoids and antioxidant vitamins in patients after burn injury. *J Burn Care Rehabil* May-Jun 1997, 18 (3) p269-78; discussion 268

The role of IGFs in catabolism. *Bailliere's Clinical Endocrinology and Metabolism* (UK), 1997, 11/4 (679-697)

Antioxidant defense of the brain: A role for astrocytes. *Canadian Journal of Physiology and Pharmacology* (Canada), 1997, 75/10-11 (1149-1163)

Parenteral nutritional treatment. *Anaesthesist* (Germany), 1997, 46/5 (371-384)

Influence of large intakes of trace elements on recovery after major burns. *Nutrition* (United States) 1994, 10/4 (327-334+352)

Proline metabolism in adult male burned patients and healthy control subjects. *American Journal of Clinical Nutrition* 1991, 54/2 (408-413)

Magnesium- deficiency syndrome in burns. *Lancet* (England) Nov 30 1968, 2 (7579) p1156-8

Reversal of postburn immunosuppression by the administration of vitamin A. *Surgery* 1984, 96/2 (330-335)

Serum carotene, vitamin A, retinol-binding protein and lipoproteins before and after jejunoileal bypass surgery. *Int J Obes* (England) 1982, 6 (5) p491-7

Bypass phrynoderma. Vitamin A deficiency associated with bowel-bypass surgery. *Arch Dermatol* Jul 1984, 120 (7) p919-21

Effect of dietary vitamin C on compression injury of the spinal cord in a rat mutant unable to synthesize ascorbic acid and its correlation with that of vitamin E. Japan *Spinal Cord* (UK), 1996, 34/4 (234- 238)

Effect of allopurinol, sulphasalazine, and vitamin C on aspirin induced gastroduodenal injury in human volunteers. *United Kingdom Gut* (UK), 1996, 38/4 (518-524

Hemodynamic effects of delayed initiation of antioxidant therapy (beginning two hours after burn) in extensive third-degree burns. *Journal of Burn Care and Rehabilitation,* 1995, 16/6 (610-615)

Dietary intake and plasma levels of antioxidant vitamins in health and disease: A hospital-based case-control study. *Journal of Nutritional and Environmental Medicine* (UK), 1995, 5/3

Vitamin C and pressure sores. *Journal of Dermatological Treatment* (UK), 1995, 6/3

Supplementation with vitamins C and E suppresses leukocyte oxygen free radical production in patients with myocardial infarction. *European Heart Journal* (UK), 1995, 16/8 (1044-1049)

Antioxidant therapy using high dose vitamin C: Reduction of postburn resuscitation fluid volume requirements. *World Journal of Surgery,* 1995, 19/2 (287-291)

Vitamin C reduces ischemia-reperfusion injury in a rat epigastric island skin flap model. *Ann. Plast. Surg.*, 1994, 33/6 (620-623)

An experimental study on the protection against reperfusion myocardial ischemia by using large doses of vitamin C. *Chin. J. Cardiol.* (China), 1994, 22/1 (52-54+80)

Vitamins as radioprotectors in vivo. I. Protection by vitamin C against internal radionuclides in mouse testes: Implications to the mechanism of damage caused by the auger effect. *USA Radiat. Res.*, 1994, 137/3 (394-399)

Experimental studies on the treatment of frostbite in rats. *Indian J. Med. Res. Sect. B Biomed. Res. Other Than Infect. Dis.* (India), 1993, 98/AUG. (178-184)

The effects of high-dose vitamin C therapy on postburn lipid peroxidation. *USA J. Burn Care Rehabil.*, 1993, 14/6 (624- 629)

Effect of antioxidant vitamin supplementation on muscle function after eccentric exercise. *Eur. J. Appl. Physiol. Occup. Physiol.* (Germany), 1993, 67/5 (426-430)

Vitamin C as a radioprotector against iodine-131 in vivo. *J. Nucl. Med.*, 1993, 34/4 (637-640)

Effects of high-dose vitamin C administration on postburn microvascular fluid and protein flux. *Rehabil.*, 1992, 13/5 (560-566)

Modification of the daily photoreceptor membrane shedding response in vitro by antioxidants. *Invest. Ophthalmol. Visual Sci.*, 1992, 33/10 (3005-3008)

Ascorbate treatment prevents accumulation of phagosomes in RPE in light damage. *Invest. Ophthalmol. Visual Sci.*, 1992, 33/10 (2814-2821)

Topical vitamin C protects porcine skin from ultraviolet radiation-induced damage. *Br. J. Dermatol.* (UK), 1992, 127/3 (247-253)

The synergism of gamma-interferon and tumor necrosis factor in whole body hyperthermia with vitamin C to control toxicity. *Med. Hypotheses* (UK), 1992, 38/3 (257- 258)

Tirilazad mesylate protects vitamins C and E in brain ischemia- reperfusion injury. *J. Neurochem.*, 1992, 58/6 (2263-2268)

Vitamin C supplementation in the patient with burns and renal failure. *J. Burn Care Rehabil.*, 1992, 13/3 (378-380)

High-dose vitamin C therapy for extensive deep dermal burns. *USA Burns* (UK), 1992, 18/2 (127-131)

Metabolic and immune effects of enteral ascorbic acid after burn trauma. *Burns* (UK), 1992, 18/2 (92-97)

Reduced fluid volume requirement for resuscitation of third-degree burns with high-dose vitamin C. *J. Burn Care Rehabil.*, 1991, 12/6 (525-532)

Biochemical basis of ozone toxicity. *Free Radic. Biol. Med.*, 1990, 9/3 (245-265)

Decreases in tissue levels of ubiquinol-9 and -10, ascorbate and alpha-tocopherol following spinal cord impact trauma in rats. *USA Neurosci. Lett.* (Netherlands), 1990, 108/1-2 (201-206)

Nutritional considerations for the burned patient. *Surg. Clin. North Am.*, 1987, 67/1 (109-131)

Ascorbic acid metabolism in trauma. *Indian J. Med. Res.* (India), 1982, 75/5 (748-751)

Multiple pathologic fractures in osteogenesis imperfecta. *Orthopade* (Germany, West), 1982, 11/3 (101-108)

Effect of zinc supplementation in fracture healing. *Indian J. Orthop.* (India), 1980, 14/1 (62-71)

Treatment results of spinal cord injuries in the Swiss paraplegic centre of Basle. *Paraplegia* (Edinb.) (Scotland), 1976, 14/1 (58-65)

Effect of piracetam on electroshock induced amnesia and decrease in brain acetylcholine in rats. *Indian J. Exp. Biol.* (India), 1993, 31/10 (822-824)

Use of piracetam in treatment of head injuries. Observations in 903 cases. *Clin. Ter.* (Italy), 1985, 114/6 (481-487)

Urinary Tract Infections

History, clinical findings, sexual behavior and hygiene habits in women with and without recurrent episodes of urinary symptoms. *Acta Obstet Gynecol Scand* (Denmark) Jul 1998, 77 (6) p654-9

Acupuncture in the prophylaxis of recurrent lower urinary tract infection in adult women. *Scand J Prim Health Care* (Norway) Mar 1998, 16 (1) p37-9

[Can acupuncture prevent cystitis in women?]. *Tidsskr Nor Laegeforen* (Norway) Mar 30 1998, 118 (9) p1370-2

Urinary tract infections in children: Why they occur and how to prevent them. *American Family Physician*, 1998, 57/10 (2440-2446)

Urogenital aging—A hidden problem. *American Journal of Obstetrics and Gynecology,* 1998, 178/5 (S245-S249)

Herbal urinary antiseptics—Still up-to-date? *Zeitschrift fur Phytotherapie* (Germany), 1998, 19/2 (90-95)

Effect of cranberry juice on urinary pH in older adults. *Home Health Nurse* Mar 1997, 15 (3) p198-202

Cranberry juice and its impact on peri-stomal skin conditions for urostomy patients. *Ostomy Wound Manage* Nov-Dec 1994, 40 (9) p60-2, 64, 66-8

Infection control. The therapeutic uses of cranberry juice. *Nurs Stand* (England) May 17-23 1995, 9 (34) p33-5

Urinary problems after formation of a Mitrofanoff stoma. *Prof Nurse* (England) Jan 1995, 10 (4) p221-4

New support for a folk remedy: cranberry juice reduces bacteriuria and pyuria in elderly women. *Nutr Rev* May 1994, 52 (5) p168-70

An examination of the anti-adherence activity of cranberry juice on urinary and nonurinary bacterial isolates. *Microbios* (England) 1988, 55 (224-225) p173-81

Inhibitory activity of cranberry juice on adherence of type 1 and type P fimbriated Escherichia coli to eucaryotic cells. *Antimicrob Agents Chemother* Jan 1989, 33 (1) p92-8

Inhibition of bacterial adherence by cranberry juice: potential use for the treatment of urinary tract infections. *J Urol* May 1984, 131 (5) p1013-6

Knight-Ridder Info. Effect of cranberry juice on urinary pH. *Nurs Res* Sep-Oct 1979, 28 (5) p287-90

First-time urinary tract infection and sexual behavior. *Epidemiology* Mar 1995, 6 (2) p162-8

Anti-Escherichia coli adhesin activity of cranberry and blueberry juices [letter]. *N Engl J Med* (1991 May 30) 324(22):1599

Effect of cranberry juice on urinary pH. *Nurs Res* (1979 Sep-Oct) 28(5):287-90

Bladder Conditions

Unconventional treatment of superficial bladder carcinoma. *Urologe Ausg. A*, 1994, 33/6 (553-556)

Relative importance of risk factors in bladder carcinogenesis: Some new results about Mediterranean habits. *Cancer Causes Control*, 1994, 5/4 (326-332)

Megadose vitamins in bladder cancer: A double-blind clinical trial. *J. Urol.*, 1994, 151/1 (21-26)

Carcinogen-induced tissue vitamin A depletion: Potential protective advantages of beta-carotene. *Ann. New York Acad. Sci.*, 1993, 686/- (203-212)

Vitamin A, beta-carotene, and the risk of cancer: A prospective study *J. Natl. Cancer Inst.*, 1987, 79/3 (443-448)

The current role of vitamines (A, E, C, D), folates and selenium in the chemical prevention and treatment of malignant tumours. *Minerva Med.*, 1987, 78/6 (377-386)

Serum vitamin levels and the risk of cancer of specific sites in men of Japanese ancestry in Hawaii. *Cancer Res.*, 1985, 45/5 (2369-2372)

Vitamin A levels in human bladder cancer. *Int. J. Cancer,* 1982, 30/2 (143-145)

Vitamin A and retinol-binding protein in patients with myelomatosis and cancer of epithelial origin. *Eur. J. Cancer Clin. Oncol.*, 1982, 18/4 (339-342)

A study on the etiological factors of bilharzial bladder cancer in Egypt: IV. beta-carotene and vitamin A level in serum. *Tumori*, 1982, 68/1 (19-22)

Diet and cancer of the esophagus. *Nutr. Cancer,* 1981, 2/3 (143-147)

Herbal urinary antiseptics—Still up-to-date? *Zeitschrift fur Phytotherapie*, 1998, 19/2 (90-95)

Risk factors for bladder cancer: a case-control study in northeast. *Eur J Cancer Prev* Aug 1997, 6 (4) p363-9

Carbogen and nicotinamide in the treatment of bladder cancer with radical radiotherapy. *Br J Cancer* 1997 , 76 (2) p260-3

Valvular Insufficiency/Heart Valve Defects

[Doppler echocardiography of heart valve defects in the dog]. *Tierarztl Prax* (Germany) Apr 1996, 24 (2) p177-89

Also, refer to references under Congestive Heart Failure/Cardiomyopathy

Vertigo

Multicenter study with standardized extract of Ginko-Biloba EGB 761 in the treatment of memory alteration, vertigo and tinnitus. *Investigacion Medica Internacional* (Mexico) 1997, 24/2 (31-39)

[Hydergine in pathology of the inner ear]. *An Otorrinolaringol Ibero Am* 1990;17(1):85-98

Dimethyl sulfoxide therapy in subjective tinnitus of unknown origin. *Ann N Y Acad Sci* 1975 Jan 27;243:468-74

The effectiveness of piracetam in vertigo. *Pharmacopsychiatry* 1999 Mar;32 Suppl 1:54-60

The treatment of minocycline-induced brainstem vertigo by the combined administration of piracetam and ergotoxin. *Acta Otolaryngol Suppl* (Stockh) 1989;468:171-4

[Clinical trial of the use of the combination of piracetam and dihydroergocristine in vertigo from different causes]. *An Otorrinolaringol Ibero Am* 1989;16(3):271-9

The use of piracetam in vertigo. *S Afr Med J* 1985 Nov 23;68(11):806-8

Piracetam in the treatment of post-concussional syndrome. A double-blind study. *Eur Neurol* 1978;17(1):50-5

How to use cerebral vasodilators and metabolic activators. *Tokai Journal of Experimental and Clinical Medicine* (Tokai J. Exp. Clin. Med.) (Japan) 1998, 23/4 (187-192)

Beneficial effect of vinpocetine on cerebral blood flow, measured with ^{123}I-IMP SPECT, and clinical symptoms in patients with chronic cerebral infarction. *Japanese Pharmacology and Therapeutics* (Jpn. Pharmacol. Ther.) (Japan) 1997, 25/12 (81-88)

Nootropics: Pharmacological properties and therapeutic use. *Polish Journal of Pharmacology* (Pol. J. Pharmacol.) (Poland) 1994, 46/5 (383-394)

Clinical analysis of Vinpocetine (Calan(R) Tablet) on dizziness. Vertebral blood flow volume and clinical effect. *Equilibrium Research* (Japan) 1987, 46/4 (387-393)

Clinical study of vinpocetine in the treatment of vertigo. *Japanese Pharmacology and Therapeutics* (Japan) 1986, 14/2 (577-589)

Prospects of using Cavinton in Meniere's disease. *Vestnik Oto-Rino-Laringologii* (Russia) 1980, 42/3 (18-22)

Cavinton and Lucidril in the treatment of auditory damage of various origins. *Therapia Hungarica* (Hungary) 1979, 27/1 (28-30)

Mental decline in the elderly: pharmacotherapy (ergot alkaloids versus papaverine). *J Am Geriatr Soc* Apr 1975, 23 (4) p169

A clinical trial comparing 'Hydergine' with placebo in the treatment of cerebrovascular insufficiency in elderly patients. *Curr Med Res Opin* (England) 1973, 1 (8) p463-8.

[Effect of hydergine on the functional manifestations of encephalic vasomotricity]. *Lyon Med* (France) Jun 13 1971, 225 (11) p1177-82.

Hydergine in inner ear pathology. *Anales Otorrinolaringologicos Ibero-Americanos* (Spain) 1990, 17/1 (85-98)

The nootropic concept and its prospective implications. *Drug Development Research* 1982, 2/5 (441-446)

Double-blind study of the clinical efficacy of hydergin administered by two schedules: 1 x 4.5 mg and 3 x 1.5 mg per day. *Revue Medicale de la Suisse Romande* (Switzerland) 1981, 101/2 (157-163)

Relieving select symptoms of the elderly. *Geriatrics* (1975, 30/3 (133-142)

Dihydroergotoxin (Hydergine) in the treatment of cerebral circulatory disorders, including arteriosclerosis. *Praxis* 1974, 63/21 (660-665)

Dihydroergotoxine ('hydergine') in the treatment of the symptoms of cerebrovascular insufficiency. *Noro-Psikiyat.Ars.* 1973, 10/2 (117-123)

Our experience from the treatment of vestibular cochlear symptoms due to schemia with piracetam.International Congress Series; Vertigo, nausea, tinnitus and hearing loss in central and peripheral vestibular diseases. *International Congress Series* (1087):p189-192 1995

Efficacy of aniracetam in the treatment of labyrinthine disorders. *Adv Ther* 3 (4). 1986. 185-192.

[Hemorheologic therapy of asystematic vertigo]. *Vasa Suppl* (Switzerland) 1991, 33 p169-70

[Evaluation of the therapeutic effectiveness of a piracetam plus dihydroergocristine combination in the treatment of vertigo]. *Acta Otorrinolaringol Esp* (Spain) Jul-Aug 1988, 39 (4) p287-8.

[Treatment of vertigo syndrome with Nootropil]. *Otolaryngol Pol* (Poland) 1988, 42 (5) p312-7.

The efficacy of piracetam in vertigo. A double-blind study in patients with vertigo of central origin. *Arzneimittelforschung* (Germany, West) 1980, 30 (11) p1947-9.

The balancing outcome of a pharmacological treatment by vertiginous patients. *Anales Otorrinolaringologicos Ibero-Americanos* (Spain) 1999, 26/3 (271-291)

Dizziness and dizzy feeling in the elderly: Treatment. *Revue de Geriatrie* (France) 1997, 22/7 (457-462)

Disabling acute vertigo attack. *Revista Brasileira de Otorrinolaringologia* (Brazil) 1994, 60/4 (326)

Vertigo. *Revista Brasileira de Medicina* (Brazil) 1993/1994, 50/Spec. Iss. Dec. (193-202)

Hemorheologic therapy of vertigo. *Vasa—Journal of Vascular Diseases* (Switzerland) 1991, 20/Suppl. 33 (169-170)

Vertigo, dysarthria and hemiparesis in a 71 year-old woman. *Revue Neurologique* (France) 1991, 147/11 (752-758)

Drugs for dizziniess; exploitation of medical incapability. *Nederlands Tijdschrift voor Geneeskunde* (Netherlands) 1991, 135/14 (599-603)

Vertigo syndrome treatment by nootropil. *Otolaryngologia Polska* (Poland) 1988, 42/5 (312-317)

Clinic assay on the assocation piracetam and dihydroergocristine in vertigo of several etiologies. *Anales Otorrinolaringologicos Ibero-Americanos* (Spain) 1989, 16/3 (271-279)

Treatment of vertigo with piracetam: Comparison with placebo in 50 cases. *Gazette Medicale* (France) 1986, 93/28 (67-70)

Current concepts in management. *Drugs* (Australia) 1985, 30/3 (275-283)

Thc cffcct of piracctam (Nootropil, UCB 6215) upon thc latc symptoms of patients with head injuries. *Journal of International Medical Research* 1975, 3/5 (352-355).

Piracetam in patients with chronic vertigo. Results of a double-blind,placebo-controlled study. *Clinical Drug Investigation* (New Zealand), 1996, 11/5 (251-260)

Nootropics: Efficacy and tolerability of products from three active substance classes. *Journal of Drug Development and Clinical Practice* (UK), 1996, 8/2 (77-94)

The effect of ginkgo biloba glycoside on the blood viscosity and erythrocyte deformability. *Clinical Hemorheology*, 1996, 16/3 (271-276)

[Clinical trial of the use of the combination of piracetam and dihydroergocristine in vertigo from different causes]. *An Otorrinolaringol Ibero Am* (Spain) 1989, 16 (3)

Treatment of vertigo syndrome with Nootropil]. *Otolaryngol Pol* (Poland) 1988, 42 (5) p312-7

The use of piracetam in vertigo. *S Afr Med J* (South Africa) Nov 23 1985, 68 (11) p806-8

Piracetam in the treatment of post-concussional syndrome. A double-blind study. *Eur Neurol* (Switzerland) 1978, 17 (1) p50-5

[The elimination of chemotherapy side effects in pulmonary tuberculosis patients]. *Vrach Delo* (USSR) Apr 1990, (4) p71-3

The treatment of minocycline-induced brainstem vertigo by the combined administration of piracetam and ergotoxin. *Acta Otolaryngol Suppl* (Stockh) (Sweden) 1989, 468

[Clinical trial of the use of the combination of piracetam and dihydroergocristine in vertigo from different causes]. *An Otorrinolaringol Ibero Am* (Spain) 1989, 16 (3)

Viral Meningitis

Herpes simplex virus infection as a cause of benign recurrent lymphocytic meningitis. *Ann Intern Med* 1994 Sep 1;121(5): 334-8

Herpes simplex virus type 2: unique biological properties include neoplastic potential mediated by the PK domain of the large subunit of ribonucleotide reductase. *Front Biosci* 1998 Feb 15;3:D237-49

Benign recurrent aseptic meningitis (Mollaret's meningitis): case report and clinical review. *Arch Neurol* 1979 Oct;36(10):657-8

Twenty-eight years of benign recurring Mollaret meningitis. *Arch Neurol* 1983 Jan;40(1):42-3

Mollaret's meningitis associated with acute Epstein-Barr virus mononucleosis. *Arch Neurol* 1987 Nov;44(11):1204-5

Mollaret's meningitis. A variant of recurrent hereditary polyserositis, both provoked by metaraminol. *Arch Neurol* 1988 Aug;45(8):926-7

Mollaret's meningitis and differential diagnosis of recurrent meningitis. Report of case, with review of the literature. *Am J Med* 1972 Jan;52(1):128-40

Recurrent aseptic meningitis secondary to intracranial epidermoid cyst and Mollaret's meningitis: two distinct entities or a single disease? A case report and a nosologic discussion. *Am J Med* 1990 Dec;89(6):807-10

Central nervous system epidermoid cyst: a probable etiology of Mollaret's meningitis. *Am J Med* 1990 Dec;89(6):805-6

Mollaret meningitis: report of a case with recovery after colchicine. *Ann Neurol* 1980 Dec;8(6):631-3

Isolation of herpes simplex virus type 1 in recurrent (Mollaret's) meningitis. *Trans Am Neurol Assoc* 1981;106:37-42

Mollaret's meningitis: a case with increased circulating natural killer cells. *Ann Neurol* 1986 Sep;20(3):359-61

Herpes simplex virus type 1 DNA in cerebrospinal fluid of a patient with Mollaret's meningitis. *N Engl J Med* 1991 Oct 10;325(15):1082-5

Recurrent aseptic meningitis secondary to intracranial epidermoids. *Can J Neurol Sci* 1984 Aug;11(3):387-9

Mollaret's meningitis: a case report and literature review. *Chung Hua I Hsueh Tsa Chih* (Taipei) 1992 Apr;49(4):289-93

Mollaret's meningitis: an unusual disease with a characteristic presentation. *Am J Med Sci* 1984 Jan-Feb;287(1):52-3

Mollaret's meningitis: CSF-immunocytological examinations. *J Neurol* 1987 Feb;234(2):103-6

Failure of colchicine in the treatment of Mollaret's meningitis. *Arch Intern Med* 1984 Nov;144(11):2265-6

Mollaret's meningitis responding to phenylbutazonum. A case report. *Clin Neurol Neurosurg* 1985;87(2):127-30

Mollaret's meningitis revisited. Report of a case with a review of the literature. *Clin Neurol Neurosurg* 1988;90(2):163-7

Benign aseptic (Mollaret's) meningitis after genital herpes. *Lancet* 1991 Jun 1;337(8753):1360-1

Benign recurrent aseptic meningitis (Mollaret's meningitis). A case report. *S Afr Med* J 1983 May 7;63(19):741-2

Mollaret's meningitis: Differential diagnosis and diagnostic pitfalls. *Neurology* 1962; 12: 745-753

Bacterial meningitis—A review of selected aspects : 1. General clinical features, special problems and unusual meningeal reactions mimicking bacterial meningitis. *[No Journal Listed]* 1965; 272: 842-848.

Weight Loss

See references under Obesity.

Wound Healing (Surgical Wounds, Trauma, Burns)

Role of pantothenic and ascorbic acid in wound healing processes: in vitro study on fibroblasts. *Int J Vitam Nutr Res* 1988;58(4):407-13

Nutrition and the immune response—a review. *Int J Vitam Nutr Res* 1979;49(2):220-8

Effects of pantothenic acid on fibroblastic cell cultures. *Res Exp Med* (Berl) 1988;188(5):391-6

Effect of pantothenic acid and ascorbic acid supplementation on human skin wound healing process. A double-blind, prospective and randomized trial. *Eur Surg Res* 1995;27(3):158-66

In vitro effect of ascorbic acid on the proliferation of bovine scleral and Tenon's capsule fibroblasts. *Eur J Ophthalmol* 1998 Jan-Mar;8(1):37-41

Can the wound healing process be improved by vitamin supplementation? Experimental study on humans. *Eur Surg Res* 1996 Jul-Aug;28(4):306-14

[Improvement in the healing of colonic anastomoses by vitamin B5 and C supplements. Experimental study in the rabbit]. *Ann Chir* 1990;44(7):512-20

Oxygen free radicals impair wound healing in ischemic rat skin. *Ann Plast Surg* 1997 Nov;39(5):516-23

Depletion of reduced glutathione, ascorbic acid, vitamin E and antioxidant defence enzymes in a healing cutaneous wound. *Free Radic Res* 1997 Feb;26(2):93-101

Studies on wound healing: effects of calcium D-pantothenate on the migration, proliferation and protein synthesis of human dermal fibroblasts in culture. *Int J Vitam Nutr Res* 1999 Mar;69(2):113-9

Prevention of ongoing lipid peroxidation by wound excision and superoxide dismutase treatment in the burned rat. *Am J Emerg Med* 1994 Mar;12(2):142-6

Copper deficiency alters collagen types and covalent cross-linking in swine myocardium and cardiac valves. *Am J Physiol* 1993 Jun;264(6 Pt 2):H2154-61

Impaired mechanical strength of bone in experimental copper deficiency. *Ann Nutr Metab* 1993;37(5):245-52

Vitamin C and copper interactions in guinea-pigs and a study of collagen cross-links. *Br J Nutr* 1997 Feb;77(2):315-25

Successful treatment of radiation-induced fibrosis using liposomal Cu/Zn superoxide dismutase: clinical trial. *Radiother Oncol* 1994 Jul;32(1):12-20

Use of magnet therapy to heal an abdominal wound: a case study. *Ostomy Wound Manage* May 1998, 44 (5) p24-9

Immunological status of septic and trauma patients. I. High tumor necrosis factor alpha serum levels in septic and trauma patients are not responsible for increased mortality; a prognostic value of serum interleukin 6. *Arch Immunol Ther Exp* (Warsz) (Poland) 1997, 45 (2-3) p169-75

Burn injuries benefit from massage therapy. *J Burn Care Rehabil* May-Jun 1998, 19 (3) p241-4

The impact of Helicobacter pylori eradication on peptic ulcer healing. *Am J Gastroenterol* Jul 1998, 93 (7) p1080-4

Ascorbic acid in the prevention and treatment of cancer. *Altern Med Rev* Jun 1998, 3 (3) p174-86

Factors influencing wound healing after surgery for metastatic disease of the spine. *Spine* Mar 15 1998, 23 (6) p726-32; discussion 732-3

Pharmacological nutrition after burn injury. *J Nutr* May 1998, 128 (5) p797-803

Treatment of the seriously burned infant. *J Burn Care Rehabil* Mar-Apr 1998, 19 (2) p115-8

Is tissue oxygen tension during esophagectomy a predictor of esophagogastric anastomotic healing? *J Surg Res* Feb 1 1998, 74 (2) p161-4

Effect of mechanical treatment on healing after third molar extraction. *Int J Periodontics Restorative Dent* Jun 1997, 17 (3) p250-9

Nutritional intake and physical activity in leg ulcer patients. *J Adv Nurs* (England) Mar 1997, 25 (3) p571-8

Enteral nutrition for the burn patient. *Nutr Clin Pract* Feb 1997, 12 (1 Suppl) pS43-5

Recombinant human granulocyte-macrophage colony-stimulating factor as treatment for chronic leg ulcers. *Revista de Investigacion Clinica* (Mexico), 1997, 49/6 (449-451)

The effect of hyperbaric oxygen therapy on a burn wound model in human volunteers. *Plastic and Reconstructive Surgery*, 1997, 99/6 (1620-1625)

Autolytic debridement of chronic wounds by means of alginate containing hydrogel. *Vasomed* (Germany), 1997, 9/1 (26-34)

Preventing symblepharon formation with a gelatin sponge in the eye of a patient with an alkali burn. *American Journal of Ophthalmology*, 1997, 123/4 (552-554)

Healing by secondary intention in relation to anatomical subunits of the middle face. *Hautarzt* (Germany), 1997, 48/2 (110-112)

Basal nutrition promotes human intestinal epithelial (Caco-2) proliferation, brush border enzyme activity, and motility. *Critical Care Medicine*, 1997, 25/1 (159-165)

Inflammation and growth factors. *Journal of Urology*, 1997, 157/1 (303-305)

Analysis of p53 gene mutations in keloids using polymerase chain reaction-based single-strand conformational polymorphism and DNA sequencing [see comments]. *Arch Dermatol* Aug 1998, 134 (8) p963-7

Pharmacological nutrition after burn injury. *J Nutr* May 1998, 128 (5) p797-803

The role of nitric oxide synthase isoforms and arginase in the pathogenesis of diabetic foot ulcers: possible modulatory effects by transforming growth factor beta 1. *Diabetologia* 1999 Jun;42(6):748-57

Necrotizing fasciitis: case study of a nursing dilemma. *Ostomy Wound Manage* Jun 1997, 43 (5) p30-4, 36, 38-40.

Aloe vera: magic or medicine? *Nurs Stand* (England) Jul 1-7 1998, 12 (41) p49-52, 54

Role of nitric oxide in the angiogenic response in vitro to basic fibroblast growth factor. *Circulation Research*, 1998, 82/9 (1007-1015)

Arginine: Wound healing, immune and endocrine functions. *Cahiers de Nutrition et de Dietetique* (France), 1998, 33/1 (19-24)

What is left of the concept of essential amino acid? *Nutrition Clinique et Metabolisme* (France), 1998, 12/2 (129-136)

TGF-beta 1 stimulates cultured human fibroblasts to proliferate and produce tissue-like fibroplasia: a fibronectin matrix-dependent event. *J Cell Physiol* Jan 1997, 170 (1) p69-80

Doxorubicin-induced inhibition of prolidase activity in human skin fibroblasts and its implication to impaired collagen biosynthesis. *Polish Journal of Pharmacology* (Poland), 1998, 50/2 (151-157)

[Phytotherapy in chronic dermatoses and wounds: what is the evidence]? *Forsch Komplementarmed* 1999 Apr;6 Suppl 2:5-8

Acemannan hydrogel dressing versus saline dressing for pressure ulcers. A randomized, controlled trial. *Adv Wound Care* 1998 Oct;11(6):273-6

Influence of Aloe vera on collagen turnover in healing of dermal wounds in rats. *Indian J Exp Biol* 1998 Sep;36(9):896-901

Influence of Aloe vera on collagen characteristics in healing dermal wounds in rats. *Mol Cell Biochem* 1998 Apr;181(1-2): 71-6

Influence of aloe vera on the healing of dermal wounds in diabetic rats. *J Ethnopharmacol* 1998 Jan;59(3):195-201

Influence of Aloe vera on the glycosaminoglycans in the matrix of healing dermal wounds in rats. *J Ethnopharmacol* 1998 Jan;59(3):179-86

Effect of the combination of Aloe vera, nitroglycerin, and L-NAME on wound healing in the rat excisional model. *J Altern Complement Med* 1997 Summer;3(2):149-53

Beneficial effect of Aloe on wound healing in an excisional wound model. *J Altern Complement Med* 1996 Summer;2(2):271-7

An overview of the topical management of wounds. *Aust Vet J* 1997 Jun;75(6):408-13

Inhibition of nitric oxide synthesis in wounds: pharmacology and effect on accumulation of collagen in wounds in mice. *Eur J Surg* 1999 Mar;165(3):262-7

Patients with Chronic Leg Ulcers Show Diminished Levels of Vitamins A and E, Carotenes, and Zinc. *Dermatol Surg* 1999 Aug;25(8):601-604

Prevalence of magnesium and zinc deficiencies in nursing home residents in Germany. *Magnes Res* 1999 Sep;12(3):181-9

Nutritional intake and status of clients in the home with open surgical wounds. *J Community Health Nurs* 1990, 7 (2)

High-dose vitamin C therapy for extensive deep dermal burns. *Burns* (England) Apr 1992, 18 (2)

Yeast Infections

Refer to references under Candida Infection.

INDEX

A

B

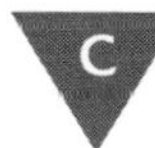
C

D

F

G

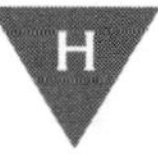
H

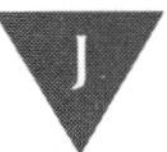
J

K

L

M

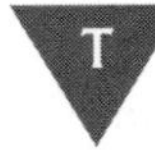
T

U

V

W

X

Y

Z

Notes

Notes

Notes

Notes

Notes

Notes

Notes

Notes

Notes

Notes

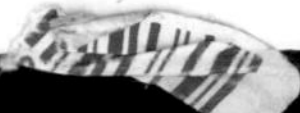

Notes